In the last two decades, the field of cultural psychology has come of age. A growing body of research explores how culture influences the ways people think, feel, and behave, and, conversely, how human psychological processes shape our social and cultural environments. This definitive handbook provides a comprehensive overview of where cultural psychology is today and where it may be headed in the future. With contributions from leading authorities who demonstrate how culture affects nearly every aspect of human functioning, this is a timely, authoritative, and immensely thought-provoking work.

The *Handbook* begins by reviewing the history of the field and explicating major theories and methods, including both experimental and ethnographic approaches. Subsequent sections delve into how topics fundamental to psychology—for example, identity and social relations, the self, cognition, emotion and motivation, and development—are influenced by cultural meanings and practices. In all, more than 60 contributors have written 36 chapters covering such diverse areas as love, religion, intelligence, memory, multicultural identities, language, attachment, psychopathology, morality, narratives, food, and work. Going beyond cross-cultural comparisons, the volume focuses on the basic processes and mechanisms that underlie cultural differences and similarities. Included is cutting-edge research on the evolutionary underpinnings of cultural stability and change. Contributors also examine how the field has emerged out of more traditional models of psychological and anthropological inquiry, and address conceptual and methodological challenges that remain.

Unique in the breadth and depth of its coverage, this handbook is an indispensable reference for researchers in cultural, social, developmental, and cognitive psychology, as well as cultural anthropology, and will also be of interest to readers in sociology and communication. Students in these fields will find it a stimulating, highly informative text.

HANDBOOK OF CULTURAL PSYCHOLOGY

Handbook of
Cultural
Psychology

Edited by

SHINOBU KITAYAMA
DOV COHEN

THE GUILFORD PRESS
New York   London

© 2007 The Guilford Press
A Division of Guilford Publications, Inc.
72 Spring Street, New York, NY 10012
www.guilford.com

Printed in the United States of America

This book is printed on acid-free paper.

Last digit is print number: 9   8   7   6   5   4   3   2   1

Library of Congress Cataloging-in-Publication Data

Handbook of cultural psychology / edited by Shinobu Kitayama and Dov Cohen.
   p. cm.
  Includes bibliographical references and indexes.
  ISBN-13: 978-1-59385-444-7   ISBN-10: 1-59385-444-7 (cloth: alk. paper)
  1. Ethnopsychology.   I. Kitayama, Shinobu.   II. Cohen, Dov.
  GN502.H36 2007
  155.8′2—dc22

                                           2006102547

*In memory of Giyoo Hatano
for his enormous contribution
to the study of culture and psychology*

About the Editors

Shinobu Kitayama, PhD, is Professor of Psychology and Director of the Culture and Cognition Program at the University of Michigan. He received his doctorate from the University of Michigan, where he has been teaching since 2003. Prior to joining the faculty there, Dr. Kitayama taught at the Universities of Oregon and Chicago and at Kyoto University. He serves as an Associate Editor of the *Personality and Social Psychology Bulletin*. Throughout his career Dr. Kitayama has studied cultural variations of self, emotion, and cognition and has presented his work in the books *Emotion and Culture: Empirical Studies of Mutual Influences* (with Hazel Markus) and *The Heart's Eye: Emotional Influences in Perception and Attention* (with Paula Niedenthal), as well as in such leading journals as *Psychological Review, Psychological Science,* and the *Journal of Personality and Social Psychology.*

Dov Cohen, PhD, received his doctorate from the University of Michigan and taught at the University of Waterloo, Ontario, Canada, and the University of Illinois, where he is currently a faculty member. His research interests relate to cultural continuity and change, within-culture variability, and the way people position themselves with respect to dominant cultural ideals. Dr. Cohen has conducted research on the cultural syndromes of honor, dignity, and face, as well as on cross-cultural similarities and differences in the experience of self. He coauthored the book *Culture of Honor* (with Richard Nisbett) and coedited *Culture and Social Behavior* (with Richard Sorrentino, James Olson, and Mark Zanna).

Contributors

Nalini Ambady, PhD, Department of Psychology, Tufts University, Medford, Massachusetts

Scott Atran, PhD, National Center for Scientific Research, Paris, France; Department of Psychology, University of Michigan, Ann Arbor, Michigan; Department of Sociology, John Jay College of Criminal Justice, New York, New York

Robert Boyd, PhD, Department of Anthropology, University of California, Los Angeles, Los Angeles, California

Marilynn B. Brewer, PhD, Department of Psychology, The Ohio State University, Columbus, Ohio

Joan Y. Chiao, PhD, Department of Psychology, Northwestern University, Evanston, Illinois

Chi-yue Chiu, PhD, Department of Psychology, University of Illinois, Urbana–Champaign, Champaign, Illinois

Incheol Choi, PhD, Department of Psychology, Seoul National University, Seoul, South Korea

Dov Cohen, PhD, Department of Psychology, University of Illinois, Urbana–Champaign, Champaign, Illinois

Michael Cole, PhD, Department of Communication, University of California, San Diego, La Jolla, California

Ed Diener, PhD, Department of Psychology, University of Illinois, Urbana–Champaign, Champaign, Illinois

Sean Duffy, PhD, Department of Psychology, Rutgers–Camden, State University of New Jersey, Camden, New Jersey

Alan P. Fiske, PhD, Department of Anthropology, University of California, Los Angeles, Los Angeles, California

Susan T. Fiske, PhD, Department of Psychology, Princeton University, Princeton, New Jersey

Heidi Fung, PhD, Institute of Ethnology, Academia Sinica, Nankang, Taipei, Taiwan

MarYam G. Hamedani, PhD, Department of Psychology, Stanford University, Stanford, California

Giyoo Hatano, PhD, (deceased) Keio University, Tokyo, Japan

Elaine Hatfield, PhD, Department of Psychology, University of Hawaii at Manoa, Honolulu, Hawaii

Steven J. Heine, PhD, Department of Psychology, University of British Columbia, Vancouver, British Columbia, Canada

Lawrence A. Hirschfeld, PhD, Departments of Anthropology and Psychology, New School University, New York, New York

Ying-yi Hong, PhD, Department of Psychology, University of Illinois, Urbana–Champaign, Champaign, Illinois

Shinobu Kitayama, PhD, Department of Psychology, University of Michigan, Ann Arbor, Michigan

Melvin Konner, PhD, Department of Anthropology, Emory University, Atlanta, Georgia

Michele Koven, PhD, Department of Speech Communication, University of Illinois, Urbana–Champaign, Champaign, Illinois

Letty Kwan, MA, Department of Psychology, University of Illinois, Urbana–Champaign, Champaign, Illinois

Fiona Lee, PhD, Department of Psychology, University of Michigan, Ann Arbor, Michigan

Spike Wing-Sing Lee, BA, Department of Psychology, University of Michigan, Ann Arbor, Michigan

Janxin Leu, PhD, Department of Psychology, University of Washington, Seattle, Washington

Angela K-y. Leung, PhD, School of Social Sciences, Singapore Management University, Singapore

Robert W. Levenson, PhD, Department of Psychology, University of California, Berkeley, Berkeley, California

Robert A. LeVine, PhD, Graduate School of Education, Harvard University, Cambridge, Massachusetts

Shu-Chen Li, PhD, Max Planck Institute for Human Development, Center for Lifespan Psychology, Berlin, Germany

Hazel Rose Markus, PhD, Department of Psychology, Stanford University, Stanford, California

Lise D. Martel, PhD, Department of Psychology, University of Hawaii at Manoa, Honolulu, Hawaii

Anthony J. Marsella, PhD, Department of Psychology, University of Hawaii at Manoa, Honolulu, Hawaii

Douglas L. Medin, PhD, Department of Psychology, Northwestern University, Evanston, Illinois

Rodolfo Mendoza-Denton, PhD, Department of Psychology, University of California, Berkeley, Berkeley, California

Batja Mesquita, PhD, Department of Psychology, University of Leuven, Leuven, Belgium

Joan G. Miller, PhD, Department of Psychology, New School University, New York, New York

Peggy J. Miller, PhD, Departments of Psychology and Speech Communication, University of Illinois, Urbana–Champaign, Champaign, Illinois

Walter Mischel, PhD, Department of Psychology, Columbia University, New York, New York

Gilda A. Morelli, PhD, Department of Psychology, Boston College, Chestnut Hill, Massachusetts

Lesley Newson, PhD, School of Psychology, University of Exeter, Exeter, United Kingdom

Richard E. Nisbett, PhD, Department of Psychology, University of Michigan, Ann Arbor, Michigan

Sun No, MA, Department of Psychology, University of Illinois, Urbana–Champaign, Champaign, Illinois

Ara Norenzayan, PhD, Department of Psychology, University of British Columbia, Vancouver, British Columbia, Canada

Daphna Oyserman, PhD, Department of Psychology, University of Michigan, Ann Arbor, Michigan

Kaiping Peng, PhD, Department of Psychology, University of California, Berkeley, Berkeley, California

Nnamdi Pole, PhD, Department of Psychology, University of Michigan, Ann Arbor, Michigan

Richard L. Rapson, PhD, Department of History, University of Hawaii at Manoa, Honolulu, Hawaii

Peter J. Richerson, PhD, Department of Environmental Science and Policy, University of California, Davis, Davis, California

Michael Ross, PhD, Department of Psychology, University of Waterloo, Waterloo, Ontario, Canada

Fred Rothbaum, PhD, Eliot–Pearson Department of Child Development, Tufts University, Medford, Massachusetts

Paul Rozin, PhD, Department of Psychology, University of Pennsylvania, Philadelphia, Pennsylvania

Jeffrey Sanchez-Burks, PhD, Stephen M. Ross School of Business, University of Michigan, Ann Arbor, Michigan

Carmi Schooler, PhD, Section on Socio-Environmental Studies, National Institute of Mental Health, Bethesda, Maryland

Richard A. Shweder, PhD, Department of Comparative Human Development, University of Chicago, Chicago, Illinois

José Soto, PhD, Department of Psychology, The Pennsylvania State University, University Park, Pennsylvania

Robert J. Sternberg, PhD, Department of Psychology, Tufts University, Medford, Massachusetts

William Tov, MA, Department of Psychology, University of Illinois, Urbana–Champaign, Champaign, Illinois

Harry C. Triandis, PhD, Department of Psychology, University of Illinois, Urbana–Champaign, Champaign, Illinois

Yukiko Uchida, PhD, Department of Psychology, Koshien University, Takarazuka, Japan

Sara J. Unsworth, MA, Department of Psychology, Northwestern University, Evanston, Illinois

Ching Wan, PhD, Division of Psychology, Nanyang Technological University, Singapore

Qi Wang, PhD, Department of Human Development, Cornell University, Ithaca, New York

Ann Marie Yamada, PhD, School of Social Work, University of Southern California, Los Angeles, California

Masaki Yuki, PhD, Department of Behavioral Science, Hokkaido University, Sapporo, Japan

Preface

Although it has many important predecessors in related disciplines such as anthropology, linguistics, and sociology, the field of cultural psychology as we know it today has only recently become a major force in the discipline of psychology. In its initial stage, during the 1980s, the field received a substantial boost from Richard Shweder's admonition, "Culture and psyche make each other up." By this, he meant that culture is not a "thing" out there; rather, it is a loosely organized set of interpersonal and institutional processes driven by people who participate in those processes. By the same token, the psyche is also not a discrete entity packed in the brain. Rather, it is a structure of psychological processes that are shaped by and thus closely attuned to the culture that surrounds them. Accordingly, culture cannot be understood without a deep understanding of the minds of people who make it up and, likewise, the mind cannot be understood without reference to the sociocultural environment to which it is adapted and attuned. In significant ways, the field has since evolved by exploring the nature of the mutual constitution of culture and the psyche.

Because many of us who engaged in this exploration were committed empirical psychologists, substantial effort was devoted to the questions of how culture might foster and even create different forms of psychological processes and how one could identify demonstrable consequences of such cross-culturally divergent psychological processes. These questions were raised and addressed with respect to some central topics of psychology, including self, identity, cognition, emotion, motivation, and interpersonal relationships.

Sometimes, initial efforts were guided by a rather simple heuristic of finding out specific ways in which the contemporary theories in psychology might be seen as culturally bound, and were largely confined to middle-class, young, Western samples. In retrospect, this might seem reactive, because it searched for limitations and problems with "mainstream psychology." Curiously, however, the empirical effort designed to show limitations of "mainstream theories" did in fact have more positive, proactive consequences. It enabled the researchers to extend existent theories, elaborate on them, and thus refine them as full-fledged theories of the interactions between sociocultural processes and psychological processes. In large part because of this, we believe that the field of cultural psychology has emerged from the periphery of the discipline to establish itself as a mainstay of contemporary psychology. Culture, then, has become an indispensable way to enrich basic theories of psychology. Here the current cultural approach in psychology differs most significantly from its cousins both in the past and the present.

This handbook represents an overview of the field of cultural psychology as it exists today. It starts with historical and disciplinary backgrounds of the field (Part I, "The Discipline and Its History"), followed by discussions of some theoretical perspectives and methodological advances (Part II, "Theory and Methods"). The main body of the handbook comprises more than 20 reviews of the diverse areas the field encompasses. The major themes include "Identity and Social Relations" (Part III), "Acquisition and Change of Culture" (Part IV), "Cognition" (Part V), and "Emotion and Motivation" (Part VI). We have compiled a total of 36 chapters, written by more than 60 top-notch researchers who pursue a diverse array of questions about culture.

We are very happy and proud of what has come out as a major reference volume for the field. We believe that one virtue of any endeavor of this magnitude is to encourage our colleagues and new generations of researchers to reflect on our current shortcomings and drawbacks, which in reality constitute a fertile source of ideas, visions, and empirical hypotheses for further expansions and elaborations of the field. The best contribution this handbook makes, then, may be to provide a moment of such critical self-appraisals. If it can meet this modest aspiration, we may also hope that it will be remembered as a noteworthy stepping stone by succeeding generations of researchers on culture and the human mind.

Contents

III. IDENTITY AND SOCIAL RELATIONS

IV. ACQUISITION AND CHANGE OF CULTURE

V. COGNITION

VI. EMOTION AND MOTIVATION

VII. COMMENTARIES FROM TWO PERSPECTIVES

VIII. EPILOGUE

PART I

THE DISCIPLINE AND ITS HISTORY

CHAPTER 1

Sociocultural Psychology

The Dynamic Interdependence among Self Systems and Social Systems

HAZEL ROSE MARKUS
MARYAM G. HAMEDANI

The word *cultural* has modified psychology throughout its history. Cole (1990) calls cultural psychology "a once and future discipline," Shweder (1990, 2003) notes that cultural psychology's time has arrived "once again," and J. G. Miller (1999) contends that psychology is and "always has been cultural." Despite important and often heated arguments about differences among the areas designated by the terms "cultural psychology," "cross-cultural psychology," "sociocultural psychology," "psychological anthropology," and "situated cognition" (Atran, Medin, & Ross, 2005; Berry, 2000; Keller et al., 2006; Keller & Greenfield, 2000; Kim & Berry, 1993; Markus & Kitayama, 1991; Matsumoto, 2001; Nisbett, 2003; Norenzayan & Heine, 2005; Shweder & Sullivan, 1990, 1993; Triandis, 1989; Veroff & Goldberger, 1995; Vygotsky, 1978; Wertsch, 1991), the joint reemergence of these terms and the robust interest they have generated is a significant developmental marker for the field of psychology. The theory

and research produced under these flags reveal a new and mature appreciation for an old and powerful idea. Expressed in a wide variety of ways, the core of this historically elusive and empirically challenging notion is that people and their social worlds are inseparable: They require each other.

The psychological—typically defined as patterns of thought, feeling, and action, sometimes also called the mind, the psyche, the self, agency, mentalities, ways of being, or modes of operating—is grounded in and also fosters the sociocultural. The sociocultural—or patterns in the social world, sometimes called socialities, sociocultural contexts, social systems, the environment, social structure, or culture—is grounded in and fosters the psychological. Thus, in a process of ongoing *mutual constitution*, the psychological and the cultural "make each other up" (Shweder, 1990, p. 24), and are most productively analyzed and understood together (Adams & Markus, 2001; Kashima, 2000; Wertsch & Sammarco, 1985).

The history of what we label here as "sociocultural psychology" is a story characterized by both a persistent attraction to the idea that culture and psyche make each other up, and an equally strong resistance to this idea, set up by the pervasive individualist representation—particularly densely distributed in North American contexts—that "it's what's inside" the person and not the "context" that matters the most. The current wave of rapidly expanding interest among social scientists regarding how behavior is socially and culturally constituted is driven, we suggest, by a confluence of several factors: (1) a robust set of empirical findings that challenge many of psychology's signature theories, and are thus not easily interpreted with dominant or mainstream frameworks; (2) a growing realization among psychologists that the capacity for culture making and culture sharing is at the core of what it means to be human, and that this capacity is a clear evolutionary advantage of the human species (Bruner, 1990; Carrithers, 1992; Kashima, 2000; Mesquita, 2003; Schaller & Crandall, 2004; Tomasello, 1999); and (3) an increasing sophistication in how to conceptualize both the cultural and the psychological, such that the nature of their mutual and reciprocal influence can be examined.

We have organized our review and integration of the sociocultural perspective in psychology around a set of questions:

1. Mutual constitution—what does it mean?
2. A sociocultural approach—what is it?
3. A sociocultural approach—where does it come from?
4. What does a sociocultural approach add to psychology?
5. What definition of culture is suitable for psychology?
6. Assessing mutual constitution—what are the current approaches?
7. Sociocultural psychology—what next?

MUTUAL CONSTITUTION—WHAT DOES IT MEAN?

Sociocultural psychologists begin their theorizing with the person and several key observations. People exist everywhere in social networks, in groups, in communities, and in relationships. They are chronically sensitive and attuned to the thoughts, feelings, and actions of others. Their actions (i.e., their ways of being an agent in the world, their identities, their *selves*) require, reflect, foster, and institutionalize these sociocultural affordances and influences. Thus, as people actively construct their worlds, they are made up of, or "constituted by," relations with other people and by the ideas, practices, products, and institutions that are prevalent in their social contexts (i.e., environments, fields, situations, settings, worlds). The people whose thoughts, feelings, and actions are included in this circuit of mutual constitution include the individuals' contemporaries, the individual him or herself, and many others who have gone before and left their respective worlds replete with representations, products, and systems reflecting prior thoughts, feelings, and actions.

The major focus of the last two decades of research in sociocultural psychology has been to discover just how mutual constitution proceeds. What does it mean about the brain, the mind, and behavior to say that they are cultural or socioculturally constituted? For some researchers, the goal has been to show that ideas, practices, and products are not separate from "experience" or applied *after* behavior. The sociocultural is not "overlaid" on a set of *basic* or *fixed* psychological processes. Instead, ideas, practices, and products are active and incorporated in the very formation and operation of psychological processes (e.g., Cole, 1996; Markus, Mullally, & Kitayama, 1997; J. G. Miller, 1994; Nisbett, 2003; Wertsch, 1991). The goal of other researchers has been to show that the context is not separate or external to the person but is, in fact, the psychological externalized or materialized (D'Andrade & Strauss, 1992; Kitayama, Markus, Matsumoto, & Norasakkunkit, 1997; Markus, Uchida, Omoregie, Townsend, & Kitayama, 2005; Shore, 1996). In the terms of Shweder (1995), who has pioneered the theoretical development of modern cultural psychology, the goal is to find ways to talk about the psychological and about the cultural such that neither "is by nature intrinsic or extrinsic to the other" (p. 69).

Our intent in this chapter's title is to signal our focus on theories and research that examine the structure and patterning inherent in various social worlds, how this patterning continually shapes psychological functioning, and how people (selves or agents) require and depend on these patterns as they become meaning-*full* participants in their social worlds. The patterning of social worlds includes ideas and images, as well as the embodiment, animation, and realization of these ideas and images in social practices, material products, and institutions (here called "social systems").

We use the word *sociocultural* rather than the term *cultural* to emphasize that a sociocultural analysis includes within its scope both the conceptual and the material. Thus, it includes both *meanings*—ideas, images, representations, attitudes, values, prototypes, and stereotypes—and what is often termed the *sociostructural*—cultural products, interpersonal interactions, institutional practices and systems—and person–situation contingencies, all of which embody, as well as render material and operable, normative patterns prevalent in a given context. We invoke the term *interdependence* to convey the sense that as people are involved in the processes of mutual constitution, they are not passive recipients of culture. Instead they are active agents who are socioculturally shaped *shapers* of themselves and their worlds. The causal arrows between social and psychological formation are bidirectional; the constitution is mutual.

Finally, we use the term *dynamic* to signal that sociocultural patterns of ideas, practices, and products are not fixed, but are open and complex networks or distributions of mental and material resources that are often, although not always, linked with significant, in the sense of psychologically meaningful (socially, politically, historically), constructed categories such as ethnicity, race, religion, gender, occupation, political party, social class, caste, sect, tribe, or region of the country or world. These categories are elements of the repertoire of symbolic resources that people themselves invoke, or that are invoked by others, to render the social world meaningful. Such sets of ideas, practices, products, and institutions are constantly in flux and undergoing transformation as they are engaged—appropriated, incorporated, contested—by selves acting or being in the world. Others' ways of categorizing the sociocultural context that are less well-instituted in existing contexts and map less well onto existing social categories (e.g., high or low gross domestic product [GDP] nations, red or blue America, mountainous or flat habitats) are also important to investigate.

A SOCIOCULTURAL APPROACH—WHAT IS IT?

The emerging sociocultural psychology reflects the most recent and most specific realization within psychology of the theory that being a person is fundamentally a social transaction (Asch, 1952; Baldwin, 1911; Lewin, 1948; Mead, 1934; for a review, see Cross & Markus, 1999) Moreover, it is an effort to extend and to elaborate empirically the view that social formations and psychological formations are fully interdependent, both contemporaneously and historically (Berger & Luckmann, 1966; Bourdieu, 1990; Moscovici, 1988; Shweder, 1990; Wundt, 1916).

From a sociocultural perspective, individuals are biological entities (as well as genetic, neuronal, chemical, hormonal entities), and all behavior has a biological, as well as an evolutionary, foundation. Yet individuals are also ineluctably social and cultural phenomena. The option of being *a*social or *a*cultural, that is, living as a neutral being who is not bound to particular practices and socioculturally structured ways of behaving, is not available. People eat, sleep, work, and relate to one another in culture-specific ways. As the rapidly expanding volume of theoretical and empirical studies has made clear, people also think and feel and act in culture-specific ways—ways that are shaped by the particular meanings and practices of their lived experiences (for reviews see Cole, 1996; Fiske, Kitayama, Markus, & Nisbett, 1998; Greenfield & Cocking, 1994; Heine, Lehman, Markus, & Kitayama, 1999; J. G. Miller, 1997; Nisbett & Cohen, 1996; Shweder, 1990, 2003; Shweder & LeVine, 1984; Smith & Bond, 1993). Becoming a mature, competent adult necessitates that an individual successfully engage the systems of meanings, practices, and institutions that configure the contexts of her particular everyday life (Bruner, 1990; Geertz, 1975; Markus et al., 1997; Shweder, 1982, 1990).

The sociocultural engagement that is an essential and constant process of human life is an *active* process that transforms the biological being into a social individual—a person with a self and a set of context-contingent identities. In the process of this cultural engagement, "others"—their language; their ideas of what is good, true, and real; their understandings of why and how to attend to, engage with, and operate within various worlds—become part of a dynamic self that mediates and regulates behavior. The patterns and processes of individuals' social contexts condition their behavior and give form to the interpretive systems that organize the behavioral system. As people participate in their respective contexts, settings, and environments, they are constantly in the process of making meaning and reflecting these meanings in their actions by building them into products and practices in their worlds (Bruner, 1990; Hallowell, 1955; Markus & Kitayama, 1994; Shweder, 1990).

As Shweder (1990) postulates, the intentional person, or psyche, is interdependent with the intentional world, or culture. Intentional worlds are worlds of meanings—human artifactual worlds, populated with products of our own design. An intentional world, Shweder says, is replete with events such as "stealing" or "taking communion"; processes such as "harm" or "sin"; stations such as "in-law" or "exorcist"; practices such as "betrothal" or "divorce"; visible entities such as "weeds" and invisible entities such as "natural rights" (p. 42). These cultural products are not just expressions, correlates, or residue of behavior. Human behavior is premised on and organized by these taken-for-granted meanings and categorizations of social reality that are objectified in material objects and institutionalized in social relations and social systems.

For example, many urban, middle-class adults in North American contexts reveal high levels of self-esteem, self-efficacy, optimism, and intrinsic motivation; express a desire for mastery, control, and self-expression; and show preferences for uniqueness (Kim & Markus, 1999; Snibbe & Markus, 2005). This robust set of psychological tendencies is not, however, an expression of universal human nature. The middle-class contexts of North America are replete with choices; with requirements for self-expression and feeling good about the self; and with opportunities for focusing on the self, mastering, and controlling one's environment, and constructing the self as the primary source of action.

What is readily apparent from a comparative approach is that North American psychological tendencies have in many significant ways been created, fostered, and maintained by widely distributed ideas—such as the importance of individual achievement—and have been reinforced and instituted by dense networks of everyday practices—such as complimenting and praising one another for individual performance by a frequent distribution of awards and honors in classrooms and workplaces, and by situations such as job applications and interviews that require people to focus on their good features and explain their life outcomes in terms of their own actions and decisions. These psychological tendencies and everyday practices further structure worlds through intentional products such as coffee mugs, bumper stickers, cars, medications, and cigarette advertisements that declare "You're the best," or exhort people to "Be a star," "Take control," "Never follow," and "Resist homogenization." Such practices and products foster material and behavioral environments in which self-serving and self-interested actions are valued and normative. These cultural resources thereby condition characteristic ways of being and are themselves the result of previous conditioned responding.

As we analyze the process of sociocultural transformation, two facts become apparent: (1) Individuals are not separate from social contexts, and (2) social contexts do not exist apart from or outside of people. Instead, contexts are the products of human activity: They are repositories of previous psychological activity, and they afford psychological activity. As a consequence, social contexts do more than what psychology typically labels "influence." Instead, they "constitute," as in create, make up, or establish, these psychological tendencies. The mental processes and behavioral tendencies that are the subject of study in psychology, then, are not separate from, but are fundamentally realized through, cultural ideas and practices.

As researchers and theorists turn toward a sociocultural approach, they take seriously Bruner's (1990) claim that it is impossible to "construct a human psychology on the basis of the individual alone" (p. 12). Developing a sociocultural psychology requires spanning the divides created by the many familiar and foundational psychological binaries, that is, person–situation, individual–environment, culture–social structure, and self–society, that conceptualize people as separate from their "surrounding" contexts. Moreover, there is a need to bridge the many disciplinary barriers that separate sociology, anthropology, and history from psychology.

Given the theorized interdependence of mind and sociocultural context, the assumption of a sociocultural psychology is that the psychological nature of human beings can vary with time and space (Shweder, 2003). Thus, two central goals of sociocultural psychology are to examine variation in modes of psychological functioning across sociocultural contexts, and to specify the varied cultural meanings and practices with which they are linked (Fiske et al., 1998; Graumann, 1986; Markus, Kitayama, & Heiman, 1996; Moscovici, 1981; Shweder, 1990, 2003; Wundt, 1916). The field, however, is often identified with (and criticized for) the search for differences in subjectivities, as well as with what Shweder (1990) calls the "rejection of psychic unity." In conjunction with this goal, however, sociocultural psychology seeks (1) to discover systematic principles underlying the diversity of culturally patterned socialities and psyches, and (2) to describe the processes by which all humans are constituted as fundamentally social beings.

Notably, the behavior of all individuals engaged in a particular (e.g., middle-class, European American) context is by no means uniform or identical, revealing that sociocultural contexts may constitute, in the sense of shape or condition, people in a variety of ways as they engage differently with their contexts. Contexts do not "determine," in the sense of definitively settle or fix, the limits or forms of human behavior. People engage with and respond to the ideas and practices of a given context in somewhat variable ways, with variable intents and purposes. These varieties of engagement depend on the person's own particular set of orienting, mediating, and interpretive frameworks, which themselves are the result of a host of other individual and situational differences, and also shape a person's mode of being in the world. People, then, are never monocultural, because they are always interacting with multiple contexts (e.g., those delineated by gender, ethnicity, socioeconomic status, region, sexual orientation, occupation). Cultural contexts are therefore not monolithic: Various combinations of cultural ideas and practices intersect within individuals, so that individuals may have different reactions to the same context. Furthermore, as psychological tendencies are realized and expressed, they not only foster and reinforce but also sometimes change the contexts in which they are grounded. The consequences of cultural engagement on behavior, although systematic and predictable in many aspects, are never monolithic and invariable.

A SOCIOCULTURAL APPROACH— WHERE DOES IT COME FROM?

The major ideas of a sociocultural perspective, as we have sketched it here, have multiple overlapping sources throughout the social sciences and philosophy. They can be traced to Herder and to Vico in philosophy (Shweder, 2003; Taylor, 1997; see also Triandis, Chapter 3, this volume); to Boas, Hallowell, Kroeber, and Kluckholn in anthropology (see LeVine, Chapter 2, this volume); to sociology (Berger & Luckmann, 1966; Bourdieu, 1991; Moscovici, 1991, 1998); and to a variety of psychological theorists, such as Wundt, Mead, Baldwin, Sullivan, G. Kelly, Asch, Lewin, and Bruner, all of whom emphasized meaning and the role of intersubjectively shared understandings in creating and maintaining reality. In general, sociocultural psychologists can be identified by their appreciation for the interdependence of the individual with the social, the material, and the historical, and by their view of people as active meaning makers and world makers.

Thinking Beyond the Person

Common to many approaches classified as sociocultural psychology is a belief that the sources of mind and behavior cannot all be located within the brain, the head, or the body. The sources of mind and behavior are distributed, existing both internally in the mind and externally in the world. This commitment to the ways in which psychological processes are made up of, or made by, the social elements of one's contexts is revealed in some of psychology's earliest theorizing, although the term *cultural* was not explicitly invoked. Wundt believed that no thought, judgment, or evaluation could be methodologically isolated from its sociocultural base (Graumann, 1986). More explicitly, Lewin (1948) wrote:

> The perception of social space and the experimental and conceptual investigation of the dynamics and laws of the processes in social space are of fundamental and theoretical and practical importance. . . . The social climate in which a child lives is for the child as important as the air it breathes. The group to which the child belongs is the ground on which he stands. (p. 82)

Similarly, Allport (1948) noted that:

> the group to which the individual belongs is the

ground for his perceptions, his feelings, and his actions. Most psychologists are so preoccupied with the salient features of the individual's mental life that they are prone to forget it is the ground of the social group that gives to the individual his figured character. Just as the bed of a stream shapes the direction and flow of water, so does the group determine the current of an individual's life. The interdependence of the ground and the figured flow is inescapable, intimate, dynamic, but is also elusive. (p. vii)

Extending these ideas, Wertsch and Sammarco (1985) argue forcefully, like Bruner, that to explain the individual one must go beyond the individual. They invoke the words of Luria (1981):

> In order to explain the highly complex forms of human consciousness, one must go beyond the human organism. One must seek the origins of conscious activity and "categorical" behavior not in the recesses of the human brain or in the depths of the spirit, but in the external conditions of life. Above all, this means that one must seek these origins in external processes of social life, in the social and transhistorical forms of human existence. (p. 25)

Meaning Making as Basic Process

Another defining element of the sociocultural approach is the idea that, whereas the world suggests itself and can attract and bind attention, the person is not simply a passive recipient of what the social world has to offer, but is instead an active, intentional agent. From a sociocultural–psychological perspective, an essential element of behavior is an *engagement*, or a coming together, an encounter, of a person making sense of a world replete with meanings, objects, and practices (Asch, 1952; Bruner, 1990; Geertz, 1973).

Most recently, in summarizing several decades of research, Bruner (1990; see also Markus, Kitayama, & Heiman, 1996), invoked these now century-old claims about the social and cultural nature of the mind, then extended them. He specified how cultural systems give form and direction to our lives. It is culture, he contends, that

> shapes human life and the human mind, that gives meaning to action by situating its underlying intentional states in an interpretive system. It does this by imposing the patterns inherent in the culture's symbolic systems—its language and dis-

course modes, the forms of logical and narrative explication, and the patterns of mutually dependent communal life. (p. 34)

WHAT DOES A SOCIOCULTURAL APPROACH ADD TO PSYCHOLOGY?

In short, the social systems that the self systems engage derive from previous psychological activity and provide the resources and blueprints for meaning-making and action. The organizing theme of a sociocultural approach, and of this chapter, is that people and their social worlds are inseparable: They fundamentally require each other. A comprehensive social-psychological science requires mapping the range of ways that the social world can be made meaningful, and analysis of the processes by which this meaning making and world making occur (Bruner, 1990; Markus, Kitayama, & Heiman, 1996; Shweder, 1990, 2003). Just as neuroscientists scan the brain, seeking to produce a neural mapping of the mind, so must psychologists scan the sociocultural environment to generate a sociocultural mapping of the mind. Attaching a wide-angle lens to the current psychological camera so as to encompass more fully the sociocultural (as well as the historical) will allow researchers to identify the meaningful contexts that ground and organize the cognitive, emotional, and behavioral tendencies observed in psychological studies.

Analyzing intentional worlds simultaneously as both products and shapers of psychological activity is challenging. Many features of the social environment—schools, churches, theaters, marriage, as well as many other social objects, roles, practices, and relations generated in the process of mutual constitution—are understandable only in terms of their social settings and functions. As Asch (1952) noted, "A chair, a dollar bill, a joking relative are social things; the most exhaustive physical, chemical and biological analysis will fail to reveal this most essential property" (p. 178).

Meanings

One category of the context that is central to understanding how the sociocultural and psychological make each other up is what Bruner (1990) and Shweder (1990) call "meanings," or what Sperber (1985) and Moscovici (1981) call "representations." Meanings or representations are useful units of mutual constitution, because they refer to constructed entities that cannot be located solely in the head of the meaning maker or solely in the practices or products of world; they are always distributed across both. Once ideas and images or other symbolic resources are instituted in actions and in the world, they are simultaneously forms of social knowledge and social practices (Moscovici, 1981). For example, the meanings associated with phenomena such as person, self, group, family, sex, marriage, friendship, enemyship, society, mind, emotion, consciousness, time, the future, the past, life, luck, death, goodness, evil, and human nature provide the substratum of images and assumptions that are essential for understanding sociocultural contexts. Some of these meanings are created, distributed, and instituted in response to critical—perhaps universal—problems of ethnicity, maturity, hierarchy, autonomy, and morality. Others speak to particular concerns and are more historically contingent or locally selected and derived.

One important goal of sociocultural psychology is to analyze the complex of meanings that have been naturalized and taken for granted as basic human drives, needs, or psychological processes, but that may be quite context-specific. Until recently, most psychologists have been Europeans and North Americans who have analyzed middle-class European and North American college students. The dense and extensive set of representations that are foundational for and specific to this context (including representations of independence, individual responsibility, self-determination, self-esteem, control, freedom, equality, choice, work, ability, intelligence, motivation, success, influence, achievement, power, and happiness), which lend structure and coherence to behavior, have been largely invisible and have gone unmarked (Jost & Major, 2001; Markus & Kitayama, 1994; Quinn & Crocker, 1999). Identifying the vast system of meanings that affords agency in middle-class European and North American contexts underscores the possibility of marked differences in agency in other contexts.

Substantial differences in these meanings in terms of how they are conventionalized and publically expressed in the environment (e.g., what is self, what is the group, what is emotion, what is life–death), and in how they are distributed, provide useful ways of distinguishing among cultural contexts. Often these meanings are linked to meanings of socially and historically significant categories such as ethnicity, region of the world, or religion. Sociocultural psychologists have begun to systematically extract divergent meanings from various contexts (those associated with region of the country or world, religion, ethnicity, race, gender, age, sexual preference, social class, and occupation). They have identified multiple meanings for concepts that are psychological staples—concepts of self and identity, cognition, emotion, motivation, morality, well-being, friendship, family, and group. They have identified such broad concepts as independence and interdependence that are evident in some form in almost every context, but that differ in their prevalence, dominance, or in how densely they are elaborated and distributed in a given context. They have identified concepts such as happiness, control, and choice that appear to organize middle-class American psyches and contexts but that are not particularly prevalent or salient in other contexts. They have also distinguished many more specific concepts that can be understood and identified but are not emphasized or foregrounded in the middle-class North American perspective that still provides the unmarked framework of reference for most work in psychology. These include concepts such as honor, shame, adjustment, face, compassion, serenity, enemyship, hierarchy, respect, deference, propriety, moderation, balance, silence, divinity, restraint, and relativism, as well as a growing set of concepts such as *amae* or *simpatía* that can be translated but do not have simple English counterparts. Many sociocultural studies produce findings that are surprising and that pose questions for common middle-class North American understandings. For example, in Japanese contexts, happiness includes sadness (Uchida, Norasakkunkit, & Kitayama, 2004); in West African contexts, enemies are part of everyday life (Adams, 2005); in Latin American contexts, work requires socializing (Sanchez-Burks & Mor Barak, 2004), and in Taiwanese contexts, feeling good is more likely to be identified with feeling calm and tranquil than with feeling energized or excited (Tsai, Knutson, & Fung, 2006). These different ideas about what is normative or of value imply worlds and psyches organized in different ways from middle-class North American ones.

Practices

Cultural contexts are identified and maintained by not only shared subjective elements but also particular ways of acting and interacting in the recurrent episodes of everyday life. Thus, another category of the sociocultural context that can be analyzed is practices. As with meanings, a focus on practices is an effort to move beyond the individual considered in isolation (Cole, 1995; Kitayama et al., 1997; P. J. Miller & Goodnow, 1995; Rogoff, 1991). An emphasis on practices bridges the divide between thinking and other parts of psychological activity typically called "doing" or "being." Participation in routine activities, such as talking to a friend, going shopping, going to the bank, attending a meeting, parenting, or teaching, expresses in concrete form what a given context communicates about how to be a normatively appropriate person, as well as what is regarded as "good," "right," or "real." Practices, therefore, are not neutral behavior, but rather are those that "reflect a social and moral order" (Miller & Goodnow, 1995, p. 10). Practices, or what Bruner (1990) calls "acts," are behaviors that reflect intention or meaning. Practices, then, are not just behavior; they are meaning-*full* acts that coordinate the actions of individuals with those of others and maintain the social context. A practice perspective has been used to analyze, for example, processes of self-esteem maintenance (Heine et al., 1999; Kitayama et al., 1997; P. J. Miller & Goodnow, 1995), sleeping arrangements/sleeping behaviors (Shweder, Balle-Jensen, & Goldstein, 1995), hiring decisions (D. Cohen & Nisbett, 1997), prayer and religious activity (A. B. Cohen, Malka, Rozin, & Cherfas, 2006; J. L. Tsai, Miao, & Seppala, in press), talking (H. S. Kim, 2002), and health promotion (Markus, Curhan, & Ryff, 2006).

Products

Within psychology, Cole (1990) has focused on cultural contexts as defined by a continual flow of constructed activity. He describes the material flow of culture and stresses that humans enter a world that is transformed by "the accumulated artifacts of previous generations." Culture, then, is history in the present. Cole, who traces his thinking to the writings of Vygotksy, Luria, and Leontiev, claims that the main function of the cultural artifact is to inte-grate people with the world and with each other. Cultural products can be conceptualized as the psychological externalized, or as the social order objectified. As noted by Asch (1952), such products have powerful effects on action. For example, products such as an abacus, a magazine advertisement, a child's book, a song, the iPod on which said song is played, and, perhaps most obviously, the Internet are simultaneously conceptual and material. They carry with them past interactions, and they mediate the present. These products reflect the ideas, images, understandings, and values of particular contexts, and are therefore a good source of these meanings. Simultaneously, as people engage with these products, they re-present and institutionalize these ideas and values. In the last few years, a growing number of psychologists have analyzed cultural products, including song lyrics, television commercials, television news coverage, children's storybooks, Web advertisements, want ads, personals ads, newspaper articles and headlines, photographs, school and university mission statements, and social networking sites (Aaker & Williams, 1998; H. Kim & Markus, 1999; Plaut & Markus, 2005; Rothbaum, Weisz, & Snyder, 1982; Snibbe & Markus, 2005; J. Tsai, Knutson, & Fung, 2006).

The goal of a sociocultural analysis is to analyze more of what is called "the situation" or "the environment," and to expand psychology's understanding of the role of individual in maintaining the situations that influence them. A sociocultural approach adds to psychology a focus on the content and function of meanings, practices, and products. Such a focus succeeds in analyzing "more" of the situation, providing a wider, and at the same time, a more in-depth view.

WHAT IS A DEFINITION OF CULTURE SUITABLE FOR PSYCHOLOGY?

Most of the research we are categorizing under the rubric of sociocultural psychology has concentrated on the psychological, leaving the patterning or the distribution or the coherence of the *sociocultural* mostly unspecified, and the workings of the process of mutual constitution unelaborated. For example, early cultural psychology investigations by J. G. Miller (1984), Triandis (1989), and Markus and Kitayama (1991) revealed detailed representations and normative practices associated with observed differences in psychological tendencies. Most subsequent references to these studies, however, report the cultural differences observed as those between types of people—"individualists" and "collectivists," or "independents" and "interdependents," or "Westerners" and "Easterners." This type of description locates the sources of the behavioral differences in some internal attributes or traits of the *individuals* rather than in some aspects of the cultural contexts, or in the *transaction* between the individual and the context.

Cultural Psychology as Stereotyping 101?

Although it is easier to say "East Asians" or "interdependents" than to say "people participating in the ideas and practices that are pervasive in East Asian cultural contexts," the labels, even if it is only a shorthand, repeatedly reinforce the sense that observed psychological tendencies (e.g., a prevalent tendency to be aware of the preferences and expectations of close others and to correctly anticipate these preferences) derive from some properties or *traits* of interdependence or collectivism rather than from persistent engagement in a world that is structured in specific ways, and that requires and fosters a particular type of attention to others.

One of the formidable stumbling blocks on the road to a systematic sociocultural psychology has been the failure to articulate a definition of "culture" or "the sociocultural" that fits the idea that the psychological and sociocultural are dynamically making each other up. Without specific definitions, most observers, laypersons, and social scientists alike have gravitated toward the simple and widely distributed idea of culture as a collection of traits that define particular groups or collections of people. The commonsense idea reflected here is that a group is like a big person, and that "culture" is the group's "personality" or "character."

In everyday discourse, people make statements such as "He has visited 34 cultures," suggesting that cultures are specified by geographical boundaries. Other seemingly commonsense statements include "Members of Chinese culture are family oriented," or "Members of Mexican culture are hierarchical." Such statements can easily imply the view that cultures are monolithic and can be understood as discrete, categorical groups that are "internally homogeneous, externally distinctive objects" (Hermans & Kempen, 1998, p. 1113). As noted by Adams and Markus (2004), such statements also suggest that culture is an entity, or some defining cultural essence that groups "have." From this perspective, culture is often understood as something extra that "other" groups "have," and is less often used to make sense of ingroup behavior.

Culture as Patterns

Most recent scientific definitions of culture conceptualize it very differently, departing markedly from the idea of culture as a bundle of traits or as a stable set of beliefs or norms, and are less likely to be vulnerable to the stereotyping charge. Instead, *culture* is defined as patterns of representations, actions, and artifacts that are distributed or spread by social interaction. Under this definition, the conceptual location of culture shifts from the interior of a person to the often-implicit patterns that exist simultaneously in people and in the world with which they necessarily engage in the course of any behavior. For example, Atran et al. (2005), in a recent description of the cultural mind, defines *culture* as "causally distributed patterns of mental representations, their public expression, and the resultant behaviors in given ecological contexts" (p. 751).

Among the hundreds of definitions of culture (Kroeber & Kluckhohn, 1952), many theorists (Adams & Markus, 2004; Shweder, 2003) developing sociocultural theory have returned to the insights of Kroeber and Kluckhohn (1952):

> Culture consists of explicit and implicit *patterns* of historically derived and selected ideas and their embodiment in institutions, practices, and artifacts; cultural patterns may, on one hand, be considered as products of action, and on the other as conditioning elements of further action. (as summarized by Adams & Markus, 2004, p. 341; emphasis in original).

Using this type of definition, the focus is not on studying culture as collections of people, but is instead on how psychological process may be implicitly and explicitly shaped by the worlds, contexts, or cultural systems that people inhabit. Culture, then, is not about groups of people—the Japanese, the Americans, the whites, the Latinos; thus, it is not groups themselves that should be studied. Rather, the focus should be on the implicit and explicit patterns of meanings, practices, and artifacts distributed throughout the contexts in which people participate, and on how people are engaged, invoked, incorporated, contested or changed by agents to complete themselves and guide their behavior. These ideas, practices, and artifacts, although not a fixed or coherent set and not shared equally by all in a given context, create and maintain the social level of reality that lends coherence to behavior and renders actions meaningful within a given cultural context.

A recent program of research on cognitive dissonance in East Asian and European American contexts (Kitayama, Snibbe, Markus, & Suzuki, 2004) is an example of a "culture as patterns" approach. These studies, along with earlier ones by Heine and Lehman (1997), demonstrate that people in East Asian cultural contexts did not show dissonance when tested in the standard dissonance conditions. In these studies participants rank-ordered a set of compact discs (CDs) according to their own preferences. Later, they were offered a choice between the fifth- and sixth-ranked CDs. When asked to give a second ranking of the 10 CDs, North Americans, but not East Asians, showed a strong justification effect; that is, they rated the CD that they had chosen more highly than the unchosen CD. Demonstrating one such difference between people engaging in two different cultural contexts was not the end, however, but rather the beginning of this series of studies. The goal was to account for the observed difference in terms of different patterns of ideas and practices relevant to choice, and furthermore, to understand what meanings and functions choice had in the two cultural contexts. In a series of subsequent studies, the situation was manipulated such that North American and East Asian participants made either a "public" or "private" choice. In the public condition, respondents were asked to consider the preferences of others or were exposed to the schematic faces of others. In these conditions East Asians, but not North Americans, revealed a tendency to justify their choices.

A careful analysis of the patterns of meaning and practices relevant to choice in East Asian and North American contexts explains these sharp differences in behavior. For North Americans, prevalent models of agency suggest that choices should express individual preferences and be free from influence by others. In contrast, in East Asian cultural contexts, choice—like many actions—is an interpersonal phenomenon, an expression of one's public stance, and is subject to social evaluation and criticism. As a consequence of this very different culturally shared and practiced model of agency, making a choice in public renders people vulnerable to a loss of face, honor, or reputation.

Together these studies examining variation in patterns of attention to self and other in the two contexts show that when choices are public, where the scrutiny of others is possible, rather than private, people in East Asian cultural contexts are likely to justify their actions. Other studies varying the nature of the other invoked during the choice situation—a liked versus disliked other—revealed that participants in East Asian contexts were particularly sensitive to the interpersonal nature of the situation compared with those in European American contexts. An analysis of this type illuminates context differences in normative patterns of how to be a person, and when and how to reference others. Still other studies by researchers focusing on choice as a prototypical agentic act (Iyengar & DeVoe, 2003; Savani, Markus, & Snibbe, 2006; Stephens, Markus, & Townsend, 2006) show that because choice in North American contexts is a signature of authentic agency and functions as a powerful schema for organizing behavior, people organize their own behavior and that of others in terms of choices and make inferences about behavior in terms of choice. By focusing on the behavioral patterns affording choice and analyzing how choice is understood and practiced in the two contexts, these studies underscore that differences in behavior among North Americans and Japanese are neither a result of something they "have" nor a matter of divergent traits or attributes. Instead, these differences are a function of something they do, of differences in their actions that result from engaging different symbolic resources and social systems.

ASSESSING MUTUAL CONSTITUTION: WHAT ARE THE CURRENT APPROACHES?

How are psychologists empirically examining the dynamic interdependence between sociocultural context and mind? One important issue to consider is how researchers conceptualize the psychological system with which the sociocultural system is interacting. Psychologists have typically carved up the psychological space into cognition, emotion, and motivation, and it is the cognitive system that has been the most elaborated in recent decades (Wierzbicka, 1994). These psychological systems have typically been assumed to function similarly across all people, but the database of psychological research has been based "almost completely on findings from samples of less than 10–15% of the populations on the face of the earth" (Rozin, 2001, p. 13), such as North America, Western Europe, and other regions in the English-speaking world (see also Gergen & Davis, 1985; Sears, 1986). This reliance on such a limited sampling of the human population may have led psychologists to conceptualize the psychological system in a fashion more congruent with their sample and with the cultural contexts most familiar to them.

Psychologists studying the dynamic interdependence between mind and culture have confronted the following questions in their research approach:

1. What counts as the psychological?
2. What counts as the sociocultural?
3. What is the nature of the mutually constituting relationship linking the two together?

Whether or not the psychological system functions similarly across all humans has been a central issue for psychologists assuming a sociocultural approach. Some would argue that the psychological system is universal, that it is made up from the same basic bits in the same fundamental fashion—in terms of cognition, emotion, and motivation—across all sociocultural contexts. Others ask why the psychological system has been carved up in this particular way, and whether or not it should be conceptualized in the same manner across all social worlds in which people engage.

Wierzbicka (1994), for example, notes that typical categories of emotion used in most psychological research may "constitute cultural artifacts of Anglo culture reflected in, and continually reinforced by, the English language" (p. 135). Rozin (2001), for example, identifies food, religion, ritual, leisure, sports, music, drama, money, and work as the major domains of human social life, thus contending that "there is no doubt that food, work, and leisure are the three most time consuming waking activities of human beings, and are all deeply so-

cial" (p. 13). He asks why psychologists have not organized their study of the psychological with these, or other, particular bits.

Surveying current empirical work in the field of sociocultural psychology, five major approaches emerge from the literature, offering perspectives on how to capture the dynamic interdependence between the psychological and the sociocultural. These five approaches are outlined first in this section. They are not mutually exclusive, although researchers utilizing them often attempt to conceptualize and investigate empirically the psychological study of sociocultural constitution in different ways. What varies among them is how they theoretically conceptualize and empirically investigate the psychological, the sociocultural, and the constituting relationship between the two. For each approach, this review focuses on its previous or prototypical, rather than prospective, contributions.

Following this description of the five approaches, some of the proposed central mechanisms and mediating processes that fashion the relationship between the cultural and the psychological are discussed. Finally, at the end of this chapter, an important distinction emerging in cultural psychological research is highlighted: conceptualizing culture as a constituting process versus a method of social influence.

Figure 1.1 summarizes and organizes the perspectives articulated by the five approaches. The schematics associated with each approach represent graphically how each approach conceptualizes the link between the psychological and the sociocultural. Each schematic contains a P, which represents the various structures and processes of the psychological system, and an SC, which represents elements of the various sociocultural contexts with which the psychological system engages. The size of the Ps relative to the SCs vary to indicate the relative emphasis placed on the psychological or the sociocultural in each approach's theoretical and empirical work. In each schematic, the arrows represent how the sociocultural and the psychological are considered to interact with one another, and we reflect this by varying the direction of the arrows and whether they are solid or dashed. A solid arrow indicates that the relationship is relatively well specified, while a dashed arrow indicates that the relationship is relatively less well specified in each approach's theoretical and empirical work. Three of the schematics include additional terms (*dimension*, *ecology*, and *situation*) be-

APPROACH	EMPIRICAL GOAL	MECHANISM OF CONSTITUTION	EXAMPLE
Dimensional SC ↓ Dimension 1 ⟶ Dimension 2 ⟶ **P** Dimension *n*	Specify the dimensions of culture that explain differences in attitudes, beliefs, values, and behaviors.	Worldviews, beliefs, values, attitudes translate the sociocultural into the psychological.	Horizontal–vertical relationships dimension
Models SC ⟷ **P**	Specify models that organize the links between the sociocultural and self systems.	Psychological tendencies, meanings, practices, and products reflect, foster, and sustain one another.	Influencing–adjusting models of agency
Cognitive Toolkit SC ⟶ **P**	Specify how cultural meanings and practices can influence basic cognitive tendencies.	Attention and perception are guided by cognitive tools or sets of interpretive tools.	Holistic–analytic cognition
Ecocultural Ecology → SC → **P**	Specify how ecological and sociopolitical factors influence psychological adaptation to a context.	Cultural adaptation and transmission shape the development and display of basic human characteristics.	Variations in cognitive competence
Dynamic Constructivist Situation ↓ SC ⟶ **P**	Specify the situational factors and boundary conditions that govern cultural influence.	Particular knowledge structures/implicit theories are activated by situational cues in a given situation.	Bicultural frame switching

FIGURE 1.1. Current approaches in psychology to studying the dynamic interdependence between the cultural and the psychological. *SC* indicates the sociocultural system, and *P* indicates the psychological system.

cause they are focal concepts explicitly theorized in each perspective.

Five Major Approaches

The Dimensional Approach: A Focus on Quantifying Differences

Several cross-cultural researchers (e.g., Hofstede, 1980, 1990; Leung, 1987; Schwartz, 1990; Triandis, 1989, 1990, 1995) explain the source of cultural psychological variation by identifying certain key dimensions along which cultural contexts may differ. They argue that, for culture to function as a useful explanatory variable, it should be conceptualized as a complex, multidimensional structure that can be evaluated along a set of particular dimensions. Cultural differences may reflect underlying basic value orientations, beliefs, and worldviews prevalent in a context; however, these differences can be best and most parsimoniously captured by identifying and describing cultures according to where they fall along a series of

dimensions. Thus, each context's distribution of behavior patterns, norms, attitudes, and personality variables can be measured and compared (Triandis, 1989). Triandis (1996) terms this series of dimensions *cultural syndromes*, which are "dimensions of cultural variation that can be used as parameters of psychological theories" (p. 407), are composed of attitudes, beliefs, norms, roles, self-definitions, and values shared by members in a given cultural context and can be organized around a series of central themes. The effect of the sociocultural on the psychological is therefore assumed to be "defined" by where a specific combination of people engaging in that culture, on average, "score" along a series of dimensions, thereby creating a particular patterning or cultural profile (i.e., syndrome). The dimensional approach, therefore, attempts to capture the ways the sociocultural may constitute the psychological by organizing potential sources of difference along a series of dimensions.

Some examples of these dimensions are power distance, uncertainty avoidance, masculinity–femininity, and individualism–collectivism (Hofstede, 1980); tightness, complexity, active–passive, honor, collectivism–individualism, and vertical–horizontal relationships (Triandis, 1989, 1990, 1995, 1996); and mastery, hierarchy, conservatism, affective autonomy, intellectual authority, egalitarian commitment, and harmony (Schwartz, 1990). An example of how these dimensions function is that although both Sweden and Germany are individualistic contexts, (or contexts privileging a notion of personhood as independent, autonomous, and personally motivated), Sweden is a horizontally individualistic context, emphasizing egalitarian social relations, while Germany is a vertically individualistic context, emphasizing a hierarchical conception of relations between people and groups (Triandis, 1995). Thus, Swedish and German contexts, and their corresponding constitution of the psychological, can be more accurately characterized by utilizing both dimensions, and potential cultural psychological effects can be more precisely understood.

In this approach, therefore, the cultural dimension is the way of capturing how the sociocultural and the psychological interact. The dimensional approach places emphasis upon providing a parsimonious organizing structure by which a wide array of cultural elements and their effects on the psychological can be measured and compared; thus, they can be understood as dimensions of constitution. These dimensions of constitution can thereby be systematically organized around a particular set of effects. Furthermore, this approach creates a common metric by which different contextual influences on the psychological may be compared along a discrete number of elements.

The dimensional approach, however, places little emphasis on the process by which the sociocultural and the psychological mutually constitute one another. It focuses on organizing the effects of the sociocultural on the psychological, but as of yet has little to say about *how* this relationship functions. For the most part, this approach has not focused on how psychological values and attitudes might be translated into social institutions, conventions, and habitual psychological tendencies. For this reason, the schematic for this approach (Figure 1.1) highlights that the dimensional perspective focuses on quantifying the ways in which *SC* may interact with *P*, without examining the constituting processes

themselves. Thus, *SC* is connected to *P* only through particular *dimensions*, and *SC* and *P* are not treated with equal emphasis. The dimensional approach thereby offers a method of conceptualizing what can be considered "meta-constitution," or a method of organizing the effects of mutual constitution without focusing on constituting processes themselves. Furthermore, this approach has not yet attempted to address the dynamic, changing nature of culture and its interdependence with the psychological, and can appear to view this relationship as rather static.

The Sociocultural Models Approach: A Focus on the Interacting Self System and Sociocultural System

Sociocultural models can be defined as culturally derived and selected ideas (both implicit and explicit) and practices (both informal and formal) about what is real, true, beautiful, good, and right—and what is not—that are embodied, enacted, or instituted in a given context (Markus & Kitayama, 2004; Shweder, 2003). Thus, sociocultural models give form and direction to individual experience, for example, perception, cognition, emotion, motivation, action. For example, models of agency provide implicit guidelines for "how to be," reflecting both descriptive and normative understandings of how and why people act (Kitayama & Uchida, 2005; Markus et al., 2005). Sociocultural models are dynamic, in that they both contribute to the *mutual* constitution of culture and mind, and remain mutable over time (Fiske et al., 1998). The concept of sociocultural models derives from cultural and cognitive anthropology, as well as sociocultural psychology (D'Andrade, 1990; Fiske et al., 1998; Holland & Quinn, 1987; Shore, 1996; Shweder, 1990; Shweder et al., 1998; Strauss, 1992).

Shared meaning is central to their existence, in that a sociocultural model can be described as an intersubjective cognitive schema (D'Andrade, 1990). Cultural schemas, furthermore, "are presupposed, taken for granted models of the world that are widely shared (though not to the exclusion of other alternative models) by the members of a society and that play an enormous role in their understanding of the world and their behavior in it" (Holland & Quinn, 1987, p. 4). Sociocultural models are frequently imperceptible to the minds that engage them, because they are represented at the private, internal, mental level and function by providing blueprints for how to think, feel, and act—how to *be*—in the world.

Particularly important to the sociocultural models approach is that models not only exist in the minds of people participating in a particular context but also structure the worlds in which people live. Culture is understood as public and exists before individuals participate in it (J. G. Miller, 1999). Shore (1996) emphasizes the point that cultural models exist not only as "cognitive constructs 'in the mind' of members of a community" (p. 44) but also as public artifacts and institutions "in the world" (see Berger & Luckmann, 1966). Hence, cultural models are also represented at the public, external, social, material level. This approach thereby focuses on how culture exists both "in the head" and "in the world," demonstrating that culture not only interacts with the psychological via the "heads" of people engaging in a particular context but also via the material worlds that people inhabit.

The existence of cultural models is dynamic and mutually constituted by person and environment, contingent upon and negotiated through "endless social exchanges" (Shore, 1996). The theory of social representations (Moscovici, 1981), deriving from sociology and social psychology, is another articulation of a sociocultural models approach, emphasizing that systems of values, ideas, practices, and products serve as orienting devices that allow people to successfully navigate their social worlds. Furthermore, social representations enable effective communication to take place among members existing in the same context through engagement with shared meanings (Moscovici, 1981).

The sociocultural models approach has been utilized to examine phenomena such as self systems (Heine et al., 1999; Markus & Kitayama, 1991; Markus et al., 1997), agency (Kitayama & Uchida, 2005; Markus & Kitayama, 2004; Markus et al., 2005; Snibbe & Markus, 2005), modes of being (Kitayama, Duffy, & Uchida, Chapter 6, this volume), emotion (Mesquita, 2003; J. L. Tsai, Chentsova-Dutton, Freire-Bebeau, & Przymus, 2002), motivation (H. Kim & Markus, 1999), cognitive and social development (Cole, 1985, 1992; Cole, Gay, Glick, & Sharp, 1971; Greenfield & Childs, 1977a, 1977b; Maynard & Greenfield, 2003; Moiser & Rogoff, 2003; Rogoff, 1991, 1995;

Wertsch, 1991), morality (J. D. Miller, Bersoff, & Harwood, 1990; Shweder, Much, Mahapatra, & Park, 1997), food and eating behavior (Rozin, 1996), intergroup relations (Plaut & Markus, 2005), education (Fryberg & Markus, 2006; Li, 2003), work ethic (Sanchez-Burks, 2002), honor (D. Cohen, Nisbett, Bowdle, & Schwarz, 1996; Nisbett & Cohen, 1996), hierarchy (A. Y. Tsai & Markus, 2006), relationships (Adams, 2005; Fiske, 1991, 1992), and well-being (Markus, Curhan, & Ryff, 2006; Plaut, Markus, & Lachman, 2002).

For example, people engaging in working-class (WK) contexts are more likely to inhabit social and material worlds that afford fewer resources, less opportunities for control and choice, and more interdependence with family and kin than do people engaging in middle-class (MD) contexts (Markus et al., 2005; Snibbe & Markus, 2005). As a consequence, people in WK contexts are less disturbed than those in MD contexts when others usurp their ability to make a choice, because choice making, and the self-expression and control over environmental contingencies that it affords, does not structure what it means to have a good and normatively appropriate self in WK contexts (Snibbe & Markus, 2005). Moreover, WK ideas about the right way to be in the world are more likely to foster a model of well-being focused on interdependent relations with close others (predominantly family and kin), and adjusting to obligations rather than a model of well-being focused on developing and expressing the self—the model most prevalent in MD contexts (Markus et al., 2005). Most importantly, these differences are reflected not only in the psychological processes of those engaging in MD and WK contexts but also in everyday cultural products—including, for example, popular song lyrics and magazine advertisements—that contribute to the structuring of WK and MD worlds, replete with different meanings, practices, and structures communicating how to be and what kinds of self and life are normal, valued, and good.

Sociocultural models organize the interplay between the more discrete elements of the sociocultural and the psychological systems identified in the mutual constitution model of culture and psyche (see Fiske et al., 1998) and described previously. For this reason, the schematic reflecting this approach contains one large, bidirectional arrow linking *P* and *SC* (Figure 1.1). Through the bidirectionality of this large arrow, we represent the theoretical and empirical attention paid to the mutual constitution process itself by researchers utilizing this approach. The center of the arrow is composed of several lines, intended to represent the variety of ways in which difference levels of the sociocultural systems (i.e., pervasive cultural ideas and the institutions, products, and everyday practices that reflect and promote these ideas) and the psychological system sustain and foster one another. Since the cultural models approach attempts to delineate the process of mutual constitution by organizing how cultural patterns both exist and necessarily depend upon how they are manifested and made real both "in the head" and "in the world," this approach focuses on the constitution process itself. Additionally, the relative emphasis placed on *SC* and *P* in this approach is comparable.

Like the tool kit approach we discuss next, the models perspective contests the content–process distinction, in that culture does not enter the psychological by influencing the basic psychological system, but rather is deeply involved in the constitution of the psychological itself. What is universal, from this perspective, is that humans are most fundamentally social beings whose psychological processes are interdependent with and dependent upon the social worlds with which they engage. The models approach, however, does need to specify more clearly the mechanisms by which the mutual constitution of the cultural and the psychological occur, which researchers have largely addressed thus far only at fairly broad levels. It also needs to empirically specify how the cultural and psychological systems exist in dynamic interaction with one another. Though this approach emphasizes this point theoretically, it should further address empirically how people engaging in contexts also shape the cultural, as well as how these constituting systems change over time. Furthermore, the models approach needs to outline more clearly and empirically test the relationship between the material products that structure sociocultural contexts and the minds that engage them.

The Tool Kit Approach:
A Focus on Culture and Cognition

Culture can also be thought of as an interpretive tool, or set of interpretive tools, that guide the ways individuals perceive and construct meaning in the world. The "culture as tools" approach builds on the early work of Sapir (1956) and Whorf (1956). The tool kit of any given culture, explains Bruner (1990), "can be described as a set of prosthetic devices by which human beings can exceed or even redefine the 'natural limits' of human functioning" (p. 21). Culture may be best conceptualized as a cognitive tool kit in three primary ways (Nisbett, Peng, Choi, & Norenzayan, 2001). The first is that even if all cultural contexts

> possessed essentially the same basic cognitive processes as their tools, the tools of choice for the same problem may be habitually very different. People may differ markedly in their beliefs about whether a problem is one requiring use of a wrench or pliers, in their skill in using the two types of tools, and in the location of particular tools at the top or the bottom of the toolkit. Moreover, members of different cultures may not see the same stimulus situation "in need of repair." (Nisbett et al., 2001, p. 306)

The second is that "cultures may construct composite cognitive tools out of the basic universal tool kit, thereby performing acts of elaborate cognitive engineering" (p. 306). Nisbett and colleagues (2001) offer Dennett's (1995) characterization of culture as a "crane-making crane," citing the transformation of ancient Chinese ideas about yin and yang into more complex dialectical concepts about change, moderation, relativism, and the necessity of multiple viewpoints.

A third perspective that Nisbett and colleagues (2001) promote, is a "situated cognition" view of the cultural tool kit, citing Resnick's (1994) claim that "tools of thought . . . embody a culture's intellectual history" and that these tools of thought "have theories built into them, and users accept these theories—albeit unknowingly—when they use these tools" (pp. 476–477, as cited in Nisbett et al., 2001). For example, people who participate in Western contexts, propose Nisbett and colleagues, have chronically been exposed to an intellectual history, beliefs, and theories about how the world is structured that emphasize object discreteness and attributes, the development of rule-based categorization systems, individual agency, personal freedom, control, causality, and abstraction. Alternatively, people who engage in East Asian contexts have been chronically exposed to intellectual history, beliefs, and theories about how the world is struc-

tured that emphasize object continuity and relationships, as well as identify systemic
interconnection, collective agency, social obligation, harmony, intuition, and practical em-
piricism. Thus, one consequence of the continued influence of this contextual variation is
that East Asians tend to adopt a more holistic
cognitive style, which directs attention toward
continuity, context, and a focus on similarities
and relationships, whereas Westerners tend to
adopt a more analytic cognitive style, which directs attention toward discreteness, focal objects, and a focus on categories and rules.

In a particularly intriguing example of the
mutual constitution of cultural patterns and
perceptual tendencies, Miyamoto, Nisbett and
Masuda (2006) demonstrated that Japanese
street scenes are more ambiguous and contain
more elements than American street scenes.
The implication is that Japanese physical environments may thus encourage a more holistic
processing than American scenes. A study exploring this idea found that, when primed with
Japanese as opposed to American scenes, both
Americans and Japanese attended more to contextual information.

The tool kit approach has also been applied
to studies on predictions of change (Ji, Nisbett,
& Su, 2001), context sensitivity (Masuda &
Nisbett, 2001), reasoning about contradiction
(Choi & Nisbett, 2000; Peng & Nisbett, 1999),
preferences for formal versus intuitive reasoning (Norenzayan, Smith, Kim, & Nisbett,
2002), and judgments of causal relevance
(Choi, Dalal, Kim-Prieto, & Park, 2003). The
recent work of Medin, Atran, and colleagues
(Atran et al., 2005; Medin & Atran, 2004),
with its emphasis on the role of inferential and
developmental cognitive processes in preparing
people to participate in cultural life, also fits
the culture as tool kit approach.

The tool kit approach, which is not entirely
separate from the sociocultural models approach, focuses primarily on how culture—
broadly construed—shapes the cognitive and
perceptual systems. The mechanism of constitution in this approach is how culture functions
as an interpretive tool or set of interpretive
tools that guide attention and perception (Figure 1.1). This approach challenges the notion
that perceptual and other such fundamental
cognitive processes are uniformly part of the
"basic" human mind by demonstrating that
culture can guide such basic processes, rendering the content-process distinction extremely

problematic. Culture, therefore, does not function as an overlay on basic cognitive processes;
rather, it is involved from the bottom up and
may significantly shape even the most fundamental psychological processes.

Although offering a perspective on the cultural constitution of basic cognitive processes,
the tool kit approach does not focus on specifying how the broad sociohistorical patterns that
researchers identify to account for observed
differences are made current or are continually
and dynamically manifested in the institutions,
practices, products, and daily experiences of
people participating in present contexts. Although researchers utilizing this approach certainly attend to characterizing contexts by
identifying prevalent, broad sociohistorical
patterns, they frequently move directly to as-
certaining very specific psychological effects.
Thus this perspective has been criticized for a
lack of attention to the constitution process itself, which could lead to an interpretation of
this research as essentializing differences even
though this is not the intent. It is for these reasons that the schematic representing this approach (see Figure 1.1) does not comprise one
large, multilevel arrow encompassing *SC* and *P*.
The arrow from *SC* to *P* is bold because this aspect of constitution has been highlighted much
more than the ways in which the psychological
constitute the cultural (represented by the
dashed arrow) though this direction of constitution has been the target of some theorizing.

The tool kit approach primarily focuses on
investigating how culture may interact with the
cognitive system, rather than also examining
the affective, motivational, and behavioral systems, thereby privileging the notion that the
sociocultural interacts with the psychological
via the cognitive system. In the schematic reflecting this approach, therefore, the *P* representing the psychological is large relative to the
SC. This indicates that the tool kit approach
appears to locate culture as more "inside the
head" of the person rather than as engaged in
constant and dynamic interaction with present
social contexts, material worlds, and the psychological system.

The Ecocultural Approach: A Focus on Adaptations to Ecological and Sociopolitical Contexts

Another approach related to the models perspective, though somewhat different in scope,
emphasis, and empirical methods, is the eco-

cultural approach. Proponents of the ecocultural approach, primarily developed by Berry (1976, 1979, 2000), and related ecological perspectives on culture (e.g., Bronfenbrenner, 1979; Whiting & Whiting, 1975), aim to understand how cultural and psychological processes interact by examining how two particular aspects of cultural context—ecological and sociopolitical factors—and a set of variables that connect these factors to psychological processes—cultural and biological adaptation at the population level, as well as several transmission processes at the individual level (e.g., enculturation, socialization, acculturation)—affect psychological functioning and behavioral variation. The ecocultural framework accounts for both cultural and psychological diversity among humans as adaptations—both collective and individual—to particular contexts (Berry, Poortinga, Segall, & Dasen, 2002; Georgas, van de Vijver, & Berry, 2004). Thus, ecological and sociopolitical environments are employed as specific, independent context variables that can be utilized to capture the continuous and interactive process by which sociocultural variables interact with a variety of psychological variables (Berry, 2004). The ecocultural approach is based on both a universalist assumption that basic psychological processes are shared across all humans, and an adaptive assumption that cultural variation arises from adaptations to objective requirements of the physical and social habitat, which allow for effective functioning in particular environments (Berry, 2000). Particular attention is paid to the transmission and developmental processes that link ecological and sociopolitical factors to individual psychological functioning (Berry, 2004; Berry et al., 2002).

The ecocultural approach has been utilized to study topics such as variations in the development of cognitive competence and adaptation (Berry, 1976, 2004; Berry et al., 1986), cultural competence (Lonner & Hayes, 2004), spatial orientation (Dasen & Wassmann, 1998; Mishra, Dasen, & Niraula, 2003), acculturation (Berry, 2003), relationships between ecosocial indicators and psychological variables (Georgas et al., 2004), and cognitive processes (e.g., Berry, Irvine, & Hunt, 1988). An example of this approach is a study of how ecology and language affect performance on spatial cognitive tasks (Mishra et al., 2003). Variations in spatial orientation systems, and the language that corresponds to such variations, are adap-

tive to the ecological conditions that arise in particular contexts (Mishra et al., 2003). Thus, the predominant spatial orientation style utilized in a flatland village near Varanasi, India, where cardinal directions are employed; in a mountainous village in Nepal, where relative directions are employed; and in the city of Varanasi, India, where a variety of spatial references are employed in response to the more complex environment, differentially affect performance on spatial cognitive tasks. Furthermore, the emergence of these tendencies can be traced developmentally, as children progressively learn the normative adult system.

Several research programs that are best classified as examples of the cultural models approach, because of their attention to meanings as reflected in cultural norms and psychological tendencies, might also be included as examples of the ecocultural approach. These programs include the work of Cohen, Nisbett, and colleagues (D. Cohen & Nisbett, 1994; Nisbett & Cohen, 1996; Vandello & Cohen, 1999) on a culture of honor in the American South and that of Kitayama, Ishii, and Imada (2006) on voluntary settlement patterns in Japan and the United States. A focus on the ways in which behavior patterns emerge as adaptations to both the physical and the social environment is an explicit feature of both research programs.

The ecocultural approach aims to link specific aspects of context (ecological and sociopolitical factors) to psychological processes through particular transmission processes. Though the cultural models approach emphasizes this focus as well, researchers utilizing the ecocultural approach have striven to concentrate on delineating the effects of particular aspects of the context on the psychological system. Furthermore, the attention paid to cultural transmission processes—also emphasized in cultural models theory, but significantly needing more consideration and clarification—is foregrounded. The ecocultural approach, however, assumes that "basic human characteristics are common to all members of the species (i.e., constituting a set of psychological givens), and that culture influences the development and display of them (i.e., culture plays different variations on these underlying themes)" (Berry, 2004, pp. 6–7). Common underlying universal psychological processes are thereby taken as a set of psychological givens, because expressive variation leads to some cultural differences in psychological functioning depending on environmental influence (Berry, 2000). Culture is therefore allowed to constitute some of the psychological system, but it does not go "all the way down."

Although criticized earlier for being environmental determinists who conceive of culture in a largely static fashion, ecocultural perspective theorists now conceptualize people as agents who actively interact with and change their dynamic environments, as ecological adaptation functions as both a continuous and an interactive process (Berry, 2004). Proponents of the ecocultural approach also utilize the notion of context variables (e.g., ecological and sociopolitical factors) as a means to conceptualize culture as an independent variable. Problems with conceptualizing culture as an independent variable have been argued extensively elsewhere (Fiske et al., 1998; Shweder, 1990), and although their goal of specifying how particular aspects of a context may interact with the psychological is important, the idea of culture as a complex, mutually reinforcing, multicomponential system should not be lost. In this approach's schematic (Figure 1.1), *ecology* is highlighted as shaping how SC and P may constitute one another. The arrow representing how P constitutes SC is dashed because this aspect of the ecocultural perspective has not yet been underscored in theory and research. P is also somewhat larger than SC because ecocultural theorizing has placed more relative emphasis on conceptualizing P.

The Dynamic Constructivist Approach: A Focus on Culture's Situational Influence

Researchers who adopt a dynamic constructivist approach aim to emphasize that culture resides in the mind in the form of a loose network of knowledge structures, mental constructs, and representations that are widely shared within a given context, and that these internalized constructs do not continuously guide our information processing but rather do so only when activated (Hong, Benet-Martinez, Chiu, & Morris, 2003; Hong & Chiu, 2001; Hong, Morris, Chiu, & Benet-Martinez, 2000). Culture therefore affects cognition when, in particular social situations, the relevant implicit theories or shared assumptions are available, accessible, salient, and applicable in the situation (Hong et al., 2003; Hong & Chiu, 2001; Hong et al., 2000). Hong and Chiu (2001) propose that cultural influences on cognition are "mediated by

the basic principles of social cognition" and activated in specific domains across particular situations; thus, they "seek to identify when well-documented cultural differences in cognitions would surface, disappear, or even reverse" (p. 183). Participants engaging in East Asian contexts, for example, did not differ from participants engaging in American contexts in their propensity to compromise in a decision-making task, unless they were asked to provide reasons for making their decisions (Briley, Morris, & Simonson, 2000). Cultural differences in choice behavior therefore resulted only when participants were required to provide an explanation for their decisions, because "reasons for choices depend on the cultural norms as to what is acceptable and persuasive" (Briley et al., 2000, p. 161).

Expanding on the tool kit idea, described previously, researchers adopting a dynamic constructionist approach emphasize that the applicability of context-based interpretive tools depends upon a specific combination of factors or boundary conditions. Applying a "culturally shared cognitive tool" may be more likely when a person is under high cognitive load or when quick decisions are required, for example, because a spontaneous reaction, rather than deliberative consideration, is more likely to emerge in those types of situations (Hong & Chiu, 2001). When exposed to such conditions, "perceivers are likely to draw on the well learned, widely shared, highly accessible cultural theories to guide their judgments" because perceivers will possess "less cognitive resources and a high need for closure" (Hong & Chiu, 2001, p. 189). Several studies support this idea that cognitive busyness and the need for spontaneous responses augment the potential to observe cultural differences (Chiu, Morris, Hong, & Menon, 2000; Knowles, Morris, Chiu, & Hong, 2001; Zàrate, Uleman, & Voils, 2001).

In this approach, the sociocultural interacts with the psychological when a particular knowledge structure, among a loose network of knowledge structures, is activated in accordance with the tenets of basic social cognition principles (see Figure 1.1). The dynamic constructivist approach thereby provides a precise, mechanistic account of cultural influence, with a particular emphasis on variation due to the situational factors and boundary conditions of cultural effects. Thus, P in this schematic is quite large relative to SC because of the centrality of basic social cognitive theory in this perspective. *Situation* is also highlighted because the situational must first activate *SC*, as presented by the solid vertical arrow pointing to the solid horizontal arrow linking *SC* and *P*. Situation will influence *P*, then, only when situational conditions are ripe. The other four approaches consider issues of situational dynamism fairly infrequently, and in order to have a more complete understanding of how the cultural and the psychological interact, it is important to understand how such factors play a role in modifying cultural influence on the psychological. The focus of this approach, however, is on cultural *influence* more so than the process of mutual *constitution*, because its aim is to specify the conditions under which the cultural influences the psychological, rather than focusing on the processes by which the cultural and the psychological constitute one another.

Thus, this approach aims to promote the notion that "dramatic effects can involve comparable processes," in that "while concrete aspects of process differ qualitatively, more abstract aspects of process operate similarly across cultures" (Chiu et al., 2000, p. 257). Chiu and colleagues thereby propose that contrasting cultural variations and universal processes are less productive than modeling the dynamic interplay of culture and mind. Yet with what sort of "mind" is "culture" interacting? Though proponents of the tool kit and models approaches, which focus primarily on constituting processes (though in different fashions), are by no means "merely relativistic," both do argue for the notion that the psychological system at very basic levels is shaped by the sociocultural. Alternatively, proponents of the dynamic constructivist approach seem to imply that the psychological system is, at core, basic and universal. The dynamic constructivist perspective therefore appears to propose that there is a basic psychological system present with which culture sometimes interacts. This is another reason why the *P* in the dynamic constructivist schematic is relatively large. Moreover, by conceptualizing culture mainly as an interplay between cognitive processes, this approach appears to locate culture primarily "in the head" of the person. The mind is therefore connected to the context only when the social-cognitive conditions are ripe, and that mind seems likely to be a "basic human mind" rather than a "socioculturally contingent mind."

Comparing Approaches: An Example

The previous section identified and briefly sketched some features of five major approaches to capturing the dynamic interdependence between the psychological and the sociocultural. The approaches have various strengths and weaknesses, and their usefulness is likely to depend on the problem under study. Whether one approach will prove superior to others or whether the approaches will be eventually amalgamated as researchers have a better grasp of both *P* and *SC* is an unanswered empirical question. Analyzing a single problem from the perspective of all five approaches can highlight their differences. A current problem of both theoretical and practical significance is how to understand the differences in academic performance of students with different racial and ethnic associations. In some California schools, but not others, white students and Asian students perform strikingly better in terms of grades and standardized test scores than black and Latino students (Steele et al., 2006). Importantly, in some schools matched for socioeconomic status and curriculum, such disparities are attenuated; thus, differences in performance are primarily or only about differences in relevant skills. Most researchers who are aware of the literature on racial and ethnic gaps in performance would begin with one sociocultural approach or another, assuming that the explanation for these differences is to be found in the interdependence among selves and social systems.

A *dimensional* approach to this problem might be the most straightforward and easiest to assume. It would hypothesize that differences in academic performance result from differences in underlying beliefs, attitudes, and behaviors, and would develop a questionnaire with some well-validated measures to be given to these students. Based on previous research (Katz, 1987), such a study would likely reveal no important differences among these groups of students in how education is valued; almost all students in every context value education and believe in its importance for upward mobility. Questionnaires assessing self-construal, individualism–collectivism, mastery, control, or psychological well-being may reveal differences in how students generally think about themselves. To explain which aspects of culture have produced these differences, investigators might examine the attitudes and values of teachers or peers toward the students and schooling.

A *sociocultural models* approach would be likely to examine how students are thinking about themselves, their school, their teachers, and the other students. A focus in this analysis would be on the prevalent meanings or implicit norms that are structuring agency and guiding action. Questions might assess what school means to the students and what academic performance means to their views of themselves. Investigators taking this approach might also assess how teachers, parents, or other students are thinking and feeling about the students. A models approach is more likely than other approaches to begin with collecting qualitative data—with not only observations of students in the classroom but also open-ended questions that would allow students to construct their performance in their own terms, using their own words. The assumption of a cultural models approach would be that the school climate does not afford all students a sense of self as normatively good or appropriate; thus, the performance of some students is impaired. A qualitative approach might be combined with the use of vignettes or experimental techniques that would manipulate how students understand themselves or what students believe others understand about them. A models approach might also include an analysis of cultural products such as curricula, school mission statements, assignments, materials on display in the school, teacher practices, and social relations in the classroom. The assumption behind these analyses would be the need to assess the public and private meanings that are prevalent in the school, and to assume that these meanings cannot merely be reduced to or explained in terms of any other factors.

A *tool kit* approach would attend to the attentional and cognitive styles of students, hypothesizing that because of the ideas about learning in their respective contexts, or because of the habitual tasks to which they have been exposed, students from different racial or ethnic groups may have different tools in their tool kit, or may differ in how accessible their tools are. Researchers would be likely to administer a variety of tests to determine how the cognitive processing or attentional skills of the students vary. This approach would work reasonably well for explaining some of these differences. White and Asian students, compared with black and Latino students, are likely to have relatively higher socioeconomic status, and thus more experience in settings with people who have had more formal schooling, and with tasks and activities that would develop the type of tools required by formal schooling. Investigators might study how various habitual practices in home or previous school environments have given rise to these differences in tools for high grades and test scores.

An *ecocultural* approach would begin with careful attention to the details of the classroom and school situation, perhaps noting classroom size and layout, school size, and ethnic and racial composition of the school and neighborhood. Such an analysis might collect data on the economic level of the school, determining, for example, how many children receive free lunch or other aid. Furthermore, such an approach might also assess the level of teacher preparation in the schools and per-pupil level of school funding, and even the political climate in the neighborhood of the school or the region, including racial and ethnic attitudes. The assumption behind these analyses would be that differential academic performance is a function of how effectively students adapt or are helped to adapt to relevant sets of ecological and sociopolitical factors.

A *dynamic constructivist* approach would not use the wide-angle lens of the ecoculturalist, but would instead zoom in on the immediate situation in the classroom. Such an analysis might begin with the assumption that the differences among students relate to something that happens in the classroom either at the time of the test or at the time of completing or grading the assignment—the situation. Like much research in mainstream social psychology, it is this situation that activates and makes salient different ideas or knowledge, which then produce differences in performance. A dynamic constructivist approach might assume that something is happening in the classroom around academic performance. Perhaps some set of situational factors is producing contingencies between school performance and identity, such that some students feel threatened, devalued, or limited in the classroom and do not perform well. The source of the differences among racial and ethnic groups for the dynamic constructivists would be in some details of the situation and the knowledge structures this situation primes. Proponents of this approach would assume that these group differences would not be observed at other times in other situations. Dynamic constructivists might experiment with creating different types of situations or with making different ideas, knowledge structures, and self or other conceptions salient, then observing performance.

All five approaches could be useful for the analysis of this problem. None are irrelevant, and the best results are likely to come from using a variety of approaches in combination. All of the approaches could be used to illuminate the full cycle of mutual constitution, but most have yet to attend carefully to how the sociocultural and the psychological interact. Some investigators taking a sociocultural models approach have made some effort to demonstrate how the practices and products generated by people in particular contexts foster particular psychological tendencies, but the other approaches have yet to focus on how culturally shaped people *shape* their contexts. For example, the dimensional approach has not examined how the expression of particular attitudes and values creates and maintains particular contexts. Several other points of tension among the approaches are obvious. An ecocultural approach assumes that the psychological is universal, and that differences among people result from differences in how successfully people have adapted to the various structural characteristics of their situations. A cultural models approach insists that meaning cannot be reduced to the structural, and that it is its own independent level that requires analysis. For example, for students to benefit from a structural variable such as small class size or a factor such as teacher attention, they must attach the relevant meaning to this act; they must construct it as a sign of attention or an indication of high expectations, and they must value such an expression. Such constructions are not automatic; they are contingent on prior constructions. Just as meanings must be expressed in practice or institutionalized in structures before they are powerful, so must structures be animated by particular meanings before they have particular effects.

Among other differences, dynamic constructivists are likely to investigate the details of the classroom. Some students, for example, may perform better when collaborating rather than when working independently, and changing the configuration of the classroom may be one possible route to improved performance. Yet if a relational way of being involves a complex of attitudes, values, practices, activities, and behavioral orientations, changing behavior may require more than activating a interdependent mind-set or set of knowledge structures relevant to interdependence. At the same time, dimensionalists may fail to see how different situations could in fact prime different norms or values and produce changes in performance. Moreover, the approaches differ somewhat in how likely they are to locate the source of performance in the student. The tool kit approach is probably particularly likely to do so, even though the particulars of the tools depend on the context. The ecocultural and sociocultural models approaches are less likely to do so. All of these approaches could directly assess the views that others have about the students and locate at least some of the performance differences in the eyes of others or in what students perceive as the expectations that others hold for them. Such measures may be more powerful predictors of performance than measures taken of the students' views of themselves.

A key aspiration of a sociocultural perspective, regardless of the particular approach to mutual constitution, is to go beyond the person in explaining the person. Many important effects are likely to be located in intersubjective space and are the result of what the target person is thinking that another person(s) is thinking about her or him. Finally, although these approaches have so far been identified by different methods, all of the approaches to mutual constitution could profitably use all methods.

A Note on Mechanism and Mediation: Toward Specifying How It Works

Mutual Constitution Mechanisms

What are the mechanisms that fashion the interplay between the sociocultural and the psychological? In a broad sense, repeated mere exposure (Zajonc, 1968) certainly applies, in that particular contexts afford exposure to certain meanings, practices, and institutions that constitute the fabric of our social worlds, and in that exposure leads us to construct these certain meanings, practices, and institutions as familiar, normal, and good. Sperber (1996) further contends that representations that are "repeatedly communicated," while being "minimally transformed" in a given context, end up "belonging" to a culture. Thus, exposure to meanings and practices prevalent in a given context can provide a network of implicit and explicit associations to guide what it means to be a good person and competent social actor in that context, such as models of agency (Markus & Kitayama, 2003) or models of self (Markus et al., 1997). Kitayama and colleagues (Chapter 6, this volume) suggest that, in particular, the patterning of social relations prevalent in a context affords a particular principle of action regulation, such as goal directedness versus responsiveness to social contingencies, which then guides an array of related psychological tendencies and behaviors. Thus, social relations in East Asian contexts, oriented toward interdependence and collectivism, direct people participating in such contexts to attend to the external contingencies of relating with others, such as others' expectations, desires, and needs, as well as particular features of the social situation, such as whether one is situated in a work or home context. Therefore, to behave as a competent social actor, individuals are motivated to respond to such social contingencies, adjusting their behaviors accordingly.

Cultural models, therefore, seek to organize how certain meanings and practices that are pervasive in a context structure the individual's psychological world. Individuals engaging in particular contexts in turn embody, reproduce, contest, and transform these prevalent contextual patterns. Thus, both the psychological and the contextual are conceptualized as interacting systems: The context is a system that comprises meanings, practices, institutions, and daily experiences, whereas the psychological is a system of behavioral, cognitive, affective, and motivational processes, often organized as a self-system. Even the act of contesting or rebelling against a prevalent cultural pattern, such as choosing to devote one's self to the hyperindividualistic teachings of Ayn Rand despite growing up and currently living in a relatively collectivistic Japanese context, nevertheless involves a deep level of engagement with that particular cultural pattern. Though much cultural patterning of the person does takes place at the implicit level, to engage with and be shaped by a cultural model does not imply that an individual does so as a mindless automaton.

Acquired attentional strategies are another broad-level mechanism by which the cultural and the psychological interact (Nisbett et al., 2001). Such strategies, which derive from the interplay between context-specific, naive metaphysical and epistemological systems and cognitive processes, can serve to direct individuals' perceptual processes, thereby shaping (at least in part) the cognitive tool kit available to people participating in given contexts. These acquired strategies guide the information about the world on which the perceptual system focuses, and thereby the information available for cognitive processing (e.g., Hong & Chiu, 2001; Hong et al., 2000; Ji et al., 2001; Kitayama, Duffy, Kawamura, & Larsen, 2003; Masuda & Nisbett, 2001; Nisbett et al., 2001). Nisbett and colleagues, for example, propose that enduring differences in the cognitive styles of people participating in Western versus East Asian contexts support the interplay between cognitive processes and historically derived beliefs and theories about how the world is structured. These differences both render and reinforce distinct systems of thought.

These attempts at delineating the mutual constitutional mechanisms that guide how the dynamic interdependence between the sociocultural and psychological functions have in common an attempt to capture how the cultural and the psychological exist in constant, dynamic interaction with one another. They attempt to organize how the sociocultural and the psychological shape and require one another. The cultural models approach and the tool kit approach tend to focus on broad constitutional mechanisms of exposure and attentional orientation, with the intent of identifying how mutual constitution takes place. The cultural models approach tries to organize how different levels of the cultural system (core cultural ideas and representations, institutions, practices, products, and daily experiences) interact with different levels of the self-system (affect, cognition, motivation, and behavior). Researchers employing the tool kit approach predominantly do not focus on how the cultural and the psychological are mutually constituted through the different levels of the cultural system; rather, they focus on how sociohistorical differences in context may be reflected in the most basic levels of the cognitive system.

Mechanisms That May Mediate the Relationship between the Cultural and the Psychological

In further attempts to clarify how the cultural and the psychological work together, researchers have also aimed to specify some of the mediating mechanisms by which the cultural and the psychological interact. Hong and colleagues (Hong et al., 2000, 2003; Hong & Chiu, 2001) suggest that culture interacts with the psychological in a situational manner, according to the basic social-cognitive principles of availability, accessibility, saliency, and applicability. According to the dynamic constructivist approach, culture, at the psychological level, resides in the mind in the form of domain-specific knowledge structures or implicit theories; thus, "cultural differences are mediated by the activation of cultural theories" and cultural differences in self-cognitions and social behaviors "emerge only when relevant cultural theories are activated" (Hong, Ip, Chiu, Morris, & Menon, 2001, p. 260). In a formal mediation analysis framework, for example, Briley and colleagues (2000) found that the content of participants' reasons for a decision—whether the reason was compromise-oriented or not—mediated the relationship between consumer cultural background and their preference for compromise alternatives. Furthermore, individualism–collectivism and conflict resolution style, both individual difference or dispositional measures, were not found to mediate the cultural effect (Briley et al., 2000).

Moreover, the effects of culture on the psychological may be attenuated or enhanced due to particular boundary conditions on cultural influence (Hong & Chiu, 2001), such as need for closure (NFC; Chiu et al., 2000). Whether existing chronically (Chiu et al., 2000), or induced via time pressure (Chiu et al., 2000) or cognitive load (Knowles et al., 2001), people high in NFC demonstrate magnified cultural differences. Thus, "another kind of evidence for cultural differences in chronic accessibility hinges on the interaction of accessible constructs with epistemic motives" (Hong et al., 2003, p. 454), in that the desire or need for a clear answer to a question and a dislike for ambiguity lead the individual to rely on well-learned, repeatedly rehearsed, highly accessible—and thereby potentially cultural—constructs (Chiu et al., 2000). Thus timing, when culture influences the psychological, is a central theme characterizing this stream of research.

The moderating effects of NFC, suggest Chiu and colleagues (2000), may be mediated by the immediacy principle, or the epistemic

need to reach any decision quickly regarding an ambiguous issue. Because cultural theories are not the only way an individual understands the social world, and "do not emerge out of a motivational vacuum," people engaging in various contexts can "develop and apply a cultural theory to meet their epistemic needs" when necessary (Chiu et al., 2000, p. 10). Epistemic needs may generally derive from the individual's attempt to make sense of the reality of daily life, which is often ambiguous (Adams & Markus, 2004; Richter & Kruglanski, 2004). Another articulation of how cultural influence may be the result of motivated cognition comes from terror management theory, in that cultural theories help people make sense out of the "big questions," such as the meaning of life (Pyszczynski, Greenberg, Solomon, Arndt, & Schimel, 2004). Religion, for example, is a cultural institution that offers solutions for the potentially paralyzing, existential terror induced by the awareness of one's mortality. People are thus motivated both to construct and to engage in such institutions that embody particular cultural patterns (Solomon, 2004).

Self-construal, another significant mechanism proposed to mediate and cause cultural effects, was originally proposed as an organizing device, able to capture the interplay among cognitive, affective, and motivational systems that may comprise how a person in a given context construes the self, and how the self relates to others in similar or differing modes across cultural contexts (Markus & Kitayama, 1991). Although some researchers have maintained studying the self in a systems framework (Cross & Madson, 1997; Heine et al., 1999; Kitayama et al., 1997; Markus & Kitayama, 2003; Markus et al., 1997), and have directed their research at understanding the mutual constitution of context and self, others have adopted more social-cognitive approaches geared toward delineating the causal role of self-construal as a cognitive mechanism in producing and/or mediating particular psychological effects. Shifts in self-construal (either priming aspects of independence–individualism or interdependence–collectivism) have been found, for example, to mediate shifts in values and judgments of obligation (Gardner, Gabriel, & Lee, 1999), increase the retrieval of self-cognitions relating to the aspect of the self primed (Trafimow, Triandis, & Goto, 1991), guide whether a context-dependent versus context-independent mode guides cognition

(Kühnen, Hannover, & Schubert, 2001; Kühnen & Oyserman, 2002), determine whether attentiveness to others is a self-defining goal and thereby an enhanced tendency (Haberstroh, Oyserman, Schwartz, Kühnen, & Ji, 2002), determine the consequences of social comparison (Stapel & Koomen, 2001), elicit modes of regulatory focus (Lee, Aaker, & Gardner, 2000), and influence mimicry behavior (van Baaren, Maddux, Chartrand, de Bouter, & van Knippenberg, 2003). These findings often appear to mirror analogous effects observed between unprimed people engaging in different contexts (e.g., North American and East Asian, suggesting that the proposed cultural effects are actually due to some aspect of self-construal; see Cohen, Chapter 8, this volume).

Although the manipulation of self-construal helps researchers strengthen the causal argument in support of interdependent constitution between mind and context, it is unclear whether such cognitive priming effects are truly comparable to chronic contextual effects (see Cohen, Chapter 8, this volume, for an extended discussion). Moreover, in citing previous work, those who have interpreted "selves" to mean explicit concepts that can be assessed directly through attitude or value scales appear to miss the significant point that the self is not a particular set of attitudes, or conscious verbal propositions about the self, that are accessible or even activated reliably on a conscious level; instead, the self is a set of implicit and explicit modes of operating in the world. For example, in an independent mode of operating in the world, behavior is organized and made meaningful primarily by reference to one's own internal repertoire of one's own thoughts, feelings, and actions. In contrast, in an interdependent mode, behavior is organized and made meaningful to a large extent by reference to the thoughts and feelings of others in their encompassing social networks. These orienting patterns that guide thought, feeling, and action do not necessarily translate into explicit concepts that can be assessed directly through attitude or value scales (Markus & Kitayama, 2003; Heine & Norenzayan, 2006), though this work is attractive because it "uncomplicates" the complexities of thinking of self and culture as multifaceted interacting systems, and is therefore relatively easy to use (Kitayama, 2002).

Responses to self-report attitudinal scales are not necessarily valid or accurate indices of cultural constitution, often demonstrating a host of measurement biases and inconsistencies with cultural effects demonstrated on other types of measures (Chen, Lee, & Stevenson, 1995; Heine, Lehman, Peng, & Greenholtz, 2002; Peng, Nisbett, & Wong, 1997), and the primes utilized to induce self-construal effects may not serve as very meaningful proxies for cultural constitution or influence (for recent discussions, see Kitayama, 2002; Heine & Norenzayan, 2006). Furthermore, relatively few precise mediating mechanisms have been identified besides cognitive self-construal (Heine & Norenzayan, 2006), so researchers in the field should be careful not to overprivilege this one potential mechanism.

Also, it remains unclear whether or not self-construal priming in and of itself has the same effects on people engaging in different contexts. Although the researchers cited earlier appear to demonstrate that this may be the case to a certain degree (e.g., Gardner et al., 1999; Trafimow et al., 1991), others have suggested that it may not (Oyserman, Coon, & Kemmelmeier, 2002). Hong et al., (2001), however, found that although priming the individual self ("I") versus the collective self ("we") among Chinese and American participants affected spontaneous self-concept, the effect was manifested differently between the two groups. When the collective self was activated for Chinese participants, their awareness of duties was also increased, though this was not the case for American participants. On the other hand, when the individual self was activated for American participants, their awareness of individual rights was also increased, though this was not the case for Chinese participants. The authors propose that because duties are emphasized in Chinese contexts, they are central to the notion of the collective self, but because rights are not emphasized, they are not salient in the individual self-concept. Alternatively, because rights are emphasized in American contexts, they are central to the individual self, but because duties are not emphasized, they are not associated with the collective self-concept. Hong et al. conclude that "although the 'I' or 'we' manipulation can enhance individualistic or collectivistic orientations regardless of participants' cultural background, how such manipulation affects spontaneous self-cognitions may depend to a large extent on what constitutes the individual and collective selves in the culture" (p. 260). It is important to disentangle how situational priming interacts with chronic contextual influence.

Whereas other researchers are beginning to offer accounts that specify the mediating mechanisms that structure the relationship between the cultural and the psychological, such as choice-making perceptions and goals (Iyengar & DeVoe, 2003) and social beliefs (Bond, 2005), the question of how the cultural and the psychological interact is still very open in the field, leaving much room for further exploration. Cohen (Chapter 8, this volume) offers an account of both the advantages and disadvantages of applying formal mediation analysis to cultural-psychological research, which should be considered carefully due to the current emphasis on performing mediation analyses in social and personality psychology. A consideration Cohen (Chapter 8, this volume) highlights that deserves particular attention, is that typical conceptions of the mediation method locate culture within the individual, particularly "inside the head" of the individual. This approach thereby underemphasizes how culture also exists "outside of the person," built into the sociocultural environments that we inhabit. Cultural researchers also need to consider the possibility of external factors that may mediate the relationship between the sociocultural and the psychological. The worlds that people inhabit are *themselves* cultural products; they are meaning-saturated repositories of the psychological activity of those who preceded us (Adams & Markus, 2004; Bourdieu, 1990; Cole, 1996; Shore, 1996). We need to delineate how meaning-saturated everyday worlds that comprise institutions, practices, experiences, products, and representations mediate how the cultural works on the psychological.

Moreover, it is important to point out that failing to *directly* measure hypothesized causal mechanisms is not unique to the study of sociocultural psychology; in fact this is true in many of the phenomena studied in social psychology (Heine & Norenzayan, 2006). For example, the "dissonance" in cognitive dissonance theory (Festinger, 1957), the "terror" in terror management theory (Pyszczynski et al., 2004), the "threat" in stereotype threat theory (Steele & Aronson, 1995), and the particular computational mechanisms underlying the biases and heuristics that lead people to commit the conjunction fallacy and base-rate neglect

(Kahneman & Tversky, 1973) all deal with hypothesized constructs that have as yet been directly assessed or captured either rarely or not at all through measurement techniques (Heine & Norenzayan, 2006). Thus, sociocultural psychology does not uniquely confront challenges associated with measurement precision, and should not incur special criticism for this issue (Matsumoto & Yoo, 2006).

Culture as "Process" versus Culture as "Social Influence"

Reflecting on the field as a whole, one important distinction that can be drawn regarding the current empirical approaches to studying the relationship between the cultural and the psychological is whether researchers seem to conceptualize culture as *process* or as *social influence*. Conceptualizing culture as process entails emphasizing that it functions as a "constituent process that is implicated in explaining what are considered basic psychological phenomena," a "source of patterning" for psychological processes themselves (J. G. Miller, 1999, p. 85; 2002). Researchers who view culture as process tend to focus on how one becomes and exists as a cultural being, emphasizing that the cultural and the psychological, the environmental and the individual, cannot be separated. Culture is a symbolically structured environment (Greenfield, 1997), wherein the sociocultural and the psychological exist in mutual interdependence with one another. Thus, neither the sociocultural nor the psychological can be reduced to or extracted from the other (J. G. Miller, 1999).

J. G. Miller (1999) points out that manipulating individualism–collectivism in the lab, for example, does not replicate the nature of cultural constitution that arises from engaging in collectivist contexts, because "cultural variation in psychological functioning arises not merely from individuals maintaining contrasting schematic understandings but also from their involvement in contrasting cultural activities and practices" (p. 89). Researchers who conceptualize culture as a means of social influence, alternatively, may assume that the psychological system is at core basic, universal, and unstructured by the sociocultural; thus, the psychological is influenced by culture only when the appropriate situational conditions arise. This way of conceptualizing culture relies on more typically social-psychological understandings of social influence (discussed previously) that do not recognize the full extent of the sociocultural constitution of the psychological. The field will need to address the implications of conceptualizing culture as influence or as process, and delineate what can be learned from each perspective to elucidate the dynamic interdependence between the sociocultural and the psychological.

THE SOCIOCULTURAL APPROACH—WHAT NEXT?

Together the studies reviewed here are successful in illuminating some of the ways in which people and their social world make each other up. These studies are a significant start in establishing an empirical foundation for the theoretical vision of some of psychology's earliest theorists. As the sociocultural approach is elaborated, two ideas emerge clearly: (1) Many theoretical and methodological challenges still have to be met, and (2) the sociocultural approach can be extended productively to other areas within psychology.

Conceptual Challenges

The application of a sociocultural approach to psychology makes clear that the dualistic notions of "inside and outside the head" and of "the person and the situation" are frameworks that, though useful in the past, may now impede theorizing. Behavior is not the function of "the person" and "the situation" as separate entities, but is rather the consequence of the dynamic relationship and basic constitutive interdependence between the two.

Persistent Dualisms

The ideology of individualism has been the powerful perspective that has dominated psychology, forcing a divide between "person" and "context," "inside" and "outside." Typically, the actor in a psychological interaction is cast as an entity separate from the external contextual stage, and that actor's internal psychological system is then moved or influenced by the external immediate situation "performed" on that stage. Many theories in psychology conceptualize the person as a bounded, autonomous, independent being who aims to move through the world unfettered by

group ties or situational pressures (for a discussion of these ideas, see Baumeister, 1987; Bellah, Madsen, Sullivan, Swidler, & Tipton, 1985; Farr, 1991; Guisinger & Blatt, 1994; Markus & Kitayama, 1994; Sampson, 1985, 1988; Shweder & Bourne, 1984).

Psychology has thereby taken as normal and natural a fundamentally *asocial* model of the person. The implicit notion that the individual is an a priori separate and self-contained (as well as rational and self-interested) social actor, who must resist or be on guard with respect to control or influence by others, is a key idea in all areas of psychology. A sociocultural approach challenges psychology to consider a more social model of the person, in which the person exists in a dynamic and inextricable bond with her or his context. There is no "neutral" or "natural" person that exists apart from her or his context, or apart from the social construction of her or his existence as a fully functioning self. Similarly, as noted earlier, the situations that are often cast as separate from people cannot be understood as separate from their affording cultural contexts.

These context-contingent patterns of meanings, practices, and products *cannot be isolated from* basic psychological processes and behavior. Despite the clear understanding of the constructed nature of social reality evinced by most early theorists, over subsequent decades psychologists have often described the social world as if it existed independently of the perceiver's standpoint, and was there for perceivers to apprehend either adeptly or speciously. Sapir (1924), arguing against the notion of an external reality existing outside the person, claimed that "the worlds in which different societies live are distinct worlds, not merely the same world with different labels attached" (p. 409). Likewise, Goodman (1984) asserted, "One might say there is only one world but this holds for each of the many worlds" (p. 278).

More recently, some programs of research have begun to move closer to empirically illustrating the many worlds that exist within the one world and to carefully track the ways the idea that the individual and the social world exist in a fundamentally contingent relationship. Nisbett (2003) and colleagues, in the studies we reviewed earlier, have shown that those engaging in European American contexts and those engaging in East Asian cultural contexts *see* the same stimulus in very different ways, and that the products they produce reflect these differences. Markus et al. (2005) have shown that perceivers in Japanese and American contexts are likely to understand agency in different ways, and their social worlds are constructed accordingly. Thus, perceivers in American contexts saw the performance of Olympic athletes as a function of various athletic strengths and skills, whereas perceivers in Japanese contexts saw the performance of Olympic athletes as equally reflective of athletic strengths, past training, and experience. These differences were not just a matter of different construals of the same athletic performance. The constructed social world also reflected these differences. The respective television coverage of the Olympics (one type of cultural product) incorporated these different understandings of behavior. American coverage contained many more observations of athletic strength by commentators, reporters, and athletes themselves than did the Japanese coverage. Additionally, the Japanese coverage contained more observations about the critical role of training and past experience than did the American coverage.

Universals, Yes; Universalistic Fallacies, No!

One aim of a sociocultural approach is to contest universalistic fallacies and the empirically false assertion that people are more or less the same psychologically, regardless of their historical and sociocultural circumstances. Multiple worlds and multiple psychologies are attuned to reproduce and foster these worlds. Yet all is not relative: A world exists. The distinct worlds that lend structure and meaning to experience in particular and specifiable ways are indeed part of one world, and these distinct ways make contact and have consequences for each other. Thus, identifying some ideas and practices that cross-cut contexts and specify some human universals is also a goal: Similarities and differences have meaning only in the context of each other. For example, with respect to agency, people everywhere experience agency and behave agentically; they act in the world or regulate their own behavior. The psychological system of agency is universal, but the form it takes is culture-specific, because the actual workings of the system are contingent on and afforded by particular symbolic resources and social systems. Agency, then, in its phenomeno-

logical form, is very much socioculturally tailored and sanctioned.

Whereas people engaging in North American contexts experience agency as an autonomous self, intrinsically motivated and engaged in control, influence, and self-expression, people in East Asian cultural contexts are likely to experience agency as an interdependent self, actively adjusting to others' expectations to realize various relational goals and to maintain interpersonal harmony. Whereas the word *doing* seems the best and obvious gloss for agency in North American contexts, the word may carry with it a sense of direct action or of work in the world that may not be equally appropriate in Asian contexts. In these latter contexts, the word *be-ing* may be a better gloss that more accurately reflects the psychological state that accompanies agency. Both modes of doing and being in the world are agentic; however, each context affords a divergent structure for agency—thus, what "counts" as agentic differs.

Much of psychology has been very quick to universalize findings in many domains, doing so before any data that would allow such generalizations exist. Even the division among cognition, emotion, and motivation that comprise the deep structure of the field may in the fullness of time and careful empirical research emerge as a culture-specific commitment that derives from the particular Western philosophical assumptions built into American psychology. Psychology will improve as a science as it assumes a sociocultural approach across the field. Thus, for example, before looking for the evolutionary or the genetic underpinnings of a given behavior, it would seem wise, and also scientifically sound, to determine whether a given observed behavior can still be observed once the context shifts. For the most part, there is no allergy to universals among sociocultural psychologists. Regardless of their particular approach, they are alike in hoping to avoid the premature generalizations and universalistic fallacies that still pervade much of psychology.

Extending a Sociocultural Approach

The Example of Social Identity Research

Many areas within psychology might be more fully theorized and well understood with an approach that explores the interdependencies among self systems and social systems. A good example of a body of research that addresses many of the same content areas that we have been considering with a sociocultural approach, and could benefit from study under this approach, is the literature on social identity, stereotyping and prejudice. Social identity theories, for example, focus on how selfhood and identity are affected by the groups to which people belong. These studies reveal the ways in which the sociocultural is crucial to identity. In a dynamic process, people categorize and identify with some groups and contrast themselves against other groups. By creating groups (e.g., dot overestimators and dot underestimators) in the laboratory, thus producing a microcosm of the world, social identity researchers have been able to illuminate some of the ways in which social identity is powerfully contingent on the sociocultural context (e.g., Ellemers, Spears, & Doosje, 2002; Tajfel & Turner, 1979).

Being classified as a dot overestimator, for example, creates for the participant some important aspects of the group experience. Yet the laboratory microcosm is better at modeling some aspects of social identity negotiation than others. The fact that the social categorization can be produced easily in the laboratory is theoretically important, but it means that the category being examined is not a category saturated with social meaning and manifest in multiple social practices. Once branded an "overestimator" by the experimenter, the participant will experience an affinity with others so branded, and indeed reveal ingroup bias. This process is critically important for understanding some of the sources of social identity. Yet a given individual will not "be" a dot overestimator in the sense that he or she is recognized, treated, and judged as such by others in a way that has important life consequences. Nor will this categorization carry with it many ideas about what is right, good, true, and normatively appropriate for overestimators across many domains of behavior and social interaction.

The sources of social identity, its societal affordances, and its role in regulating behavior are also critical in research on stereotype threat. In these studies of social identity the psychological is indeed linked to the context; however, it is primarily linked to immediate variations in the configuration of the sociocultural context (i.e., whether one is solo or not, whether one feels safe in the context or instead feels implicitly or explicitly threatened

e.g., see Steele, Spencer, & Aronson, 2002; Taylor et al., 2004). These studies reveal, for example, that being exposed to a commercial with a stereotypical image of a woman—as flighty, emotional, and concerned about the home—is related to reduced performance and aspirations in women (Davies, Spencer, & Steele, 2005). The focus of such research is on specifying the process, in particular, the cognitive process by which threats to social identity alter performance and group identification. Indeed, many features of this process are similar whether the threat is initiated because of gender, ethnicity, age, or weight.

What could be usefully added to such analyses of the social context's influence are (1) the source and meaning of the threat, and (2) how pervasive, chronic, and well-instituted the threat is in the practices, policies, and products of the larger sociocultural context. The stereotype threat studies persuasively demonstrate that singling out or devaluing some aspect of one's identity matters for psychological functioning. They clearly link the social with the psychological. Being branded as an intense New Yorker by one's laid-back Silicon Valley coworkers is a threat to group belongingness to be sure, but is likely to have powerfully different consequences than trying to live a normal life as a gay individual in the U.S. military, where the threat is instituted as official policy. A combination of research on social identity, stereotyping, and prejudice with a sociocultural approach would not only facilitate a more specific and comprehensive understanding of these processes but also extend their applicability and utility.

Links to Stereotyping and Implicit Associations Research

Similarly, the recent surge of interest in implicit attitudes and biases could also be productively harnessed to sociocultural theorizing. Powerful implicit associations, such as those between white and American (Devos & Banaji, 2005) and those between black and criminal (Eberhardt, Goff, Purdie, & Davies, 2004), are extremely common, because they are built into our everyday worlds in multiple incarnations. Such findings locate some of the sources of discrimination and prejudice in the content of the worlds that people inhabit. They offer the optimistic view that important changes in behavior can be produced by changing the meanings, practices, and products prevalent in the various contexts that originally prompted the behavior. For example, some implicit association test (IAT) findings suggest that the associational space can be rearranged and other associations (black and good) and can be made more available (Richeson & Trawler, 2005). A sociocultural approach would caution, however, that although possible, successful interventions would require considerable sustained effort and resources, because these associations need to be embedded in meanings, practices, and products that are pervasively and chronically distributed throughout everyday worlds to truly change the associational structure of the people who inhabit them.

Links to Racial Formation Theory

Whereas prejudice, stereotyping, racial attitudes, and the effects of categorization by race are among the most important and well-developed areas of research in social psychology, seldom is the phenomenon of race itself directly approached. Most research is silent on what race is or how it has come to be. Nor is there typically discussion about the content of racial categories and ethnic identities. Saying "Race is real," in the sense of mutually constituted as "real in the world," invokes a long and pernicious history of essentialism and biological racism. As a result the ways in which race has been constituted and instituted have been largely ignored in social psychology, a field identified from its inception with overcoming stereotyping, and with distancing itself from describing and discussing group differences; it is not surprising that scholars would focus on the consequences of racial ascription rather than confront ideas of how race is constructed and made real in everyday social worlds. Instead, the focus has been on stereotypes, with the implicit assumption that if people could be purged of their negative racial attitudes and implicit biases, all would be well, because racism "is in the head."

Yet a sociocultural approach to race reveals that even if people's heads were free of racial prejudice, what would be left is the material world—a world replete with prejudicial representations, practices, policies and products, such as popular movies and television, saturated with stereotypical images, racial profiling, segregated housing, biased hiring practices, and unequal credit policies and opportunities to secure loans. These stubborn social facts would continue to exert their effects on the psychological and would soon reconstitute the familiar implicit and explicit prejudicial processes.

Race, then, can be understood as a sociocultural context itself—a matter of social structure and cultural representation that can be productively analyzed using a sociocultural approach. Sociologists (Omi & Winant, 1994) who began such an analysis of race have analyzed race as a "sociohistorical process by which racial categories are created, inhabited, transformed, and destroyed" (p. 55). Racial formation, they argue, "is a process of historically situated *projects* in which human bodies and social structures are represented and organized" (p. 56; emphasis in original). In their theorizing they connect meanings (i.e., what race means) with status and power, and the ways in which social structures and everyday experiences are organized based upon such meanings. In short, extending the sociocultural approach to race is useful because it highlights the central idea of this chapter. Phenomena such as stereotyping, discrimination, and racism cannot be located either solely in stereotypes inside individual heads or solely in inert social structures.

CONCLUDING COMMENTS

We have explained in this chapter that a sociocultural approach is signaled by the view that people and their social worlds require each other and should be analyzed together. The signature of this approach is not a particular method, set of methods, but rather an emphasis on interdependences among the person and the sociocultural system. Defining features of this approach include a concern with thinking beyond the person and attending to meaning-making processes and how meanings are manifested and maintained in the worlds people inhabit. Notably, a sociocultural approach does not require an explicit comparison between two or more contexts. Such a comparison affords an appreciation of the role of the symbolic resources and social systems in constituting selves and action, but it is not essential to all sociocultural questions. Once an understanding of the ways in which psychological systems are grounded in, and afforded by, meanings, practices, and products is achieved, this approach can applied to the analysis of any problem (e.g., aggression, violence, obesity, depression).

Psychological functioning, being a self or an actor in the world, is contingent on the symbolic resources and the patterns of social life distributed among the various sociocultural contexts in which a person engages. The precise nature of this contingency remains to be empirically determined, but a sociocultural approach highlights that this contingency is the nature of human beings. Very important insights into human functioning are being produced rapidly, for example, by current neuroscience methods, but no matter how precise and well-specified, a focus on the person will tell only half the story. In closing, this review of the principal sociocultural approaches, and the promising research generated by these approaches, convincingly supports Bruner's (1990) assertion that it will be impossible to construct a comprehensive psychology on the basis of the human alone. The radical vision of some of psychology's original thinkers—specifying how biological beings become *human* beings through their engagement with the meanings and practices of their social world—is becoming a well-grounded empirical reality.

REFERENCES

Aaker, J. L., & Williams, P. (1998). Empathy versus pride: The influence of emotional appeals across cultures. *Journal of Consumer Research, 25*, 241–261.

Adams, G. (2005). The cultural grounding of personal relationship: Enemyship in North American and West African worlds. *Journal of Personality and Social Psychology, 88*, 948–968.

Adams, G., & Markus, H. R. (2001). Culture as patterns: An alternative approach to the problem of reification. *Culture and Psychology, 7*, 283–296.

Adams, G., & Markus, H. R. (2004). Toward a conception of culture suitable for a social psychology of culture. In M. Schaller & C. S. Crandall (Eds.), *The psychological foundations of culture* (pp. 335–360). Mahwah, NJ: Erlbaum.

Allport, G. W. (1948). Foreword. In G. W. Lewin (Ed.), *Resolving social conflicts: Selected papers on group dynamics* (pp. vii–xiv). New York: Harper & Row.

Asch, S. (1952). *Social psychology*. Englewood Cliffs, NJ: Prentice-Hall.

Atran, S., Medin, D. L., & Ross, N. O. (2005). The cultural mind: Environmental decision making and cultural modeling within and across populations. *Psychological Review, 112*, 774–776.

Baldwin, J. M. (1911). *The individual and society*. Boston: Boston Press.

Baumeister, R. F. (1987). How the self became a problem: A psychological review of historical research. *Journal of Personality and Social Psychology, 52*, 163–176.

Bellah, R. N., Madsen, R., Sullivan, W. M., Swidler, A., & Tipton, S. M. (1985). *Habits of the heart: Individualism and commitment in American life*. New York: Harper & Row.

Berger, P. L., & Luckmann, T. (1966). *The social construction of reality: A treatise in the sociology of knowledge*. Garden City, NY: Doubleday.

Berry, J. W. (1976). *Human ecology and cognitive style: Comparative studies in cultural and psychological adaptation*. New York: Wiley.

Berry, J. W. (1979). Research in multicultural societies: Implications of cross-cultural methods. *Journal of Cross-Cultural Psychology, 10*, 415–434.

Berry, J. W. (2000). Cross-cultural psychology: A symbiosis of cultural and comparative approaches. *Asian Journal of Social Psychology* [Special issue], *3*, 197–205.

Berry, J. W. (2003). Origin of cross-cultural similarities and differences in human behavior: An ecocultural perspective. In A. Toomela (Ed.), *Cultural guidance in the development of the human mind* (pp. 97–109). Westport, CT: Ablex.

Berry, J. W. (2004). An ecocultural perspective on the development of competence. In R. J. Sternberg & E. L. Grigorenko (Eds.), *Culture and competence: Contexts of life success* (pp. 3–22). Washington, DC: American Psychological Association.

Berry, J. W., Irvine, S. H., & Hunt, E. B. (Eds.). (1988). *Indigenous cognition: Functioning in cultural context*. Dordrecht, The Netherlands: Nijhoff.

Berry, J. W., Poortinga, Y. H., Segall, M. H., & Dasen, P. R. (2002). *Cross-cultural psychology: Research and applications* (2nd ed.). New York: Cambridge University Press.

Berry, J. W., van de Koppel, J. M. H., Sénéchal, C., Annis, R. C., Bahuchet, S., Cavalli-Sforza, L. L., et al. (1986). *On the edge of the forest: Cultural adaptation and cognitive development in Central Africa*. Lisse, The Netherlands: Swets & Zeitlinger.

Bond, M. H. (2005). A cultural-psychological model for explaining differences in social behavior: Positioning the belief construct. In R. M. Sorrentino, D. Cohen, J. M. Olson, & M. P. Zanna (Eds.), *Cultural and social behavior: The Ontario symposium* (Vol. 10, pp. 31–48). Mahwah, NJ: Erlbaum.

Bourdieu, P. (1990). *The logic of practice*. Stanford, CA: Stanford University Press.

Bourdieu, P. (1991). *Language and symbolic power*. Cambridge, MA: Harvard University Press.

Briley, D. A., Morris, M. W., & Simonson, I. (2000). Reasons as carriers of culture: Dynamic versus dispositional models of cultural influence on decision making. *Journal of Consumer Research, 27*, 157–178.

Bronfenbrenner, U. (1979). Contexts of child rearing: Problems and prospects. *American Psychologist, 34,* 844–850.

Bruner, J. S. (1990). *Acts of meaning.* Cambridge, MA: Harvard University Press.

Carrithers, M. (1992). *Why humans have culture: Explaining anthropology and social diversity.* New York: Oxford University Press.

Chen, C., Lee, S.-Y., & Stevenson, H. W. (1995). Response style and cross-cultural comparisons of rating scales among East Asian and North American students. *Psychological Science, 6,* 170–175.

Chiu, C., Morris, M. W., Hong, Y., & Menon, T. (2000). Motivated cultural cognition: The impact of implicit cultural theories on dispositional attribution varies as a function of need for closure. *Journal of Personality and Social Psychology, 78,* 247–259.

Choi, I., Dalal, R., Kim-Prieto, C., & Park, H. (2003). Culture and judgment of causal relevance. *Journal of Personality and Social Psychology, 84,* 46–59.

Choi, I., & Nisbett, R. E. (2000). Cultural psychology of surprise: Holistic theories and recognition of contradiction. *Journal of Personality and Social Psychology, 79,* 890–905.

Cohen, A. B., Malka, A., Rozin, P., & Cherfas, L. (2006). Religion and unforgivable offenses. *Journal of Personality, 74,* 85–117.

Cohen, D., & Nisbett, R. E. (1994). Self-protection and the culture of honor: Explaining Southern violence. *Personality and Social Psychology Bulletin* [Special issue], *20,* 551–567.

Cohen, D., & Nisbett, R. E. (1997). Field experiments examining the culture of honor: The role of institutions in perpetuating norms about violence. *Personality and Social Psychology Bulletin, 23,* 1188–1199.

Cohen, D., Nisbett, R. E., Bowdle, B. F., & Schwarz, N. (1996). Insult, aggression, and the southern culture of honor: An "experimental ethnography." *Journal of Personality and Social Psychology, 70,* 945–960.

Cole, M. (1985). The zone of proximal development: Where culture and cognition create each other. In J. V. Wertsch (Ed.), *Culture, communication, and cognition: Vygotskian perspectives* (pp. 146–161). Cambridge, UK: Cambridge University Press.

Cole, M. (1990). Cultural psychology: A once and future discipline? In R. A. Dienstbier & J. Berman (Eds.), *Nebraska Symposium on Motivation: Vol. 37. Current theory and research in motivation* (pp. 279–335). Lincoln: University of Nebraska Press.

Cole, M. (1992). Culture in development. In M. H. Bornstein & M. E. Lamb (Eds.), *Developmental psychology: An advanced textbook* (3rd ed., pp. 731–789). Hillsdale, NJ: Erlbaum.

Cole, M. (1995). Culture and cognitive development: From cross-cultural research to creating systems of cultural mediation. *Culture and Psychology, 1,* 25–54.

Cole, M. (1996). *Cultural psychology: A once and future discipline.* Cambridge, MA: Harvard University Press.

Cole, M., Gay, J., Glick, J. A., & Sharp, D. W. (1971). *The cultural context of learning and thinking.* New York: Basic Books.

Cross, S. E., & Madson, L. (1997). Models of the self: Self-construals and gender. *Psychological Bulletin, 122,* 5–37.

Cross, S. E., & Markus, H. R. (1999). The cultural constitution of personality. In L. Pervin & O. John (Eds.), *Handbook of personality: Theory and research* (2nd ed., pp. 378–396). New York: Guilford Press.

D'Andrade, R. G. (1990). Some propositions about the relations between culture and human cognition. In J. W. Stigler, R. A. Shweder, & G. Herdt (Eds.), *Cultural psychology* (pp. 65–129). New York: Cambridge University Press.

D'Andrade, R. G., & Strauss, C. (Eds.). (1992). *Human motives and cultural models.* Cambridge, UK: Cambridge University Press.

Dasen, P. R., & Wassmann, J. (1998). Balinese spatial orientation: Some empirical evidence of moderate linguistic relativity. *Journal of the Royal Anthropological Institute, 4,* 689–711.

Davies, P. G., Spencer, S. J., & Steele, C. M. (2005). Clearing the air: Identity safety moderates the effects of stereotype threat on women's leadership aspirations. *Journal of Personality and Social Psychology, 88,* 276–287.

Dennett, D. C. (1995). Do animals have beliefs? In H. L. Roitblat & J.-A. Meyer (Eds.), *Comparative approaches to cognitive science. Complex adaptive systems* (pp. 111–118). Cambridge, MA: MIT Press.

Devos, T., & Banaji, M. R. (2005). American = White? *Journal of Personality and Social Psychology, 88,* 447–466.

Eberhardt, J. L., Goff, P. A., Purdie, V. J., & Davies, P. G. (2004). Seeing black: Race, crime, and visual processing. *Journal of Personality and Social Psychology, 87,* 876–893.

Ellemers, N., Spears, R., & Doosje, B. (2002). Self and social identity. *Annual Review of Psychology, 53,* 161–186.

Farr, R. M. (1991). Individualism as a collective representation. In A. Aebischer, J. P. Deconchy, & M. Lipiansky (Eds.), *Ideologies et representations sociales* (pp. 129–143). Cousset (Fribourg), Switzerland: Delval.

Festinger, L. (1957). *A theory of cognitive dissonance.* Stanford, CA: Stanford University Press.

Fiske, A. P. (1991). *Structures of social life: The four elementary forms of human relations.* New York: Free Press.

Fiske, A. P. (1992). The four elementary forms of sociality: Framework for a unified theory of social relations. *Psychological Review, 99,* 689–723.

Fiske, A. P., Kitayama, S., Markus, H. R., & Nisbett, R. E. (1998). The cultural matrix of social psychology. In D. T. Gilbert, S. T. Fiske, & G. Lindzey (Eds.), *Handbook of social psychology* (4th ed., pp. 915–981). San Francisco: McGraw-Hill.

Fryberg, S., & Markus, H. R. (in press). Models of education in American Indian, Asian American, and European American contexts. *Social Psychology of Education.*

Gardner, W. L., Gabriel, S., & Lee, A. Y. (1999). "I" value freedom, but "we" value relationships: Self-construal priming mirrors cultural differences in judgment. *Psychological Science, 10,* 321–326.

Geertz, C. (1973). *The interpretations of cultures.* New York: Basic Books.

Geertz, C. (1975). On the nature of anthropological understanding. *American Scientist, 63,* 47–52.

Georgas, J., van de Vijver, F. J. R., & Berry, J. W. (2004). The ecocultural framework, ecosocial indices, and psychological variables in cross-cultural research. *Journal of Cross-Cultural Psychology, 35,* 74–96.

Gergen, K., & Davis, K. (1985). *The social construction of the person.* New York: Springer-Verlag.

Goodman, N. (1984). Notes on the well-made world. *Partisan Review, 51,* 276–288.

Graumann, C. F. (1986). The individualization of the social and desocialization of the individual: Floyd H. Allport's contribution to social psychology. In C. F. Graumann & S. Moscovici (Eds.), *Changing conceptions of crowd mind and behavior* (pp. 97–116). New York: Springer-Verlag.

Greenfield, P. M. (1997). You can't take it with you: Why ability assessments don't cross cultures. *American Psychologist, 52,* 1115–1124.

Greenfield, P. M., & Childs, C. P. (1977a). Understanding sibling concepts: A developmental study of kin terms in Zinacantan. In P. Dasen (Ed.), *Piagetian psychology: Cross-cultural contributions* (pp. 335–358). New York: Gardner Press.

Greenfield, P. M., & Childs, C. P. (1977b). Weaving, color terms and pattern representation: Cultural influences and cognitive development among the Zinacantecos of Southern Mexico. *Inter-American Journal of Psychology, 11,* 23–48.

Greenfield, P. M., & Cocking, R. R. (1994). *Cross-cultural roots of minority child development.* Hillsdale, NJ: Erlbaum.

Guisinger, S., & Blatt, S. J. (1994). Individuality and relatedness: Evolution of a fundamental dialect. *American Psychologist, 49,* 104–111.

Hallowell, A. I. (1955). *Culture and experience.* Philadelphia: University of Pennsylvania Press.

Heine, S. J., & Lehman, D. R. (1997). Culture, dissonance, and self-affirmation. *Personality and Social Psychology Bulletin, 23,* 389–400.

Heine, S. J., Lehman, D. R., Markus, H. R., & Kitayama, S. (1999). Is there a universal need for positive self-regard? *Psychological Review, 106,* 766–794.

Heine, S. J., Lehman, D. R., Peng, K., & Greenholtz, J. (2002). What's wrong with cross-cultural comparisons of subjective Likert scales?: The reference-group effect. *Journal of Personality and Social Psychology, 82,* 903–918.

Hermans, H. J. M., & Kempen, H. J. G. (1998). Moving cultures: The perilous problems of cultural dichotomies in a globalizing society. *American Psychologist* [Special issue], *53,* 1111–1120.

Hofstede, G. (1980). *Culture's consequences.* Beverly Hills, CA: Sage.

Hofstede, G. (1990). A reply and comment on Joginder P. Singh: "Managerial culture and work-related values in India." *Organization Studies, 11,* 103–106.

Holland, D., & Quinn, N. (Eds.). (1987). *Cultural models in language and thought.* New York: Cambridge University Press.

Hong, Y., Benet-Martinez, V., Chiu, C., & Morris, M. W. (2003). Boundaries of cultural influence: Construct activation as a mechanism for cultural differences in social perception. *Journal of Cross-Cultural Psychology, 34,* 453–464.

Hong, Y., & Chiu, C. (2001). Toward a paradigm shift: From cross-cultural differences in social cognition to social-cognitive mediation of cultural differences. *Social Cognition, 19,* 181–196.

Hong, Y., Ip, G., Chiu, C., Morris, M. W., & Menon, T. (2001). Construction of the self: Collective duties and individual rights in Chinese and American cultures. *Social Cognition, 19,* 251–268.

Hong, Y., Morris, M. W., Chiu, C., & Benet-Martinez, V. (2000). Multicultural minds: A dynamic constructivist approach to culture and cognition. *American Psychologist, 55,* 709–720.

Iyengar, S. S., & DeVoe, S. E. (2003). Rethinking the value of choice: Considering cultural mediators of intrinsic motivation. In V. Murphy-Berman & J. J. Berman (Eds.), *Cross-cultural differences in perspectives on the self: Nebraska Symposium on Motivation* (Vol. 49, pp. 146–191). Lincoln: University of Nebraska Press.

Ji, L.-J., Nisbett, R. E., & Su, Y. (2001). Culture, change, and prediction. *Psychological Science, 12,* 450–456.

Jost, J. T., & Major, B. (Eds.). (2001). *The psychology of legitimacy: Emerging perspectives on ideology, justice, and intergroup relations.* New York: Cambridge University Press.

Kahneman, D., & Tversky, A. (1973). On the psychology of prediction. *Psychological Review, 80,* 237–251.

Kashima, Y. (2000). Conceptions of culture and person for psychology. *Journal of Cross-Cultural Psychology, 31,* 14–32.

Katz, M. B. (1987). *Reconstructing American education.* Cambridge, MA: Harvard University Press.

Keller, H., Bettina, L., Monika, A., Relindis, Y., Borke, J., Jensen, H., et al. (2006). Cultural models, socialization goals, and parenting ethnotheories: A multicultural analysis. *Journal of Cross-Cultural Psychology, 37,* 155–172.

Keller, H., & Greenfield, P. M. (2000). History and future of development in cross-cultural psychology. *Journal of Cross-Cultural Psychology, 31,* 52–62.

Kim, H., & Markus, H. R. (1999). Deviance or uniqueness, harmony or conformity?: A cultural analysis. *Journal of Personality and Social Psychology, 77,* 785–800.

Kim, H. S. (2002). We talk, therefore we think?: A cultural analysis of the effect of talking on thinking. *Journal of Personality and Social Psychology, 83,* 828–842.

Kim, U., & Berry, J. W. (1993). *Indigenous psychologies: Research and experience in cultural context.* Newbury Park, CA: Sage.

Kitayama, S. (2002). Culture and basic psychological processes—toward a system view of culture: Comment on Oyserman et al. *Psychological Bulletin, 128,* 189–196.

Kitayama, S., Duffy, S., Kawamura, T., & Larsen, J. T. (2003). Perceiving an object and its context in different cultures: A cultural look at New Look. *Psychological Science, 14,* 201–206.

Kitayama, S., Ishii, K., & Imada, T. (2006). Voluntary settlement and the spirit of independence: Evidence from Japan's "Northern Frontier." *Journal of Personality and Social Psychology, 91,* 369–384.

Kitayama, S., Markus, H. R., Matsumoto, H., & Norasakkunkit, V. (1997). Individual and collective processes in the construction of the self: Self-enhancement in the United States and self-criticism in Japan. *Journal of Personality and Social Psychology, 72,* 1245–1267.

Kitayama, S., Snibbe, A. C., Markus, H. R., & Suzuki, T. (2004). Is there any "free" choice?: Self and dissonance in two cultures. *Psychological Science, 15,* 527–533.

Kitayama, S., & Uchida, Y. (2005). Interdependent agency: An alternative system for action. In R. M. Sorrentino, D. Cohen, J. M. Olson, & M. P. Zanna (Eds.), *Cultural and social behavior: The Ontario Symposium* (Vol. 10., pp. 137–164). Mahwah, NJ: Erlbaum.

Knowles, E. D., Morris, M. W., Chiu, C., & Hong, Y. (2001). Culture and process of person perception: Evidence for automaticity among East Asians in correcting for situational influences on behavior. *Journal of Personality and Social Psychology, 27,* 1344–1356.

Kroeber, A. L., & Kluckhohn, C. (1952). *Culture: A critical review of concepts and definitions.* New York: Vintage Books.

Kühnen, U., Hannover, B., & Schubert, B. (2001). The semantic–procedural interface model of the self: The role of self-knowledge for context-dependent versus context-independent modes of thinking. *Journal of Personality and Social Psychology, 80,* 397–409.

Kühnen, U., & Oyserman, D. (2002). Thinking about the self influences thinking in general: Cognitive consequences of salient self-concept. *Journal of Experimental Social Psychology, 38,* 492–499.

Lee, A., Aaker, J. L., & Gardner, W. (2000). The pleasures and pains of distinct self-construals: The role of interdependence in regulatory focus. *Journal of Personality and Social Psychology, 78,* 1122–1134.

Leung, K. (1987). Some determinants of reactions to procedural models for conflict resolution: A cross-national study. *Journal of Personality and Social Psychology, 53,* 898–908.

Lewin, K. (1948). *Resolving social conflicts: Selected papers on group dynamics.* New York: Harper & Row.

Li, J. (2003). U.S. and Chinese cultural beliefs about learning. *Journal of Educational Psychology, 95,* 258–267.

Lonner, W. J., & Hayes, S. A. (2004). Understanding the cognitive and social aspects of intercultural competence. In R. J. Sternberg & E. L. Grigorenko (Eds.), *Culture and competence: Contexts of life success* (pp. 89–110). Washington, DC: American Psychological Association.

Luria, A. R. (1981). *Language and cognition* (J. V. Wertsch, Trans.). New York: Wiley.

Markus, H. R., Curhan, K., & Ryff, C. D. (2006). *Educational attainment and models of well-being in America: A sociocultural analysis.* Unpublished manuscript, Stanford University.

Markus, H. R., & Kitayama, S. (1991). Culture and the self: Implications for cognition, emotion, and motivation. *Psychological Review, 98,* 224–253.

Markus, H. R., & Kitayama, S. (1994). A collective fear of the collective: Implications for selves and theories of selves. *Personality and Social Psychology Bulletin, 20,* 568–579.

Markus, H. R., & Kitayama, S. (2003). Culture, self, and the reality of the social. *Psychological Inquiry, 14,* 277–283.

Markus, H. R., & Kitayama, S. (2004). Models of agency: Sociocultural diversity in the construction of action. In V. Murphy-Berman & J. Berman (Eds.), *Cross-cultural differences in perspectives on self: Nebraska Symposium on Motivation* (Vol. 49, pp. 1–57). Lincoln: University of Nebraska Press.

Markus, H. R., Kitayama, S., & Heiman, R. (1996). Culture and "basic" psychological principles. In E. T. Higgins & A. W. Kruglanski (Eds.), *Social psychology: Handbook of basic principles* (pp. 857–913). New York: Guilford Press.

Markus, H. R., Mullally, P. R., & Kitayama, S. (1997). Selfways: Diversity in modes of cultural participation. In U. Neisser & D. A. Jopling (Eds.), *The conceptual self in context: Culture, experience, self-understanding* (pp. 13–61). New York: Cambridge University Press.

Markus, H. R., Uchida, Y., Omoregie, H., Townsend, S. S. M., & Kitayama, S. (2005). Going for the gold: Models of agency in Japanese and American contexts. *Psychological Science, 17,* 103–112.

Masuda, T., & Nisbett, R. E. (2001). Attending holistically versus analytically: Comparing the context sensitivity of Japanese and Americans. *Journal of Personality and Social Psychology, 81,* 922–934.

Matsumoto, D. (Ed.). (2001). *The handbook of culture and psychology*. Oxford:, UK Oxford University Press.

Matsumoto, D., & Yoo, S. H. (2005). Culture and applied nonverbal communication. In R. E. Riggio & R. S. Feldman (Eds.), *Applications of nonverbal communication* (pp. 255–277). Mahwah, NJ: Erlbaum.

Matsumoto, D., & Yoo, S. H. (2006). Toward a new generation of cross-cultural research. *Perspectives on Psychological Science, 1*, 234–250.

Maynard, A. E., & Greenfield, P. M. (2003). Implicit cognitive development in cultural tools and children: Lessons from Maya Mexico. *Cognitive Development, 18*, 489–510.

Mead, G. H. (1934). *Mind, self, and society*. Chicago: University of Chicago Press.

Medin, D. L., & Atran, S. (2004). The native mind: Biological categorization and reasoning in development and across cultures. *Psychological Review, 111*, 960–983.

Mesquita, B. (2003). Emotions as dynamic cultural phenomena. In R. J. Davidson, H. Goldsmith, & P. Rozin (Eds.), *Handbook of the affective sciences* (pp. 871–890). Oxford, UK: Oxford University Press.

Miller, J. D., Bersoff, D. M., & Harwood, R. L. (1990). Perceptions of social responsibilities in India and in the United States: Moral imperatives or personal decisions? *Journal of Personality and Social Psychology, 58*, 33–46.

Miller, J. G. (1984). Culture and the development of everyday social explanation. *Journal of Personality and Social Psychology, 46*, 961–978.

Miller, J. G. (1994). Cultural diversity in the morality of caring: Individually oriented versus duty-based interpersonal moral codes. *Cross-Cultural Research, 28*, 3–39.

Miller, J. G. (1997). Cultural conceptions of duty: Implications for motivation and morality. In J. Schumaker, D. Munro, & S. Carr (Eds.), *Motivation and culture* (pp. 178–193). New York: Routledge.

Miller, J. G. (1999). Cultural psychology: Implications for basic psychological theory. *Psychological Science, 10*, 85–91.

Miller, J. G. (2000). Vertragen sich gemeinschaft mit autonomie? Kulturelle ideale und empirische wirklichkeiten. In W. Edelstein & G. Nunner-Winkler (Eds.), *Moral im Kontext* (pp. 337–362). Frankfurt am Main, Germany: Suhrkam.

Miller, J. G. (2002). Bringing culture to basic psychological theory—Beyond individualism and collectivism: Comment on Oyserman et al. (2002). *Psychological Bulletin, 128*, 97–109.

Miller, P. J., & Goodnow, J. J. (1995). Cultural practices: Toward an integration of culture and development. In J. J. Goodnow, P. J. Miller, & F. Kessel (Eds.), *Cultural practices as contexts for development* (Vol. 67, pp. 5–16). San Francisco: Jossey-Bass.

Mishra, R. C., Dasen, P. R., & Niraula, S. (2003). Ecol-

ogy, language, and performance on spatial cognitive tasks. *International Journal of Psychological Science, 38*, 366–383.

Miyamoto, Y., Nisbett, R. E., & Masuda, T. (2006). Culture and the physical environment: Holistic versus analytic perceptual affordances. *Psychological Science, 17*, 113–119.

Moiser, C. E., & Rogoff, B. (2003). Privileged treatment of toddlers: Cultural aspects of individual choice and responsibility. *Developmental Psychology, 39*, 1047–1060.

Moscovici, S. (1981). On social representations. In J. Forgas (Ed.), *Social cognition: Perspectives on everyday understanding* (pp. 181–210). London: Academic Press.

Moscovici, S. (1988). Notes towards a description of social representations. *European Journal of Social Psychology, 18*, 211–250.

Moscovici, S. (1991). Experiment and experience: An intermediate step from Sherif to Asch. *Journal for the Theory of Social Behaviour, 21*, 253–268.

Moscovici, S. (1998). The history and actuality of social representations. In U. Flick (Ed.), *The psychology of the social* (pp. 209–247). Cambridge, MA: Cambridge University Press.

Nisbett, R. E. (2003). *The geography of thought: How Asians and Westerners think differently . . . and why*. New York: Free Press.

Nisbett, R. E., & Cohen, D. (1996). *Culture of honor: The psychology of violence in the South*. Boulder, CO: Westview Press.

Nisbett, R. E., Peng, K., Choi, I., & Norenzayan, A. (2001). Culture and systems of thought: Holistic versus analytic cognition. *Psychological Review, 108*, 291–310.

Norenzayan, A., & Heine, S. J. (2005). Psychological universals: What are they and how can we know? *Psychological Bulletin, 131*, 763–784.

Norenzayan, A., Smith, E. E., Kim, B. J., & Nisbett, R. E. (2002). Cultural preferences for formal versus intuitive reasoning. *Cognitive Science, 26*, 653–684.

Omi, M., & Winant, H. (1994). *Racial formation in the United States: From the 1960s to the 1990s*. New York: Routledge.

Oyserman, D., Coon, H. M., & Kemmelmeier, M. (2002). Rethinking individualism and collectivism: Evaluation of theoretical assumptions and meta-analyses. *Psychological Bulletin, 128*, 3–72.

Peng, K., & Nisbett, R. E. (1999). Culture, dialectics, and reasoning about contradiction. *American Psychologist, 54*, 741–754.

Peng, K., Nisbett, R. E., & Wong, N. Y. C. (1997). Validity problems comparing values across cultures and possible solutions. *Psychological Methods, 2*, 329–344.

Plaut, V. C., & Markus, H. R. (2005). The "inside" story: A cultural-historical analysis of being smart and motivated, American style. In A. J. Elliot & C. S. Dweck (Eds.), *Handbook of competence and motivation* (pp. 457–488). New York: Guilford Press.

Plaut, V. C., Markus, H. R., & Lachman, M. E. (2002). Place matters: Consensual features and regional variation in American well-being and self. *Journal of Personality and Social Psychology, 83,* 160–184.

Pyszczynski, T., Greenberg, J., Solomon, S., Arndt, J., & Schimel, J. (2004). Why do people need self-esteem?: A theoretical and empirical review. *Psychological Bulletin, 130,* 435–468.

Quinn, D. M., & Crocker, J. (1999). When ideology hurts: Effects of belief in the Protestant ethic and feeling overweight on the psychological well-being of women. *Journal of Personality and Social Psychology, 77,* 402–414.

Resnick, L. B. (1994). Situated rationalism: Biological and social preparation for learning. In L. A. Hirschfeld & S. A. Gelman (Eds.), *Mapping the mind: Domain specificity in cognition and culture.* (pp. 474–493). New York: Cambridge University Press.

Richeson, J. A., & Trawler, S. (2005). On the categorization of admired and disliked exemplars of admired and disliked racial groups. *Journal of Personality and Social Psychology, 89,* 517–530.

Richter, L., & Kruglanski, A. (2004). Motivated closed mindedness and the emergence of culture. In M. Schaller & C. S. Crandall (Eds.), *The psychological foundations of culture* (pp. 101–121). Mahwah, NJ: Erlbaum.

Rogoff, B. (1991). The joint socialization of development by young children and adults. In M. Lewis & S. Feinman (Eds.), *Social influence and socialization in infancy* (pp. 253–280). New York: Plenum Press.

Rogoff, B. (1995). Observing sociocultural activity on three planes: Participatory appropriation, guided participation, apprenticeship. In J. V. Wertsch, P. D. Rio, & A. Alvarez (Eds.), *Sociocultural studies of mind* (pp. 139–164). New York: Cambridge University Press.

Rothbaum, F., Weisz, J. R., & Snyder, S. S. (1982). Changing the world and changing the self: A two-process model of perceived control. *Journal of Personality and Social Psychology, 42,* 5–37.

Rozin, P. (1996). Towards a psychology of food and eating: From motivation to module to model to marker, morality, meaning, and metaphor. *Current Directions in Psychological Science, 5,* 18–24.

Rozin, P. (2001). Social psychology and science: Some lessons from Solomon Asch. *Personality and Social Psychology Review, 5,* 2–14.

Sampson, E. E. (1985). The decentralization of identity: Toward a revised concept of personal and social order. *American Psychologist, 40,* 1203–1211.

Sampson, E. E. (1988). The debate on individualism: Indigenous psychologies of the individual and their role in personal and societal functioning. *American Psychologist, 43,* 15–22.

Sanchez-Burks, J. (2002). Protestant relational ideology and (in)attention to relational cues in work settings. *Journal of Personality and Social Psychology, 83,* 919–929.

Sanchez-Burks, J., & Mor Barak, M. (2004). Interpersonal relationships in a global work context. In M. Mor Barak (Ed.), *Managing diversity in the age of globalization: Toward a worldwide inclusive workplace* (pp. 114–168). Thousand Oaks, CA: Sage.

Sapir, E. (1924). Culture: Genuine and spurious. *American Journal of Sociology, 24,* 401–429.

Sapir, E. (1956). *Culture, language and personality* (Vol. 207). Berkeley: University of California Press.

Savani, K., Markus, H. R., & Snibbe, A. (2006). Do people always choose what they like: The relationship between preferences and choices in Indian and American contexts. Unpublished manuscript, Stanford University.

Schaller, M., & Crandall, C. S. (Eds.). (2004). *The psychological foundations of culture.* Mahwah, NJ: Erlbaum.

Schwartz, S. H. (1990). Individualism–collectivism: Critique and proposed refinements. *Journal of Cross-Cultural Psychology, 21,* 139–157.

Sears, D. (1986). College sophomores in the laboratory: Influences of a narrow data base on social psychology's view of human nature. *Journal of Personality and Social Psychology, 51,* 515–530.

Shore, B. (1996). *Culture in mind: Cognition, culture and the problem of meaning.* New York: Oxford University Press.

Shweder, R. A. (1982). Beyond self-constructed knowledge: The study of culture and morality. *Merrill–Palmer Quarterly, 28,* 41–69.

Shweder, R. A. (1995). Cultural psychology: What is it? In N. R. Goldberger & J. B. Veroff (Eds.), *the culture and psychology reader* (pp. 41–86). New York: New York University Press.

Shweder, R. A. (2003). *Why do men barbecue?: Recipes for cultural psychology.* Cambridge, MA: Harvard University Press.

Shweder, R. A., Balle-Jensen, L., & Goldstein, W. (1995). Who sleeps by whom revisited: A method for extracting the moral goods implicit in praxis. In P. J. Miller, J. J. Goodnow, & F. Kessell (Eds.), *A practices approach to child development: New directions to child development* (pp. 21–39). San Francisco: Jossey-Bass.

Shweder, R. A., & Bourne, L. (1984). Does the concept of the person vary cross-culturally? In R. A. Shweder & R. A. LeVine (Eds.), *Culture theory: Essays on mind, self, and emotion* (pp. 158–199). New York: Cambridge University Press.

Shweder, R. A., Goodnow, J., Hatano, G., LeVine, R. A., Markus, H. R., & Miller, P. (1998). The cultural psychology of development: One mind, many mentalities. In W. Damon & R. M. Lerner (Eds.), *Handbook of child psychology: Vol. 1. Theoretical models of human development* (5th ed., pp. 865–937). Hoboken, NJ: Wiley.

Shweder, R. A., & LeVine, R. A. (1984). *Culture theory: Essays on mind, self, and emotion.* New York: Cambridge University Press.

Shweder, R. A., Much, N. C., Mahapatra, M., & Park, L. (1997). The "big three" of morality (autonomy, community, divinity), and the "big three" explanations of suffering. In A. Brandt & P. Rozin (Eds.), *Morality and health* (pp. 119–169). Stanford, CA: Stanford University Press.

Shweder, R. A., & Sullivan, M. A. (1990). The semiotic subject of cultural psychology. In L. A. Pervin (Ed.), *Handbook of personality: Theory and research* (pp. 399–418). New York: Guilford Press.

Shweder, R. A., & Sullivan, M. A. (1993). Cultural psychology: Who needs it? *Annual Review of Psychology, 44,* 497–523.

Smith, P. B., & Bond, M. H. (1993). *Social psychology across cultures: Analysis and perspectives.* New York: Harvester Wheatsheaf.

Snibbe, A. C., & Markus, H. R. (2005). You can't always get what you want: Educational attainment, agency, and choice. *Journal of Personality and Social Psychology, 88,* 703–720.

Solomon, J. L. (2004). Modes of thought and meaning making: The aftermath of trauma. *Journal of Humanistic Psychology, 44,* 299–319.

Sperber, D. (1985). Anthropology and psychology: Towards an epidemiology of representations. *Man, 20,* 73–89.

Sperber, D. (1996). *Explaining culture: A naturalistic approach.* Oxford, UK: Blackwell.

Stapel, D. A., & Koomen, W. (2001). I, we, and the effects of others on me: How self-construal level moderates social comparison effects. *Journal of Personality and Social Psychology, 80,* 766–781.

Steele, C. M., & Aronson, J. (1995). Stereotype threat and the intellectual test performance of African Americans. *Journal of Personality and Social Psychology, 69,* 797–811.

Steele, C. M., Spencer, S. J., & Aronson, J. (2002). Contending with group image: The psychology of stereotype and social identity threat. In M. P. Zanna (Ed.), *Advances in experimental social psychology* (Vol. 34, pp. 379–440). San Diego: Academic Press.

Steele, D. M., Steele, C. M., Markus, H. R., Green, F., Lewis, A. E., & Davis, P. G. (2006). *How identity safety improves students achievements.* Unpublished manuscript, Stanford University.

Stephens, N. M., Markus, H. R., & Townsend, S. S. M. (2006). *Models of agency and divergent meanings of choice in working class and middle class contexts.* Manuscript submitted for publication.

Strauss, C. (1992). Models and motives. In R. D'Andrade & C. Strauss (Eds.), *Human motives and cultural models.* Cambridge, UK: Cambridge University Press.

Tajfel, H., & Turner, J. (1979). An integrative theory of intergroup conflict. In W. G. Austin & S. Worchel (Eds.), *The social psychology of intergroup relations* (pp. 33–47). Monterey, CA: Brooks/Cole.

Taylor, S. E. (1997). The social being in social psychology. In D. Gilbert, S. Fiske, & G. Lindsey (Eds.), *The handbook of social psychology* (pp. 58–95). New York: McGraw-Hill.

Taylor, S. E., Sherman, D. K., Kim, H. S., Jarcho, J., Takagi, K., & Dunagan, M. S. (2004). Culture and social support: Who seeks it and why? *Journal of Personality and Social Psychology, 87,* 354–362.

Tomascello, M. (1999). *The cultural origins of human cognition.* Cambridge, MA: Harvard University Press.

Trafimow, D., Triandis, H. C., & Goto, S. G. (1991). Some tests of the distinction between the private self and the collective self. *Journal of Personality and Social Psychology, 60,* 649–655.

Triandis, H. C. (1989). The self and social behavior in differing cultural contexts. *Psychological Review, 93,* 506–520.

Triandis, H. C. (1990). Cross-cultural studies of individualism and collectivism. In J. Berman (Ed.), *Nebraska Symposium on Motivation, 1989: Vol. 3. Cross-cultural perspective* (pp. 41–133). Lincoln: University of Nebraska Press.

Triandis, H. C. (1995). *Individualism and collectivism.* Boulder, CO: Westview Press.

Triandis, H. C. (1996). The psychological measurement of cultural syndromes. *American Psychologist, 51,* 407–415.

Tsai, A. Y., & Markus, H. R. (2006). *Equality or propriety: A cultural models approach to understanding social hierarchy.* Unpublished manuscript, Stanford University, Stanford, CA.

Tsai, J., Knutson, B., & Fung H. H. (2006). Cultural variation in affect valuation. *Journal of Personality and Social Psychology, 90,* 288–307.

Tsai, J. L., Chentsova-Dutton, Y., Freire-Bebeau, L., & Przymus, D. E. (2002). Emotional expression and physiology in European Americans and Hmong Americans. *Emotion, 2,* 380–397.

Tsai, J. L., Louie, J., Chen, E. E., & Uchida, Y. (2006). Learning what feelings to desire: Socialization of ideal affect through children's storybooks. *Personality and Social Psychology Bulletin, 32,* 1–14.

Tsai, J. L., Miao, F., & Seppala, E. (in press). Good feelings in Christianity and Buddhism: Religious differences in ideal affect. *Personality and Social Psychology Bulletin.*

Uchida, Y., Norasakkunkit, V., & Kitayama, S. (2004). Cultural constructions of happiness: Theory and empirical evidence. *Journal of Happiness Studies, 5,* 223–239.

van Baaren, R. B., Maddux, W. W., Chartrand, T. L., de Bouter, C., & van Knippenberg, A. (2003). It takes two to mimic: Behavioral consequences of self-construals. *Journal of Personality and Social Psychology, 84,* 1093–1102.

Vandello, J. A., & Cohen, D. (1999). Patterns of individualism and collectivism across the United States. *Journal of Personality and Social Psychology, 77,* 279–292.

Veroff, J. B., & Goldberger, N. R. (1995). What's in a name?: The case for "intercultural." In N. R. Goldberger & J. B. Veroff (Eds.), *The culture and psychology reader* (pp. 3–24). New York: New York University Press.

Vygotsky, L. S. (1978). *Mind in society: The development of higher psychological processes*, Ed. M. Cole, V. John-Steiner, S. Scribner, & E. Souberman. Cambridge, MA: Harvard University Press.

Wertsch, J. V. (1991). *Voices of the mind: A sociocultural approach to mediated action*. Cambridge, MA: Harvard University Press.

Wertsch, J. V., & Sammarco, J. G. (1985). Social precursors to individual cognitive functioning: The problem of units of analyses. In R. A. Hinde, A. N. Perret-Clermont, & J. Stevenson-Hinde (Eds.), *Social relationships and cognitive development* (pp. 276–293). Oxford, UK: Oxford University Press.

Whiting, B. B., & Whiting, J. W. (1975). *Children of six cultures: A psycho-cultural analysis* (Vol. 237). Oxford, UK: Harvard University Press.

Whorf, B. L. (1956). *Language, thought, and reality: Selected writings*. Cambridge, MA: MIT Press.

Wierzbicka, A. (1994). Emotion, language, and "cultural scripts." In S. Kitayama & H. R. Markus (Eds.), *Emotion and culture: Empirical studies of mutual influence* (pp. 133–196). Washington, DC: American Psychological Association.

Wundt, W. (1916). *Elements of folk psychology: Outlines of a psychological history of the development of mankind*. London: Allen & Unwin.

Zajonc, R. B. (1968). Attitudinal effects of mere exposure. *Journal of Personality and Social Psychology, 9*, 1–27.

Zàrate, M. A., Uleman, J. S., & Voils, C. I. (2001). Effects of culture and processing goals on the activation and binding of trait concepts. *Social Cognition, 19*, 295–323.

CHAPTER 2

Anthropological Foundations of Cultural Psychology

ROBERT A. LeVINE

This chapter examines the roots of cultural psychology in the anthropology of the 20th century and explores the varied ways in which contemporary social anthropologists approach problems relating culture and psychology. Contemporary cultural psychology is partly an outgrowth of the American anthropology of the mid-20th century (1925–1975), which formulated, explored, and investigated the concept of culture, relationships between psychological and cultural characteristics, and culture-specific conceptions of person, self, mental processes and psychopathology, using ethnographic, linguistic and clinical methods. In this chapter I review some of this history, particularly to call attention to a little-known, earlier literature that dealt with conceptual and methodological issues that remain problematic in current research.

My focus is on the emergence of fundamental concepts, the controversy over the individual or collective locus of culture, and the methodological division between "objective" and "subjective"—or statistical versus clinical—approaches to psychocultural phenomena. I argue that the intellectual fault lines that developed in anthropology during the 1930s grew wider in successive decades and challenged

psychological anthropologists to build the bridges represented by recent interdisciplinary work.

Although my historical narrative gives primary attention to the intellectual legacy of Franz Boas and Edward Sapir, as it affected later generations of American anthropologists, this limitation does not represent a judgment that the British influences of W. H. R. Rivers, C. G. Seligman, and Bronislaw Malinowski (Stocking, 1995) or the development of cognitive anthropology documented and interpreted by Roy D'Andrade (1995) are unimportant. My primary concern is to present the Boas–Sapir legacy in the terms made possible by the historical research of George Stocking (e.g., 1968, 1992), Regna Darnell (1990, 2001), and Judith Irvine (Sapir, 1993), who have retrieved and illuminated this line of thought from documents and oral history. My account is also affected by my personal communications in the generations following Sapir with anthropologists who attempted to translate his approach into empirical research (John and Beatrice Whiting, Clyde Kluckhohn, A. Irving Hallowell, Melford E. Spiro, George DeVos, William Caudill, Anthony F. C. Wallace, George and Louise Spindler, Gananath Obeyesekere). The aim is to give cultural psychologists a historical perspective on their own work through an intellectual genealogy in which they can locate themselves as the heirs to problems and methods framed by pioneers of 20th-century anthropology.

BOAS AND SAPIR: THE PSYCHOLOGY OF CULTURE

Franz Boas (1859–1942) and Edward Sapir (1884–1939) laid the most important anthropological foundations for cultural psychology, even though they published little on the subject. In Boas's writings, the theory of culture and psychology is largely implicit. Sapir wrote explicitly but at his death had published only a few papers in this area. Their influence, however, was enormous, and it is mainly through the work of historians and biographers that we have come to understand their thought and how it affected research in psychological anthropology.

Boas is known largely as the leader of American anthropology early in the 20th century and the teacher of those who founded "culture and personality studies" (as psychological anthropology was called up to 1960), namely, Edward Sapir, Ruth Benedict, Margaret Mead, Abram Kardiner, and A. Irving Hallowell. Boas's own writings, however, were mainly on specialized topics in physical anthropology, linguistics, material culture, and folklore, and within those areas, on problems that were at issue before 1914, mostly in Native American studies. Furthermore, most of the many published pages of "ethnography" Boas left behind at his death were unannotated Native American texts recorded for the study of language and folklore (Berman, 1996). Where is the psychology in his publications, apart from the titles of some of his works, such as his famous book *The Mind of Primitive Man* (1911)? George Stocking (1992), the preeminent Boas scholar, has attempted to answer this question.

Boas, as Stocking tells us, was well versed in German psychology before his immigration to the United States in 1887 (when he was 28 years old), and he had published pieces on Fechnerian psychophysics in 1882 (Stocking, 1968). From early in his career, Boas was a radical empiricist who avoided what he regarded as speculative generalization in his writing, so that his publications focused on specific empirical problems, without spelling out his basic

premises concerning culture and its relationship to human psychology. Underlying these particularistic concerns, however, was a grand plan: to replace the speculative theories that abounded in the human sciences during the late 19th century with empirical data drawn from the diversity of conditions—cultural, linguistic, ecological, and historical—in which humans lived.

Boas had a special interest in methods and measurement, and was drawn to research fields in which a corpus of reliable data could be collected, both to falsify a priori speculations and to indicate how diverse environments produced diverse outcomes. Trained in anthropometric methods by Rudolf Virchow, the Berlin biomedical pioneer, in 1883, Boas adopted both Virchow's concept of plasticity as a basic biological principle and his skepticism about theories ungrounded in empirical fact. In Virchow's obituary in *Science* in 1902, Boas denied the charge that Virchow did not accept Darwinian evolution through natural selection. It is undeniable, however, that the skeptical attitude Boas admired in Virchow led the younger man not only to oppose evolutionary proposals in the social sciences but also to rule out the cross-cultural comparisons that he believed led to false generalizations.

Boas saw himself as a biological scientist initiating studies of human variation. At Clark University (1889–1892), where he was hired by G. Stanley Hall, Boas taught a course on statistical methods in anthropology in the anthropology division of Hall's psychology department. Later, when analyzing physical growth data on immigrants to the United States, Boas—who had met Francis Galton, the inventor of correlational analysis—improvised his own forms of correlation, analysis of variance and factor analysis, and corresponded with the statistician Karl Pearson (Howells, 1959; Tanner, 1959). Boas also learned and accepted Mendelian genetics and viewed the physical growth of children as a joint outcome of genetic and (largely unspecified) environmental factors.

Boas believed that historical research on the borrowing of customs (cultural diffusion) could identify a selective core of cultural ideas that determined which customs would be borrowed and which rejected, and that understanding this core should be high on the agenda for future anthropological research. His students sought to achieve this goal through culture and personality studies, but in doing so they engaged in speculations—including psychoanalytic ones—he would not endorse. In the last book he edited, *General Anthropology* (1938), Boas included chapters by Sapir, Mead, and Benedict, but none on culture and personality, though the field was developing rapidly at the time (Stocking, 1992).

There is no doubt that Boas had a phenomenological side based on neo-Kantian philosophy that was expressed in his teaching and greatly influenced his students. From a contemporary perspective, he did not consistently distinguish between the "cultural" and the "mental"; rather, he saw them as fused. Stocking (1992, p. 312) points out that as late as 1907, Boas divided the whole discipline of anthropology into two parts, "biological anthropology" and "psychological anthropology," apparently intending the latter title to designate what we now call "cultural anthropology." This seems also to be the case with *The Mind of Primitive Man*, his magnum opus of 1911, in which "mind" refers to both cultural and mental phenomena.

In attempting to understand Boas as an ancestor of cultural psychology, we have to begin with his goal of falsifying the anthropological theories that divided the human species into hereditary racial types determining each individual's bodily form, mental characteristics, and behavior, measurable through the cephalic index (the cranial height:width ratio). Boas focused first on the cephalic index itself: If one could demonstrate that it was highly variable within a population, as well as variable across generations raised under differing environmental conditions (when parents moved from rural to urban areas or from Europe to America), then the fixity of racial types was called into question and with it, the genetic determination of mental characteristics and behavior. Boas (1912) left no doubt, however, that his demonstrations of plasticity in physical growth implied that mental and behavioral attributes also varied in accordance with "social and geographical" factors. His strategy was to undermine racial formalism with a statistical approach to bodily characteristics, but this was only the first step.

In other works, Boas showed that the Native American languages and cultures exhibit qualities of order, complexity, and historical change incompatible with their characterization as "primitive" in older anthropological formulations, particularly those of an evolutionary cast. Here, again, he focused on qualities that could be empirically assessed (though not quantitatively measured) to challenge theories of Western superiority with indisputable evidence. If it could be shown, for example, that the Native American languages were not deficient in their sound systems (phonology) compared to Western languages, but just different, and that the apparent deficiency was in the method used by early linguistic investigators (Boas, 1889), then the notion of Native American inferiority was undermined. But whereas the linguistic evidence showed the Native Americans to be *mentally capable* of speaking and transmitting a language equivalent in complexity and order to Western languages, it did not address directly the question of their other mental—as distinct from cultural—characteristics. Indeed, this is a question that Boas did not address himself—possibly because he could see no answer that would satisfy his radical empiricist scruples—but left to his students.

The lack of differentiation between the cultural and the mental in American social science discourse came to an end in 1917, when W. I. Thomas (the Chicago sociologist, later a collaborator of Sapir) and Florian Znaniecki published the first volume of their classic *The Polish Peasant in Europe and America* (1917/ 1927), with its introduction distinguishing between (social) "values" and (personal) "attitudes." That same year, within the circle of Boasian anthropology, A. L. Kroeber, who had been Boas's first student at Columbia, published "The Superorganic" in *American Anthropologist*, arguing that culture was in a realm of its own and not reducible to psychology or biology, and Sapir (1917) published a rejoinder, "Do We Need a Superorganic?" This debate—anticipated by the French sociologist Émile Durkheim's (1895/1982) argument that society was *sui generis*, and that social facts were distinct from, and not reducible to, psychological facts—made it virtually impossible for social scientists to presume that a distinction between cultural and mental phenomena was unnecessary. The two realms might be related—in which case, how?—or unrelated—in which case, why?—but the problem was now unavoidable. This brings us to the contributions of Edward Sapir.

Sapir received his PhD with Boas at Columbia in 1909, and went on to become a founder of anthropological linguistics and a leading researcher on Native American languages, before turning his attention to the study of culture and personality. In 1921 he published an influential book for the general public, *Language: An Introduction to the Study of Speech*. Sapir taught at the University of Chicago from 1925 to 1931 and thereafter at Yale. At both institutions he lectured on the psychology of culture—indeed, his Chicago course in 1926 was probably the first on this subject at an American university—but his planned book on that topic was not completed at the time of his death in 1939. More than 50 years later, students' lecture notes were compiled, and a book, *The Psychology of Culture*, edited by Judith Irvine, was published in 1993. (Some of his influential essays on culture and personality had been reprinted earlier in David Mandelbaum's [1949] *Selected Writings of Edward Sapir*.) Sapir also exerted an influence on behalf of culture and personality studies at the National Research Council, and at conferences sponsored by the Rockefeller Foundation and the Social Science Research Council. In these forums and organizations, he worked with and influenced younger anthropologists, such as A. Irving Hallowell and Clyde Kluckhohn, and other social scientists, such as Harold Lasswell, John Dollard, and W. I. Thomas. Sapir was widely admired as an intellectual leader and a fascinating lecturer. Thus, with relatively few publications on the subject, Sapir became known as the leading theoretical influence in culture and personality studies. The distinctive nature of this influence on Hallowell, Kluckhohn, and their students is of particular relevance here.

Sapir's model of culture and psychology was shaped not only by his training with Boas and his experience as an investigator of Native American languages but also by his friendship with the psychiatrist and psychoanalyst Harry Stack Sullivan, dating from 1926 (Darnell, 1990; Perry, 1982). Sapir incorporated Sullivan's (1947) theory of interpersonal relations (as the source of order and disorder in the mental development of the individual) in his own conception of culturally organized interpersonal relations as the source of meanings for individuals raised in a particular symbolic environment. In other words, children learn culture-specific symbols through their interpersonal experience, itself shaped by cultural conventions. The focus on the individual in Sullivan's psychiatric account was compatible with Boas's focus on the development of the in-

dividual human organism and with Sapir's own work with linguistic informants. Cultural meanings were transmitted from one individual to another through symbolic communication in interpersonal relations; the meanings, according to Sapir, had no life apart from the individuals who communicated them.

This last proposition represented a theoretical break with Kroeber's (1917) "superorganic" view of culture, which Sapir considered a reification (i.e., a form of what Merton would later call "misplaced concreteness"), and with other attempts to define anthropology as an academic discipline that owed little or nothing to psychology. The culture and personality movement initiated by Sapir, Mead, and Benedict attempted to counter the stronger current of disciplinary separateness that characterized the social sciences as they strove to establish themselves at universities in the first half of the 20th century.

The boundaries of Sapir's psychology of culture were marked by his disagreements with colleagues in the culture and personality movement, particularly Ruth Benedict and John Dollard. In his lectures on the psychology of culture at Yale, 1934–1937, Sapir made the following statements:

> The term "cultural psychology" is ambiguous, and there has been much confusion between two types of psychological analysis of social behavior. The one is a statement of the general tendencies or traits characterizing a culture, such as the pattern of self-help in our culture; [as we have pointed out,] different cultures do have certain delineating factors, [including attitudes and] psychological standards about emotional expression. The other is a statement of certain kinds of actual behavior, [by actual individuals] related to these cultural patterns. [In other words, it is a statement of] the individual's psychology and the problem of individual adjustment [to a cultural setting.] . . .
>
> [If the idea of a cultural psychology is so tangled, ought we to speak of such a thing at all? In a sense perhaps we ought not. Strictly speaking,] culture, in itself, has no psychology; only individuals [have a psychology.
>
> On the cultural plane] there is only [what I call] the "as-if psychology." That is to say, there Is a psychological standard in each culture as to how much emotion is to be expressed, and so on. This is the as-if psychology, which belongs to the culture itself, not with the individual personality. . . .
>
> Ruth Benedict's book, *Patterns of Culture*, is a brilliant exposition of as-if psychology, but with confusion about the distinction made here. She is

not clear on the distinction between the as-if psychology she is discussing and the psychology of the individual. A culture cannot be paranoid. . . . You have to know the individual before you know what the baggage of his culture means to him.

In itself, culture has no psychology. It is [just] a low-toned series of rituals, a rubber stamping waiting to be given meaning by you. (1993, pp. 182–183)

This position reflected a breach between Sapir and Benedict, who had previously been close as friends and in their approach to the study of culture and personality. And since Margaret Mead adopted (or at least defended) Benedict's position, it also represented a split among the pioneers of the culture and personality movement. In my view, several of the younger anthropological researchers in that movement (e.g., Hallowell, Kluckhohn, Cora DuBois, and John Whiting, joined later by Beatrice Whiting and the students of Hallowell's students) followed Sapir on this issue. Benedict and Mead had little support among anthropologists altogether. But *Patterns of Culture*, published in 1934, became one of the best-selling social science books of all time, as did Mead's books, making Mead and Benedict the most famous American anthropologists of the century—not only in the 1930s but for decades thereafter, when their books were required reading at American colleges. Sapir's views, on the other hand, were delivered only to a classroom of Yale graduate students and to certain scholars who attended interdisciplinary conferences. For many within anthropology, and almost everyone outside it, culture and personality research was seen as representing Benedict's as-if psychology, not Sapir's critique and his more complex cultural psychology.

Sapir's disagreement with John Dollard was over other issues. The two had met in the late 1920s at the University of Chicago, where Dollard was a graduate student in sociology and Sapir, a senior professor of anthropology; their common interest was psychoanalysis. After finishing his doctorate, Dollard spent a year in training at the Berlin Psychoanalytic Institute and was brought to Yale by Sapir in 1931. At Yale, Dollard moved away from his mentor and joined an interdisciplinary group of psychologists and other social scientists exploring ways of testing Freudian theory through rigorous experiments, and applying the "learning theory" of Clark L. Hull (later called "behavior theory" and based on drive-reduction experiments with animals) to human personality development and psychotherapy (Dollard, Doob, Miller, Mowrer, & Sears, 1938; Miller & Dollard, 1941; Dollard & Miller, 1949). (John W. M. Whiting and Allison Davis worked with Dollard during this period.) This type of social science, with its formal experiments, quantitative evidence, and reductionism, was anathema to Sapir, who saw his psychology of culture as exploring the complex symbolic worlds of human cultures through naturalistic methods used in ethnographic, linguistic, and clinical–psychiatric research.

Sapir was too much of an empirical scientist to accept the casual psychologizing of Benedict's ethnographic portraiture but also too much the humanist to accept the scientism of Dollard and the Yale learning theorists. I believe he was right on both counts, but Sapir faced insuperable obstacles in translating his sound ideas about cultural psychology into a research program: There were no relevant precedents in Boas's work, in ethnography or in his own linguistic research; his conception of the individual was drawn from psychiatry (Sullivan), which was itself struggling to find satisfactory methods of research; he never conducted psychological or psychocultural research himself and had no students who did during his life, which rapidly came to an end when he was 57.

Sapir's vision of a cultural psychology gave some substance and direction to Boas's general ideas about plasticity in human mental development. Having followed Boas in seeing the individual as the locus of culture, Sapir turned away from the statistical approach Boas had used to analyze the distribution of individual characteristics in a population, but without proposing a clear alternative. Like the cultural and personality movement he helped bring into being, Sapir's cultural psychology was a promising theoretical framework—focused on interpersonal experience as the basis for the individual's acquisition of cultural meanings—but it lacked a practical prescription for research. Nevertheless, the problems Sapir faced in his painful disagreements with Benedict and Dollard foreshadowed issues that remain critical in cultural psychology: the distinction between normative and idiosyncratic versions of culture (and their location) and the question of how to assess or measure psychologically salient cultural ideas.

Sapir left a long list of publications on linguistics but only six articles on culture and personality and the unpublished lectures that were to have become his book on the psychology of culture. Had he lived longer, the book would have been published and it would no doubt have inspired others to conduct research on cultural psychology. In fact, A. Irving Hallowell (1892–1974) and Clyde Kluckhohn (1905–1960) had worked with Sapir in interdisciplinary seminars and had already been inspired to do field research during the 1930s and thereafter. Their studies and theoretical ideas are described in the following sections.

INDIVIDUAL VARIATION IN CULTURAL CONTEXT: HALLOWELL AND KLUCKHOHN

Most of Sapir's students at Yale became linguistic anthropologists; others became cultural anthropologists not concerned with psychology (David Mandelbaum) or psychological anthropologists more closely associated with Dollard and his methods (John and Beatrice Whiting). But Hallowell and Kluckhohn, though trained at the University of Pennsylvania and Harvard, respectively, were specialists in Native American cultures (Ojibwa and Navajo, respectively) who allied themselves with Sapir during the 1930s and sought to implement his ideas in their research.

Hallowell, as a student of the Boasian anthropologist Frank Speck at the University of Pennsylvania, had attended Franz Boas's seminar at Columbia (with Ruth Benedict) in 1922, and studied also with Alexander Goldenweiser, an early student of Boas, who was interested in psychoanalysis. By 1931, when Sapir led meetings on psychology and anthropology for the National Research Council, he picked Hallowell to be *rapporteur*. They worked closely during this period.

Kluckhohn, who had studied at Harvard and Oxford in the late 1920s, visited Sapir in New Haven weekly during the year 1936–1937 for lessons in the Navajo language (Stocking, personal communication, 2005). His writings at that time and later show him to be an admirer and follower of Sapir.

Both Hallowell and Kluckhohn developed working relationships with personality psychologists—the former with Bruno Klopfer, the Rorschach analyst, and the latter with Henry A. Murray, coinventor of the Thematic Apperception Test—and wrote articles during the 1930s arguing and illustrating Sapir's points that culture should be conceptually distinguished from the individual psyche, that cultural patterns can be realized only in individual behavior, and that individual behavior (informed by culture) varies widely within a community or population.

In 1938 Hallowell published the article "Fear and Anxiety as Cultural and Individual Variables in a Primitive Society" in the *Journal of Social Psychology* (reprinted in 1955 as Chapter 13 of *Culture and Experience*). In it Hallowell used ethnographic evidence from his Ojibwa field studies to make the case against confusing personal adherence to conventional standards of thought and feeling with personal psychopathology.

> Once we relegate commonly motivated fears to their proper frame of reference—cultural tradition—a fundamental etiological distinction can be made between fears of this category and those which arise in individuals from conditions primarily relevant to the circumstances of their own personal history. The *genuine* neurotic, in addition to sharing the culturally constituted fears of his fellows, as Horney says, "has fears which in quantity or quality deviate from those of the cultural pattern." Any comparison, then, between the fears and defenses of such individuals and the culturally constituted fears and institutionalized defenses of whole human societies is not only superficial, it is actually misleading, since no account is taken of differences in etiological factors. . . . To seriously maintain that the culturally constituted fears and defenses of primitive peoples are evidence of "cultural neuroses" which are of the same order as the neurosis of individuals in Western civilization, is just such a fallacy. Manifest surface analogies are compared whereas the underlying differences in the dynamic factors that produced them are ignored. (1955, p. 259; italics in original)

Although Ruth Benedict is not mentioned in the article, no reader in 1938 could miss the implied rebuke to her claim in *Patterns of Culture* (1934) that "culture is personality writ large" and her characterization of the Kwakiutl and Dobuan peoples in terms derived from psychopathology. Hallowell's quotation from the neo-Freudian psychoanalyst Karen Horney and his citation in a footnote of a personal communication with Harry Stack Sullivan, leave no doubt that he was articulating and defending Sapir's position against that of Benedict.

Hallowell's terms "institutionalized defenses" and "culturally constituted fears" pointed to a more complex and promising understanding of person–culture interactions than is usually attributed to the culture and personality studies of the 1930s and 1940s. Except for a small group of specialists, however, the Benedict book—together with the books of Margaret Mead and Geoffrey Gorer (Gorer & Rickman, 1949)—overshadowed Hallowell and Sapir as the image of culture and personality theory and research for decades to come. Despite the respect he received as a North American Indian specialist, and his election to the presidency of the American Anthropological Association in 1949, Hallowell was only "discovered" as a theorist after the publication in 1955 of his *Culture and Experience*, in which many of his earlier essays were reprinted.

Kluckhohn also published an article in 1938 that made the point of differentiating between the individual and cultural forms. His article "Participation in Ceremonials in a Navaho Community," published in *American Anthropologist*, focused not on mental states and processes but on individual behavior: specifically, religious behavior. By counting the number of times individuals in a particular community performed a certain ceremonial activity, it was possible to move beyond generalized statements such as "the Navaho are a ceremonial people." The reported frequency of their religious acts would provide a more accurate description of Navajo ceremonialism. Kluckhohn's approach was based on the assumption that customary practices attributed to an entire community are actually variable among them, as Sapir had argued, but his quantitative method resembled sociology or psychology rather than linguistics:

> Now our problem may be phrased as follows: To what extent does an inductive analysis of the behaviors of the individuals making up a particular Navaho group support the generalization that a preferred Navaho mode of reacting is ceremonial? (Kluckhohn, 1938, p. 360)

> In short, the evidence which has been presented seems to create a strong presumption in favor of the hypothesis that ceremonials are a focal point of the actions of this Navaho society (p. 368)

Thus, Kluckhohn was implicitly presenting to anthropologists a radical methodological proposal, namely, that a crucial step in assessing the psychological salience of a discretionary or optional, though culturally organized, activity is to observe and record its frequency in a particular community. He also advocated assessing the economic costs of ceremonies and the amount of time spent doing them, as well as repeating these measurements over time to discover whether participation in ceremonials was increasing or decreasing. In other words, to avoid speculation about the "preferred mode of reaction" of a people, the anthropologist must measure individuals' reactions in observable situations and reportable activities in the aggregate. Kluckhohn offered this empirical and frankly reductive approach as necessary (though not sufficient) for psychocultural understanding, and, as with Hallowell's article, the implicit contrast with Benedict's *Patterns of Culture* could not have been sharper and would not have been missed by readers in 1938. Kluckhohn and Hallowell were both attempting to define the terms of a cultural psychology based on Sapir's critique of Benedict's approach as "as-if psychology."

However, behaviorist Kluckhohn's approach in that 1938 article also embraced two cardinal features of American anthropology (then and now): ethnographic knowledge and the concept of culture. The article on Navajo ceremonial participation, though focused on the counting of activities and behaviors, was framed—and made possible—by Kluckhohn's ethnographic knowledge of Navajo ceremonials and their contexts in Navajo culture and social life. And the following year, Kluckhohn (1939) published an article on the acquisition of culture by individuals in which he coined the term *culturization* ("an admittedly horrid word") as a counterpart to *socialization*, as used by sociologists and social psychologists.

The 1939 article presents Kluckhohn's recommendations for conducting research on a process that Sapir had, in his lectures, recognized as crucial to the psychology of culture. Kluckhohn's emphasis, however, was on the "empirical method" to be used, and on his argument that "if we are to deal with any problem (such as that of the acquisition of culture by individuals) in a way that is reducible to actual human behaviors, generalizations must be given a quantitative basis" (1939, p. 103). (Sapir, though emphasizing individual variability in a population, would not have agreed that the acquisition of culture is reducible to behaviors; in any event, Sapir's focus was on the mental processes of "the culture-acquiring child" rather than the behavior of children and their parents.) Kluckhohn presented the topical outline and methods of his own study of Navajo children and his systematic sampling procedures, anticipating in many details the six cultures study of Whiting et al. (1966) 15 years later. He accused Malinowski and others of representing communities as a whole through contextualized "anecdotes" concerning their typical behavior, while ignoring individual variations. Benedict is not mentioned, though the criticisms obviously apply to her work as well. But Kluckhohn does not address in this article the question of what comprises the culture that is being acquired.

KLUCKHOHN'S SEMIOTIC VIEW OF CULTURE

Kluckhohn spent much of his subsequent career developing and refining the culture concept. Although he urged anthropologists to ground their descriptive statements about behavior in quantifiable observations, he had not abandoned Sapir's notions of cultural meanings and patterns. In 1945, he and W. H. Kelly published an article, "The Concept of Culture," in the form of a Socratic dialogue between an anthropologist and his colleagues and companions. The dialogue format enabled them to display a variety of viewpoints about culture, but Kluckhohn's preferred position emerged quite clearly: Culture is a historically created design or blueprint for living; it consists of both signs and symbols organized as patterns of and for behavior. This formulation is remarkably close in its metaphors as well as underlying ideas to the influential conception of culture for which Clifford Geertz (who was a student of Kluckhohn) has been known since the publication of his book, *The Interpretation of Cultures*, in 1973.

The following quotations from the Kluckhohn and Kelly dialogue indicate key features of the culture concept for which they are arguing.

Culture is not, strictly speaking, the visible act, the speech, or the product of these things. It is a *way* of thinking, feeling, believing. It is the knowledge stored up (in memories of men, in books and ob-

jects) for future use—patterns for doing certain things in certain ways, not the doing of them. (Kluckhohn, 1962, p. 25, italics in original)

The conception of one single, unchanging "human nature" is a reassuring fiction of folklore. When it comes to details, there are "human natures." (p. 36)

The notion of defining culture, in a descriptive sense, as a set of blueprints for action (including feeling, of course) is very attractive. And it is probably sound . . . (p. 53)

By "culture" we mean all those historically created designs for living, explicit and implicit, rational, irrational, and nonrational, that exist at any given time as potential guides for the behavior of men (p. 54) and that tend to be shared by all or specially designated members of a group. (p. 56, italics in original)

A culture is made up of overt, patterned ways of behaving, feeling, and reacting. But it also includes a characteristic set of unstated premises or hypotheses that vary greatly in different societies. (p. 58)

A language is not merely an instrument for communication and rousing the emotions. Every language is also a device for categorizing experience. (p. 59)

Social life among humans never occurs without a system of "conventional understandings" that are transmitted more or less intact from generation to generation. (p. 67)

Every culture is also a structure of expectancies. If we know a culture, we know what various classes of individuals within it expect from each other—and from outsiders of various categories. We know what types of activity are held to be inherently gratifying. (p. 69)

Thus, Kluckhohn's concept of culture was articulated in 1945 as a set of conventional, historically derived ideas that influence behavior, feeling, and thinking in a particular human group, a set of blueprints that shape interpersonal communication and expectancies, as well as other activities. Culture in this concept is both cognitive (knowledge) and normative (guiding action). It is not to be confused with behavior or artifacts produced under cultural influence. There is no suggestion that it could be reduced to quantifiable form.

This concept, which I would call "semiotic," is consistent with the concept of Sapir that inspired it and that of Geertz that followed later, though Kluckhohn was far more concerned than either of them to connect it to the interests of psychologists, biologists, and policymakers. In this regard, it is noteworthy that Sapir's proposed cultural psychology was based on clinical psychiatry as he had learned it through Harry Stack Sullivan, not on academic psychology. Kluckhohn, on the other hand, when he published the 1945 article, was already working with two academic psychologists (Henry A. Murray and Gordon Allport) and a sociologist (Talcott Parsons) in founding the Harvard Department of Social Relations, and he had written an article on culture and personality with the psychologist O. H. Mowrer (Kluckhohn & Mowrer, 1944). He did not reject their methods and approaches, but tried to relate his approach to theirs. From Kluckhohn's point of view, Sapir's opening to clinical psychiatry, which failed to address the question, for example, of the representativeness of individual cases, was not adequate for anthropology as a social science.

As for Geertz, however much Kluckhohn's 1945 concept of culture was compatible with his viewpoint (initially developed when he was a graduate student in the Social Relations Department at Harvard), he found much to disagree with by the 1950s. Kluckhohn's published monograph with A. L. Kroeber on definitions of culture (Kroeber & Kluckhohn, 1952) retreated somewhat from the purely ideational concept of culture, seeking an ecumenical consensus definition that admitted products and practices under the cultural umbrella. In response, Geertz (2000) became determined to "shrink" the culture concept by his own work. Furthermore, Kluckhohn continued to insist on the importance of human cultural universals rooted in biological and situational constraints and to speculate on what the universals might be (Kluckhohn, 1953), whereas Geertz (1973, p. 29) developed the viewpoint that "it's culture all the way down," that cultural inquiry can reveal only the patterns of a particular symbolic system, and only if it is not burdened by the assumption that all systems, sharing universal constraints, must be comparable with another.

Kluckhohn (personal communication, 1953–1954) saw Sapir's work on the phoneme—a universal biosocial category permitting language-specific variations—as the model for conceptualizing culture in general, and in this sense his semiotic viewpoint resembled that of the linguist Kenneth Pike (1954), who extended the linguistic division between phonemic and phonetic analysis to the description of particular cultures in the emic–etic distinction. But Geertz, approaching culture through phenomenological philosophy, hermeneutics, and literary criticism, apparently saw this as a form of scientism that led away from the deeper understanding of particular cultures. As of this writing, Geertz has not dealt directly with the psychology of culture (LeVine, 2005).

Although it is not explicitly stated in Kluckhohn's posthumously published book of essays, *Culture and Behavior* (1962), which was incomplete when he died, it seems clear that the title represents his recommendations for a cultural psychology: Culture is to be studied as a set of ideas—knowledge and norms—constituting a partly shared symbolic system that the anthropologist describes holistically. The behavior of individuals in a particular community is to be recorded and aggregated to permit quantitative description. The investigator then searches for correspondences between cultural ideas and behavioral profiles or distributions (e.g., in the central tendencies of behavior in two communities of different cultures), predicting behavioral tendencies from cultural differences. This seems to have been Kluckhohn's preferred cultural psychology at the time of his death in 1960 at the age of 55. (He was also, as mentioned, searching for the universals in which the cultural variations in behavior were grounded.) Of course, this method had a precedent in Émile Durkheim's (1895/1951) *Suicide*, which Alex Inkeles (1959) referred to as correlating a state and a rate, and it was used in many comparative studies throughout the 20th century, including those of recent cultural psychology (e.g., Markus & Kitayama, 1991).

Kluckhohn may not have acknowledged the Durkheim precedent, but his unfinished work represents a pioneering mid-20th-century effort to realize Sapir's dream of a cultural psychology—not in the way Sapir imagined it, but by connecting ethnography with empirical (and quantitative) psychology. The book of readings Kluckhohn edited with Murray in 1948, *Personality in Nature, Culture and Society*, represented this interdisciplinary connection in a sophisticated and mature phase that was often forgotten in subsequent criticisms of the culture and personality movement. Working in parallel to Kluckhohn, Hallowell mounted another pioneering effort to extend Sapir's ideas and translate them into a research program.

HALLOWELL'S CONCEPT OF THE SELF

Most of Hallowell's psychocultural papers were reprinted in his 1955 book *Culture and Experience* (which is still in print), which includes his articles on Rorschach testing among the Ojibwa, his presidential address to the American Anthropological Association on personality and human evolution, and his new thinking on the self in culture. The latter seems particularly important as a precursor to contemporary cultural psychology, though it was not appreciated in anthropology for perhaps another two decades.

Hallowell's lengthy article, "The Self and Its Behavioral Environment," is divided into two chapters in the book, one with the original title and the other titled "The Ojibwa Self and Its Behavioral Environment," wherein he outlines and illustrates his comparative framework for studying the self cross-culturally. Far from claiming originality, Hallowell (who was a pioneering historian of anthropology) indicates his predecessors in exploring the self, including Ernst Cassirer in philosophy; William James, James Mark Baldwin, and Gardner Murphy in psychology; George Herbert Mead and C. H. Cooley in sociology; and Marcel Mauss (1938) and Dorothy Lee (1950) in anthropology. His framework is original, however, in several respects.

Hallowell begins to present his assumptions and hypotheses by emphasizing that the self-awareness of humans is not only a "social product" but also "culturally constituted."

If it is possible to view the self as culturally constituted and known to the individual in the same frame of reference as we view the culturally constituted world in which the individual must act, this preliminary step may enable us to apprehend with greater clarity both the essential role of culture in relation to a generic human attribute and to define with more precision some of the constant and variable factors that structuralize the psychological field of behavior for the individual in different societies. (Hallowell, 1955, p. 81)

For the acquisition and use of a particular language, the specific content that is given to an articulated world of objects that is built up *pari passu* with self-awareness, and the integration of personal experience with a concept of the nature of the self as traditionally viewed, are among the necessary conditions that make possible the emergence and functioning of human awareness. . . . At the same time, such cultural constituents give various colorings to this unique psychological attribute of man. (p. 82)

Culture may be said to play a constitutive role in the psychological adjustment of the individual to his world. (p. 89)

Hallowell makes clear in this chapter that the culturally constituted self of which he writes is not simply a collective representation or an aspect of a disembodied culture but is essential to and part of individual psychodynamics. He also proposes a set of universal dimensions for the mental contents of the self: self-orientation, object orientation, spatiotemporal orientation, motivational orientation, and normative orientation. He argues the plausibility of these hypothesized orientations with ethnographic data (especially his own from the Ojibwa) and quotations from developmental psychologists and philosophers whose observations have led them to believe they are universal.

The orientations, as Hallowell expounds them, are what Kluckhohn at about the same time called "universal categories of culture"— "the invariant points of reference" (1953, p. 522)—within which cultural variability occurs. Thus, the normative orientation means that a moral order of some kind is universal in human societies; it does not mean that any particular morality is common to more than members of a particular community. Hallowell's orientations are psychological parameters or dimensions along which culturally constituted selves vary widely. This way of reconciling the ethnographers' perceptions of cultural variation with the assumption of species-wide, biologically grounded human attributes—whether or not it reflects the influence of Sapir and his concept of the phoneme—seemed to Hallowell and Kluckhohn to be as the foundation for research into cultural psychology in the 1950s.

Hallowell's conceptual suggestions for cultural psychology did not end with the five orientations of the self; the essays reprinted in

Culture and Experience also pointed to a cultural psychodynamic. When Hallowell referred to "culturally constituted fears and institutionalized defenses" in the passage quoted earlier from his 1938 article (Chapter 13 in *Culture and Experience*), his primary goal was to distinguish such fears and defenses from their phenotypically similar symptoms in the psychiatric diagnosis of mentally ill individuals. Thus, in a behavioral environment constituted according to Ojibwa cultural standards, believing in witchcraft and sorcery is conventional and not to be equated with the phobic or paranoid beliefs of mentally ill patients, who stand out as different among the Berens River Ojibwa as they do elsewhere. But how are we to understand the nonpathological belief in witchcraft and sorcery? In Chapter 14 (originally published in 1941), he asserts that "the whole magico-religious apparatus of the Salteaux [Ojibwa] is a complex anxiety-reducing device" (1955, p. 276). Traditional beliefs about disease arouse the anxieties of the ordinary person, but customary therapeutic practices operate symbolically to reduce them, in a theoretical model analogous to that of the psychodynamics of symptom formation in psychoanalysis.

Later, Melford E. Spiro (1961, 1965) explicated the concept of "culturally constituted defenses" in theoretical terms and with ethnographic examples, advancing the cultural psychodynamics implicit in Hallowell's writings. Spiro (1961) wrote that cultural practices can be functional for the individual, whose forbidden impulses are allowed disguised expression that might otherwise lead to psychosis, and for the society, which tames or contains its members' potential disorderly behavior. Thus, the description and analysis of culturally constituted defenses become central to the understanding of society, culture, and personality in terms of a psychosocial functionalism, combining Freudian psychodynamics with the social–structural functionalism of Talcott Parsons (homeostatic models of psychic and societal equilibrium). Obeyesekere (1990), who sees Kardiner's works (1939, 1945) as originating the concept of culturally constituted defenses in his formulations concerning "projective systems," critically reviews Spiro's use of the concept in the latter's analysis of Burmese Buddhist monks, finding it unnecessary to assume, as Spiro does, that the defenses substitute for psychoses. Obeyesekere's (1981) own research in

Sri Lanka exemplifies an approach in which defenses drawing on religious imagery play a crucial role in the psychodynamics of religious specialists without making that assumption.

Hallowell therefore laid the conceptual foundation for not only the ethnographic and psychological study of the self in diverse cultures but also the future study of cultural psychodynamics, with culturally constituted defenses as its central concept. If that possibility has remained largely unrealized, it is probably due to the lack of an empirical research program on which psychological anthropologists after Hallowell could agree. This in turn seems to be a function of (1) doubts about the cross-cultural validity of projective tests and other personality assessment methods that arose in psychology (e.g., Lindzey, 1961) during the 1960s; (2) unresolved issues regarding cultural particularism versus Freudian universalism and clinical versus statistical approaches among the psychological anthropologists who might have been expected to construct such a program; and (3) the unstated recognition in anthropology that collecting valid data about culturally constituted defenses without the use of personality tests is extremely difficult for a foreign anthropologist to do.

Whatever the research after 1960 that followed the writings of Kluckhohn and Hallowell, it is now possible to appreciate their contributions to the foundations of cultural psychology. They elaborated Sapir's distinction between culture and the individual. They implemented that distinction in their studies of the Navajo and Ojibwa, respectively, explicitly following Boas in their use of samples and statistical methods. Kluckhohn revived attention to the concept of culture and suggested the ideational approach that eventually became dominant. Hallowell formulated the self as an object of ethnographic inquiry, and initiated interest in culturally constituted defenses as a key concept for the cultural study of psychodynamics.

ETHNOPSYCHOLOGY

In the late 20th century, many diverse strands of anthropological theory and research were seen as foundations of cultural psychology. For example, in the year 1973 alone, the following five books were published in the United States: *Socialization for Achievement: The Cultural Psychology of the Japanese* by George A.

DeVos, *The Anatomy of Dependence* (English translation) by Takeo Doi, *The Interpretation of Cultures* by Clifford Geertz, *Culture, Behavior and Personality: An Introduction to the Comparative Study of Psychosocial Adaptation* by Robert A. LeVine, and *Tahitians: Mind and Experience in the Society Islands* by Robert I. Levy. It would take another chapter to do justice to the analyses and evidence in all of these works, but several of them are particularly relevant to this chapter.

Ethnopsychology as a field of research was prominent in the anthropological literature during the 1970s and 1980s, and represents an important aspect of and problem for cultural psychology. An ethnopsychological account is a description of the psychological categories (i.e., concerning emotion, cognition, behavior, and development) indigenous to a particular language and culture. Ethnopsychological descriptions raise the questions of the extent to which those categories can be translated into Western psychological concepts, whether the latter provide a basis for understanding persons in non-Western contexts, and whether psychology as we know it is only of many culture-specific conceptualizations rather than a scientific theory of universal validity. At the same time, an ethnopsychological account calls attention to the issue of whether experience, individual and collective, can be adequately understood in terms of indigenous cultural categories alone or requires the assumption of universal mental processes for a satisfactory explanation. These are issues of fundamental import to cultural psychology.

Tahitians, by Robert I. Levy, who became an anthropologist after a career in clinical psychiatry, then did 26 months of field work in Tahiti, played an important role in bringing these issues to the fore and stimulating ethnopsychological research during the 1970s and later. His book elevated the standards for understanding psychological experience in a culture other than our own and stands as a model for such investigations 32 years after its publication. Levy did not use the word *ethnopsychology* in the book and did not classify his own work among previous studies in that field.

Ethnopsychology had been independently invented by various field-workers who encountered people in another culture using vernacular terms to describe and explain what we would call their mental processes or subjective experience. Many 20th-century ethnographers

assumed that the cultures of the world have diverse points of view on many phenomena, including thought, emotion, and personal development. Before the 1970s, most anthropologists did not use the term *ethnopsychology* or cite earlier studies of a similar sort. A good example is the 1959 article by Hildred Geertz, "The Vocabulary of Emotion: A Study of Javanese Socialization Processes." It seems that the earliest use of the term *ethnopsychology* as a body of knowledge equivalent to ethnobotany and other "ethnosciences" was in the 1950 (third) edition of *The Outline of Cultural Materials* by Murdock et al., the volume that provides the categories for the Human Relations Area Files as an archive of ethnographic data. The ethnographic monographs that took an ethnopsychological approach before *Tahitians* are George Devereux's (1961) *Mohave Ethnopsychiatry and Suicide* and Jean Briggs's (1970) *Never in Anger.*

Devereux's book is unfortunately flawed by a disorganized and opinionated presentation; the Mohave voice is there, but it is drowned out by lengthy commentaries. Briggs's *Never in Anger: Portrait of an Eskimo Family* is well known as an ethnographic masterpiece that generates psychocultural insights from a detailed account of the anthropologist's relationship with one family. But it was also a landmark in ethnopsychology, providing a glossary of emotion terms used in the text and a 55-page appendix explaining the meanings of these terms and the normative contexts that specify their use in everyday life. This was an exemplary, though circumscribed, demonstration of the ethnographic depth and microscopic attention needed to translate emotional experience from one culture to another.

Levy's *Tahitians* (1973) was another such demonstration, but on a larger canvas and with a broader set of goals. Levy sought to convey in convincing detail how Tahitian psychological concepts were collective and personal at the same time. He coined terms such as "shared privacy," which seems to embody a contradiction, that he judged were needed to frame a description of communication as inevitably social and psychological, conventional and idiosyncratic. This theoretical frame, derived in part from Gregory Bateson (to whom the book is dedicated), provides the structure for relating cultural symbols and personal experience through the communicative contexts of social interaction. A person-centered ethnography of over 500 pages, it provides an unusually rich combination of ideational and behavioral material, a critical and self-critical questioning of descriptive generalizations, and meticulous attention to the justification of inferences concerning connections between observable behavior and subjective experience. It remains unsurpassed as an ethnopsychological description of a community, for at least five reasons:

1. Levy's ethnopsychology provides a contextual and pragmatic account rather than a formal taxonomy. Although a glossary of Tahitian psychological terms is included and their meanings are examined, their practical contexts and functions in Tahitian social life, and in the lives and actions of participants, are the focus rather than the cognitive relationships of the terms.

2. The historical situation is part of the ethnopsychological portrait. The Tahitians with whom Levy worked had lost most of the rituals and other aspects of public culture described in travelers' accounts from the 19th century, but some meanings lived on, in altered forms, in the sphere of interpersonal relations and the subjective experience of individuals. Levy's detailed historical documentation thus provides a dynamic dimension that is often missing in descriptive ethnopsychology.

3. The text of the study involves a gradual movement from the observable social surface of interpersonal relations to inferences about personal experience and psychodynamics at greater depth and abstraction. This movement embodies in ethnographic work the approach of a careful psychoanalytic clinician—without, however, requiring a prior commitment to psychoanalytic theory.

4. Levy's concepts of *hypocognized* and *hypercognized* feelings introduced the dimensions of psychological salience and awareness into ethnopsychological description, which can otherwise treat all terms as equally salient. This distinction is Levy's restrained and empiricist way of dealing with the issues of psychic censorship and repression that Freud (1900/1958, 1913/1958) introduced in *The Interpretation of Dreams* and applied to culture in the early chapters of *Totem and Taboo*. As Levy recognized, it moves ethnopsychology into the field of psychodynamic interpretation, requiring clinical investigation but gaining deeper illumination of social behavior.

5. The organization of experience in cultural representations and personality is deliberately included. Levy assumed that an understanding of Tahitians' experience could not end with a description of the lexicon in which their experience was encoded but had to include the ways ideas and behavior were organized, and disorganized, and the style that characterized their behavior. The characterization of organization in culture or personality involves another set of inferences that can reflect illusory correlations or at least systematic distortion—as Shweder and D'Andrade (1980) have warned—but which Levy was prepared to justify with empirical evidence from multiple sources.

Thus, *Tahitians* provides the lesson that ethnopsychology, however necessary as an instrument of cultural and psychological understanding, is insufficient without investigation of the communicative contexts, both personal and social, that give the lexicon of thought and feeling its meanings. He includes the results of clinical interviews designed to illustrate the various ways Tahitian categories of experience work out in individual lives. On the whole, however, Levy resists depth interpretations and perhaps leaves questions a reader might have about Tahitian personality unanswered; the implication is that they are unanswerable through the ethnographic research of an outsider.

As mentioned earlier, Geertz's *The Interpretation of Cultures* was also published in 1973. In his chapter on person, time, and conduct in Bali (originally published in 1966), Geertz said:

> What we want and do not yet have is a developed method of describing and analyzing the meaningful structure of experience (. . . the experience of persons) as it is apprehended by representative members of a particular society at a particular point in time—in a word, a scientific phenomenology of culture. (1973, p. 364)

It is ironic that these words were reprinted during the same year that Robert Levy actually offered such a method in *Tahitians*. For psychological anthropologists, Levy's multifaceted work in Tahiti was an admired model, difficult to emulate; but for anthropologists outside of our subfield it was easier (and more in keeping with disciplinary orthodoxy) to expunge "psychologizing" even from the study of such obviously mental contents as thought, emotion, and self-concepts.

But another book published (in its English translation) in 1973 pointed in a more promising direction. Takeo Doi's *The Anatomy of Dependence* presented an analysis of Japanese relationships in home, work, and therapeutic settings through the extended description of a single Japanese vernacular term, *amae*. Doi is a Japanese psychiatrist partly trained in the United States, where he was exposed to psychoanalysis and American culture before beginning clinical work in Japan. Like Levy, he had years of clinical experience and a healthy skepticism about orthodox Freudian theory before embarking on cultural study. Unlike Levy, however, Doi was explicating his own culture, albeit in comparison with American culture as he experienced it, and interpreting the behavior of individuals from the same cultural background as himself. His insights into normal and pathological development in Japan are deep and illuminating, and they are convincing in a way that is hard (though not impossible) for an outsider to achieve. This suggests an alternative to the difficult challenge of matching Levy's masterful accomplishment in *Tahitians*, namely, turning the kind of ethnopsychology it exemplifies into a research program by scholars of diverse backgrounds instead of a method in which Westerners describe, translate, and interpret the terms of non-Western experience.

Doi (1962, 1973) translated the Japanese term *amae* as "to presume upon the benevolence of others" and argued for its pervasiveness in Japanese interpersonal relations (including formal bureaucratic relationships), its individual origins in a culture-specific pattern of mother–child interactions, and its involvement in forms of neurosis occurring among the Japanese. His evidence is anecdotal but drawn from his clinical observations and his experience as a Japanese man. It has the authority of the insider's judgment combined with Doi's awareness of how the patterns he describes differ from those he experienced in the United States. He followed the first book with a second, *The Anatomy of Self* (Doi, 1986), which extends his ethnopsychological description of Japanese experience into the social world of typical individuals in Japan and also contains comparative observations. Doi's writings influenced others investigating psychological issues in Japan (e.g., Lebra, 1976, 1994; Schwalb &

Schwalb, 1996) and provided a powerful example of how culturally specific expectations concerning psychologically significant phenomena can be embedded in the verbal idioms of a particular language. Doi himself remains convinced that although the Japanese have their own way of thinking, feeling, and talking about themselves, their ways are but a particular version of universal aspects of human experience.

A number of subsequent ethnopsychological studies carried out in Oceania are presented in the books by White and Kirkpatrick (1985) and Lutz (1988); a thoughtful review by White appeared in 1992. Ethnopsychology forces us to confront the drastically different terms in which peoples of diverse cultures conceptualize their experience: They may locate emotions in parts of their bodies or in invisible spirits rather than in their conscious or unconscious selves, and in that sense it is fundamental to cultural psychology. Yet ethnopsychological research, though necessary to reconstruct the insider's experience, is only the first step toward understanding and explaining that experience.

EPISTEMOLOGICAL ISSUES IN PSYCHOLOGICAL ANTHROPOLOGY

I have long believed that the culture and personality movement of the period 1925–1960 generated new, important, and basically sound theoretical ideas but failed to achieve consensus on a research program, on methods to be used to test and elaborate the theory, or even on what body of knowledge it was attempting to construct through its research. Many of those issues remain unresolved. In this section I offer my own efforts to address these issues, particularly during the 1970s, as exemplifying this lack of resolution.

My view of the tasks of culture and personality research was based on Spiro's (1961) distinction between culture as *explanans* and culture as *explanandum* (i.e., culture as an explanatory factor in the analysis of personality and behavior, and individual motivation as explanatory in the analysis of culture). Spiro argued that anthropologists had focused on showing that culture helps account for cross-population variations in the distribution of psychological and behavioral characteristics (as in Kluckhohn's "culture and behavior" model mentioned earlier), but tended to neglect the ways in which individual motivational factors influence cultural stability and change. Insofar as culture and personality interact with and mutually affect each other (as originally suggested by Thomas and Znaniecki in the introduction to the 1917 edition of their volumes, *The Polish Peasant in Europe and America*), both types of research and analysis were equally necessary. I accepted this imperative and explored it in my 1973 book, *Culture, Behavior and Personality.*

On the side of culture as an explanatory variable, I proposed a "population psychology" resembling population genetics, epidemiology, and other statistical sciences of populations to investigate specific cultural influences on behavioral/psychological variations across populations. This was not an original idea but seemed an obvious implication of earlier social research from Durkheim's (1895/1951) study of suicide to the formulations of my teachers Gordon W. Allport (1954) and Alex Inkeles (1959), and I had already presented it myself in articles (LeVine, 1966, 1970). (Dan Sperber, in 1985, proposed an "epidemiology of representations.")

As I envisioned this approach, variations across populations in phenotypic behaviors (i.e., behavioral indicators of individual emotional and cognitive dispositions) would be described in terms of their statistical distributions, then related to the cultural and institutional environments inhabited by the individuals of differing populations. This "culture and behavior" approach based on population studies often leaves an intervening "black box" of hypothesized dispositions that are only indirectly assessed through behavioral indicators and require deeper investigation to uncover the psychosocial processes that mediate the influence of culture and institutions on observable behaviors. The approach is also susceptible to the "ecological fallacy" in which covariations across populations are taken to be causally related, when they might be the results of historical accident or unmeasured determinants. Thus, the initial analysis of statistical distributions would have to lead to further research—clinical, developmental, and neurophysiological—designed to clarify what the mediating dispositions are and how they operate in the processes and contexts of social life.

On the other side—that of the psychological analysis of culture—I made a more innovative proposal that would prove far more controversial. When psychological factors are taken as underlying causes of a social process, as in all motivational theories, the need for valid measurement of those factors is even greater than when psychological factors are hypothesized as outcomes. But how are the deep psychological causes of cultural stability and change to be measured? For Spiro (1970), as for his teacher Hallowell, the answer was to be found in the Rorschach test. But I found not only great disagreement among psychologists about how to analyze Rorschach responses but also a powerful cross-cultural critique of projective techniques by Gardner Lindzey (1961) that had never been answered in subsequent research. In addition, collaborating with the social psychologist Donald T. Campbell (LeVine & Campbell, 1972) had acquainted me with the devastating critiques of personality tests and experimental assessment procedures that had created a validity crisis within personality and social psychology during the 1960s. As an anthropologist shopping for a means of assessing the psychological causes of cultural patterns, I was looking for something more valid than academic psychology seemed to offer.

Having completed my training at the Chicago Institute for Psychoanalysis in 1971, I tried to rethink cross-cultural personality measurement from an epistemological perspective on the clinical situation in psychoanalysis. I argued that, as a long-term series of observations free of the pressure to reach final diagnostic judgments, psychoanalysis offered methodological advantages over the shortcut procedures of projective tests and psychometric personality measurement, advantages that might generate more valid methods usable among the illiterate majority of humans. For this I was pilloried by some personality psychologists: The review of my book by H. J. Eysenck was titled "Commit It to the Flames." Yet I knew that my concerns about validity were shared by many other psychologists concerned only with Western populations. Anthropologists as fieldworkers had a deep-seated aversion to imported rapid assessments that seemed not to capture what they saw in the field, but their criticisms (and mine) were not entirely alien to those of thoughtful social psychologists and psychometricians.

In the book, I made a number of tentative suggestions about how to adapt psychoanalytic clinical method to field situations, including the "bicultural collaboration" of an insider social scientist (who had acquired a particular culture in childhood) with the conventional anthropologist approaching that particular culture and its patterns of experience from the outside, using the tools of ethnography. Rather than specifying methods in advance, I recommended criteria for the development of methods in the field. Soon after the book was published, however, I embarked on a 2-year collaborative study of infant care among the Gusii of Kenya, and my primary attention has been on issues of early child development ever since (LeVine et al., 1994). Thus my project of constructing a new, psychoanalytically influenced, approach to personality assessment in diverse cultures was never brought to completion.

In the second edition of the book (LeVine, 1982), I added a chapter, "The Self in Culture," that recognized the emergence during the previous decade of anthropological field studies focused on experience, to which I gave the label "person-centered ethnography":

> Taken together, these . . . tendencies comprise a new attack on subjective experience in other societies—its indigenous cultural constituents, its form and content in individual lives and its problematic role in the investigative relationship. This new attack operates without an explicit consensus on methods of data collection or comparative analysis. It is a development of and from the ethnographic tradition in anthropology: a person-centered ethnography, taking the individual perspective on culture and experience rather than that of a collective system or external observer. Standard ethnography produces a cultural description analogous to a map or aerial photograph of a community; person-centered ethnography tells us what it is like to live there—what features are salient to its inhabitants. Like other anthropological field workers, person-centered ethnographers often aspire to "thick description" (Geertz, 1973)—accounts of sufficient detail and diversity to reveal the meanings that lie behind behavior. This is a modest step toward generalization compared to cross-cultural hypothesis-testing, but it represents the conviction that greater ambitions cannot be fulfilled without data of better quality. (p. 293)

In the remainder of that chapter, I proposed an ethnographic approach to the self through the narratives embedded in local conventions of interpersonal communication: conventions of face-to-face interaction, ritual, and autobiographical discourse that contain narratives of a culturally constituted self. Having retreated from a direct attempt to plumb the depths of personality, I found in the focus on self a way of uniting Hallowell's cultural phenomenology with the psychoanalytic self psychology of Heinz Kohut (1971, 1977). By exploring continuities and discontinuities—repetitions and dialectical tensions—between cultural narratives of interaction and those of the imagination in a given community, it would be possible, I argued, to identify the culturally constituted representations of self (including defenses) characteristic of a local population. This approach remains to be elaborated in future work.

My approaches to the assessment of socially significant aspects of individual psychology, like those of many other anthropologists, have been to "complexify" its assessment, in contrast to the psychologist's typical simplifying and reductive approach. In the aforementioned chapter, I made the following argument, which can serve as the conclusion of my work to date:

> A major lesson from research in personality and social psychology of the past two decades is that there can be no psychological X-ray that bypasses contextual analysis, no way of tapping "pure" dispositional competence uninfluenced by the conditions surrounding its observable performance—any more than it is possible to speak without speaking a particular language. . . . Deprived of the illusion of "independent" and "direct" personality assessment, the psychological anthropologist has no choice but to ground psychological investigation in an ethnographic analysis of communicative contexts. (LeVine, 1982, p. 295)

CONCLUSIONS

This selective review of anthropological foundations of cultural psychology has taken a historical approach, revealing that American anthropologists between 1925 and 1975 concerned themselves with some of the basic topics of contemporary cultural psychology. Their formulations—on the nature of culture; the relationships of cultural ideas and practices to individual mental processes; the self-concept as culturally variable, culturally constituted defenses; and the translation of indigenous psychological terminology—were grounded in ethnographic fieldwork with native North Americans, Pacific Islanders and other non-Western peoples. Their writings remain instructive, not only in terms of revealing the emergence and evolution of concepts and research agendas during the 20th century but also in terms of understanding earlier efforts to grapple with fundamental issues that continue to affect cultural psychology.

Edward Sapir, in the 1920s and 1930s, saw the need for a cultural psychology that studied the relationships between cultural symbols and the individual psyche, and he attempted to ground it in clinical psychiatry rather than in academic psychology, or any other discipline that took a statistical approach to individual variation. The culture and personality movement he cofounded did not achieve a consensus on this issue or on issues of universalism versus relativism and the use of psychological tests versus ethnographic and clinical approaches to capture the individual psyche as distinct from but influenced by culture. When the movement came to an end after 1950 and transformed itself into "psychological anthropology" (see LeVine, 2001), a consensus on these issues remained elusive, and though increasingly sophisticated theoretical and empirical studies followed, the field as a whole continues to have an exploratory and provisional character. We still struggle with problems of validity that need to be solved to translate Sapir's dream of a cultural psychology into an effective interdisciplinary research program.

REFERENCES

Allport, G. W. (1954). *The nature of prejudice*. Cambridge, MA: Addison-Wesley.

Benedict, R. (1934). *Patterns of culture*. Boston: Houghton Mifflin.

Berman, J. (1996). "The culture as it appears to the Indian himself": Boas, George Hunt, and the methods of ethnography. In G. W. Stocking (Ed.), Volksgeist *as method and ethic: Essays on Boasian ethnography and the German anthropological tradition* (pp. 215–256). Madison: University of Wisconsin Press.

Boas, F. (1889). On alternating sounds. *American Anthropologist, 2,* 47–53.

Boas, F. (1911). *The mind of primitive man*. New York: Macmillan.

Boas, F. (1912). Instability of human types. In G. Spiller (Ed.), *Papers on interracial problems communicated to the First Universal Races Congress Held at the University of London, July 26–29, 1911* (pp. 99j103). Boston: Ginn & Co. Reprinted 1974 in G. Stocking (Ed.), *A Franz Boas reader: The shaping of American anthropology, 1883–1911* (pp. 214–218). New York: Basic Books.

Boas, F. (Ed.). (1938). *General anthropology*. Boston: D.C. Heath & Co.

Briggs, J.(1970). *Never in anger: Portrait of an Eskimo family*. Cambridge, MA: Harvard University Press.

D'Andrade, R. G. (1995). *The development of cognitive anthropology*. New York: Cambridge University Press.

Darnell, R. (1990). *Edward Sapir: Linguist, anthropologist, humanist*. Berkeley: University of California Press.

Darnell, R. (2001). *Invisible genealogies: A history of Americanist anthropology*. Lincoln: University of Nebraska Press.

Devereux, G. (1961). *Mohave ethnopsychiatry and suicide*. Washington, DC: Bureau of American Ethnology.

DeVos, G. A. (1973). *Socialization for achievement: The cultural psychology of the Japanese*. Berkeley: University of California Press.

Doi, T. (1962). "Amae": A key concept for understanding Japanese personality structure. In R. J. Smith & R. K. Beardsley (Eds.), *Japanese culture: Its development and characteristics* (pp. 253–287). New York: Wenner-Gren Foundation for Anthropological Research.

Doi, T. (1973). *The anatomy of dependence*. New York: Kodansha International.

Doi, T. (1986). *The anatomy of self: The individual versus society*. Tokyo: Kodansha.

Dollard, J., Doob, L., Miller, N. L., Mowrer, O. H., & Sears, R. R. (1938). *Frustration and aggression*. New Haven, CT: Yale University Press.

Dollard, J., & Miller, N. L. (1949). *Personality and psychotherapy*. New Haven, CT: Yale University Press.

Durkheim, É. (1951). *Suicide*. Glencoe, IL: Free Press. (Original work published 1895)

Durkheim, É. (1982). *The rules of sociological method* (S. Lukes, Ed., & W. D. Halls, Trans.). New York: Free Press. (Original work published 1895)

Freud, S. (1958). The interpretation of dreams. In J. Strachey (Ed.), *The standard edition of the complete psychological works of Sigmund Freud* (Vol. IV, pp. 1–338; Vol. V, pp. 339–625). London: Hogarth Press. (Original work published 1900)

Freud, S. (1958). Totem and taboo. In J. Strachey (Ed.), *The standard edition of the complete psychological works of Sigmund Freud* (Vol. XIII, pp. 1–162). London: Hogarth Press. (Original work published 1913)

Geertz, C. (1973). *The interpretation of cultures*. New York: Basic Books.

Geertz, C. (2000). *Available light: Anthropological reflections on philosophical topics*. Princeton, NJ: Princeton University Press.

Geertz, H. (1959). The vocabulary of emotion: A study

of Javanese socialization processes. *Psychiatry, 22*, 225–237.

Gorer, G., & Rickman, J. (1949). *The people of Great Russia.* London: Crescent Press.

Hallowell, A. I. (1955). *Culture and experience.* Philadelphia: University of Pennsylvania Press.

Howells, W. W. (1959). Boas as statistician. In W. Goldschmidt (Ed.), *The anthropology of Franz Boas: Essays on the centennial of his birth* (Memoir No. 89). Washington, DC: American Anthropological Association.

Inkeles, A. (1959). Personality and social structure. In R. K. Merton, L. Broom, & L. Cottrell (Eds.), *Sociology today* (pp. 249–276). New York: Basic Books.

Kardiner, A. (1939). *The individual and his society.* New York: Columbia University Press.

Kardiner, A. (1945). *The psychological frontiers of society.* New York: Columbia University Press.

Kluckhohn, C. K. M. (1938). Participation in ceremonials in a Navaho community. *American Anthropologist, 40*, 359–369.

Kluckhohn, C. K. M. (1939). Theoretical bases for an empirical method of studying the acquisition of culture by individuals. *Man, 39*, 98–103.

Kluckhohn, C. K. M. (1953). Universal categories of culture. In A. L. Kroeber (Ed.), *Anthropology today* (pp. 507–523). Chicago: University of Chicago Press.

Kluckhohn, C. K. M. (1962). *Culture and behavior: The collected essays of Clyde Kluckhohn.* New York: Free Press.

Kluckhohn, Clyde K. M., & Kelly, W. H. (1945). The concept of culture. In R. Linton (Ed.), *The science of man in the world crisis* (pp. 78–105). New York: Columbia University Press.

Kluckhohn, C. K. M., & Mowrer, O. H. (1944). Culture and personality: A conceptual scheme. *American Anthropologist, 46*, 1–29.

Kluckhohn, C. K. M., & Murray, H. A. (Eds.). (1948). *Personality in nature, culture and society.* New York: Knopf.

Kohut, H. (1971). *The analysis of the self.* New York: International Universities Press.

Kohut, H. (1977). *The restoration of the self.* New York: International Universities Press.

Kroeber, A. L. (1917). The superorganic. *American Anthropologist, 19*, 163–213.

Kroeber, A. L., & Kluckhohn, C. K. M. (1952). *Culture: A critical review of concepts and definitions* (Papers of the Peabody Museum, Vol. 47, No. 1). Cambridge, MA: Harvard University.

Lebra, T. S. (1976). *Japanese patterns of behavior.* Honolulu: University of Hawaii Press.

Lebra, T. S. (1994). Mother and child in Japanese socialization: A Japan–U.S. comparison. In P. M. Greenfield & R. R. Cocking (Eds.), *Cross-cultural roots of minority child development* (pp. 259–274). Hillsdale, NJ: Erlbaum.

Lee, D. D. (1950). Notes on the conception of the self among the Wintu Indians. *Journal of Abnormal and Social Psychology, 45*, 538–543.

LeVine, R. A. (1966). (1966). Toward a psychology of populations: The cross-cultural study of personality. *Human Development, 9*, 30–46.

LeVine, R. A. (1970). Cross-cultural study in child psychology. In P. H. Mussen (Ed.), *Carmichael's manual of child psychology* (Vol. II, pp. 559–612). New York: Wiley.

LeVine, R. A. (1973). *Culture, behavior and personality: An introduction to the comparative study of psychosocial adaptation.* Chicago: Aldine.

LeVine, R. A. (1982). *Culture, behavior and personality* (2nd ed.). New York: Aldine.

LeVine, R. A. (2001). Culture and personality studies, 1918–1960: Myth and history. *Journal of Personality, 69*(6), 803–818.

LeVine, R. A. (2005). Coded communications: Symbolic psychological anthropology. In R. A. Shweder & B. Good (Eds.), *Clifford Geertz by his colleagues* (pp. 24–27). Chicago: University of Chicago Press.

LeVine, R. A., & Campbell, D. T. (1972). *Ethnocentrism: Theories of conflict, ethnic attitudes, and group behavior.* New York: Wiley.

LeVine, R. A., Dixon, S., LeVine, S., Richman, A., Leiderman, P. H., Keefer, C. H., et al. (1994). *Child care and culture: Lessons from Africa.* New York: Cambridge University Press.

Levy, R. I. (1973). *Tahitians: Mind and experience in the Society Islands.* Chicago: University of Chicago Press.

Lindzey, G. (1961). *Projective techniques and cross-cultural research.* New York: Appleton-Century-Crofts.

Lutz, C. A. (1988). *Unnatural emotions: Everyday sentiments on a Micronesian atoll and their challenge to Western theory.* Chicago: University of Chicago Press.

Mandelbaum, D. (Ed.). (1949). *Selected writings of Edward Sapir in language, culture and personality.* Berkeley: University of California Press.

Markus, H., & Kitayama, S. (1991). Culture and self: Implications for cognition, emotion and motivation. *Psychological Review, 98*, 224–253.

Mauss, M. (1938). Une categorie de l'esprit humain: La notion de personne celle de "moi." *Journal of the Royal Anthropological Institute, 48*, 263–281.

Miller, N. L., & Dollard, J. (1941). *Social learning and imitation.* New Haven, CT: Yale University Press.

Murdock, G. P., Ford, C. S., Hudson, A. E., Kennedy, R., Simmons, L. W., & Whiting, J. W. M. (1950). *Outline of cultural materials* (3rd ed.). New Haven, CT: Human Relations Area Files, Inc.

Obeyesekere, G. (1981). *Medusa's hair: An assay on personal symbols and religious experience.* Chicago: University of Chicago Press.

Obeyesekere, G. (1990). Culturally constituted defenses and the theory of collective motivation. In D. K. Jordan & M. J. Swartz (Eds.), *Personality and the cultural construction of society: Papers in honor of Melford E. Spiro.* Tuscaloosa: University of Alabama Press.

Perry, H. S. (1982). *Psychiatrist of America: The life of Harry Stack Sullivan.* Cambridge, MA: Harvard University Press.

Pike, K. (1954). *Language in relation to a unified theory of human behavior.* The Hague: Mouton.

Sapir, E. (1917). Do we need a "superorganic"? *American Anthropologist, 19,* 441–447.

Sapir, E. (1921). *Language: An introduction to the study of speech.* New York: Harcourt Brace.

Sapir, E. (1993). *The psychology of culture* (J. Irvine, Ed.). New York: Mouton.

Shwalb, D. W., & Shwalb, B. J. (Eds.). (1996). *Japanese childrearing: Two generations of scholarship.* New York: Guilford Press.

Shweder, R. A., & D'Andrade, R. G. (1980). The systematic distortion hypothesis. In R. Shweder (Ed.), *Fallible judgment in behavioral research* (New Directions for Methodology of Social and Behavioral Research No. 4, pp. 37–58). San Francisco: Jossey-Bass.

Sperber, D. (1985). Anthropology and psychology: Toward an epidemiology of representations. *Man, 20,* 73–87.

Spiro, M. E. (1961). An overview and a suggested reorientation. In F. L. K. Hsu (Ed.), *Psychological anthropology* (pp. 459–492). Homewood, IL: Dorsey Press.

Spiro, M. E. (1965). Religious systems as culturally constituted defense mechanisms. In *Context and meaning in anthropology* (pp. 100–113). New York: Free Press.

Spiro, M. E. (1970). *Buddhism and society.* Berkeley: University of California Press.

Stocking, G. (1968). *Race, culture and evolution: Essays in the history of anthropology.* New York: Free Press.

Stocking, G. (1992). Polarity and plurality: Franz Boas as psychological anthropologist. In T. Schwartz, G. M. White, & C. A. Lutz (Eds.), *New directions in psychological anthropology* (pp. 311–323). New York: Cambridge University Press.

Stocking, G. (1995). *After Tylor: British social anthropology, 1888–1951.* Madison: University of Wisconsin Press.

Sullivan, H. S. (1947). *Conceptions of modern psychiatry.* New York: William Alanson White Memorial Foundation.

Tanner, J. M. (1959). Boas' contributions to knowledge of human growth and form. In W. Goldschmidt (Ed.), *The anthropology of Franz Boas: Essays on the centennial of his birth* (Memoir No. 89). Washington, DC: American Anthropological Association.

Thomas, W. I., & Znaniecki, F. (1927). *The Polish Peasant in Europe and America.* New York: Knopf. (Original work published 1917)

White, G. (1992). Ethnopsychology. In T. Schwartz, G. W. White, & C. A. Lutz (Eds.), *New directions in psychological anthropology* (pp. 21–46). New York: Cambridge University Press.

White, G., & Kirkpatrick, J. (Eds.). (1985). *Person, self and experience: Exploring Pacific ethnopsychologies.* Berkeley: University of California Press.

Whiting, J. W. M., Child, I. L., Lambert, W. W., Fischer, A. M., Fischer, J. L., Nydegger, C., et al. (1966). *Field guide for a study of socialization.* New York: Wiley.

CHAPTER 3

Culture and Psychology
A History of the Study of Their Relationship

HARRY C. TRIANDIS

The history of the study of the relationship between culture and psychology has been presented in considerable detail by Jahoda (1993). Other histories have been published by Klineberg (1980) and Jahoda and Krewer (1997). Furthermore, Cole (1996) included much historical material in the first section of his *Cultural Psychology*. What follows is my integration of these publications, supplemented by personal observations, because I was somewhat involved in this history during the last half-century. I also try to assess the future of the relationship of culture and psychology by examining how historical trends in psychology have shaped current work and will shape future work in this field.

EARLY HISTORY

Students of psychological processes in antiquity and the Middle Ages usually contrasted the assumed universal psychological processes found in their location with "inferior" psychological processes found among "inferior" groups (Jahoda & Krewer, 1997). One exception was Herodotus (460–359 B.C.), who realized that people in all cultures are ethnocentric.

They see themselves as the centers of the world, and processes that are common in their location are "good," whereas processes that are different are "bad." Thucydides (about 455–395 B.C.) was a boy when he heard Herodotus recite from *The Histories* at the Olympic Games. He was so moved that he wept (Thucydides, 1934). Later when he wrote his *History of the Peloponnesian War*, Thucydides provided a surprisingly modern account of psychological processes. He argued that there were differences in the fertility of soils in ancient Greece, and humans gravitated toward the fertile soils. To hold these fertile soils people had to fight, so they developed war-like attributes. However, those who did not like fighting moved to the Athens area, because it was not fertile. As a result, a highly heterogeneous population comprising people from all over Greece settled in Athens. These people had different ways of perceiving the world, but because they did not like to fight they debated with considerable frequency to reach agreements. Democratic behavior patterns and institutions were generated as a result of these debates (Thucydides, 1934).

Thus, the ancient Greek historians had two insights: (1) People in all cultures are ethnocentric, and (2) ecology leads to reciprocal relationships among personality, culture, and social institutions. This view emerged again in psychological anthropology (Whiting, 1973/1977, 1994) and in modern psychology (Berry, 1976, 2003; Cohen, 2001; Nisbett, 2003; Triandis, 1972).

Ethnocentrism is a universal human attribute (Herskovits, 1955; Triandis, 1990). It is inevitable because most people start life by knowing only their own culture, and see themselves as being located in the center of the world. Thus, for instance, the Ancient Greeks thought that the center of the earth was located in Delphi, and they even specified the exact spot, which they called the *omphalos*—meaning the belly button of the world. Everyplace to the east of Delphi was called East, and everyplace to the west of Delphi was called West. The Romans adopted this terminology, which then entered into the European languages, so that even today we talk about "the Middle East" and "the Far East," as well as "the West." The Ancient Assyrians, who wrote on the tablets now in the Pergamon Museum in Berlin, were quite explicit that they were the center of the world, and their king, Sargon II, was "King of the universe." Herskovits (1955, p. 356) noted that "the ethnocentrism of nonliterate peoples . . . is manifest in many tribal names whose meaning in their respective languages signifies 'human being.' " The Chinese called their country "the central kingdom." In 1793 the Chinese Emperor Ch'ien Lung wrote to George III of England as follows: "We possess all things. I set no value on objects strange or ingenious, and have no use for your country's manufactures" (Klineberg, 1980, p. 31).

Only people who are in touch with many cultures, as was the case with Herodotus, who visited about 30 cultures in all directions around Greece, see that ethnocentrism is due to ignorance. Vico (1744/1970) established an "axiom" that stated, "It is another property of the human mind, that whenever men can form an idea of distant and unknown things, they judge them by what is familiar and at hand" (p. 18). This, Vico pointed out, is an inexhaustible source of errors for judging other cultures.

A consequence of ethnocentrism is the perception of what goes on in "our culture" is "natural," "normal," and "correct," whereas what goes on in other cultures is "unnatural," "immoral," and "incorrect" (Brewer & Campbell, 1976). Ingroup customs are perceived as universally valid. Ingroup norms, role definitions, and values are "obviously correct."

With very few exceptions up to about 1900, most studies of the relationship of culture and psychology were ethnocentric. Even in the 20th century, most psychologists thought that their discoveries were "universal laws" and "eternally valid." This view became less and less acceptable as cultural psychology developed. In the 1970s, a few psychologists abandoned the universalistic view and after Markus and Kitayama (1991) published "Culture and Self," universalism became a minority view.

During the Renaissance (15th and 16th centuries), the universality of psychological processes was assumed, but increasing diversity became apparent as trade and exploration resulted in diverse peoples' meeting. Some writers, such as De Las Casas and Montaigne (Jahoda, 1993, p. 8), questioned the universality of moral principles and started a debate on universalism. But for most writers ethnocentrism was endemic. Also, it was assumed that cultures went through a linear evolution from "savage" to "civilized." Vico (1744/1970) identified three stages of the evolution of cultures—the divine, the heroic, and the humane. The divine required submission to the authority of gods; the heroic, submission to the aristocracy; and the humane, submission to human-made laws. Interestingly, the current emphasis on return to *shariah* laws, advocated by Muslim fundamentalists, is a return to the most "primitive" form of society according to Vico's analysis. The assumption of stages of development of cultures continued until the 20th century (e.g., Wundt, 1900–1914, trans. 1916). The concept of culture as shared norms and customs or shared mentalities was used to explain the diversity among the people encountered. This concept is found also in the 20th century, with Geertz (1973) defining *culture* as shared meanings.

By the 18th century, Vico (1744/1970) used the concept of culture (he called it "nation") to include language, myth, art, custom, religion, and so on. Culture interacted with "mind" to produce what researchers in the 20th century called "context-specific competencies" (Laboratory of Comparative Human Cognition, 1983) and "multiple realities" (Shweder, 1990).

Cultural relativism began very tentatively at the end of the 18th century when Herder

(1784/1969) argued that psychological processes depend on time and place. Linguistic analyses were incorporated in a *Völkerpsychologie* that started with von Humboldt (1820/1969), who argued that there was a close relationship between language and thought, a position that later became known as the Sapir–Whorf hypothesis. But by advocating the study of collective mental phenomena, Lazarus and Steinthal (1860) were the "real" founders of *Völkerpsychologie*. The new discipline was to occupy a position intermediate between the humanities and the natural sciences. They argued that a psychology without a historical framework is bound to remain incomplete. In 1860, Lazarus occupied the First Chair of Psychology in Bern, Switzerland, as "Professor of *Völkerpsychologie*" (Jahoda, 1993). Steinthal (1858) advocated the study of language as central to psychology and the key to understanding of the "souls" of the people who are its speakers. In addition, folklore and religion would provide the data needed to understand psychology in a broader framework.

Wilhelm Wundt's 10-volume opus on the subject (Wundt, 1900–1914) was the most impressive presentation of *Völkerpsychologie*. He considered the study of language, myth, religion, and the like to have similar significance for understanding collective consciousness, just as cognition, feeling, and will are significant for understanding individual consciousness. Wundt derived culture from psychology, which may have been a mistake, though it is half of contemporary cultural psychology that sees "culture and psyche making each other up" (Shweder, 1990, p. 24). Berry (1983) thought that perhaps interest in Wundt would increase because of developments in contemporary psychology. For example, the substantial recent interest is the study of religion (Tarakeshwar, Stanton, & Pargament, 2003; Triandis, 2006) was an important component in Wundt's work.

The 19th century produced many race-related theories of differences in customs and the like (Jahoda, 1993, Chapter 6). Some claimed that there was a resemblance between a Negro brain and that of an ape. Others claimed that civilization was entirely the product of an "Arian" race. Because race explained cultural differences, these authors had nothing to say about culture.

A contrasting view proclaimed the "psychic unity of mankind" (Waitz, 1859, trans. 1863). Waitz's *magnum opus*, in six volumes, was his *Anthropologie der Naturvölker* (1859). Similar to Pritchard (1843/1848), who stated that the "same inward and mental nature is to be recognized in all the races of man" (p. 546), he emphasizes the similarities in human institutions and mental characteristics. Waitz argued that there is tremendous variability within groups, an argument that can be found more recently in Minturn and Lambert's (1964) empirical demonstration of more within- than between-cultures variance. Empirical support for the psychic unity of mankind thesis was provided by Bastian (1860), who visited several cultures in the South Pacific and the Americas. He argued that some elementary ideas can be found in all cultures. Recent empirical support of this view was obtained by Osgood, May and Miron (1975), who found that in all the cultures tested, meaning was reflected in evaluation, potency, and activity judgments.

Empirical developments were started in 1799 by the Observateurs de l'Homme (Jahoda, 1993), who formulated detailed manuals for how to collect data in other cultures. However, practical difficulties made competent data collection rare.

By the end of the 19th century, Tylor provided a broad definition of culture: " . . . the complex whole which includes knowledge, belief, art, morals, law, custom, and many other capabilities and habits acquired by man as a member of society" (1871, p. 1). Tylor (1889) for the first time also correlated two attributes of culture (avoidance patterns among relatives, e.g., husband and mother-in-law; and residence patterns, such as living in the same household) across 350 societies. He showed that there was a positive correlation. This was the first holocultural study (see Naroll, Michik, & Naroll, 1980), a type of research that is carried out today by many members of the Society for Cross-Cultural Research. When Tylor presented this method, Francis Galton (Darwin's cousin), who was in the audience, pointed out that the computation of the significance of a correlation requires that the data be independent, and cultural diffusion can make them nonindependent. This is now called "Galton's problem," and can be solved in several ways (Naroll et al., 1980), such as making sure that the cultures sampled are geographically distant from each other.

Also at the end of the 19th century, expeditions were undertaken to obtain "mental measurements" (Rivers, 1901, 1905). Rivers obtained evidence that some natives studied during his expedition were *less* susceptible to some and *more* susceptible to other visual illusions than were Europeans. This finding anticipated the work of Segall, Campbell, and Herskovits (1966). In the late 19th century the framework provided by Darwin's theory of evolution started influencing psychology and has remained influential (Campbell, 1975).

THE 20TH CENTURY

Boas (1911/1938) emphasized that ethnocentrism must be replaced with an appreciation of each culture. His students were most influential and included Sapir (1921), who formulated the Sapir–Whorf hypothesis, which I discus later; Benedict (1934/1959), who viewed cultures as integrated wholes; Mead (1928), who became famous for her studies of Samoa and New Guinea (1930), and argued that much that passes as biologically determined is in fact culturally determined (Mead, 1935); and Herskovits (1948, 1955), who was a most articulate exponent of cultural relativism. Thurnwald (1912, mentioned by Jahoda, 1993) advocated the intensive study of particular cultures, a position that later in the century was advocated by indigenous and cultural psychologists.

Bartlett (1932/1950) produced a classic work when he studied memory among the Swazi and argued that cross-cultural investigations yield important results of both theoretical and practical significance.

The mid–20th century included intensive discussions of culture and personality. However, these discussions were assessed by Bruner (1974) as "magnificent failures." This observation reflects in part the lower status of psychoanalysis in contemporary psychology, and the observation that data at the cultural and individual levels of analysis are often independent of each other (Hofstede, 1980). More recent discussion of the topic took very different directions, focusing on dimensions of cultural variation and cultural syndromes (Triandis, 1997; Triandis & Suh, 2002). It is too early to tell whether these directions will be influential.

An important influence on social psychology, in the middle of the 20th century was Kluckhohn's (1954) chapter, "Culture and Behavior," in the *Handbook of Social Psychology* and Klineberg's (1954) text, which used much cultural material. Both publications were studied with much care and quoted extensively by the cross-cultural psychologists who emerged in the 1960s and 1970s. Klineberg (1980) provided an account of why he included so much anthropological material in his social psychology text. He had become "converted" in interaction with Boas, Sapir, Benedict, and Mead.

Anthropologists have been debating for more than a century the best way to define "culture." They are still discussing this problem (Borowsky, Barth, Shweder, Rodseth, & Stolzenberg, 2001). Some define it as shared "practices" (what people do) and others, as shared "meanings." Shweder, in Borowsky et al., favored the definition by Redfield (1941): "Culture is shared understandings made manifest in act and artifact" (p. 1). Herskovits (1948, 1955), defined "culture" as the human-made part of the environment. Based on that definition, Triandis (1972) distinguished objective and subjective culture. "Objective culture" includes concrete and observable elements such as artifacts (e.g., tools, bridges), institutions and social structures. "Subjective culture" includes categorizations (language), evaluations, beliefs, attitudes, stereotypes, expectations, norms, ideals, roles, task definitions, and values. Psychological methods were proposed to study these constructs, and examples were provided with the study of stereotypes, roles, and values. The data for these studies came from Greece, India, Japan, and the United States. A recent publication influenced by this approach is that of Adamopoulos and Kashima (1999).

The 20th century has been characterized by multiple definitions of culture. Among the most interesting are the following: "Culture is to society what memory is to individuals" (Kluckhohn, 1954). It includes what "worked" in the experience of a society, so that it was worth transmitting to future generations. Sperber (1996) used the analogy of an epidemic: A useful idea (e.g., how to make a tool) is adopted by more and more people and becomes an element of culture. Barkow, Cosmides, and Tooby (1992) distinguished three kinds of culture: metaculture, evoked culture, and epidemiological culture. They argued that "psychology underlies culture and society, and biological evolution underlies psychology" (p. 635). The biology that has been common to all humans, as a species distinguishable from other species, results in a "metaculture" that corresponds to panhuman mental contents and organization. Baumeister (2005), in *The Cultural Animal*, explicitly states that he is talking about the metaculture, and is therefore not interested in cultural differences. Biology in different ecologies results in "evoked culture" (e.g., a hot climate leads to light clothing), which reflects domain-specific mechanisms triggered by local circumstances and leads to within-group similarities and between-groups differences. Sperber's (1996) conception of culture was called "epidemiological culture" by Barkow et al. (1992).

Klineberg's (1980) history of social psychology covers several topics that were important before 1960. Is thought influenced by language? The so-called Whorfian hypothesis was the focus of much interest before 1960, and a weak version of the theory has received some empirical support even recently (see review in Triandis, 1994). For example, people who have a language that does not have terms for "green" and "blue" show less differentiation among color chips that include these colors than English speakers when making multidimensional scaling judgments.

Klineberg (1980) also discussed perception and memory; the application of projective techniques; psychoanalysis; Piaget's contributions, modified by the cross-cultural work of Dasen (1972); the application of tests, the problem of national character; the study of national stereotypes, psychopathology, authoritarianism, leadership, field-dependence, acculturation, and the achievement motive.

A theme detectable across all this work is the mutual influence of anthropology and psychology. Psychological statements that are supposedly universal were challenged by anthropologists. For example, Freud's suggestion of the universality of the Oedipus complex was challenged by Malinowski (1927a, 1927b), who argued that there is among the Trobrianders a "matrilineal complex" in which boys show a repressed hatred for their mother's brother, who is the main source of discipline, authority, and executive power in that society. Statements made by anthropologists were criticized by psychologists (e.g., that they disregard individual differences within culture when they study only a few "informants" to learn about a culture).

An important achievement of early studies of the relationship between culture and psychology was the demonstration that even a basic process such as perception is influenced by culture (Segall et al., 1966). This was followed by work on the relationship between culture and cognition, such as that of Witkin and Berry (1975). During the early part of the 21st century, important work on culture and cognition was done by Nisbett (2003) and his students. Berry's work on culture and cognitive differentiation did not have much impact, because Berry became disappointed when his predictions were not supported by some data he collected in Africa, and he turned to other research topics. Cronbach and Drenth (1972) outlined how mental tests may be adapted to other cultures.

Much of the work up to 1978 or so was summarized in the first edition of the *Handbook of Cross-Cultural Psychology* (Triandis, General Editor, 1980–1981), which included volumes with coeditors on perspectives (William W. Lambert), methodology (John Berry), basic processes (Walter Lonner), developmental psychology (Alastair Heron and Elke Kroeger), social psychology (Richard Brislin), and psychopathology (Juris Draguns). A second edition of this handbook was published in 1997 in three volumes by Berry and his coeditors. Munroe, Munroe, and Whiting (1981) published the *Handbook of Cross-Cultural Human Development*.

Some discussions of culture have focused on specific elements or processes. For example, Triandis (1994) stressed shared standard operating procedures, unstated assumptions, norms, values, habits about sampling the environment, and the like. Because perception and cognition depend on the information sampled from the environment and are fundamental psychological processes, this culturally influenced sampling of information is of particular interest to psychologists. Cultures develop conventions for sampling information from the environment (Triandis, 1989), and also implicit agreements about how much to weigh the sampled elements. For example, people in hierarchical cultures are more likely to sample clues about hierarchy than clues about aesthetics.

CONTEMPORARY VIEWS

There are many definitions of *culture* (Kroeber & Kluckhohn, 1952), but almost all researchers see certain aspects as characteristics of culture. First, culture emerges in adaptive interactions between humans and environments. Second, culture consists of shared elements. Third, culture is transmitted across time periods and generations. Consider each of these aspects of culture in turn.

Humans Interact with Environments

As people interact with others in their physical and social environments, they reach agreements about how to behave together. The psyche develops through interaction with the social environment (Nisbett, 2003). Social relationships are internalized and become part of human psychology (Vygotsky, 1978, 1987). Parts of culture, such as words and tools, become internalized, and as a result the mind is shaped by culture. Thus, humans are expressions of their culture.

This view of culture as adaptive to environmental context has a long history (Jahoda, 1995). Even now (e.g., Berry, 2003), it considers that culture is both constrained and shaped by a group's habitat, leading to the use of the term *ecocultural* to describe it. People develop language, writing, tools, skills, and definitions of concepts. They determine ways of organizing information, symbols, evaluations, and patterns of behavior; intellectual, moral, and aesthetic standards; knowledge, religion, and social patterns (e.g., marriage, kinship, inheritance, social control, sports); systems of government, systems of making war; and expectations and ideas about correct behavior that are more or less effective (functional) in adapting to their ecosystem.

One way to think of cultural evolution (Boyd & Richerson, 1985) is to think of Darwinian mechanisms (Campbell, 1965); that is, people try this and that and some of what they try works, so they select it for transmission to their children and friends. Elements of culture that were effective (e.g., that resulted in satisfying solutions to everyday problems of existence), became shared and were transmitted to others (e.g., the next generation of humans).

These elements often reflect unstated assumptions and result in standard operating procedures for solving the problems of everyday life. Thus, they become aspects of culture. However, circumstances keep changing, and what was functional in one historical period (e.g., having six children when infant mortality was very high) can become dysfunctional in another. But members of cultures do not shed easily the dysfunctional elements. Thus, many elements of culture are dysfunctional (Edgerton, 1992). For instance, Friedl (1964) described a phenomenon called "lagging emulation": As lower status people acquire enough wealth, they emulate the obsolete customs of higher status people! We might argue that this is not functional, but we must remember that people may derive satisfaction even from behaviors that are no longer functional. Many of our behaviors, clothes, features of our houses, and so forth, are no longer functional.

Shared Elements

Two kinds of shared elements are important: shared practices and shared meanings.

One issue of importance in the study of culture and psychology is how to specify the limits of culture. One way of doing this is to look for shared elements. For example, do people share a language? It is also useful to consider shared time and place. People who share a language, a time period, and a geographic region are most likely to be able to interact, and to develop shared meanings (i.e., to belong to the same culture). Granted, interactions can also take place among individuals who do not share a language (e.g., via interpreters), time (e.g., reading a book written centuries earlier), or place (e.g., via satellite). But most interactions occur when people share a language, time, and place. Diffusion and acculturation are also important ways that cultures influence each other (see below). Furthermore, what has worked in one historical period is often used in other historical periods.

Common fate and other factors resulting in easy interaction among individuals can also result in the formation of cultures or subcultures. Thus, nations, occupational groups, social classes, genders, "races," religions, tribes, corporations, clubs, and social movements may become the bases of specific subcultures.

How many cultures are there? "Hundreds of thousands" is probably a correct answer. The question of the definition of the boundary of a culture has been discussed in anthropology, in which one proposal is to use a double boundary; that is, culture is delimited when people on both sides of a boundary do not understand the language spoken on the other side of the boundary (Naroll, 1971). Thus, because laypeople do not understand the language of medicine does not make medicine a separate culture, because physicians do understand the language of laypeople.

Although there are thousands of cultures, fortunately for the purpose of studying them there are similarities among different cultures. For example, Europe and North America, when viewed from a global perspective, are relatively similar; Africa South of the Sahara, South Asia, East Asia, Polynesia, and different regions of the Americas, where Native Americans can be found, have more elements of culture in common than elements that are different. Thus, anthropologists talk about "cultural regions" such as Africa South of the Sahara (Burton, Moore, Whiting, & Romney, 1996). Of course, there are thousands of cultures in Africa, yet they have some elements in common, so we can consider Africa South of the Sahara a cultural region. There is disagreement among anthropologists concerning how many cultural regions there are, but the consensus of opinion seems to be between six (Murdock et al., 1950) and 10 (Burton et al., 1996).

Even within a culture there is a tremendous variation in personalities, yet there are some things that most English people, for example, have in common, so we can call England (with a distinct language, history, food, dress, etc.) a culture that is different from, say, France or Germany.

Thus, we can conceive of a tree with its trunk comprising the metaculture (universal elements; Barkow et al., 1992), six to 10 major branches, and each branch having scores of minor branches, with the leaves represented by thousands of subcultures.

Attributes such as nationality, religion, "race," or occupation are not appropriate criteria for defining cultures. The use of a single criterion is likely to lead to confusion, as would happen if all people who eat pizza were placed in one category. Culture is a complex whole, and it is best to use many criteria to discriminate between one culture and another. Most modern states comprise many cultures; most corporations have unique subcultures; and most occupations have distinct subcultures.

Cultures are in constant flux, but the change tends to be slow. Some elements of culture do not change much. For instance, whether people drive to the right or left usually does not change. Other elements change slowly, requiring one or two generations before there is a major transformation. Still other elements change quickly. The meaning of some terms changes in years or decades rather than in centuries. For example, what was called "cool" in 1950 and in 2000 is rather different.

Transmission to Others

Cultural elements are transmitted to a variety of others, such as the next generation, coworkers, colleagues, family members, and a wide range of publics through a process of *enculturation*. A distinction has been made between three forms of cultural transmission: *vertical*, *horizontal*, and *oblique* (Berry, Poortinga, Segall, & Dasen, 2002). Vertical transmission takes place from parents to offspring, thus paralleling that of genetic forms of transmission. These two forms of transmission are usually entwined, so that their relative contributions to behavior in the second generation cannot be allocated easily. In horizontal transmission, human behavior is influenced by peers (within generations) and is more of a mutual process than is parent–child (vertical) cultural transmission. Finally, oblique transmission takes place when social institutions (e.g., schools, media) that already preexist an individual in a society influence the developing individual. These latter two forms are entirely cultural and have no genetic aspects (Berry & Triandis, 2004).

Another form of transmission takes place from outside a person's own cultural group as a result of direct contact (e.g., colonization, migration) or indirect influence (e.g., telemedia or books). This form of cultural transmission, termed "acculturation" (Chun, Balls-Organista, & Marin, 2002), is responsible for changing existing behaviors and introducing new ones. Thus, rather than providing a basis for cultural continuity (as enculturation does), acculturation serves as a cultural source of discontinuity, and even disruption in some cases (Berry & Triandis, 2004).

These considerations led to the most satisfying definition of *culture*: "Culture consists of explicit and implicit patterns of historically derived and selected ideas and their embodiment in institutions, practices, and artifacts; cultural patterns may, on one hand, be considered as products of action, and on the other as conditioning elements of further action" (Adams & Markus, 2004, p. 341).

Concepts and Methods

The post-1970 period resulted in the development of concepts and methods especially appropriate for cross-cultural and cultural psychology. Emic and etic concepts are an example. *Emics* are concepts that are unique to one culture. *Etics* are concepts that can be found in most, if not all, cultures. Pike (1967), developed these terms, inspired by the difference between phon*etics* and phon*emics* (for details, see Triandis, 1964; Berry, 1999). Some students of culture assume that every culture is unique. In some sense, every object in the world is unique. However, science is an attempt to understand the world as simply or as parsimoniously as possible. The glory of science is that very diverse phenomena can be understood by identifying the underlying similarity. For example, Newton "showed that the same force that pulls an apple to Earth keeps the Moon in its orbit and accounts for the revolutions of the then recently discovered moons of Jupiter in their orbits about that distant planet" (Sagan, 1980, p. 69).

Thus, the core issue is whether a scientist is interested in the specific (emic) elements of culture and/or the elements that are broadly shared (etic elements). In psychology this is not a simple dichotomy. There are elements of culture found only in one culture, in a cultural region, and across cultures. For example, there are cultural elements found only in one particular hunter-gathering culture, such as a tribe in the Kalahari Desert (e.g., DeVore & Konner, 1974); elements that are shared among hunters and gatherers, such as low hierarchical differentiation when there is no way to accumulate and preserve food; and elements that are common across cultures, such as collectivism or individualism (Triandis, 1995). Carpenter (2000) discovered the tendency for tight cultures to be more collectivist by correlating materials from the Human Relations Area Files across cultures.

Many of the elements of culture, such as ideas, patterns of behavior, and standards of evaluation, are specific to each culture, but they are often of limited interest. Many cross-cultural psychologists find of greater interest the common or etic elements observed in cultural patterns. But, as argued by Pike (1967), emics can be systematically related to etics. For instance, the concept of "social distance" is an etic. In all cultures people feel close to some other people and far from others (e.g., members of the same family feel close to each other and far from people on another continent). But the way that concept is expressed differs from culture to culture. In the northern United States, in 1900, the distance between whites and blacks was large, and a reliable clue of social distance was barring blacks from the neighborhood. In the 21st century, that clue is

no longer valid as a measure of social distance. Nowadays, a better clue might be rejection from a club or job discrimination. In India, the same idea is expressed by rejecting people from one's kitchen, because the concept of ritual pollution specifies that one should not allow people of a lower caste to touch one's earthenware. Thus, different emics can be used to reflect the same etic.

Methodologically, we can ask people in different cultures to tell us where a particular emic behavior is located on a social distance scale that ranges from "to marry" to "to kill." Then we can empirically obtain the scale value of the emic behavior in each culture (Triandis, 1992). That is the first step. In the second step, we study a new sample and use the previously obtained scale values for each behavior item. For example, we might present a particular social stimulus, such as "An African American physician" to people from different cultures, and ask them to indicate whether they are likely to use each of the previously scaled behaviors toward that stimulus person. The participants in each culture respond to emic behaviors of their own culture when making these judgments. But because we know the scale value of each emic behavior on the etic scale, we can compute the social distance in etic units of measurement, so we can compare the cultures. We can, for example, say that an African American physician is more acceptable in one culture than in another (Triandis, 1967, 1992).

In short, when we study cultures for their own sake we may well focus on emic elements, but when we compare cultures we have to work with the etic cultural elements.

Berry et al. (2002) outlined three theoretical orientations to the relationships between culture and psychology: *absolutism*, *relativism*, and *universalism*. The *absolutist* position assumes that human phenomena are basically the same (qualitatively) in all cultures (e.g., any personality trait found in one culture is exactly the same as that personality trait in all other cultures; any mental illness is exactly the same in all cultures). From the absolutist perspective, culture is thought to play little or no role in either the meaning or the display of human characteristics. Assessments of such characteristics are made using standard instruments (perhaps with linguistic translation), and interpretations are made easily, without taking into account alternative, culturally based views.

In sharp contrast, the *relativist* approach assumes that all human behavior is culturally patterned. It seeks to avoid ethnocentrism by trying to understand people "the way the natives see the world." Explanations of human diversity are sought from within the cultural context in which people have developed. Assessments typically employ the values and meanings that a cultural group gives to a phenomenon. Comparisons are judged to be problematic and ethnocentric, and are therefore virtually never made.

A third perspective lies between absolutism and relativism. *Universalism* assumes that basic psychological processes are common to all members of the species (i.e., constituting a set of psychological givens), and that culture influences the development and display of these processes (i.e., culture plays different variations on these underlying themes). Assessments are based on the underlying process (etics), but measures are developed in culturally meaningful versions (emics). Comparisons are made cautiously and employ a wide variety of methodological principles and safeguards (Triandis & Berry, 1980), whereas interpretations of similarities and differences take alternative, culturally based meanings into account (Berry & Triandis, 2004).

Up to the 18th century, the absolutist perspective was dominant. In the last part of the 18th century, some support for the relativist perspective emerged and became strong in the 19th century, and especially in the early 20th century. The third perspective emerged in the middle of the 20th century. Currently all three perspectives can be found, though the relativist and universalist perspectives are now dominant.

While few today advocate a strictly absolutist view, the relativist/emic position has given rise both to "indigenous psychology" (Kim & Berry, 1993; Yang, 1981), and "cultural psychology" (Shweder, 1990). An important element in one kind of cultural psychology is intensive ethnographic work; it emerged from anthropology. Another kind of cultural psychology uses experimental methods, with random assignment of participants, in more than one culture (e.g., Hong, Morris, Chiu, & Benet-Martinez, 2000). This development emerged from social and experimental psychology.

Indigenous psychology examines the meaning systems of a particular culture, with emic concepts and methods. For example, Yang (1981) examined the interplay between traditional Chinese culture and modernity in Taiwan. Most indigenous psychologists study their own culture but have been trained in the West. The goal of indigenous psychology is to convert the "folk psychological theory" of that culture into a scientific psychological theory. The methods tend to be standard psychological methods, and university students are the most common participants. Berry et al. (2002) and Berry and Kim (1993) claimed that indigenous psychologies, although valuable in their own right, serve an equally important function as useful steps on the way to achieve a universal psychology.

Some cultural psychology focuses on one culture and uses mostly ethnographic methods, such as observations, interviews, focus groups, and analyses of texts in intensive accounts of that culture. The researcher, usually from a Western culture, studies a village culture. Thus, the participants are often nonliterate members of a culture, which makes the use of most psychological methods inappropriate. This perspective is favored particularly by developmental psychologists (e.g., Greenfield, 2000; Rogoff, 1990) while examining how the culture of the parents becomes incorporated in the culture of the children. In other kinds of cultural psychology (e.g., Hong et al., 2000) participants are assigned randomly to two conditions. For example, after participants receive a prime from a collectivist or individualist culture, their responses on some individualism–collectivism scale are assessed. A typical finding is that participants from collectivist cultures give collectivist responses, but this tendency is augmented when they receive the collectivist prime; similarly, participants from individualist cultures give individualist responses, but they are more extreme when they receive an individualist prime. The important point is that participants can temporarily "change culture" when they receive the appropriate prime. This tells us that both the stimuli received from the environment and culturally shaped internally wired-in factors determine the responses.

A related issue is whether culture should be conceptualized inside or outside the person. Triandis (1980) introduced the *Handbook of Cross-Cultural Psychology* with the definition: "Cross-cultural psychology is concerned with the systematic study of behavior and experience as it occurs in different cultures, is influenced by culture, or results in changes in existing cultures" (p. 1). The first part of this definition makes explicit that culture is outside the person. In that case, culture is represented by an *index* rather than by a *process* (Greenfield, 2000). The last part of the definition suggests that people may change the culture, so that "culture and psyche make each other up" (Shweder, 1990, p. 24). Culture is now viewed as meanings embodied in cultural artifacts. Thus, it emerges when the inside meets the outside.

Up to about 1950, the dominant view in both anthropology and psychology was that culture is outside the person. At that time, culture was considered as a kind of experimental treatment (Strodtbeck, 1964). In the 1980s, many researchers started emphasizing that culture is also inside the person (Shweder & LeVine, 1984). In other words, the recent view is that the internalization of aspects of culture has influenced all psychological processes (Vygotsky, 1987); this view is held especially by "cultural psychologists" (e.g., Cole, 1996) and indigenous psychologists. Currently, those identified as "cross-cultural psychologists" accept both perspectives (e.g., Berry, 2000; Triandis, 1972, 1980, 2000).

In my opinion, the differences between cross-cultural and cultural psychology are small. There is considerable variability among the studies that can be classified as one or the other psychology. For example, both questionnaire studies and studies that use the Human Relations Area Files qualify as cross-cultural psychology. Ethnographic and experimental studies can be found in cultural psychology. But Triandis (1972) included not only a chapter on values, with data from Japan, India, Greece, and the United States, that fits the definition of cross-cultural psychology, but also a chapter that focuses on meanings in Greece (Triandis & Vassiliou, 1972), which most psychologists would consider cultural psychology.

In fact, the differences are of emphasis rather than of qualitative substance. Specifically, cross-cultural psychologists emphasize content more than context, and cultural psychologists emphasize context more than content. Cross-cultural psychologists emphasize that culture is outside the person, and cultural psychologists, that it is inside the person. But in fact it is both inside and outside.

Cross-cultural psychologists tend to study attributes of culture that do not change much over time. For instance, Bond and Smith (1996) found that conformity is high in collectivist cultures; Carpenter (2000) found that collectivist

cultures are tight; Diener, Diener, and Diener (1995) found higher levels of well-being in individualist cultures.

Cultural psychologists tend to study less stable attributes, such as meanings or conceptions, for example, how the "self" is conceived in different cultures.

Cross-cultural psychologists are more likely to use questionnaires and collect data in many cultures, whereas cultural psychologists are more likely to use intense ethnographic work or experiments and collect data in a few cultures. As a result, cross-cultural psychologists consider differences in meaning barriers to overcome with elaborate psychometric methods, whereas cultural psychologists focus their research on differences of meaning (Cole, 1996; Shweder, 1990).

Cole characterized cultural psychology by its emphasis on mediated action; its inclusion of historical, ontogenetic, and microgenetic levels of analysis; and its grounding in everyday life events. Mind emerges in the interactions of people. Individuals are active agents of their own development. Cultural psychology, according to Cole (1995) draws methodologies from the humanities, as well as from the social and biological sciences, and rejects cause–effect explanations in favor of analyses that emphasize the emergent nature of mind in activity, which requires interpretations of events that have different meanings.

There is also a difference that reflects the topics under study. Cross-cultural psychologists are often industrial/organizational or political psychologists, whereas cultural psychologists are more often developmental or social psychologists. Developmental psychologists are especially likely to study very different (e.g.. exotic) cultures, with ethnographic methods (e.g., Greenfield's work in 1990 on how children learn to weave in Zinacanteco culture), whereas organizational psychologists study highly developed cultures with psychometric instruments. For example, Huang and Van de Vliert (2004), who examined the job satisfaction of 129,087 respondents in 39 countries, found that those who had higher job status were more satisfied, but this occurred only in the individualist countries and when jobs provided individuals the opportunity to use their skills and abilities.

Each of these approaches has advantages and disadvantages (Triandis, 2000), so it seems desirable to combine the approaches, to use multimethod approaches, and to look for the convergence of findings across approaches.

Recent reviews of the literature, such as that of Lehman, Chiu, and Schaller (2004), have sections on empirical studies supporting both the cross-cultural and cultural psychology perspectives. In short, culture is both outside the person (a set of practices shared by the group, and existing prior to any particular individual) and inside the person (influencing a person's behavior by providing interpretive perspectives for making sense of reality as a result of enculturation). Indigenous and cultural psychologists favor the view that culture is inside the person, in the sense that most psychological processes are shaped by culture. They try to develop a psychology that is satisfactory for understanding a particular culture. Indigenous psychologists do this by identifying categories and linguistic elements that are more or less unique in a particular culture. For example, the Japanese concept called *amae* means something like "indulgent dependency" (Doi, 1973), one interpretation of which is "to tolerate the other person's dependence." This concept does not exist as a single word (monoleximic) in other languages. Monoleximics tell us that the idea is used frequently in a culture (Zipf, 1949), and that it is really important in that culture. The fact that there is no monoleximic term in European languages that means the equivalent of *amae* means that the concept is a Japanese emic. The judgment that *amae* is important in Japan is in agreement with expert analyses of Japanese psychology (Doi, 1986). In short, indigenous psychologists have a way of getting at the *most important ways of thinking* in a particular culture.

Cultural psychologists study most intensively a few cultures and look for the way psychological processes are influenced by culture. For example, Kitayama, Markus, Matsumoto, and Norasakkunkit (1997) generated 400 Japanese and 400 American situations, and found that the Japanese situations tend to decrease self-esteem, whereas the American situations tend to increase it. A variant of cultural psychology, ethnopsychology, looks at different theories of the mind in various ethnic groups (Lillard, 1998).

Still another issue is whether culture should be conceived as consisting of an arbitrary code or an organized configuration of elements. Culture has been discussed as both an arbitrary code (D'Andrade & Romney, 1964), and as a configuration of cultural elements organized around a theme. For instance, Triandis (1996) proposed that "cultural syndromes" can be identified, such as individualism, collectivism, verticality, horizontality, tightness (or uncertainty avoidance), and masculinity (Hofstede, 1980, 2001), in which cultural elements are interrelated so as to form coherent wholes centered around the importance of the individual, the collective, rank, equality, close observance of norms, and gender differentiation, respectively.

Triandis (1995) argued that corresponding to each cultural syndrome are personality patterns. *Idiocentrics* behave and feel like most people in individualist cultures; *allocentrics* behave and feel like most people in collectivist cultures. However, although collectivism and individualism are opposite cultural patterns, idiocentrism and allocentrism are orthogonal to each other. People in all cultures have both idiocentric and allocentric cognitions, but they use them more or less depending on the situation. Thus, when idiocentrics and allocentrics were randomly assigned to situations that were collectivist or individualist (an experimental treatment that simulated the two types of culture), the allocentrics in collectivist situations were most cooperative, whereas the idiocentrics were not cooperative, and even the allocentrics in individualist situations were not especially cooperative (Chatman & Barsade, 1995). Thus, neither personality nor situation predict behavior. Rather the interaction between two cognitions—one derived from personality shaped by culture and the other reflecting the situation—results in behavior. Furthermore, an as yet unpublished psychiatric study found that allocentric Americans and idiocentric Turks have poor mental health. Americans who are moderately idiocentric and Turks who are allocentric have good mental health. Thus, if there is a good fit between personality and culture, individuals are mentally healthy. Finally, allocentrics who spend several years in an individualist culture have very high levels of both allocentrism and idiocentrism (Yamada & Singelis, 1999).

It is also important to think of some aspects of culture as enduring even though the people who created them are no longer alive (Kroeber, 1917). Individuals come and go, but cultures remain more or less stable. For example, a behavior pattern such as driving on the left side does not change even though the people who started it are no longer alive.

Functions of Culture

Recent reviews of the literature, such as that by Lehman et al. (2004), emphasize that culture has functions such as allowing people to understand their position in the cosmos. This reminds us of Katz (1960), who identified four functions of attitudes. Cultures have parallel functions, and Katz identified four functions:

1. The *adjustment* function allows people, in the course of interaction with the environment, to maximize the rewards and minimize the penalties. Many culture theorists (e.g., Whiting, 1973/1977, 1994) have emphasized that cultures help individuals adjust to their ecology. Certainly, cultures provide norms, which furnish guidance for behavior and maximize the chances that people will receive appropriate rewards.

2. The *ego-defensive* function allows the individual to protect the self from uncomplimentary truths. Because members of all cultures are ethnocentric (discussed earlier), they compare themselves to other cultures in ways that increase their self-esteem. High self-esteem is functional because it protects individuals from becoming devastated when they are criticized.

3. The *value expressive* function allows people to derive pleasure by expressing their basic values. Values are a central element of culture (Schwartz, 1992) that function to provide guidance in life.

4. The *knowledge* function allows people to understand their position in the universe and to predict events. Religion is an aspect of culture (Tarakeshwar et al., 2003) and one of its main functions is to provide an understanding of the relationship between humans and the cosmos (Swanson, 1960). The epistemic function of culture is emphasized by Lehman et al. (2004), who reviewed empirical research supporting it.

Biology constrains the development of culture. Certain aspects of culture develop more readily, and other aspects develop with great difficulty because biology interacts with the development of culture.

Recent Examples of the Impact of the Concept of Culture on Psychology

The study of the relationship of culture and psychology in the second half of the 20th century went through four phases: (1) the culture and personality work, (2) the emphasis on universalism, (3) the emphasis on cultural syndromes, and (4) the integration of the cultural perspectives with work in mainstream psychology and the other social sciences. I comment about each of these below.

Culture and Personality

This phase occurred primarily between 1950 and 1970. Bruner (1974) called it a "magnificent failure," because one cannot measure personality out of context, then use the information to characterize a culture. He argued also that after 30 years of work on this topic, no reliable findings were widely accepted.

Universalism

This phase was observed especially in the period between 1970 and 1980. In the previous phase there was much emphasis on relativism. In this phase the stress was placed on universalism. Work by Ekman (1972) and Osgood et al. (1975) emphasized universal categories of emotion or meaning. However, Shweder and Bourne (1982) were skeptical about this kind of universalism, because it used a very high level of abstraction, so that both "God" and "ice cream" are good, potent, and active.

Cultural Syndromes

This phase had its peak in the period between 1980 and 2000. The focus was on cultural syndromes (Triandis, 1996) such as cultural complexity (Draper, 1973), tightness, and especially collectivism and individualism (Triandis, 1994, 1995). Such dimensions result in a psychological phenomenon being different in cultures with high or low incidence on a syndrome. For example, the way the "self" is defined is different when the culture is collectivist rather than individualist (Triandis, 1989). People in individualist cultures (Western Europe, United States, Canada, Australia, New Zealand) sample with high probability elements of the personal self (e.g., "I am busy," "I am kind") and internal processes (e.g., attitudes, beliefs, personality) as predictors of behavior. People from collectivist cultures (many traditional cultures, the cultures of East Asia), tend to sample mostly elements of the collective self (e.g., "My family thinks I am too busy," "My coworkers think I am kind") and aspects of the external environment (e.g., group memberships, norms, social pressures, roles) as predictors of behavior (Triandis, 1995; Triandis, McCusker, & Hui, 1990; Trafimow, Triandis, & Goto, 1991). The self has much social content in collectivist cultures (e.g., "I am an uncle," "I am a member of the communist party") and little such content in individualist cultures (e.g., "I am hardworking," "I am happy"; Triandis et al., 1990). Much research (e.g., Triandis & Suh, 2002) focuses on individualism and collectivism and the presence of an independent or relational or interdependent self (Kagitçibasi, 1996; Markus & Kitayama, 1991) having a particular form in certain kinds of culture. Other conceptions have examined culture-sensitive taxonomies of activities (Cole, 1995) or action in action-in-context (Eckensberger, 1995).

Integration of Culture and Mainstream Psychology

This phase started about 1985 and continues to the present. The main emphasis is that the fundamental principles of psychology may depend on culture. Much of the work employs experimental methods, and shows that culture modifies an important psychological process that was hitherto considered to be universal. Representative publications include those by Choi, Nisbett, and Norenzayan (1999), Cole (1995, 1996), Hong et al. (2000), Iyengar, Lepper, and Ross (1999), Kitayama and Markus (1994), Kitayama et al. (1997), Markus and Kitayama (1991), Miller (1984), Nisbett (2003), and Shweder (1990).

Overview of the Various Phases

As we look at the four-phase development of the field, a major theme has been that psychological processes are probably shared features of our species, but behavioral expression must be understood in the context of the culture in which a person develops. There are some psychological universals (Lonner, 1980), but they deal with phenomena that are at a high level of abstraction and serve as a basis for making cross-cultural comparisons. Other phenomena, at intermediate and low levels of abstraction, are more enveloped by culture, making comparisons more difficult. Thus, there are both universalistic and context-specific views of the development of cognition (Laboratory of Comparative Human Cognition, 1983), perception (Segall et al., 1966), learning (Brislin & Horvath, 1997; Tweed & Lehman, 2002), affective meaning (Osgood et al., 1975), emotion

(Kitayama & Markus, 1994; Mesquita, 2001), facial expression of emotion (Ekman, 1992), motivation (Markus & Kitayama, 1991), thinking (Nisbett, 2003), personality (e.g., McClelland, 1961; Triandis, 1997) and other basic processes (Berry, Dasen, & Saraswathi, 1997), communication (e.g., Gudykunst, 1991), and social behavior (Miller, 1984; Fiske, 1990; Berry, Segall, & Kagitçibasi, 1997). Many theoretical perspectives that include culture, such as evolutionary approaches, and the stress on indigenous psychologies (Berry, Poortinga, & Pandey, 1997) evolved after 1980. In fact, up to that point, most cross-cultural psychology was concerned with methods (Triandis & Berry, 1980). As the field matured, the multimethod approaches that developed found consistencies among ethnographic, survey, and experimental methods (e.g., Nisbett, 2003).

Much of pre-1980 psychology was shaped by the fact that the participants, the researchers, and editors of the major journals were members of Western individualistic cultures. A universal psychology requires expansion to include the perspectives found in all cultures.

Fortunately, after 1960, a number of psychologists born outside the West produced work that reflected their own cultures. Only the most prominent examples can be mentioned here. Chinese culture was represented by Cheung and Leung (1998), Ho (1996), Hui and Yee (1994), Hwang and Yang (2000), and Yang (2000), among others. India was reflected in the work of Pandey (1988), D. Sinha (1986), and J. B. P. Sinha (1980). Japan was studied by Kashima and Yamaguchi (e.g., Kashima et al., 1995), Kitayama (e.g., Kitayama & Markus, 1994), and Misumi (1985). Korea has been described by Kim (e.g., Kim & Berry, 1993), Choi (e.g., Choi et al., 1999), and Suh (2000). Mexico was studied by Diaz-Guerrero (1963, 1975, 1990). His son Diaz-Loving (1998) has been a strong proponent of an indigenous psychology. Turkey has been represented by Kagitçibasi (1990, 1996). The Philippines has been represented by Enriques (1990). Venezuela has been discussed by Salazar (1984).

Probable Fifth Phase

As the field matures there should be more cooperation between cultural and cross-cultural psychologists. As they jointly design projects, collect data with multimethod approaches, and write up their findings in joint papers, there will be a natural synthesis of the various approaches. But studies already combine the two approaches. For example, Greenfield (2000) argues that individualism–collectivism is the "deep structure" of cultural differences, and "knowing that a culture is in the individualist family tells about the overall shape and meaning of the culture; this primes you for the specifics" (p. 230). She found that collectivism allowed her to place many specifics of Zinacanteco culture into a single cultural framework. She also reports an empirical study that used both psychometric and ethnographic methods. This maybe the best example of the fifth phase.

The next phase may also include greater emphasis on religion. Religion emerges under the influence of some universal psychological mechanisms (Hinde, 1999), such as the tendency to understand the world in terms of cause–effect relationships, to learn from others, and to develop self-efficacy. Most important maybe the need to control the environment, reflected in experiments in which participants prefer strong electric shocks that they control to weak electric shocks that they do not control (Averill, 1973). Furthermore, there are universal dimensions of social behavior (Triandis, 1978): association versus dissociation, and superordination versus subordination. Most primates show social behaviors that have corresponding structures, associate with members of the band, reject those who are not members of the band from their territory, and have pecking orders. Religions provide means of associating with coreligionists and dissociating (avoiding or even fighting) from those who do not belong to the ingroup. In most cultures "good gods" are in heaven and "bad gods" are below. Finally, as Freud (1964) has pointed out, though religion is an illusion, it provides wish fulfillment—"We do not die, we go to paradise"; "We are the chosen people"; "The gods are protecting us"—that is most satisfying.

It is perhaps inevitable that the study of religion will again become an important part of cultural psychology. After all, Wundt made it central to his *Völkerpsychologie*, and we might well go back to the beginning of the field and do a better job than was done previously.

ACKNOWLEDGMENT

I am grateful for critical comments on an earlier version of this chapter by John Berry, Roy D'Andrade, Gustav Jahoda, Shinobu Kitayama, and Lee Munroe.

REFERENCES

Adamopoulos, J., & Kashima, Y. (1999). *Social psychology and cultural context*. Thousand Oaks, CA: Sage.

Adams, G., & Markus, H. (2004). Toward a conception of culture suitable for a social psychology of culture. In M. Schaller & C. S. Crandall (Eds.), *The psychological foundations of culture* (pp. 335–360). Mahwah, NJ: Erlbaum.

Averill, J. R. (1973). Personal control over aversive stimuli and its relationship to stress. *Psychological Bulletin, 80*, 286–303.

Barkow, G., Cosmides, L., & Tooby, J. (Eds.). (1992). *The adapted mind: Evolutionary psychology and the generation of culture*. New York: Oxford University Press.

Bartlett, F. C. (1950). *Remembering*. Cambridge, UK: Cambridge University Press. (Original work published 1932)

Bastian, A. (1860). *Der Mensch in der Geschichte* (Vols. I–III). Leipzig: Wigand.

Baumeister, R. (2005). *The cultural animal: Human nature, meaning, and social life*. New York: Oxford University Press.

Benedict, R. F. (1959). *Patterns of culture*. New York: Mentor. (Original work published 1934)

Berry, J. W. (1976). *Human ecology and cognitive style*. Beverly Hills, CA: Sage.

Berry, J. W. (1979). A cultural ecology of human behavior. In L. Berkowitz (Ed.), *Advances in experimental social psychology* (Vol. 12, pp. 177-207). New York: Academic Press.

Berry, J. W. (1983). Advances in historiography of psychology. In G. Eckardt & L. Sprung (Eds.), *Contributions to a history of developmental psychology* (pp. 3–23). Berlin: VEB Deutscher Verlag der Wissenschaften.

Berry, J. W. (1999). Emics and etics: A symbiotic conception. *Culture and Psychology, 5*, 165–171.

Berry, J. W. (2000). Cross-cultural psychology: A symbiosis of cultural and comparative approaches. *Asian Journal of Social Psychology, 3*, 197–205.

Berry, J. W. (2003). Origin of cross-cultural similarities and differences in human behaviour: An ecocultural perspective. In A. Toomela (Ed.), *Cultural guidance in the development of the human mind* (pp. 97–109). Westport, CT: Ablex.

Berry, J. W., Dasen, P. R., & Saraswathi, T. S. (1997). *Handbook of cross-cultural psychology* (2nd ed., Vol. 2). Boston: Allyn & Bacon.

Berry, J. W., & Kim, U. (1993). The way ahead: From indigenous psychologies to a universal psychology. In *Indigenous psychologies* (pp. 277–280). Newbury Park, CA: Sage.

Berry, J. W., Poortinga, Y. H., & Pandey, J. (1997).

Handbook of cross-cultural psychology (2nd ed., Vol. 1). Boston: Allyn & Bacon.

Berry, J. W., Poortinga, Y. H., Segall, M. H., & Dasen, P. R. (2002). *Cross-cultural psychology: Research and applications* (2nd ed.). New York: Cambridge University Press.

Berry, J. W., Segall, M. H., & Kagitçibasi, C. (1997). *Handbook of cross-cultural psychology* (2nd ed., Vol. 3). Boston: Allyn & Bacon.

Berry, J. W., & Triandis, H. C. (2004). Cross-cultural psychology: Overview. In C. Spielberger (Ed.), *Encyclopedia of applied psychology.* (Vol. 1, pp. 527–538). New York: Elsevier.

Boas, F. (1911/1938). *The mind of primitive man.* New York: Macmillan.

Bond, R., & Smith, P. B. (1996). Culture and conformity: A meta-analysis of studies using Asch's (1952b, 1956) line judgment task. *Psychological Bulletin, 119,* 111–137.

Borowsky, R., Barth, F., Shweder, R. A., Rodseth, L., & Stolzenberg, N. M. (2001). When: A conversation about culture. *American Anthropologist, 103,* 432–446.

Boyd, R., & Richerson, P. J. (1985). *Culture and the evolutionary process.* Chicago: University of Chicago Press.

Brewer, M. B., & Campbell, D. T. (1976). *Ethnocentrism and intergroup attitudes: East African evidence.* New York: Halsted/Wiley.

Brislin, R. W., & Horvath, A. M. (1997). Cross-cultural training and multicultural education. In J. W. Berry, M. H. Segall, & C. Kagitçibasi (Eds.), *Handbook of cross-cultural psychology* (2nd ed., Vol. 3, pp. 327–370). Boston: Allyn & Bacon.

Bruner, J. (1974). Concluding comments and summary of conference. In J. L. M. Dawson & W. J. Lonner (Eds.), *Readings in cross-cultural psychology* (pp. 381–391). Hong Kong: University of Hong Kong Press.

Burton, M. L., Moore, C. C., Whiting, J. W., & Romney, K. (1996). Regions based on social structure. *Current Anthropology, 37,* 87–123.

Campbell, D. T. (1965). Variation and selective retention in socio-cultural evolution. In J. R. Barringer, G. Blanksten, & R. Mack (Eds.), *Social change in developing areas* (pp. 19–49). Cambridge, MA: Schenkman.

Campbell, D. T. (1975). On the conflicts between biological and social evolution and between psychology and moral tradition. *American Psychologist, 30,* 1103–1126.

Carpenter, S. (2000). Effects of cultural tightness and collectivism on self-concept and causal attributions. *Cross-Cultural Research, 34,* 38–56.

Chatman, J. A., & Barsade, S. G. (1995). Personality, organizational culture, and cooperation: Evidence from a business simulation. *Administrative Science Quarterly, 40,* 423–443.

Cheung, F., & Leung, K. (1998). Indigenous personality measures: Chinese examples. *Journal of Cross-Cultural Psychology, 29,* 233–248.

Choi, I., Nisbett, R., & Norenzayan, A. (1999). Cultural attribution across cultures: Variation and universality. *Psychological Bulletin, 125,* 47–63.

Chun, K., Balls-Organista, P., & Marin, G. (Eds.). (2002). *Acculturation: Advances in theory, measurement and applied research.* Washington: American Psychological Association Press.

Cohen, D. (2001). Cultural variation: Considerations and implications. *Psychological Bulletin, 127,* 451–471.

Cole, M. (1995). Culture and cognitive development: From cross-cultural research to creating systems of cultural mediation. *Culture and Psychology, 1,* 25–54.

Cole, M. (1996). *Cultural psychology: A once and future discipline.* Cambridge, MA: Harvard University Press.

Cronbach, L. J., & Drenth, P. J. D. (1972). *Mental tests and cultural adaptation.* The Hague, Netherlands: Monton.

D'Andrade, R., & Romney, A. K. (1964). Summary of participants' discussion: Transcultural studies in cognition. *American Anthropologist, 66,* 230–242.

Dasen, P. R. (1972). Cross-cultural Piagetian research: A summary. *Journal of Cross-Cultural Psychology, 3,* 23–39.

DeVore, I., & Konner, M. J. (1974). Infancy in hunter-gatherer life: An ethnographic perspective. In N. F. White (Ed.), *Ethology and psychiatry* (pp. 113–141). Toronto: University of Toronto Press.

Diaz-Guerrero, R. (1963). Sociocultural premises, attitudes, and cross-cultural research. *Anuario de Psicologia, 2,* 31–45.

Diaz-Guerrero, R. (1975). *Psychology of the Mexican: Culture and personality.* Austin: University of Texas Press.

Diaz-Guerrero, R. (1990). Mexican ethnopsychology. In U. Kim & J. W. Berry (Eds.), *Indigenous psychologies: Experience and research in cultural context* (pp. 44–55). Newbury Park, CA: Sage.

Diaz-Loving, R. (1998). Contributions of Mexican ethnopsychology to the resolution of the etic–emic dilemma in personality. *Journal of Cross-Cultural Psychology, 29,* 104–118.

Diener, E., Diener, M., & Diener, C. (1995). Factors predicting the subjective well-being of nations. *Journal of Personality and Social Psychology, 69,* 851–864.

Doi, T. (1973). *The anatomy of dependence.* Tokyo: Kodansha International.

Doi, T. (1986). *The anatomy of conformity: The individual versus society.* Tokyo: Kodansha International.

Draper, P. (1973). Crowding among hunter-gatherers: The !Kung bushmen. *Science, 182,* 301–303.

Eckensberger, L. H. (1995). Activity or action: Two different roads towards an integration of culture into psychology? *Culture and Psychology, 1,* 67–80.

Edgerton, R. (1992). *Sick societies: Challenging the myth of primitive harmony.* New York: Free Press.

Ekman, P. (1972). Universals and cultural differences in facial expressions of emotions. In J. Cole (Ed.), *Ne-*

braska Symposium on Motivation (pp. 207–218). Lincoln: University of Nebraska Press.

Ekman, P. (1992). Facial expression of emotion: New findings, new questions. *Psychological Science, 3,* 34–38.

Enriques, V. G. (Ed.) (1990). *Indigenous psychologies.* Quezon City, The Philippines: Psychological Research and Training House.

Fiske, A. P. (1990). *Structures of social life: The four elementary forms of human relations.* New York: Free Press.

Freud, S. (1964). *The future of an illusion.* New York: Doubleday Anchor.

Friedl, E. (1964) Lagging emulation in post-peasant society. *American Anthropologist, 66,* 569–586.

Geertz, C. (1973). *The interpretation of cultures.* New York: Basic Books.

Greenfield, P. M. (2000). Three approaches to the psychology of culture: Where do they come from? Where can they go? *Asian Journal of Social Psychology, 3,* 223–240.

Gudykunst, W. (1991). *Bridging differences.* Newbury Park, CA: Sage.

Herder, J. G. (1969). Herder's Werke (5 vols.). Berlin: Aufbau. (Original work published 1874)

Herodotus (1966). *The histories.* New York: Norton.

Herskovits, M. J. (1948). *Man and his works.* New York: Knopf.

Herskovits, M. J. (1955). *Cultural anthropology.* New York: Knopf.

Hinde, R. A. (1999). *Why Gods persist.* London: Routledge.

Ho, D. Y. F. (1996). Filial piety and its psychological consequences. In M. H. Bond (Ed.), *Handbook of Chinese psychology* (pp. 155–165). Hong Kong: Oxford University Press.

Hofstede, G. (1980). *Culture's consequences.* Beverly Hills, CA: Sage.

Hofstede, G. (2001). *Culture's consequences* (2nd ed.). Thousand Oaks, CA: Sage.

Hong, Y., Morris, M. W., Chiu, C. Y., & Benet-Martinez, V. (2000). Multiple minds: A dynamic constructivist approach to culture and cognition. *American Psychologist, 55,* 709–720.

Huang, Y., & van de Vliert, E. (2004). Job level and national culture as joint roots of job satisfaction. *Applied Psychology: An International Review, 53,* 329–348.

Hui, C. H., & Yee, C. (1994). The shortened individualism–collectivism scale: Its relationship to demographic and work related variables. *Journal of Research in Personality, 28,* 409–424.

Hwang, K. K., & Yang, C. F. (2000). Indigenous, cultural and cross-cultural psychologies. *Asian Journal of Social Psychology, 3,* 183–293.

Iyengar, S. S., Lepper, M. R., & Ross, L. (1999). Independence from whom? Interdependence from whom? Cultural perspectives on ingroups versus outgroups. In D. A. Prentice & D. T. Miller (Eds.), *Cultural di-*

vides: Understanding and overcoming group conflict (pp. 273–301). New York: Russell Sage.

Jahoda, G. (1993). *Crossroads between culture and mind.* Cambridge, MA: Harvard University Press.

Jahoda, G. (1995). The ancestry of a model. *Culture and Psychology, 1,* 11–24.

Jahoda, G., & Krewer, R. (1997). *History of cross-cultural and cultural psychology.* In J. W. Berry, Y. H. Poortinga, & J. Pandey (Eds.), *Handbook of cross-cultural psychology* (2nd ed., pp. 1–42). Boston: Allyn & Bacon.

Kagitçibasi, C. (1990). Family and socialization in cross-cultural perspective: A model of change. In J. Berman (Ed.), *Nebraska Symposium on Motivation* (pp. 135–200). Lincoln: University of Nebraska Press.

Kagitçibasi, C. (1996). *Family and human development across cultures: A view from the other side.* Hillsdale, NJ: Erlbaum.

Kashima, Y., Yamaguchi, S., Kim, U., Choi, S. C., Gelfand, M., & Yuki, M. (1995). Culture, gender, and self: A perspective from individualism-collectivism research. *Journal of Personality and Social Psychology, 69,* 925–937.

Katz, D. (1960). The functional approach to the study of attitudes. *Public Opinion Quarterly, 24,* 163–204.

Kim, U., & Berry, J. W. (Eds.). (1993). *Indigenous psychologies: Research and experience in cultural context.* Newbury Park, CA: Sage.

Kitayama, S., & Markus, H. R. (Eds.). (1994). *Emotion and culture: Empirical studies of mutual influence.* Washington, DC: American Psychological Association.

Kitayama, S., Markus, H. R., Matsumoto, H., & Norasakkunkit, V. (1997). Individual and collective processes in the construction of the self: Self-enhancement in the United States and self-criticism in Japan. *Journal of Personality and Social Psychology, 72,* 1245–1267.

Klineberg, O. (1954). *Social psychology* (2nd ed.). New York: Holt, Rinehart & Winston.

Klineberg, O. (1980). Historical perspectives: Cross-cultural psychology before 1960. In H. C. Triandis & W. W. Lambert (Eds.), *Handbook of cross-cultural psychology* (Vol. 1, pp. 31–68). Boston: Allyn & Bacon.

Kluckhohn, K. (1954). Culture and behavior. In G. Lindzey (Ed.), *Handbook of social psychology* (Vol. 2, pp. 921–976). Cambridge, MA: Addison-Wesley.

Kroeber, A. L. (1917). *Zuni kin and clan.* New York: Trustees.

Kroeber, A. L., & Kluckhohn, C. (1952). *Culture: A critical review of concepts and definitions.* Cambridge, MA: Peabody Museum.

Laboratory of Comparative Human Cognition. (1983). Culture and cognitive development. In P. H. Mussen (Ed.), *Handbook of child psychology* (Vol. 1, 4th ed., pp. 295–356). New York: Wiley.

Lazarus, M., & Steinthal, H. (1860). Einleitende

Gedanaken über Völkerpsychologie, als Einladung für Völkerpsychologie und Sprachwissenschaft. *Zeitschrift für Völkerpsychologie und Sprachwissenschaft*, *1*, 1–73.

Lehman, D. R., Ciu, C., & Schaller, M. (2004). Psychology and culture. *Annual Review of Psychology*, *55*, 689–714.

Lillard, A. (1998). Ethnopsychologies: Cultural variations in theories of mind. *Psychological Bulletin*, *123*, 3–32.

Lonner, W. J. (1980). The search for psychological universals. In H. C. Triandis & W. W. Lambert (Eds.), *Handbook of cross-cultural psychology* (Vol. 1, pp. 143–204). Boston: Allyn & Bacon.

Malinowski, B. (1927a). *Sex and repression in savage society*. London: Routledge & Kegan Paul.

Malinowski, B. (1927b). *The father in primitive psychology*. New York: Norton.

Markus, H., & Kitayama, S. (1991). Culture and self: Implications for cognition, emotion and motivation. *Psychological Review*, *98*, 224–253.

McClelland, D. C. (1961). *The achieving society*. Princeton, NJ: Van Nostrand.

Mead, M. (1928). *Coming of age in Samoa*. New York: Morrow.

Mead, M. (1930).*Coming of age in New Guinea*. New York: Morrow.

Mead, M. (1935). *Sex and temperament in three primitive societies*. New York: Morrow.

Mesquita, B. (2001). Emotions in collectivist and individualist contexts. *Journal of Personality and Social Psychology*, *80*, 68–74.

Miller, J. G. (1984). Culture and the development of everyday social explanation. *Journal of Personality and Social Psychology*, *46*, 961–978.

Minturn, L., & Lambert, W. W. (1964). *Mothers of six cultures*. New York: Wiley.

Misumi, J. (1985). *The behavioral science of leadership*. Ann Arbor: University of Michigan Press.

Munroe, R. H., Munroe, R. L., & Whiting, B. B. (Eds.). (1981). *Handbook of cross-cultural human development*. New York: Garland STPM Press.

Murdock, G. P., Ford, C. S., Hudson, A. E., Kennedy, R., Simmons, L. W., & Whiting, J. W. M. (1950). *Outline of cultural materials* (3rd ed., rev.). New Haven, CT: Human Relations Area Files.

Naroll, R. (1971). The double language boundary in cross-cultural surveys. *Behavioral Science Notes*, *6*, 95–102.

Naroll, R., Michik, G. L., & Naroll, F. (1980). Holocultural research methods. In H. C. Triandis & J. W. Berry (Eds.), *Handbook of cross-cultural psychology* (Vol. 2, pp. 479–521). Boston: Allyn & Bacon.

Nisbett, R. (2003). *The geography of thought*. New York: Free Press.

Osgood, C. E., May, W., & Miron, M. (1975). *Cross-cultural universals of affective meaning*. Urbana: University of Illinois Press.

Pandey, J. (Ed.). (1988). *Psychology in India: State of the art*. New Delhi: Sage.

Pike, K. L. (1967). *Language in relation to a unified theory of the structure of human behavior*. The Hague: Mouton.

Pritchard, J. C. (1843/1848). *The natural history of man* (3rd ed.). London: Baillière.

Redfield, R. (1941). *The folk culture of the Yucatan*. Chicago: University of Chicago Press.

Rivers, W. H. R. (1901). Primitive color vision. *Popular Science Monthly*, *59*, 44–58.

Rivers, W. H. R. (1905). Observations on the senses of the Todas. *British Journal of Psychology*, *1*, 321–396.

Rogoff, B. (1990). *Apprenticeship in thinking: Cognitive development in social context*. New York: Oxford University Press.

Sagan, C. (1980). *Cosmos*. New York: Random House.

Salazar, J. M. (1984). The use and impact of psychology in Venezuela. *International Journal of Psychology*, *19*, 113–122.

Sapir, E. (1921). *Language*. New York: Harcourt Brace.

Schwartz, S. H. (1992). Universals in the content and structure of values: Theoretical advances and empirical tests in 20 countries. In M. Zanna (Ed.), *Advances in experimental social psychology* (Vol. 25, pp. 1–66). New York: Academic Press.

Segall, M. H., Campbell, D. T., & Herskovits, M. J. (1966). *Influence of culture on visual perception*. Indianapolis, IN: Bobbs-Merrill.

Shweder, R. A. (1990). Cultural psychology—what is it? In J. W. Stigler, R. A. Shweder, & G. Herdt (Eds.), *Cultural psychology* (pp. 1–46). Cambridge, UK: Cambridge University Press.

Shweder, R. A., & Bourne, E. J. (1982). Does the concept of person vary cross-culturally? In A. J. Marsella & G. M. White (Eds.), *Cultural conceptions of mental health and therapy* (pp. 97–137). London: Reidel.

Shweder, R. A., & LeVine, R. A. (1984). *Culture theory*. Cambridge, UK: Cambridge University Press.

Sinha, D. (1986). *Psychology in a Third World country: The Indian experience*. New Delhi: Sage.

Sinha, J. B. P. (1980). *The nurturant leader*. New Delhi: Concept.

Sperber, D. (1996). *Explaining culture: A naturalistic approach*. Oxford, UK: Blackwell.

Steinthal, H. (1858). *Der Ursprung der Spache* [The origins of language]. Berlin: Dümmler.

Strodtbeck, F. (1964). Considerations of meta-method in cross-cultural studies. *American Anthropologist*, *66*, 223–229.

Suh, E. M. (2000). Self, the hyphen between culture and subjective well-being. In E. Diener & E. M. Suh (Eds.), *Culture and subjective well-being* (pp. 63–87). Cambridge, MA: MIT Press.

Swanson, G. E. (1960). *The birth of Gods: The origin of primitive beliefs*. Ann Arbor: University of Michigan Press.

Tarakeshwar, N., Stanton, J., & Pargament, K. I. (2003). Religion: An overlooked dimension of cross-cultural psychology. *Journal of Cross-Cultural Psychology, 34,* 377–394.

Thucydides. (1934). *The complete writings of Thucydides.* New York: Modern Library.

Trafimow, D., Triandis, H. C., & Goto, S. (1991). Some tests of the distinction between private self and collective self. *Journal of Personality and Social Psychology, 60,* 640–655.

Triandis, H. C. (1964). Cultural influences upon cognitive processes. In L. Berkowitz (Ed.), *Advances in experimental social psychology* (pp. 1–48). New York: Academic Press.

Triandis, H. C. (1967). Towards an analysis of the components of interpersonal attitudes. In C. Sherif & M. Sherif (Eds.), *Attitudes, ego involvement and change (pp. 227–270). New York: Wiley.*

Triandis, H. C. (1972). *The analysis of subjective culture.* New York: Wiley.

Triandis, H. C. (1978). Some universals of social behavior. *Personality and Social Psychology Bulletin, 4,* 1–16.

Triandis, H. C. (1980). Introduction. In H. C. Triandis & W. W. Lambert (Eds.), *Handbook of cross-cultural psychology* (Vol. 1, pp. 1–14). Boston: Allyn & Bacon.

Triandis, H. C. (1989). The self and social behavior in different cultural contexts. *Psychological Review, 96,* 269–289.

Triandis, H. C. (1990). Theoretical concepts of use to practitioners. In R. Brislin (Ed.), *Cross-cultural applied psychology* (pp. 34–55). Thousand Oaks, CA: Sage.

Triandis, H. C. (1992). Cross-cultural research in cultural psychology. In D. Granberg & G. Sarup (Eds.), *Social judgment and intergroup relations: Essays in honor of Muzafer Sherif* (pp. 229–244). New York: Springer-Verlag.

Triandis, H. C. (1994). *Culture and social behavior.* New York: McGraw-Hill.

Triandis, H. C. (1995). *Individualism and collectivism.* Boulder, CO: Westview Press.

Triandis, H. C. (1996). The psychological measurement of cultural syndromes. *American Psychologist, 51,* 407–415.

Triandis, H. C. (1997). Cross-cultural perspectives on personality. In R. Hogan, J. Johnson, & S. Briggs (Eds.), *Handbook of personality psychology* (pp. 440–465). San Diego: Academic Press.

Triandis, H. C. (2000). Dialectics between cultural and cross-cultural psychology. *Asian Journal of Social Psychology, 3,* 185–195.

Triandis, H. C. (2006). *Simple self-deceptions in everyday life.* Manuscript in preparation.

Triandis, H. C., & Lambert, W. W. (Eds.). (1980). *Handbook of cross-cultural psychology* (Vol. 1). Boston: Allyn & Bacon.

Triandis, H. C., McCusker, C., & Hui, C. H. (1990).

Multimethod probes of individualism and collectivism. *Journal of Personality and Social Psychology, 59,* 1006–1020.

Triandis, H. C., & Suh, E. M. (2002). Cultural influences on personality. *Annual Review of Psychology, 53,* 133–160.

Triandis, H. C., & Vassiliou, V. (1972). A comparative analysis of subjective culture. In H. C. Triandis (Ed.), *The analysis of subjective culture* (pp. 299–338). New York: Wiley.

Tweed, R. G., & Lehman, D. R. (2002). Learning considered within a cultural context. *American Psychologist, 57,* 89–99.

Tylor, E. B. (1871). *Primitive culture.* New York: Harper.

Tylor, E. B. (1889). On a method of investigating the development of institutions. *Journal of the Royal Anthropological Institute of Great Britain and Ireland, 18,* 245–272.

Vico, G. (1970). *The new science* (T. G. Bergin & M. H. Fish, Trans.). Ithaca, NY: Cornell University Press. (Original work published 1744)

von Humbolt, W. (1969). *Schriften zur Sprachphilosophie* [Writings on the philosophy of language]. Berlin: Dümmler. (Original work published 1820)

Vygotsky, L. S. (1978). *Mind in society.* Cambridge, MA: Harvard University Press.

Vygotsky L. S. (1987). *The collected works of L. S. Vygotsky* (R. W. Rieber & A. S. Carton, Eds.). New York: Plenum Press.

Waitz, T. (1863). *Introduction to anthropology.* London: Anthropological Society. (Original work published 1859)

Whiting, J. W. M. (1973, November 29). *A model for psychological research.* Distinguished lecture to the American Anthropological Association, New York. Reproduced (1994) as Chapter 3 in E. H. Chasdi (Ed.), *Culture and human development* (pp. 89–101). New York: Cambridge University Press.

Witkin, H. A., & Berry, J. W. (1975). Psychological differentiation in cross-cultural perspective. *Journal of Cross-Cultural Psychology, 6,* 4–87.

Wundt, W. (1900–1914). *Völkerpsychologie.* Leipzig: Engelmann.

Yamada, A., & Singelis, T. (1999). Biculturalism and self-construal. *International Journal of Intercultural Relations, 23,* 697–709.

Yang, K. S. (1981). Social orientation and international modernity among Chinese students in Taiwan. *Journal of Social Psychology, 113,* 159–170.

Yang, K. S. (2000). Monocultural and cross-cultural indigenous approaches. *Asian Journal of Social Psychology, 3,* 241–263.

Zipf, G. K. (1949). *Human behavior and the principle of least effort.* Cambridge, MA: Addison-Wesley.

CHAPTER 4

Evolutionary Foundations of Cultural Psychology

MELVIN KONNER

In the 1980s and 1990s, with considerable enthusiasm, some psychologists announced that they had discovered culture. Influenced explicitly by the psychologist Lev Vygotsky, who had a brief but brilliant career in the Soviet Union in the 1920s and 1930s, they held that culture pervades every aspect of mind—that mind is in its essence "dialogic"—and that it is foolish to try to understand cognition without recognizing that it is cultural, as it were, "all the way down." The developmental psychologists among them traced their basic theoretical stance to the year that Vygotsky's (1962) work was published in English. Anthropologists were puzzled, because this stance in its essence was part of the bedrock of our discipline, and had been written about and taught for almost a century.

For example, E. B. Tylor, in the first sentence of his 1871 book *Primitive Culture*, strongly hinted at the concept when he wrote, "Culture . . . taken in its wide ethnographic sense, is that complex whole which included knowledge, belief, art, morals, law, custom, and any other capabilities and habits acquired by man as a member of society" (p. 1). By 1934, when Ruth Benedict wrote her classic *Patterns of Culture*, it was firmly established that

the life history of the individual is first and foremost an accommodation to the patterns and standards traditionally handed down in his community. From the moment of his birth the customs into which he is born shape his experience and behavior. By the time he can talk, he is a little creature of his culture, and by the time he is grown and able to take part in its activities, its habits are his habits, its beliefs his beliefs, its impossibilities his impossibilities. (Benedict, 1934, pp. 3–4)

And Alfred Kroeber, in the 1948 edition of his textbook, the model for all subsequent ones, wrote, "The mass of learned and transmitted motor reactions, habits, techniques, ideas, and values—is what constitutes *culture*" (p. 8; italics in original).

Of course, Vygotsky and his intellectual descendants added much to these generalizations: Concepts such as self-directed (private), then internalized speech, intersubjectivity, scaffolding, and the zone of proximal development served important functions in analyzing the role of the social and cultural context in mental development (Fernyhough, 1997; Wertsch & Sohmer, 1995). These psychological concepts have had great value in specifying more clearly some of the processes of what anthropologists call "socialization" and "enculturation." Furthermore, cultural psychology (and not just the developmental kind) came along at the right moment in the history of anthropology. Many cultural anthropologists, including many psychological anthropologists, were smitten by postmodernism, which led some to reject the entire enterprise of the scientific study of culture (Greenfield, 2000). Psychological anthropology stumbled, and the banner of scientific method was largely dropped, just when continued adoption of psychological methods could have had the greatest impact. So it is fortunate that cultural psychology picked up the banner by applying standardized and sophisticated methods cross-culturally.

However, anthropologists have also always recognized that some features of human behavior and culture are universal, have definable evolutionary origins, and may be tied to biology. Other features, although not universal across all cultures, are characteristic of human groups that subsist by hunting and gathering. This means that they may have been needed in the human environment of evolutionary adaptedness, and even though other cultures have departed from them in the course of history, there may be costs to these divergences that are presently unknown. This model, known as "the discordance hypothesis," posits that in the long course of human evolution our genome formed in response to certain external conditions, and that departures from these conditions may in some cases have been too rapid and extensive for our genes to have responded; thus, there may be a discordance between our current environment and our genes, the latter being not much changed since the hunting-gathering era.

This model has proved very fruitful in evolutionary medicine, which holds that changes in diet, physical activity, and exposure to microbes and parasites have left us with widespread chronic diseases that were uncommon in our remote ancestors (atherosclerosis, diabetes, and asthma, among others). Although it is more speculative to cite changes in social and cultural aspects of the environment as grist for this mill, it is possible that these nonphysical aspects of our ancestral environment have left us with behavioral and psychological characteristics that are not perfectly adapted to current environments.

For example, attention-deficit/hyperactivity disorder (or at least the diagnosis of it) has become endemic in the United States, and we know that it most often comes to light as poor adaptation to school. Some of the features of the disorder, at least in its milder forms, were probably innocuous or even adaptive in our ancestral environments, and although extreme forms of the disorder would be maladaptive anywhere, it is fairly clear that the line between normal and abnormal would be drawn in a different place in a hunter–gatherer culture. Another example might be the consequences of social isolation, which is rare in hunter-gatherer cultures but more common in industrial cultures. Could this change have implications for the prevalence of mood or anxiety disorders? This domain of questions about adaptation and cultural change, and the corresponding approach to human behavior, is the primary subject of this chapter.

SOME RELEVANT HISTORY

The transformation of anthropology during the late 20th century included an increasing focus on large-scale and developed societies, a new emphasis on hearing the voices of the people being studied, recognition of variation within cultures, and an increasingly sophisticated application of quantitative methods (D'Andrade, 1991, 1992, 2001)—even as postmodernist theory has raised questions (sometimes valid, sometimes very exaggerated) about the distortions that such "objectification" of culture and behavior may produce.

Recent decades have also led to a new emphasis on biology as a window on human behavior and culture, not as a strategy for explaining differences among human groups (it cannot) but as an aid to finding common ground among them. As both Alfred L. Kroeber and Margaret Mead, great pioneers in cultural anthropology, recognized by the 1950s, the delineation of cross-cultural variety also inevitably reveals *invariant* features of human behavior and mental life. This proved to be a prescient observation, because the description of universals of language, culture, facial expression, parent–offspring interaction, and many other aspects of human life would soon become possible (D. E. Brown, 1991). These universals constitute a part of what is meant by "human nature," a term that must be considered again, after decades of disfavor, as having scientific legitimacy (Konner, 2002).

A brief historical review may be useful. In the late 19th century it was not unusual for treatises on aspects of human psychology to refer to ethnographic data. Darwin's seminal book (1998) on the expression of emotion cited the occurrence of certain expressions in primitive societies as evidence for their biological basis and attempted to relate them to emotional expressions in nonhuman animals in an evolutionary sequence. Edward Westermarck, whose theory of incest aversion has survived modern tests (Wolf, 1995), appealed to ethnographic evidence to illuminate a deeper psychodynamic process he considered to be as universal as certain facial expressions. In the late 19th century it was common for prominent anthropologists to attempt to array nonindustrial societies in an evolutionary sequence, whether of social complexity, religion, or language. And in the early years of the 20th century ethnological expeditions tested members of small-scale, nonindustrial societies for the presence of proposed perceptual universals.

These trends, which might be seen as early efforts to characterize human nature and its origins, were transformed by the development of modern social and cultural anthropology and by the parallel emergence of psychoanalysis. Anthropologists came to reject evolutionary sequencing of cultures, replacing this effort with descriptive characterization of cultures as independent units. Proposed universals of human behavior or mental function were met with equal skepticism, and anthropologists to this day delight in the opportunity to say, "Not among my people they don't," a kind of statement that has been aptly called the anthropological veto.

Early generalizations by Piaget and others were tested cross-culturally (Mead, 1932), but none elicited the sort of enthusiasm for such testing as psychoanalysis. The British social anthropologist Bronislaw Malinowski attempted to demolish the universality of the Oedipus complex by describing a separation of male authority (vested in the mother's brother) from the object of male jealousy (the biological father) in "his" society in the Trobriand Islands (an argument persistently debated; Malinowski, 1964; Spiro, 1982). With the skeptical encouragement of Franz Boas, the dean of American cultural anthropology, disciples such as Margaret Mead attempted not only to undermine certain psychoanalytic convictions by means of cross-cultural comparison

(Mead, 1935, 1949) but also to use psychoanalytic and other psychodynamic theory to *explain* culture (Kardiner & Linton, 1939, 1945).

The fundamental theorem of this school was that cultures are distinctive because of distinctive patterns of child rearing, and that a unified approach combining psychoanalysis and cultural anthropology could explain culture and elucidate laws of psychological development simultaneously (LeVine, 2001; Spindler, 1979). During World War II this approach reached its height with speculations about the "national character" of Russians, Japanese, Germans, and Americans, relating them to unscientific observations of infant and child care. Freud's method, difficult at best when applied to a single patient studied for hundreds of hours over several years, was thus adopted for a completely distinct task for which it was clearly not intended.

By the 1950s the approach had generated research that to some extent transcended it through refinement and measurement. Both the assessment of adult psychological disposition and the objective description of child training were made quantitative, the first through projective testing and the second through direct behavior observation, with interview methods supporting both approaches. DuBois (1944) and Wallace (1952) showed through projective testing and interviews that even small-scale, seemingly homogeneous cultures do not have something properly called basic personality (an entity corresponding to the "national character" of large-scale societies). Rather, individual variation in personality and character is great in every known culture, however small-scale or "primitive." At best there is perhaps a "modal personality" shared by a substantial minority of a culture's members (as shown by Wallace for two distinctive Native American groups), and in any case a culture must derive its distinctiveness from the particular mutual articulation of its various personality types, and the opportunities it provides for their expression, rather than from fundamental tendencies shared by a majority—a sort of symphony orchestra model of culture and personality, in which each culture provides a series of scores.

Meanwhile, John Whiting and Beatrice Whiting were trying to place the cross-cultural study of child training on a scientific foundation. A landmark study by John Whiting and Irvin Child (1953) demonstrated that aspects of childhood experience of interest to psychoanalysts are correlated with certain themes in religion, folklore, and other cultural expressions (which they pointedly called "projective systems") in a large cross-cultural sample. However, they recognized that such correlations might not imply causality and that childhood experience needed to be measured much more rigorously. The Whitings devoted the next three decades to such measurement in a number of societies around the world and developed a model of the influence of fundamental features of society—such as ecology, economy, and vulnerability to external attack—on child training practices, which in turn might give rise to certain consistent adult predispositions (B. B. Whiting & Edwards, 1988; B. B. Whiting & Whiting, 1975; J. W. M. Whiting, Child, & Lambert, 1966). But it was rarely possible to establish such relationships beyond the level of correlations.

In addition to the Whitings' work, that of LeVine, Melford Spiro, and others helped bring this strand of psychological anthropology into maturity in terms of both theory and methods (LeVine, 1982, 1998; LeVine et al., 1994; Spindler, 1979; Spiro, 1987, 1999). Overall, the psychological processes of interest to these anthropologists have been those suggested by psychodynamic or personality theory, such as parental behavior, childhood relationships, sex differences, aggression, and nurturance, and they sometimes used cross-cultural studies to challenge prevailing wisdom about these dimensions of behavior (Spiro, 1954, 1979, 1982). It was also sometimes friendly to the overall project of elucidating human nature through the study of cross-cultural differences and similarities in psychological processes (Schlegel & Barry, 1991; Spiro, 1987, 1999).

A parallel development relevant to cross-cultural psychology was the attempt to study systematically the incidence of psychiatric disorders cross-culturally (Murphy, 1976, 1981). This effort was useful but was beset by doubts about the cross-cultural validity of diagnostic categories. Recent attempts to rationalize diagnostic categories at the international and even national level reveal similar obstacles to cross-cultural diagnosis (Summerfield, 2002). Nevertheless three still-valid conclusions emerged from this work.

First, both the general category of psychological deviance and at least several distinct syndromes (depression, bipolar disorder, anxiety spectrum disorders, and schizophrenia) are characteristic of all cultures in which they have been sought (Kleinman, 2003; Murphy, 1976, 1994). These core disorders appear in the face of marked variation in social organization, religious beliefs, gender relations, child-rearing methods, and even of some genetic variation, and appear to be part of the human condition.

Second, although the traditional designation "culture-bound syndrome" is often too strong, some psychiatric disorders in one way or another do appear to be relatively culture-specific. This includes *susto* in Latin America, *amok* in Indonesia, *hikikomori* (social withdrawal) in Japan, *dhat* (semen "loss") in India, and bulimia (and, to some extent, attention-deficit/hyperactivity disorder) in the United States (Chowdhury, 1996; Keel & Klump, 2003; Levine & Gaw, 1995; Perme, Ranjith, Mohan, & Chandrasekaran, 2005; Sakamoto, Martin, Kumano, Kuboki, & Al-Adawi, 2005; Weller et al., 2002; Westermeyer, 1985). Cultural differences in where the line is drawn between normal and abnormal and between different syndromes may be thought of as "soft" manifestations of the cultural specificity of illnesses. Even if some of the "culture-bound" syndromes are mainly different ways of conceptualizing parts of a cross-culturally universal symptom spectrum, such differences in labeling may be very significant because of the interactive process between symptoms and cognition that plays a role in all mental illness.

Third, given the diagnostic challenges, it is extremely difficult to compare incidence or prevalence of most disorders cross-culturally, much less to draw conclusions about the etiology of hypothesized cross-cultural differences in prevalence. This is particularly true in the developing world, where differential mortality can delete many victims of illness before the survey is done, and in small-scale societies of classic anthropological interest, where the number of individuals suffering any serious mental illness would be expected to be small.

Finally, a separate strand of the psychological approach to culture began rather ignobly, with an attempt to characterize what early 20th-century anthropologists called "the primitive mind." There was also a belief among psychologists that some contemporary human cultures represented earlier levels of mental functioning, corresponding to alleged earlier stages of mental evolution (Werner, 1948). There was no evidence, but barriers of language and cultural differences prevented some psychologists from appreciating the quality and level of mental functioning in nonindustrial cultures. Actual studies of "primitive" language and thought revealed it to be complex and sophisticated (Lévi-Strauss, 1962; Shore, 1996). There is no evidence that different human groups have evolved at different rates, or that any are at earlier stages of physical or mental evolution. In fact, because of the flow of genes among human populations around the world, there has been little opportunity for different human groups to evolve separately (Mayr, 1963; Cavalli-Sforza, Menozzi, & Piazza, 1994). But it took sophisticated methods of cross-cultural cognitive study to establish the complexity of "primitive" thought.

So, two inferences about culture and mind emerged from early 20th century anthropology: First, there is no evolutionary sequence of thought from traditional to modern cultures; second, some basic patterns of human cognition and its development are universal. In addition to universals of language, Franz Boas, Claude Lévi-Strauss, and others posited a psychic unity of the human species and attempted to unveil some of its features. To take one example, Lévi-Strauss (1962) identified a universal dualistic or polarizing tendency in human thought, already studied by Robert Hertz (1960) in the early 20th century and subsequently well demonstrated from ethnological materials subsequently (Almagor, 1989). Dichotomies such as right–left, good–evil, black–white, village–bush, cultured–savage, and us–them typically exaggerate contrasts in what is really a continuum, and this tendency is so widespread cross-culturally as to suggest that a distaste for ambiguity may be inherent in human thought. In the realm of the social, it has been shown experimentally that children and adults embrace the "us against them" dichotomy all too readily (Robinson & Tajfel, 1997; Sherif, Harvey, White, Hood, & Sherif, 1961; Tajfel, 1982)

The late 20th century brought many further changes, both within anthropology and in the emerging field of cultural psychology. Although some cultural anthropologists drifted out of the stream of science, finding their affinities with "postmodern" literary criticism and philosophy (Greenfield, 2000), others became increasingly quantitative, scientific, and to some extent biological (Betzig, 1997; D'Andrade, 1995; Harris, 1968, 1979; John-

son & Earle, 1987; Plattner, 1989; Shore, 1996; Spiro, 1987, 1999). The four subfields of traditional American anthropology—cultural anthropology, archaeology, linguistics, and biological anthropology—became for many anthropologists reunified in an enterprise that had been moribund since the late 19th century: the characterization of human nature, its cultural variety, and its evolutionary origins.

This enterprise advanced on at least eight fronts: (1) the adoption, extension, and testing of evolutionary theory, including applications to behavior; (2) the characterization of human origins in an ever-improving fossil record; (3) the systematic description and analysis of the behavior of nonhuman primates, to test evolutionary theory and to make inferences about the behavior of our ancestors; (4) the study of contemporary and recent hunter–gatherer cultures, with a view toward making inferences about behavior and social organization in the varied environments of human evolutionary adaptedness; (5) the rise of scientific archeology, which reconstructs the demographic and social worlds of past societies; (6) the corresponding attempt by cultural anthropologists to understand ecological influences on contemporary nonindustrial societies; (7) the ongoing documentation of the spectrum of cultural variation; and (8) the characterization of cross-cultural universals of language, nonverbal behavior, and culture.

A very ambitious intellectual program of this kind was proposed by Wilson (1998) in his book *Consilience*, the title of which refers to the merging of different disciplines in a seamless fabric of human understanding. But anthropology, which is inherently interdisciplinary, has a century-long head start on this project. Some cultural anthropologists remain aloof from this unified enterprise, but they admit to being aloof from science as a whole. The many anthropologists who work within it are laying the foundations of a science of human nature (Betzig, 1997; Konner, 2002; Shore, 1996; Sperber, 1996; Spiro, 1987, 1999), whether or not they use the term explicitly, the results of which have proved to be of great and increasing interest to psychology (Barkow, Cosmides, & Tooby, 1992; Buss, 1984, 1989; Cosmides & Tooby, 2000; Crawford & Krebs, 1998; Tooby & Cosmides, 2000).

Cultural psychology, despite its appropriate focus on variation, cannot proceed much further without a deeper understanding of the evolutionary origins, biological underpinnings, and cross-cultural constants that form the context for this variation. Paradoxically, evolutionary principles are even relevant to the cultural variation itself, not because of cross-population genetic differences, which are minimal, but because some of the cultural variation is canalized by underlying norms of reaction that ensure, or at least promote, adaptation in each of the varieties. Applications of this concept, also called facultative adaptation, to human development have already proved fruitful (Belsky, 1997, 1999; Belsky, Steinberg, & Draper, 1991; Chisholm, 1993; Chisholm, 1999; Hrdy, 1992, 1999).

BIOLOGICAL AND BEHAVIORAL EVOLUTION

The fossil evidence for human evolution has accumulated steadily for 150 years and no one familiar with it doubts the reality and continuity of that evolution. The first specimen recognized as a separate species, a Classic Neandertal, was discovered in 1856; human-related (hominid) fossils have accumulated at an accelerating rate, and now there are thousands, covering a period of 6 million years. But new discoveries each year change the details of the picture; biochemical taxonomy and, in the last few years, direct taxonomy of genomes have added new dimensions. Controversies remain. It is clear, for example, that the bonobo (*Pan paniscus*) and the common chimpanzee (*Pan troglodytes*) are our closest relatives—each shares more than 98% of our gene sequences—but the behavior of these two species differs markedly, although their estimated time of divergence from each other (1–2 million years ago) is much more recent than that of the human from the ape line (6–8 mya). Chimpanzees are very aggressive, and males markedly dominate females, whereas highly sexual bonobo females assert their relative equality by means of strong coalitions that limit male violence (de Waal, 1989; Wrangham, 1993).

It is also clear that there were more contemporaneous species of hominid than we thought a generation ago, but it is not yet known just how many there were (Wood, 2000; Wood & Richmond, 2000). And it is clear that upright posture was established before most of human brain evolution took place, but the lag between the two, and the role of tool using or tool-

making in brain evolution, remain controversial (Ambrose, 2001). For our purposes, there is no need to resolve these debates, but there is much to be gained from understanding (1) the general higher primate background of human evolution; (2) the environment of human evolutionary adaptedness, that of hunting and gathering; and (3) the principles of evolutionary adaptation as applied to behavior and reproduction. Some propositions in these three categories of knowledge are likely to be relatively insensitive to disruption by future discoveries.

THE HIGHER PRIMATE BACKGROUND

All higher primates (monkeys, apes, and humans) are social animals with great learning capacity, and with the mother–offspring bond at the center of social life (Smuts, Cheney, Seyfarth, Wrangham, & Struhsaker, 1987; Strier, 2000). This bond is prolonged compared with that of most mammals, as are the anatomical and behavioral courses of development, including the lifespan as a whole (Martin, 1990, 1995). Laboratory and field studies demonstrate complex social cognition and social learning, including transmission of social rank, tool using techniques, and knowledge of location of food sources. Play, especially social play, is characteristic of all primate species, particularly during development, and is an important opportunity for learning. The higher primate emphasis on both the mother–infant bond and on play is an intensification of the pattern established by early mammals, and is essential to the understanding of the phylogeny of the limbic system and the emotions (MacLean, 1985, 1993).

Primate groups include a core of genetically related individuals with associated nonrelatives. In most instances, especially among the Old World monkeys more closely related to us, that core is matrilineal, stable over the life course of individuals; but in a few species, including our very close relative the common chimpanzee, the core is patrilineal, and the females are unrelated migrants—although here, too, our equally close relative the bonobo takes the matrilineal tack (Strier, 1994). Acts of social support, mutual defense, and generosity are directed preferentially toward genetic relatives (Altmann et al., 1996; Kurland, 1977), and individuals recognize their relatives from an early age and have a complex cognitive understanding of their relationships (H. Gouzoules & Gouzoules, 1990; S. Gouzoules & Gouzoules, 1987). Despite this bias, monkeys and apes do aid nonrelatives and often receive reciprocal aid in return. Cooperation is ubiquitous, but so is competition, and one of the major purposes of cooperation is mutual defense against members of the same species. Conflict is frequent, with both sexes participating, but with males generally exhibiting more aggression than females (Hrdy, 1981; Wrangham & Peterson, 1996), including sometimes substantial aggression *against* females (Smuts & Smuts, 1993).

Beyond these broad generalizations great variation exists in social organization between and within species. Monogamy is found, although variably, in some South American monkeys and in gibbons, but larger group associations that subsume more temporary associations between individual males and individual females are the rule in most species. Despite orangutans' (*Pongo pygmaeus*) relatively close genetic relationship to humans, the usual social grouping is a lone female with her offspring, living separately from solitary males. In chimpanzees and some New World monkey species, females change groups after puberty, whereas in most others, males change groups, which is a very dangerous process and therefore an opportunity for natural selection. The causes of this variation in higher primate social organization remain uncertain.

Some generalizations may also be made about the nature and social context of individual development among monkeys and apes. Because the New World monkeys separated from the Old World Monkeys and the apes between 40 and 25 mya, some of these generalizations do not apply to all New World monkeys. However, they do approximate the course of development in all the *catarrhines*, a category that subsumes all Old World higher primates, including monkeys, apes, and—with modifications to the developmental pattern—humans. (The rationale for including humans is proposed in the next section.) The *catarrhine* mother–infant complex (Table 4.1) is characterized by a hemochorial placenta, with exceptionally intimate maternal–fetal circulation; singleton birth, with rare and usually unsuccessful twinning; 24-hour physical contact, mainly with the mother, for at least the first few

TABLE 4.1. The Catarrhine Mother–Infant Complex

1. Hemochorial placenta
2. Singleton birth
3. Twenty-four-hour physical contact in first weeks
4. Twenty-four-hour proximity until weaning
5. Nursing more than three times per hour while awake
6. Night nursing until weaning
7. Weaning at around 30% of the age of first ovarian cycles
8. Transition to multiage play group
9. Variable but low adult male care
10. Separation from mother → protest, then dejection
11. Isolation rearing → dysfunctional behavior

weeks; staying within a few feet of the mother continuously until weaning; frequent nursing, at least three times per hour, throughout the waking hours; waking to nurse at least once a night for most of the nursing period; late weaning, at around 25–30% of the age at first estrus or menses; gradual transition to a multiage play group; and variable but low involvement of adult males in most species.

In addition, although there are species variations, it may be said that higher primates are generally sensitive to significant perturbations of the early social environment. Mother–infant separations result in protest by the infant, sometimes lasting days, followed by dejection or grief, although in some species, removing the infant from the mother can be much less distressing than removing the mother (Hinde & Davies, 1972a, 1972b; Rosenblum & Kaufman, 1968). More serious and prolonged interventions, such isolation rearing or repeated, involuntary mother–infant separation, give rise to abnormalities of sexual, maternal, and aggressive behavior that in humans would be viewed as psychopathology (Suomi, 1997, 1999). Furthermore, the extended, direct mother–infant physical contact characteristic of these species may be important to the formation of the relationship (Maestripieri, 2001).

In a number of species, isolation rearing gives rise to stereotyped behavior such as rocking and self-directed aggression, and even deprivation of contact with peers during development has produced abnormal behavior in some experiments. Apparent human analogues of these causal relationships, although difficult to interpret, have encouraged the use of primate models. These primate experiments greatly enhance the interpretive value of field studies of higher primate behavior and emphasize the extent to which the normal development of behavior in such animals has come to depend, in the course of evolution, on an intact social matrix.

Natural variation in stable, individual behavior patterns corresponding to personality or temperament occurs in free-ranging monkey and ape groups, and extends to variants that would be considered pathological if seen in humans, such as hyperaggressive, isolative, phobic, or depressed behavior. It is rarely possible to explore the etiology of such variants, but most cannot result from specific abnormalities of social rearing such as the ones deliberately instituted in laboratory experiments. They are probably both genetic and environmental in etiology, and recent research has found an important interaction; rhesus monkeys carrying the short allele of the gene for the serotonin transporter are vulnerable to being reared with peers but without mothers, whereas individuals carrying the long allele show no evident behavioral abnormalities after being reared in this condition (C. S. Barr et al., 2004), a phenomenon with a remarkable parallel in humans (Caspi et al., 2003). (This set of studies comprises the first clear demonstration at the molecular level of the kind of genotype–environment interaction that many psychologists have long proposed.) Some reactions, such as severe depression, as in the case of an 8-year-old wild chimpanzee after the death of its mother, may be incompatible with survival (Goodall, 1986). Others, however, such as hyperaggressiveness (as in the case of two female chimpanzees that systematically and repeatedly killed the infants of other females) may actually enhance reproductive adaptation for the abnormal individual. This theoretical possibility is discussed in greater detail below.

HUNTER–GATHERER ADAPTATIONS

The previous generalizations apply to the social and psychological world of Old World higher primate species for a period of 25 to 40 million years. Against this background, hominids evolved during the last few million years, culminating in the emergence of our species within the last few hundred thousand years, and finally in the appearance of truly modern *Homo*

sapiens about 100,000 years ago (Ambrose, 2001; Cavalli-Sforza & Feldman, 2003).

In the mid-20th century, anthropologists became interested in modeling the circumstances in which our species evolved by reference to studies of extant hunter–gatherers (Lee & DeVore, 1968a). Such studies attempted to document their subsistence ecology and social organization during the limited time in which they were likely to resist modernization. Classical studies included those of Australian aborigines, Eskimo, Amazonian hunter-gatherers such as the Siriono, and many others on all continents (Lee & DeVore, 1968a). More systematic, multidisciplinary, quantitative studies were subsequently done on the Hadza of Tanzania (Hawkes, 1991; Hurtado, Hawkes, Hill, & Kaplan, 1985), the Aché of Paraguay (Hill & Hurtado, 1999), the Agta of the Philippines (Griffin & Estioko-Griffin, 1985), the Efe Pygmies of Zaire (Bailey, 1991; Peacock, 1991), and the Bushmen of South Africa (Lee, 1979; Silberbauer, 1981), among others (Lee & Daly, 1999). These populations have been viewed as representing the environment of evolutionary adaptedness (EEA), although given the variation among them and among the past populations they may represent, the phrase should be pluralized to *environments* of evolutionary adaptedness, or EEAs. The phrase implies that this was the range of contexts for which natural selection prepared us, and from which we have departed only in the past 10,000 years, a very short time in evolutionary terms. (The Industrial Revolution, in the same terms, began just a minute ago.) No one claims that the whole spectrum of EEAs is observable among recent hunter–gatherers, who have occupied only some of the wide range of ecological situations available to our ancestors. However, we also have extensive archaeological, paleodemographic, and paleopathological evidence (Keenleyside, 1998; Reinhard, Fink, & Skiles, 2003) that—with the studies of recent hunter–gatherers—leads to reasonable models of life during human evolution (Kelly, 1995; Winterhalder & Smith, 1981).

From many studies of recent and current hunter–gatherers, combined with archeological evidence of those of the distant past, certain generalizations are possible:

1. Groups were usually small, ranging in size from 15 to 40 people related through blood

or marriage (but could be larger in ecologically rich settings).

2. They were usually nomadic, moving with changing subsistence opportunities, and flexible in composition, size, and adaptive strategies, although they could be sedentary in richer settings.

3. Daily life involved physical challenge, vigorous exercise, and occasional hunger, but with a usually dependable food base from a moderate work effort (less than in most agricultural societies), and with a marked division of labor by gender.

4. Disease, mainly infectious and acute rather than chronic and degenerative, produced high rates of mortality especially in infancy and early childhood, with consequent frequent experience of loss.

5. Almost all of their life activities occurred in a highly social context with people they knew well—often the same people for different activities.

6. Privacy was limited, but creative expression in the arts was frequently possible.

7. Conflicts and problems were dealt with through extensive group discussions, but these did not always work, in which event conflict could escalate to assault and even to homicide.

These generalizations describe the contexts in which almost all of human evolution and history have occurred, so it is often said that we are, in effect, hunter–gatherers in skyscrapers.

However, the environments of evolutionary adaptedness were variable. In some times and places, especially in the last stages of human evolution, populations were larger, denser, and more sedentary (Kelly, 1995). These would probably have afforded the opportunity for social stratification and division of labor, along the lines of the cultures of the Native Americans of the Northwest Coast (Kwakiutl, Tlingit, and others). Such cultures, although based on hunting (including fishing) and gathering, would have prefigured the kinds of social and political arrangements that became common after the advent of agriculture.

In the more basic cultures of human foragers and in some of the more complex ones, whether in the fossil or the ethnographic record, hunting was of major importance. Most of the stone tools that have survived archaeologically were used in hunting or butchering,

and the demands caused by this activity have long been held to be central to the emergence of human intelligence and social organization (Lee & DeVore, 1968b; Stanford, 2002). Some stone used for this purpose had to be traded over long distances, implying unexpectedly complex social networks among our ancestors 2 million years ago. Furthermore, even chimpanzees share meat after a kill (but not plant foods), and among human hunter–gatherers, following elaborate regulations for such sharing of meat may have been a life-and-death matter. Finally, with one important exception (the Agta of the Philippines, where women routinely hunted) all hunting and gathering societies in the ethnographic record had a division of labor by sex, with men doing almost all the hunting and providing meat for women and children, and women providing most of the plant foods. For these reasons, among others, it is believed that some peculiarly human aspects of social life are due to the advent of hunting but were grafted onto an already complex social life characteristic of nonhuman higher primates.

However, this is at most half of the story (Dahlberg, 1981). In many hunting and gathering societies, plant foods gathered by women constituted much more than half of the diet. Plant foods were shared in these societies (although not beyond the immediate family), whereas they were not shared in nonhuman primates. Postweaning mortality is much higher in nonhuman primate juveniles than in human children, and it has been suggested that the provision of children with plant foods by human mothers accounts for this difference (Lancaster & Lancaster, 1983) and that the long postreproductive life of human mothers is what allowed not only this process but the so-called "grandmother effect," in which postmenopausal women serve the same function for their grandchildren (Hawkes, O'Connell, & Jones, 2003; Hawkes, O'Connell, Jones, Alvarez, & Charnov, 1998). Even the early advent of upright posture may have had more to do with women's need to carry plant foods, as well as infants, to a base camp than with any advantage upright posture conferred in hunting, and it may be that among the first tools invented were digging sticks and carrying devices for plants or infants—tools that, however crucial, would not be preserved in archaeological assemblages and would most likely have been invented by women (Tanner, 1987; Zihlman, 1981).

Baby and child care were also distinctive in such societies (Konner, 2005) although there were significant variations (Blurton Jones, 1993; Griffin & Estioko-Griffin, 1985; Hewlett, 1991; Marlowe, 2005; Tronick, Morelli, & Ivey, 1992) and included the following: (1) frequent breast-feeding (up to four times an hour); (2) late weaning (at least age 2, and up to age 4); (3) close mother–infant contact, including extensive skin-to-skin carrying and adjacent sleeping until weaning; (4) prompt response to infant crying and indulgent response to other infant and child demands; (5) the opportunity for maternal primacy in attachment; (6) more father involvement than in most societies; (7) a gradual transition from an intense mother–infant bond to a multiage mixed-sex play group; (8) usually less assignment of responsibility in the sense of chores or formal education in middle childhood, with learning taking place through observation and play; (9) liberal premarital sexual mores compared with non-hunter–gatherers, with sex play in middle childhood gradually giving rise to adolescent sexuality; (10) late menarche, limiting opportunities for childbearing until the late teens or early 20s. These generalizations about hunter–gatherer infancy and childhood have withstood the test of time and of excellent new research in at least five hunter–gatherer societies (Konner, 2005).

Humans, like Old World monkeys and apes, are catarrhines, but they can only be included in the catarrhine mother–infant complex if the mother–infant relationship in the human EEAs conforms to it, because departures are very evident in other ecological settings. The question of whether the mother–infant relationship in the EEAs can be subsumed under the general catarrhine model hinges in turn on the validity of the hunter–gatherer childhood (HGC) model already discussed. Unlike the catarrhine mother–infant complex (CMIC), this model goes substantially beyond infancy. Table 4.2 lists the main features of the HGC model as originally proposed (for references, see Konner, 2005).

Each feature of the model was originally derived from observations of the !Kung, supported by descriptive accounts of other hunter–gatherers in the older ethnographic literature. The generalizations were presented as hypotheses for further study, in the hope that others

TABLE 4.2. Features of !Kung Infancy and Childhood: The First HGC Model

1. Prolonged close physical contact with the mother
2. High indulgence of dependent needs and demands
3. Frequent nursing (four times per hour) throughout waking hours
4. Mother and infant sleep on same bed or mat; night nursing
5. Weaning after age 3 and 4-year birth spacing[a]
6. Strong separation and stranger protest until late ages[b]
7. Dense social context that seems to reduce pressure on mother
8. Nonmaternal care much less than maternal care until second year[a]
9. Paternal care much less than maternal care, but more than in most cultures
10. Transition to multiage, mixed-gender child play group
11. Minimal childhood responsibility for subsistence or baby care[a]
12. Minimal restrictions on childhood or adolescent sexuality

[a] An important challenge comes from new research.
[b] There is too little information in other studies to generalize.

would do serious HGC research. This hope was realized, and subsequent studies have been excellent.

New quantitative studies have focused on infancy and childhood in at least five hunter–gatherer cultures: the Hadza, the Efe, the Aka, the Aché, and the Agta. Each of these groups has been described as departing in one way or another from the HGC model as originally presented based on studies of the !Kung and reviews of older literature on other hunter–gatherers (Konner, 1981). We can now place these departures in context with a systematic comparison.

Table 4.3 (Konner, 2005) shows the findings of recent studies regarding key features of the HGC model, suggesting a high level of support for most of the original generalizations: frequent nursing, mother–infant cosleeping, high physical contact, high overall indulgence (possibly excepting the Hadza), substantial to high nonmaternal care and father involvement, maternal primacy, transition to a multiage child group, a relatively carefree childhood (except the Hadza), low restriction of premarital sex, and strong adolescent initiation rites. Only the Aka match the !Kung in age at weaning and

TABLE 4.3. The HGC Model in Six Cultures

	Frequent nursing	Weaning age/interbirth interval (mo)	Sleeping with mother	Physical contact, all	Overall indulgence	Nonmaternal care	Father involvement	Maternal primacy	Multiage child group	Carefree childhood	Premarital sex
!Kung	+++	42/48	+++	+++	+++	++	++	+++	+++	+++	+++
Hadza	+++	30/38	+++	+++	+	++	++	++	+++	+	+++
Efe	+++	30/38	++	+++	+++	+++	+	++	++	++	++
Aka	+++	42/48	+++	+++	+++	+++	+++	++	+++	++	++
Aché	+++	25/37	+++	+++	++	+	++	+++	+++	+++	+++
Agta	+++	27/36	+++	+++	+++	++	+	+++	+++	+	+++

Note. From published data and descriptions supplemented by personal communications. +, present; ++, strongly present; +++, very strongly present. For explanation and references, see text and Konner (2005).

interbirth interval, but the other three cultures have weaning ages over 2 years and interbirth intervals over 3 years. This is at the upper end of the range for nonindustrial cultures and sustains the generalization that hunter–gatherers have relatively late weaning and long birth spacing.

However, the HGC model does represent an important departure from the CMIC. Two- or even 3-year birth spacing is not 25–30% of the age at female sexual maturity, which in hunter–gatherer societies (and most other traditional cultures) is about age 16. The great apes may in fact depart in the other direction from the basic catarrhine pattern, nursing until age 4 or 5, with a female age at sexual maturity of 9. The shortening of the length of nursing is one of the key changes in human evolution, making possible more rapid population growth; it is in turn made possible by the practice of postweaning provisioning, unknown in other primates (Hawkes et al., 1998; Lancaster & Lancaster, 1983). In hunter–gatherers, as in nonhuman carnivores, meat is offered to children after or even before weaning. However, human hunter–gatherers also provide children with plant foods appropriately prepared as weaning foods; despite the long and solicitous mother–offspring relationships that occur in all catarrhines, providing the young with food occurs only in humans.

To place these generalizations in a broader phylogenetic context, the care of infants and juveniles in Old World monkeys and apes (in contrast to that of human hunter-gatherers) is characterized by not only (proportionately) somewhat later weaning age and interbirth interval but also by variable and species-specific importance of nonmaternal care, minimal father involvement except in gibbons, the absence of postweaning provisioning (the basis of a relatively carefree childhood), mixed-sex play groups that may be same-age groups in seasonal breeders, and the absence of initiation rites. But other HGC features *are* present in most higher primates, including frequent nursing, late weaning, mother–infant cosleeping, high overall indulgence, maternal primacy, and adolescent sexuality. The wide distribution of these features in monkeys and apes suggests that they are common features of the catarrhines and may have been present in the common ancestor, which lived between 30 and 40 million years ago (Martin, 1990).

However, although it is not strictly a part of child rearing, the great majority of hunter-gatherer children experienced loss and grief through the death of siblings, parents, or other loved ones, and many had life-threatening illnesses themselves. Largely because of morbidity and mortality, the hunter–gatherer pattern of childhood experience was far from idyllic, although frustration and loss came mainly from inadvertent features of the environment rather than from parentally imposed stresses. Still, physical punishment and ridicule were occasionally used by parents among the !Kung (Shostak, 1981), children were required to forage for themselves among the Hadza (Blurton Jones, 1993), and the experience of loss was virtually universal.

As for the outcome of these child care practices, we cannot infer causality, but the limits of any protective effect are suggested by the fact that both major and minor mental illnesses were present in such societies, and that all of them experienced some level of violent conflict up to and including homicide, which may have exceeded levels in American cities in some groups (Lee, 1979). Normal human behaviors usually considered undesirable, such as selfishness, deceit, adolescent rebellion, adultery, desertion, and child abuse, occurred in such societies, although it is impossible to compare the rates of such behaviors to those in large-scale industrial states. Although fluid and flexible in many ways, life in such societies was restricted to a much smaller number of people than in our own, and the lack of privacy and inability to get away from those people could have been stressful, just as crowding and high levels of contact with strangers may be stressful for us. (Relationship problems tended to be everybody's business, discussed at length around the fire at night, and it may not be far from the truth to consider much of the Paleolithic—at least after the evolution of language—one interminable encounter group.) And, of course, the stresses of morbidity and mortality, as well as the stresses and uncertainties of the daily food quest, must have taken their toll. It is possible that the very common generalized anxiety disorders of our present world are the evolutionary legacy of a world in which mild, recurring fear was adaptive (Nesse & Lloyd, 1992).

War was rare or unknown in hunter–gatherers in recent generations, although ambushes did occur, and deadly intervillage raids are described in some historical material. Conflicts were often resolved by the sharing of food and other goods, and by talking well into the night, sometimes for weeks on end. Few social or economic distinctions were known, nor could they be maintained, because the ethic of sharing strongly pressured a person to part with any accumulated wealth as soon as such wealth became visible (Wiessner, 1982, 1996). Stinginess was in general a serious offense, punished by social ostracism; in cultures where mutual aid is central to survival, no one can suffer ostracism for long. However, ample evidence suggests that in times and places where the food base was rich enough to allow higher population densities (e.g., the cultures of the northwestern United States and western Canada), economic distinctions and social stratification did emerge.

CROSS-CULTURAL UNIVERSALS OF HUMAN BEHAVIOR, MIND, AND CULTURE

We have considered what may be distinctive about psychological aspects of culture among recent hunter–gatherers, with a view toward establishing a baseline of adaptations characteristic of our species in its environments of evolutionary adaptedness. Although these features are arguably more "natural" than those in other cultural adaptations, and departures from them could conceivably have interesting psychological consequences, they do not have the more privileged status of cross-cultural universals, which are more likely to reflect underlying biological tendencies. Although the main enterprise of cultural anthropology in general and of psychological anthropology in particular, as well as of cultural psychology, has been the description and analysis of cross-cultural variation, that enterprise has always had an inevitable, if tacit, complement: characterizing features of human behavior that vary relatively little or not at all.

The concept of universals has, however, at least five different meanings: (1) behaviors, such as coordinated bipedal walking or smiling in some social greetings, that are exhibited by all normal members of every known society; (2) behaviors that are universal within an age or sex class, such as the Moro reflex in all normal neonates or the muscle contraction patterns of orgasm in all postpubertal males; (3) central tendencies that apply to all populations but not all individuals, such as the sex difference in physical aggressiveness; (4) universal features of culture rather than of behavior, such as taboos against incest and homicide, the variable but always present institution of marriage, or the social construction of illness and attempts at healing; and (5) characteristics that, although unusual or even rare, are found at some level in every population, such as homicidal violence, thought disorder, depression, suicide, or incest.

The list of characteristics that fill these five categories is a very long one, much longer than the prominent anthropologists of the early heyday of cross-cultural study might have predicted. It includes remarkable constancies in not only nonverbal communication (Eibl-Eibesfeldt, 1971, 1989) and its interpretation (Ekman et al., 1987; Ekman & Rosenberg, 1997), and the semantic domains of words used to describe basic emotions (Heider, 1991), but also in social arrangements and many features of culture (D. E. Brown, 1991). The search for societies that have no violence, no gender differences that go beyond childbearing, or no mental illness, or that lack basic skills, such as making and using effective tools and fire, has been a vain one. Although there is convincing documentation of variation in the incidence or context of expression of most human behaviors, the existence of such a large core of constantly present, if variable, features constitutes a demonstration of the reality of human nature and its validity as a scientific construct. These universals are fundamental to the nature of our species in a deeper way than the features found in human hunter–gatherers and from which later forms of society departed; universals are found in all societies regardless of environment or subsistence ecology, and thus may be intrinsic to human nature.

Traditional cultural anthropologists frequently have shown little or no interest in such universals, viewing them as trivial or outside their subject matter, but the elucidation of universal features of human behavior and culture is increasingly being recognized as a central task of the discipline, and one likely to enhance the study of cultural variation. Some cultural anthropologists—most prominently Claude Lévi-Strauss—have attempted to delineate such universals as symbol systems and mental structures whose common underlying characteristics link widely disparate surface manifestations in art, language, and ritual (Lévi-Strauss, 1962, 1963; Shore, 1996). This intellectual strategy owes much to that of comparative linguists, who have found a variety of common functional features of all languages that transcend their specific manifestations (C. H. Brown & Witkowski, 1981; Chomsky, 1988; Comrie, 1989).

A model of the role of phylogeny and its consequences for human nature in the generation of cross-cultural differences is shown in Figure 4.1. It is based on a model presented by B. B. Whiting and J. W. M. Whiting (1975), which did not include an explicit role for phylogeny but did recognize a universal course of psychological development at the center of the psychocultural dynamic. It also gave a privileged place to the ecological situation of cultures in shaping their psychosocial realities;

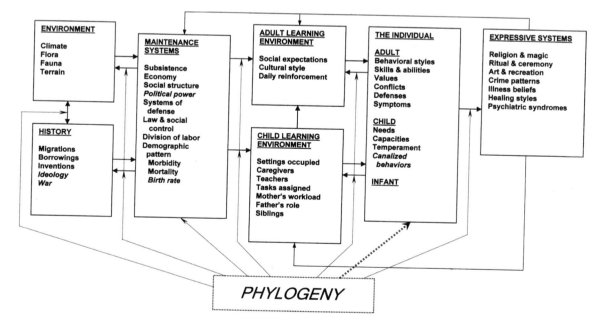

FIGURE 4.1. A model of the influence of phylogeny on psychocultural adaptations. Modified from Whiting and Whiting (1975). Substantive additions are italicized.

that is, it took what anthropologists would call both a materialist and a functionalist position, arguing that people and cultures must adapt to ecological circumstances in historical context, and that cultural psychology is best understood as an adaptation or consequence of other adaptations. In this model, history and culture are not driven by ideas; rather, ideas emerge as part of human responses to situations and needs. However, this modified version of the model does contain more feedback than the Whiting model, which relied almost entirely on unidirectional causal flow.

The modified version suggests that describing universal features of human behavior is central to understanding the effects of phylogeny, which are shown in dotted lines in the diagram. Phylogeny is shown directly to affect one of the boxes, that representing the individual— not only the "innate needs, capacities, and temperament" but also the relatively fixed elements of cognitive and psychosocial development. But most phylogenetic effects on the system are modeled as occurring through evolution's influence on other arrows; that is, natural selection operating on organisms ancestral to ourselves created not only individuals with certain needs, capacities, temperaments, and canalized maturational plans, but also equations—if . . . then . . . statements—relating the environment to the social system, the social system to the individual, and so on. These are the facultative adaptations familiar to evolutionary biologists that set limits on plasticity by guiding the organism's responses to environmental variation: plasticity, yes, but canalized plasticity.

Referring again to the example of husband–wife intimacy (J. W. M. Whiting & Whiting, 1975), phylogeny appears to have given us a system such that separating men from women and small children enhances men's effectiveness as warriors. This is not to say that men must be warriors or that they must be aloof from their wives, but that choosing aloofness may increase effective belligerency, and/or that the reverse may be true. The universal feature here is not a phenotypic characteristic, but an underlying mechanism relating two phenotypic continuums to each other. This example (irrespective of its empirical validity) clearly shows that a Darwinian explanation of a social adaptation is fully compatible with a psychological explanation of its development, the latter serving as the means to achieve the adaptation in

our long-lived, slowly growing, highly cultural species. In recent years Darwinian theory has been extended to encompass this possibility, in which a particular causal relationship between childhood experience and adult behavior *is* the adaptation (Belsky, 1997, 1999; Belsky et al., 1991; Chisholm, 1993, 1999; Hrdy, 1992, 1999).

In the past few decades the application of neo-Darwinian or sociobiological theory to ethnological materials has produced some findings that at first glance seem to bypass complex questions of the relationships among society, culture, and individual development (for a helpful critique, see Symons, 1992). For example, societies in which young men inherit land from their mothers' brothers are more lax about the control of women's sexuality than are those in which young men inherit from their fathers (Hartung, 1982); in societies that allow polygyny, wealthier men tend to have more wives, the extreme being despots with as many as hundreds (Betzig, 1986, 1992); and in small-scale societies in which adoption of children is common, it tends to follow patterns predicted by genetic relatedness (Silk, 1980, 1987). Investigators making these findings usually do not claim any direct genetic basis for these variations in human cultural practices; indeed, some of the most unfortunate confusion stems from a failure to appreciate this distinction between the propositions of neo-Darwinian theory and those of behavioral genetics.

Even in a nonhuman species such as the red-winged blackbird, males singing on richer territories mate with several females instead of one. But the mechanism of this flexible adaptive system—an example of facultative adaptation—may be quite different in blackbirds than that of the functionally parallel flexibility in human beings. The wings of insects come from thorax, the wings of birds from forearm structures, the wings of bats from fingers, and the wings of humans from technology. These four solutions to the adaptive challenge of flight serve similar functions with extremely different points of origin. The same will prove to be true of subtler adaptations in social behavior.

For example, evolutionary psychologists (like classical evolutionists and geneticists before them) predicted that incest would be avoided in most sexually reproducing species to prevent maladaptive homozygous recessive conditions. But adults seeking mates must recognize close kin. In insects, and in some vertebrates, such recognition depends on pheromones (L. Greenberg, 1979; Manning, Wakeland, & Potts, 1992), but the unlikelihood of that mechanism in humans has led to a search for other ontogenetic explanations. The anthropologist Arthur Wolf, motivated more by psychological than evolutionary considerations, has shown conclusively that in traditional China, where young girls sometimes live with the families of their intended spouses (also still children), the resulting marriages had a much higher rate of failure and infertility than did other arranged marriages, and has also identified a sensitive period of contact required for the effect (Wolf, 1995). Similar findings emerge from studies of the marriage rate among Israeli kibbutz cohort members (Shepher, 1971).

These studies support the "familiarity breeds contempt" hypothesis of incest, first introduced by Edward Westermarck in the 19th century. The implication is that human beings achieve inbreeding avoidance through a psychological mechanism partly dependent on cultural choice, even though the evolutionary effects (the adaptation) may ultimately be functionally equivalent to those in species that rely on pheromones for their own incest avoidance. In analyses such as these, the purposes and methods of cultural anthropology, cultural psychology, and evolutionary psychology are joined, and the study of human behavior in general is much better served than it is by sterile debates about nature and nurture.

UNIVERSALS AND VARIATIONS IN PSYCHOSOCIAL GROWTH

Freud postulated, and present-day psychodynamic psychology continues to accept in altered and disputed forms, a universal sequence of emotional development upon which the social dynamic of the family was said to produce enduring emotional traits. Beyond some very general elements—the formation of an attachment to a primary caregiver who is usually the mother, for example, or the ubiquity of conflicts and jealousies within the family—this hypothesized universal sequence has found little empirical support. But cross-cultural studies of human behavioral and psychological development have produced extensive evidence supporting some different, more empirically

grounded proposed universals of psychosocial growth. In the absence of knowledge of neuropsychological development, psychoanalytic theory postulated a crude libidinal theory of neural development. Now, the growing body of knowledge of neural and neuroendocrine development can begin to serve a parallel function in relation to the more empirically supported, newer studies of psychosocial growth.

Among the well-established cross-cultural universals of psychosocial development, the following are the best supported and can in most cases be plausibly related to possible underlying neural or neuroendocrine maturation:

1. The emergence of sociality, as heralded by social smiling and mutual gaze, between 2 and 4 months of age, in parallel with the maturation of basal ganglia and cortical motor circuits (Konner, 1991; Yakovlev & Lecours, 1967).

2. The emergence of strong attachments, as well as of fears of separation and of strangers, in the second half of the first year of life (van IJzendoorn & Sagi, 1999), in parallel with the maturation of the major fiber tracts of the limbic system (Konner, 1991; van IJzendoorn & Sagi, 1999).

3. The emergence of language during and after the second year (Bates & Marchman, 1987), in parallel with the maturation of the thalamic projection to the auditory cortex, among other circuits (Lecours, 1975).

4. The emergence of a sex difference in physical aggressiveness in early and middle childhood, with boys on average exceeding girls (Maccoby, 1998; B. B. Whiting & Edwards, 1988), a consequence in part of prenatal androgenization of the hypothalamus (Collaer & Hines, 1995).

5. Growth beyond the emotional lability of early childhood in the 5- to 7-year shift, with its major cognitive advances including advanced perspective taking, concrete operations, and metacognition, enabling years of complex enculturation (Rogoff, Sellers, Pirrotta, Fox, & White, 1975; White, 1970, 1996), a transition that may be due to the peak of both synapse number and brain metabolic rate in this age range.

6. The onset of adult sexual motivation and functioning in adolescence (Schlegel & Barry, 1991), in parallel with and following the maturation of the hypothalamic–

pituitary–gonadal axis at puberty (Ebling, 2005; Halpern, Udry, & Suchindran, 1997, 1998), against the background of the prenatal androgenization of the hypothalamus, as well as continuing maturation of brain white matter (Paus et al., 2001).

There are other likely cross-cultural developmental universals, such as the rise and fall of distress crying over the first 3 months (R. G. Barr, 1990; R. G. Barr, Konner, Bakeman, & Adamson, 1991), increased babbling in the second half of the first year (Locke, 1989), the attainment of the false-belief task at approximately age 4 (Callaghan et al., 2005), and progress through the first three or perhaps four of the six stages in Lawrence Kohlberg's scheme of moral development in childhood (Edwards, 1981). But these are neither as well established nor as plausibly related to underlying maturational events as are the six universals proposed earlier. Although their underlying neurobiology is at an early stage of elucidation, their cross-cultural universality is well established, and there is in each case extensive experimental evidence to support the maturational nature of the process in behavioral development. Thus they constitute a first approximation of the true structural basis of psychosocial development.

They also constitute a basis for future understanding of how variations in social experience interact with maturing psychosocial competence to produce potentially stable variations. In each of the six processes mentioned, cross-cultural differentiation of the maturing competence begins almost as soon as the maturation occurs, or even during the maturation process itself. In some cases there is sufficient evidence to state provisional rules relating environment to differentiation, for example, "Infants whose smiles are favorably responded to will smile more" or "All children will acquire languages with similar cognitive and social functions, but with whatever arbitrary semantic content is presented, and with much less arbitrary variation in syntactic features." In others, such as the differentiation of the strength, duration, and multiplicity or exclusiveness of attachment in different cultures, it has been difficult to demonstrate causal relationships to the characteristics of the social and emotional world that preceded the attachment. Thus, some important developmental events and trends remain refractory to explanation, whether biological,

psychological, or cultural. However, the acceptance and increasingly detailed and reliable description of the maturational constants underlying cultural variations in psychosocial growth will provide a steadily firmer place on which to stand while attempting to grasp the role of cultural and individual experience.

NEO-DARWINIAN THEORY OF BEHAVIORAL ADAPTATION

Since the late 1960s an influential new field of evolutionary study has emerged, known variously as *neo-Darwinian theory, evolutionary psychology, Darwinian social science*, or *sociobiology*, although these names are not exact equivalents. It has been quickly adopted by most investigators who study animal behavior under natural conditions and has also influenced many anthropologists and psychologists. Briefly summarized, the principles are as follows.

1. An organism is a gene's way of making another gene (Dawkins, 1978, 1989). More strictly, it is a way thousands of cooperating genes make copies of themselves. If nature is physicochemical, then continued membership in an ongoing genetic line is the ultimate purpose served by any gene. To the extent that a gene influences behavior, it can only continue in the line if it maintains or enhances, through the behavior, the number of copies of itself in the next generation's gene pool.

2. Genes persist or increase by enhancing reproductive success. Where survival and reproductive success are in conflict, reproductive success prevails. "Fitness" in evolutionary theory means only the relative frequency of genes (Lewontin, 1974). It is a tautological dimension of reproductive success and has nothing necessarily in common with medical, social, or athletic definitions of fitness, all of which can be achieved without an increase, or even with a decrease, in technically defined fitness.

3. Fitness is *inclusive*, meaning that genes influence their frequency through not only the reproductive success of the individual carrying them but also that of close relatives who may carry the same gene through common descent. This is the concept introduced by W. D. Hamilton (1964) using the mathematics of evolutionary genetics, to account for the altruism in ani-

mals, which previously seemed as if it should be culled by natural selection (1964). It led to a newly defined subprocess of natural selection, *kin selection* (Dawkins, 1979). If I die to save my identical twin, then the frequency of any gene that helped predispose me to that action will (all else being equal) be unaffected by my death. In general terms, genes predisposing me to self-sacrifice for a relative, should be favored when $b/c > 1/r$, where b is the benefit to the recipient, c the cost to the altruist, and r the degree of genetic relatedness, or likelihood that a gene is found in two individuals by common descent. This helps explain the self-sacrifice of soldier ants, the alarm calls of birds and ground squirrels, and nepotism in human beings, among other phenomena. Other theories bearing on the problem of altruism are reciprocal altruism (Trivers, 1971) and the prisoner's dilemma model of cooperation (Axelrod & Dion, 1988; Axelrod & Hamilton, 1981), neither of which requires that the altruist and the recipient be related.

4. As argued by Trivers based on an observation by Darwin, in species with two sexes that differ in the energy invested in offspring, the sex that invests more is a scarce resource over which the other competes (Trivers, 1972). In mammals and in most birds, females invest more, but direct male parental investment is very high in some species. Species in which investment is high tend to have long-lasting pairing of a breeding male and female, and low levels of sexual dimorphism, male–male competition for females, and male variability in reproductive success. These pair-bonding species, including 8,000 species of birds but only a few mammals, may be contrasted with so-called "tournament" species, in which there are annual seasonal breeding events where males compete intensely for females. These species often have high sexual dimorphism for fighting or display (e.g., antlers and peacock feathers), low levels of pair formation and male parental investment in offspring, and high variability in male reproductive success. Human beings are near but not at the pair-bonding end of the continuum, as indicated by sexual dimorphism, degree of direct male involvement in child care cross-culturally, and the known distribution of human marriage forms (Daly & Wilson, 1983). Polygyny (one man marrying two or more women) is allowed in most cultures in the anthropological record (708 of 849, or 83%), whereas the converse, polyandry, is rare (4 of 849), and a double standard of sexual restriction is common (Murdock, 1949). Still, most human marriages have probably been monogamous, at least in intent.

5. A neo-Darwinian model of parent–offspring conflict (Trivers, 1974) has important implications for the nature of the family. Weaning conflict is common in mammals, and equivalent phenomena among birds even include tantrum behavior. If the evolutionary purposes of mother and offspring were identical, then they would "agree" (shorthand for "would have been selected to act as if they agreed," not implying conscious intent) that a given level and duration of investment is necessary and sufficient, after which the mother should produce another offspring. However, the offspring's gain will be two or four times as great (depending on whether the siblings share a father) if it acts selfishly. Eventually the offspring's diminishing need is outweighed by the inclusive fitness advantage gained through the sibling's birth, but this comes later for the offspring than for the mother.

6. Competition among unrelated individuals can be extreme (Daly & Wilson, 1988). Almost all adequately studied animal species exhibit violence, up to and including killing, in the wild. One particularly noteworthy phenomenon is competitive infanticide, already alluded to in chimpanzees. The paradigmatic case is the Hanuman langur monkey of India, *Presbytis entellus* (Hrdy, 1977). Langur troops comprise a core of related females, their offspring, and unrelated males, sometimes challenged by new males. If the new males drive the previous ones away, they systematically kill all infants under 6 months of age. The mothers then come into estrus again, much sooner than if they had continued to nurse, and are impregnated by the new males. Controversy over whether this is normal behavior or a response to crowding or other stress misses the point: It enhances the reproductive success of the new males at the expense of the old, and so can be expected to be favored by natural selection, whether or not we call it "normal." Life and evolution are stressful, and responses to stress determine ultimate outcomes. Similar phenomena have been observed in many species (Hausfater & Hrdy, 1984).

Overall, these principles necessitate rejection of a naive model of the family, which assumes that it functions as a harmonious unit under ideal conditions. It was not so designed and is instead an association of individuals with overlapping but distinct evolutionary interests. Its members naturally pursue goals that are sometimes at odds with each other's ultimate purposes, and their relations are naturally conflictual rather than harmonious. Rather than being the result of friction in what should be a smoothly functioning system, much conflict is intrinsic.

This is even truer of communities, societies, and cultures, each of which is a collection of individuals, families, and larger kinship units engaged in short- or long-term cooperation for the pursuit of individual and inclusive fitness goals. If it is true that societies or cultures as a whole are adapted (Harris, 1979, 1997), limits to this collective adaptation are imposed by individuals and kin groups that take advantage of the collective, favoring their own inclusive fitness. The well-known "tragedy of the commons" is only one example. Cultures with slaves, castes, hierarchies of ethnic groups, racism, sexism, and even mere social classes may be in some sense adapted *as cultures*, because they are surviving and reproducing, but such cultures enable some groups to enhance their reproductive success at the expense of others. These arrangements may be stable over time, but that does not make them adaptive for all members of the culture. Furthermore, this statement is true of not only cultures that encourage competition (e.g., the United States) but also those that encourage cooperation (e.g., Japan), although the mechanisms of exploitation may differ greatly.

A CULTURAL ACQUISITION DEVICE

Despite human universals and guided adaptations, and in part because of them, the particulars of culture invade and affect the developing mind. But how?

This question is best answered by reference to a much broader range of psychological processes than is conventionally considered by cultural psychologists. The acquisition of culture, like the acquisition of language, is basically a human adaptation, protocultural (and protolinguistic) achievements of other animals notwithstanding. But if there is a language acquisition device (LAD), as proposed by Chomsky, Lenneberg, and others, it remains quite mysterious. The cultural acquisition device (CAD),

on the other hand, comprises elements that are fairly well understood by psychologists and anthropologists. A proposed version of the CAD is presented in Table 4.4.

The CAD consists of 17 processes loosely divided into four categories; the italicized processes are probably unique to the human species. The first category, reactive processes, comprise the most basic mechanisms of behavior modification that occur inevitably in growing up in a certain context (J. W. Whiting, 1941). The second, facilitative processes, includes social processes that rely on intersubjectivity, the ability to take the perspective of the other, at least in one direction. The third, emotional enculturation, includes processes that are inherently based on strong emotions designed by evolution to shape behavior. The fourth and last category, symbolic processes, rests on uniquely human capacities for the formation of symbols and their integration into culturally significant schemas. Brief definitions of the processes follow.

TABLE 4.4. A Proposed CAD

Reactive processes (cultural habitus)
  Habituation (response decrement)
  Classical conditioning (including emotions)
  Associative conditioning (perceptual learning)
  Instrumental conditioning (cultural selection of actions)
  Social facilitation (relaxation of inhibition)

Facilitative processes (social learning)
  Local enhancement (ad hoc scaffolding)
  Imitation (nontargeted modeling)
  Instruction (Contingently responsive scaffolding)
  Collaboration (Co-construction of knowledge)

Psychodynamic processes (emotional enculturation)
  Attachment (recruitment for socialization)
  Positive identification (focused modeling)
  Fear of strangers (the comfort of the familiar)
  Negative identification (us–them polarization)
  Emotion management (the comfort of ritual)

Symbolic processes (cognitive enculturation)
  Cultural construction of perception (collective assimilation)
  Cultural schematization (collective accommodation)
  Narrative construction (narrative meaning)
  Cultural coherence (overarching themes)

Note. Freely adapted from theoretical discussions in Whiting (1941), LeVine, (1982), Tomasello, Kruger, and Ratner (1993), and Shore (1995). Processes unique to humans are italicized.

Reactive Processes (Cultural Habitus)

Habituation

Habituation, or response decrement, is a classic ethological concept referring to a usually adaptive waning or disappearance of an inborn response that is repeatedly elicited by the environment without serving a function. For maturational reasons 8- to 10-month-olds show wariness of strangers, but in American culture, with its high frequency of encounters with strangers, the response wanes over weeks to months, whereas in !Kung culture, where strangers are rare, it does not.

Classical Conditioning

Children are bathed in stimuli that occur in association with a much more restricted initial group of unconditioned stimuli, linked through innate neural circuits to reflexive responses. Suppose that the calming effect of being held by a calm mother is innate. If being in church calms the mother, then this setting will gain the power to calm the child, because the unconditioned stimulus (calm mother) becomes associated with conditioned stimuli such as liturgical music.

Associative Conditioning

This ubiquitous process engrains expectations as to the spatial and temporal contiguity of stimuli, and so establishes patterns or schemas even in the absence of action. In Samoa, a welcoming ritual places an orderly set of sights, sounds, actions, and utterances before a child, who does not need to participate to learn the pattern.

Instrumental Conditioning

In all societies some naturally occurring behaviors are rewarded (reinforced), and others are punished. From infancy !Kung children are socially rewarded for sharing, a fundamental cultural value and pattern, but punished for approaching a fire, and the behaviors wax or wane, respectively.

Social Facilitation

A child observes others performing an action for which there is a tendency already present, but which is released from inhibition by the observation, the simplest example being yawning. This is probably the main process involved in the acquisition of culturally specific dietary patterns.

Facilitative Processes (Social Learning)

Local Enhancement

In a kind of "scaffolding," or enhancement of the child's opportunity to learn, the ordinary course of events in the life of one individual of necessity brings the child into situations that make learning by trial and error easier. A berry-picking expedition, for example, brings a child into a setting where the reward of eating berries and the punishment of encountering thorns shape the child's behavior.

Imitation

This general process by which observing another's behavior allows the child to shorten greatly the time required for learning by matching the actions and/or the goals of the other does not necessarily require a relationship or an identification (see below), but it does require the child to take the perspective of the other. It differs from social facilitation in that it is not an internally driven response under inhibition before the observation.

Instruction

Unique or almost unique to humans, instruction involves *inter*subjectivity (Tomasello et al., 1993); not only must the child take the other's perspective but the other must also take the child's and engage in deliberate scaffolding that tailors the learning process to the child's current ability—in other words, teach. In addition to its obvious role in the cultural transmission of complex skills such as weaving (Greenfield, 1999), instruction functions very widely in human cultures in the service of different kinds of cultural transmission (Kruger & Tomasello, 1996).

Collaboration

This process involves two learners of approximately equal skill and cognitive capacity in relation to the problem at hand. Rather than one teaching the other, they co-construct a solution by learning interactively (Kruger, 1992, 1993;

Kruger & Tomasello, 1986). As with true instruction, collaboration requires two-way perspective taking, such that each learner can see the problem as the other sees it. (This is sometimes attributed to "theory of mind," although that designation seems to imply something much more elaborate than perspective taking.)

Psychodynamic Processes (Emotional Enculturation)

Attachment

Attachment to a primary caregiver and then to other individuals, both human and nonhuman, provides the foundation for ongoing social interaction fundamental to social learning and ultimately to socialization. Social skills emerge and are practiced in this emotionally rich context, reinforced by emotional rewards and punishments. In human cultures, this process not only socializes the young but also forms a major part of enculturation.

Positive Identification

This emotional process organizes imitative tendencies by focusing them on one or more individuals to which the child feels similar, likes, and/or admires. This process is involved in the formation of gender-specific behavior in all cultures, as well as behavior specific to a clan, a class, or to the cultural group itself.

Fear of Strangers

Xenophobia, or fear of strangers, sets a limit very early in life on the outward reach of identification and imitation. It drives infants and children toward primary caregivers and makes within-family identification stronger.

Negative Identification

Xenophobia may (and does in most cultures) develop by middle childhood into prejudice against an outgroup. This may entail hatred, disgust, and/or fear, and these strong emotions form the basis of a desire to be different from the outgroup, thus reinforcing ingroup cultural identity.

Emotion Management

Because unsettling inner experiences, including anxiety, fear, grief, rage, hunger, lust, and falling in love, among others, are pervasive in life, human cultures provide rules and rituals that calm the anxieties associated with such experiences. This transforms a highly intense individual experience into a collective one, and it changes an experience that feels idiosyncratic and disturbing to one that is and has been shared by others.

Symbolic Processes (Cognitive Enculturation)

Cultural Construction of Perception

Because the brain routinely sets the sensitivity of sense organs, selecting and shaping input, the opportunity arises in human experience for culture to shape perception by shaping cognition. Thus the cultures whose languages make no phonemic distinction between *l* and *r* produce toddlers who never again attend to the distinction, although making it is a trivial matter for 2-year-olds in other cultures. Culture also shapes many other forms of perception (Sapir, 1994).

Cultural Schematization

Cultures do more than filter perception at the sense organs. They actively build schemas (models) to represent the complexities of the world and give structure to thought (Shore, 1996). Thus, in cultures such as those of highland New Guinea, goods and services flow toward one man who commands the respect of others, and who then can be (more or less) relied on to redistribute them (as well as other goods and services) in ways that are culturally appropriate. There is a strong tendency in these cultures to see all of economic and social life in terms of this model or schema.

Narrative Construction

The human propensity for creating narratives orders life in a temporal dimension much like that of the life course itself, with a beginning, a middle, and an end (Bruner, 2003; Bruner & Feldman, 1996). Stories can be true or invented, funny or sad, instructive or baffling, cynical or edifying, and end happily or tragically, but every one of them helps to order life events in a way that is meaningful and at least somewhat comprehensible. Just as the narrative of one's own life, accurate or not, gives it meaning and orders future events against its background, so the narrative of a culture's history—suffering and the overcoming of it for the Jews, independence and pioneering for Americans—functions for a people.

Cultural Coherence

Cultures appear to have themes (usually more than one), and these may organize many schemas into a linked web of cognitive function (Durham, 1991; Shore, 1996). Warlike toughness may have been such a theme for the Plains Indians and the Yanomamo, cooperation for the Japanese, competition for Americans, and positive attitude for the Balinese. Although at best gross oversimplifications, they may make the large array of symbols and schemas in any culture cohere to some extent, and make them easier to learn.

IMPLICATIONS FOR CULTURAL PSYCHOLOGY

Postmodernist skepticism about human universals notwithstanding, research has progressed along many lines, including neo-Darwinian approaches to human culture (Barkow et al., 1992; Betzig, 1997), D. E. Brown's (1991) survey of universals (Brown, 1991), and Shore's (1996) attempt to place psychological anthropology on a foundation of recent cognitive science. As Shore notes, "A kind of cognitive romanticism . . . has begun to crystallize" (p. 35) in cultural anthropology, founded on the fallacy that "if cultural practices or beliefs are not fully determined or universally shared . . . then they must be arbitrary and thus infinitely variable" (p. 37). This extreme position, itself ironically an example of the human mind's universal dualizing tendency, has been espoused by Richard Schweder: "The mind, according to cultural psychology, is content-driven, domain specific, and constructively stimulus bound; and it cannot be extricated from the historically variable and cross-culturally diverse intentional worlds in which it plays a constitutive part" (as quoted by Shore, p. 36).

This strong version of the claim is clearly false; in large part, the mind can be so extricated, as shown by work of Darwin, Eibl-Eibesfeldt, Ekman, Tooby, Cosmides, and many others in evolutionary psychology, and by the work of Boas, Lévi-Strauss, D'Andrade, Shore, and other cultural anthropologists who accept in some form the reality of a universal

human cognitive apparatus. Even if cognition is inherently dialogic, that does not rule out important universal characteristics of the dialog shared among different cultures and even different social species. The weak version of the statement has always been embraced by anthropologists and now, thanks to cultural psychology, psychologists accept it as well. Except in extreme pathological instances, no human child can develop without culture, and so all human behavior, thought, and feeling is tinged or brushed or saturated with cultural color, and this color is different in different traditions. More importantly, much of the content of mental life is different, in the same sense that different languages have different content but for the most part serve similar functions and even share many fundamentals of structure. Finally, behavior is regulated by culture in myriad ways that allow us to feel protected and accepted, and to fend off the anxiety that would come with having an infinite range of choices every moment of every day.

Yet behavior too shows universal features that are far from trivial, and somehow almost all cultures direct behavior, thought, and feeling toward final common pathways of survival and reproduction. Some developmental psychologists have also run the risk of cognitive romanticism, claiming that Vygotskian cultural psychology should largely supplant the discoveries of Jean Piaget and others about universal processes in human mental function and its development (Bruner, 1999; Fernyhough, 1997; Rogoff, 1990; Rogoff, Baker-Sennett, Lacasa, & Goldsmith, 1995). That a limited number of mainly observational studies in this field could have so revolutionary an effect seems implausible, and, indeed, the claim is not sustained by the evidence, but it finds a comfortable place in the postmodernist rhetoric of recent and even current academia—a "hegemonic discourse" in its own right.

In fact, although learning to weave in a Mayan community in Highland Guatemala has been cited as support for Vygotskian models of mental development (Rogoff, 1990, Chapter 6), the same process in a village in Zinacantan, Mexico has been shown to support a Piagetian approach (Greenfield, 2005, Chapter 2). Not only are the developmental patterns compatible with Piagetian models but also the "Zinacantecs' implicit theory of development corresponds to Piagetian theory" (pp. 48–49). Teaching is important, of course, as are the tools of instruction, but they do not take the place of maturation. Indeed, "the tools show us specific cultural expressions of universal stages of development while simultaneously showing us the Zinacantecs' implicit conceptions of these stages. They reveal that a theory of cognitive development and a developmental theory of instruction are built into the culture" (p. 49). In other words, even culture-specific models of teaching and learning are constrained by universal facts of maturation.

Again, there is a weaker form of the claim that cannot be denied—enculturation is an important aspect of mental development—but the strong form, in which there are few or no universals of mental function and its development, is demonstrably false. But, of course, cultural psychology has an important subject matter even when its claims are not exaggerated: the real variation in psychological processes across cultures and the understanding of how culture affects cognitive function (Lehman, Chiu, & Schaller, 2004). Equally important, it has filled a gap left by the postmodernist rejection of scientific method in much of cultural anthropology. What relevance does evolution have for this important enterprise? I answer this question in four ways.

First, since psychological processes have evolved, the starting point for cultural psychology must be the cognitive apparatus brought forward from our higher primate background. These capabilities evolved under selective pressures, increasingly accessible to investigation, that explain much of human behavior and mental life. Cultural variation follows particular paths that begin with the hunter-gatherer baseline and diverge in ways that are sometimes predictable from neo-Darwinian principles. It may be that Japanese and other East Asian cultures have a corporate or collective bias compared with the individualistic bias in the United States (Markus & Kitayama, 1991; Triandis, 2001), although even this widely accepted generalization is open to challenge (Voronov & Singer, 2002). But an anthropologist might argue that this collective bias is present in all hunter-gatherers and most traditional societies in the anthropological record. So the question may be not "How do East Asian cultures bring about this distinctive cultural bias?" but "Why did the United States and a few other Western cultures abandon a pattern that had previously been a central part of the human adaptation?"

Second, psychological processes are instantiated in the brain, and any cognitive models, cultural or not, must come to terms with rapidly advancing knowledge of higher brain function. Quite soon, the brain will be the standard cognitive model. Plasticity is substantial, but it has both firm limits and favored pathways with which culture must come to terms as it influences the mind. Lévi-Strauss (1962, 1963) showed that so-called "primitive" cultures all tend to dichotomize the social world and to represent the respective halves with potent totems or symbols whose relationship to each other mirrors that of the social groups. Modern states, or collections of states, also fit this pattern, as in the confrontations of the Cold War or the war on terror, perceived by many as a conflict between Christianity and Islam. If this is a widespread or universal human mental tendency—Lévi-Strauss would have said that dualities are "good to think"—then it would be interesting to know why in terms of brain function, and it would be especially interesting to understand the cultural psychology—and the cultural psychobiology—of people (e.g., Norwegians or Tibetans) who seem to transcend this tendency better than do others.

Third, the study of cultural variation always reveals invariant properties of behavior and mind. Not only cross-cultural universals, of which there are many, but also cross-cultural biases—departures from a random distribution of variation—often reveal evolved properties of mind instantiated in the brain. In the realm of language, cross-cultural hierarchical regularities in color naming, phonetics, and grammar set firm limits on the observable variation (Berlin & Kay, 1969; J. H. Greenberg, 1975), and this is undoubtedly true of other dimensions of culture. For example, compared with the North, the Southeastern United States may have a "culture of honor" (Cohen et al., 1996; Nisbett, 1993), but so do inner-city gang members reacting to what they perceive as a disrespectful glance, and hunter-gatherers experiencing a presumed insult in the process of meat distribution. The question therefore is not "What is unique about Southern cultural psychology?" but "What do the many cultures of honor have in common psychologically that distinguishes them from those in which honor is less important?"

Finally—culture notwithstanding—the course of human development is first of all maturational, proceeding according to a plan set and guided by the genes. This plan may provide opportunities for culture to be especially effective in shaping mind, and it would be useful to understand these opportunities and when they occur. For example, does the widespread tendency of traditional cultures (including Japan) to have infants sleep in the same bed, or at least in the same room, with their mothers provide some kind of psychological foundation for the collective bias of their cultures, or does the causal arrow go the other way? Does the American practice of letting a baby cry itself to sleep in its own room until it gets used to sleeping alone foster independence, or is it just a by-product of our culture of independence? Or both? At this point in the history of this science, whether we call it psychological anthropology or cultural psychology, we simply do not know.

CONCLUSION

Cultural psychology represents the realization by psychologists of something that psychological anthropologists have known and investigated for a century: Culture has profound influences on mind that go beyond habitual or customary behavior, and mind in turn may help explain the uniqueness of cultures. This is a welcome development, because these phenomena merit study, and anthropology does not have the resources to do justice to all of them, nor, in the wake of the postmodernist revolution (Greenfield, 2000), does it usually approach them with the kinds of quantitative methods psychologists use. However, there are many exceptions (D'Andrade, 1992, 2001; Heider, 1991; LeVine, 1999, 2002; LeVine et al., 1994). Better communication between the two groups might be of value, along with greater recognition by cultural psychologists of the history of their much older sister discipline. Also, cultural psychology has been slow to recognize the contributions of biological anthropology and evolutionary psychology. These approaches explain the baseline from which cultural divergences depart, as well as indicate some predictable ways those divergences are distributed. Behavior is adaptation, and culture aids or impedes adaptation in different ways for different human groups. In the future, neurobiological studies will help us to understand both the constancies and varieties of human minds as they develop in different cultures. It is often said that nothing in biology makes sense except in the light of evolution. Little in behavior, mind, or culture makes much sense except in the same light.

REFERENCES

Almagor, U. (1989). Dual organization reconsidered. In D. Maybury-Lewis & U. Almagor (Eds.), *The attraction of opposites: Thought and society in the dualistic mode* (pp. 19–32). Ann Arbor: University of Michigan Press.

Altmann, J., Alberts, S. C., Haines, S. C., Dubach, J., Muruthi, P., Coote, T., et al. (1996). Behavior predicts gene structure in a wild primate group. *Proceedings of the National Academy of Sciences USA, 93,* 5797–5801.

Ambrose, S. H. (2001). Paleolithic technology and human evolution. *Science, 291,* 1748–1753.

Axelrod, R., & Dion, D. (1988). The further evolution of cooperation. *Science, 242,* 1385–1390.

Axelrod, R., & Hamilton, W. D. (1981). The evolution of cooperation. *Science, 211,* 1390–1396.

Bailey, R. C. (1991). *The behavioral ecology of Efe Pygmy men in the Ituri Forest, Zaire* (Vol. 86). Ann Arbor: Museum of Anthropology, University of Michigan.

Barkow, J. H., Cosmides, L., & Tooby, J. (Eds.). (1992). *The adapted mind: Evolutionary psychology and the generation of culture.* New York: Oxford University Press.

Barr, C. S., Newman, T. K., Lindell, S., Shannon, C., Champoux, M., Lesch, K. P., et al. (2004). Interaction between serotonin transporter gene variation and rearing condition in alcohol preference and consumption in female primates. *Archives of General Psychiatry, 61*(11), 1146–1152.

Barr, R. G. (1990). The normal crying curve: What do we know? *Developmental Medicine and Child Neurology, 32,* 368–374.

Barr, R. G., Konner, M., Bakeman, R., & Adamson, L. (1991). Crying in !Kung San infants: A test of the cultural specificity hypothesis. *Developmental Medicine and Child Neurology, 33,* 601–610.

Bates, E., & Marchman, V. A. (1987). What is and is not universal in language acquisition. In F. Plum (Ed.), *Language, communication, and the brain* (pp. 19–38). New York: Raven Press.

Belsky, J. (1997). Attachment, mating, and parenting: An evolutionary interpretation. *Human Nature, 8*(4), 361–381.

Belsky, J. (1999). Modern evolutionary theory and patterns of attachment. In J. S. P. R. Cassidy (Ed.), *Handbook of attachment: Theory, research, and clinical applications* (pp. 141–161). New York: Guilford Press.

Belsky, J., Steinberg, L., & Draper, P. (1991). Childhood experience, interpersonal development, and reproductive strategy: An evolutionary theory of socialization. *Child Development, 62,* 647–670.

Benedict, R. (1934). *Patterns of culture.* Boston: Houghton Mifflin.

Berlin, B., & Kay, P. (1969). *Basic color terms: Their universality and evolution.* Berkeley: University of California Press.

Betzig, L. (1992). Roman polygyny. *Ethology and Sociobiology, 13,* 309–349.

Betzig, L. (Ed.). (1997). *Human nature: A critical reader.* New York: Oxford University Press.

Betzig, L. L. (1986). *Despotism and differential reproduction: A Darwinian view of history.* New York: Aldine.

Blurton Jones, N. (1993). The lives of hunter-gatherer children: Effects of parental behavior and parental reproductive strategy. In M. E. Pereira & L. A. Fairbanks (Eds.), *Juvenile primates: Life history, development, and behavior* (pp. 309–326). New York: Oxford University Press.

Brown, C. H., & Witkowski, S. R. (1981). Figurative language in a universalist perspective. *American Ethnologist, 8,* 596–615.

Brown, D. E. (1991). *Human universals.* Philadelphia: Temple University Press.

Bruner, J. (1999). Prologue to the English edition of *The collected works of L. S. Vygotsky.* In P. Lloyd & C. Fernyhough (Eds.), *Lev Vygotsky: Critical assessments: Future directions* (Vol. IV, pp. 421–441). London: Routledge.

Bruner, J. (2003). The narrative construction of reality. In M. Mateas & P. Sengers (Eds.), *Narrative intelligence* (pp. 41–62). Amsterdam: Benjamins.

Bruner, J., & Feldman, C. F. (1996). Group narrative as a cultural context of autobiography. In D. C. Rubin (Ed.), *Remembering our past: Studies in autobiographical memory.* New York: Cambridge University Press.

Buss, D. (1989). Sex differences in human mate preferences: Evolutionary hypotheses tested in 37 cultures. *Behavioral and Brain Sciences, 12,* 1–49.

Buss, D. M. (1984). Evolutionary biology and personality psychology: Toward a conception of human nature and individual differences. *American Psychologist, 39,* 1135–1147.

Callaghan, T., Rochat, P., Lillard, A., Claux, M. L., Odden, H., Itakura, S., et al. (2005). Synchrony in the onset of mental-state reasoning: Evidence from five cultures. *Psychological Science, 16*(5), 378–384.

Caspi, A., Sugden, K., Moffitt, T. E., Taylor, A., Craig, I. W., Harrington, H., et al. (2003). Influence of life stress on depression: Moderation by a polymorphism in the 5-HTT gene [see comment]. *Science, 301,* 386–389.

Cavalli-Sforza, L., Menozzi, P., & Piazza, A. (1994). *The history and geography of human genes.* Princeton, NJ: Princeton University Press.

Cavalli-Sforza, L. L., & Feldman, M. W. (2003). The application of molecular genetic approaches to the study of human evolution. *Nature Genetics, 33*(Suppl.), 266–275.

Chisholm, J. S. (1993). Death, hope, and sex: life-history theory and the development of reproductive strategies. *Current Anthropology, 34,* 1–24.

Chisholm, J. S. (1999). *Death, hope and sex: Steps to an evolutionary ecology of mind and morality.* New York: Cambridge University Press.

Chomsky, N. (1988). *Language and problems of knowledge: The Managua lectures.* Cambridge, MA: MIT Press.

Chowdhury, A. N. (1996). The definition and classification of Koro. *Culture, Medicine and Psychiatry, 20*(1), 41–65.

Cohen, D., Nisbett, R. E., Bowdle, B. F., & Schwartz, N. (1996). Insult, aggression, and the southern culture of honor: An "experimental ethnography." *Journal of Personality and Social Psychology, 70*(5), 945–959.

Collaer, M. L., & Hines, M. (1995). Human behavioral sex differences: A role for gonadal hormones during early development? *Psychological Bulletin, 118*(1), 55–107.

Comrie, B. (1989). *Language universals and linguistic typology: Syntax and morphology* (2nd ed.). Chicago: University of Chicago Press.

Cosmides, L., & Tooby, J. (2000). The cognitive neuroscience of social reasoning. In M. Gazzaniga (Ed.), *The new cognitive neurosciences* (2nd ed., pp. 1259–1270). Cambridge, MA: MIT Press.

Crawford, C., & Krebs, D. L. (Eds.). (1998). *Handbook of evolutionary psychology.* Mahwah, NJ: Erlbaum.

Dahlberg, F. (Ed.). (1981). *Woman the gatherer.* New Haven, CT: Yale University Press.

Daly, M., & Wilson, M. (1988). *Homicide* (2nd ed.). New York: Aldine de Gruyter.

Daly, M., & Wilson, M. (1983). *Sex, evolution and behavior* (2nd ed.). Boston: Willard Grant Press.

D'Andrade, R. (1991). The identification of schemas in naturalistic data. In M. J. Horowitz (Ed.), *Person schemas and maladaptive interpersonal patterns* (pp. 279–301). Chicago: University of Chicago Press.

D'Andrade, R. (1995). *The development of cognitive anthropology.* Cambridge, UK: Cambridge University Press.

D'Andrade, R. (2001). A cognitivist's view of the units debate in cultural anthropology. *Cross-Cultural Research: Journal of Comparative Social Science, 35*(2), 242–257.

D'Andrade, R. G. (1992). Cognitive anthropology. In T. Schwartz, M. White, & C. A. Lutz (Eds.), *New directions in psychological anthropology* (p. 47–52). Cambridge, UK: Cambridge University Press.

Darwin, C. (1987). Notebook M, August 16, 1838. In P. H. Barrett, P. J. Gautrey, L. Herbert, D. Kohn, & S. Smith (Eds.), *Charles Darwin's notebooks, 1836–1844; Geology, transmutation of species, metaphysical inquiries* (p. 359). Ithaca, NY: Cornell University Press.

Darwin, C. (1998). *The expression of the emotions in man and animals: Introduction, afterword, and com-

mentaries by Paul Ekman (3rd ed.). New York: Oxford University Press.

Dawkins, R. (1978). Replicator selection and the extended phenotype. *Zeitschrift für Tierpsychologie, 47*, 61–76.

Dawkins, R. (1979). Twelve misunderstandings of kin selection. *Zeitschrift für Tierpsychologie, 51*, 184–200.

Dawkins, R. (1989). *The selfish gene, new edition.* New York: Oxford University Press.

de Waal, F. B. M. (1989). Behavioral contrasts between bonobo and chimpanzee. In P. G. Heltne & L. A. Marquardt (Eds.), *Understanding chimpanzees* (pp. 154–175). Cambridge, MA: Harvard University Press/Chicago Academy of Sciences.

DuBois, C. (1944). *The people of Alor.* New York: Harper.

Durham, W. H. (1991). *Coevolution: Genes, culture, and human diversity.* Stanford, CA: Stanford University Press.

Ebling, F. J. P. (2005). The neuroendocrine timing of puberty. *Reproduction, 129*(6), 675–683.

Edwards, C. P. (1981). The comparative study of the development of moral judgement and reasoning. In R. H. Munroe, R. L. Munroe, & B. B. Whiting (Eds.), *Handbook of cross-cultural human development* (pp. 501–528). New York: Garland STPM Press.

Eibl-Eibesfeldt, I. (1971). Zur Ethologie menschlichen Grussverhaltens: II. Das Gruss verhalten und einige andere Muster freundlicher Kontaktaufnahme der Waika-Indianer (Yanoama). *Zeitschrift für Tierpsychologie, 29*, 196–213.

Eibl-Eibesfeldt, I. (1989). *Human ethology.* New York: Aldine de Gruyter.

Ekman, P., Friesen, W. V., O'Sullivan, M., Chan, A., Diacoyanni-Tarlatzis, Heider, K., et al. (1987). Universals and cultural differences in the judgements of facial expressions of emotion. *Journal of Personality and Social Psychology, 53*, 712–717.

Ekman, P., & Rosenberg, E. L. (Eds.). (1997). *What the face reveals: Basic and applied studies of spontaneous expression using the facial action coding system (FACS).* New York: Oxford University Press.

Fernyhough, C. (1997). Vygotsky's sociocultural approach: Theoretical issues and implications for current research. In S. Hala (Ed.), *The development of social cognition* (pp. 65–92). East Sussex, UK: Psychology Press.

Goodall, J. (1986). *The chimpanzees of Gombe: Patterns of behavior.* Cambridge, MA: Harvard University Press.

Gouzoules, H., & Gouzoules, S. (1990). Matrilineal signatures in the recruitment screams of pigtail macaques, *Macaca nemestrina. Behaviour, 115*(3–4), 327–347.

Gouzoules, S., & Gouzoules, H. (1987). Kinship. In B. B. Smuts, D. L. Cheney, R. M. Seyfarth, R. W. Wrangham, & T. T. Struhsaker (Eds.), *Primate societies* (pp. 299–305). Chicago: University of Chicago Press.

Greenberg, J. H. (1975). Research on language universals. *Annual Review of Anthropology, 4*, 75–94.

Greenberg, L. (1979). Genetic component of bee odor in kin recognition. *Science, 206*, 1095–1097.

Greenfield, P. M. (1999). Historical change and cognitive change: A two-decade follow-up study in Zinacantan, a Maya community in Chiapas, Mexico. *Mind, Culture, and Activity, 6*, 92–108.

Greenfield, P. M. (2000). What psychology can do for anthropology, or why anthropology took postmodernism on the chin. *American Anthropologist, 102*(3), 564–576.

Greenfield, P. M. (2005). *Weaving generations together: Evolving creativity in the Maya of Chiapas.* Santa Fe, NM: School of American Research.

Griffin, P. B., & Estioko-Griffin, A. (Eds.). (1985). *The Agta of Northeastern Luzon: Recent studies.* Cebu City, Philippines: San Carlos Publications.

Halpern, C. T., Udry, J. R., & Suchindran, C. (1997). Testosterone predicts initiation of coitus in adolescent females. *Psychosomatic Medicine, 59*(2), 161–171.

Halpern, C. T., Udry, J. R., & Suchindran, C. (1998). Monthly measures of salivary testosterone predict sexual activity in adolescent males. *Archives of Sexual Behavior, 27*(5), 445–465.

Hamilton, W. D. (1964). The genetical evolution of social behavior, I and II. *Journal of Theoretical Biology, 7*, 1–52.

Harris, M. (1968). *The rise of anthropological theory: A history of theories of culture.* New York: Crowell.

Harris, M. (1979). *Cultural materialism: The struggle for a science of culture.* New York: Random House.

Harris, M. (1997). *Culture, people, nature: An introduction to general anthropology* (7th ed.). New York: Longman.

Hartung, J. (1982). Polygyny and inheritance of wealth. *Current Anthropology, 23*, 1–12.

Hausfater, G., & Hrdy, S. B. (Eds.). (1984). *Infanticide: Comparative and evolutionary perspectives.* New York: Aldine de Gruyter.

Hawkes, K. (1991). Hunting income patterns among the Hadza: Big game, common goods, foraging goals, and the evolution of the human diet. *Philosophical Transactions of the Royal Society of London B, 334*, 243–251.

Hawkes, K., O'Connell, J. F., & Jones, N. G. (2003). Human life histories: Primate trade-offs, grandmothering socioecology, and the fossil record. In P. M. Kappeler & M. E. Pereira (Eds.), *Primate life histories and socioecology* (pp. 204–227). Chicago: University of Chicago Press.

Hawkes, K., O'Connell, J. F., Jones, N. G. B., Alvarez, H., & Charnov, E. L. (1998). Grandmothering, menopause, and the evolution of human life histories. *Proceedings of the National Academy of Sciences USA, 95*(3), 1336–1339.

Heider, K. (1991). *Landscapes of emotion: Mapping*

three cultures of emotion in Indonesia. New York: Cambridge University Press.

Hertz, R. (1973). The pre-eminence of the right hand: A study in religious polarity. In R. Needham (Ed.), *Right and left: Essays in dual symbolic classification* (pp. 3–31). Chicago: University of Chicago Press. (Original work published 1909)

Hewlett, B. S. (1991). *Intimate fathers: The nature and context of Aka Pygmy paternal infant care.* Ann Arbor: University of Michigan Press.

Hill, K., & Hurtado, M. (1999). The Aché of Paraguay. In R. B. Lee & R. Daly (Eds.), *The Cambridge encyclopedia of hunters and gatherers* (pp. 92–96). Cambridge, UK: Cambridge University Press.

Hinde, R. A., & Davies, L. (1972a). Removing infant rhesus from mother for 13 days compared with removing mother from infant. *Journal of Child Psychology and Psychiatry, 13,* 227–237.

Hinde, R. A., & Davies, L. M. (1972b). Changes in mother–infant relationship after separation in rhesus monkeys. *Nature, 239,* 41–42.

Hrdy, S. B. (1977). *The langurs of Abu: Female and male strategies of reproduction.* Cambridge, MA: Harvard University Press.

Hrdy, S. B. (1981). *The woman that never evolved.* Cambridge, MA: Harvard University Press.

Hrdy, S. B. (1992). Fitness tradeoffs in the history and evolution of delegated mothering with special reference to wet-nursing, abandonment, and infanticide. *Ethology and Sociobiology, 13*(5–6), 409–442.

Hrdy, S. B. (1999). *Mother nature: A history of mothers, infants, and natural selection.* New York: Pantheon.

Hurtado, A. M., Hawkes, K., Hill, K., & Kaplan, H. (1985). Female subsistence strategies among Aché hunter-gatherers of Eastern Paraguay. *Human Ecology, 13,* 1–27.

Johnson, A. W., & Earle, T. (1987). *The evolution of human societies: From foraging group to agrarian state.* Stanford, CA: Stanford University Press.

Kardiner, A., & Linton, R. (Eds.). (1939). *The individual and his society.* New York: Columbia University Press.

Kardiner, A., & Linton, R. (Eds.). (1945). *The psychological frontiers of society.* New York: Columbia University Press.

Keel, P. K., & Klump, K. L. (2003). Are eating disorders culture-bound syndromes?: Implications for conceptualizing their etiology. *Psychological Bulletin, 129*(5), 747–769.

Keenleyside, A. (1998). Skeletal evidence of health and disease in pre-contact Alaskan Eskimos and Aleuts. *American Journal of Physical Anthropology, 107*(1), 51–70.

Kelly, R. L. (1995). *The foraging spectrum: Diversity in hunter-gatherer lifeways.* Washington, DC: Smithsonian Institution Press.

Kleinman, A. (2003). Introduction: common mental disorders, primary care, and the global mental health research agenda. *Harvard Review of Psychiatry, 11*(3), 155–156.

Konner, M. (1991). Universals of behavioral development in relation to brain myelination. In K. R. Gibson & A. C. Petersen (Eds.), *Brain maturation and cognitive development: Comparative and cross-cultural perspectives* (pp. 181–223). New York: Aldine de Gruyter.

Konner, M. (2005). Hunter-gatherer infancy and childhood: The !Kung and others. In B. S. Hewlett & M. E. Lamb (Eds.), *Hunter-gatherer childhoods: Evolutionary, developmental and cultural perspectives.* New Brunswick, NJ: Aldine Transaction.

Konner, M. J. (1981). Evolution of human behavior development. In R. H. Munroe, R. L. Munroe, & B. B. Whiting (Eds.), *Handbook of cross-cultural human development* (pp. 3–51). New York: Garland STPM Press.

Konner, M. J. (2002). *The tangled wing: Biological constraints on the human spirit* (2nd ed.). New York: Holt/Times Books.

Kroeber, A. L. (1948). *Anthropology.* New York: Harcourt Brace.

Kruger, A. C. (1992). The effect of peer and adult–child transactive discussions on moral reasoning. *Merrill–Palmer Quarterly, 38*(2), 191–211.

Kruger, A. C. (1993). Peer collaboration: Conflict, cooperation, or both. *Social Development, 2*(3), 165–182.

Kruger, A. C., & Tomasello, M. (1986). Transactive discussions with peers and adults. *Developmental Psychology, 22,* 681–685.

Kruger, A. C., & Tomasello, M. (1996). Cultural learning and learning culture. In D. Olson & N. Torrance (Eds.), *Handbook of education and human development: New models of learning, teaching, and schooling* (pp. 369–387). Oxford, UK: Basil Blackwell.

Kurland, J. (1977). *Kin selection in the Japanese monkey* (Vol. 12). Basel: Karger.

Lancaster, J. B., & Lancaster, C. S. (1983). Parental investment: the hominid adaptation. In D. Ortner (Ed.), *How humans adapt* (pp. 35–56). Washington, DC: Smithsonian Institution Press.

Lecours, A. R. (1975). Myelogenetic correlates of the development of speech and language. In E. Lenneberg & E. Lenneberg (Eds.), *Foundations of language development* (Vol. 1, pp. 121–135). New York: Academic Press.

Lee, R. B. (1979). *The !Kung San: Men, women and work in a foraging society.* Cambridge, UK: Cambridge University Press.

Lee, R. B., & Daly, R. (Eds.). (1999). *The Cambridge encyclopedia of hunters and gatherers.* Cambridge, UK: Cambridge University Press.

Lee, R. B., & DeVore, I. (1968a). *Man the hunter.* Chicago: Aldine.

Lee, R. B., & DeVore, I. (1968b). Problems in the study of hunters and gatherers. In *Man the hunter* (pp. 3–12). Chicago: Aldine.

Lehman, D. R., Chiu, C.-Y., & Schaller, M. (2004). Psychology and culture. *Annual Review of Psychology,* 55, 689–714.

LeVine, R. A. (1982). *Culture, behavior, and personality* (2nd ed.). Chicago: Aldine.

LeVine, R. A. (1998). Child psychology and anthropology: An environmental view. In C. Panter-Brick (Ed.), *Biosocial perspectives on children* (pp. 102–130). Cambridge, UK: Cambridge University Press.

LeVine, R. A. (1999). An agenda for psychological anthropology. *Ethos,* 27(1), 15–24.

LeVine, R. A. (2001). Culture and personality studies, 1918–1960: Myth and history. *Journal of Personality,* 69(6), 803–818.

LeVine, R. A. (2002). Populations, communication and child development. *Human Development,* 45(4), 291–293.

LeVine, R. A., Dixon, S., LeVine, S., Richman, A., Leiderman, P. H., Keefer, C. H., et al. (1994). *Child care and culture: Lessons from Africa.*

Levine, R. E., & Gaw, A. C. (1995). Culture-bound syndromes. *Psychiatric Clinics of North America,* 18(3), 523–536.

Lévi-Strauss, C. (1962). *The savage mind.* London: Weidenfeld & Nicholson.

Lévi-Strauss, C. (1963). *Totemism* (R. Needham, Trans.). Boston: Beacon Press.

Lewontin, R. C. (1974). *The genetic basis of evolutionary change.* New York: Columbia University Press.

Locke, J. L. (1989). Babbling and early speech: Continuity and individual differences. *First Language,* 9, 191–206.

Maccoby, E. E. (1998). *The two sexes: Growing up apart, coming together.* Cambridge, MA: Harvard University Press.

MacLean, P. D. (1985). Brain evolution relating to family, play, and the separation call. *Archives of General Psychiatry,* 42(4), 405–417.

MacLean, P. D. (1993). Cerebral evolution of emotion. In M. Lewis & J. M. Haviland (Eds.), *Handbook of emotions* (pp. 67–83). New York: Guilford Press.

Maestripieri, D. (2001). Is there mother–infant bonding in primates? *Developmental Review, 21(1),* 93–120.

Malinowski, B. (1964). *Sex and repression in savage society.* Cleveland, OH: Meridian Books/World.

Manning, C. J., Wakeland, E. K., & Potts, W. K. (1992). Communal nesting patterns in mice implicate MHC genes in kin recognition. *Nature,* 360, 581–583.

Markus, H. R., & Kitayama, S. (1991). Culture and the self: Implications for cognition, emotion, and motivation. *Psychological Review,* 98(2), 224–253.

Marlowe, F. W. (2005). Who tends Hadza children? In B. S. Hewlett & M. E. Lamb (Eds.), *Hunter-gatherer childhoods: Evolutionary, developmental and cultural perspectives* (pp. 177–190). New Brunswick, NJ: Aldine Transaction.

Martin, R. (1990). *Primate origins and evolution: A phylogenetic reconstruction.* Princeton, NJ: Princeton University Press.

Martin, R. D. (1995). Phylogenetic aspects of primate reproduction: The context of advanced maternal

care. In R. D. Martin, C. R. Pryce, & D. Skuse (Eds.), *Motherhood in human and nonhuman primates: Biosocial determinants* (pp. 16–26). Basel: Karger.

Mayr, E. (1963). *Animal species and evolution.* Cambridge, MA: Harvard University Press.

Mead, M. (1932). An investigation of the thought of primitive children, with special reference to animism. *Journal of the Royal Anthropological Institute,* 62, 173–190.

Mead, M. (1935). *Sex and temperament in three primitive societies.* New York: Morrow.

Mead, M. (1949). *Male and female.* New York: Morrow.

Murdock, G. P. (1949). *Social structure.* London: Macmillan.

Murphy, J. (1976). Psychiatric labelling in cross-cultural perspective. *Science,* 191, 1019–1028.

Murphy, J. M. (1981). Abnormal behavior in traditional societies: Labels, explanations, and social reactions. In R. H. Munroe, R. L. Munroe, & B. B. Whiting (Eds.), *Handbook of cross-cultural human development* (pp. 809–826). New York: Garland STPM Press.

Murphy, J. M. (1994). Anthropology and psychiatric epidemiology. *Acta Psychiatrica Scandinavica, Supplementum,* 385, 48–57.

Nesse, R. M., & Lloyd, A. T. (1992). The evolution of psychodynamic mechanisms. In J. H. Barkow, L. Cosmides, & J. Tooby (Eds.), *The adapted mind: Evolutionary psychology and the generation of culture* (pp. 601–624). New York: Oxford University Press.

Nisbett, R. E. (1993). Violence and U.S. regional culture. *American Psychologist,* 48(4), 441–449.

Paus, T., Collins, D. L., Evans, A. C., Leonard, G., Pike, B., & Zijdenbos, A. (2001). Maturation of white matter in the human brain: R review of magnetic resonance studies. *Brain Research Bulletin,* 54(3), 255–266.

Peacock, N. R. (1991). Rethinking the sexual division of labor: Reproduction and women's work among the Efe. In M. di Leonardo (Ed.), *Gender at the crossroads of knowledge: Feminist anthropology in the postmodern era* (pp. 339–360). Berkeley: University of California Press.

Perme, B., Ranjith, G., Mohan, R., & Chandrasekaran, R. (2005). *Dhat* (semen loss) syndrome: A functional somatic syndrome of the Indian subcontinent? *General Hospital Psychiatry,* 27(3), 215–217.

Plattner, S. (Ed.). (1989). *Economic anthropology.* Stanford, CA: Stanford University Press.

Reinhard, K., Fink, T. M., & Skiles, J. (2003). A case of megacolon in Rio Grande Valley as a possible case of Chagas disease. *Memorias do Instituto Oswaldo Cruz,* 98(Suppl. 1), 165–172.

Robinson, P., & Tajfel, H. (Eds.). (1997). *Social groups and identities: Developing the legacy of Henri Tajfel.* London: Butterworth-Heinemann.

Rogoff, B. (1990). *Apprenticeship in thinking: Cognitive development in social context.* New York: Oxford University Press.

Rogoff, B., Baker-Sennett, J., Lacasa, P., & Goldsmith, D. (1995). Development through participation in sociocultural activity. In J. J. Goodnow, P. J. Miller, & F. Kessel (Eds.), *Cultural practices as contexts for development* (Vol. 67, pp. 45–65). San Francisco: Jossey-Bass.

Rogoff, B., Sellers, M. J., Pirrotta, S., Fox, N., & White, S. H. (1975). Age of assignment of roles and responsibilities to children: A cross-cultural survey. *Human Development, 18,* 353–369.

Rosenblum, L. A., & Kaufman, I. C. (1968). Variations in infant development and response to maternal loss in monkeys. *American Journal of Orthopsychiatry, 38*(3), 418–426.

Sakamoto, N., Martin, R. G., Kumano, H., Kuboki, T., & Al-Adawi, S. (2005). Hikikomori, is it a culture-reactive or culture-bound syndrome?: Nidotherapy and a clinical vignette from Oman. *International Journal of Psychiatry in Medicine, 35*(2), 191–198.

Sapir, E. (1994). *The psychology of culture: A course of lectures.* Berlin: de Gruyter.

Schlegel, A., & Barry, H., III (Eds.). (1991). *Adolescence: An anthropological inquiry.* New York: Free Press.

Shepher, J. (1971). Mate selection among second generation kibbutz adolescents and adults: Incest avoidance and negative imprinting. *Archives of Sexual Behavior, 1,* 293–307.

Sherif, M., Harvey, O. J., White, B. J., Hood, W. R., & Sherif, C. W. (1961). *Intergroup conflict and cooperation: The Robbers Cave experiment.* Norman, OK: Institute of Group Relations.

Shore, B. (1996). *Culture in mind: Cognition, culture, and the problem of meaning.* New York: Oxford University Press.

Shostak, M. (1981). *Nisa: The life and words of a !Kung woman.* Cambridge, MA: Harvard University Press.

Silberbauer, G. B. (1981). *Hunter and habitat in the central Kalahari Desert.* Cambridge, UK: Cambridge University Press.

Silk, J. (1987). Adoption and fosterage in human societies: Adaptations or enigmas? *Cultural Anthropology, 2,* 39–49.

Silk, J. B. (1980). Adoption and kinship in Oceania. *American Anthropologist, 82,* 799–820.

Smuts, B. B., Cheney, D. L., Seyfarth, R. M., Wrangham, R. W., & Struhsaker, T. T. (Eds.). (1987). *Primate societies.* Chicago: University of Chicago Press.

Smuts, B. B., & Smuts, R. W. (1993). Male-aggression and sexual coercion of females in nonhuman-primates and other mammals: Evidence and theoretical implications. *Advances in the Study of Behavior, 22,* 1–63.

Sperber, D. (1996). *Explaining culture: A naturalistic approach.* Oxford, UK: Blackwell.

Spindler, G. D. (1979). *The making of psychological anthropology.* Berkeley: University of California Press.

Spiro, M. E. (1954). Is the family universal? *American Anthropologist, 56,* 839–846.

Spiro, M. E. (1979). *Gender and culture: Kibbutz women revisited.* Durham: Duke University Press.

Spiro, M. E. (1982). *Oedipus in the Trobriands.* Chicago: University of Chicago Press.

Spiro, M. E. (1987). *Culture and human nature.* Chicago: University of Chicago Press.

Spiro, M. E. (1999). Anthropology and human nature. *Ethos, 27,* 7–14.

Stanford, C. B. (2002). The ape's gift: Meat-eating, meat-sharing, and human evolution. In F. B. M. de Waal (Ed.), *Tree of origin: What primate behavior can tell us about human social evolution* (pp. 95–117). Cambridge, MA: Harvard University Press.

Strier, K. B. (1994). Myth of the typical primate. *Yearbook of Physical Anthropology, 37,* 233–271.

Strier, K. B. (2000). *Primate behavioral ecology.* Boston: Allyn & Bacon.

Summerfield, D. (2002). ICD and DSM are contemporary cultural documents. *British Medical Journal, 324,* 914.

Suomi, S. J. (1997). Early determinants of behaviour: Evidence from primate studies. *British Medical Bulletin, 53*(1), 170–184.

Suomi, S. J. (1999). Attachment in rhesus monkeys. In J. Cassidy & P. R. Shaver (Eds.), *Handbook of attachment: Theory, research, and clinical applications* (pp. 181–197). New York: Guilford Press.

Symons, D. (1992). On the use and misuse of Darwinism in the study of human behavior. In J. H. Barkow, L. Cosmides, & J. Tooby (Eds.), *The adapted mind: Evolutionary psychology and the generation of culture* (pp. 137–162). New York: Oxford University Press.

Tajfel, H. (1982). *Social identity and intergroup relations.* New York: Cambridge University Press.

Tanner, N. M. (1987). The chimpanzee model revisited and the gathering hypothesis. In W. G. Kinzey (Ed.), *The evolution of human behavior: Primate models* (pp. 3–27). Albany: State University of New York Press.

Tomasello, M., Kruger, A. C., & Ratner, H. H. (1993). Cultural learning. *Behavioral and Brain Sciences, 16,* 495–452.

Tooby, J., & Cosmides, L. (2000). Toward mapping the evolved functional organization of mind and brain. In M. S. Gazzaniga (Ed.), *The new cognitive neurosciences, second edition* (pp. 1167–1178). Cambridge, MA: MIT Press.

Triandis, H. C. (2001). Individualism-collectivism and personality. *Journal of Personality, 69*(6), 907–924.

Trivers, R. L. (1971). The evolution of reciprocal altruism. *Quarterly Review of Biology.*

Trivers, R. L. (1972). Parental investment and sexual selection. In B. Campbell (Ed.), *Sexual selection and the descent of man, 1871–1971* (pp. 136–179). Chicago: Aldine.

Trivers, R. L. (1974). Parent–offspring conflict. *American Zoologist, 14,* 249–264.

Tronick, E. Z., Morelli, G. A., & Ivey, P. K. (1992). The Efe forager infant and toddler's pattern of social relationships: Multiple and simultaneous. *Developmental Psychology, 28*(4), 568–577.

Tylor, E. B. (1871). *Primitive culture: Researches into the development of mythology, philosophy, religion, language, art and custom.* London: Murray.

van IJzendoorn, M. H., & Sagi, A. (1999). Cross-cultural patterns of attachment: Universal and contextual dimensions. In J. Cassidy & P. R. Shaver (Eds.), *Handbook of attachment: Theory, research, and clinical applications* (pp. 713–734). New York: Guilford Press.

Voronov, M., & Singer, J. A. (2002). The myth of individualism–collectivism: A critical review. *Journal of Social Psychology, 142*(4), 461–480.

Vygotsky, L. (1962). *Thought and language.* Cambridge, MA: MIT Press.

Wallace, A. F. C. (1952). The modal personality structure of the Tuscarora Indians as revealed by the Rorschach test. *Bulletin, Bureau of American Indian Ethnology, 150.*

Weller, S. C., Baer, R. D., de Alba Garcia, J. G., Glazer, M., Trotter, R., Pachter, L., et al. (2002). Regional variation in Latino descriptions of *susto. Culture, Medicine and Psychiatry, 26*(4), 449–472.

Werner, H. (1948). *Comparative psychology of mental development.* Chicago: Follet.

Wertsch, J. V., & Sohmer, R. (1995). Vygotsky on learning and development. *Human Development, 38,* 332–337.

Westermeyer, J. (1985). Psychiatric diagnosis across cultural boundaries. *American Journal of Psychiatry, 142*(7), 798–805.

White, S. (1970). Some general outlines of the matrix of developmental changes between five and seven years. *Bulletin of the Orton Society, 20,* 41–57.

White, S. H. (1996). The child's entry into the "age of reason." In A. J. Sameroff & M. M. Haith (Eds.), *The five to seven year shift: The age of reason and responsibility* (pp. 17–30). Chicago: University of Chicago Press.

Whiting, B. B., & Edwards, C. P. (1988). *Children of different worlds: The formation of social behavior.* Cambridge, MA: Harvard University Press.

Whiting, B. B., & Whiting, J. W. M. (1975). *Children of six cultures: A psychocultural analysis.* Cambridge, MA: Harvard University Press.

Whiting, J. W. (1941). *Becoming a Kwoma.* New Haven, CT: Yale University Press.

Whiting, J. W. M., & Child, I. L. (1953). *Child training and personality: A cross-cultural study.* New Haven, CT: Yale University Press.

Whiting, J. W. M., Child, I. L., & Lambert, W. W. (1966). *Field guide for a study of socialization* (Vol. 1). New York: Wiley.

Whiting, J. W. M., & Whiting, B. B. (1975). Aloofness and intimacy between husbands and wives. *Ethos, 3,* 183–207.

Wiessner, P. (1982). Risk, reciprocity and social influences on !Kung San economics. In E. Leacock & R. B. Lee (Eds.), *Politics and history in band societies* (pp. 61–84). Cambridge, UK: Cambridge University Press.

Wiessner, P. (1996). Leveling the hunter: Constraints on the status quest in foraging societies. In P. Wiessner & W. Schiefenhövel (Eds.), *Food and the status quest: An interdisciplinary perspective* (pp. 171–191). Providence: Berghahn Books.

Wilson, E. O. (1998). *Consilience: The unity of knowledge.* New York: Knopf.

Winterhalder, B., & Smith, E. A. (Eds.). (1981). *Hunter-gatherer foraging strategies: Ethnographic and archeological analyses.* Chicago: University of Chicago Press.

Wolf, A. P. (1995). *Sexual attraction and childhood association: A Chinese brief for Westermarck.* Stanford, CA: Stanford University Press.

Wood, B. (2000). Investigating human evolutionary history. *Journal of Anatomy, 197*(Pt. 1), 3–17.

Wood, B., & Richmond, B. G. (2000). Human evolution: Taxonomy and paleobiology. *Journal of Anatomy, 197*(Pt. 1), 19–60.

Wrangham, R. (1993). The evolution of sexuality in chimpanzees and bonobos. *Human Nature, 4,* 47–79.

Wrangham, R. W., & Peterson, D. (1996). *Demonic males: Apes and the origins of human violence.* Boston: Houghton Mifflin.

Yakovlev, P. I., & Lecours, A. R. (1967). The myelogenetic cycles of regional maturation of the brain. In A. Minkowski (Ed.), *Regional development of the brain in early life* (pp. 3–70). Oxford, UK: Blackwell Scientific.

Zihlman, A. L. (1981). Women as shapers of the human adaptation. In F. Dahlberg (Ed.), *Woman the gatherer* (pp. 75–120). New Haven, CT: Yale University Press.

PART II

THEORY AND METHODS

CHAPTER 5

Cultural–Historical Activity Theory
Integrating Phylogeny, Cultural History, and Ontogenesis in Cultural Psychology

MICHAEL COLE
GIYOO HATANO

This chapter presents an approach to cultural psychology that broadens the issue of culture and *ontogeny* to place the study of culture and human nature in a broad evolutionary and historical framework. We take as our theoretical starting point the position developed by L. S. Vygotsky and his colleagues that human psychological processes can be understood as the emergent outcome of four "genetic domains"—phylogeny, cultural history, ontogeny, and microgenesis (Vygotsky, 1977; Vygotsky & Luria, 1930/1993; Wertsch, 1985). Although the work of the early cultural–historical psychologists is in some respects out of date and can be faulted on various grounds, their emphasis on the constitutive role of culture in development and their broadly inclusive evolutionary framework provide an advantageous foundation upon which to build an integrative cultural psychology.

The expansion of cultural psychology in the direction proposed by early Russian cultural–historical psychologists is an important contemporary task for several reasons. Whereas

those who consider themselves cultural psychologists would not deny that human nature is heavily constrained by our species' phylogenetic heritage, examination of the relationship between phylogeny and culture in ontogeny has, with some notable exceptions, been marginal to development of the field. (For examples of such exceptions see Greenfield, 2004, and Tomasello, 1999, whose work falls under the scope of our present concerns.)

For example, Shweder and his colleagues (1998) explicitly state that human beings are creatures with a long, common phylogenetic past that provides constraints on ontogenetic development. They also invoke ideas about the influence of experience on development that come directly from neuroscience. However, they do not explore how these phylogenetic factors are linked to human ontogeny, restricting themselves to pointing out that whatever these primeval, shared, characteristics are, they "only gain character, substance, definition and motivational force . . . when they are translated and transformed into, and through, the concrete actualities of some particular practice, activity setting, or way of life" (p. 871). In a similar manner, Rogoff (2003) also presupposes, but does not analyze, species-specific phylogenetic foundations of cognitive development, focusing instead on historical changes in cultural practices and shifting modes of participation within and between cultural practices during ontogeny as the cornerstone of her approach.

In light of contemporary evidence, we adopt a version of the early cultural–historical psychologists' approach that can be briefly described as a "skeletal constraints plus cultural practices" view of cultural psychology. This perspective has won a number of adherents in recent years, among both psychologists who typically do not invoke culture as a constituent of development (e.g., Gelman & Kalish, 2006) and those who do (Shweder et al., 2006). This position makes contact with increasingly popular work in the fields of evolutionary developmental psychology and comparative developmental evolutionary psychology, which do focus on the relationship between phylogeny and ontogeny but unfortunately pay little attention to the role of cultural history (e.g., Bjorklund & Pellegrini, 2002; Parker, 2003). Our overall goal is to bring culture–history into the study of human ontogeny without abandoning a commitment to an evolutionary perspective.

BASIC IDEAS OF THE EARLY CULTURAL–HISTORICAL PSYCHOLOGISTS

The Russian cultural–historical school was founded on the assumption that the structural uniqueness and developmental course of human psychological processes emerge in the process of humanity's culturally mediated, historically developing, practical activity (Leontiev, 1981; Luria, 1979; Vygotsky, 1987). Each term in this formulation plays a role in how we conceive of the interplay of phylogeny and cultural history in ontogeny.

Cultural Mediation

According to this approach, characteristically human psychological processes emerged in phylogeny simultaneously with a new form of behavior in which material objects are modified as a means of regulating their interactions with both the physical world and each other. It

was common at the time to refer to such mediational devices as *tools*, but we adopt the more inclusive concept, *artifact*, for reasons that will become clear later.

The basic idea of tool (artifact) mediation of human experience is clearly expressed by Alexander Luria (1928) in the first publication of the idea in English: "Man differs from animals in that he can make and use tools . . . [that] not only radically change his conditions of existence, they even react on him in that they effect a change in him and his psychic condition" (p. 493).

The consequence of tool creation/use for the basic structure of behavior is "that instead of applying directly its natural function to the solution of a particular task, the child *puts between that function and the task a certain auxiliary means . . .* by the medium of which the child manages to perform the task" (Luria, 1928, p. 495, italics in original).[1]

This idea of tool mediation is, of course, not original to early Russian cultural–historical psychologists. It was also central to the ideas of many thinkers at the turn of the 20th century, who emphasized not only tool use but also the creation of tools that generated the idea of *homo faber* (see Cole, 1996, for an extended discussion).

Historical Development

Vygotsky and Luria (1930/1993) included both the history of the human species and historical change following the emergence of modern *Homo sapiens* in their approach to ontogeny. They asserted that the evolutionary, the historical, and the ontogenetic–genetic domains each has its own "turning point" in which *something new* is introduced into the process of development.

Their proposed turning point in phylogeny is the appearance of tool use in apes. The turning point in human history is the appearance of labor and symbolic mediation. The major turning point in ontogeny is the coming together of culture–history and phylogeny with the acquisition of language. The products of these fusions of different "streams of history" are the distinctly human, higher psychological functions.

The overall story concerning the processes of change went something like this: With the higher apes one reaches a point of anthropoid evolution in which tool use is observed (they based the bulk of these ideas on Kohler's work), bespeaking the phylogenetic development of practical intelligence. But there is more to the specifically human form of development than tool use.

> In spite of the fact that the ape displays an ability to invent and use tools—the prerequisite for all human cultural development—the activity of labor, founded on this ability,[2] has still not even minimally developed in the ape. . . . This form of behavior [tool use] does not constitute the main form of adaptation for them. We cannot say that the ape adapts itself to its environment with the help of tools. (Vygotsky & Luria, 1930/1993, p. 74)

Tool use among humans has a different character:

> The entire existence of an Australian aborigine depends upon her machines. Take the boomerang away from the aborigine, make him a farmer, then out of necessity he will have to completely change his life style, his habits, his entire style of thinking, his entire nature. (p. 74)

The crucial difference that distinguishes ape and human ability to use tools and human labor is the involvement of language and symbolic mediation, "tools for the mastery of behavior," as well as nature. This combination produces a qualitatively new form of mediation, one in which tools and languages unite in the artifact. At this point "primitive man" emerges.

Vygotksy and Luria (1930/1993) note that the concept of "primitive man" is an abstraction, "the starting point of historical development" (p. 82). Yet, they argue, data about prehistoric humans ("the lowest rung of cultural development") and people from different contemporary cultures can both provide evidence about the psychology of primitive man.

By their account, historical change from the original humans to modern adult humans occurs along two dimensions. First, there is an increasing use of cultural/mediated/higher functions in place of natural/unmediated/lower functions. Second, there is development in the complexity of the mediational means themselves.

In one of their favorite examples, Vygotsky and Luria (1930/1993) argued that in primitive cultures natural remembering, such as eidetic imagery, is dominant. Incidental memory concerning participation in various events, what we might call "everyday memory," also qualified as natural remembering, a process in which humans record the world but do not actively use their memories to transform it.

This sort of "natural" (to humans) form of everyday memory is built upon phylogenetically evolved, "elementary" psychological processes that are assumed to be universal across cultures and historical periods. "Cultural" memory develops through the elaboration of the "mediational means" by which memory is accomplished and the cultural practices that incorporate these new mediators. Tying a knot around one's finger to control one's memory from the outside and the Inca *quipu* provided clear examples of what Vygotsky and Luria (1930/1993) meant by the "cultural form of behavior."

In short, according to this view, culture undergoes both quantitative change in terms of the number and variety of artifacts, and qualitative change in terms of the new forms of mediated behavior potentials that they embody. As a consequence, both culture and human thinking develop.

In summary, culture, according to this perspective, can be understood as the entire pool of artifacts (including language, norms, customs, tools, values) accumulated by the social group in the course of its historical experience. It is the species-specific *medium* of human development. The capacity to develop within this medium and to arrange for its reproduction in succeeding generations is *the* distinctive characteristic of our species.

Practical Activity

The third basic premise of the cultural–historical approach, adopted from Hegel by way of Marx, is that the analysis of human psychological functions must be grounded in everyday activities. A. N. Leontiev (1981) asserted the primacy of everyday activities with respect to cultural–historical psychology in the following vivid terms:

> . . . human psychology is concerned with the activity of concrete individuals, which takes place either in a collective—that is, jointly with other people—or in a situation in which the subject deals directly with the surrounding world of objects—for example, at the potter's wheel or the writer's desk. . . . With all its varied forms, the hu-

man individual's activity is a system in the system of social relations. It does not exist without these relations. The specific form in which it exists is determined by the forms and means of material and mental social interaction. (p. 11)

Additional principles of the cultural–historical approach to cultural psychology follow from the three already mentioned.

First, because phylogeny, culture–history, and ontogeny are all processes that occur over time and for which change is the central phenomenon to be explained, a developmental approach is required. It is for this reason that Vygotsky often invoked the idea that "to understand behavior we must understand the history of behavior" (Vygotsky & Luria, 1993, p. 79).

Second, this perspective gives a special importance to the *social origins* of human thought processes. As Vygotsky (1929) argued, all means of cultural behavior (*artifacts* in our terminology) are social in their essence: "Social relations or relations among people genetically underlie all higher functions and their relationships" (Vygotsky, 1981, p. 163). This view of social origins arises because of the special role of adults as bearers of the cultural resources of the social group. It does *not* imply a passive child; recall from Luria's earlier statement that incorporating tools (cultural artifacts) into ongoing efforts to master one's environment is the essential marker of the "cultural form of behavior." From this perspective, the biologically maturing child and the socially organized, culturally mediated, social environment "co-construct" development.

A MODERN PERSPECTIVE ON PHYLOGENY AND DEVELOPMENT: HOMIZATION AND PRIMATOLOGY

In deciding to take the phylogenetic past of *H. sapiens* as a starting point for cultural psychology, two errors need to be avoided. First, as Wertsch (1985) pointed out, Vygotsky and his followers, in keeping with their contemporaries in the West (e.g., Kroeber, 1917), adopted a "critical point" theory of phylogeny–culture relations. A critical point theory assumes that at some moment in the distant past, culture arose as a "sudden, all-or-none type of occurrence in the phylogeny of the primates" (Geertz, 1973, pp. 62–63). There is, however, a

good deal of evidence to support Geertz's famous assertion of the *coevolution* of phylogeny and cultural history in the development from the early common ancestor of *H. sapiens* and its nonhuman primate "cousins." Because the human brain developed over millennia during which culture became an ever-more-essential part of human life, it seems necessary to take seriously Geertz's colorful assertion that

man's nervous system does not merely enable him to acquire culture, it positively demands that he do so if it is going to function at all. Rather than culture acting only to supplement, develop, and extend organically based capacities logically and genetically prior to it, it would seem to be ingredient to those capacities themselves. A cultureless human being would probably turn out to be not an intrinsically talented, though unfulfilled ape, but a wholly mindless and consequently unworkable monstrosity. (p. 68)

Contemporary paleological evidence indicates that culture is not an "add on" to a primal, biological human nature. Culture is a biological prerequisite to the normal functioning of the human brain (Plotkin, 2001).

A second problem with the early Russian cultural psychologists' treatment of phylogeny with respect to ontogeny was that it was only minimally developed (Wertsch, 1985). As indicated earlier, their basic idea was that phylogenetic ("natural") contributions to ontogeny are reflected in elementary, unmediated forms of behavior manifested in various psychological realms, including memory, attention, numeracy, and language. For example, with respect to concept formation, a topic of special concern in this chapter, they assumed that the phylogenetic contribution to ontogenetic change was restricted to general cognitive capacities that might change during ontogeny owing to maturation but that the development of systematic category systems depend upon participation in formal schooling, which itself evolved as a cultural institution in connection with the advent of writing. Current evidence, however, indicates that various cognitive capacities once thought to arise entirely from general learning mechanisms and maturation are present at birth, or at least well before the appearance of grammatical language and formal schooling. So a reexamination of the culture and phylogeny relationship with respect to fundamental processes of conceptual development is required to avoid immediate dismissal by contemporary psychologists.

Our treatment of phylogeny, culture, and ontogenetic development is divided into three sections. The first discusses nonhuman primates' cognition and culture from a comparative cognitive science perspective. This discussion is closely related to what is called "phylogenetic development," but instead of examining primates' biological evolution based on archeological evidence, we exploit information from currently living species of nonhuman primates, especially chimpanzees, as our evolutionary neighbors. As will be seen, the reconstructed picture of phylogenesis using such evidence indicates that culture plays a minor, though significant, role in behavioral development and change among nonhuman primates.

The second section covers the process of hominization. It is generally agreed that human beings and chimpanzees/bonobos shared a common ancestor some 6 million years ago (Noble & Davidson, 1996). The successors to the common ancestor that lead to *H. sapiens sapiens* (some 20 species of which have subsequently disappeared) underwent massive changes not only in the brain and in physical morphology of the body (bipedalism; the structure of the arms, hands, fingers, vocal tract, etc.) but also in physical ecology, cognitive capacities, and the accumulation of the products of the past in the form of human culture. By contrast, there is no evidence that the anatomy, body size, physical morphology, behavior, cognitive abilities, and modes of life have changed markedly over the past several million years among chimpanzees or bonobos.

The third section covers the period of history following the "great leap forward," when human cultural capacities were clearly present. Change during this period has been particularly rapid; cultural–historical–social change is much faster than biological evolution, because our experiences can be accumulated and revised in the form of increasingly elaborated artifacts. In turn, human intellectual achievements are unique, because humans accumulate their experiences in the form of culture, so that offspring can access and incorporate them through language or other mediational means.

Taken together, the discussion in this section provides the essential context within which to consider human ontogeny and its relationship to human culture in evolutionary context, the topic for the last section.

Cognition and Culture among Nonhuman Primates

In the middle of the 20th century, Darwin's views to the contrary, Anglo-American scholars who considered culture a significant contributor to human development adopted the idea of "human exceptionalism," the belief that the human species is distinguishable by its cognitive capacities, which in turn owe their special powers to the involvement of culture in their operation. Despite challenging cognitive abilities shown by Kohler's apes and parallel experiments in Russia documenting apes' problem-solving skills, researchers have maintained that, in many crucial respects, human beings are not only quantitatively but also qualitatively different than other species in both their cognitive abilities and their use of culture as a medium of human life (these views are summarized in Cole, 1996). This view was not universal. For example, in Japan, where wild monkeys live, both professionals and laypeople regard them as human-like, though with several notable differences (e.g., the hairy body, a tail, slightly less intelligence).

The antiexceptionalism (continuity) side of this controversy, Darwinian saltation of cognitive capacity or cultural characteristics (producing a change in degree not kind), was revolutionized by such scientific milestones as DNA comparisons between humans and chimpanzees (Marks, 2002) and the ethnographic/ecological observations of communities of chimpanzees pioneered by Jane Goodall (1968). Such achievements made it more manageable to think of bonobos and chimpanzees as genetically and psychologically very similar to humans. Matt Ridley (2003) summed up the shifting conceptions of chimpanzee mental, social, and cultural capacities when he referred to Goodall's descriptions of chimpanzee behavior in the wild as "simian soap operas." Goodall's chimps deceived each other; "cheated" on each other, and even killed each other. They also used leaves and sticks to fish for ants, and their offspring seemed to learn from seeing them do this.

We first examine current evidence concerning tool use and cognitive abilities, consider evidence for the presence of culture among nonhuman primates. Then we turn to the question of culture–cognition relations in these species and the questions those relations pose for scholars interested in culture–cognition relations in human ontogeny.

Acquisition and Use of Tools

At least from the time of Kohler's classic studies of problem solving, a great deal of attention has focused on chimpanzee tool use and tool creation. McGrew's (1998) summary regarding tools clearly indicates the nature of current claims for chimpanzee tool use and toolmaking capabilities:

> Each chimpanzee population has its own customary tool kit, made mostly of vegetation, that functions in subsistence, defense, self-maintenance, and social relations. . . . Many have tools sets, in which two or more different tools are used as composites to solve a problem. . . . The same raw material serves multiple functions: A leaf may be a drinking vessel, napkin, fishing probe, grooming stimulator, courtship signaler, or medication. . . . Conversely, a fishing probe may be made of bark, stem, twig, vine, or the midrib of a leaf. An archeologist would have no difficulty classifying the cross-cultural data in typological terms, based on artifacts alone; for example, only the far western subspecies . . . uses stone hammers and anvils to crack nuts. . . . Given this ethnographic record, it is difficult to differentiate, based on material culture, living chimpanzees from earliest *Homo* . . . or even from the simplest living human foragers. (pp. 317–318)

In at least one case it has been claimed that chimpanzees carry different tools with them to accomplish different goals (Boesch & Boesch, 1984). The chimpanzees in question encountered two kinds of nuts in their foraging, one with hard shells, the other with softer shells. For the harder nuts, they transported harder, heavier hammers (mostly stones) from their home base. They seemed to remember the location of stones and to choose the stones so as to keep the transport distance minimal.

Boesch and Boesch (1984) concluded that these chimpanzees possess a representation of Euclidian space that allows them to measure and remember distances; to compare several such distances so as to choose the stone with the shortest distance to a goal tree; to locate a new stone location with reference to different trees; and to change their reference point to measure the distance to each tree from any stone location. In a study with the bonobo Kanzi, raised in captivity, Savage-Rumbaugh and her colleagues obtained a similar result using lexigrams for location (Menzel, Savage-Rumbaugh, & Menzel, 2002).

Some tool use is reported also among monkeys. For example, Japanese macaques can be trained to use tools skillfully, though they seldom do so in their natural environment. The monkeys, using a rake, can pull closer food that is placed beyond their reach after 2 weeks or so of training (Ishibashi, Hihara, & Irik, 2000). Interestingly, in these trained monkeys, "bimodal" neurons in the intraparietal cortex respond to visual stimuli not only near the hand but also surrounding the tool, suggesting that the tool becomes literally an extension of the body part. The monkeys can also be trained to use two tools successively, that is, to use first a nearby short rake to pull closer a long rake, then to pull closer food that can be reached only by the long rake. Moreover, they can learn to monitor the movement of their hand and tool on a video screen (Iriki, Tanaka, Obayashi, & Iwamura, 2001). The authors claim that though higher-order cognitive abilities such as tool use do not emerge spontaneously, this capacity exists and begins to manifest itself when there is external pressure to exploit it.

Culture among Monkeys and Apes

Belief in a narrow, quantitative gap between human and nonhuman primate cognition is paralleled by belief in a narrow gap with respect to culture (Wrangham, McGrew, de Waal, & Heltne, 1994). However, in making such claims, one must be mindful of the fact that the researchers adopt what might be called a "minimalist" definition of their object of study by focusing on culture as behavioral traditions spread or maintained by nongenetic means through processes of social learning. This kind of definition is useful because it does not presuppose characteristics that are themselves arguably specifically human (e.g., religious beliefs, aesthetic values, social institutions, etc.); hence, the analyst can remain agnostic with respect to culture–cognition relationships. It allows examination of the extent to which cognitive characteristics claimed to be necessary for acquisition of human culture are present in displays of nonhuman primate behavioral traditions (cultures) such as deliberate teaching or toolmaking and use. And it leaves open the question of how similar the cultures of humans and apes might be.

The textbook example of a tradition for which we know the origin and have data on its spread comes from sweet potato washing by Japanese macaque monkeys on Koshima Island. In 1953 a juvenile female monkey was observed washing a muddy sweet potato in a stream. This behavior first spread to peers and then to older kin. Ten years later, it was observed among more than 50% of the population and 30 years later, by 71%. A few years later the same monkey invented a form of "wheat sluicing" in which wheat that had been mixed with sand was cast upon water, so that the floating bits of wheat could be easily sorted from the sinking sand. Within 30 years, 93% of the group engaged in this behavior. It is not clear whether this shared behavioral tradition was based on monkeys' observational learning or imitation in the strict sense, or on the availability of environmental cues, including other members' behaviors that attract their attention (Matsuzawa, 2003).

Such cultural traditions do not remain entirely static and need not bear any discernable relation to subsistence activities. A group of monkeys living in the far north adopted the tradition of bathing in warm springs in winter; initially the mothers left their offspring on the edge of the pools, but the young monkeys began to swim under water. Several groups of macaques routinely handle small stones in a variety of ways (rolling, rubbing, piling) that are not related to any discernable adaptive function. These observations blunt attempts to find restrictions of the observed cultural behaviors to subsistence constraints.

Chimpanzees have provided the most extensive evidence on nonhuman culture based not only on specially provisioned populations, such as the Koshima macaques, but also on several dozen wild populations and long-term studies in zoos and laboratories. The behavioral traditions involved have included ways of using probes for termites and ants, nut cracking by using sticks and stones in various ways, hunting strategies, nest building, and styles of grooming behavior (McGrew, 1998; Matsuzawa, 2001; Whitten, 2000; Wrangham et al., 1994). (Interestingly, in light of their importance in discussions of both primate language and cognition, bonobos in the wild appear to display no evidence of tool use. This species difference should serve to block any simple equation between tool use and either cognitive development or the existence of cultural traditions.)

Among chimpanzees, some tools may be left over and used again by other members of a group. In a sense, leftover tools constitute culture as a set of socially inherited artifacts. In fact, Hirata and Morimura (2000) found that leftover tools serve as environmental cues enhancing chimps' observational learning of honey fishing (an experimental simulation of ant/termite fishing found in the wild). Naive chimpanzees often observed their experienced partners after their own failed first attempts and also used the leftover tools of the experienced ones. Hirata and Celli (2003) further suggested that infant chimpanzees in captivity acquire honey fishing behaviors earlier than recorded in the wild not only by repeatedly observing the behaviors of experienced mothers but also by using selectively the tools often used by mothers.

In summary, this evidence indicates that there must be some evolutionary continuity between humans and other apes and monkeys in potential competencies. However, for the potentialities to be actualized, "a human-like social-cognitive environment," or even human intensive teaching, appears necessary (Tomasello, 1994).

Culture and Hominization

A few relatively uncontroversial "facts" serve as anchors for more accounts of hominid evolution prior to the advent of modern human beings. The best available evidence is found with respect to morphological changes and to changes in material artifacts. More speculative is the evidence concerning the evolution of language and cognition.

Brain Size and Other Morphological Changes

There is a marked increase in the size of the brain in the sequence of species leading to *H. sapiens sapiens*. The most frequent way of calculating this increase is to represent brain size in relation to overall body size, which is referred to as an encephalization quotient (EQ; Falk & Gibson, 2001). The EQ of modern humans is almost three times that of the chimpanzee and other great apes. More interestingly, this growth appears to have been especially pronounced in the frontal and prefrontal cortices, hippocampus, and cerebellum, all heavily implicated in cognitive changes both in phylogeny and ontogeny. Of special interest has been the appearance, derived from endocasts (moldings of the inside of skulls) of increased brain volume in Broca's area that appears with the advent of *Homo erectus*, because of the relationship of Broca's area to language in normally developing modern humans.

Also widely studied have been morphological changes in other parts of the body that are associated with species changes following divergence from the common ancestor. Such changes include bipedalism and various changes in anatomy, with significance for hominization such as changes in the hand implicated in fine motor control (especially the opposable thumb), the pelvic region (which is crucial to the timing of birth and the length of infancy), and the vocal apparatus necessary for rapid a fluent speech (see Lewin & Foley, 2004, for a summary).

Bipedalism is often considered to be the first step toward hominization, because whereas the EQ of members of *Australopithecus* was about the same as that of present-day chimpanzees, there is clear evidence that some of them were bipedal walkers. Bipedalism required radical morphological changes that might have endangered early ancestors' lives in the trees, where they were relatively safe. Moreover, bipedalism was *not* absolutely necessary in the wood-savanna mosaic region where they initially lived. Its direct advantage was that bipedalism in the upright posture was more economical in the use of energy for long-distance locomotion, thus enabling bipedal creatures to get food from a relatively wide geographical area. Bipedalism changed selection pressure, because different morphological characteristics became adaptive.

Changes in Material Artifacts

Data relevant to the cultural sphere, particularly the evidence of changes in material artifacts, are perhaps the second most reliable source of evidence concerning cognition–culture relations (Foley & Lahr, 2003). *Australopithecus*, or even the common ancestor, can be assumed to have used stone tools because chimpanzees do so, but they may not have made clearly identifiable artifacts. The first, crude tools are usually said to appear with *Homo habilis*, the earliest *Homo*. These tools, called Oldowan artifacts, were made of stone according to most interpreters, and appear to have been made by shattering small rocks to make sharp-edged implements (choppers) and additional tools, such as knives made by chipping off flakes from the remaining stone core. Although they were not very sophisticated, producing them seems beyond bonobo's capability (Toth, Schick, Savage-Rumbaugh, Sevcik, & Rumbaugh, 1993). The tools were used, it is believed, mainly for cutting dead animals into small pieces, because, unlike *Australopithecus*, which was mostly herbivorous, *H. habilis* was a scavenger who ate the animal protein needed to grow and maintain its enlarged brain.

H. erectus is generally believed to provide evidence of a quantum increase in size and the complexity of the cultural tool kit. According to this line of interpreting the fossil record, tools now included hand axes with two cutting edges, which required a much more complex manufacturing process.

With respect to the way of living, which is inferred from the tools and the uses to which they were presumably put (e.g., cutting up large animals for meat, and skins used as clothing), as well as evidence of group size and patterns of food consumption, *H. erectus* appears to have been a "critical turning point." For the first time there is evidence of creatures who lived in relatively permanent base camps, had stone tools that clearly differed from any claimed for other species, and ventured out to hunt and gather. *H. erectus* revealed a reduced sex difference in size, implying changes in male–female relationships—for example, a male may have helped a female who had to take care of an infant for an extended period of time because it was born in an immature state. *H. erectus* had molar teeth reduced in size, which suggests that the species had to masticate less owing to the use of fire for cooking. It was also *H. erectus* that ventured out of Africa and made its appearance in Asia and Europe.

It should be noted that, initially, change in the hominid tool kit was exceedingly slow, lasting perhaps a million years. The rate of change, the variety, and the complexity of tools increased in the course of human evolution, although the timing of changes is disputed (Foley & Lahr, 2003; Lewin & Foley, 2004). This fact has potentially important implications. First, cumulative cultural evolution, or the "ratchet effect" (Tomasello, 1999) is not always clearly observed; culture as a set of shared artifacts may have been inherited by the following generations almost unchanged. Second, insofar as culture is stable and enduring, it often induces selection pressure for particular types of competence (e.g., for designing and manufacturing an axe). Generally speaking, when there are genetically transmitted variations among group members in a number of properties, which ones are adaptive (i.e., advantageous for having many offspring) is determined by not only the natural but also the sociocultural environment.

Evolution of Language and Cognition

When we get to *H. erectus*, some scholars argue that language was one constituent of a pattern of increased cognitive and cultural complexity (Bickerton, 1990; Deacon, 1997; Dunbar, 2004). Others argue that language came later, or with the advent of *H. sapiens sapiens*, owing to the development of a specialized vocal tract that could produce rapid speech (Lieberman, 1984). We believe that these conflicting views can be reconciled by assuming a few stages in the evolution of language. For example, protolanguage (Jackendoff, 1994), which mainly relies on two-word combinations, may have appeared early and functioned well, because even pidgin is quite useful for communication within a small and familiar group. In contrast, syntactically more sophisticated language may have appeared fairly late, as more precise and detailed information had to be communicated in a larger group. Whether early or late in hominization, symbolic language is agreed to be essential to the emergence of modern humans.

Suggestions for important cognitive changes that may have accompanied language include increased ability to coordinate motor and spatial processing (Stout, Toth, Schick, Stout, & Hutchins, 2000; Wynn, 1989), increased ability to cooperate with others over extended periods of time to produce standardized products (Foley & Lahr, 2003), and increased ability to imitate the behavior of others (Donald, 1991, 2000; for discussion of Donald's views, pro and con, see Renfrew & Scarre, 1998).

An intriguing puzzle in the story of hominization is the apparent "great cognitive leap forward" that seems to have occurred approximately 45,000 years ago. V. S. Ramachandran (2000) succinctly describes this discontinuous change in the following way:

> The hominid brain grew at an accelerating pace until it reached its present size of 1500 cc about 200,000 years ago. Yet uniquely human abilities such the invention of highly sophisticated "standardized" multi-part tools, tailored clothes, art, religious belief and perhaps even language are thought to have emerged quite rapidly around 40,000 years ago—a sudden explosion of human mental abilities and culture that is sometimes called the "big bang." If the brain reached its full human potential—or at least size—200,000 years ago why did it remain idle for 150,000 years? (p. 4)

Whereas some posit a genetic mutation to account for these changes (Berlim, Mattevi, Belmonte-de-Abreu, & Crow, 2003), as Ramachandran points out, it appears most likely that rapid environmental changes brought together heretofore isolated hominid groups, creating the conditions for the emergence of those cultural innovations that make us uniquely human. This position has been bolstered by evidence of a great many species whose remains have been found in Africa, bespeaking the presence of various elements of the "human revolution" (new technologies, long-distance trading, systematic use of pigment for art and decoration) tens of thousands of years earlier than previously thought but never fully developed in one place (McBreaty & Brooks, 2000). By this latter account, the "human revolution" was simply "human evolution" in which many isolated changes in different species came together with the changes in climate and population that brought disparate peoples together 40,000 years ago in Europe.

Still another interpretation is in terms of increased fluidity among domain-specific knowledge systems (Mithen, 1996). Mithen claims that whereas Neanderthal's stone toolmaking, social skills, and natural history knowledge were as advanced as those of modern humans, they were unable to integrate the knowledge located within each of these domains. In contrast, modern humans could produce, for example, artistic cave drawings and tools well suited to their target use, by integrating needed pieces of information across domains.

We refer briefly to mirror neurons in this context. Mirror neurons are activated both when an animal observes and when it executes a specific action. Such neurons have been observed in the premotor area of monkeys (Rizzolatti & Craighero, 2004) and are assumed to exist in the corresponding area of human and other great apes' brains. The neurons seem to serve as the basis of the understanding and imitation of others' actions (Brass & Heyes, 2005; Rizzolatti, Fadiga, Fogassi, & Gallese, 2002). Some researchers (e.g., Ramachandran, 2000) speculate that mirror neurons provided primates with the foundation for the development of the theory of mind, language, and culture.

It is certainly premature to attribute any definite role to mirror neurons in the formation of these characteristically human competencies.

We would suggest a more conservative view than the authors cited in the preceding paragraph, because although mirror neurons may facilitate, they cannot be the sufficient condition for a social-cognitive development such as imitation. Monkeys, and even chimpanzees in the wild, seldom imitate. Having mirror neurons is at best a genetic potential, the realization of which needs the right ecological conditions. Mirror neurons are probably not the necessary condition either, because there can be other routes for the acquisition of socio-cognitive skills (e.g., "emotional reactivity"; Hare & Tomasello, 2005).

A Tentative Conclusion

If we seek to rise above the myriad disagreements among those who attempt to synthesize analyses and interpretations regarding the processes of hominization, the most important conclusion for our purposes is that the relations between biological, cultural, and cognitive change are reciprocal. The "virtuous circle" that the evidence most strongly supports is that changes in anatomy (increased relative brain volume) is linked to a change in diet, in particular, greater intake of protein from the killing and ingestion of animals. The ability to kill and eat animals was in turn linked to concomitant anatomical changes (the ability to run long distances that evolved following the evolution of the ability to walk upright, which also freed the hands and was accompanied by greater dexterity of the fingers). These biological changes were both cause and result of increased sophistication of the cultural tool kit, including the control of fire (a clearly cultural practice, but one whose origins are disputed across a million year margin). The development of a richer diet, and the way of life associated with it, enabled the growth of new cognitive capacities, which further enriched the cultural tool, which in turn further supported growth of the brain, and so on. As Henry Plotkin (2001) emphasized, human evolution and cultural evolution are two-way streets of causal interactions.

CULTURAL HISTORY

Although there are innumerable differing explanations for the causes of the transition to *H. sapiens sapiens* (a genetic change; a change in climate enabling increased interactivity among

groups of *H. sapiens*, creating a critical mass of cultural isolates; some combination of the above; etc.), there is reasonable agreement that the following key features indicating the presence of genetically modern *H. sapiens* were observable between 40,000 and 50,000 years ago, the "high Paleolithic" period of paleontology:

1. Semeiosis, or the act of creating signs that stand for objects and number.
2. Production of second-order tools to create a variety of new tools, such as points, awls, needles, pins, and spear throwers.
3. An ability to visualize the complex action of tools or simple machines.
4. Complex spatial–structural organization of living sites.
5. Long-distance transport of raw materials such as stones and shells over tens or even hundreds of kilometers.
6. Rapid expansion of human populations into territories previously occupied by earlier, developed forms of humans and rapid replacement of the indigenous populations.
7. Further expansion into territories not previously inhabited by humans.
8. An increase in population densities to levels comparable to those of hunting and gathering societies of historical times (Cheyne, n.d.).

Here, it appears, is the beginning of modern humans, the "cavemen" and "hunter–gatherers" of anthropological, paleontological, and historical lore.

A number of sources present a roughly agreed-upon story of changes following the emergence of biologically modern humans over the next 35,000 to 40,000 years (cf. Diamond, 1997; Donald, 1991; Gellner, 1988). Some of the hunter–gatherers who inhabited parts of the earth and lived in small bands went on to engage in sedentary agriculture. Among some agriculturalists there emerged in some places aggregations of people into city-states and a marked increase in sociocultural complexity (Feinman, 2000). Among others, older ways of life continued in very much the same way for millennia.

A defining characteristic of the Paleolithic period was the appearance of external systems of symbolic, representational cave art, statuary, and perhaps elementary counting devices (Donald, 2001). According to Damerow (1998), it seems most reasonable to consider the many millennia between the beginning of the Paleolithic period and the Neolithic period around 8,000 B.C. (when people began to domesticate plants and animals, and live in permanent villages) as a historical equivalent of the transition from sensorimotor to preoperational thinking. If, as McGrew (1987) argues, such societies approximate the level encountered in small, face-to-face societies during the European age of exploration, it provides evidence in favor of the assumption that the cognitive processes of such peoples are best characterized as preoperational (Hallpike, 1979).

According to both Damerow (1998) and Donald (1991, 2001), the urban revolution coinciding with the smelting of copper, and then bronze, and the elaboration of tools, weapons, and agricultural techniques, marks the transition from preoperational to operational thinking in human history. Two important lessons for contemporary studies of culture and human ontogeny are emphasized by this literature. First, when concrete operational thinking begins to make an appearance, it is tightly bound to particular domains of culturally organized activity. Second, the causal relations between the development of culture and the historical development of cognition were reciprocal. Like Plotkin (2001), quoted earlier, who was referring to the process of hominization, Donald (2000) is emphatic in his conclusion that the brain and culture "have evolved so closely that the form of each is greatly constrained by the other" (p. 25). Moreover, with the advent of literacy especially, "culture actually configures the complex symbolic systems needed to support it by engineering the functional capture of the brain for epigenesis" (p. 23).

However intriguing, the difficulty with using prehistoric and even historical materials that have survived only in images and stone artifacts is that we have too little information about their contexts of use to make refined inferences about culture and cognitive development in ontogeny. Moreover, the notion that people in small, face-to-face, nonliterate societies had the cognitive capabilities of 3- to 5-year-old children living in industrialized societies has been rejected on both theoretical and empirical grounds (cf. Laboratory of Comparative Human Cognition, 1983). For these reasons, studies enabled by rapid cultural–historical change in most parts of the world over the past several decades are particularly valuable. Conditions of rapid cultural–historical change make it easier to tease apart

relations between cultural–historical and ontogenetic change, because there are coexisting generations close to each other in age that engaged in markedly different culturally organized activities but were phylogenetically speaking, contemporaries.

Cross-Sectional Cultural–Historical Comparisons

Perhaps the most well-known study to focus on the relation of rapid cultural–historical change to cognitive change was carried out by Alexander Luria (1976) in the early 1930s. Luria studied a cohort of people under conditions of rapid change in remote parts of the Kyrgyzstan and Uzbekistan.

The historical occasion, the collectivization of agricultural labor under state control, brought with it changes, such as formal schooling, modern labor, and exposure to bureaucratic state agencies, during what can fairly be described as a revolutionary period in that part of the world. Luria concluded that the new modes of life deeply affected the dominant modes of thought, such that the "premodern" group was restricted to a form of "graphical/functional" reasoning based on common experience, while modernization brought with it access to scientific concepts that replaced graphical/functional thinking.

Luria's conclusions are open to at least two criticisms. First, according to the basic methodology underlying his theory, Luria's data should have come from either direct observation of people engaged in identifiable indigenous activities (or schools and collective farms) or experimental models of those activities. Instead, he used the results from psychological tasks originating in studies of developmental changes, or the effects of brain damage, among Europeans. The interview situation itself was an alien form of activity to the traditional pastoralists who served as subjects in Luria's experiments, so that their responses may have reflected as much the alien nature of the modes of discourse as the influence of their own cultural experience employed in indigenous activities. Second, the failure to gather data from the theoretical site of change, the activities themselves, made it difficult to grasp the change processes at work and made it appear that the changes from concrete–graphic to theoretical thinking were of a general nature.

Subsequent research replicating Luria's results in different parts of the world confirmed his basic empirical observations but cast doubt on his conclusions of general cognitive change associated with schooling or involvement in modern economic enterprises. Tulviste (1979), Scribner (1977) and Scribner and Cole (1981), among others, found that a few years of schooling increased dramatically the tendency of people to respond to syllogistic reasoning problems "theoretically," that is, in terms of the logic of the problem as presented, whereas those with little or no schooling responded in terms of their empirical knowledge about the contents of the problems presented. But these same authors presented evidence of theoretical reasoning among nonschooled people, whereas others have shown that even highly educated people are likely to depend upon their empirical knowledge of the contents of the problem presented in many cases (D'Andrade, 1989). The result has been a convergence on the conclusion that cultural–historical variations in cognition (i.e., verbal syllogistic reasoning) arise from, and are closely related to, the introduction of new forms of activity (Tulviste, 1999). New forms of reasoning become general only insofar as the activities giving rise to them are general in the society in question.

Research by King Beach (1995) in an area of Nepal undergoing rapid historical change appears to overcome some of the uncertainties of Luria's approach and its replications by including indigenous activities discovered through ethnographic observation in psychological problem-solving tasks that were themselves modeled on the activities observed. Beach studied changing forms of arithmetic calculations in a Nepalese village that underwent rapid socioeconomic and cultural change in the 1960s and 1970s. As roads from India moved closer to the village, schooling was introduced for the first time and continued to expand over ensuing decades. Shops that exchanged merchandise for money appeared during the same period and rapidly increased in number.

At the time Beach initiated this research in the late 1980s, two coexisting generations of Nepalese men had experienced different relations between their experience of traditional farming and new cultural institutions such as shopkeeping and schooling. All groups shared some experience with subsistence agriculture and the need to buy and sell in the shops using traditional nonmetric units to measure a given length of cloth, then calculate their price in terms of meters and centimeters, to which the monetary price was linked. However, whereas the traditional system relied on using the length from the elbow to the tip of the middle finger, the newly introduced system involved use of a ruler and the metric system.

Some senior high school students were apprenticed to shopkeepers in the village, whereas some shopkeepers who had never had the opportunity to attend school were enrolled in an adult literacy/numeracy class. Farmers who had never attended school or worked in a shop also completed a shopkeeping apprenticeship or were enrolled in the adult education class. The transitions between education and work activities induced as a part of Beach's (1995) study simulated larger-scale changes taking place in rural Nepalese society.

Some of the mathematical problems posed by Beach (1995) to track changes in arithmetic during the shop apprenticeship involved purchases requiring translation and calculation between the two measurement systems. Arithmetic problems presented to those enrolled in the adult education class were the kind typically encountered in school mathematics classes.

Traditionally, shopkeepers used indigenous arithmetic forms that bear little surface relationship to either metric measurement (arm lengths vs. a metric measuring stick) or to the methods of calculating amounts and prices (the use of objects and other artifacts, as well as traditional decomposition strategies, vs. the use of paper and pencil to write equations and calculate with column algorithms). Those students becoming shopkeepers continued to use the written form they had learned in school after they entered the shops, even though reliable traditional methods long in use were prevalent there. Over time and with much pressure from the shopkeeper and customers, the students adapted their written form to the calculation strategies used by the shopkeepers. Those who began as shopkeepers and were studying in the adult education class initially used their arms and traditional measurement objects to carry out their calculations but eventually adopted a flexible approach, sometimes using traditional measurement units and calculation strategies, and at other times doing written calculations adapted to the problem.

From interviews with the participants, Beach (1995) was able to determine that students who were becoming shopkeepers viewed themselves as engaged in two activities that initially contradicted each other—school learning and shopkeeping. The status of schooling and of "being educated" made it difficult for them give up the written form of calculation, though the speed and adaptability of the shopkeepers' calculations eventually induced them to adapt their written form to the shopkeepers' calculation strategies. In this way their status as formally educated adults was retained, marked by their use of writing, but they could use the written form to do the calculations they needed to do as shopkeepers more quickly and accurately. Even though they were in an evening school, the shopkeepers always thought of themselves as engaged in shopkeeping activities (their own shopkeeping activities) and shifted over to the school-based system only when they saw that it facilitated their ongoing work as shopkeepers. By virtue of both the tasks he presented and the way he presented them, Beach verified the links between cultural–historical and ontogenetic change that depended on both the history of relations between the activities and the individuals' developmental history when they began to participate in those activities. Beach's results point to a process of culturally inflected ontogenesis that is much more variable and more content–artifact–activity-specific than Luria's results would suggest.

Longitudinal Studies of Cultural–Historical Change

Despite differences in methods, the research by Beach (1995) and Luria (1976) involved people with different amounts of exposure to new cultural practices. The studies are, in this sense, cross-sectional developmental studies.[3] In the longitudinal studies briefly sketched in this section the same developmentalist returned after many years to the same cultural group, so that it is possible to document the course of cognitive development under changed sociocultural conditions at two disparate historical times.

Historical Change and Cognitive Change in Zinacantan

In the late 1960s, Greenfield and Childs (1977) went to a Mayan community in the state of Chiapas, Mexico, where they began to study the cognitive and social consequences of learning to weave. Their work included experimental tests of categorizing ability by both boys and girls, careful descriptions of the weaving process of women and young girls being apprenticed into weaving, and analysis of the products produced. In the 1990s they returned to the same village and conducted parallel observations of parents (former child subjects) inducting their children into weaving and the products of this work (Greenfield, 1999; Greenfield, Maynard, & Childs, 2000).

In recent written comparisons of the relation among cultural change, modes of weaving, and modes of weaving instruction, Greenfield has emphasized the interconnectedness of historical change in economic activity, exposure to new products and practices resulting from contact with people representing the modern sector of Mexican society, changed socialization practices (in particular, modes of socializing girls into weaving), and changed cognitive processes involving the mental representation of the patterns in woven cloth (Greenfield, 2002, 2004; Greenfield et al., 2000). These changes are viewed as interconnected.

The analysis begins with historical changes in general modes of living. In contrast with the late 1960s, by the mid-1990s this Mayan community had shifted from an economy based primarily on subsistence agriculture and relative seclusion from the modern state to one based more heavily on involvement in the money economy, trade, and much more frequent interaction with people and trade from outside the village and the local region.

The instructional mode characterizing the mother–child weaving sessions in 1970 emphasized a long process of socialization involving many roles preparatory to weaving itself. When children first began to weave, mothers hovered close by and guided children with their own hands and bodies, using little verbal instruction. The entire system appeared to focus on maintenance of tradition that Greenfield and her colleagues (2000) characterized as "interdependent cultural learning."[4] In the 1990s, mothers who were more involved in the modern economy (e.g., by weaving products for sale) instructed their children verbally from a distance, sometimes using older siblings to take over instruction, and the children learned by a process that Greenfield and her colleagues characterize as "independent cultural learning," characterized by a good deal more trial and error and self correction of errors.

The variety of products also changed. In the late 1960s, the variety of products was limited, reflecting a very small set of "right ways to weave cloth." By the 1990s there was no longer a small set of simple, "correct" patterns, but an efflorescence of patterns, indicating the increased respect paid to individual innovation that comes with a trial-and-error approach to learning. This proliferation in turn depended upon, and contributed to, changes in weaving practices.

Accompanying these historical changes were changes in the way children represented weaving patterns in an experimental task by inserting sticks of varying width and color into a rack to reproduce model patterns from woven models. Instead of using, for example, three white sticks to represent a broad band of white cloth, they were more likely to use a single broad white stick in the later historical period, and those who attended school were more likely to be able to create novel patterns. Importantly these historical changes were accompanied by an unchanging pattern of representational development related to age: Older children in both historical periods were more able than younger children to represent more complex visual patterns, a fact that Greenfield et al. (2000) interpret as an indication of universal developmental processes accompanying culturally contingent ones.

Based on her decades-long involvement with a Mayan community in the Yucatan, Suzanne Gaskins (1999, 2000, 2003) notes the same kinds of economic changes observed by Greenfield and her associates (2000) but provides a different, although compatible, explanation of the causal factors involved. Gaskins focuses on how the changing economic circumstances change maternal work patterns, suggesting that reduced time spent on traditional chores (e.g., hauling water because there is running water, or having a longer day because of electricity) and in the commercial sector outside the home shifts the division of labor inside the house in a variety of ways that reduce direct parental involvement with children's socialization in general, not just with respect to specific practices such as weaving.

Differences in interpretation of underlying process notwithstanding, the Greenfield et al. (2000) multigenerational study brings a whole new range of data to bear on the question of the mechanisms of cultural change and accumulation, suggesting a strong link between cultural change resulting from the interaction of cultures and the development of new means of teaching and learning that accompanies the shift to more intensively commercially mediated forms of life.

The Cultural Evolution of Arithmetic in New Guinea

A second "longitudinal cultural–historical" study was begun in the late 1970s by Geoffrey Saxe and his colleagues, who conducted a number of developmental studies among the Oksapmin from a remote area in the highlands of central New Guinea (Saxe, 1982, 1994). The number system used by the Oksapmin became the subject of longitudinal cultural–historical comparisons.

Traditionally, the Oksapmin use a 27-digit counting system based upon body parts, beginning with the pinky of the right hand and ending at the pinky of the left hand. When Saxe first arrived, he found the traditional number system in wide use, but that people who had traveled to earn money at nearby tea and copra plantations were likely to bring back a taste for not only some of the goods they encountered there but also money (a heretofore unknown phenomenon), which could be exchanged for those desirable consumer goods. Moreover, the outside world had penetrated Oksapmin life sufficiently for there to be schools whose teachers taught in an English-related pidgin language, in which children learned base-10 arithmetic and the standard calculation procedures.

More than two decades later, Saxe and Esmonde (2005) returned to the Oksapmin. As one means for studying population variations associated with various schooling experience or the use of money (which was now much more prevalent in the area because of increased trade in agricultural products and the introduction of mining in not-too-distant areas), Saxe and Esmonde traced the cultural history of a single lexical item, *fu*, demonstrating that it underwent a number of changes during the period between 1978 and 2001. When Saxe first went to New Guinea, traditional Oksapmin, who had not yet learned pidgin, used *fu* to refer to the completion of counting a set of objects, as in "1 . . . 27, done." During the ensuing 20 years, the English system of 20 shillings to the pound, which was relatively new to the Oksapmin when Saxe was first there, was replaced by a national Papua New Guinea (PNG) base-10 system, in which 10 units that functioned like shillings summed to 1 PNG denomination called a *kuan*. People used the same term to refer to a 2-*kuan* note as that used to refer to a pound. In both cases, the number 20 is of exceptional importance. Saxe and Esmonde found that the number 20, which is at the left elbow, became a privileged site in the body counting system, and at the same time, *fu* took on the new function of referring to completion of a count of shillings/2 PNG *kuan*.

As a result of treating developmental change over a cultural–historical epoch as a focus of interest, Saxe and Esmonde (2005) were faced with the possibility that the changing meanings of *fu* were not the result of conscious human effort to create a more powerful arithmetic. Rather, this "cognitive development" emerged as a by-product of the mixture of ways Oksapmin use their language and their bodies to represent number through their participation in the ever-changing, and ever-more-commercialized social and economic exchange practices in which people engaged.

Although examples of research that combine the study of cultural–historical and ontogenetic change remain scarce, each example justifies the general assumption that cultural–historical change is an important constituent of ontogenetic change, justifying the basic assumption that the traditional dialectic between phylogeny and ontogeny must be expanded to include cultural change as an essential ingredient to the process of human development.

CULTURE AND BIOLOGY IN ONTOGENY: CORE DOMAINS AND CULTURAL PRACTICES

Contemporary accounts of cognitive development point to the need to combine two active areas of research if we are to provide a synthetic account that does justice to both the phylogenetic and the cultural–historical constraints from which the ontogeny of cognitive development emerges. The first area emphasizes phylogenetic contributions to cognitive development that manifest themselves particularly in infancy and young childhood, and, according to some, at birth. The second area focuses on cultural practices characteristic of the social group into which the child is born.

Phylogenetic Contributions

Early-appearing phylogenetic contributions to ontogeny are of two general kinds. The first are psychological processes organized in terms of "core," or "privileged" domains. Such processes display characteristic domain boundaries and task specificity. Each represents a particular class of entities for a particular set of

purposes (Spelke, 2000). Widely accepted candidates for such core domains supporting naive, domain-specific theories include naive physics, naive psychology (theory of mind), and naive biology (Wellman & Gelman, 1998).

In addition to such domain-specific constraints, researchers have also identified powerful general learning mechanisms. Even infants are able to identify sequential dependencies in the speech stream (Saffran, Aslin, & Newport, 1996) or in the mechanical movement that occurs when one object collides with another (Baillargeon, 1994). Moreover, humans early on are conceptual learners. They are able (1) to build concepts coherent within a larger system (Mandler, 2004); (2) to understand a set of antecedent–consequent pairs in terms of unobservable, mediating forces (Tomasello, 1999); and (3) to "bootstrap" (i.e., create a new system of representation that is more powerful than those present; Carey, 2004).

These general learning mechanisms are also products of evolution, but not in response to task-specific adaptation. They are heavily dependent on enlarged frontal and prefrontal cortices that may have evolved through uniquely human ways of living, such as posing and solving complex interpersonal and social problems, learning and using culturally inherited artifacts, adapting the natural environment to their needs, and so on (Quartz & Sejnowski, 2002).

Cultural Contributions

Whatever the initial constraints that characterize knowledge acquisition in core domains, such knowledge is woefully inadequate to normal adult human functioning; they are skeletal, not structurally complete (Gelman, 2000; Hatano & Inagaki, 2002). Consequently, ontogenetic development of the human mind requires repeated participation in culturally organized practices. Cultural practices are a bridge between phylogeny and ontogeny. On the one hand, the cultural history of a child's social group provides the kinds of practices that are available, their relative frequency, and their accessibility as proximal environments for development. On the other hand, developing individuals increasingly have at least limited freedom to choose the practices in which they engage and to change the features of these practices through their participation. Even when participants have no choice but to participate in a cultural practice, and have no desire to improve their skills, repeated participation enhances the cognitive, social, and physical skills needed to perform well in these practices.

Practices vary greatly both within and between social groups. In some cases people acquire skills to perform competently only in a specific practice, whereas in other cases they acquire a rich and well-structured body of knowledge and associated skills as well. Among these knowledge-rich domains, they may further acquire conceptual knowledge that helps them to modify known procedures flexibly, to invent new procedures, and to employ their knowledge in a wide variety of practices. Gaining cognitive competence may require years of experience in solving problems in the domain and often takes the form of "deliberate practice" requiring sustained concentration (Ericsson, Krampe, & Tesch-Romer, 1993); alternatively, it may be achieved readily and promptly, based on a small number of experiences (Wellman, 2003).

The amount of time and effort required to gain expertise in a given cultural practice or with respect to a particular cognitive domain (depending upon whether one is dealing with a core domain and its skeletal principles or a domain of social practice for which no obvious skeletal principles appear) is currently uncertain. It seems plausible that when dealing with core domains, acquisition to a level broadly characteristic of the adult population should be relatively rapid and effortless, whereas acquisition of cultural practices that bear no clear relation to any known core domain would be slower, more effortful, and require specialized arrangements. So, for example, natural languages appear to be acquired rapidly, without any explicit instruction (in fact, young language learners may acquire a natural language even when doing so is discouraged, as in the case of deaf children placed in oralist schools run by hearing people; Padden & Humphries, 1988). By contrast, learning to read English, or to fly an airplane, is rarely accomplished without explicit instruction and a great deal of practice. Human beings evolved to speak natural languages. Tens of thousands of years were required for them to invent written languages or to construct and fly airplanes, and to this day, such knowledge is not universal.

As Keil (2003, p. 369) commented, "Most people seem to live in worlds of the artificial," which immediately poses a problem. Although people may be able to make inferences about

function from observing someone using an artifact, and inferences about their intentions, there appear to be no straightforward, domain-specific "core principles" that will help them draw proper inferences about the categories of artifacts involved and the functions they fulfill outside of core domains. Gelman and Lucariello (2002) made this point using examples such as learning to play chess, history, algebra, economics, literature, and so on. They argued that learning in the absence of support from core domains presents considerable challenges

> because there is no domain-relevant skeletal structure to start the learning ball rolling. The relevant mental structures must be acquired de novo, which means that learners acquire domain-relevant structures as well as a coherent knowledge base of domain-relevant knowledge about the content of the domain. . . . It is far from easy to assemble truly new conceptual structures and it usually takes a very long time. Something resembling formal instructions is often required and still this is not effective unless there is extended practice and effort on the part of the learner. (p. 399)

Within the framework presented here, deliberate instruction is a subset of the general category of historically evolved cultural practices. Consequently, the constraints that arise from the patterned forms of interaction that structure a great variety of cultural activities may serve to enable concept formation in non-core domains. Unfortunately, to date, relatively little developmental research has been conducted with these issues in mind, beyond the social practices associated with various forms of formal schooling, although some relevant research can be gleaned from what has come to be known as the study of "everyday cognition" (Rogoff & Lave, 1984; Schliemann, Carraher, & Ceci, 1997). The work of Greenfield (2004; Greenfield et al., 2000) on changes in classification associated with apprenticeship in weaving provides one such example. This work implicates a variety of general learning mechanisms, including the ability to detect sequential dependencies, imitation, and intent observation (Rogoff, Paradise, Arauz, Correa-Chavez, & Angelillo, 2003).

Knowledge acquisition in non-core domains also requires particular forms of social organization that are likely, as Gelman and Lucariello (2002) suggest, to require more elaborate forms of sociocultural organization than in cases where skeletal principles provide a "leg up" on the acquisition process. We return to this issue below. Because knowledge and skills, whether or not anchored in core domains, are acquired in particular cultural practices, their cognitive consequences tend to be specific to that practice and the cognitive domain(s) with which it is associated. However, at least some domain-general development can also be expected as the consequence of experience with different practices. Such broad experience is primarily due to the fact that some activities occur across so many different settings and/or some artifacts are used so widely that they can have cognitive consequences well beyond particular domains. Narratives, orthography, and measurement are just a few examples of such activities and associated artifacts. Such general learning is also aided by cultural models that indicate the relevance of one activity to another, thereby stimulating generalization across settings/activities (Laboratory of Comparative Human Cognition, 1983). To the extent that there is coherence in culture, it is because of the commonality of contents, forms of the activities, ethnotheories of the linkages between different activities, and generally useful artifacts that characterize the lifeworlds of the people involved.

Because human life involves a broad range of cultural practices, each of which may involve a mixture of privileged and nonprivileged domains, and a concomitant mixture of domain-specific and general learning mechanisms, it is not possible to specify a single path of ontogenetic cognitive development independent of the domains and cultural practices in which individuals engage. We can, however, determine how processes of learning and development differ in cases where the domains and cultural practices are relatively well known to get an idea of the range of processes at work. We begin with a case where privileged domains and cultural practices are closely associated and proceed to a case where the cultural practice, while involving a core domain, involves rich knowledge and complex skills well beyond those specified by the core domain in question.

Complementarity of Domain-Specific Constraints and Cultural Practices

As we have noted, knowledge systems in privileged domains occur under constraints that direct developing individuals' attention and cod-

ing, simultaneously restricting the range of their interpretations of observed connections, allowing them to be acquired to at least a modest level of complexity early and without difficulty. Such cognitive developments can be expected to be relatively universal across cultures. But this does not mean that cultural mediation plays no role in their development.

The emergence of naive biology provides a good example for purposes of exposition, because the presence innate, domain-specific constraints in relation to naive theories and later development has been the subject of considerable research (Inagaki & Hatano, 2002). Our fundamental assumption is threefold. First, we assume that innate constraints for the acquisition of a naive theory of biology are skeletal principles that allowed our ancestors to survive (e.g., avoid dangers from other animals, find food). We do not assume that humans are born with propositional forms of biological knowledge, because constraints as dispositions can effectively mitigate learnability problems, and because it is hard to believe that specific biological knowledge can be genetically transmitted or neurally prewired. Moreover, because the process of evolution is very slow, possessing specific pieces of innate knowledge may be detrimental when ecological environments change.

Second, though we use the term "innate," we might more precisely say "present at birth or acquired very early." It is almost impossible using behavioral studies to show convincingly that a given domain-specific tendency or bias is innate in the sense of being manifested at birth. We can reasonably assume that such a bias is innate, however, when it emerges very early in infancy, without any seemingly responsible experience, when is observed universally both across and within cultures, or when its absence can be attributed to the deficit of a particular part of the brain.

Third, although we use the expression "domain-specific," we are not sure whether a particular core domain constraint is applicable to just one naive theory. We do not know yet how infants and young children divide their knowledge into domains. So by "domain-specific," we mean only to claim that the constraint is highly relevant to the acquisition of a theory in the particular domain.

These basic assumptions imply, first of all, that humans can readily acquire knowledge in core domains, although they are not born with these bodies of knowledge. In other words, innate constraints greatly enhance learning but do not make learning unnecessary. A number of domain-specific and general learning mechanisms may be involved.

For example, humans tend to pay attention to those aspects of animals that serve to distinguish them from nonanimals (e.g., they differentiate those that move spontaneously from those that do not). There is evidence indicating that even infants make the animate–inanimate distinction on this basis (Mandler, 2004). Humans also have tendencies to attend to certain features, states, and behaviors of animals: They classify animals based on their size and ferocity (Atran, 1998); they pay attention to whether animals are active, hungry, and so on; and animals' eating and excretion are often eye-catching—all of which seem adaptive for humans in the "wild environment" (Toda, 2000).

Plants share with animals the fact that they are alive. Human attention may also be directed to plants in order to find food. It would be important for hunters-gathers to be able to use subtle cues by which they could distinguish plants and their products (that are potentially edible) from nonliving natural objects (e.g., pieces of clay or rocks). It is also important for farmers to pay attention to the states of their plants, such as whether they are healthy, growing vigorously, producing fruits and seeds, or catching some disease, and so on.

Humans also display preferences for antecedent–consequent pairings or causal attribution, in other words, a set of constraints that serves to eliminate in advance a large number of logically possible interpretations or hypotheses about events. Whereas some of these constraints work in highly specific situations, others work in a variety of settings. Many animals, including humans, display a tendency to search among a variety of foods for one that has made them ill, so that only a single trial (assuming they survive), even with a considerable delay between ingestion and painful symptoms, is sufficient to learn to avoid foods that have made them sick (Revusky & Garcia, 1970).

Nonetheless, participation in cultural practices is central to the development of rich knowledge about plants and animals. This kind of developmental process is illustrated by Inagaki (1990), who arranged for 5-year-old Japanese children to raise goldfish at home, whereas as a comparison group had no such experience. The goldfish raisers soon displayed far richer knowledge about the development of fish than their counterparts who had not raised fish. They could even generalize what they had learned about fish to frogs when asked, for example, "Can you keep the frog in its bowl forever?" They answered, "No, we can't, because goldfish grow bigger. My goldfish were small before and now they are big" (quoted in Inagaki & Hatano, 2002, p. 144).

Additional evidence in favor of cultural involvement in the development of biological knowledge comes from the work of Atran and his colleagues on the growth of biological classifications (Medin, Ross, Atran, Burnett, & Blok, 2002; Ross, Medin, Coley, & Atran, 2003). Working among Yucatecan farmers, Native American rural dwellers, and a variety of urbanized people, these researchers found that factors such as density of experience and local ecological significance contribute to the development of biological understanding beyond early childhood.

Another piece of evidence is that whereas Israeli children tend to be underinclusive in their categorization of living species, separating out plants, Japanese children tend to be overinclusive. The difference, it is proposed, reflects the presence of different narratives in particular cultures: Israeli culture contains a well-known Biblical passage in which plants are described as created to provide food for animals, birds, and insects, whereas Japanese culture contains a number of stories that encourage the perception of many inanimate objects as possessing life (Hatano et al., 1993; Stavy & Wax, 1989).

Development in Cultural Practices That Amplify Core Domain Abilities

As noted earlier, whereas knowledge in privileged domains may be present in an elementary form early in life, the development of high levels of knowledge and skill, what is ordinarily termed *expertise*, requires repeated participation in culturally organized practices. The domain of number provides interesting examples of the way that cultural factors enter into the process of development beyond their rudimentary forms.

Studies of numerical reasoning in early childhood indicate that it builds upon these early starting conditions in an orderly fashion. Thus, for example, Zur and Gelman (2004) report that when 3-year-olds who had not attended preschool viewed the addition or subtraction of N objects from a known number were asked to predict the answer, then check their predictions, they provided reasonable cardinal values as predictions and accurate counting procedures. Such rapid learning in the absence of explicit instruction, they argue, supports the idea that there are "skeletal mental structures that expedite the assimilation and use of domain-relevant knowledge" (p. 135). Such data, despite uncertainties about mechanism, support the argument for number reasoning as a core domain, and, hence, a human universal.

Evidence from number development in other cultures, however, leaves little doubt that Hatano and Inagaki (2005) are correct in arguing that because innately specified knowledge is still skeletal, it is essential to study the ways cultural experience interacts with phylogenetic constraints to produce adult forms of numerical reasoning. Many societies in the world appear to have at most a few count words on the order of "one, two, many" (Gordon, 2004; Pica, Lemer, Izard, & Dehaene, 2004). For example, Gordon (2004) has recently reported that Pirahã adults living in a remote area of the Amazon jungle have a restricted number vocabulary of this type, and that cultural practices involving number are virtually nonexistent. They display elementary arithmetic abilities for very small arrays of objects, but their performance quickly deteriorates with larger numbers. Saxe (1982) reports similar findings for the Oksapmin of New Guinea, who rarely used their base-27 number system as part of traditional systems of exchange of farm surplus.

Expertise in abacus operation nicely illustrates how domain-specific cognitive skills develop when a society creates artifacts and cultural practices to support more complex cognitive achievements (Hatano, 1997). An abacus, an external memory and computational device, can register a number as a configuration of beads, and one can find the answer to a given calculation problem, in principle, by manipulating them. It is no longer used widely in day-to-day commercial activity in Japan, but the abacus still constitutes a significant aspect of Japanese culture because it survives as a special artifact, and skilled use of it is valued in circles of enthusiasts. It survives also as an instructional tool: Quite a number of children go to private after-school instruction for abacus training, and a few of these become enthusi-

asts. To put it differently, abacus operation is embedded in two kinds of practices, educational and hobby.

People can learn how to operate a (real) abacus in an elementary but serviceable manner in a few hours when they participate in deliberate instruction. Advanced training is geared almost entirely to accelerating the speed of the operations involved. Cultural values respecting the speed of calculation are shared among abacus operators.

As a result of extensive training, abacus operation tends to be gradually interiorized to such a degree that most abacus masters can calculate accurately, and even faster without a physical abacus present, than with the instrument itself. During mental calculation, it appears that they can represent an intermediate, resultant number on their "mental abacus," in the form of a mental image of the configuration of beads onto which (mentally) they enter, or from which they remove, the next input number. In other words, abacus experts can solve calculation problems by mentally manipulating the mental representation of abacus beads. The interiorization of the operation is an important mechanism for accelerating the speed of calculation, because the mental operation is not constrained by the speed of muscle movement. Thus, expert abacus operators use the real abacus only when they deal with very large numbers that cannot be represented on their mental abacus.

Some abacus operators calculate extraordinarily rapidly (Hatano, 1997). When mixed addition and subtraction problems (e.g., $957 + 709{,}143 + 386 + 2{,}095 - 810 - 91{,}748 + 105$ . . .) are presented in print, experts manipulate 5–10 digits per second. Remarkable speed is also observed for multiplication and division. Experts give, for example, an answer for 3×3 or 4×2 digit multiplication within 5 seconds. When they use a real abacus, they are basically error-free. Their mental calculation is not entirely free from errors, but their accuracy is quite respectable.

As might be expected, abacus experts' calculation is highly automatic. Experienced abacus operators can converse during calculation, even without the instrument. The conversation cannot be very demanding—usually, just a short and simple factual or preferential question–answer exchange is required. However, this feat is remarkable considering the fact that we generally ask people around us to be quiet when we calculate, especially when we do so without paper and pencil.

Expertise in mental abacus operation also induces changes at the neuronal level. For example, using event-related functional magnetic resonance imaging (fMRI), Tanaka, Michimata, Kaminaga, Honda, and Sadato (2002) showed that whereas ordinary people retain series of digits in verbal working memory (revealed as increased activation in the corresponding cortical areas, including Broca's area), mental abacus experts hold them in visuospatial working memory, showing activations in the bilateral superior frontal sulci and the superior parietal lobe. Hanakawa, Honda, Okada, Fukuyama, and Shibasaki (2003) demonstrated, using fMRI, that the posterior superior parietal cortex is significantly more activated while mental additions are performed among mental abacus experts than among nonlearners of the abacus.

The case of gaining expertise in abacus operation (both material and mental) exemplifies the sociocultural nature of expertise (Hatano, 1997). Pupils who attend abacus lessons are usually first sent there by their parents, while the children are in elementary school. The parents often believe that the exercise will foster children's diligence and punctiliousness, as well as enhance their calculation and estimation ability. Young pupils are motivated to learn abacus skills to get parental praise, especially by passing an exam for increasing qualification ranks. Like many other out-of-school domains of learning in Japan, abacus learning has an elaborate qualification system and frequent exams. It nicely fits with, or even is encouraged by, the fact that Japanese culture emphasizes effort rather than ability (Sato, Namiki, Ando, & Hatano, 2004).

The students' motivation changes when they join an abacus club at school or become a representative of the abacus school, in other words, when the operation is embedded in a different kind of practice. Abacus enthusiasts compete in matches and tournaments, just as tennis or chess players do. Also like these players, abacus club members not only engage in exercise at least a few hours every day but also seek knowledge of how to improve their skills. Their learning is strongly supported by the immediate social context of the club and the larger community of abacus operators. Formal and informal relationships with an instructor and peers organize their way of life, and sanc-

tions from other players regulate their daily activities. Moreover, they may participate in the community of abacus operators by taking an administrative role in players' organizations, as well as by serving as an examiner or a judge at matches and tournaments. They participate more and more fully by assuming more and more significant responsibilities in the community.

Abacus operators are also socialized in terms of their values, for example, regarding the importance of abacus skills and their status in general education, as well as their respect for the speed of calculation mentioned earlier. In fact, the community of abacus educators and players constitutes a strong pressure group in the world of education in Japan. In this sense, gaining expertise is far from purely cognitive. It is a social process (Lave & Wenger, 1991) that involves changes in values and identities (Goodnow, 1990). The experts' values and identities are undoubtedly forms of "culture in mind," acquired through internalization. They serve as the source of motivation for experts to excel in the target domain.

Interactive Sociocultural Constraints

As clearly shown by these examples, we can reasonably assume that most, if not all, forms of cognitive development, whether or not their content is focused on (or implicates) core domains, are induced through participation in culturally organized practices. Participants in these practices are motivated to perform well because the process and product are interesting and/or significant, and positively sanctioned by the culture. Moreover, inclusion in such practices is facilitated owing to interactive sociocultural constraints that make it possible for novices/newcomers to participate in roles that are appropriate to their level of expertise, so that what should be done for the activity as a whole can be done by flexible arrangements of the division of labor.

This kind of sociocultural arrangement is often referred to as a "zone of proximal development" or "legitimate peripheral participation," each of which indexes interactional dynamics that provide sociocultural constraints on, and supports for, development (Lave & Wenger, 1991; Vygotsky, 1978). These constraints are realized when other people who have extensive prior experience and shared physical, symbolic, and social tools help novices/newcomers/developing individuals acquire knowledge and skills through continuous interpersonal interaction.

For example, imitation plays an important role in the initial phase of learning to operate an abacus, and more mature members of the abacus learner community, in addition to serving as role models, give hints and suggestions for improving the skills. The construction of an abacus itself adds useful constraints, often specifying what should be done next—for instance, something different has to be done when there is not a sufficient number of beads left to enter a new addend.

This kind of process is illustrated in a different way when children raise an animal at home (Inagaki, 1990). In one likely scenario, children acquire knowledge from their parents or older siblings who already know how to raise the animal of interest. The children are likely to learn the procedures involved promptly, because their observation and choice of procedures are directed by joint attention with, or by imitation of, their more mature partners. In addition, active engagement in raising animals may lead children to acquire conceptual knowledge or a mental model of the animals being raised, often helped by guided comprehension activity engaged in for the sake of the animals. The children tend to be more competent when they engage in a joint activity than in a solitary activity, and they construct and elaborate on relevant pieces of knowledge more promptly (see also Rogoff, 2003).

The artifacts (including the routines) used in raising animals also serve to direct children's attention and narrow the range of procedures and interpretations they consider. For example, the manual for raising goldfish and other pets may include some information that is understandable to the children. A fish tank or a cage may suggest what kind of care the animal needs. Special food may be available, so that the procedure for feeding the animals can readily be standardized. Although the enabling constraints offered by such artifacts are primarily for the practical purpose of successfully raising the animals, they tend to enhance the acquisition of knowledge as well.

To generalize, when interacting with other people, our cognition and learning are constrained in the following ways (Hatano & Inagaki, 2005; Tomasello, Call, & Hare, 1993): What we observe is not randomly selected out of an almost infinite range of information but is directed by joint attention; what

we try to do is not to choose randomly a chosen chain of responses from our repertoire but is often triggered by imitation; and how we interpret a set of observations is influenced by guided comprehension activity. Tools also serve to direct our attention and narrow the range of procedures and interpretations we consider. For example, a machine helps us realize how to use it properly, because it does not respond when our actions are incorrect or are performed in the wrong order. In short, sociocultural constraints enable us not only to be competent but also to acquire knowledge and skills readily.

Even young children acquire knowledge and skills in a uniquely human way, in other words, through participating in practices. Their learning is helped by interactive sociocultural constraints, the operation of which is based on children's ability to represent other people's mental representations mentally (Tomasello et al., 1993).

Domain Characteristics and Cultural Support for Innovation

The case of expertise in mental abacus operation is informative, because it shows without a doubt that a set of cognitive skills is a form of culture in mind, derived from skills using an artifact that initially exists outside the mind. It is also clear that cognitive growth in a domain is associated with the development of corresponding values, identity, and status in the community of practitioners. However, the domain of abacus operation does not represent many other knowledge-rich domains that require learners to solve new problems using the knowledge in an adaptive and creative fashion.

First, abacus experts do not learn much about entities in the world or theoretical notions. It is true that they have constructed a mental model of a physical abacus, but it represents only highly restricted aspects of the physical device by which they may be able to find solutions to a limited range of problems very quickly. Second, abacus experts are characterized by their efficiency in applying acquired procedures and/or running an impoverished mental model in rather fixed ways. Therefore, their expertise is basically reproductive in nature; that is, they do not enrich the culture of the entire community of abacus operators.

In contrast, experts in domains such as science and everyday problem solving (e.g., cooking, arts, and interactive games like chess) often acquire, in addition to skills for using solution procedures or routines, conceptual knowledge in the form of cultural–mental models of both concrete and abstract entities, as well cultural–mental scripts (event schemas) that can be used to run mental simulations, much as the mental abacus can simulate actions with a material abacus (Collins & Gentner, 1982). Relying on a mental model of the target object, experts in these domains can understand the meaning of each step of solution routines, modify the routines flexibly, and predict what will occur in novel situations.

Experts in cooking, for example, when deciding what to do next, are no longer heavily dependent on other people's knowledge or knowledge given in an externalized, symbolic form (e.g., a printed recipe or the advice of an experienced cook; Hatano & Inagaki, 2005). They are less dependent on devices and materials, though the physical environment, such as a frying pan filled with oil, may serve as a reminder. The expert cook can often tell which steps have to be performed in the prescribed order and which do not, add different ingredients from those called for in the standard recipe, choose different cooking tools when needed, and still make essentially the same or equally delicious dish. Their conceptual knowledge is both an individual construction and a form of culture in mind, because it reflects the knowledge shared by experienced members participating in the practice that has been manifested in prior joint activity. Moreover, problem solving in these knowledge-rich domains also involves considerable exploration and search, in other words, processes to generate a variety of new ideas and to evaluate how well these ideas work. Therefore, it is not rare that individuals, after gaining expertise, contribute to the cultural change. Expert cooks may invent new dishes by mentally combining a variety of materials and modes of cooking. The invented dishes may be incorporated into the culture of cooking, if their taste attracts a number of members constituting the community of cooks.

To put it differently, in these domains, culture can remediate itself by allowing (or even encouraging) its members to deviate from tradition. Innovations can be realized with resources that are available in the culture but not extensively used by a majority of its members, as in the case of an ethnic or local food's gaining popularity. Alternatively, the new knowledge can be produced through nonconventional individual construction based on the database the culture provides. In either case, the cultural sanction enhances or inhibits innovation, either directly or indirectly. As we have seen, as the variety of products increased to attract tourists who visit Zinacantan, the process of production and learning changed toward the increased respect paid to individual innovation (Greenfield, 2004). Early childhood education practices in China have changed dramatically in the past 20 years toward emphasizing creativity because of the national goal of raising entrepreneurs who can be successful in the world economy (Hsueh, Tobin, & Karasawa, 2004).

CONCLUSION

In recent years one encounters an increasing number of programmatic claims that human ontogeny is the emergent outcome of phylogenetic, cultural–historical, and moment-by-moment (microgenetic) processes (Engeström, 1987; Rosa, Vega, & Gomila, 2004; Wertsch & Tulviste, 1992; Vygotsky, 1978). But since the early work of Vygotsky and his students (e.g., Vygotsky & Luria, 1930/1993), there has been little systematic effort to flesh out this programmatic statement, in terms of existing empirical data, from the many disciplines involved. At the same time, Vygotsky's name is often associated with cultural psychology (e.g., Nisbett, Peng, Choi, & Norenzayan, 2001; Shweder et al., 1998). Our major goal in writing this chapter has been to assess the viability of an approach to cultural psychology that retains the early commitments of cultural–historical psychology to an integrated evolutionary, historical, developmental approach to the problem of culture in mind.

The one part of the cultural–historical program on which we have not focused in this chapter has been the study of microgenetic processes. Microgenesis is present, of course, in all of the studies that use ethnographic and experimental methods to make their claims about culture and human psychological processes, but owing to lack of space, we have kept our discussion of culture and ontogeny at a fairly general level. Readers are invited to consult research such as Beach's (1995) study of arithmetic in shops, Coles' work (1996) on early reading instruction, or Greenfield's (2004) study of Zinacantecan weaving practices, for a more appropriate level of detail, as well as formulations by the mainstream developmentalists who have incorporated sociocultural factors into their research (e.g., Granott & Parziale, 2002).

Within the limits imposed by the existing data, limits of space, and our own intellects, we believe we have found ample reason to adopt the original programmatic claim when considering the topic of culture and cognitive development.

First, it is clear that rudimentary forms of culture-as-behavioral-tradition can be found in chimpanzees, whose brains are approximately the size of the presumed common ancestor shared by humans and chimpanzee. At the same time, evidence on language acquisition and problem solving among nonhuman primates suggests that under some conditions (often, as a result of living with and being trained by humans), chimpanzee and bonobo symbolic and cognitive capacities reach a threshold approximated by the capacities of 24- to 36-month-old children. Consequently, strong claims for human uniqueness based on the presence of culture or tool use appear untenable, although culture appears to play a notably more restricted role in chimpanzee cognitive and social life (Latour, 1996).

Evidence from studies of hominization indicates that the differentiation between human and nonhuman primates, which began approximately 6 million years ago, has resulted from a dialectical interaction that takes place in the line leading to *H. sapiens sapiens* and can be briefly summarized as follows: Changes in morphology and behavior result in changes in the cultural tool kit that result in changes in nutrition, that in turn result in changes in morphology, that in return result in changes in the cultural tool kit in a never-ending spiral of development.

The evidence from analysis of extant cross-historical research focused on cultural change indicates an uneven process of increasing complexity in societies' "cultural tool-kits," some of which appear to have relatively restricted consequences for cognitive change bound to particular cultural practices, and some of which appear applicable to a broad range of practices producing equally broad cognitive changes (e.g., the development of writing systems). However, levels of cultural complexity are never uniform within societies and do not inexorably undergo increases in complexity. There is, to modify Tomasello's (1999) metaphor, "slippage" in the "ratchet effect" that often characterizes human cultural change.

For the study of culture and ontogeny in modern humans, an approach that combines study of domain-specific and domain-general phylogentic factors in combination with culturally practice-specific and culturally general factors, appears to provide a systematic way to approach the role of culture in ontogenetic cognitive development. As appropriately pointed out by Keil (2003), it is undeniable that some phylogenetic constraints on development are domain-general. As noted earlier, we also believe that some cultural tools, ideas, tendencies, preferences, and so on serve as constraints across a large number of practices.

When we focus on microgenetic development, that is, cognition and learning at particular phases of ontogenetic development, relevant prior knowledge and general processing mechanisms (e.g., changes in memory capacity, studied by Robbie Case, and operational logic, studied by Jean Piaget) seem to serve as the most powerful constraints. Thus, a number of cognitive developmentalists (e.g., Keil, 2003) assume a 2×2 table of innate–acquired by specific–general processes, which is compatible with the combinations of phylogenetic–cultural and specific–general processes we have adopted here. However, within our framework, prior knowledge and processing mechanisms are emerging products of the interaction between innate and cultural constraints.

An important task for the future is to generalize this approach to a broader range of behaviors, including the connections between cognitive, social, and emotional aspects of development, all of which, we believe, are subject to the general principles invoked in this chapter.

NOTES

1. The wording of this passage reveals an important commonality between the words *means* and *medium* in Russian. The Russian word translated here as *medium* in the phrase "by the medium of which" was almost certainly *sredstvo*, judging from similar statements in other articles written at this time. *Sredstvo* is often translated as "means," particularly in the phrase "by means of which." We note this convergence because the intimate relation between means and media is one of the central theoretical assumptions of the cultural–historical approach.

2. Labor involves more than tool use to overcome barriers to a goal: "In short, the animal merely *uses* external nature, and brings about changes in it simply by his presence; man by his changes makes it serve his ends,

masters it. This is the final, essential distinction between man and other animals, and once again it is labor that brings about this distinction" (Engels, 1960, pp. 290–291, quoted in Vygotsky & Luria, 1993, p. 76; italics in original).

3. Although Beach's students were in their early 20s and his shopkeepers, in their 40s, this age difference was not the object of his research, and all were treated as adults.

4. The importance of getting an early start on learning to weave reveals itself in the fact that when American psychologists such as Greenfield and Rogoff have sought to learn to weave, one of the major hurdles is the great difficulty they experience being able to maintain the postural position required. This pervasively experienced fact is a clear reminder of how cultural practice shapes biological capacity during ontogeny.

REFERENCES

Atran, S. (1998). Folk biology and the anthropology of science: Cognitive universals and cultural particulars. *Behavioral and Brain Sciences*, 21(4), 547–609.

Baillargeon, R. (1994). How do infants learn about the physical world? *Current Directions in Psychological Sciences*, 3, 133–140.

Beach, K. (1995). Activity as a mediator of sociocultural change and individual development: The case of school–work transition in Nepal. *Mind, Culture, and Activity*, 2, 285–302.

Berlim, M. T., Mattevi, B. S., Belmonte-de-Abreu, P., & Crow, T. J. (2003). The etiology of schizophrenia and the origin of language: Overview of a theory. *Comprehensive Psychiatry*, 44(1), 7–14.

Bickerton, D. (1990). *Language and species*. Chicago: University of Chicago Press.

Bjorklund, D. F., & Pellegrini, A. D. (2002). *The origins of human nature: Evolutionary developmental psychology*. Washington, DC: American Psychological Association.

Boesch, C., & Boesch, H. (1984). Mental map in wild chimpanzees: An analysis of hammer transports for nut cracking. *Primates*, 25, 160–170.

Brass, M., & Heyes, C. M. (2005). Imitation: Is cognitive neuroscience solving the correspondence problem? *Trends in Cognitive Sciences*, 9, 489–495.

Carey, S. (2004, Winter). Bootstrapping and the origin of concepts. *Daedalus*, pp. 1–10.

Cheyne, J. A. (n.d.). Signs of consciousness: Speculations on the psychology of paleolithic graphics. Available online at *www.arts.uwaterloo.ca/~acheyne/signcon.html*.

Cole, M. (1996). *Cultural psychology*. Cambridge, MA: Harvard University Press.

Collins, A., & Gentner, D. (1982). Constructing runnable mental models. In *Proceedings of the 4th Annual Conference of the Cognitive Science Society* (pp. 86–89). Ann Arbor: University of Michigan Press.

Damerow, P. (1998). Prehistory and cognitive development. In J. Langer & M. Killen (Eds.), *Piaget, evolution and development* (pp. 247–270). Mahwah, NJ: Erlbaum.

D'Andrade, R. G. (1989). Culturally based reasoning. In A. Gellatly, D. Rogers, & J. A. Sloboda (Eds.), *Cognition and social worlds: Keele cognition seminars* (Vol. 2, pp. 132–143). New York: Clarendon Press/Oxford University Press.

Deacon, T. W. (1997). *The symbolic species: The co-evolution of language and the brain*. New York: Norton.

Diamond, J. (1997). *Guns, germs, and steel: The fates of human societies*. New York: Norton.

Donald, M. (1991). *Origins of the modern mind: Three stages in the evolution of culture and cognition*. Cambridge, MA: Harvard University Press.

Donald, M. (2000). The central role of culture in cognitive evolution: A reflection on the myth of the "isolated mind." In L. P. Nucci, G. B. Saxe, & E. Turiel (Eds.), *Culture, thought, and development* (pp. 19–40). Mahwah, NJ: Erlbaum.

Donald, M. (2001). *A mind so rare: The evolution of human consciousness*. New York: Norton.

Dunbar, R. I. (2004). *The human story: A new history of mankind's evolution*. London: Faber & Faber.

Engels, F. (1960). *The dialectics of nature*. New York: International.

Engeström, Y. (1987). *Learning by expanding: An activity theoretical approach to developmental research*. Helsinki: Orienta-Konsultit Oy.

Ericsson, K. A., Krampe, R. T., & Tesch-Romer, C. (1993). The role of deliberate practice in the acquisition of expert performance. *Psychological Review*, 100, 363–406.

Falk, D., & Gibson, K. (Eds.). (2001). *Evolutionary anatomy of the primate cerebral cortex*. Cambridge, UK: Cambridge University Press.

Feinman, G. M. (2000). Cultural evolutionary approaches and archeology: Past, present, and future. In G. M. Feinman & L. Manzanilla (Eds.), *Cultural evolution: Contemporary viewpoints* (pp. 3–12). New York: Kluwer.

Foley, R., & Lahr, M. M. (2003). On stony ground: Lithic technology, human evolution, and the emergence of culture. *Evolutionary Anthropology*, 12(3), 109–122.

Gaskins, S. (1999). Children's daily lives in a Mayan village: A case study of culturally constructed roles and activities. In A. Göncü, (Ed.), *Children's engagement in the world: Sociocultural perspectives* (pp. 25–60). New York: Cambridge University Press.

Gaskins, S. (2000). Children's daily activities in a Mayan village: A culturally grounded description. *Cross-Cultural Research*, 34(4), 375–389.

Gaskins, S. (2003). From corn to cash: Change and continuity within Mayan families. *Ethos*, 31(2), 248–273.

Geertz, C. (1973). *The interpretation of culture*. New York: Basic Books.

Gellner, E. (1988). *Plough, sword and book: The structure of human history.* London: Collins Harvill.

Gelman, R. (2000). Domain specificity and variability in cognitive development. *Child Development, 71*(4), 854–856.

Gelman, R., & Lucariello, J. (2002). The role of learning in cognitive development. In H. Pashler & R. Gallistel (Eds.), *Steven's handbook of experimental psychology, 3rd ed.: Vol. 3. Learning, motivation, and emotion* (pp. 395–443). New York: Wiley.

Gelman, S., & Kalish, C. W. (2006). Conceptual development. In D. Kuhn & R. S. Siegler (Eds.), *Handbook of child psychology: Vol. 2. Cognition, perception, and language* (pp. 687–733). New York: Wiley.

Goodall, J. (1968). *The behaviour of free-living chimpanzees in the Gombe Stream Reserve.* London: Baillière, Tindall, & Cassell.

Goodnow, J. J. (1990). Using sociology to extend psychological accounts of cognitive development. *Human Development, 33,* 81–107.

Goodnow, J. J. (1990). The socialization of cognition: Acquiring cognitive values. In J. Stigler, R. Shweder, & G. Herdt (Eds.), *Culture and human development* (pp. 259–286). Chicago: University of Chicago Press.

Gordon, P. (2004). Numerical cognition without words: Evidence from Amazonia. *Science* [Special Issue]. *306*(5695), 496–499.

Granott, N., & Parziale, J. (Eds.). (2002). *Microdevelopment: Transition processes in development and learning.* Cambridge, UK: Cambridge University Press.

Greenfield, P. M. (1999). Historical change and cognitive change: A two-decade follow-up study in Zinacantan, a Maya community in Chiapas, Mexico. *Mind, Culture, and Activity, 6*(2), 92–108.

Greenfield, P. M. (2002). The mutual definition of culture and biology in development. In H. Keller, Y. H. Poortinga, & A. Schölmerick (Eds.), *Between culture and biology: Perspectives on ontogenetic development* (pp. 57–76). New York: Cambridge University Press.

Greenfield, P. M. (2004). *Weaving generations together: Evolving creativity in the Maya of Chiapas.* Santa Fe, NM: School of American Research.

Greenfield, P. M., & Childs, C. P. (1977). Weaving, color terms and pattern representation: Cultural influences and cognitive development among the Zinacantecos of southern Mexico. *Inter-American Journal of Psychology, 11,* 23–28.

Greenfield, P. M., Maynard, A. E., & Childs, C. P. (2000). History, culture, learning, and development. *Cross-Cultural Research: Journal of Comparative Social Science, 34*(4), 351–374.

Hallpike, C. R. (1979). *The foundations of primitive thought.* New York: Clarendon Press.

Hanakawa, T., Honda, M., Okada, T., Fukuyama, H., & Shibasaki, H. (2003). Neural correlates underlying mental calculation in abacus experts: A functional magnetic resonance imaging study. *NeuroImage, 19,* 296–307.

Hare, B., & Tomasello, M. (2005). Human-like social skills in dogs? *Trends in Cognitive Science, 9,* 439–444.

Hatano, G. (1997). Commentary: Core domains of thought, innate constraints, and sociocultural contexts. In H. M. Wellman & K. Inagaki (Eds.), *The emergence of core domains of thought: Children's reasoning about physical, psychological, and biological phenomena* (pp. 71–78). San Francisco: Jossey-Bass.

Hatano, G., & Inagaki, K. (2005). The formation of culture in mind: A sociocultural approach to cognitive development. *Bulletin of Faculty of Education, Chiba University.*

Hatano, G., & Inagaki, K. (2002). In W. W. Hartup & R. K. Silbereisen (Eds.), *Growing points in developmental science: An introduction* (pp. 123–142). Philadelphia, PA: Psychology Press. 53, 91–104.

Hatano, G., Siegler, R., Richards, D., Inagaki, K., Stavy, R., & Wax, N. (1993). The development of biological knowledge: A multi-national study. *Cognitive Development, 8*(1), 47–62.

Hirata, S., & Celli, M. L. (2003). Role of mothers in the acquisition of tool-use behaviours by captive infant chimpanzees. *Animal Cognition, 6,* 235–244.

Hirata, S., & Morimura, N. (2000). Native chimpanzees' (*Pan troglodytes*) observation of experienced conspecifics in a tool-using task. *Journal of Comparative Psychology, 114,* 291–296.

Hsueh, Y., Tobin, J., & Karasawa, M. (2004). The Chinese kindergarten in its adolescence. *Prospects: Quarterly Review of Comparative Education, 34,* 457–469.

Inagaki, K. (1990). Children's use of knowledge in everyday biology. *British Journal of Developmental Psychology, 8*(3), 281–288.

Iriki, A., Tanaka, M., Obayashi, S. & Iwamura, Y. (2001) Self-images in the video monitor coded by monkey intraparietal neurons. *Neuroscientific Research, 40,* 163–173.

Ishibashi, H., Hihara, S., & Iriki, A. (2000). Acquisition and development of monkey tool-use: Behavioral and kinematic analyses. *Canadian Journal of Physiology and Pharmacology, 78,* 958–966.

Jackendoff, R. (1994). *Patterns in the mind: Language and human nature.* New York: Basic Books.

Keil, F. (1989). *Concepts, kinds, and cognitive development.* Cambridge, MA: MIT Press.

Keil, F. (2003). That's life: Coming to understand biology. *Human Development, 46*(6), 369–377.

Kroeber, A. (1917). The superorganic. *American Anthropologist, 19,* 163–213.

Laboratory of Comparative Human Cognition. (1983). Culture and development. In P. H. Mussen (Series Ed.), & W. Kessen (Vol. Ed.), *Handbook of child psychology: Vol. 1. History, theory, and methods* (pp. 295–356). New York: Wiley.

Latour, B. (1996). On interobjectivity. *Mind, Culture, and Activity, 3*(4), 228–243.

Lave, J., & Wenger, E. (1991). *Situated learning: Legiti-*

mate peripheral participation. Cambridge, UK: Cambridge University Press.

Leontiev, A. N. (1981). *Problems in the development of the mind.* Moscow: Progress.

Lewin, R., & Foley, R. A. (2004). *Principles of human evolution.* Malden, MA: Blackwell.

Lieberman, P. (1984). *The biology and evolution of language.* Cambridge, MA: Harvard University Press.

Luria, A. R. (1928). The problem of the cultural development of the child. *Journal of Genetic Psychology, 35,* 493–506.

Luria, A. R. (1976). *Cognitive development.* Cambridge, MA: Harvard University Press.

Luria, A. R. (1979). *The making of mind.* Cambridge, MA: Harvard University Press.

Mandler, J. M. (2004). *The foundations of mind: Origins of conceptual thought.* New York: Oxford University Press.

Marks, J. (2002). *What it means to be 98% chimpanzee: Apes, people, and their genes.* Berkeley: University of California Press.

Matsuzawa, T. (Ed.). (2001). *Primate origins of human cognition and behavior.* Tokyo: Springer-Verlag.

Matsuzawa, T. (2003). The Ai project: Historical and ecological contexts. *Animal Cognition, 6,* 199–211.

McBreaty, S., & Brooks, A. S. (2000). The revolution that wasn't: A new interpretation of the origin of modern human behavior. *Journal of Human Evolution, 39*(5), 453–563.

McGrew, W. C. (1987). Tools to get food: The subsistants of Tasmanian aborigines and Tanzanian chimpanzees compared. *Journal of Anthropological Research, 43*(3), 247–258.

McGrew, W. C. (1998). Culture in nonhuman primates? *Annual Review of Anthropology, 27,* 301–328.

Medin, D. L., Ross, N., Atran, S., Burnett, R. C., & Blok, S. V. (2002). Categorization and reasoning in relation to culture and expertise. In B. H. Ross (Ed.), *The psychology of learning and motivation: Advances in research and theory* (Vol. 41, pp. 1–41). San Diego: Academic Press.

Menzel, R. C., Savage-Rumbaugh, E. S., & Menzel, E. W., Jr. (2002). Bonobo (*Pan paniscus*) spatial memory in a 20-hectare forest. *International Journal of Primatology, 23*(3), 601–619.

Mithen, S. (1996). *The prehistory of the mind: A search for the origins of art, religion and science.* London: Thames & Hudson.

Nisbett, R. E., Peng, K., Choi, I., & Norenzayan, A. (2001). Culture and systems of thought: Holistic versus analytic cognition. *Psychological Review, 108*(2), 291–310.

Noble, W., & Davidson, I. (1996). *Human evolution, language, and mind.* Cambridge, UK: Cambridge University Press.

Padden, C., & Humphries, T. (1988). *Deaf in America: Voices from a culture.* Cambridge, MA: Harvard University Press.

Parker, S. (2003). Teaching the new baby to talk with biologists! *Human Development, 46*(5), 282–287.

Pica, P., Lemer, C., Izard, V., & Dehaene, S. (2004). Exact and approximate arithmetic in an Amazonian indigenous group. *Science, 306*(5695), 499–503.

Plotkin, H. (2001). Some elements of a science of culture. In E. Whitehouse (Ed.), *The debated mind: Evolutionary psychology versus ethnography* (pp. 91–109). New York: Berg.

Quartz, S. R., & Sejnowski, T. J. (2002). *Liars, lovers, and heroes: What the new brain science reveals about how we become who we are.* New York: Morrow.

Ramachandran, V. S. (2000). Mirror neurons and imitation learning as the driving force behind "the great leap forward" in human evolution. *Edge, 69.*

Renfrew, C., & Scarre, C. (Eds.). (1998). *Cognition and material culture: The archeology of symbolic storage* (McDonald Institute for Archeological Research, Cambridge University). Oxford, UK: Oxbow Books.

Revusky, S., & Garcia, J. (1970). Learned associations over long delays. In G. Bower & J. Spence (Eds.), *Psychology of learning and motivation: Advances in research and theory* (Vol. 4, pp. 1–84). New York: Academic Press.

Ridley, M. (2003). *Nature via nurture: Genes, experience and what makes us human.* New York: HarperCollins.

Rizzolatti, G., & Craighero, L. (2004). The mirror-neuron system. *Annual Review of Neuroscience, 27,* 169–192.

Rizzolatti, G., Fadiga, L., Fogassi, L., & Gallese, V. (2002). From mirror neurons to imitation, facts, and speculations. In A. N. Meltzoff & W. Prinz (Eds.), *The imitative mind: Development, evolution, and brain bases* (pp. 247–266). Cambridge, UK: Cambridge University Press.

Rogoff, B. (2003). *The cultural nature of human development.* New York: Oxford University Press.

Rogoff, B., & Lave, J. C. (1984). *Everyday cognition: Its development in social context.* Cambridge, MA: Harvard University Press.

Rogoff, B., Paradise, R., Arauz, R. M., Correa-Chavez, M., & Angelillo, C. (2003). Firsthand learning through intent participation. *Annual Review of Psychology, 54,* 175–203.

Rosa, A., Vega, J., & Gomila, Y. A. (2004). Evolution of the mind: Some methodological and substantive considerations. *Estudios de Psicología, 25*(2), 205–215.

Ross, N., Medin, D., Coley, J. D., & Atran, S. (2003). Cultural and experimental differences in the development of folkbiological induction. *Cognitive Development, 18,* 25–47.

Saffran, J. R., Aslin, R. N., & Newport, E. L. (1996). Statistical learning by 8-month old infants. *Science, 274,* 1926–1928.

Sato, T., Namiki, H., Ando, J., & Hatano, G. (2004). Japanese conception of and research on human intelligence. In R. J. Sternberg (Ed.), *International handbook of psychology of human intelligence* (pp. 302–324). New York: Cambridge University Press.

Saxe, G. B. (1982). Developing form of arithmetical

thought among the Oksapmin of Papua New Guinea. *Developmental Psychology, 18,* 583–595.

Saxe, G. B. (1994). Studying cognitive development in sociocultural contexts: The development of practice-based approaches. *Mind, Culture, and Activity, 1*(1), 135–157.

Saxe, G. B., & Esmonde, I. (2005). Studying cognition in flux: A historical treatment of Fu in the shifting structure of Oksapmin mathematics. *Mind, Culture, and Activity, 12*(3–4), 171–225.

Schliemann, A., Carraher, D., & Ceci, S. J. (1997). Everyday cognition. In J.W. Berry, P. R. Dasen, & T. S. Sarawathi (Eds.), *Handbook of cross-cultural psychology: Vol. 2. Basic processes and human development* (2nd ed., pp. 177–226). Needham Heights, MA: Allyn & Bacon.

Scribner, S. (1977). Modes of thinking and ways of speaking: Culture and logic reconsidered. In P. N. Johnson-Laird & P. C. Wason (Eds.), *Thinking: Readings in cognitive science* (pp. 483–500). Cambridge, UK: Cambridge University Press.

Scribner, S., & Cole, M. (1981). *The psychology of literacy.* Cambridge, MA: Harvard University Press.

Shweder, R. A., Goodnow, J., Hatano, G., LeVine, R. A., Markus, H., & Miller, P. (1998). The cultural psychology of development: One mind, many mentalities. In R. M. Lerner (Ed.), *Handbook of child psychology: Vol 1. Theoretical models of human development* (pp. 865–938). New York: Wiley.

Shweder, R. A., Goodnow, J., Hatano, G., LeVine, R. A., Markus, H., & Miller, P. (2006). The cultural psychology of development: One mind, many mentalities. In W. Damon & R. M. Lerner (Editors-in-Chief) & R. M. Lerner (Vol. Ed.), *Handbook of child psychology: Vol. 1. Theoretical models of human development* (6th ed., pp. 716–792). New York: Wiley.

Spelke, E. S. (2000). Core knowledge. *American Psychologist, 55*(11), 1233–1243.

Stavy, R., & Wax, N. (1989). Children's conceptions of plants as living things. *Human Development, 32*(635), 1–11.

Stout, D., Toth, N., Schick, K., Stout, J., & Hutchins, G. (2000). Stone tool-making and brain activation: Positron tomography (PET) studies. *Journal of Archeological Science, 27*(12), 1215–1233.

Tanaka, S., Michimata, C., Kaminaga, T., Honda, M., & Sadato, N. (2002). Superior digit memory of abacus experts: An event-related functional MRI study. *NeuroReport, 13*(17), 2187–2191.

Toda, M. (2000). Emotion and social interaction: A theoretical overview. In G. Hatano, N. Okada, & T. Tanabe (Eds.), *Affective minds* (pp. 3–12). Amsterdam: Elsevier.

Tomasello, M., Call, J., & Hare, B. (1993). Chimpanzees understand psychological states: The question is "Which ones and to which extent?" *Trends in Cognitive Sciences, 7,* 153–156.

Tomasello, M. (1994). The question of chimpanzee culture. In R. W. Wrangham, W. C. McGrew, F. B. M. de Waal, & P. Heltne (Eds.), *Chimpanzee cultures*

(pp. 301–317). Cambridge, MA: Harvard University Press.

Tomasello, M. (1999). *The cultural origins of human cognition.* Cambridge, MA: Harvard University Press.

Toth, N., Schick, K. D., Savage-Rumbaugh, E. S., Sevcik, R. A., & Rumbaugh, D. M. (1993). Pan the tool-maker: Investigations into the stone tool-making and tool-using capabilities of a bonobo (*Pan paniscus*). *Journal of Archaeological Science, 20,* 81–91.

Tulviste, P. (1979). On the origins of theoretic syllogistic reasoning in culture and the child. *Quarterly Newsletter of the Laboratory of Comparative Human Cognition, 1*(4), 73–79.

Tulviste, P. (1999). Activity as an explanatory principle in cultural psychology. In S. Chaiklin, M. Hedegaard, & U. J. Jensen (Eds.), *Activity theory and social practice* (pp. 66–78). Aarhus, Denmark: Aarhus University Press.

Vygotsky, L. S. (1929). The problem of the cultural development of the child, II. *Journal of Genetic Psychology, 36,* 415–432.

Vygotsky, L. S. (1977). *The collected works of L. S. Vygotsky: Problems of general psychology.* New York: Plenum Press.

Vygotsky, L. S. (1978). *Mind in society.* Cambridge, MA: Harvard University Press.

Vygotsky, L. S. (1981). The genesis of higher mental functions. In J. V. Wertsch (Ed.), *The concept of activity in Soviet psychology* (pp. 144–240). Armonk, NY: Sharpe.

Vygotsky, L. S. (1987). *The collected works of L. S. Vygotsky: Vol. 1. Problems of general psychology* (R. W. Rieber & A. S. Carton, Eds.). New York: Plenum.

Vygotsky, L. S., & Luria, A. R. (1993). *Studies on the history of behavior: Ape, primitive, and child.* Mahwah, NJ: Erlbaum. (Original work published 1930)

Wellman, H. M., & Gelman, S. A. (1998). Knowledge acquisition in foundational domains. In H. M. Wellman, S. A. Gelman, & W. Damon (Eds.), *Handbook of child psychology: Vol. 2. Cognition, perception, and language* (pp. 523–573). New York: Wiley.

Wertsch, J. (1985). *Vygotsky and the social formation of mind.* Cambridge, MA: Harvard University Press.

Wertsch, J., & Tulviste, P. (1992). L. S. Vygotsky and contemporary developmental psychology. *Developmental Psychology, 28*(4), 548–557.

Whitten, A. (2000). Primate culture and social learning. *Cognitive Science, 24*(3), 477–508.

Wrangham, R. W., McGrew, W. C., de Waal, F. B. M., & Heltne, P. G. (Eds.) (1994). *Chimpanzee cultures.* Cambridge, MA: Harvard University Press.

Wynn, T. (1989). *The evolution of spatial competence.* Champaign: University of Illinois Press.

Zur, O., & Gelman, R. R. (2004). Young children can add and subtract by predicting and checking. *Early Childhood Quarterly Review, 19,* 121–137.

CHAPTER 6

Self as Cultural Mode of Being

SHINOBU KITAYAMA
SEAN DUFFY
YUKIKO UCHIDA

Culturally inspired approaches to psychology have flourished during the last two decades (Bruner, 1990; Cole, 1996; D'Andrade, 1995; Fiske, Kitayama, Markus, & Nisbett, 1998; Greenfield, Keller, & Fuligni, 2003; Lehman, Chiu, & Shaller, 2004; Markus & Kitayama, 1991; Shore, 1996; Shweder, 2003; Triandis, 1995). These approaches have covered a wide range of territory from basic perception and attention (Nisbett, Peng, Choi, & Norenzayan, 2001), emotion and motivation (Kitayama & Markus, 1994; Mesquita & Frijda, 1992), and all the way up to social institutions and organizational behavior (Earley, 1989; Nisbett & Cohen, 1996). Although cultural issues are traditionally studied by anthropologists using ethnography as a primary method, in more recent years they have been examined in increasing quantity and quality by psychologists with their traditional methods of cross-cultural surveys and experiments (e.g., Nisbett & Cohen, 1996). Although informed significantly by ethnographic knowledge, these methods bring to the field more rigorous and consensually verifiable means by which to assess hypotheses suggested by in-depth observations of culture and, moreover, to determine certain boundary conditions for the hypotheses (Cohen, Chapter 8, this volume).

From the very outset of this psychologically oriented work on culture, the notion of self has been central in defining issues, formulating questions, and theoretically integrating a great variety of empirical findings (e.g., Markus & Kitayama, 1991; Marsella, DeVos, & Hsu, 1985; Shweder & Bourne, 1982; Triandis, 1989). Two fundamental insights have emerged from this analysis. The first is the time-honored idea of the self as a *social product* (Cooley, 1902/1922; Mead, 1934). Humans, in this view, are social and cultural animals (Aronson, 1992; Baumeister, 2005); that is, the self is made possible through symbolically mediated, collaborative social interaction among many individuals in a given cultural community. Second, researchers have begun to realize that the self is best conceptualized as a psychological system for behavioral regulation (Kitayama & Duffy, 2004; Markus & Kitayama, 2004). This system, moreover, is not merely an organization of conceptual schemas on which to reflect back. More importantly, it is providing a principle for one's spontaneous behavioral organization or his or her *modus operandi*. In other words, the self is a matter of "I" as well as "me" (Mead, 1934).

MUTUAL CONSTITUTION OF CULTURE AND SELF

The idea that "I"—the active agent—is a social product can be articulated most clearly by referring to earlier theorists in the symbolic interactionist school of social psychology such as Mead (1934) and Cooley (1902/1922), according to whom the self is seen as a set of behavioral response tendencies that are coordinated with response tendencies of social others in the cultural community. In early years of life, before children reach school age, social others are limited largely to mothers and other caregivers. But once in school, the child's world is dramatically expanded to include peers. This added dimension of sociality is likely to serve as a much needed impetus to achieve a generalized conception of how social others in general (i.e., the generalized other; Mead, 1934) act and respond to the self. Patterns of others' responses are recognized, and response tendencies of the self are thereby coordinated and gradually attuned to the perceived social patterns. From this point on, there is a continuous process of assimilation and accommodation between the self and social others. This interaction between self and others is often mediated by linguistic symbols. It can therefore take the form of dialogue (Hermans, Rijks, & Kempen, 1993). But more generally, this interaction is more behavioral, grounded in daily practices and routines carried out at both verbal and nonverbal levels, and often nondeliberate, and even automatic and unconscious, although it is still fully mediated by symbols.

An outcome of this symbolically mediated social interaction between self and other is the development of a system of action—or agency—that is shaped by and thus closely coordinated with the surrounding cultural environment. Each individual self is very much a collaborative output of the entire cultural community, which provides a matrix of generalized patterns of responses to the self.

The notion that cultural ideas are both reflected in and justified in terms of relevant social practices and institutions is quite old (see LeVine, Chapter 2, this volume, for a historical review). Over a century ago, Max Weber (1904–1906/1958) pointed out that much of the contemporary capitalist social system and the individualistic ethos associated with it can be traced back to Protestant varieties of Christianity. Referring to this social system as an "iron cage" (p. 123), Weber emphasized the invisible yet highly objective nature of the cultural environment that is socially and historically constructed throughout the modern West. This cultural environment comprises a set of implicit rules that specify, for example, what it means and what it will actually take to succeed or even to survive. People's behaviors are governed by these rules, thereby transforming the rules into a "brutal" reality of life that in turn constrains and affords people's further behaviors. Characteristics of the behaviors that are afforded in this way by the Protestant Ethic and the resultant ethos of capitalism include, for example, hard work, personal goal orientation, and task focus. Because these mental features are literally required to survive in the capitalist environment, they are further fostered and reinforced by this environment.

Likewise, Giddens (1984), a British sociologist, proposed a structuration theory of society, wherein the social structure is an emerging property of the minds shaped by that social structure. This mutual influence between society and the mind is also a recurring theme of a theoretical writing of Bourdieu—a French sociologist (1977). More recently, the same idea has been elaborated by Shweder (1991), who reminded us that "psyche and culture . . . make each other up" (p. 73). Likewise a number of psychologists and anthropologists who follow the lead of Vygotsky and his Russian colleagues have argued for the fundamentally social nature of human thought and, by extension, individual agency in general (Cole & Hatano, Chapter 5, this volume), and have analyzed how this agency is constituted by myriad social practices, with a frequent emphasis on linguistic practices and use (e.g., Ochs, 1988).

This diverse array of proposals and analyses in various social science disciplines has converged to suggest that once socialized in a given cultural community, individuals will gradually develop a psychological system of regulating their own thoughts, feelings, and actions in attunement with myriad characteristics of the surrounding sociocultural environment. This psychological system of self-regulation constitutes the person's *mode of being*—his or her generalized pattern of thought, feeling, and action or standard operating procedures (Triandis, Chapter 3, this volume) employed for these psychological functions (Kitayama & Duffy, 2004; Markus & Kitayama, 2004). The "mode of being," therefore, can be defined as a psychological system for action, or simply as agency. These terms are therefore used interchangeably hereafter. Each individual's mode of being is both constantly afforded and constrained by behaviors, expectations, or evaluations of others.[1] More generally, it is maintained by generalized societal response tendencies or norms shared by others in the community. The emerging patterns of interdependence between one's mode of being and the generalized responses of the society at large provide the basis for anticipating substantial cross-cultural variations in the mode of being.

DEFINING CULTURE

To begin our analysis of the mode of being, it is necessary to have some tentative agreement about what culture is. Over the course of social science literature, culture has been variously defined (Kroeber & Kluckhorn, 1952/1966; see Borofsky, Barth, Shweder, Rodseth, & Stolzenberg, 2001, for a recent debate on the issue). Yet common in many of the definitions is the notion that culture is a whole set of symbolic resources of a given community, such as lay theories, icons, scripts, and schemas (Adams & Markus, 2004). The symbolic resources of culture are accumulated and transmitted across generations and are usually externalized into social practices and social institutions (D'Andrade, 1995). For example, the cultural idea of God-given human rights is constitutive of many Western democratic social institutions. The same idea is also central in daily practices that emphasize choice (Iyengar & Lepper, 1999). These symbolic resources of culture—both ideas and practices—inform members of the pertinent cultural community of what we referred to earlier as the more general societal response tendencies or norms shared by others in the community.

Culture is dynamic in that cultural ideas and practices are invented, accumulated, and systematically changed over time, both within and across generations (Moscovici, 1984). Culture is also dynamic because cultural ideas and practices have multiple meanings that are constantly in flux, negotiated, manipulated, and arbitrated for a variety of reasons by all individuals who participate in a cultural community. For example, practices and ideologies of people of power are often imitated by people of lower rank (Richerson & Boyd, 2005), enabling the former to initiate major cultural, political, and societal changes.

One particularly powerful type of symbolic resources of culture specifies the nature of self and its relationship with others. These ideas, called models of self and relationship (Markus, Mullally, & Kitayama, 1997), deserve special attention in psychology, because they are directly implicated in all psychological processes that constitute the self as agent and its relations with the surrounding social environment. As we have already noted, one cultural model of self and social relations that is especially influential in mainstream American middle-class culture can be traced back to the Protestant Ethic (Kitayama & Markus, 1999). This model distinguishes between the domains of work and social life. Originally, the distinction was grounded in the theological notion of calling—a mission assigned personally by God to the self. The notion of work as calling required the segregation of this domain from other domains, including social relations. Today, however, this segregation of work from social life is conventionalized as a social routine that represents a secular, mostly North American, middle-class work ethic of professionalism (Sanchez-Burks, 2005).[2] This model and the associated moral imperatives then foster a variety of social behaviors that are highly individualistic, task-oriented, and relatively impervious to socioemotional cues in work settings, and that behaviors become highly consensual within a group of people who share the model.

One important consequence of the fact that cultural models are externalized in social practices is that relevant behaviors are regarded as normative and consensual (D'Andrade, 1995). Thus, they are often taken for granted. Rarely can any doubt be raised about the practices and their underlying assumptions. This applies not only to laypeople but also to the researchers who study them. Comparative methods are therefore imperative in cultural psychological research (Cohen, Chapter 8, this volume). For example, only when a comparison is drawn between middle-class American practices and those in other cultural groups do the historical roots and cultural groundings of the Protestant relational ideology become evident. Only through such comparison can the uniqueness of this cultural model be identified and delineated. In the absence of such explicit comparisons, culture is typically invisible. Yet, it can be very powerful. As Durkheim (1938/1964) noted, "Air is no less heavy because we do not detect its weight" (p. 5).

CHAPTER OUTLINE

In this chapter, we elaborate on the thesis that cross-culturally divergent modes of being are contingent on cultural ideas and practices. Our emphasis is twofold. First, we hope to articulate two broad types of modes of being, independence and interdependence. Second, we also hope to delineate variable manifestations of these modes of being as a function of regions, social class, and other relevant sociocultural and historical factors and forces. The chapter consists of three parts.

First, we set up a theoretical framework. We argue that culturally sanctioned patterns of social relations encourage two divergent principles of action organization, which in turn foster correspondingly divergent modes of being; that is, independent social patterns encourage self-directedness, which in turn leads to (1) influence-oriented style of action, (2) self-centricity in self–other representations, and (3) analytic cognition. In contrast, interdependent social patterns encourage social responsiveness, which in turn leads to (1) adjustment-oriented style of action, (2) other-centricity in self–other representation, and (3) holistic cognition.

Second, we review evidence for psychological tendencies associated with the respective modes of being. Our review is organized around three components of the mode of being (i.e., style of agency, self–other representations, and cognition). We show that the three components tend to cohere together when one examines cultures that are historically highly independent (e.g., North American middle-class cultures) or highly interdependent (mainstream East Asian cultures).

In the third part of this chapter we examine developmental and social antecedents of the two modes of being. We first review evidence for systematic cultural shaping of the model of being through socialization, then examine cultures that are neither strongly independent nor strongly interdependent. We argue that the three components of the mode of being are distinct and thus dissociable. The analysis here is necessarily preliminary, because pertinent data are lacking. Yet we suggest that future effort along this line will allow us to take a focused look at antecedent conditions for the mode of being.

Altogether, we seek to advance a thesis that, through socialization, culture's symbolic resources are incorporated or appropriated to form a system of behavioral regulation. This system—called the "cultural mode of being"—is thus symbolically mediated, both behavioral and mental, and, moreover, it is an integral part of a larger collective process by which culture is created, preserved, and changed. Thus, a dynamic process of mutual constitution emerges between culture and self. After examining some critical appraisals of the current approach to culture and self, we conclude with some suggestions for future work on the cultural mode of being.

THEORETICAL FRAMEWORK: SOCIAL RELATIONS AND ACTION REGULATION

Our theoretical framework is presented in Figure 6.1. We assume that cultures vary substantially in what patterns of social relations are valued, encouraged, and appropriated to construct daily social interactions at many different levels and spheres. Because the culturally typical pattern of social relations requires disparate principles of behavioral regulation, it promotes correspondingly divergent ways in which social actions are organized, resulting in cross-culturally variable modes of being. It should be kept in mind that the causal sequence may go in the other direction. Thus, a given mode of being highlights the corresponding principle of action organization, which in turn may encourage the respective social relational patterns. In Figure 6.1, this possibility is acknowledged by dotted arrows (for earlier versions of the conceptualization, see, e.g., Kitayama & Markus, 1994, 1999; Markus et al., 1997).

Pattern of Social Relations

Gesellschaft and Gemeinschaft

It goes without saying that there are many different social relations. However, these relations are likely to be classified into a relatively small number of types (Fiske, 1992). According to one prominent line of analysis, there are two

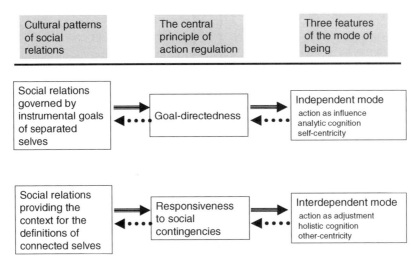

FIGURE 6.1. The theoretical framework: patterns of social relations, the principle of action regulation, and features of the mode of being.

fundamentally different forms of sociality. These forms were referred to by Tönnies (1887/1998)—one of the first proponents of this view—as *gesellschaft* and *gemeinschaft*, respectively. *Gessellschaft* is a form of sociality maintained by instrumental goals of participating individuals, whereas *gemeinschaft* is derived from inherent connectedness of participating individuals. A society created by the consent of like-minded individuals is a typical example of *gesellschaft*, and family and other small-size communities are typical of *gemeinschaft*.

Whereas Tönnies suggested that the two forms of sociality define the most fundamental types, Fiske (1992) has argued for four basic models of social relations. Fiske's first type, called "communal sharing," is analogous to *gemeinschaft*. Equality matching encompasses reciprocal exchanges, which can take place in both *gemeinschaft* and *gesellschaft*. Authority ranking implies hierarchical relations, which can also take place in both *gemeinschaft* and *gesellschaft*. Finally, his market pricing focuses on instrumental social relations and thus resembles *gesellschaft*. It would appear, then, that Fiske's framework adds elements of exchange and hierarchy to the scheme suggested by Tönnies.

Yet another important theoretical scheme by Shweder, Much, Mahapatra, and Park (1997) has proposed that three important classes of moral codes are used to organize social life. The morality of autonomy rests on the idea

that each individual has an inherent value and comes with a set of "God-given" rights. It depicts the person as independent and both fully responsible for his or her own action and valuable in his or her own right. According to this morality, social relations are seen as derivative and thus largely instrumental. They are thus analogous to *gesellschaft* (or Fiske's market pricing). The morality of community is derived from the idea that community is primary, and duties and obligations vis-à-vis the community are the ultimate arbiter of values and judgments. Therefore, this morality entails social relations that are given or that preexist prior to the emergence or definition of each individual participant, similar to Tönnies's *gemeinschaft* (or Fiske's communal sharing).

What is unique in the Shweder et al. (1997) scheme is inclusion of the third class of morality called "divinity," which emphasizes sacred values associated with supernatural being(s) found in many religions of the world (Atran, Chapter 17, this volume). This third class of morality is distinct from both autonomy and community; moreover, it is associated with a distinct set of emotions (Rozin, Lowery, Imada, & Haidt, 1999). Yet in terms of social relations, it is not clear whether this moral system is instrumental in forging any unique class of worldly social relationships.

In short, it is a reasonable first approximation to suggest that *gesellschaft* and *gemeinschaft* are two of the most basic types of social relations. In fact, analogous typologies have been repeatedly proposed. Thus, models of so-cial relations analogous to *gesellschaft* have been called independent (Markus & Kitayama, 1991), autonomous (Sampson, 1988), self-oriented (Parsons & Shils, 1951), egocentric (Shweder & Bourne, 1982), exchange (Clark & Mills, 1979), and individualist (Hofstede, 1980; Triandis, 1989). Given this class of mod-els, social relations are formed on the basis of instrumental goals of participating individuals. The other class of models is based on a con-trasting assumption that the self is fundamen-tally connected with others and is in fact em-bedded and made meaningful within social relationships. These models are referred to as interdependent, connected, socially oriented, sociocentric, communal, and collectivist.

It is important to emphasize that both inde-pendent, instrumental, and goal-directed prac-tices, values, and ideas and interdependent, communal, and group-oriented ones are avail-able in all cultures (Fiske, 1992). Moreover, in all cultures, some types of relations (e.g., busi-ness transactions) are mostly construed to be goal-oriented and guided by self-interests, whereas some other types of relations (e.g., friendship relations) are mostly construed as communal and relation-centered (Fiske, 1992; Kitayama & Uchida, 2004). However, these two models of social relations are unevenly dis-tributed, and differentially sanctioned and val-ued across cultures. Thus, the overarching hy-pothesis is that there is a substantial cross-cultural variation in the relative significance and prevalence of the two forms of social rela-tions.

Cross-Cultural Variation
in Predominant Forms of Social Relations:
Evidence from Cross-Cultural Value Surveys

Whereas the foregoing classifications are largely theoretical, during the last three de-cades there have been numerous attempts to measure cultural values. This literature has discussed the distinction between *gesellschaft* and *gemeinschaft* under the rubric of individ-ualism and collectivism (Hofstede, 1980; Triandis, 1989), and has provided an impor-tant clue to the question of whether cultural groups might vary systematically in terms of their relative emphasis on the two values re-lated to both self and social relations (for reviews, see Kağitçibaşi, 1997; Smith & Schwartz, 1997).

In 1980 Hofstede published *Culture's Conse-quences*. In this influential monograph, Hofstede reports results from a survey con-ducted on 117,000 IBM employees in 40 na-tions. In one part of the survey, participants were asked to report how important each of 14 work-related values was to them. The re-searcher first controlled for acquiescence re-sponse bias (a tendency to provide affirmative answers regardless of question contents; Smith 2004). By factor-analyzing the mean country scores for the 14 values, Hofstede identified two factors, the first of which is of interest here. This factor had high positive loadings on the tendencies to value (1) personal time out-side of work, (2) freedom to choose different approaches in job, and (3) challenges in work. It also had high negative loadings on the ten-dencies to value (1) training opportunities in work, (2) good physical conditions in work, and (3) full use of one's work skills (Hofstede, 1980, p. 220). One problem with this work is that some of the items have no obvious connec-tions to either individualism or collectivism. Hofstede (1991) argues, however, that *within the work environment in which the survey was conducted*, the discovered dimension can be seen as representing individualism (i.e., a value placed on both personal freedom work obliga-tion and personal initiatives at work) on the one hand, and collectivism (i.e., a value placed on the work environment and, thus, on IBM—the company) on the other.

The Hofstede measure has several problems. First, as already mentioned, not all items would seem obviously related to the constructs unless considered and interpreted in the specific con-text in which the survey was conducted—IBM workers responding on their work values with-in the context of their own work environment. Second, country-level indicators of values are enormously noisy; hence, they are unlikely to be completely valid. Third, reported values and attitudes are, after all, what people think and say. But culture's practices, symbols, and insti-tutions are much more than each person's thought contents (Kitayama, 2002). Fourth, some important artifacts can potentially distort survey results. These artifacts include ref-erence group effect (Heine, Lehman, Peng, & Greenholtz, 2002), acquiescence bias (Schimmack, Oishi, & Diener, 2005), and ab-sence of any one-to-one relationship between social values or norms and personal values (Peng, Nisbett, & Wong, 1997). Hence, there is good reason to be cautious in interpreting the results from cross-cultural value and attitude surveys.

Nevertheless, the Hofstede measure has proved to be valid, often highly correlated with certain cultural or societal characteristics. For example, it is related to other country-level measures of values (Bond, 1988; Ingelhart & Baker, 2000; Triandis et al., 1986; Schwartz, 1992). Moreover, it is positively correlated with the Gross National Product (GNP; Smith & Schwartz, 1997), democratization (Ingelhart & Baker, 2000), national means of subjective well-being (Diener & Diener, 1995), and even certain linguistic features such as pronoun drop (Kashima & Kashima, 2003; see Diener & Suh, 2000, for a review). It is also important that these country scores correspond closely to expert judgments (Peng et al., 1997). We regard this empirical convergence as impressive, which provides a basis to assume that the Hosftede score of individualism (vs. collectivism) is basically valid as a country-level indicator of individualism and collectivism.

For the present purposes, then, this dimension may be seen as an index of predominant forms of social relations sanctioned in varying cultural contexts. Thus, both Western European countries and the United States are high in individualism (thus *gesellschaft*, or instrumental relations, are encouraged and culturally sanctioned) and many Asian and South American countries are high in collectivism (thus *gemeinschaft*, or communal relations, are encouraged and culturally sanctioned).

In summary, the classic dimension of *gemeinschaft* (collectivism and interdependence) and *gesellschaft* (individualism and independence) has been identified, albeit often implicitly, by numerous researchers in the past as crucial in understanding cultural values (Hofstede, 1980; Ingelhart & Baker, 2000; Schwartz, 1992), morality (Shweder et al., 1997), social behavior (Triandis, 1995), social institutions (Parsons & Shils, 1951), and self (Markus & Kitayama, 1991). Moreover, despite some recent claims to the contrary (Oyserman, Coon, & Kemmelmeier, 2002; Matsumoto, 1999; Takano & Osaka, 1999), the cultural variation along this dimension appears both systematic and substantial, often correlated strongly with some distinct cultural characteristics, including GNP, linguistic features, and overall levels of subjective well-being (Hofstede, 1980; Schimmack et al., 2005).

Among others, these data provide evidence that Western Europeans and North Americans are considerably more oriented toward independence and individualism, whereas Asians are considerably more oriented toward interdependence and collectivism.

Principle of Action Regulation

The two forms of social relations discussed earlier authenticate very different principles of action regulation. To participate in instrumental social relations, individuals have to know their goals, desires, needs, and plans, appraise the attendant social situation with respect to these internal attributes of the self, then direct themselves in accordance with the relevant attributes of the self. The central principle of action organization, then, is goal directedness. In contrast, to participate in communal social relations, individuals have to be vigilant with respect to external contingencies, including expectations, desires, and needs of others, as well as a variety of other nonpersonal elements in the attendant social situation, then actively act to adjust their own behaviors to such contingencies. The central principle, then, is responsiveness to social contingencies.

At first glance, self-directedness might seem to give rise to war-like interpersonal states where egocentric Machiavellian strategists try to deceive one another to promote their own interests without mercy for others, whereas social responsiveness might appear to encourage benign welfare-oriented social utopias. This initial impression is both naive and deceptive. In fact, within an instrumental social relationship, individuals have to be chosen by others to benefit from social relations. Social rejection is just as damaging in instrumental relations as in communal relations (Baumeister & Leary, 1995). Moreover, social rejection may present a realistic threat, especially in instrumental relations, because, unlike communal relations, instrumental relations are relatively easy to terminate. Thus, one important class of goals in instrumental social interactions is to be liked and respected by others. In contrast, within a communal social relationship, individuals can be confident that others in the relationship are attentive to their actions, and even their thoughts and feelings. Yet this attentiveness need not be benign. In many interdependent, collectivist societies, therefore, the worst enemy is often imagined to be among one's best friends (Adams & Plaut, 2003). Thus, in many instances, general trust that people experience and report in respect to social others or the society in general is bound to be higher in independent, individualist societies than in interdependent, collectivist societies (Fukuyama, 1992; Ingelhart & Baker, 2000; Putnam, 1993; Yamagishi & Yamagishi, 1994).

Mode of Being

We propose that the cross-culturally divergent principles of action organization (self-directedness and social responsiveness) give rise to differences in three components of self-regulation. In organizing and regulating one's own actions, one has to represent the surrounding environment in which action takes place (*cognition*). Within this environment, one then has to represent both the self and other relevant people (*self–other representation*). On the basis of both the general situational construal and the representation of both the self and others, one then regulates his or her own behaviors (*style of action*). These three elements of self-regulation are coordinated with one another. Yet they are distinct and partially independent. This idea is illustrated in Figure 6.2, where the components are denoted by overlapping circles. Within the respective mode of being, the most typical case can be found at the center, where the three circles overlap. Yet there are many other cases in which one or even two of the elements are missing. We argue later that this analysis allows us to cover a wide range of cultures that are neither strongly independent nor interdependent.

Independent Mode

When culture emphasizes independent, goal-oriented, instrumental practices and ideas in organizing social relations (i.e., *gesellschaft*), one's predominant form of action tends to be the use of his or her own goals, desires, judgments, and other internal attributes in an effort to cause changes in the environment. This form of action has been sometimes called "primary control" (Weisz, Rothbaum, & Blackburn, 1984). Typical examples include behaviors oriented toward personal achievement and attempts at persuading others. Morling, Kitayama, and Miyamoto (2002) have called this mode of action "influence" to emphasize that it involves an effort to cause changes in the environment. Of course, within the influence mode of action, social others are important. But they are considered important only to the extent that they are seen as instrumental in achieving one's own goals and desires. Accordingly, the representations of the self tend to be more emphasized, elaborated, and/or valued than the representations of others. This mode of self–other representation may be said to be self- or egocentric (Shweder & Bourne, 1982) or self-oriented (Parsons & Shils, 1951). Moreover, goal-directedness is likely to foster focused attention toward a goal-relevant object in the environment. This may be the case even when the object at issue is another individual. When a single object is picked up and detached from the immediate context, it is likely to be scrutinized "for its own sake," categorized in terms of a general taxonomic system. In person perception, for example, a focal person is likely to be categorized in terms of personality taxon-

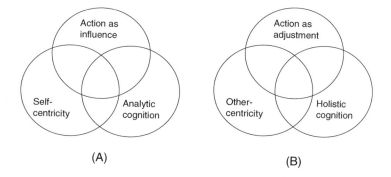

(A)   (B)

FIGURE 6.2. Varieties of independence (A) and interdependence (B): The respective modes of being comprise three primary features—agency, self–other representation, and cognition. The three features tend to go together, but there may be many exceptions.

omy. Likewise, in object perception, a focal stimulus is likely to be understood in terms of a relevant semantic category. This mode of thought is called "analytic" (Nisbett et al., 2001). In short, the independent mode of being is associated with (1) action as influence, (2) self-centricity in self–other representations, and (3) analytic mode of thought.

There is a general consensus in the literature that the view of the self as independent and the corresponding form of social relation (*gesellschaft*) have their origins in the modern period in Western Europe, although many of the ideas of the modern West can be traced back to the Greek civilization (Nisbett, 2003). Reformation of the Catholic Church and the resulting Calvinist varieties of Protestantism had a major influence on the emergence of the independent view of person (Sanchez-Burks, 2005). So did numerous philosophers of the Enlightenment, including Rousseau, Locke, and Voltaire (Taylor, 1989). Once transplanted in North America through initial waves of Western European immigrants and espoused by the Founding Fathers of the United States, the independent view of the self has since become a cornerstone of mainstream American culture (Bellah, Madsen, Sullivan, Swidler, & Tipton, 1985). As Geertz (1975) noted, North Americans are wedded to the view of the person as "a bounded, unique, more or less integrated motivational and cognitive universe, a dynamic center of awareness, emotion, judgment, and action organized into a distinctive whole and set contrastively both against other such wholes and against its social and natural background" (p. 48). Today this view of the person is embodied in numerous cultural artifacts, mundane practices of daily life, social institutions, and personal values.

Nevertheless, there is likely to be substantial variation within North America in the degree to which people subscribe to the independent view of the self. One can expect considerable ethnic variations, such that the independent mode of being may be most clearly identified among Americans of Western European descent. Moreover, to the extent that self-direction is related to job complexity (Schooler, Chapter 15, this volume), the independent mode of being may be less pronounced for working-class people, whose jobs are bound to be more routinized, not requiring flexible thought, and are thus less complex. Moreover, the same consideration might suggest that the independent mode of being may be identified in many other regions of the world. For example, middle-class individuals in industrialized societies may show some sign of independence in part because their jobs require a greater extent of self-directedness, flexible thinking, and autonomy.

Interdependent Mode

When culture emphasizes interdependent, other-oriented communal practices and ideas in organizing social relations (i.e., *gemeinschaft*), one's predominant form of action tends to be the consideration of expectations, desires, and needs of others in an effort to adjust one's own actions to these intentional states attributed to the others. This form of action, most typically characterized in terms of its responsiveness to concerns and expectations of others, and more generally to a variety of social contingencies, has sometimes been called "secondary control" (Weisz et al., 1984). Typical examples include behaviors oriented toward concerns of others and attempts at conforming to and gratifying others. Morling and colleagues (2002) have called this mode of action "adjustment" to emphasize the fact that this mode involves an effort to accommodate one's own behaviors in accordance with contingencies that present themselves in social relations.

Within the adjustment mode of action, others are centrally important. In fact, selves are often defined and made meaningful in respect to such others. For example, most social roles, such as child, parent, teacher, and student, can be defined only in reference to pertinent social others. Likewise, even seemingly purely private attributes, such as opinions and judgments, may also be defined in such relational terms. For example, one might agree or disagree with others. Or one might identify him- or herself with someone else in a particular domain. Interdependence does not necessarily imply obedience and conformity. In fact, many forms of rebellion also presume a tightly knit relationship with powerful others. In all these cases, because the self is defined in reference to social others, the cognitive representations of these others are likely to be at least as elaborated, highlighted, and often valued as the cognitive representations of the self. In this sense, this mode may be said to be sociocentric (Shweder & Bourne, 1982) or socially oriented (Parsons & Shils, 1951). Moreover, responsiveness to social contingencies is likely to foster holistic attention—that is, attention that is dispersed to many potentially significant elements of the environment. This may be the case even when the elements at issue are other individuals. When individuals attend to many such elements simultaneously, they are likely to be understood within a holistic scheme. Instead of characterizing each of many individuals involved in terms of their unique personality traits, one may come up with a broader schema of the relationship or the group as a whole that encompasses all the individuals involved. This mode of thought is called "holistic" (Nisbett et al., 2001). In short, the interdependent mode of being is associated with (1) action as adjustment, (2) sociocentricity in self–other representations, and (3) holistic mode of thought.

It is generally agreed that in many societies outside the West, the self is inherently more social, connected with others and immediate communities. In fact, throughout much of the history of human existence, social relations have predominantly been kin-based and relatively stable (Brewer, 2004; Richerson & Boyd, 2005; Konner, Chapter 4, this volume); moreover, they are limited to relatively small groups of up to 80 at most (Dunbar, 1996). These considerations suggest that the interdependent mode of being, which is defined primarily in terms of its connectedness with others and its immersion in a community, may have been common for much of its history for the human species (Konner, Chapter 4, this volume). If true, this substantially reduces the burden of explaining the origins of cultural differences, with a main emphasis to be placed on the emergence of the independent mode out of the interdependent mode. Some possible hypotheses include modernization (Inglehart & Baker, 2000), voluntary settlement (Kitayama, Ishii, Imada, Takemura, & Ramaswamy, 2006), and wealth (Triandis, 1995).

Nevertheless, even if the interdependent mode is primordial, defining some sort of default form of sociality for humans, this by no means implies that cultures outside of the modern West are entirely homogeneous. To the contrary, it is likely that different types of interdependence existed throughout history and over different geographic regions (Fiske et al., 1998). For example, a deep commitment to immediate family of Chinese is clearly different than the Moroccan way of defining the self in terms of birthplaces (Geertz, 1973). Likewise, whereas a founding ideology for Chinese society, Confucianism, emphasizes virtues of adhering to hierarchical social relations, there is a much stronger egali-

tarian, communal emphasis in hunter–gatherer groups in Africa (Fiske, 1992) and Australia (Myers, 1986). Moreover, collectivism of Confucian cultures regards personal positive affect as a hindrance of social harmony, but collectivism of Latin cultures appears to use positive affect as a glue of social relations (Cohen, Chapter 8, this volume). Nevertheless, in all these cases, the primary commitment is to a social unit of which the self is part. The self is ascribed to the unit and often is deeply connected and attached to it. The self's belongingness to the group is taken largely as given, not as chosen for his or her own instrumental goals or considerations. Accordingly, along with massive differences, a set of common themes or features may cut across many of the interdependent societies and communities.

EAST–WEST DIFFERENCES IN MODE OF BEING

Much of the evidence for the two modes of being comes from systematic cross-cultural comparisons between North American middle-class populations and East Asian populations. This evidence suggests that whereas East Asians show a predominantly interdependent mode of being, middle-class North Americans exhibit a predominantly independent mode of being. These two cultures can be characterized by the completely overlapping area of Figure 6.2. In what follows, we review evidence for each of the three components of the mode of being. Our review is more thorough and comprehensive for the style of action component than for either the self–other representation or the cognition, because the latter two domains are covered in full in other chapters by Heine (Chapter 29, this volume) and Norenzayan et al. (Chapter 23, this volume), respectively.

Style of Action

The first component of the mode of being involves a style of action as either influence or adjustment. Whereas self-directedness fosters influence, social responsiveness promotes adjustment.

Prevalence and Consequences of Influence and Adjustment

In an influential article, Weisz and colleagues (1984) reviewed a variety of cultural practices and customs of both American and Japanese cultures. In North America, many more practices highlight the self (thereby allowing one to stand out and act in accordance with one's own judgments), and the corresponding values and beliefs in self-directedness and active effort to cause changes to happen in the environment (called "primary control"). In contrast, in Japan many more practices encourage the self to conform to expectations or needs of others (thereby adjusting oneself to these expectations or needs), and the corresponding values and beliefs in social sensitivity and attunedness (called "secondary control"). *Secondary control* is a misnomer, because this mode of action is just as agentic as the mode called primary control; moreover, it is no less primary in Japan. Morling, Kitayama, and Miyamoto (2002) therefore call the two styles of action "influence" and "adjustment," respectively.

To see whether this cultural difference is prevalent in practices involving influence and adjustment, Morling and colleagues (2002) asked both North Americans and Japanese to remember the most recent instance in which they either "influenced the surrounding" or "adjusted themselves to the surrounding." They then asked the participants to indicate how recently the remembered event took place. If a given class of events is frequent, they should occur in the more recent past. As predicted, the latest influencing episode was less than a day old in the United States, but it was several days old in Japan. This cross-cultural difference was completely reversed for the adjusting episodes.

What are the consequences of acts of influence or adjustment relative to self-perception? Two dimensions of self-perception are especially relevant. First, efficacy, esteem, or power of the self (or self-esteem) is a central defining feature of the sense of the self as independent (Heine, Lehman, Markus, & Kitayama, 1999). Because the act of influencing is an expression of self-esteem, it may be predicted that individuals would feel empowered and thus report enhanced self-esteem when they engage in an act of influence. This effect, however, may depend on culture. Because influencing behaviors are culturally sanctioned in North America to a far greater extent than in Japan, the effect of an influencing act on self-esteem may be predicted to be more pronounced in North America than in Japan. The second relevant dimension of self-perception concerns the sense of connectedness to others. Because an act of adjusting is an expression of one's commitment to a relationship and the value one attaches to it, it may be predicted that individuals feel more connected when they engage in an act of adjustment. Moreover, because adjusting behaviors are more culturally sanctioned in Japan than in North America, this effect of adjustment on perceived connectedness of self may be predicted to be greater in Japan than in the United States.

These predictions received support in another study by Morling and colleagues (2002), who first collected many episodes of both influencing and adjusting from both American and Japanese participants. New groups of both American and Japanese participants were then presented with a randomly selected subset of the episodes thus collected. They were asked to imagine that they engaged in each act described in each episode, and to report how they would feel on dimensions of (1) self-esteem (self-efficacy, esteem, and power) and (2) perceived connectedness with others. The results lend support to the preceding analysis. When engaging in American-made influencing acts, Americans felt quite empowered, reporting enhanced self-esteem. Although a comparable empowering effect of influence was found in Japan, the effect was much weaker. In contrast, when engaging in Japanese-made adjusting acts, Japanese participants reported a strongly enhanced sense of interpersonal connectedness. Furthermore, in line with the foregoing analysis, a comparable connection-enhancing effect of adjustment was virtually nonexistent in the United States.

Interestingly, Americans reported an enhanced sense of connectedness when they engaged in American-made influencing acts. This latter finding suggests that acts of influencing in North America provide a culturally sanctioned way to interpersonally relate to others. Americans often relate to others by arguing or debating, persuading, and proactively helping others. Persuasion defines a major genre of interpersonal relations in all spheres of American life. Even conflicts and interpersonal tensions are often believed to be generative (Rothbaum, Pott, Azuma, Miyake, & Weisz, 2000). These acts are obviously interpersonal, yet they involve a form of influence. Influence thus provides a way in which separated selves are related to one another without compromising the ever-important sense of the self as independent and separate. There was no evidence that influence has such a connecting function in Japan.

The thesis that Americans use social influences to connect to others has received additional support from recent research by Taylor and colleagues (2004), who show that Americans are much more likely than Asians and Asian Americans to seek support. The explicit solicitation of support is a form of influence; thus, it fits neatly into the default mode of social relations for Americans. Notice that as long as support is explicitly sought, any helpful acts Americans might receive as a consequence are unlikely to compromise their sense of self as independent and self-sufficient. Instead, they are likely to signify the self's interpersonal efficacy, as shown by Morling et al. (2002) in the previously cited work. In contrast, Taylor and colleagues (2004) suggest that Asians do not explicitly seek support from others because of relational concerns, such as causing trouble to the others.

All research available to date on influence is concerned with relations involving peers and friends. It might seem plausible that Asians also seek to influence others as long as these others are lower in social status and rank. Alternatively, even in hierarchical relationships, Asians might seek to avoid explicit forms of influence in part because those in lower in status or rank (e.g., subordinates, children, etc.) might willingly adjust to the expectations of those higher in status and rank. At present, no empirical work exists on this question.

Self-Images and Dissonance

Influence and adjustment as alternative principles of agency may result in quite different concerns about the self. Whereas individuals operating on the principle of independence and influence are concerned with efficacy, competence, moral integrity, and other internal qualities of the self, those operating on the principle of interdependence and adjustment are concerned with what social others might think about the self's qualities. Recently, this analysis has been applied to cognitive dissonance.

Drawing on theories of dissonance process that emphasize the role of self (Aronson, 1968; Steele, Spencer, & Lynch, 1993), Kitayama, Snibbe, Markus, and Suzuki (2004) suggested that dissonance can take cross-culturally divergent forms, because cultures emphasize different aspects of self. In independent cultural contexts, such as North American cultures, private self-images, such as the self's competence and moral integrity, are highlighted; as a consequence, individuals are hypothesized to experience dissonance when their behavioral choice

poses a threat to a certain private self-image they wish to sustain. For example, a choice between two equally attractive cars can raise a threat to one's competence as a wise decision maker and consumer, because the chosen car might have negative features and/or the rejected car might have positive features. Kitayama and colleagues have called this "personal dissonance." In contrast, in interdependent cultural contexts, such as many Asian cultures, public self-images, such as the self's reputations and social acceptance, are highlighted; as a consequence, individuals experience dissonance when their behavioral choice poses a threat to a certain public self-image they hope to maintain. For example, having chosen to buy a luxurious German car might raise a concern about what one's colleagues and neighbors might think about the self. This has been called interpersonal dissonance.

Whether personal or interpersonal, dissonance is an aversive emotional state that motivates the person to justify the original choice (Festinger, 1957). Thus, once induced to experience dissonance, individuals are motivated to justify the act of positively choosing one item by increasing their liking for it and/or justifying the act of giving up another item by decreasing their liking for it. Nevertheless, the foregoing theoretical framework suggests that, depending on the cultural contexts of the person at issue, the dissonance is likely to be aroused under quite different circumstances.

One critical variable is an awareness of "eyes of others" watching and closely monitoring the self (Imada & Kitayama, 2006; Kitayama et al., 2004). Because personal dissonance hinges on what one's choice would mean to one's private self-image, it should happen in total privacy, in the absence of the eyes of others. In contrast, interpersonal dissonance hinges on what one's choice might mean to one's public self-image. For this dissonance to arise, the choice would have to be perceived as public. In fact, if the choice is believed to be completely private, it entails no ramifications for one's public self-image. Under these conditions, there should be little or no dissonance effect.

To test these ideas, Kitayama and colleagues (2004; Imada & Kitayama, 2006) had both American (mostly white, middle class) and Japanese participants (living in Kyoto) choose between two equally attractive CDs and examined the degree to which liking for the chosen CD increased and that for the rejected CD decreased. A key manipulation involved a poster that, seemingly prepared for a conference presentation, contained several schematic faces that were "watching" whoever was seated right in front of it. In an eyes-of-others condition, this poster was surreptitiously placed so that participants were exposed to the schematic faces. Although no one raised any suspicions about the poster, Kitayama and colleagues (2004) drew on previous work on automatic information processing (e.g., Baldwin, Carrell, & Lopez, 1990), and predicted that the watching eyes of others would covertly, yet powerfully, evoke public self-image concerns among Japanese. In a control condition, no poster was placed before participants.

In support of the foregoing analysis, Japanese participants did not show any dissonance effect in the control condition, but they did show a reliable dissonance effect in the "eyes-of-others" condition. This suggests that in making a choice, the Japanese worry mostly about what the choice might mean to their public self-image. A dissonance effect for them can therefore happen only when these public self-image concerns are engaged. In contrast, Americans showed a strong dissonance effect in the control condition. But this effect was reduced in the eyes-of-others condition. Imada and Kitayama (2006) replicated this effect and proposed that Americans assume that others try to influence them and, as a consequence, watching eyes of others are perceived to constrain their choice. Alternatively, the eyes might have provoke a degree of reactance (Brehm, 1966). In either case, choice under these conditions is perceived as externally constrained and less free, entailing a lesser threat to one's private self-images and a lesser need for self-justification. In support of this proposal, Imada and Kitayama have shown that a strong dissonance effect remains even when faces are presented, as long as the faces look weak and submissive (thus, unlikely to exert any unwanted influences). This pattern of findings suggests that in making a choice, Americans worry mostly about what the choice might mean to their private self-image. Only to the extent that this anxiety affects one's private self does a dissonance effect accrue for Americans.

Another recent series of studies has provided further evidence for the present analysis. Hoshino-Browne and colleagues (2005) proposed that a strong interpersonal dissonance (an interpersonal worry resulting from a threat to one's public image) can result from a choice one makes for one's friend. But this effect should be observed only for those who hold quite strong public self-image concerns (e.g., Asians), not for those who do not worry much about public self-images (e.g., European Canadians). As predicted, a justification effect subsequent to a choice made for a friend was significantly larger for Asian Canadians and Japanese than for European Canadians.

Researchers have argued that dissonance represents a threat to the personal self; thus, an affirmation of the personal self should readily eliminate self-justification (Steele, 1988). This prediction has been borne out in many studies. Yet, if the dissonance experienced by Asian Canadians is interpersonal rather than personal in nature, the affirmation must be directed at the interpersonal (rather than personal) self for it to be effective in eliminating the dissonance. In a typical self-affirmation manipulation, participants are asked to circle all values that they personally shared. In addition to this personal affirmation manipulation, Hoshino-Browne and colleagues (2005) used an interpersonal affirmation manipulation in which participants were to circle values their families shared. As predicted, the dissonance effect of Asian Canadians in the friend choice condition was significantly weaker in the interpersonal affirmation condition than in a no-affirmation control. The finding from the personal affirmation condition was quite noteworthy. It turned out that this affirmation manipulation was quite effective if the Asian Canadians were fully acculturated in Canada and identified themselves with the Canadian mainstream culture. No such effect was evident among nonacculturated Asian Canadians.

Intrinsic Motivation

The personal dissonance process just discussed suggests that choice is an integral part of behavioral motivations for Americans. In agreement with this analysis, self-determination theory has suggested that through choice and autonomous engagement in an activity, one's intrinsic motivation is enhanced (Deci & Ryan, 1985; Lepper & Greene, 1978). For interdependent agents, however, it may be choice made by ingroup members that engages the intrinsic motivation of the person at issue. Such a choice conveys to the person high expectations and hopes held by the others with regard to the performance of this person. Consistent with this analysis, several observers of Asian cultures have noted that achievement in Asia is often motivated by feelings of indebtedness to parents. Thus, a desire to return obligations to them and to erase any sense of guilt or shame is a major source of personal strivings for excellence (DeVos, 1983; Yang, 1986).

In support of this analysis, Iyengar and Lepper (1999) had European and Asian American children work on a video game involving spaceships. One group of children were allowed to choose the color of their own spaceship. A second group of children were assigned one color by the experimenter; finally, a third group of children were told that their mother chose the color of the spaceship for them. As may be predicted by both our analysis of independent agency and self-determination theory, white children performed much better when they made the choice by themselves than when the color was assigned by the experimenter. Their performance was worst when their mothers made the choice for them. In contrast, as predicted by our analysis on interdependent agency, Asian American children performed better when their mothers made the choice than when either they made their own choice or the experimenter assigned the color.

The motivation to improve the self to meet high expectations held by significant others has been called "self-improvement" (Kitayama, Markus, Matsumoto, & Norasakkunkit, 1997), which involves identification of one's own shortcomings and deficits via-à-vis collectively shared high expectations and standards, and an assessment of one's own performance in comparison to such high expectations or standards. It is the experience of deficit or shortcoming that strongly motivates the person to improve. In a recent series of experiments, Heine and colleagues (2001) observed that in an intellectual competence task, Japanese participants were most motivated to persist in the task when they were led to believe they had failed rather than succeeded in a similar task. This pattern was in stark contrast with the pattern observed for Americans, who persisted much more after success than after failure.

Lay Theories of Agency

Do individuals have naive beliefs about actions that are in line with their respective modes of being as independent or interdependent? Our

analysis suggests that North Americans would see another person's act as a form of influence and, as a consequence, would look for internal events that motivated the person to engage in the act. A voluminous social psychology literature on causal attribution has provided ample evidence for the American tendency to focus on internal cause of action, while ignoring potentially available external causes. This effect is so pervasive that it has been called the "fundamental attribution error" (Nisbett & Ross, 1980; Ross, 1977). In contrast, Asians would see another person's act as a form of adjustment and, as a consequence, would immediately look for external events that prompted the person to engage in that act. Hence, the fundamental attribution error may be attenuated or even nonexistent in cultures organized around an alternative view of the self as interdependent (Markus & Kitayama, 1991; Nisbett, 2003).

Since a pioneering study by Miller (1984), this cross-cultural prediction has received substantial support (Choi, Nisbett, & Norenzayan, 1999; Norenzayan, Choi, & Peng, Chapter 23, this volume). Morris and Peng (1994), for example, presented to both American and Chinese respondents various pictures of a number of fish swimming in different formations. When asked for reasons explaining the movement of a central fish, Americans were more likely to refer to internal factors of the fish (e.g., its psychological dispositions) than to factors external to it (e.g., movements of other fish that are present) as a causal factor underlying the fish's movement. In contrast, Chinese respondents were more likely to refer to external factors than to internal factors in the same task. The same cross-cultural difference has been observed in content analyses of media materials (Morris & Peng, 1994) and commentaries on professional sports events (Lee, Hallahan, & Herzog, 1996).

The dispositional bias in attribution implies that individuals are relatively impervious to external or situational factors. Thus, when observing another person behaving under a social constraint, individuals may be expected to ignore the social constraint and instead infer directly from the person's behavior a disposition that corresponds to the behavior (Jones, 1988). This bias, called the "correspondence bias," has been demonstrated among Americans even when the social constraint is quite salient, or when the action is seemingly nondiagnostic at all of the disposition at hand (Gilbert & Jones, 1986). Under these conditions, however, Asians show very little evidence for correspondence bias (Choi & Nisbett, 1998; Masuda & Kitayama, 2004; Miyamoto & Kitayama, 2002).

For example, Masuda and Kitayama (2004) tested participants in pairs. One participant was assigned an inducer role and the other, an observer role. The task of the inducer participant was to choose one of two essays and give it to a third participant, who in turn read the essay. Both the inducer and the observer were to observe the third participant read the essay and report an impression of him or her. The inducer participant was then given two alternative essays that argued for one or another position on a socially controversial issue at the time (e.g., the nuclear testing France carried out in the Mururoa Coral Reef), and asked to choose one and to give it to the third participant. Both the inducer and the observer subsequently saw a video of the third participant reading the essay and estimated the real attitude of this person on the social issue at hand. Notice that under these conditions, it is very clear that the third participant did not actively choose the essay; nor did he or she write it. Moreover, the social pressure the inducer exerted on the target person is also very clear. Conceptually replicating an earlier study by Gilbert and Jones (1986), Masuda and Kitayama (2004) found that Americans still inferred that the target person's attitude corresponded to the essay content. This very strongly illustrates how robust this dispositional bias in fact is among Americans. As predicted, however, Japanese respondents showed no correspondence bias. They acknowledged the nature of social constraints imposed on the target person and made adjustments for them in estimating his or her real attitude.

Lay Theories of Happiness

If the mode of being is different along with common lay theories of agency that go with it, people may appraise their lives in the correspondingly divergent fashion. Accordingly, although happiness as a general positive emotional state is widely acknowledged in all known cultures (Mesquita & Fridja, 1992), underneath this general proposition might be profound cross-cultural differences in lay under-standings about happiness. Kitayama and Markus (2000) have suggested that in North America, happiness is typically construed as a personal achievement. Thus, individuals strive to attain happiness and, once obtained, happiness affirms the worth of the internal, private self. In contrast, according to Kitayama and Markus, happiness in Japan is more socially anchored. It is seen as a realization of social harmony or state of mutual sympathy and understanding.

Evidence for this proposal comes from a recent study by Uchida and Kitayama (2006), who asked both American and Japanese participants to describe as many "features, effects, or consequences of happiness" as they could. A large number of features collected in the respective cultures were printed on separate index cards. A stack of cards was then presented to another group of participants within each culture. These participants were asked to sort the cards according to perceived similarities of the descriptions. On the basis of these data, Uchida and Kitayama computed the likelihood of each pair of descriptions to be classified into the same pile. This likelihood (an index of perceived similarities among the features of happiness, varying between 0 and 1) was used to compute a multidimensional scaling solution. In both cultures, three types of descriptions were commonly found: general hedonic states (e.g., joy, excitement, and positive attitude), personal achievement (e.g., getting a good grade, getting a job) and interpersonal harmony (e.g., getting along with others, having a party for a friend).

In support of the Kitayama and Markus (2000) hypothesis, Uchida and Kitayama (2006) observed in the American sorting data that the descriptions related to personal achievement were much more likely to be classified into the general hedonic state pile than were those related to interpersonal harmony. This suggests that positive hedonic experience of happiness is most closely associated with personal achievement for Americans. In contrast, the Japanese associated the general hedonic state of happiness to a far greater extent with social harmony than with personal achievement. Thus, social harmony and interdependence are the crucial element of the Japanese understanding of happiness. Results of several studies that examine correlates of happiness and life satisfaction (e.g., Kitayama, Markus, & Kurokawa, 2000; Kwan, Bond, &

Singelis, 1997; Oishi & Diener, 2003) are consistent with this analysis (see Diener & Tov, Chapter 28, this volume; Uchida, Norasakkunkit, & Kitayama, 2004 for reviews; also see the section on health and well-being).

Emotional Consequences of Style of Action

Kitayama and colleagues (2000; Kitayama, Markus, & Matsumoto, 1995; Kitayama, Mesquita, & Karasawa, 2006) pointed out that some emotions are closely associated with either independence or interdependence. Emotions associated with an accomplishment of independence (including pride, self-confidence, and feelings of superiority) are called "socially disengaging positive emotions." Emotions associated with a failure in independence and an attendant motivation to restore the tarnished independence (including anger, frustration, and sulky feelings) are called "socially disengaging negative emotions." Likewise, socially engaging emotions include both positive emotions, which result from success in tasks of interdependence (e.g., friendly feelings, close feelings, and respect), and negative emotions, which result from a failure in tasks of interdependence and accompany a motivation to restore tainted interdependence (e.g., guilt, shame, and feelings of indebtedness).

In a recent series of studies, Kitayama, Mesquita, and Karasawa (2006) asked both American and Japanese participants to report how intensely they experienced a number of emotions in each of many different social situations. They found, as should be predicted, that emotions are intensely experienced only when they share the pleasantness with the attendant situations. But more importantly, among the emotions matched in pleasantness to the situations, the intensity of experience depended very much on each emotion's social orientation (engaged vs. disengaged). As predicted by the notion that Americans and Japanese seek independence and interdependence, respectively, Americans reportedly experienced disengaged emotions more intensely than engaged emotions, but Japanese reportedly experienced engaged emotions more intensely than disengaged emotions. The cross-cultural difference was quite sizable, with Cohen's *d* ranging between 1.0 and 1.5.

Further evidence for the hypothesis that emotional experiences are organized in a way that promotes one of the two predominant modes of being comes from a recent study by Mesquita et al. (2005), who asked both Japanese and Americans (college students and adults from local communities) to provide detailed accounts of their experience of pride, humiliation, and anger. Through a systematic coding of these accounts, they found that the two cultural groups varied widely in many facets of the emotional experience. For example, when feeling pride, 80% of Americans willingly took responsibility for the positive event at issue, but only 37% of Japanese did so. Instead, a majority of Japanese (61%) in the midst of the pride episode remained self-critical by reminding themselves that there was room for further improvement—a tendency rarely observed among Americans. In anger experiences, whereas Americans tended to be strongly inclined to affirm and to justify themselves while feeling aggressive toward the offender, the Japanese were much more likely to report sympathy toward the offender. Although seemingly quite benign, this sympathy might often be close to contempt; that is, we suspect that the sympathy in a case like this might often be based on a perception of the offender as having no chance or hope for betterment, thus being unworthy of even minimal respect. This sympathy—which is close in nuance to "pity" without an overtly pejorative attitude toward the offender—might therefore be a socially desirable way of expressing the contempt. Finally, when humiliated, Americans were reportedly motivated to reaffirm the self and even to become aggressive; Japanese reportedly took responsibility for the incident and announced their intention to improve in the future. Overall, then, the experience of emotion appears to unfold in ways that establish or otherwise restore both positivity and separation of the self among Americans, but it does so in ways that further protect, and breed connectedness and better acceptance of the self by ingroup members among Japanese (Mesquita & Leu, Chapter 30, this volume).

Motivational Consequences

One classic way to assess motivation is to measure frustration that is experienced when one's motivation is blocked (Berkowitz, 1989). In a well-conducted field experiment, for example, Harris (1974) demonstrated that people in a waiting line are highly frustrated (often resulting in aggressive behaviors) when someone cuts into the line (thereby interfering with their goal attainment), and this was especially so when they were near the beginning (as opposed to the end) of the line. When people are near the beginning of the line, the goal gradient is assumed to be quite steep, and the drive toward the goal is high.

If North Americans are motivated toward independence and Asians, toward interdependence, such motivational differences should be revealed in the conditions in which people in different cultures feel constrained or frustrated; that is, people experience a degree of restraint and feel that they "cannot do what they want to do" when a key cultural motivation, such as that toward personal control and independence for Americans, and that toward social harmony and interdependence for Japanese, is blocked.

In a recent study that used a large-scale cross-cultural survey, Kitayama and colleagues (2006) measured the sense of constraint with a scale designed to assess the degree to which people chronically experience constraint (the Perceived Constraint Scale; Lachman & Weaver, 1998; Pearlin & Schooler, 1978). As predicted, Americans reported that they "could not do what they wanted," thus showing a substantive degree of constraint in their life, especially when they were low in personal control. This replicates a large body of literature that attests to the central significance of personal control (Lachman & Weaver, 1998). In contrast, Japanese subjects reported that they "could not do what they wanted," thus showing feelings of constraint, especially when they were high in relational strain. Importantly, the effect of relational strain or relational harmony was relatively weak for Americans, indicating that Americans are not motivated as much in these relational tasks. On the contrary, the effect of personal control was quite weak for Japanese subjects, showing that they are not motivated as much in this personal task.

Consequences on Health and Well-Being

Because North Americans are strongly motivated toward personal control and independence in general, they may be expected to achieve well-being and health through realizing their independence, that is, by maintaining and enhancing personal control. Although important, promotion of relational harmony or avoidance of relational strain is considered to be more discretionary. In fact, such relational

goals are often secondary, particularly when they are in direct conflict with the personal goals of attaining the sense of control and mastery (Heckhausen & Schulz, 1999). Several studies have demonstrated that a strong sense of personal control is positively predictive of well-being and health in the United States (e.g., Heckhausen & Schulz, 1999; Lachman & Weaver, 1998). In addition, the sense of personal control is likely to yield a strong sense of self-worth or high self-esteem. A large number of studies have shown that self-esteem, and an attendant tendency to self-enhance through social comparison, are major predictors of well-being among Americans (e.g., Diener & Diener, 1995; Kwan et al., 1988; Taylor & Brown, 1988; Uchida et al., 2004; Zuckerman & O'Loughlin, 2006). Likewise, positive feelings based on personal success, such as pride and feelings of superiority, are highly associated with general happiness among Americans (Kitayama et al., 2000, 2006). Additionally, Oishi and Diener (2003) reported that attaining personal goals (e.g., doing what one wants to do) leads to enhanced well-being among European Americans (see also Sheldon & Kasser, 1998).

In contrast, Japanese are motivated toward relational harmony and, therefore, interdependence in general. Thus, we may expect that they will achieve well-being and health by realizing their interdependence, that is, by promoting relational harmony and/or avoiding relational strain (Morling et al., 2002; Morling, Kitayama, & Miyamoto, 2003). Although important, attaining and maintaining the sense of personal control and mastery is not considered essential or primary. Indeed, especially when they are in direct conflict with relational concerns and goals, mastering and control must be subordinate to the ever-important interdependent concerns and goals. Those failing to subordinate them are often considered as immature and childish (Lebra, 1976; Kondo, 1990). As might be expected, well-being in East Asian contexts is strongly predicted by social relational factors, such as social harmony (Kang, Shaver, Min, & Jin, 2003; Kwan et al., 1997); attainment of relational goals (Oishi & Diener, 2003); socially engaging emotions, such as friendly feelings and communal feelings (Kitayama et al., 2000; Kitayama, Mesquita, & Karasawa, 2006); and perceived emotional support from close others (Uchida et al., 2004). The hypothesized link between relational harmony and well-being among Asians has also been suggested by the finding that attainment of relational goals (e.g., meeting expectations of significant others) is closely related to enhanced well-being among Asian Americans and Japanese but not among European Americans (Oishi & Diener, 2003).

In a recent cross-cultural survey, Kitayama, Karasawa, and colleagues (2006) tested adult, non-college-student samples in both the United States and Japan, using a large number of self-report measures in health and well-being, and provided additional evidence for the foregoing line of analysis. First, personal control proved to be a reliably more significant predictor of well-being among Americans than among Japanese. This is consistent with several recent findings that demonstrate the significance of self-esteem in predicting well-being in individualistic cultures such as the United States (Kwan et al., 1997; Uchida et al., 2004). In contrast, in Japan, the absence of relational strain most powerfully predicted the summary index of well-being. This finding is consistent with the hypothesis that in the Japanese, interdependent cultural contexts, responsiveness to others, and attendant social harmony are strongly valued and sanctioned. Interestingly, however, the researchers found that avoidance of social tension and strain, rather than promotion of social harmony per se, was most predictive of well-being. This finding is in line with a greater prevention (rather than promotion) focus demonstrated for Asians (Elliot, Chirkov, Kim, & Sheldon, 2002). For example, recent studies have indicated that behaviors of people in Japanese and other Asian contexts are strongly motivated by certain avoidance goals, such as a desire to reduce interpersonal anxiety (Kitayama et al., 2004) and to avoid failure (Heine et al., 2001).

Self, Other, and Relationship

The second of the three components of the mode of being concerns representations of self, social others, and the relationship between the two. Whereas self-directedness and the resulting propensity to influence the external environment encourages people to elaborate and value the representations of the self (their own goals, attitudes, values, and opinions), social responsiveness and the resulting tendency to adjust to the environment encourages people to elaborate and value both representations about

social others and their relationship with these others.

Self-Enhancement

If the self is more central and salient than others, the self may receive a greater symbolic value than do others. But if others are more salient and central than the self, relatively more value is given to the others than to the self. The substantial literature on positive self-uniqueness speaks to this issue. A number of studies have found that North Americans judge themselves to be positively more unique than social others (Kitayama et al., 1997; Heine et al., 1999). For example, when asked to estimate the proportion of others who are better than themselves, the average responses are consistently lower than the midpoint (50%), indicating that North Americans tend to underestimate the number of people who are better than themselves. In a review of cross-cultural studies pertaining to this effect, Heine and Hamamura (2007) observed that this effect is consistently larger for Americans than for Asians. Whenever exceptions were found for this general trend (e.g., Brown & Kobayashi, 2002; Sedikides, Gaertner, & Toguchi, 2003), researchers used a particular format of asking respondents to estimate whether the self is better than an abstract representation of social others, such as "average student" and "typical member." Yet it has been demonstrated that even other individuals are often perceived to be better than either the average other or the typical other, due perhaps to the fact that the terms *average* and *typical* are somewhat derogatory. Heine and Hamamura (2007) therefore suggest that the apparent exceptions found in the literature are entirely consistent with the general hypothesis that the positive self-uniqueness effect is substantially stronger for North Americans (those with the independent mode of being) than for Asians (those with the interdependent mode of being).

Symbolic Self-Inflation

Is the self perceived to be literally bigger than others by persons with the independent mode of being? Moreover, is such size asymmetry less common and possibly reversed for those with the interdependent mode of being? In our recent work (Duffy, Uchida, & Kitayama, 2004) we asked both American and Japanese respondents to draw a network of their friends by using circles for both the self and friends, and connecting the circles with arrows. One of the dependent variables is particularly relevant for our present purposes. We simply measured the diameter of the circles. For all of our American respondents, the self circle was bigger than the average size of the circles used to designate friends. But this was the case for only 41% of our Japanese respondents.

Further evidence for a cultural divergence in representation of self versus social others occurred in a different measure concerning popularity ratings. After participants completed their sociogram, they were asked to rate on a 0- to 10-point scale their perception of the popularity of each member of the network, including the self. Notice that this method avoids the problem, noted earlier, of using abstract terms such as *average* or *typical* other. Duffy et al. (2004) compared the average rating for all the others against participants' rating of the self's popularity. Whereas 77% of North Americans rated themselves as more popular than the average of the individual ratings for their friends, only 16% of Japanese participants did so, suggesting a significant cultural difference in subjective assessments of self versus other within the domain of popularity assessment.

Self-Uniqueness

Those with the independent mode of being not only seek a positive and somewhat inflated evaluation of the self but also they strive for uniqueness. Within independent cultures such as the United States, whereas expressing unique features of the self often signifies one's freedom and autonomy, within interdependent cultures such as Japan and Korea, doing so is usually perceived as infringing upon the ever-important value of social harmony. In agreement with this analysis, Kim and Markus (1999) have shown cross-culturally divergent preferences for uniqueness. These researchers asked Asian Americans and European Americans to choose one pen from a group of five pens as a gift for completion of a questionnaire. There were two colors of pens. In one condition, only one pen was one color (minority pen), whereas the remaining four were the same color (majority pens); in the other condition, two pens were the same color (minority pens), and the remaining three were another color (majority pens). As predicted, European

Americans in both conditions chose a minority pen more frequently (over 70%) than majority pens, whereas Asian Americans chose a majority pen more frequently than they chose minority pens (under 31%). Hence, European Americans were far more likely than Asian Americans to pursue their self-uniqueness.

Cognitive Elaboration

One cognitive task that is suitable in testing the relative salience or richness of two concepts uses a simple judgment of similarity. It has been established that perceived similarity is greater when a relatively impoverished concept, with a small number of features, is compared to a relatively rich concept, with a greater number of features, than the latter is compared to the former. For example, North Korea is typically perceived to be more similar to the former Soviet Union, because what little is known about North Korea (e.g., communist country, dictatorship, relatively low standard of living, etc.) is very much shared by the Soviet Union. But the Soviet Union by no means seems similar to North Korea, because people usually have substantially more knowledge that is unique to the Soviet Union. Applying this principle, it is possible to assess the relative salience or richness of knowledge about self and social others. Kitayama, Markus, and Kato (1989, reported in Markus & Kitayama, 1991) did this by comparing white American students with American students with an Indian cultural heritage. Replicating numerous studies conducted in North America, Kitayama et al. (1989) observed that Americans judged their friends to be less similar to themselves than they were to their friends. This suggests that for these respondents, knowledge is richer and more salient for the self than for friends. In contrast, this pattern of asymmetry in self–other similarity judgment was reversed for the Indian respondents. Thus, as predicted, for Indians, knowledge about social others is more salient or richer than knowledge about the self.

In describing one's interpersonal actions, people commonly refer to both their own action (what they did) and characteristics of the person to which the action was directed (what this person was like). Within this general scheme, the relative salience of the two types of knowledge may vary across cultures. To investigate this possibility, Kitayama, Uchida, and colleagues (2006) asked both Americans and

Japanese participants to remember an episode wherein they did something to their acquaintance who was either happy or in distress. The main dependent variation was the number of words devoted to the description of the action and the description of the other person. As predicted, Americans used substantially more words to describe the self's own action than to describe the features of the other person, but the Japanese showed a significantly reversed pattern.

Reciprocity Monitoring

If Asians value and elaborate on social relations, they might monitor reciprocal exchanges of support. As Miller and Bersoff (1994) argued, such monitoring enables Asians to return favors to others. To see whether Asians in fact closely monitor reciprocity among their friends, Kitayama, Uchida, and colleagues (2006) invited many pairs of friends to come to the lab. Mutual friends in each pair were then separated into different rooms and asked to indicate for each of many supportive acts how much support they gave to the other and how much support they received from the other. Across three independent samples of Japanese friends, Kitayama and colleagues found that one's perception of the receipt of support and the other's perception about the provision of support were highly calibrated, with a Pearson's correlation of approximately .5. In contrast, among samples of American friends, the modal correlation was zero, showing no calibration at all of reciprocal exchange of support.

Cognition

The third component of the mode of being relates to ways in which people perceive and construe the meanings of attendant situations. On the one hand, self-directed individuals tend to focus attention on one goal-relevant object at a time. The tendency to attend to focal objects at the expense of the field, and using categories, rules, and formal logic in reasoning and judgment, is called "analytic mode of thought" (Nisbett et al., 2001). On the other hand, individuals who are responsive to social contingencies tend to disperse attention to many elements available in the environment. The tendency to attend to many objects and events simultaneously, and to arrive at an understand-

ing of an encompassing event as a whole is called the "holistic mode of thought." These two divergent "systems of thought" are likely to have a number of consequences upon both relatively low-level processing of attention and perception, and relatively high-level processing of reasoning and categorization (see Norenzayan et al., Chapter 23, this volume, for a detailed review).

Attention and Perception

Several recent studies have begun to explore how cultural modes of being mediate basic attention processes (Ji, Peng, & Nisbett, 2000; Nisbett & Masuda, 2003; Kitayama & Duffy, 2004) The central idea of this literature is that what one notices about the external world determines the information available for perceptual and cognitive processing. Early socialization processes and continued engagement in cultural practices shape the aspects or elements of the world to which individuals attend (Chavajay & Rogoff, 1999). So whereas North Americans focus their attention on focal objects and their intrinsic features, Asians tend to disperse their attention more broadly among objects and their contexts.

A variety of findings are consistent with the hypothesized cultural difference in attention (e.g., Masuda & Nisbett, 2001). For instance, Masuda and Nisbett (2001) showed animated underwater vignettes to Japanese and American participants, and asked them to report what they saw. American participants tended first to describe the most salient objects in the scene. Japanese participants were much more likely to begin by describing the background or field. Japanese reported a total of 60% more background or field objects than did Americans. The cross-cultural attention difference has been observed even when very abstract geometric stimuli are used. Kitayama, Duffy, Kawamura, and Larsen (2003) developed what they call the Framed Line Test (FLT) to test cultural differences in attention. In the FLT, participants were shown a line in a square frame and asked to draw a line of either the same absolute length or relative length in another square frame that differed in size. Whereas the absolute task requires ignoring the square frames and focusing attention on the target line, the relative task requires one to incorporate information about the frame into the estimate of the original line by dispersing attention to the surrounding frames. In support of the hypothesis that Americans exhibit a focused strategy of attention, their performance on the absolute task was more accurate than performance in the relative task. Moreover, in support of the notion that the Japanese exhibit a dispersed attention strategy, they were more accurate in the relative task than in the absolute task.

It is noteworthy that analogous effects of attention have been shown for perceptual judgments, with Asians sampling information more widely from context than do Americans (Kitayama & Duffy, 2004). Such attentional differences are likely to be automatic. Thus, Ishii et al. (2003) used a Stroop interference procedure to demonstrate that whereas American's attention is automatically captured by focal verbal meanings in speech comprehension, Asian's (Japanese and Filipinos) attention spontaneously goes more to contextual vocal tones. More recently, the comparable cultural difference has been observed at the level of rapid eye movements. Chua, Boland, and Nisbett (2005) presented both Asian and Caucasian American participants with a large object (e.g., airplane) and its context (e.g., sky with clouds and many buildings in distance). Participants were simply asked to report their picture preferences. Caucasian Americans were much more likely to fixate their eyes on the central object. Asian Americans tended to show many rapid eye movements to contextual stimulus elements. Given the differences in eye movements, it is very likely that cultural differences exist from the very beginning of information processing, even when people are exposed to a seemingly identical stimulus configuration.

As might be expected from this recent series of studies that implicate lower-level cognitions, the brains of Asians and Americans appear to be activated very differently. Using functional magnetic resonance imaging (fMRI) scans, Ketay, Hedden, Aron, Markus, and Gabrieli (2006) observed that Asian Americans show greater conflict when making absolute judgments in the FLT, whereas Caucasian Americans show greater conflict when making relative judgments. Another noteworthy finding comes from a recent study by Gutchess, Welsh, Boduroglu, and Park (in press). Their use of stimulus materials similar to those of Masuda and Nisbett (2001), revealed that Americans showed more activation in object processing regions (in particular, the left lateral middle temporal cortex) than did East Asians when studying complex pictures. They also found that East Asians showed more activation of a background processing area (the left fusiform gyrus).

Reasoning and Categorization

Nisbett and colleagues (2001) have argued that the independent mode of being encourages argumentation, reliance on explicit rules, and the general art of rhetoric that was supposedly invented by Greeks to settle disputes, whereas the independent mode of being fosters more relational epistemology and dialectic ways of reasoning that lend themselves to social harmony (see Nisbett, 2003; Norenzayan et al., Chapter 23, this volume, for reviews). For example, Norenzayan, Smith, Kim, and Nisbett (2002) asked both North Americans and Asians to judge whether an object belonged to one of two categories. One of the categories was defined by dint of an explicit rule, and the other was defined by means of family resemblance. The researchers found that North Americans relied on explicit rules, but Asians tended to base their judgment on family resemblances. A similar point has been made in a classic study by Chiu (1972), and in its more recent extensions by Ji, Zhang, and Nisbett (2004).

Evidence suggests that independent people tend to emphasize logical approaches to problem solving, whereas interdependent people tend to use dialectical approaches. We believe that this difference derives from the social orientation of the respective groups of people toward either confrontation or social harmony: Logical argument is useful in settling disagreement, but dialectic reasoning is more useful in moderating or preempting disagreement. For example, when presented with apparently contradictory propositions, Americans tended to reject one in favor of the other, and even to increase their belief in the more plausible proposition when they saw it contradicted by a less plausible one (Peng & Nisbett, 1999). This "hyperlogical" pattern contrasts with the behavior of the Chinese participants, who tended to find both propositions plausible. Peng and Nisbett also found that Chinese participants showed greater appreciation of proverbs expressing contradictions than did American participants, and Chinese participants were more inclined to "split the difference" in social or intrapersonal conflicts, rather than insisting that one side or the other had to be right. Finally, they found that Chinese participants were more impressed with arguments that reflected multiple points of view than were Americans.

Summary

When wide-angle comparisons are drawn between North American and Asian cultures, there often arise a number of intriguing psychological differences. They can be readily classified into three sets, namely, style of action, self–other representations, and cognition. As shown in Figure 6.2, the independent mode of being is associated with the style of action as influence, self-centricity, and the analytic mode of cognition. In contrast, the interdependent mode of being is associated with the style of action as adjustment, other-centricity, and the holistic mode of cognition. One weakness of this literature stems from the fact that most of the reviewed studies are based on college student samples. Yet theoretically comparable findings have been observed among young children (e.g., Fernald & Morikawa, 1993), in community samples (Markus et al., 2004), and in a variety of cultural artifacts (e.g., Kim & Markus, 1999). This literature presents a reasonably strong case for the fundamental role that culture plays in the construction of the self as a mode of being.

DEVELOPMENTAL AND SOCIAL ANTECEDENTS

So far, we have discussed how social relational differences (*gesellschaft* and *gemeinschaft*) might be associated with two contrasting modes of being (independent and interdependent). Moreover, we provided evidence for this analysis by reviewing an emerging body of cross-cultural studies focused on style of action, self–other representation, and mode of thought. So far, however, this evidence leaves open a number of significant questions about the development and antecedents of the two modes of being. In this third section of the chapter, we examine some initial efforts to address these issues. We start with a review of recent theoretical analyses of socialization of independence and interdependence.

Socialization of the Mode of Being

The mode of being is a social product, fostered and shaped through socialization. Recent theoretical advancements on cultural socialization suggest that the independent mode of being is fostered by socialization practices that encourage autonomy, whereas the interdependent mode of being is promoted by those that encourage symbiotic relations.

Culture and Developmental Pathways

In their discussion on culturally variable pathways of development, Greenfield and colleagues (2003) proposed that the development of the self is contingent upon successfully resolving three universal tasks of human development: relationship formation in infancy, knowledge formation during childhood, and the balance between autonomy and relatedness in adolescence and early adulthood. Yet cultures vary along three important dimensions that mediate the strategies and, ultimately, the trajectories by which individuals resolve these important tasks. First, cultures vary in practices, such as the manner in which parents interact with their children. Second, cultures vary in ecological conditions, such as the size of families or how many people sleep together in the same room. Finally, cultures vary in meaning systems and beliefs regarding the normative and proscriptive beliefs, behaviors, action tendencies, and developmental trajectories. Each of these factors plays an important role in guiding an individual's growth along a pathway toward either independence or interdependence. In terms of relationship formation, which is most relevant to our discussion, Greenfield and colleagues point out that interdependent cultures promote the development of a symbiotic relationship between mother and child, whereas independent cultures foster children's individual autonomy.

The same theme is echoed by another important model by Rothbaum and his colleagues (2000), which proposes that in interdependent cultures such as Japan, the pathway through development is one of symbiotic harmony, whereas in independent cultures, the path is one of generative tension. More specifically, the path of symbiotic harmony entails unity in infancy, in which the distinction between mother and child is blurred, focusing on the other's expectations during childhood, maintaining stable relationships among family members during adolescence, and unconditional loyalty to partners in adulthood. The cultural practices and shared meanings along the pathway of symbiotic harmony foster allocentric attention to relationships, particularly among the kinship network, thereby promoting an interdependent mode of being. In contrast, the path of generative tension emphasizes a constructive role that interpersonal conflict plays in fostering developmental change. Along this path, infant autonomy is emphasized and actively promoted; children are expected to exhibit personal preferences and respect the preferences of others; and the transformation of affiliation from family to peers is expected and promoted during childhood. Moreover, adult relationships are based upon trust individuals confer on each other, rather than on assurance provided by formal and informed social sanctions.

Cultural Differences in Parental Practices

A variety of practices guide children toward different developmental goals. For instance, in many interdependent cultures such as India and Japan, parents co-sleep with their infants and young children, whereas in the independent cultures such as Germany and the United States, most infants sleep in separate rooms (Shweder, 2003). These practices are enforced by relevant cultural beliefs. Needless to say, a variety of ecological conditions can influence sleeping arrangements. For instance, separate sleeping arrangements may not be possible for families living in a one-room adobe hut. Yet, Shweder and colleagues (1997) found evidence that cultural preferences for different sleeping arrangements persist even when such ecological constraints are minimal.

Several studies have focused on Japan and examined cross-cultural variation in mother–infant interaction. In one of these studies, Bornstein et al. (1992) observed contents of maternal speech to infants and found marked cross-cultural differences in the frequencies of affect-salient (e.g., "The ball makes you happy!") versus information-salient maternal speech (e.g., "The ball is red!"). Japanese mothers produced more affect-salient speech, whereas U.S. mothers exhibited speech that was more information-salient and asked information-seeking questions. Similarly, Fernald and Morikawa (1993) found that, compared with their American counterparts, infant directed speech of Japanese mothers contains fewer words but a greater number of affect-salient, nonverbal vocalizations. In terms of nonverbal linguistic behavior, Bornstein et al. (1992) found that Japanese mothers are more responsive than American or French

mothers to infant's social looking. Furthermore, Japanese mothers direct infants' attention to the mother, and specifically to emotional facial expressions, whereas American mothers direct infants' attention to objects and events in the environment (Bornstein, Toda, Azuma, Tamis-LeMonda, & Ogino, 1990).

Further evidence for the cross-cultural variation in socialization practice comes from a well-replicated finding that Japanese mothers tend to exhibit greater symbiotic proximity than American mothers, spending more time in direct physical contact with their infants (see Barratt, 1993, for a review). For example, infants in Japan receive nonmaternal caregiving for about 2 hours a week, whereas American infants receive, on average, 23 hours. As might be expected, Japanese babies show a higher degree of anxiety than do American babies when separated from the mother in the Strange Situation paradigm (Miyake, Chen, & Campos, 1985). Secure and avoidant attachment styles are correspondingly less frequent in Japan. Similar cross-cultural differences persist throughout the toddler period (Zahn-Waxler, Friedman, Cole, & Mizuta, 1996). Taken as a whole, the evidence consistently suggests a systematic cultural bias in socialization practices, with Western mothers distancing the child as a little adult and directing the child's attention to his or her goal-relevant object, and Japanese mothers treating the child literally as a child, and engaging the child in an intimate symbiotic relationship.

Some more recent studies have examined cultures other than the United States and Japan. Drawing on previous evidence that mothers in interdependent cultures exhibit symbiotic or proximate parenting behaviors (which emphasize body contact and body stimulation between the caregiver and child), whereas parents in independent cultures exhibit distal behaviors (which promote face-to-face contact and object stimulation), Keller et al. (2004) proposed that whereas proximate behaviors foster an orientation toward interpersonal relatedness, distal practices create an orientation toward autonomy. To test this possibility, Keller et al. measured both proximate and distal parenting practices of mothers when their children were 3 months of age and explored behavioral consequences for the children at 18 months. The maternal styles (proximate vs. distal) were determined by a systematic coding of a 3-hour naturalistic observation. Of importance, Keller and colleagues tested an independent, urban, middle-class culture (Greeks); an interdependent, urban, middle-class culture (Costa Ricans); and an interdependent, rural farming culture (Cameroonian Nso). At 18 months, the toddlers' self-recognition (an index of independence) and compliance (an index of interdependence) were measured. Keller et al. found that children of the proximate-style Cameroonian mothers exhibited greater compliance behaviors, whereas the children of the distal-style Greek mothers exhibited greater self-recognition at 18 months. The Costa Rican mothers and children fell between these two groups. These findings support the hypothesis that cultural variations in modes of being begin to emerge at an early point in development; moreover, specific socialization practices play a significant role in this developmental change.

Voluntary Settlement

One source of within-culture variability that has received research attention of late is voluntary settlement. Cultural groups differ greatly in the degree to which they are sedentary or socially mobile. Some individuals emigrate with great effort and determination for a variety of reasons, whereas others decide to stay in the communities of their origin, under seemingly identical circumstances. Cultures may subsequently differ substantially as result of such emigration or the absence thereof. This consideration is especially important in understanding American individualism.

In the last 400 years, the United States has been a major magnet of for immigrants from all over the world. Except for African Americans who were forced to work as slaves, the vast majority of immigrants voluntarily settled in North America. Over nearly three centuries, from the 16th through the 19th century, new lands of the West were continuously exploited and settled by Americans of mostly European descent, with the frontier steadily moved westward. Does the voluntary settlement in a frontier promote an independent mode of being? A number of theorists have suggested an affirmative answer to this question (Bellah et al., 1985; Hochschild, 1995; Schlesinger, 1986; de Tocqueville, 1835/1969; Turner, 1920).

Drawing on this literature, Kitayama, Ishii, Imada, Takemura, and Ramaswamy (2006) proposed that voluntary settlement in a frontier foster independent agency by three mechanisms. First, the initial move toward settlement in new lands of freedom and opportunity requires a strong desire for independence, freedom, and economic prosperity. Hence, there may be considerable self-selection, such that settlers may be more independently disposed from the beginning. Second, frontier life is often harsh, thereby reinforcing the ethos of independence and self-directedness. Third, this ethos is institutionalized, so that the culture of independence is passed on over generations, even when the frontier no longer exists.

According to this hypothesis, there should be elements of the independent mode of being even outside of North America as long as there is a relatively recent history of economically motivated voluntary settlement. Kitayama, Ishii, and colleagues (2006) thus examined Hokkaido—a northern island of Japan—as a natural experiment for testing the voluntary settlement hypothesis. This island had been intensively settled since the 1870s over several decades, primarily by jobless samurais and, subsequently, by farmers. The motivation for the settlement was personal success and achievement in certain tangible terms. The dictum "Boys be ambitious!" broadly attributed to an American educator, Dr. William S. Clark, who served as the first vice-president of the Hokkaido University between 1876 and 1877, eloquently expresses the regional ethos of Hokkaido around that time, which supposedly has since been deeply ingrained into the regional culture.

Kitayama, Ishii, and colleagues (2006) tested three indicators of independent agency, namely, the fundamental attribution error, happiness as personal achievement, and personal dissonance. The results were quite clear: Japanese who were born and raised up in Hokkaido were more similar to Americans than to non-Hokkaido Japanese. Unlike the non-Hokkaido Japanese, the Hokkaido Japanese exhibited the fundamental attribution error. Moreover, unlike happiness for the non-Hokkaido Japanese, happiness for the Hokkaido Japanese was distinctly more personal and grounded in achievement. Finally, the Hokkaido Japanese also showed evidence of personal dissonance, which is motivated by concerns for private self-images. This Hokkaido finding on dissonance is in sharp contrast with typical findings for non-Hokkaido Japanese (Hoshino-Browne et al., 2005; Kitayama et al., 2004), in which the dissonance effect is obtained only in the presence of certain social cues or contexts that evoke public self-image concerns.

Social Class

Cultural differences that have been demonstrated are often substantial. In terms of effect size, these differences are often in the range of "moderate" to "strong" effect. For example, Miyamoto, Kitayama, and Talhelm (2006) reviewed a large number of published studies on culture and cognition, and found that the mean effect size for the West–East difference, as indicated by Cohen's d, is approximately 0.70. It goes without saying, however, that substantial individual differences are also present within each of the compared cultures. Although some of these differences are due to a variety of noises in measurement, others are likely to be more systematic. One important variable that describes such within-culture differences is social class.

"Social class" refers to a dimension defined by several, loosely correlated, value-ridden features of one's position in a society, such as education, ownership, control over the means of production, income, and associated status and prestige. Because these features are value-ridden, some positions are higher than others, resulting in a hierarchy of power, wealth, and prestige. Although some societies are highly hierarchical (e.g., India) and others are relatively egalitarian (e.g., The Netherlands), virtually all contemporary societies have some degree of such stratification (Schooler, Chapter 15, this volume). In recent years, it has become increasingly clear that different social classes foster a variety of different psychological propensities and characteristics.

Snibbe and Markus (2005) focused on one critical dimension of social class (i.e., educational attainment) and argued that college-educated and high-school-educated Americans are characterized by somewhat different models of self and agency. Whereas members of the college-educated group ground their selves in free choice and attainment of personal autonomy, the high school-educated group members emphasize protecting their integrity against adversities of the surrounding world. To examine this analysis, these researchers performed a content analysis on the various kinds of music most commonly preferred by individuals with a high school education (country music) compared to that preferred by college-educated in-

dividuals (rock music). They found that country music lyrics contain themes expressing individual integrity, self-adjustment, and resisting influence, whereas rock music lyrics express individual uniqueness, control over the environment, and influence. Snibbe and Markus provide further evidence by using the free-choice dissonance paradigm. Recall that in this paradigm participants are given a choice between two equally attractive items. Typically, Americans shift their preference for a chosen item upward, while shifting their preference for a rejected item downward. Snibbe and Markus found that this typical American pattern was found for college-educated Americans, but for the high school-educated group, only the downward shift of preference for the rejected item was observed. This finding is consistent with the overall hypothesis that working-class individuals seek to protect their integrity by justifying what they have to give up.

Another important insight into the effect of social class on identity, self, and cognition comes from a series of studies by Schooler and colleagues, who have hypothesized that individuals in positions of higher social status—those in control of the means of production—exhibit aspects of individuality, such as occupational self-direction, intrinsic motivation, and analytic modes of cognition, to a greater extent than individuals with lower social status. Schooler and colleagues link these differences to structural aspects of common working conditions among those with high- or low-status jobs. High-status jobs generally demand greater cognitive flexibility, self-directed action, and independent value orientations. Alternatively, low-status jobs generally promote interdependent thinking (e.g., teamwork), involve little self-directed action, and generally tend to involve routine actions that are part of larger processes (i.e., piecemeal work on an assembly line). Furthermore, these findings are not limited to American social structures: Schooler's general findings have been replicated in a variety of different cultural contexts, such as Poland and Japan (Kohn, Naoi, Schoenbach, Schooler, & Slomczynski, 1990; Naoi & Schooler, 1985). Additionally, Schooler and his colleagues found that differences in social status are related to child-rearing behaviors, with parents of high social status more likely than low-status parents to promote values of intellectual flexibility, self-direction, and motivation (Kohn, et al., 1990). At present, it is not clear whether self-direction, arguably associated with middle-class environments, nurtures general cognitive competences (e.g., IQ), analytic skills (e.g., focusing [vis-à-vis holistic] strategy of attention), or both. It is highly desirable to use cognitive tasks such as FLT that dissociate analytic versus holistic cognitive competencies from general cognitive competence.

Taken together, these studies suggest that social status may have an important role in shaping orientations toward the interdependent and independent dimensions of cultural modes of being. At present, it is not known whether working-class Americans are "less independent" than middle-class Americans in all three facets of independence and interdependence we have posited. Snibbe and Markus (2005) have argued that both groups are equally independent, but the specific way in which they are independent varies. Thus, whereas middle-class culture emphasizes self-reliance and self-directedness, working-class culture puts a premium on the protection of integrity. It is also possible that social classes differ in specific profiles of independence defined by the three facets. For example, Americans might have an equally strong tendency to take a style of action as influence, but their mode of thought might be dependent more on their educational attainment, with college-educated groups being much more analytical than high school-educated groups. This and other, related issues must be addressed in future work.

Cultural Affordances

Kitayama and colleagues have defined "cultural affordances" as the potential of cultural environments to evoke different sets of cognitive, emotional, and motivational responses (Kitayama & Markus, 1999; Kitayama, Mesquita, & Karasawa, 2006; see also Gibson, 1979). Cultural affordances result from a biased pool of symbolic resources of culture that are brought to bear on the construction of concrete daily situations (Kitayama et al., 1997; Morling et al., 2002). These symbolic resources are used to define general classes of events and episodes available in a given cultural context (school, exam, business, success, failure, etc.). But more importantly, they profoundly influence more subtle, yet powerful nuances and psychological meanings (pride, shame, obligation, honor, etc.) that are added to the lived experience of such events and episodes. These meanings may often be highly idiosyncratic and hardly predictable in any specific instances, yet because they are derived or fostered by a pool of symbolic resources available in a given culture, they may be systematically biased over many situations and episodes in accordance with the specific, historically crafted and accumulated contents of this pool. In this way, individual experiences may be collectively constructed through sociohistorical processes (Kitayama & Markus, 1999; Kitayama et al., 1997).

For example, "getting an A in an important course" is likely to be both positive and disengaging (causing one to feel proud) in all cultures. Nevertheless, certain engaging themes, icons, and ideas, such as smiling faces of parents who are very happy to know their daughter's performance in the course, may be more available in interdependent than in independent cultural contexts. If so, a subtle, yet distinctly engaging element or nuance may be added to the experience for those in the interdependent contexts, but such an addition of engaging nuances may be relatively unlikely for those in the independent contexts. This example illustrates how subtle the effect of cultural affordances can sometimes be. It also suggests, however, that such a subtle effect can be very powerful over time, because it is highly recurrent, present all the time, insofar as all individuals must necessarily be drawing on the pool of symbolic resources of their own culture.

Likewise, it is a common experience among many Asian sojourners in the United States to find that many of their American friends are very nice, complimenting and praising them, but they also feel the compliments and praise to be somewhat excessive. This would have been surely embarrassing in their native (Asian) contexts! After a while, however, the sojourners are resocialized in the United States; that is, they get used to the American-style friendship and, as a consequence, no longer feel their American friends' praise and compliments are unnecessarily positive, but instead will feel natural and even appropriate. Not surprisingly, Asians' self-esteem substantially goes up after some period of resocialization in North America (Heine et al., 1999). These examples illustrate that culture is not inert or passive. To the contrary, it often is an active element of psychological experience. The notion of cultural affordances highlights this potentially powerful role of culture's practices and meanings to guide psychological processes in subtle, yet highly systematic fashion.

Situation Sampling

It is reasonable that North American cultural contexts have historically incorporated a variety of cultural resources (meanings and practices) that encourage independence of the self; moreover, through enculturation, individuals become capable of recognizing and attuning themselves to the culture's affordances. Thus, Kitayama et al. (1997) proposed that "psychological tendencies . . . are importantly afforded and sustained by the ways in which the attendant social realities are collectively constructed in each cultural context" (p. 1246). It would follow, then, that North Americans and Asians should be most independent and interdependent, respectively, when exposed to social situations that are most routinely available in their own cultural contexts.

Kitayama and colleagues (1997; Morling et al., 2002) explored some implications of this collective construction theory in a series of Japan–U.S. comparison studies that use a situation-sampling method. In this method, situations that meet a certain criterion are randomly sampled according to two different cultural contexts. The situations sampled from the two cultures are then presented to respondents from both cultures. Respondents are then asked to imagine that they are in each of the situations and to estimate their own psychological responses in the situation. With this method, Kitayama and colleagues (1997) discovered that Americans feel more efficacious and esteemed (and therefore independent) when exposed to situations that are most commonly available in their own cultural contexts. In contrast, Asians are especially likely to be self-effacing when exposed to their own cultural situations.

Although Kitayama and colleagues (1997) focused on situational definitions as the primary locus in which each culture's symbolic resources play their role in shaping psychological tendencies of those engaging in the culture, it is also clear that there are many other types of cultural affordances. Indeed, the cultural affordances hypothesis amounts to the idea that culture "primes" different emotion themes (Oyserman & Lee, Chapter 10, this volume). We now turn to this literature. As will be seen, the priming research may fruitfully expand its scope to examine the entire pool of icons, lay theories, and other symbolic resources that are unevenly distributed across different cultural contexts.

Language, Cultural Icons, Ecology

First, linguistic practices serve as a powerful affordance for certain psychological processes. One case in point comes from an observation that whereas in most West European languages, including English, subject and object are obligatory in grammatically constructed sentences, they are not in most of the remaining languages in the world (Kashima & Kashima, 2003). This phenomenon is called "pronoun drop." Thus, whereas English speakers always remind the listeners that it is "I" who thinks, feels, and so forth, Asian speakers more often than not leave this aspect to the listeners' inferences. Thus, especially in Asian contexts, it is quite informative if the speaker uses pronouns even where they are reasonably inferable from context and thus ordinarily omitted. Kakuno and Ura (2002), who replicated other, related findings (e.g., Masuda & Kitayama, 2004; Miyamoto & Kitayama, 2002), showed that when asked to infer the real attitude of someone who was allegedly requested by an external authority to make a speech on a controversial political issue, Japanese subjects did not infer the attitude to closely correspond to the speech content. Although this finding may be expected to be typical in Japanese contexts, it in fact was observed only when the form of the speech allegedly made by the speaker conformed to the linguistic convention of pronoun drop. When all pronouns (especially *I*s) were inserted, Japanese participants exhibited a quite strong bias to infer that the speaker's real attitude closely corresponded to the speech content.

A second type of cultural affordance has received considerable research attention of late—a variety of cultural icons. For example, the Statue of Liberty, a football stadium packed with enthusiastic fans, Marilyn Monroe, and the like, are some of the U.S. icons, whereas dragons, Great Walls, Mao, and the like, are comparable icons in China. The respective sets of icons may induce the corresponding psychological tendencies for those who are familiar with the two cultures. In many cases, except perhaps for the Statue of Liberty relative to independence, there is nothing inherently either independent or interdependent about these icons (Why does Marilyn represent more independence than Mao?). Yet American icons such as Marilyn Monroe are associated with independence by virtue of associative connections between America and individualism. Conversely, Chinese icons such as dragons and Mao can prime interdependence by virtue of the associative links between China and collectivistic or interdependent cultural values. The best evidence so far for this possibility comes from a series of studies that examined Hong Kong Chinese, who wee expected to be equally knowledgeable about both Chinese and American culture (Hong, Wan, No, Chiu, Chapter 13, this volume). These researchers have demonstrated that the fundamental attribution error, which is more typical in American contexts, can be found even for Chinese, but only if they are exposed to American icons just before they work on the attribution task.

Third, importantly, mounting evidence indicates that some aspects of the two modes of being can be activated when the corresponding ideas or linguistic symbols of independence and interdependence are primed. In one study of this effect, Trafimow, Triandis, and Goto (1991) had American participants read either an individualistic or a collectivistic story. When asked to describe themselves in a seemingly separate study, the participants generated more individual traits in the individualistic story condition, and more group memberships in the collectivistic story condition. In another, similar attempt, Brewer and Gardner (1996) presented to American participants a story written with a number of either singular or plural first-person pronouns (*I, my, me* vs. *we, our, us*). Participants were asked to circle all the pronouns. When asked to judge themselves, the participants in the "I" condition proved to be more independent or less interdependent than their counterparts in the "we" condition. These findings have recently been extended to some cognitive effects, with more analytic or less holistic tendencies manifest after the "I" priming than after the "we" priming (e.g., Kuhnen & Oyserman, 2002). Even more intriguing, Gray, Ambady, Ishii, and Kitayama (2006) examined Americans and found that after a subliminal exposure to affiliation-related words (Lakin & Chartrand, 2003), participants become especially sensitive to vocal tone in a vocal Stroop paradigm (Ishii et al., 2003)—a marker feature of interdependence.

It is not clear whether the priming of independence and interdependence is different in kind from the priming effect demonstrated with cultural icons. It is possible that cultural icons are much more tightly embedded in a specific culture's practices and institutions, and as a consequence, priming effects due to these icons are entirely dependent on immersion in that particular cultural context.

At first glance, this consideration might seem unlikely to apply to the pronoun (*I* vs. *we*) priming effect, because this effect is grounded in the fact that every society has elements of both independence and interdependence. The relative frequency or prevalence of different pronouns may vary across cultures and societies. The story might not be so straightforward, however. If it is really true that the personal self is always defined as embedded in interpersonal contexts in Asia, the representation of the personal self (I) might have a greater overlap with the representation of the social or communal self (we). If so, the pronoun priming effect might be predicted to be much weaker in interdependent than in independent contexts. This question has yet to be addressed: There is no published work on pronoun priming outside of Western cultural contexts.

A promising way to conceptualize culture, then, is to think about it as a series of priming operations by a great many cultural artifacts, practices, discourses, and institutions, of which the specific priming manipulations examined by psychologists so far are only a few select examples. These and many other priming operations embedded in a culture's practices and meanings constitute what Kitayama, Mesquita, and Karasawa (2006) have called the "cultural affordances" of a given social setting. As we see later, it is likely that many more cultural artifacts, such as ads and textbooks, do carry images that reinforce rather than compromise the primary values of culture.

Fourth, cultural affordances may also come from cultural ecology. After all, especially in the modern world, there is no purely natural ecology (Watsuji, 1935/1961). Nature itself is already fully cultural because it has been drastically transformed through human interventions (Diamond, 1997). In a recent study, Miyamoto, Nisbett, and Masuda (2006) systematically collected photographs of scenes from several cities of differing size in both Japan and the United States, and examined both subjective and objective characteristics of the scenes. They found that, compared to their American counterparts, Japanese scenes tended to be more complex, to contain more objects, and to be more chaotic or cognitively confusing. Moreover, they went a step further and argued, using initial empirical evidence, that the relatively complex Japanese scenes may in fact induce relatively holistic cognitive styles. The attention of both American and Japanese participants became more holistic when participants were exposed to a series of scenes from Japan than when exposed to those from the United States.

Public Artifacts

The cultural ethos of independence and interdependence is likely to be incorporated into a variety of cultural artifacts, such as ads, icons, and media materials, which in turn may function as potent cues that prime the culturally sanctioned mode of being (Hong, Morris, Chiu, & Benet-Martinez, 2000). In recent years, there has been a concerted effort to demonstrate systematic cross-cultural differences in public artifacts.

For example, Markus, Uchida, Omoregie, Townsend, and Kitayama (2006) sampled actual media coverage of the 2000 and 2002 Olympics from newspapers, magazines, and television programs in the United States and Japan, and analyzed contents of the coverage, including statements of athletes, reporters, and commentators. In both Japanese and American contexts, Olympic performance was explained mainly in terms of the actions of athletes. Yet, Olympic actions (agency) were illustrated and understood differently by the athletes themselves and the media. In the American context, agency was explained as independent and disjointed (Markus & Kitayama, 2004), separate from the athlete's historical background or social and emotional experience. Rather, performance was mainly explained through positive personal characteristics and features of the competition. In Japanese contexts, however, agency was explained as interdependent or conjointed (Markus & Kitayama, 2004), strongly connected with athletes' backgrounds and others in the interpersonal relationships. For example, for Naoko Takahashi, a Japanese gold medalist in the women's marathon, media coverage almost always mentioned her relationship with her coach. Such differences, which can be seen in explanations of the nature of intentional agency in the media coverage, have same patterns as the cross-cultural differences, which can be seen in individual behavior or cognition.

Contents of ads also vary systematically across cultures. Kim and Markus (1999) analyzed how the themes of conformity and uniqueness are used in advertisements from various types of magazines (from business to youth/pop culture) in the United States and Korea. As we explained in the previous section, East Asians prefer conformity, whereas North Americans prefer uniqueness in the individual behavioral level. Consistent with that finding, Korean magazine advertisements are more likely to use conformity-related messages or appeals (95%), such as promoting group harmony or following a trend, than uniqueness-related messages (49%). In contrast, American magazine advertisements are more likely to use uniqueness-related messages or appeals (89%), such as emphasizing freedom or choices, than conformity messages (65%). Similarly, Han and Shavitt (1994) pointed out that Korean magazine advertisements use collectivistic appeals much more than do American advertisements, which in turn use individualistic appeals much more than do Korean advertisements.

Yet another example of public artifacts that potentially have the most powerful consequences for the development of culturally divergent modes of being comes from textbook materials (see also McLelland, 1985). In a recent content analysis of elementary school language textbooks in Japan and the United States, Imada (2005) found that the cultural values and beliefs used in the textbooks are significantly different across cultures. She showed that collectivistic values, such as conformity and interdependence, are more likely to be used in the Japanese textbooks than in American textbooks, whereas individualistic values, such as self-direction, achievement, and power, are more likely to be used in the American textbooks than in Japanese textbooks. Moreover, American stories have more pictures that focus only on one person and are more likely to attribute the outcomes to internal factors, such as personal characteristics or effort, than do Japanese textbooks. In contrast, Japanese stories have more pictures with two or three characters and are more likely to attribute the outcomes to external factors, such as other people's behavior or the situation.

CONCLUSIONS

Culture in the Mind

A central thesis of cultural psychology holds that psychological processes in the sense of standardized operational procedures of cognition, emotion, and motivation are socioculturally afforded; as a consequence, what initially appears to be a fully natural part of the human mind may in fact be saturated with culture (e.g., Bruner, 1990; Cole, 1996; Markus & Kitayama, 1991; Shore, 1996; Shweder, 2003). Only during the last decade or two has this point of view has taken a strong hold in the mainstream of psychology and begun to influence other social science disciplines (but see LeVine, Chapter 2, and Triandis, Chapter 3, this volume, for important historical precursors).

In fact, the idea that culture becomes part of the mind was also largely ignored in most of anthropology and sociology, where the main focus was on what Durkheim called "social facts" such as rituals and social institutions (but see LeVine, Chapter 2, this volume, for important exceptions, e.g., Sapir's elaborate view on the culture–mind interaction). Psychology was largely missing, and in its place were vaguely defined notions of "primitive minds" and "rational agents." In a way, cultural psychological investigation of the last decade rationalized primitive minds by revealing the coherent logic of them, while socializing the rational agents by specifying the sociocultural affordances for them.

Given the disciplinary history and backgrounds that placed a sharp division between culture and mind, the notion that culture and the psyche make each other up (Shweder, 1991) came as a fresh revelation to many culturally oriented psychologists and psychologically oriented anthropologists and sociologists. With this idea salvaged and returned to the center stage of the study of culture, cross-cultural comparison became something much more than a litmus test of universality.

The hypothesis of mutual constitution implies that the human mind, by its very nature, is designed to be socioculturally shaped and completed. It follows that the human mind is best understood when cast in varying contexts of different cultures and societies. Since the theoretical shift promoted by Shweder and other pioneers during the 1980s and 1990s, cross-cultural comparison has begun to be recognized as an indispensable part of all human psychology. In this emerging perspective, cross-cultural comparison can no longer be dismissed as a pastime for psychologists. To the contrary, it is an indispensable tool for theory building in all areas of human psychology.

In this chapter, we have argued that many of the recent advances in cultural psychology can be integrated by conceptualizing the self not so much as semantic or conceptual structures, but more as a mode of being, or *modus operandi*, that is, a set of standard operating procedures in major psychological functions such as cognition, emotion, and motivation. We traced the origins of the mode of operation to cross-culturally divergent structures of sociality. Moreover, we identified three facets of the mode of being, and argued that these facets are often correlated but can surely be dissociated under certain historical conditions.

Critical Appraisals

The approach to culture, delineated in this chapter, has received some concerted criticisms. In closing this chapter, it would be appropriate to discuss some of these critical appraisals. In particular, two lines of criticism against our approach are worthy comment.

Stereotyping?

First and foremost, independence or interdependence is not a label assigned to a set of psychological traits. It is often argued, however, that "independence" is defined in terms of both certain autonomous, individually oriented behaviors (e.g., choice, social mobility, and self-expression) and corresponding subjective experiences (e.g., sense of autonomy and power), whereas "interdependence" is defined in terms of cooperative and prosocial behaviors (e.g., conformity, compliance, and cooperation), and accompanying subjective experiences (e.g., harmony and trust). This argument leads to a caricature of people who fit either one or the other of these two sets of behaviors. For example, a renowned developmental psychologist recently noted:

> The characterization of cultures as individualistic or collectivist . . . is likely to be false, and it serves thereby to stereotype people and groups. . . . The idea [is] patently false for one simple reason: most groups . . . are structured hierarchically . . . and

people in positions of power in those hierarchies are often highly "individualistic." (Turiel, 2004, p. 92)

We do well to remember that personal autonomy and social relations are both significant elements of human social functions; thus, they are likely to be universally available in all cultural contexts. This means, for example, that practices, such as choice, self-expression, conformity, and cooperation, and subjective experiences, such as harmony and disagreement, are available in all cultures. Nevertheless, it is possible that any one of these practices and experiences is powerfully structured and configured in terms of an underlying model of self as either independent or interdependent. For example, there may be different ways of making a choice that are more amenable either to an independent or to an interdependent model of self (Kitayama et al., 2004). Likewise, although cooperation and trust are available and can easily be found in all cultural contexts, they can also take quite diverse forms depending on the underlying model of self as independent or interdependent (Yamagishi & Yamagishi, 1994). Whereas in the United States trust is grounded in the perceived disposition of another person, in Japan it requires specific interpersonal connections (Brewer & Yuki, Chapter 12, this volume). Cultural models of independence and interdependence provide resources and constraints for handling many universal tasks, such as choice, competition or cooperation, and agreement or disagreement.

Seen from this vantage point, the cultural analysis presented here is entirely consistent with the enormous flexibility and variability of human behaviors and cognitions. This flexibility or variability, however, is made possible by numerous cultural and largely social resources and constraints. The independent or interdependent model supplies one significant set of such social resources and constraints.

Personal Values and Beliefs?

Cultural models of self comprise many practices and public meanings that define the landscape of the cultural environment. Many of the practices and meanings are based on certain values and beliefs. For example, practices based on the Protestant relational ideology (Sanchez-Burks, 2005) were established on the basis of, and, can be traced back to certain theological ideas of Calvin and other founders of Protestantism. Nevertheless, once established, these practices comprise a collectively constituted environment of capitalism, in which each individual in the society had to survive, and with which each individual had to cope. In this particular case, whether one believes in Protestantism or values any aspects of this theological variety of Christianity would simply be irrelevant. Likewise, a cultural model of the self as interdependent is likely to have established many aspects of a cultural environment, such as communicative practices (e.g., high-context communication), interpersonal routines (e.g., various rules of etiquette), and social institutions (e.g., a company as family). To participate and even to flourish within this collective environment, however, it is not necessary to be aware of the etiology of this environment, much less to endorse personally archaic values or beliefs underlying this environment.

Traditionally, the only means available for psychologists to measure culture was attitudinal questionnaires. Thus, numerous studies were conducted to determine whether Americans are in fact more individualistic and independent, and whether Easterners are more collectivistic and interdependent. Many factors, including acquiescence bias (Schimmack et al., 2005), reference group effect (Heine et al., 2001), and culturally variable referents of abstract concepts (Peng et al., 1997), severely compromise this literature. Thus, without adequate control of these issues, whether statistical or conceptual, the results of these questionnaires can be extremely misleading. Indeed, as noted earlier, one might often get an impression that cross-cultural differences are neither strong nor systematic (Oyserman et al., 2002). From this type of observation, some researchers have immediately jumped to the conclusion that cultural variation in practices and meanings is illusory. For example, a cross-cultural psychologist stated:

> The evidence . . . overwhelmingly indicates that the Japanese are not more collectivistic than Americans; if anything, in some cases the Japanese are more individualistic than Americans. Thus, these differences cannot possibly account for differences in self-construals between the two countries. . . . (Matsumoto, 1999, p. 298)

However, once researchers adequately control for certain biasing effects of survey questionnaires (e.g., Heine et al., 2002; Schimmack et al., 2005), cross-cultural variation is quite systematic and sizable even in paper-and-pencil measures of values and beliefs. Moreover, as we have indicated, once behavioral measures are tested, cross-cultural differences that are indicative of the corresponding modes of being are bound to be even more systematic and sizable.

Toward an Implicit Measure of Independence and Interdependence

This said, however, we wish to emphasize that the field will be better served by a renewed effort to develop a more valid measure of independence and interdependence. As we mentioned earlier, to capture individual differences on this dimension, researchers have traditionally relied on several different attitudinal scales (e.g., Singelis, 1994). All these scales probe one's independence or interdependence in terms of explicit self-reports ("In general I make my own decisions" for independence and "When my opinion is in conflict with that of another person's, I often accept the other opinion" for interdependence). In addition to all the artifacts that might compromise the cross-cultural evidence based entirely on this type of measures, there is a lingering suspicion that such explicit measures of self might have an inherent limitation (Kitayama, 2002). This may be the case, because people's behavioral propensities toward independence or interdependence might be embodied, automatized, or spontaneous, and thus largely implicit; that is, they might be rarely self-reflective, deliberate, or even conscious. If there is only a limited conscious access to such behavioral propensities (Nisbett & Wilson, 1977), explicit self-report might be ill-suited as a tool for measuring them.

Many of the studies reviewed in the main body of this chapter used the notion of independent and interdependent self to predict some systematic cross-cultural variations in the pattern of cognitive, emotional, and motivational responses and behaviors. Yet, given the cumulative evidence that was reviewed, we wonder whether the converse of this standard logic might prove to be equally fruitful in future work; that is, it might be possible to use the pattern of, say, emotional responses as a means for implicit assessment of independence and interdependence.

We recently suggested, for example, that one promising measure is the extent to which engaging or disengaging positive emotions are linked to happiness (Kitayama, Mesquita, & Karasawa, 2006). Furthermore, we may also use the relative intensity of engaging versus disengaging emotions. Individuals may be said to be more independent (or interdependent) if their happiness is predicted more by disengaging positive (or engaging positive) emotions, if they experience disengaging (or engaging) emotions more, or both. Kitayama, Mesquita, and Karasawa (2006) reported initial evidence for the convergent validity of these measures and recommended that future research directly assess the predictive validity of these implicit measures of independence and interdependence with respect to a variety of cross-cultural differences in cognition, such as analytic versus holistic thought (e.g., Nisbett et al., 2001), and motivation, such as self-enhancement and self-improvement (e.g., Heine et al., 1999). To the extent that the self is embodied we suspect that many of the behavioral or online responses of the self might be better predicted by implicit measures of independence and interdependence than by their explicit counterparts, such as the one developed by Singelis (1994).

Future Directions

As we have seen, the extensive empirical studies on culture have revealed a large number of differences. Paradoxically, however, this work has also underscored an equally important set of cross-cultural similarities. Often, the same psychological function is configured or enabled in terms of culturally contingent psychological processes. Having the same psychological function, therefore, does not imply any universal psychological laws. As Richard Shweder (2003) observes, universal principles of psychology may reveal themselves more often in the diversities than in the uniformity of psychological functions. The same theme is echoed in some recent efforts to reunite evolution and culture (Konner, Chapter 4, this volume; Richerson & Boyd, 2005). Future work may therefore focus on culturally contingent solutions for carrying out many universal psychological functions or tasks (Norenzayan & Heine, 2005).

It is also important to reiterate that the work on culture and the self so far has focused mostly on adult, largely college student populations. Much more developmental work is necessary to understand how members of a cultural group may acquire the culturally contingent ways of being a person. Moreover, there is an increasing need to examine community samples. Another weakness of the field stems from the fact that much evidence so far comes from East–West comparative studies. It is a reasonable research strategy to start with groups of maximal contrast. Yet it should also be kept in mind that much of the existing variation might be masked by this particular approach. Studies on social class, voluntary settlement, and cultural affordances, summarized in this chapter, may represent one extremely important direction for future work that can fruitfully supplement the macroscopic comparisons between large cultural regions such as East and West.

Finally, culture is both inside and outside the mind. As much as psychological processes are shaped by practices and meanings of culture, they do create and perpetuate the public practices and meanings. More detailed studies on practices and meanings—including those pertaining to their origins, changes, accumulation—are very much needed. As we mentioned earlier, some notable beginnings have already been made. Yet a more systematic effort toward theorizing on what Sperber (1996) called the "epidemiology of cultural ideas" is justified, insofar as these ideas eventually constitute or complete the mind of people who engage with them. We predict that much mileage would be gained in the near future by focusing on socialization, regional variation, and related phenomena and processes discussed in this chapter.

In all these future endeavors, it will serve us well to be reminded always of the fundamental insight of G. H. Mead and his contemporaries, who argued that self is a system of (often spontaneous) behavioral regulation that is aligned to the symbolic environment of culture. According to this view, the self is simultaneously symbolic and behavioral, cognitive and emotive, and most of all, grounded in biology, yet constantly shaped by culture. Indeed, this view suggests and reinforces the conceptualization of the self as a cultural mode of being. Just as Mead anticipated nearly a century ago, we believe that, if conceptualized this way, the self will continue to be an indispensable anchor in all analyses of the interface between culture, society, and psychology.

NOTES

1. It is ironic that even what may be called "independent" behavior is strongly enforced by societal norms. In North America, for example, there is a strong moral prescription for personal control and autonomy (Lachman & Weaver, 1998). When perceived as failing to meet this cultural standard, one is strongly stigmatized and prejudiced against (Crandall et al., 2002). Nevertheless, it is possible that norms enforcing interdependence are more explicit than those enforcing independence. The latter may be manifest, as in the example earlier, only when violated; typically, they may stay dormant because they are antithetical to the very quality (i.e., freedom from norms) they try to enforce (Garfinkel, 1967).

2. It is of note that an analogous separation between the personal and the public is found in Confucian cultures such as China, Japan, and Korea (Kitayama & Markus, 1999). Because Calvinism and Confucianism may share a strong achievement orientation, a reasonable conjecture is that a tendency to focus on the focal public domain of work might be one marker of such an orientation. However, it should also be kept in mind that specific meanings and practices associated with the work/public and the social relation/private are very different between the two cultural traditions (e.g., Sanchez-Burks & Lee, Chapter 14, this volume).

REFERENCES

Adams, G., & Markus, H.R. (2004). Towards a conception of culture suitable for a social psychology of culture. In M. Shaller & S. Christian (Eds.), *The psychological foundations of culture* (pp. 335–360). Mahwah, NJ: Erlbaum.

Adams, G., & Plaut, V. C. (2003). The cultural grounding of relationship: Friendship in North American and West African worlds. *Personal Relationships, 10,* 335–349.

Aronson, E. (1968). Dissonance theory: Progress and problems. In R. P. Abelson, E. Aronson, W. J. McGuire, T. M. Newcomb, M. J. Rosenberg, & P. H. Tannenbaum (Eds.), *Theories of cognitive consistency: A source-book.* (pp. 5–27). Chicago: Rand McNally.

Aronson, E. (1992). *The social animal* (6th ed.). New York: Freeman.

Baldwin, M. W., Carrell, S. E., & Lopez, D. E. (1990). Priming relationship schematas: My advisor and the pope are watching me from the back of my mind. *Journal of Experimental Social Psychology, 26,* 435–454.

Barratt, M. S. (1993). Early childrearing in Japan: Cross-cultural and intracultural perspectives. *Early Development and Parenting, 2,* 3–6.

Baumeister, R. F. (2005). *The cultural animal: Human nature, meaning, and social life.* Oxford, UK: Oxford University Press.

Baumeister, R. F., & Leary, M. R. (1995). The need to belong: Desire for interpersonal attachments as a fundamental human motivation. *Psychological Bulletin, 117*, 497–529.

Bellah, R. N., Madsen, R., Sullivan, W. M., Swidler, A., & Tipton, S. M. (1985). *Habits of the heart: Individualism and commitment in American life*. New York: Harper & Row.

Berkowitz, L. (1989). Frustration–aggression hypothesis: Examination and reformulation. *Psychological Bulletin, 106*, 59–73.

Berry, J. W., Poortinga, Y. H., Segall, M. H., & Dasen, P. R. (1992). *Cross-cultural psychology: Research and applications*. New York: Cambridge University Press.

Bond, M. H. (1988). Finding universal dimensions of individual variation in multicultural studies of values: The Rokeach and Chinese value surveys. *Journal of Personality and Social Psychology, 55*(6), 1009–1015.

Bornstein, M. H., Tamis-LeMonda, C. S., Tal, J., Ludeman, P., Toda, S., Rahn, C. W., et al. (1992). Maternal responsiveness to infants in three societies: The United States, France, and Japan. *Child Development, 63*, 808–821.

Bornstein, M. H., Toda, S., Azuma, H., Tamis-LeMonda, C., & Ogino, M. (1990). Mother and infant activity and interaction in Japan and in the United States: II. A comparative microanalysis of naturalistic exchanges focused on the organization of infant attention. *International Journal of Behavioral Developmental Psychology, 13*, 289–308.

Borofsky, R., Barth, F., Shweder, R., Rodseth, F., & Stolzenberg, N. M. (2001). A conversation about culture. *American Anthropologist, 103*, 432–446.

Bourdieu, P. (1977). *Outline of a theory of practice* (R. Nice, Trans.). Cambridge, UK: Cambridge University Press.

Brehm, J. (1966). *A theory of psychological reactance*. New York: Academic Press.

Brewer, M. B. (2004). Taking the social origins of human nature seriously: Toward a more imperialist social psychology. *Personality and Social Psychology Review, 8*(2), 107–113.

Brewer, M. B., & Gardner, W. L. (1996). Who is this "we"?: Levels of collective identity and self representations. *Journal of Personality and Social Psychology, 71*, 83–93.

Brown, J., & Kobayashi, C. (2002). Self enhancement in Japan and America. *Asian Journal of Social Psychology, 5*, 145–167.

Bruner, J. (1990). *Acts of meaning*. Cambridge, MA: Harvard University Press.

Chavajay, P., & Rogoff, B. (1999). Cultural variation in management of attention by children and their caregivers. *Developmental Psychology, 35*, 1079–1090.

Chiu, L.-H. (1972). A cross-cultural comparison of cognitive styles in Chinese and American children. *International Journal of Psychology, 7*, 235–242.

Choi, I., & Nisbett, R. E. (1998). Situational salience and cultural differences in the correspondence bias and in the actor–observer bias. *Personality and Social Psychology Bulletin, 24*, 949–960.

Choi, I., Nisbett, R. E., & Norenzayan, A. (1999). Causal attribution across cultures: Variation and universality. *Psychological Bulletin, 125*, 47–63.

Chua, H. F., Boland, J. E., & Nisbett, R. E. (2005). Cultural variation in eye movements during scene perception. *Proceedings of the National Academy of Sciences, USA, 102*, 12629–12633.

Clark, M. S., & Mills, J. (1979). Interpersonal attraction in exchange and communal relationships. *Journal of Personality and Social Psychology, 37*, 12–24.

Cole, M. (1996). *Cultural psychology: A once and future discipline*. Cambridge, MA: Belknap Press of Harvard University Press.

Cooley, C. H. (1922). *Human nature and the social order* (rev. ed.). New York: Scribner's. (Original work published 1902)

Crandall, C. S., D'Anello, S., Sakalli, N., Lazarus, E., Wieczorkowska, G., & Feather, N. (2002). An attribution-value model of prejudice: Anti-fat attitudes in six nations. In W. A. Lesko (Ed.), *Readings in social psychology: General, classic, and contemporary selections* (5th ed., pp.). Boston: Allyn & Bacon.

D'Andrade, R. G. (1995). *The development of cognitive anthropology*. Cambridge, UK: Cambridge University Press.

Deci, E., & Ryan, R. (1985) *Intrinsic motivation and self-determination in human behavior*. New York: Plenum Press.

de Tocqueville, A. (1969). *Democracy in America* (Vol. 2, pt. 2). Garden City, NY: Anchor. (Original work published 1835).

DeVos, G. (1983). Adaptive conflict and adjustive coping: Psychocultural approaches to ethnic identity. In T. Sarbin & K. E. Scheibe (Eds.), *Studies in social identity* (pp. 204–230). New York: Praeger.

Diamond, J. (1997). *Guns, germs, and steel: The fates of human societies*. New York: Norton.

Diener, E., & Diener, M. (1995). Cross-cultural correlates of life satisfaction and self-esteem. *Journal of Personality and Social Psychology, 68*, 653–663.

Diener, E., & Suh, E. H. (Eds.). (2000). *Advances in quality of life theory and research*. Dordrecht, The Netherlands: Kluwer.

Duffy, S., Uchida, Y., & Kitayama, S. (2004). *Culture and friendship: A social network study*. Unpublished manuscript. University of Michigan, Ann Arbor.

Dunbar, R. (1996). Coevolution of neocortical size, group size, and language in humans. *Behavioral and Brain Sciences, 16*, 681–735.

Durkheim, É. (1964). *The rules of sociological method*. New York: Free Press.

Earley, P. C. (1989). East meets West meets Mideast: Further explorations of collectivistic and individualistic work groups. *Academy of Management Journal, 36*, 565–581.

Elliot, A. J., Chirkov, V. I., Kim, Y., & Sheldon, K. M.

(2002). A cross-cultural analysis of avoidance personal goals. *Psychological Science, 12,* 505–510.

Fernald, A., & Morikawa, H. (1993). Common themes and cultural variations in Japanese and American mothers' speech to infants. *Child Development, 64,* 637–656.

Festinger, L. (1957). *A theory of cognitive dissonance.* Stanford, CA: Stanford University Press.

Fiske, A. P. (1992). Four elementary forms of sociality: Framework for a unified theory of social relations. *Psychological Review, 99,* 689–723.

Fiske, A. P., Kitayama, S., Markus, H. R., & Nisbett, R. E. (1998). The cultural matrix of social psychology. In D. T. Gilbert, S. T. Fiske & G. Lindzey (Eds.), *Handbook of social psychology* (4th ed., pp. 915–981). Boston: McGraw-Hill.

Fukuyama, F. (1992). *The end of history and the last man.* New York: Free Press.

Garfinkel, H. (1967). *Studies in ethnomethodology.* Englewood Cliffs, NJ: Prentice Hall.

Geertz, C. (1973). *The interpretation of cultures.* New York: Basic Books.

Geertz, C. (1975). On the nature of anthropological understanding. *American Scientist, 63,* 47–53.

Gibson, J. J. (1979). *The ecological approach to visual perception.* Boston: Houghton Mifflin.

Giddens, A. (1984). *The constitution of society.* Berkeley: University of California, Berkeley Press.

Gilbert, D. T., & Jones, E. E. (1986). Perceiver-induced constraint: Interpretations of self-generated reality. *Journal of Personality and Social Psychology, 50,* 269–280.

Gray, H. M., Ambady, N., Ishii, K., & Kitayama, S. (2006). *Mood effects on relative attention to verbal and nonverbal cues: The role of affiliation goals.* Unpublished manuscript, Harvard University.

Greenfield, P. M., Keller, H., & Fuligni, A. (2003). Cultural pathways through universal development. *Annual Review of Psychology, 54,* 461–490.

Gutchess, A., Welsh, R., Boduroglu, A., & Park, D. C. (in press). Cultural differences in neural function associated with object processing. *Cognitive, Affective, and Behavioral Neuroscience* .

Han, S.-P., & Shavitt, S. (1994). Persuasion and culture: Advertising appeals in individualistic and collectivistic societies. *Journal of Experimental Social Psychology, 30,* 326–350.

Harris, M. B. (1974). Mediators between frustration and aggression in a field experiment. *Journal of Experimental Social Psychology, 10,* 561–571.

Heckhausen, J., & Schulz, R. (1995). A life-span theory of control. *Psychological Review, 102,* 284–304.

Heine, S. J., & Hamamura, T. (2007). In search of East Asian self-enhancement. *Personality and Social Psychology Review, 11,* 1–24.

Heine, S. J., Kitayama, S., Lehman, D. R., Takata, T., Ide, E., Leung, C., et al. (2001). Divergent consequences of success and failure in Japan and North America: An investigation of self-improving motiva-

tions and malleable selves. *Journal of Personality and Social Psychology, 81,* 599–615.

Heine, S. J., Lehman, D. R., Markus, H. R., & Kitayama, S. (1999). Is there a universal need for positive self-regard? *Psychological Review, 106*(4), 766–794.

Heine, S. J., Lehman, D. R., Peng, K., & Greenholtz, J. (2002). What's wrong with cross-cultural comparisons of subjective likert scales?: The reference-group effect. *Journal of Personality and Social Psychology, 82,* 903–918.

Hermans, H. J. M., Rijks, T. I., & Kempen, H. J. G. (1993). Imaginal dialogues in the self: Theory and method. *Journal of Personality, 61*(2), 207–236.

Hochschild, J. (1995). *Facing up to the American Dream: Race, class, and the soul of the nation.* Princeton, NJ: Princeton University Press.

Hofstede, G. (1980). *Culture's consequences: International differences in work-related values.* Beverly Hills, CA: Sage.

Hofstede, G. (1991). *Cultures and organizations: Software of the mind.* London: McGraw-Hill.

Hong, Y., Morris, M. W., Chiu, C., & Benet-Martinez, V. (2000). Multicultural minds. *American Psychologist, 55,* 709–720.

Hoshino-Browne, E., Zanna, A. S., Spencer, S. J., Zanna, M. P., Kitayama, S., & Lackenbauer, S. (2005). On the cultural guises of cognitive dissonance: The case of Easterners and Westerners. *Journal of Personality and Social Psychology, 89,* 294–310.

Imada, T., & Kitayama, S. (2006). *Dissonance and eyes of others.* Unpublished manuscript, University of Michigan, Ann Arbor.

Inglehart, R., & Baker, W. E. (2000). Modernization, cultural change, and the persistence of traditional values. *American Sociological Review, 65,* 19–51.

Ishii, K., Reyes, J. A., & Kitayama, S. (2003). Spontaneous attention to word content versus emotional tone: Differences among three cultures. *Psychological Science, 14,* 39–46.

Iyengar, S. S., & Lepper, M. R. (1999). Rethinking the value of choice: A cultural perspective on intrinsic motivation. *Journal of Personality and Social Psychology, 76,* 349–366.

Ji, L., Zhang, Z., & Nisbett, R. E. (2004). Is it culture or is it language?: Examination of language effects in cross-cultural research on categorization. *Journal of Personality and Social Psychology, 87,* 57–65.

Ji, L. J., Peng, K., & Nisbett, R. E. (2000). Culture, control, and perception of relationships in the environment. *Journal of personality and social psychology, 78*(5), 943–955.

Jones, E. E. (1988). Impression formation: What do people think about? In T. Srull & R. Wyer (Eds.), *A dual process model of impression formation* (pp. 83–89). Hillsdale, NJ: Erlbaum.

Kağitçibaşi, Ç. (1997). Human development: Cross-cultural perspectives. In J. G. Adair & D. Bélanger (Ed.), *Advances in psychological science: Vol. 1. So-*

cial, personal, and cultural aspects (pp. 475–494). Hove, UK: Taylor & Francis.

Kakuno, M., & Ura, M. (2002). *Effect of Japanese sentence subject on correspondence bias.* Paper presented at the XXV International Congress of Applied Psychology, Singapore.

Kang, S., Shaver, P. R., Min, K., & Jin, H. (2003). Culture-specific patterns in the prediction of life satisfaction: Roles of emotion, relationship quality, and self-esteem. *Personality and Social Psychology Bulletin, 29,* 1596–1608.

Kashima, Y., & Kashima, E. S. (2003). Individualism, GNP, climate, and pronoun drop: Is individualism determined by affluence and climate, or does language use play a role? *Journal of Cross-Cultural Psychology, 34*(1), 125–134.

Keller, H., Yovsi, R., Borke, J., Kärtner, J., Jensen, H., & Papaligoura, Z. (2004). Developmental consequences of early parenting experiences: Self-recognition and self-regulation in three cultural communities. *Child Development, 75*(6), 1745–1760.

Ketay, S., Hedden, T., Aron, A., Markus, H. R., & Gabrieli, J. D. (2006). *Cultural differences in neural activation during relative versus absolute perceptual judgments.* Unpublished manuscript, State University of New York, Stony Brook.

Kim, H., & Markus, H. R. (1999). Deviance or uniqueness, harmony or conformity?: A cultural analysis. *Journal of Personality and Social Psychology, 77,* 785–800.

Kitayama, S. (2002). Cultural and basic psychological processes—toward a system view of culture: Comment on Oyserman et al. *Psychological Bulletin, 128,* 189–196.

Kitayama, S., & Duffy, S. (2004). Cultural competence—tacit, yet fundamental: Self, social relations, and cognition in the United States and Japan. In R. Sternberg & E. Grigorenko (Eds.), *Culture and competence: Contexts of life success* (pp. 55–87). Washington, DC: American Psychological Association.

Kitayama, S., Duffy, S., Kawamura, T., & Larsen, J. (2003). Perceiving an object and its context in different cultures: A cultural look at new look. *Psychological Science, 14,* 201–206.

Kitayama, S., Ishii, K., Imada, T., Takemura, K., & Ramaswamy, J. (2006). Voluntary settlement and the spirit of independence: Evidence from Japan's "Northern Frontier." *Journal of Personality and Social Psychology, 91,* 369–384.

Kitayama, S., Karasawa, M., Curhan, K. B., Ryff, C., & Markus, H. R. (2006). *Independence, interdependence, and well-being: Divergent patterns in Japan and the United States.* Unpublished manuscript, University of Michigan, Ann Arbor.

Kitayama, S., & Markus, H. R. (1994). Introduction to cultural psychology and emotion research. In *Emotion and culture: Empirical studies of mutual influence* (pp. 1–19). Washington, DC: American Psychological Association.

Kitayama, S., & Markus, H. R. (1999). Yin and yang of the Japanese self: The cultural psychology of personality coherence. In D. Cervone & Y. Shoda (Eds.), *The coherence of personality: Social cognitive bases of personality consistency, variability, and organization* (pp. 242–302). New York: Guilford Press.

Kitayama, S., & Markus, H. R. (2000). The pursuit of happiness and the realization of sympathy: Cultural patterns of self, social relations, and well-being. In E. Diener & E. M. Suh (Eds.), *Culture and subjective well-being* (pp. 113–1621). Cambridge, MA: MIT Press.

Kitayama, S., Markus, H. R., & Kurokawa, M. (2000). Culture, emotion and well-being: Good feelings in Japan and the U.S. *Cognition and Emotion, 14*(1), 93–124.

Kitayama, S., Markus, H. R., & Matsumoto, H. (1995). A cultural perspective on self-conscious emotions. In J. P. Tangney & K. W. Fisher (Eds.), *Shame, guilt, embarrassment, and pride: Empirical studies of self-conscious emotions.* New York: Guilford Press.

Kitayama, S., Markus, H. R., Matsumoto, H., & Norasakkunkit, V. (1997). Individual and collective processes in the construction of the self: Self-enhancement in the United States and self-depreciation in Japan. *Journal of Personality and Social Psychology, 72,* 1245–1267.

Kitayama, S., Mesquita, B., & Karasawa, M. (2006). Cultural affordances and emotional experience: Socially engaging and disengaging emotions in Japan and the United States. *Journal of Personality and Social Psychology, 91,* 890–903.

Kitayama, S., Snibbe, A. C., Markus, H. R., & Suzuki, T. (2004). Is there any "free" choice?: Self and dissonance in two cultures. *Psychological Science, 15*(8), 527–533.

Kitayama, S., & Uchida, Y. (2004). Interdependent agency: An alternative system for action. In R. Sorrentino, D. Cohen, J.M. Olson, & M. P. Zanna (Eds.), *Culture and social behavior: The Ontario Symposium* (Vol. 10, pp. 137–164). Mahwah, NJ: Erlbaum.

Kitayama, S., & Uchida, Y. (2006). *Culture and social support.* Unpublished manuscript, Koshien University, Japan.

Kitayama, S., Uchida, Y., Nakama, D., Mesquita, B., Saitoh, K., & Morling, B. (2006). *Esteem support and reciprocity monitoring: Self and social relations in two cultures.* Unpublished manuscript, University of Michigan, Ann Arbor.

Kohn, M. L., Naoi, A., Schoenbach, C., Schooler, C., & Slomczynski, K. (1990). Position in the class structure and psychological functioning in the United States, Japan, and Poland. *American Journal of Sociology, 95,* 964–1008.

Kondo, D. (1990). *Crafting selves: Power, gender, and discourses of identity in a Japanese work place.* Chicago: University of Chicago Press.

Kroeber, A. L., & Kluckhohn, C. (1966). *Culture: A*

critical review of concepts and definitions. New York: Vintage. (Original work published in 1952)

Kuhnen, U., & Oyserman, D. (2002). Thinking about the self influences thinking in general: Cognitive consequences of salient self-concept. *Journal of Experimental Social Psychology, 38,* 492–499.

Kwan, V. S. M., Bond, M. H., & Singelis, T. M. (1997). Pancultural explanations for life satisfaction: Adding relationship harmony to self-esteem. *Journal of Personality and Social Psychology, 73,* 1038–1051.

Lachman, M. E., & Weaver, S. L. (1998). The sense of control as a moderator of social class differences in health and well-being. *Journal of Personality and Social Psychology, 74*(3), 763–773.

Lakin, J. L., & Chartrand, T. L. (2003). Using nonconscious behavioral mimicry to create affiliation and rapport. *Psychological Science, 14,* 334–339.

Lee, F., Hallahan, M., & Herzog, T. (1996). Explaining real life events: How culture and domain shape attributions. *Personality and Social Psychology Bulletin, 22,* 732–741.

Lehman, D. R., Chiu, C., & Schaller, M. (2004). Psychology and culture. *Annual Review of Psychology, 55,* 689–714.

Lepper, M. R., & Greene, D. (1978). Overjustification research and beyond: Toward a means–end analysis of intrinsic and extrinsic motivation. In M. R. Lepper & D. Greene (Eds.), *The hidden costs of reward* (pp. 109–148). Hillsdale, NJ: Erlbaum.

Letra, T. S. (1976). *Japanese patterns of behavior.* Honolulu: University of Hawaii Press.

Markus, H., & Kitayama, S. (1991). Culture and the self: Implications for cognition, emotion, and motivation. *Psychological Review, 98,* 224–253.

Markus, H. R., & Kitayama, S. (2004). Models of agency: Sociocultural diversity in the construction of action. In V. Murphy-Berman & J. J. Berman (Eds.), *Cross-cultural differences in perspectives on the self* (Vol. 49, pp. 1–57). Lincoln: University of Nebraska Press.

Markus, H. R., Mullally, P. R., & Kitayama, S. (1997). Selfways: Diversity in modes of cultural participation. In U. Neisser & D. Jopling (Eds.), *The conceptual self in context: Culture, experience, self-understanding* (pp. 13–62). Cambridge, UK: Cambridge University Press.

Markus, H. R., Ryff, C. D., Curhan, K. B., Palmersheim, K. A., Brim, O. G., & Ryff, C. D. (2004). In their own words: Well-being at midlife among high school–educated and college-educated adults. In Anonymous (Ed.), *How healthy are we?: A national study of well-being at midlife* (pp. 273–319). Chicago: University of Chicago Press.

Markus, H. R., Uchida, Y., Omoregie, H., Townsend, S. S. M., & Kitayama, S. (2006). Models of agency in Japanese and American contexts. *Psychological Science, 17,* 103–112.

Marsella, A. J., DeVos, G., & Hsu, F. L. K. (1985). *Culture and self: Asian and Western perspectives.* London: Tavistock.

Masuda, T., & Kitayama, S. (2004). Perceiver-induced constraint and attitude attribution in Japan and the U.S.: A case for the cultural dependence of the correspondence bias. *Journal of Experimental Social Psychology, 40*(3), 409–416.

Masuda, T., & Nisbett, R. E. (2001). Attending holistically versus analytically: Comparing the context sensitivity of Japanese and Americans. *Journal of Personality and Social Psychology, 81,* 992–934.

Matsumoto, D. (1999). Culture and self: An empirical assessment of Markus and Kitayama's theory of independent and interdependent self-construal. *Asian Journal of Social Psychology, 2*(3), 289–310.

McClelland, D. (1985). *Human motivation.* Glenview, IL: Scott Foresman Press.

Mead, G. H. (1934). *Mind, self, and society.* Chicago: University of Chicago Press.

Mesquita, B., & Frijda, N. H. (1992). Cultural variations in emotions: A review. *Psychological Bulletin, 112*(2), 179–204.

Mesquita, B., Karasawa, M., Haire, A., Izumi, K., Hayashi, A., Idzelis, M., et al. (2005). *Emotions as culture-specific ways of relating: A comparison between Japanese and American groups.* Unpublished manuscript, Wake Forest University, Winston-Salem, NC.

Miller, J. G. (1984). Culture and the development of everyday social explanation. *Journal of Personality and Social Psychology, 46,* 961–978.

Miller, J. G., & Bersoff, D. M. (1994). Cultural influences on the moral status of reciprocity and the discounting of endogenous motivation. *Personality and Social Psychology Bulletin, 20,* 592–602.

Miyake, K., Chen, S.-J., & Campos, J. J. (1985). Infant temperament, mother's mode of interaction, and attachment in Japan: An interim report. *Monographs of the Society for Research in Child Development, 50*(1), 276–297.

Miyamoto, Y., & Kitayama, S. (2002). Cultural variation in correspondence bias: The critical role of attitude diagnosticity of socially constrained behavior. *Journal of Personality and Social Psychology, 83,* 1239–1248.

Miyamoto, Y., Kitayama, S., & Talhelm, T. (2006, January). *A meta-analytic review of cultural differences in cognitive processes.* Poster presented at the Conference of the Society for Personality and Social Psychology, Palm Springs, CA.

Miyamoto, Y., Nisbett, R. E., & Masuda, T. (2006). Culture and the physical environment: Holistic versus analytic perceptual affordances. *Psychological Science, 17,* 113–117.

Morling, B., Kitayama, S., & Miyamoto, Y. (2002). Cultural practices emphasize influence in the United States and adjustment in Japan. *Personality and Social Psychology Bulletin, 28,* 311–323.

Morling, B., Kitayama, S., & Miyamoto, Y. (2003). American and Japanese women use different coping strategies during normal pregnancy. *Personality and Social Psychology Bulletin, 29,* 114–128.

Morris, M., & Peng, K. (1994). Culture and cause: American and Chinese attributions for social and physical events. *Journal of Personality and Social Psychology, 67,* 949–971.

Moscovici, S. (1984). The phenomena of social representations. In R. M. Farr & S. Moscovici (Eds.), *Social representation* (pp. 3–69). Cambridge, UK: Cambridge University Press.

Myers, F. (1986). *Pintupi country, Pintupi self: Sentiment, place, and politics among Western Desert Aborigines.* Washington, DC: Smithsonian Institution Press.

Naoi, A., & Schooler, C. (1985). Occupational conditions and psychological functioning in Japan. *American Journal of Sociology, 90,* 729–752.

Nisbett, R., & Cohen, D. (1996). *Culture of honor: Psychology of violence in the South.* Boulder, CO: Westview Press.

Nisbett, R., & Masuda, T. (2003). Culture and point of view. *Proceedings of the National Academy of Sciences of the USA, 100,* 11163–11170.

Nisbett, R., & Ross, L. (1980). *Human inference: Strategies and shortcomings of social judgment.* Englewood Cliffs, NJ: Prentice-Hall.

Nisbett, R. E. (2003). *The geography of thought: Why we think the way we do.* New York: Free Press.

Nisbett, R. E., Peng, K., Choi, I., & Norenzayan, A. (2001). Culture and systems of thought: Holistic vs. analytic cognition. *Psychological Review, 108,* 291–310.

Nisbett, R. E., & Wilson, D. (1977). Telling more than we know: Verbal reports on mental processes. *Psychological Review, 84,* 231–253.

Norenzayan, A., & Heine, S. J. (2005). Psychological universals: What are they and how can we know? *Psychological Bulletin, 131,* 763–784.

Norenzayan, A., Smith, E. E., Kim, B. J., & Nisbett, R. E. (2002). Cultural preferences for formal versus intuitive reasoning. *Cognitive Science, 26,* 653–886.

Ochs, E. (1988). *Culture and language development: Language acquisition and language socialization in a Samoan village.* Cambridge, UK: Cambridge University Press.

Oishi, S., & Diener, E. (2003). Culture and well-being: The cycle of action, evaluation, and decision. *Personality and Social Psychology Bulletin, 29,* 939–949.

Oyserman, D., Coon, H. M., & Kemmelmeier, M. (2002). Rethinking individualism and collectivism: Evaluation of theoretical and assumptions and meta-analyses. *Psychological Bulletin, 128,* 3–72.

Parsons, T., & Shils, E. A. (1951). *Toward a general theory of action.* Cambridge, MA: Harvard University Press.

Pearlin, L. I., & Schooler, C. (1978). The structure of coping. *Journal of Health and Social Behavior, 19,* 2–21.

Peng, K., & Nisbett, R. E. (1999). Culture, dialecticism, and reasoning about contradiction. *American Psychologist, 54,* 741–754.

Peng, K., Nisbett, R. E., & Wong, N. (1997). Validity problems of cross-cultural value comparison and possible solutions. *Psychological Methods, 2,* 329–341.

Putnam, R. D. (1993). *Making democracy work: Civic traditions in modern Italy.* Princeton, NJ: Princeton University Press.

Richerson, P. J., & Boyd, R. (2005). *Not by genes alone: How culture transformed human evolution.* Chicago: University of Chicago Press.

Ross, L. (1977). The intuitive psychologist and his shortcomings: Distortions in the attribution process. In L. Berkowitz (Ed.), *Advances in experimental social psychology* (Vol. 10, pp. 174–221). New York: Academic Press.

Rothbaum, R., Pott, M., Azuma, H., Miyake, K., & Weisz, J. (2000). The development of close relationships in Japan and the U.S.: Pathways of symbiotic harmony and generative tension. *Child Development, 71,* 1121–1142.

Rozin, P., Lowery, L., Imada, S., & Haidt, J. (1999). The CAD triad hypothesis: A mapping between three moral emotions (contempt, anger, disgust) and three moral codes (community, autonomy, divinity). *Journal of Personality and Social Psychology, 76,* 574–586.

Sampson, E. E. (1988). The debate on individualism: Indigenous psychologies of the individual and their role in personal and societal functioning. *American Psychologist, 43,* 15–22.

Sanchez-Burks, J. (2005). Protestant relational ideology: The cognitive underpinnings and organizational implications of an American anomaly. *Research in Organizational Behavior, 26,* 267–308.

Schimmack, U., Oishi, S., & Diener, E. (2005). Individualism: A valid and important dimension of cultural differences between nations. *Personality and Social Psychology Review, 9*(1), 17–31.

Schlesinger, A. M. (1986). *The cycles of American history.* Boston: Houghton Mifflin.

Schwartz, S. H. (1992). Universals in the structure and content of values. In M. P. Zanna (Ed.), *Advances in experimental social psychology* (Vol. 25, pp. 1–65). Orlando, FL: Academic Press.

Sedikides, C., Gaertner, L., & Toguchi, Y. (2003). Pancultural self-enhancement. *Journal of Personality and Social Psychology, 84*(1), 60–79.

Sheldon, K. M., & Kasser, T. (1998). Pursuing personal goals: Skills enable progress, but not all progress is beneficial. *Personality and Social Psychology Bulletin, 24,* 1319–1331.

Shore, B. (1996). *Culture in mind: Cognition, culture, and the problem of meaning.* New York: Oxford University Press.

Shweder, R. (2003). *Why men barbecue: Recipes for cultural psychology.* Cambridge, MA: Harvard University Press.

Shweder, R. A. (Ed.). (1991). *Thinking through cultures: Expeditions in cultural psychology.* Cambridge, MA: Harvard University Press.

Shweder, R. A., & Bourne, E. J. (1982). Does the concept of person vary cross-culturally? In A. J. Marsella & G. M. White (Eds.), *Cultural conceptions of mental health and therapy* (pp. 130–204). London: Reidel.

Shweder, R. A., Much, N. C., Mahapatra, M., & Park, L. (1997). The "big three" of morality (autonomy, community, divinity), and the "big three" explanations of suffering. In A. Brandt & P. Rozin (Eds.), *Morality and health* (pp. 119–169). New York: Routledge.

Singelis, T. M. (1994). The measurement of independent and interdependent self-construals. *Personality and Social Psychology Bulletin, 20*(5), 580–591.

Smith, P. B. (2004). Acquiescent response bias as an aspect of cultural communication style. *Journal of Cross-Cultural Psychology, 35*(1), 50–61.

Smith, P. B., & Schwartz, S. (1997). Values. In J. W. Berry, M. H. Segall, & Ç. Kagitçibasi (Eds.), *Handbook of cross-cultural psychology: Vol. 3. Social behavior and applications* (2nd ed., pp. 77–118). Boston: Allyn & Bacon.

Snibbe, A. C., & Markus, H. R. (2005). You can't always get what you want: Educational attainment, agency, and choice. *Journal of Personality and Social Psychology, 88*, 703–720.

Sperber, D. (1996). *Explaining culture: A naturalistic approach*. London: Blackwell.

Steele, C. M. (1988). The psychology of self-affirmation: Sustaining the integrity of the self. In L. Berkowitz (Ed.), *Advances in experimental social psychology* (Vol. 21, pp. 261–302). San Diego: Academic Press.

Steele, C. M., Spencer, S. J., & Lynch, M. (1993). Self-image resilience and dissonance: The role of affirmational recourses. *Journal of Personality and Social Psychology, 64*, 885–896.

Takano, Y., & Osaka, E. (1999). An unsupported common view: Comparing Japan and the U.S. on individualism/collectivism. *Asian Journal of Social Psychology, 2*, 311–341.

Taylor, C. (1989). *Sources of the self: The making of modern identities*. Cambridge, MA: Harvard University Press.

Taylor, S. E., & Brown, J. D. (1988). Illusion and well-being: A social psychological perspective on mental health. *Psychological Bulletin, 103*, 193–220.

Taylor, S. E., Sherman, D. K., Kim, H. S., Jarcho, J., Takagi, K., & Dunagan, M. S. (2004). Culture and social support: Who seeks it and why? *Journal of Personality and Social Psychology, 87*, 354–362.

Tönnies, F. (1988). *Community and society*. New Brunswick, NJ: Rutgers University Press. (Original published in 1887)

Trafimow, D., Triandis, H. C., & Goto, S. G. (1991). Some tests of the distinction between the private self and the collective self. *Journal of Personality and Social Psychology, 60*, 649–655.

Triandis, H. C. (1989). The self and social behavior in differing cultural contexts. *Psychological Review, 96*, 506–520.

Triandis, H. C. (1995). *Individualism and collectivism*. Boulder, CO: Westview Press.

Triandis, H. C., Kashima, Y., Shimada, E., & Villareal, M. (1986). Acculturation indices as a means of confirming cultural differences. *International Journal of Psychology, 21*, 43–70.

Turiel, E. (2004). Commentary: Beyond individualism and collectivism—a problem or progress? In M. E. Mascolo & J. Li (Eds.), *Culture and developing selves: Beyond dichotomization* (pp. 91–100). San Francisco: Jossey-Bass.

Turner, F. (1920). *The frontier in American history*. New York: Holt.

Uchida, Y., & Kitayama, S. (2006). *Happiness and unhappiness and West and East: Themes and variations*. Unpublished manuscript, Koshien University, Takaraduka, Japan.

Uchida, Y., Norasakkunkit, V., & Kitayama, S. (2004). Cultural constructions of happiness: Theory and evidence. *Journal of Happiness Studies, 5*, 223–239.

Watsuji, T. (1961). *Climate and culture*. Hokuseido Press. (Original work published 1935)

Weber, M. (1950). *The protestant ethic and the spirit of capitalism* (T. Parsons, Trans.). New York: Scribner's. (Original work published 1904–1906)

Weisz, J. R., Rothbaum, F. M., & Blackburn, T. C. (1984). Standing out and standing in: The psychology of control in America and Japan. *American Psychologist, 39*, 955–969.

Yamagishi, T., & Yamagishi, M. (1994). Trust and commitment in the United States and Japan. *Motivation and Emotion, 18*(2), 129–166.

Yang, K.-S. (1986). Chinese personality and its change. In M. H. Bond (Ed.), *The psychology of the Chinese people* (pp.106–170). New York: Oxford University Press.

Zahn-Waxler, C., Friedman, R. J., Cole, P. M., & Mizuta, I. (1996). Japanese and United States preschool children's responses to conflict and distress. *Child Development, 67*(5), 2462–2477.

Zuckerman, M., & O'Loughlin, R. E. (2006). Self-enhancement by social comparison: A prospective analysis. *Personality and Social Psychology Bulletin, 32*, 751–760.

CHAPTER 7

Integrating System Approaches to Culture and Personality
The Cultural Cognitive-Affective Processing System

RODOLFO MENDOZA-DENTON
WALTER MISCHEL

O chestnut-tree, great-rooted blossomer,
Are you the leaf, the blossom, or the bole?
O body swayed to music, O brightening glance,
How can we know the dancer from the dance?
—W. B. YEATS, *Among School Children*

As the chapters in this volume attest, the foundational premise that culture and person co-constitute one another, perhaps more than any other, characterizes contemporary cultural psychology (Cole, 1996; Kitayama, 2002; Miller, 1997; 1999; Piker, 1998; Shweder, 1990). Ironically, however, this very premise is most challenging for a cultural psychological view of personality, for "personality" has historically been, and in much cross-cultural research continues to be, conceptualized as the qualities of the individual that are separable from context

(Kitayama & Markus, 1999; Pervin, 1999; Poortinga & Hemert, 2001; Shweder, 1991).

The challenge for a cultural-psychological approach to personality remains to specify the nature of, and the mechanisms underlying, the co-constitution of person and culture. This chapter brings together insights from various theoretical and empirical lines of research (e.g., Hong & Chiu, 2001; Hong, Morris, Chiu, & Benet-Martinez, 2000; Kashima, 2001, 2004; Markus & Kitayama, 1998; Mendoza-Denton, Shoda, Ayduk, & Mischel, 1999; Cohen, 1997) that together are rising to this challenge and bringing into focus a new paradigm for the study of culture and personality. At the core of this emerging consensus are discoveries over the past 20 years in personality science and social cognition that are remarkably consistent with the premise of cultural psychology. These findings allow us to revise the long-standing assumption that situations, context, and culture are somehow "noise" or "error" that obscures the consistency of personality and obstructs the search for universals. Rather than searching for fundamental human qualities that describe people *in spite of* cultural differences, this approach focuses on the cultural differences *themselves*. Cultural differences in social behavior, in this view, are meaningful manifestations of a dynamic, culturally constituted personality system, the structure and governing principles of which may, indeed, be universal.

THE CULTURE AND PERSONALITY PARADOX

From its inception, a bedrock assumption in personality science has been that people have discernible qualities that supercede contexts and situations (Mischel, 2004; Mischel, Shoda, & Mendoza-Denton, 2002). Within this approach, a person who is high in conscientiousness should be more conscientious than most people in many different kinds of situations, and would do the appropriately conscientious thing as required by his or her culture. By the 1960s, however, it became increasingly clear that the data did not bear out this assumption, with converging data from independent investigators (Hartshorne & May, 1928; Mischel, 1968; Newcomb, 1929; Peterson, 1968; Vernon, 1964) consistently finding only modest evidence for cross-situational consistency of behavior (Mischel, 2003; Shweder, 1991; B. B. Whiting & Whiting, 1975). Bem and Allen (1974) coined the term "personality paradox" to refer to the discrepancy between the lack of strong empirical support for cross-situational consistency and our intuition that stable qualities in fact exist.

Cultural psychologists interested in the relationship between culture and personality are today faced with an analogous dilemma. On the one hand, it has been shown that for many classes of behavior, within-culture variability is greater than between-culture variability

(Barnouw, 1985; Bock, 2000; Inkeles, 1996; Kaplan, 1954; Wallace, 1961; Triandis, 1997; J. W. M. Whiting & Child, 1953; B. B. Whiting & Whiting, 1975). On the other hand, and despite the data, as perceivers and researchers we continue to have a strong intuition that some type of commonality unites the French or the Japanese, and makes them different from Argentines or the Senegalese. How does one reconcile these seemingly opposing positions? The response to the 1960s personality paradox speaks directly to the issues and alternatives faced when dealing with this "culture and personality paradox."

ONE RESPONSE: UNCOVER TRAITS THROUGH METHODOLOGICAL REFINEMENT

One reaction to the 1960s personality paradox was to assert that the findings on the variability of behavior across diverse situations simply reflect noise and error from inadequate sampling. In this view, the emergence and identification of cross-situational consistency is a matter of methodological improvement, primarily requiring better reliability through denser data sampling (Epstein, 1979), or more precise specification of the people or situations to which traits apply (Bem & Allen, 1974; Epstein & O'Brien, 1985; see Mischel & Peake, 1982, 1983; Snyder & Ickes, 1984; and Shweder, 1991, for lengthier discussions on this topic). Accordingly, no personality paradox in fact exists: One can continue to eliminate the role of situations by aggregating people's behavior across diverse situations, and by using global assessments that exclude context. At its core, then, this approach remains committed to treating situational variability as measurement error.

This response, though greeted with great enthusiasm, has paved the road for a resurgence of culture and personality research that, in spite of its methodological rigor, has not addressed the basic challenges to the paradigm's fundamental assumptions (e.g., Mischel, 1968). The consequence has been to reinforce further the metaphor shared by traditional personality and attribution theories "that construes skin as a special boundary that separates one set of 'causal forces' from another. On the sunny side of the epidermis are the external or situational forces that press inward on the person, and on the meaty side are the internal or personal forces that exert pressure outward" (Gilbert & Malone, 1995, p. 21).

Today, a principal impetus in research on culture and personality is devoted to establishing the universality of a personality trait structure, reducible to a discrete number of dimensions. This approach has largely focused on replicating the "Five-Factor Model"—open-mindedness, conscientiousness, extraversion, agreeableness, and neuroticism—across cultures (e.g., McCrae & Allik, 2002), with recent efforts aimed at "mapping" the world across the five dimensions (Allik & McCrae, 2004; McCrae, 2004). The goal of this approach is not so much in finding that the French, for example, are lower on agreeableness than Americans (McCrae, 2004), but rather that both Frenchmen and Americans can be described in terms of the five factors. Proponents of this approach cite evidence from animal studies (e.g., Gosling & John, 1999; Gosling, Kwan, & John, 2003) and heritability studies (Bouchard & Loehlin, 2001; Loehlin, McCrae, Costa, & John, 1998) as evidence for the likely biological basis of trait structure (see Triandis & Suh, 2002). It has been proposed that biological substrates underlie differences in the Big Five and, more recently, that such biological differences cause cultural differences (McCrae, 2004).

The growing literature on global traits and culture has been both ably reviewed (e.g., Triandis & Suh, 2002), and ably critiqued (e.g., Bock, 2000; Kitayama, 2002; Pervin, 1994; Shweder 1991; see also Peng, Nisbett, & Wong, 1997) elsewhere, and is not the focus of this chapter. Nonetheless, we note three important points: (1) Efforts to describe cultures in terms of a common metric assume a context-free psychic unity that cultural-psychological research is finding evidence against (e.g., Heine, Lehman, Markus, & Kitayama, 1999; Iyengar & Lepper, 1999; Norenzayan, Choi, & Peng, Chapter 23, this volume); (2) personality assessments that rely on generalized traits—including indigenously derived ones (e.g., Cheung & Leung, 1998; Church, Katigbak, & Reyes, 1996, 1998)—tacitly accept a definition of "personality" in terms of consistency across both time and situations; and (3) convergent evidence from self- and peer-ratings, or from animal studies, tell us a lot about peoples' categorization processes (Bock, 2000; Church,

2000; Morris, Nisbett, & Peng, 1995), but only a partial story about the behavioral expressions of the personality system (Borkenau, Riemann, Spinath & Angleitner, 2006; Cervone, 2004; Shoda, 1999). Our focus below is on giving a voice to the rest of that story.

A SECOND RESPONSE: TAKING VARIABILITY SERIOUSLY

To reiterate, the data over the course of a century have shown that cross-situational variability is as at least as impressive as cross-situational consistency (Mischel et al., 2002). Whereas such variability is considered error or noise within traditional approaches, research over the past 20 years has harnessed this variability, with the hunch that a new locus of personality is to be found within this variability. But how can information about behavioral variability across situations, rather than behavioral stability across situations, possibly yield information about dispositions? An analogy from automobiles is helpful (Epstein, 1994). The analogy begins with the recognition that automobiles, like people, are readily grouped in terms of their area of origin. Peugeot, for example, is different from Mitsubishi, which is different from Chrysler. It is helpful to be able to compare these different makes of car according to certain dimensions. Are they gas guzzlers or economical? Are they clunky or speedy? Silent or noisy? Such generalizations are, of course, useful in orienting buyers toward a particular brand, yet only provide distal cues about the *mechanisms* that lead to these differences—about what is going on under the hood (Cervone, 2005).

As beleaguered car owners can attest, when experts ask diagnostic questions about cars, their questions focus on the *conditions* under which certain events occur. The types of questions asked of car owners—*When* does the car make that particular screeching sound? Does the car stall only *when* it's going uphill?—can give clues to the expert about identifying the source of the surface characteristics (e.g., noisiness) and why the car does what it does. The conclusions drawn about the source of the problem, for example, will be different if the car seems to make noise when trying to accelerate (loose fan belt) as opposed to when trying to shift gears (transmission issue). In a fascinating way, then, information about how the car behaves in relation to different driving situations can be quite diagnostic about the car itself.

Similarly, identifying the conditions under which an individual displays a given behavior can be critical in understanding personal dispositions—in revealing, as it were, the engine driving the person. That is, even if two individuals display the same overall average level of behavior, depending on the pattern of *where* it is displayed, one may draw drastically different inferences about the person (Kammrath, Mendoza-Denton, & Mischel, 2005; Mendoza-Denton, 1999; Plaks, Shafer, & Shoda, 2003; Shoda & Mischel, 1993). Suppose for example, that Jack so consistently puts work above all else that his friends and family know they cannot count on him for social or family obligations. Jacques, on the other hand, is extremely dependable when it comes to interpersonal obligations, but is consistently late and sloppy when it comes to his nine-to-five job. Even though, on average, both Jack and Jacques might be seen or rated as equally dependable, their distinct patterns—if observed repeatedly and across multiple samples of situations—may be highly informative about differences in their motivations, goals, values— and importantly, their cultural background (Hong & Mallorie, 2004; Mendoza-Denton, Ayduk, Shoda, & Mischel, 1997). More than collections of ever more specific but disjointed behavior-in-context descriptions (see Shweder, 1991), these *if . . . then . . .* (if situation A, then s/he does *X*, but if situation B, then he or she does *Y*) profiles—if stable—can yield important clues about the underlying system that generates them.

Evidence for the Stability of *If . . . Then . . .* Profiles

To test for the stability and meaningfulness of *if . . . then . . .* profiles, Shoda, Mischel, and Wright (1994) analyzed the behavior of children over the course of a summer as it unfolded *in vivo* within a summer camp. The children's social behavior (e.g., verbal aggression, withdrawal, prosocial behavior) was unobtrusively observed and recorded as it occurred in relation to various interpersonal situations, with an average of 167 hours of observation per child over the course of the 6-week camp.

Nominal versus Psychological Situations

How did the researchers classify the camp situations into meaningful categories? Situations can be classified at different levels. At one level, one can describe situations *nominally*; in other words, according to their surface features (e.g., study hall, cabin meeting; see B. B. Whiting & Whiting, 1975). Unfortunately, nominal situations often contain a wide array of interpersonal psychological events for different people and different cultural groups. As an example, for one group, being "at the market" may involve quickly finding one's groceries, getting on the shortest checkout line, and leaving the store as soon as possible. For another group, being "at the market" might involve haggling with one's favorite vendor over tea, and socializing with neighbors while choosing fruit. As such, then, situations can also be meaningfully grouped according to their important psychological features, which may cut across nominal situations and settings. Such clusters have been referred to as "psychological situations" (Shoda et al., 1994).

To be able to group the situations in terms of the psychological features that seemed important to the children at the summer camp, Wright and Mischel (1988) asked those who knew the children—the camp counselors as well as the children's peers—to describe them in detail. Specifically, they were asked to imagine that the interviewer was new to the camp and the campers, and to "tell me everything you know about (target) so I will know him as well as you do." This was followed by standard prompts (e.g., "Anything else?"). This methodology yielded voluminous "thick description" (Geertz, 1973; Shweder, 1991) on the cultural group under study (in this case, the kids at the camp), with the added benefit of stemming from not one but many "cultural experts." This allowed the researchers to identify those features that the experts agreed were important to the population, rather than being idiosyncratic to any given informant. To find the common themes in these descriptions, responses were coded and subjected to cluster analysis.

Confirming the importance of traits in the language use of Americans (Church, 2000), much of the content of the descriptions consisted of trait terms. However, the data *also* revealed that these trait descriptors tended to be *hedged* spontaneously, that is, described in terms of the *conditions* under which targets displayed particular qualities (e.g., "Johnny gets aggressive *when* he gets teased about his glasses"). Clustering the types of situational hedges used to describe the targets revealed five psychological situations that seemed important to the kids at the camp: three negative situations ("peer teased, provoked, or threatened," "adult warned," and "adult punished") and two positive situations ("adult praised" and "peer approached prosocially"). The distinction between nominal and psychological situations, though subtle, has important implications, because to the degree that culture dictates the types of situations that "go together," exercises in the generalizability of nominal situations may be limited in their usefulness (Mendoza-Denton et al., 1997). In terms of assessment, identification of such psychological situations cannot be known without deep familiarity with the culture. We return to this point in the "Implications" section of this chapter.

If . . . Then . . . Profiles: Meaningful Patterns of Variability

Figure 7.1 shows illustrative profiles for two children at the camp. Their verbally aggressive behavior across the five types of psychological situations described earlier (Shoda et al., 1994) is shown in Z-scores—in other words, the children's observed level of aggression in that situation, in standard deviation units, relative to the mean of the entire sample (Z_0 on the *Y* axis). Thus, these profiles do not simply reflect the fact that situations, unsurprisingly, make a difference (e.g., on average, people tend to be more aggressive when teased than when praised). The two lines within each panel indicate the profiles based on two separate, nonoverlapping samples of situations, shown as a solid line and a dotte d line. It is worth noting here that the fact that these stability coefficients are found when reliability is high (dense data sampling) flatly contradicts the key trait assumption that variability in a person's behavior across situations is "noise" (see Mischel & Shoda, 1995; Mischel, 2004). In more recent research, the profile similarity in twins has been found to be greater than chance (Borkenau et al., 2006).

The feature of *if . . . then . . .* profiles that is important for this analysis is that they readily invite questions about the person's construals of different situations, and the relevant motivations, goals, expectations, and processing dynamics. Child 9, for example, reliably becomes

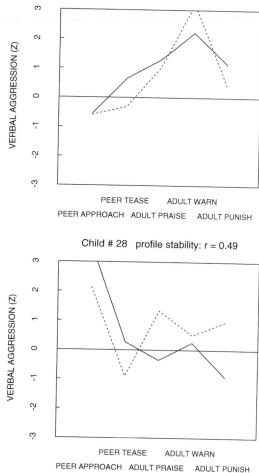

FIGURE 7.1. Illustrative *if . . . then . . .* "signatures" of verbal aggression in relation to five situations in two nonoverlapping time samples (solid and dotted lines). Data are shown in standardized scores (Z) relative to the normative levels of verbal aggression in each situation. From Mischel and Shoda (1995, p. 249). Copyright 1995 by the American Psychological Association. Reprinted by permission.

verbally aggressive when warned by adults, leading observers to consider *why* he might react in particular to being warned, and the meaning of such warnings for that individual. Perhaps the child becomes embarrassed at being "shown up" by adults in front of peers, or loves to challenge authority and see how much he can get away with. Child 28, by contrast, becomes reliably aggressive when approaches sociably by peers, inviting and suggesting a completely different set of explanations for his behavior, for how the child construes the world, for what he may consider threatening, or what goals may motivate him.

As these examples illustrate, there is not a one-to-one correspondence between the outward behavior (e.g., aggression) and the underlying disposition. Instead, such profiles require explanations of another nature, and one that perceivers seem to engage in intuitively (Kammrath et al., 2005; Plaks et al., 2003): These profiles invite questions about how the target feels, what the target thinks, and how the target perceives his or her world. In the next section, we review the theoretical account that can account for such profiles, then detail the convergences of such a model with the premises of cultural psychology.

THE CULTURALLY CONSTITUTED COGNITIVE–AFFECTIVE PROCESSING SYSTEM

Having established *if . . . then . . .* signatures as a second, reliable locus of personality coherence, the task became to generate a framework that could account for both these profiles and overall aggregate behavioral tendencies. In response to this task, Mischel and Shoda (1995, 1999) proposed a Cognitive–Affective Personality System (CAPS) framework that integrates insights about knowledge activation (Anderson, 1988; Higgins, 1996; Hong & Mallorie, 2004; Kashima, 2001), social cognition (e.g., Cantor & Kihlstrom, 1989; Downey & Feldman, 1996; Read, Jones, & Miller, 1990), and connectionism (Hinton, McClelland, & Rumelhart, 1986; Kashima, 2004; Read & Miller, 1998, 2002). We describe the framework in some detail below as one representative of a family of approaches (see Cervone, 2004; Hong & Chiu, 2001; Kashima, 2001; Pervin, 2001; see also Hong, Wan, No, & Chiu, Chapter 13, this volume) that, rather than parsing causal forces in terms of what is "dance" versus "dancer," demonstrates how personality processes and the mediating units proposed to account for them are *inherently* contextual in nature (see also Norenzayan et al., Chapter 23, this volume). Following the description of this general framework as it has been related to culture and personality (Mendoza-Denton et al., 1999), we extend and refine the framework to explicitly to take a system view of culture (Kitayama, 2002) into account.

Rather than being a theory of personality per se, CAPS theory is a general framework that outlines a set of principles. It proposes that human behavior is mediated by a set of cognitive–affective units (CAUs) organized within a stable network of activation. This network or organization, according to Mischel and Shoda (1995), constitutes the basic stable structure of the personality processing system and underlies the behavioral expressions that characterize the individual.

Common Units for Culture and Personality: CAUs

CAUs are conceptualized in terms of five relatively stable "person variables" that have been identified over a century of psychological research as playing an important role in social behavior generation (Cervone, 2004; Read et al., 1990; Mischel, 1973; Pervin, 2001). They are summarized in Table 7.1. The content of CAUs is determined through, and grounded in, the individual's cultural context—what is taught by one's family, what is valued by one's community, and what is afforded by one's culture (Kitayama, 2002; Mischel & Shoda 1995; Shoda, 1999).

CAUs provide a natural bridge to the study of culture as a result of their striking convergence with widely accepted definitions of culture. Classical, as well modern, definitions of culture consistently emphasize CAU-type constructs—

TABLE 7.1. Types of CAUs in the Personality Mediating System

1. *Encodings*: Categories (constructs) for the self, people, events, and situations (external and internal).

2. *Expectations and beliefs*: About the social world, about outcomes for behavior in particular situations, about one's self-efficacy.

3. *Affects*: Feelings, emotions, and affective responses (including physiological reactions).

4. *Goals*: Desirable outcomes and affective states, aversive outcomes and affective states; goals and life projects.

5. *Competencies and self-regulatory plans*: Potential behaviors and scripts that one can do, and plans and strategies for organizing action and for affecting outcomes and one's own behavior and internal states.

Note. From Mischel and Shoda (1995, p. 253). Copyright 1995 by the American Psychological Association. Reprinted by permission.

values, beliefs, meanings, customs, attributions, attitudes, and appraisals—as central components of the cultural heritage that is shared and transmitted among members of a given cultural group (Geertz, 1973; Obeyeskere, 1981; Schwartz, 1992; Triandis & Suh, 2002; Triandis et al., 1980; Tylor, 1871). There seems to be wide agreement that culture plays a large role in determining what is valued, what is worth pursuing, and how to interpret the world.

Given the correspondence between elements of culture and elements of a person, it is tempting to draw a one-to-one correspondence between "culture" and "person," such that a person is viewed as a culture writ small, or its converse, that culture is "personality writ large" (Benedict, 1934). A moment's thought, however, reveals a much more complicated relationship between "culture" and "person." A person cannot be a "culture" writ small, because the person can be thought of as consisting of many little cultures—people are Thai, they are men, they are family men, they are husbands, they are colleagues at work—and each of these is its own distinct culture. The mutual influence of culture and person, then, operates at multiple levels, such that each person's social circles dictate his or her unique social reality (Linton, 1936; Mendoza-Denton et al., 1999).

Culture and Principles of Knowledge Activation

As several researchers have noted (Kashima, 2001; Hong & Mallorie, 2004) principles of knowledge activation (Higgins, 1996) are helpful in thinking about the intersection between culture and personality. Members of cultural groups differ in terms of what goals, values, and beliefs are *available*. For example, whereas one culture may teach beliefs about spirit possession to its members, this notion may not be part of the explanatory repertoire for others' behavior among members of other groups. The CAPS framework also assumes that people differ in the *chronic accessibility* (Higgins, 1996; Mischel & Shoda, 1995; Shoda, LeeTiernan, & Mischel, 2002) of constructs, that is, the ease with which particular CAUs become activated. For example, a strong cultural norm of valuing others' welfare may make such a concern more chronically accessible—thus, easily activated—to individuals of that culture (e.g., Markus & Kitayama, 1991). As another example, by virtue of shared experiences, stigmatized group

members within a given culture may have concerns about discrimination more chronically accessible than nonstigmatized group members (Mendoza-Denton et al., 1997). Finally, the model also postulates that of all the beliefs, goals, values, encodings, and feelings that one can potentially experience at any given time, only those that are relevant in a given situation can become activated and influence subsequent behavior (Hong, Benet-Martinez, Chiu, & Morris, 2003). As such, CAPS makes specific the notion of *applicability*. For example, one cultural difference identified in prior research has been a greater tendency toward self-enhancement in the United States than in Japan (Heine et al., 1999), but this cultural difference is expressed in culturally defined situations and contexts. Another example comes from Kitayama, Markus, Matsumoto, and Norasakkunkit (1997), who demonstrated that European Americans are highly self-enhancing, and this is especially true for situations that European Americans spontaneously nominate as being relevant to their self-esteem. By contrast, Japanese were found to be self-critical but, again, more pronouncedly so in situations identified by the ingroup as relevant to self-esteem. As such, culture influences personality through and through—not only in terms of the goals and important beliefs but also in the way that situations are represented and what psychological features situations contain.

Thinking about a box of crayons offers a metaphor for cultural influences and principles of knowledge activation. Culture dictates what constructs or CAUs an individual has at his or her disposal to color the world. If a given crayon (CAU) is not available, the person cannot use it. "Accessibility" refers to the ease with which a person is likely to use that crayon once it is available. If we imagine a box of crayons with three rows, for example, a person is more likely to use those crayons that are more easily reachable, such as the ones in front. Finally, "applicability" refers to the rules a culture dictates about what crayons one can use and when. A spirit possession "crayon"—if available—may be applicable to explaining mental illness in certain cultures but not in others.

Interconnections among CAUs

As Kitayama (2002) notes, "It is to be anticipated that cultures should be different not only in terms of central tendencies in any given variables but also in terms of functional relations among them" (p. 93). This quote captures the second important feature of CAPS, namely, that the person is not conceptualized only as the receptacle of disjointed, unrelated CAUs. Rather, CAUs operate within an interconnected *network* whereby CAUS have excitatory and inhibitory links to each other, and in which different pathways become activated in relation to features of the situation. For any given CAU, positive (excitatory) connections to it increase that CAUs activation level, whereas negative (inhibitory) connections to it decrease its activation level. A highly simplified, schematized version of a CAPS is shown in Figure 7.2.

The large circle in the middle of Figure 7.2 represents the "person," whereas his or her stable network of CAUs is represented by the nodes and excitatory (solid lines) and inhibitory (dotted lines) links among those nodes. Al-

though the "network" of CAUs and interconnections is itself stable, as the individual moves across different situations, different mediating units and their characteristic interrelationships become activated (contingent on applicability) in relation to psychological features of those situations. The framework accounts for and is able to generate meaningfully patterned expression of behavior in relationship to situations, as well as to generalized overall tendencies in behavior (Shoda & Mischel, 1998). This is an important point, because it highlights the fact that the CAPS approach does not necessarily stand in contrast to broad differences between individuals (Mischel & Shoda, 1999).

Life experiences shared by members of a group—the teachings of elders, the experiences shared with others, the values imposed by society—generate a CAPS network that is immersed in and reflects the surrounding culture.

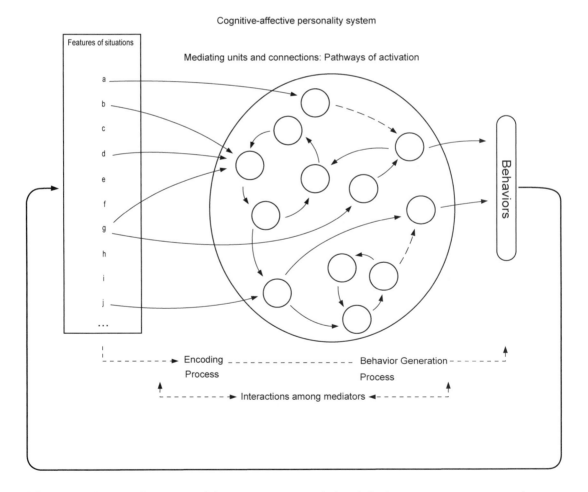

FIGURE 7.2. Schematic illustration of the CAPS. From Mischel and Shoda (1995, p. 254). Copyright 1995 by the American Psychological Association. Reprinted by permission.

If features of a situation activate this culturally shared subnetwork, an individual may generate similar reactions to that situation, without implications for the rest of the individual's distinctive processing dynamics (see also Cohen, 1997). In other words, when situations reliably activate shared networks, cultural commonalities in behavior may occur, whereas in situations that do not activate a culturally shared psychological feature, group members' responses may not converge (although they may converge with those of another group).

Consider one of the most striking examples of cultural convergence within the United States in recent memory—reactions to the 1995 verdict of the murder trial of the African American former football star and celebrity O. J. Simpson. At the time, it was clear that opinions regarding the defendant's guilt were sharply split along racial lines. An analysis of reactions to the verdict showed that, among African Americans, certain features of the case—such as the detective who planted evidence to influence a conviction—reliably activated cognitions about historically unfair police treatment toward African Americans in the United States. These cognitions, in turn, inhibited others, such as "There is a lot of evidence against the defendant." European Americans, for whom the realities of race-based discrimination are both less available and less accessible, instead focused on the evidence—and held a strong belief that Simpson should have been found guilty. Indeed, the effect of race on reactions to the verdict was mediated by the shared network of cognitions activated (Mendoza-Denton et al., 1997). Of note, reactions to verdicts of other high-profile trials are generally not split along racial lines, suggesting that members of cultural groups can share subnetworks activated in some situations but do not have to display similarity in behavior to others.

AN INTEGRATED SYSTEM VIEW OF CULTURE AND PERSON DYNAMICS

Kitayama and colleagues (Kitayama, 2002; Kitayama & Markus, 1999; Kitayama et al., 1997) have contributed a perspective that adds another layer of complexity to our understanding of the co-constitution of person and culture. Similar to how we have argued for a dynamic and flexible view of personality in favor of a static, context-free view, a systems view of *culture* stands in contrast to static treatments

of cultures as explanatory, even causal entities that "account" for group differences (cf. Betancourt & López, 1993). The influence of culture on personality is broader, and its dynamics influence the person at several levels, such that culture is not just stored "in the head" (a view perhaps taken too easily taken from the earlier CAPS analysis) but rather limits, directs, and invites culturally consonant behavior in other ways.

A systems view of culture recognizes that cultural values and belief systems shape the institutions and everyday practices of a culture, which themselves provide *cultural affordances* (Kitayama & Markus, 1999) or opportunities for the expression and reinforcement of these cultural values. A core cultural belief system such as the Protestant work ethic (Levy, West, Ramirez, & Karafantis, 2006), for example, can give rise to institutions that reinforce its very unfolding, and influence the settings and situations that people navigate in their daily lives (Vandello & Cohen, 2004). In a similar way, a belief in personal mastery over the environment, or over nature, can lead to the valuation, and construction, of gymnasiums where such mastery and discipline become practicable and true ("physical culture"; Triandis et al., 1980). At the level of the individual, these macro-level influences lead to differences in the psychological availability of certain constructs (e.g., belief in mastery over aging), the (chronic) accessibility of these belief systems (through gyms, ads, and other artifacts serving to chronically prime ideas of beauty, health, and youth), as well as the organization among the cognitions and affective evaluations. As such, then, a system view of culture reminds us that culture not only influences the content of the box of crayons people use to "color their world" but in fact also influences the coloring book itself.

A Schematized View of the C-CAPS Model

The Cultural Cognitive–Affective Processing System (C-CAPS) model is one in which a system view of culture and a system view of the person are integrated and explicitly acknowledged to influence each other. Figure 7.3 provides a schematic view of this multisystem model: This section walks the reader through Figure 7.3. We begin with the three boxes on the left-hand side—subjective culture, physical culture, and nominal situations. As a whole, they make up the cultural affordance processes that not only shape the CAPS system but also constrain the kinds of situations to which the CAPS system is exposed. "Subjective culture" is the term that Triandis and colleagues (1980) have used to refer to the cultural beliefs, values, and meaning systems that become transmitted from one generation to the next. Examples of such cultural values might be the "Protestant work ethic" (PWE; Levy et al., 2006), "social dominance orientation" (Pratto, Sidanius, Stallworth, & Malle, 1994), or "collectivism" (Triandis, 1996). Subjective culture is likely to influence directly the availability, accessibility, and network relationships of the person's own beliefs, values, and goals (arrow 1 in Figure 7.3). The cultural value referred to abstractly as "PWE," for example, might be cognitively represented in terms of concrete cognitions such as "Be all you can be," "Hard work pays off," or "No pain, no gain" (see Geertz, 1973, for a discussion of abstract value systems vs. more concrete, or "experience-near" cognitive representations). Arrow 2 captures the notion

that cultural value systems influence people's physical surroundings—the types of institutions that are built, for example, or the architectural designs that foster culturally valued types of social interaction. This arrow is bidirectional to reflect the notion that physical culture also reifies the cultural value systems that create and maintain it. As arrow 3 shows, cultural belief systems and institutions then afford group members the specific nominal situations that allow people to practice and further reinforce those belief systems as part of a shared reality. These nominal situations are more discretionary, temporally discrete instantiations of culture, such as taking an exam, running on a treadmill, or having a power lunch with a client.

Together, these first three boxes in Figure 7.3 take us from a broader "culture" to a more specific "context," to a more specific "situation," although these distinctions themselves do not have clean, easy boundaries. Although the "power of the situation" is great (see Ross

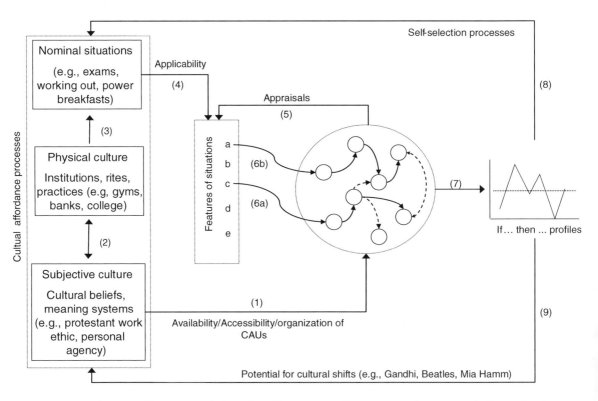

FIGURE 7.3. Schematic illustration of the culturally constituted C-CAPS. Subjective and physical culture influence the contents and organization of the individual's processing system (1), and provide the cultural affordances that form a basis for the nominal situations experienced by the person (2, 3). Psychological features of situations are influenced by both nominal situations and the person's appraisal processes (4, 5). The system yields *if . . . then . . .* signatures (6a, 6b, 7), which both influence the immediate environment of the person (8) and have the potential to enact cultural change (9).

& Nisbett, 1991), even these "situations" cannot be separated from the people who collectively, as a culture, have defined and continue to define them.

Arrows 4 and 5 in Figure 7.3 reflect the co-constitutive influence of culture and the person as reflected in the psychological situation (Shoda et al., 1994). As discussed earlier, the subjective meaning of a nominal situation is influenced by the person's existing knowledge structures through appraisal processes (arrow 5; see Cervone, 2004); however, appraisals are bound to and directed by their *applicability* to a given nominal situation (arrow 4). As in the original CAPS formulation, features of the psychological situation then activate and inhibit other CAUs (arrows 6a and 6b), following a pattern of activation and inhibition such that if . . . then . . . profiles, as well as overall behavior tendencies, are displayed (arrow 7). As various researchers have argued, these behaviors then influence the very situations in which people find themselves in (Levy, Ayduk, & Downey, 2001), creating a self-selection bias (arrow 8). For example, the person who believes in personal agency and control over aging is likely to find him- or herself working out, and encoding the experience as daily mastery against old age. Thus, culture and the person are both interpenetrating each other, mutually discernible yet inseparable.

Finally, arrow 9 in Figure 7.3 provides the possibility that people can alter subjective or physical culture. Gandhi inspired and mobilized entire groups of people toward a belief in the power of peace; the Beatles changed the meaning of music; Mia Hamm played soccer at a moment in history when a nation (in this case, the United States) was ready to get serious about women and sports. Thus, individuals can also influence the normative forces we call "culture."

TWO ILLUSTRATIONS

The stable situation–behavior profiles generated by the CAPS system lend themselves not only to the idiographic study of persons but also provide a nomothetic route to characterize cultural groups in terms of their shared subnetworks, situation–behavior signatures, and common cultural affordances. In the section that follows, we briefly illustrate some ways that a dynamic system approach to culture and personality can help shed light on cul-

tural convergences in behavior. The emphasis in these approaches is in a deeper understanding of how history, cultural meaning systems, and contextual constraints shape the thoughts, cognitions, and affects that individuals experience. We choose two examples—research on culture of honor, and on race-based rejection sensitivity—to illustrate how macro-level forces such as a herding economy or a history of discrimination against one's group shape the social-cognitive worlds of individuals.

Culture of Honor

Research on culture of honor (Cohen, 1998; Cohen, Nisbett, Bowdle, & Schwarz, 1996, Nisbett & Cohen, 1996; see also Cohen, Chapter 8, this volume) provides an in-depth analysis of how historical forces shape cultural practices and norms (cultural affordances), which in turn influence the way individuals behave in particular situations (person × situation interactions). The research provides an excellent illustration of how seemingly contradictory surface-level behaviors can be understood, and subsequently predicted, by understanding how subjective and physical culture have shaped the characteristic cognitions, affects, and encodings characteristic of a given group within the United States.

What are these contradictory surface-level behaviors? As Cohen et al. (1996) noted, "For centuries, the American South has been regarded as more violent than the North" (p. 945). Consistent with this reputation, rates in the South and West for argument-related homicides have been shown to be higher than they are in the North (Nisbett & Cohen, 1996). Despite this reputation, however, Southerners also have a reputation for being charming and polite. A recent etiquette expert ranked Charleston, South Carolina, as the nation's most polite city–for the 10th straight year. "When you pass people on the street, they will nod at you," reports a Charleston city tour guide. "People who live here are, for whatever reason, polite. Whether it's breeding or in the water, it's hard to say" (CNN, 2005). In short, the South's reputation for violence stands alongside its equally strong reputation for politeness, for that old Southern charm. How then, do we reconcile the view of a violent South with a view of a charming South?

According to the culture of honor hypothesis, a herding economy in combination with loose law enforcement in the Southern and

Western United States have led to a cultural adaptation in which honor and reputation have become critical elements in the protection of one's property and name. In the absence of adequate social control, it became important to respond quickly and affirmatively to being crossed, insulted, affronted, or stolen from, so as to communicate to the community not to "mess" with one's property and to maintain one's status. The culture of honor, characterized by strong vigilance to disrespect and ready use of violence to protect property and name, has over time affected social practices and norms. This is symbolized both in games that amount to tests of "manhood" (e.g., "chicken" games, or kicking each other in the shins) and in legal lenience toward violence instigated by affronts to honor (Cohen & Nisbett, 1994, 1997). These practices and laws are good examples of the way subjective culture influences physical culture, as illustrated by arrow 2 in Figure 7.3.

As Cohen, Vandello, Puente, and Rantilla (1999) explain, a culture of honor that rests on violent retaliation following affront dictates not only how to react when such an affront occurs, but also how to act when an affront does *not* occur. More specifically, in a culture where serious retribution is a consequence of disrespect, it is to one's best interest to be unambiguous about according respect when one is not looking for trouble. As such, then, a distinct *if . . . then . . .* pattern can be viewed as characterizing the behavior of people sharing a culture of honor.

In a laboratory-based "experimental ethnography" that provided empirical support for this culture of honor profile, Cohen and colleagues (1996, Study 3) recruited Northern and Southern white men to participate in a laboratory study generally described to be about personality. An ingenious experimental manipulation followed. Participants were brought into the lab, asked to fill out questionnaires, and then drop off the packet at the end of a long, narrow hallway. Half of the Southern and half of the Northern participants were then subjected to an affront: While walking down the hallway, they had to squeeze past an assistant (in reality, a confederate) getting something out of a cabinet. The confederate, feigning annoyance, slammed the cabinet shut, insulted the participant under his breath, and intentionally bumped the participant on his way out of the hallway. At this point, the participant still had to make his way to the end of the hallway, but

at this point a different person (also a confederate) began walking down the hall toward him. Given the width of the hallway, this in effect set the stage for a potential game of "chicken," where the point is to see who swerves out of the way first. The distance at which the participant "chickened out" or got out of the confederate's way was expected to vary both as a function of the participant's background and whether he had been bumped or not. Following this encounter, the participant finally made it to the end of the hall, where he was met by a different confederate. This confederate, blind to the regional background of the participant, rated the firmness of the participant's handshake and gave an overall impression of the participant's domineering behavior.

As expected, and corroborating prior research, Southern men who had been bumped, relative to men from the North, waited longer before stepping aside to let the second confederate through. This is consistent with the interpretation that following an affront (the bump by the first confederate), a more aggressive response to restore honor was facilitated among Southern men. Participants were also rated by the third confederate as more aggressive and dominant, and as giving a firmer handshake relative to that of Northern participants. Tellingly, however, among participants who had not been bumped, the Southern men were more "polite" than their Northern counterparts: They got out of the second confederate's way earlier, gave less firm handshakes, and were less domineering and aggressive with the third confederate.

Thus the results from this study are consistent both with the notion that Southerners are more violent, and that Southerners are more polite. Which one is correct? The answer is both—a clear *if . . . then . . .* pattern, predicted from an in-depth analysis of the historical and social influences affecting the South, as well as astute expectations as to how those macrolevel influences affect the way individuals construe and respond to situations. Importantly, a global analysis of Southern aggression without regard to the situation would miss these dynamics entirely.

Mere Recategorization, or Dynamic Complexity?

Cultural psychologists might worry about a characterization—or caricaturization—of Southern "personality" as a two-point pattern dictated by respect and affront, where the stable aspect of the person, instead of being a global adjective, is now conveniently replaced by a global belief system or even a set of folk beliefs. However, it is important to remember that the C-CAPS—the shared networks of beliefs, cognitions, affects, and actions, activated in relation to situations—exist within a broader network that may or may not be shared by other members of the group (Kashima, 2004). For example, while two men may both have grown up in the South, and may both feel physiological arousal when verbally insulted in a hallway (Cohen et al., 1996), one of these two men may consider self-control an important life value, perhaps as a result of martial arts classes, or a deep religious conviction of "turning the other cheek."

Although efforts toward a contextual analysis of behavior within cultural and cross-cultural psychology have an established history (Hoorens & Poortinga, 2000), such analyses have been criticized (Shweder, 1991) as conveniently recategorizing people into smaller and smaller groups every time a prediction goes awry (e.g., where insights about "Southern men" become insights about "Southern men who hold deep religious beliefs" and eventually "Southern men who hold deep religious beliefs but who have self-regulatory competency"). By contrast, a view of the culture–personality system as a dynamic network allows us to understand how one can reconcile both cultural homogeneity and difference *as part of the same dynamic process*. The strength of the C-CAPS lies in its recognition that an individual who can behave similarly to others in his or her cultural group, when the correct psychological features of situations are activated, can act in a completely idiosyncratic manner when a different set of features is activated, thus allowing for individuality and commonality within the same individual at different times (Mendoza-Denton et al., 1997). Thus, rather than an atheoretical recategorization of behavioral responses into smaller and smaller groups, The C-CAPS view focuses on the stability of the *if . . . then . . .* Culture–personality profiles, and their diagnostic use toward a deeper understanding of the interplay between cultural conditions and processing dynamics. The level of specificity adopted with C-CAPS is a *choice* that depends entirely on the goals for which it is used, all the way from the individual life history (McAdams, 1999) to large group and cultural comparisons.

Race-Based Rejection Sensitivity

To this point, we have provided illustrative examples of C-CAPS, such that particular features of situations (e.g., an affront to honor, or a crooked cop planting evidence) activate culturally shared dynamics that predict behavior by members of a cultural group. There is the possibility, however, of variability even in situations that seem especially relevant to cultural groups. This variability can be fruitfully harnessed to understand and map a given cultural dynamic—in other words, individual differences providing a window into psychological process (Mendoza-Denton, Page-Gould, & Pietrzak, 2006). One example of this is work on sensitivity to race-based rejection in the U.S. context, in which clear, within-group variability coexists with a dynamic predicated on particular experiences being more likely to occur to members of a particular group.

As several researchers have emphasized, the psychology of minority group members must be understood within the group's own context and historical background, an important part of which is a history of stigmatization and the continuing discrimination that exists to this day (Sellers, Caldwell, Schmeelk-Cone, & Zimmerman, 2003; Shelton, 2000). This history, as well as prior experiences, are likely to affect individuals in profound ways, affecting both the sense of self (Humphreys & Kashima, 2002; Mischel & Morf, 2003; Kashima et al., 2004) and the stable responses that the individual marshals in response to discrimination. One such mechanism, termed *sensitivity to race-based rejection* (RS-race; Mendoza-Denton, Downey, Purdie, Davis, & Pietrzak, 2002; Mendoza-Denton et al., 2005) also illustrates the intricate co-constitution of culture (societal stereotypes and prejudice), nominal situations (e.g., the university setting), and the person (RS-race dynamic).

Growing out of developmental perspectives on attachment, the construct of RS-race has its theoretical precursors in research on rejection sensitivity (Downey & Feldman, 1996; Levy et al., 2001). Based on a series of prospective, longitudinal, and experimental studies, Downey and colleagues have proposed that when people experience rejection from parents, peers, or other important figures in the form of abuse or neglect, they are vulnerable to developing anxious expectations of rejection, namely, a "hot," affectively laden expectation that future rejection lies in store in similar kinds of situations.

These anxious expectations are activated in situations where rejection is both applicable and salient (Higgins, 1996), and is a good illustration of the idea that the stable dispositional feature of the individual, namely, anxious expectations, are made accessible specifically in relation to features of the situations. Ayduk, Downey, Testa, Yen, and Shoda (1999), for example, found that when rejection-sensitive women were rejected, they retaliated by bad-mouthing the perpetrator; however, when an alternative, benign explanation for the rejection was offered, no retaliation was observed. These anxious expectations lower the threshold for perceiving the rejection and, once the rejection is perceived, activate intense, "hot" reactions to it.

To the degree that affiliation and acceptance can be considered a fundamental human motive (Fiske, 2004), people may be universally capable of developing the dynamic of rejection sensitivity (anxious expectations → ready perceptions → hot reactions) if rejected or neglected. However, the manifestation of rejection may be expressed in many different ways that are constrained by culture. Mendoza-Denton and colleagues (2002) postulated that rejection can occur on the basis of not only idiosyncratic characteristics but also devalued group membership—such as gender, sexual orientation, or race.

Cultural influences come into play at several levels. First, as has been widely recognized, stigma is context-specific: An attribute or personal characteristic that is devalued in one domain may be valued (or be neutrally valenced) in another context (Crocker, Major, & Steele, 1998). As such, the context within which a person operates can dictate the type of interpersonal experiences—and stable dynamics—that develop as a result. Second, even when two groups might be negatively stigmatized, the nature of the stigma depends on the assumptions that a given stigma carries about one's group. In the United States, for example, being African American carries a suspicion about academic inability (Steele, 1997), but not about athletic ability, whereas the reverse is true of Asian Americans (Chan & Mendoza-Denton, 2004). As such, then, although two people may be equally apprehensive concerning their status, the situations that activate their rejection concerns are different. Finally, the coping mechanisms applied in response to the rejection may be different. Again, one's cultural group provides one with culture-specific strategies, values, and culturally appropriate strategies marshaled in response to rejection.

If one takes such a cultural-psychological analysis seriously, it becomes difficult, if not impossible, to create an technique to assess status-based rejection expectations *independently* of context. Accordingly, Mendoza-Denton et al. (2002) conducted focus groups to find out the situations that activate race-based rejection concerns among African Americans, and constructed a questionnaire based specifically on those situations (this methodology parallels Kitayama et al.'s (1997) situation sampling procedure). The kinds of situations included scenarios such as a random traffic stop or being passed over for an opportunity to answer a difficult question in class—situations that contain "active ingredients" for making discrimination applicable and salient among African Americans. The researchers administered this questionnaire to a sample of African American, European American, and Asian American undergraduates. As expected, African Americans scored highest on the measure, whereas European American and Asian American participants scored low and did not differ. Individual differences in the measure predicted spontaneous attributions to race in these situations among African Americans but not among European Americans or Asian Americans (Mendoza-Denton et al., 2002). among African Americans, individual differences in anxious expectations of race-based rejection subsequently predicted, over a 3-week period, reports of rejection, and more intense feelings of alienation and rejection following the rejection. Over the course of five semesters, individual differences in RS-race among African Americans predicted students' grade point averages (GPAs). This last result in particular illustrates well how culture is both "in the head" and "out there." Individuals enact self-protective mechanisms in response to discrimination, which, at a system level, is maintained by the broader culture's subjective culture (e.g., stereotypes, system justifications), physical culture (majority-dominated college settings), and nominal settings (unequal opportunities). Rather than being a question about explaining the phenomenon either through social or personality psychology, this approach shows not only their inseparability but also the indispensability of their interplay for an understanding of the dynamic.

It may be helpful at this point to consider a hypothetical scenario in which two Americans—one black, one white—score equally highly on a measure of neuroticism, but in one case the score is capturing the individual's concerns surrounding societal discrimination, whereas in the other the score is capturing the individual's concern surrounding romantic relationships. Far from being mere "adaptations" (McCrae, 2000), not to be confused with dispositions, we argue that it is *precisely* by knowing about the trigger features, the outcomes, and the historical context surrounding the behavior of each person that one begins really to arrive at the cultural psychology underlying social behavior (Cohen, 1997; Mendoza-Denton et al., 1997). A deep understanding of people's responses to the particular predicament in question depends on cultural background, as well as cognitive-social learning history—in one case, a strong historical backdrop of oppression and discrimination (Mendoza-Denton et al., 2002) and in the other, perhaps neglect or abuse in the home (Downey & Feldman, 1996). To draw on an earlier analogy, the only way to distinguish between the two cars is by looking under the hood.

IMPLICATIONS

Assessment Issues

Having provided two illustrations of how the C-CAPS operates, we now turn to a discussion of personality assessment through a cultural-psychological lens. As noted earlier, the current dominant approach to personality assessment and comparison across cultures is the global trait approach (Triandis & Suh, 2002), which is both helpful and attractive because it provides a rigorous, methodologically driven approach to assessment. However, as we have noted, aggregating or ignoring situational variability in behavior necessarily precludes an analysis of the ways in which personality dynamics and culture influence one another.

But how should situations be grouped? This is the critical question for a viable cultural-psychological approach to personality. As reviewed earlier, this approach suggests that rather than looking at nominal situations (e.g., the marketplace, the university, a social chat around the water cooler) that are of limited generalizability (e.g., see B. B. Whiting & Whiting, 1975), people act on situations that are *psychologically* similar (e.g., contexts that

are ripe for social rejection; opportunities in which one can advance one's children's education). The distinction between nominal and psychological situations lies precisely at the heart of a cultural psychology in which the world outside is interpreted through the lens of the culture, and those interpretations are themselves facilitated through cultural affordances. To the degree that psychological situational groupings are culturally specific, it is the task of the cultural psychologist to uncover those local meanings and not be lured by outward appearances. As some of the research summarized in this chapter illustrates, personality processes as they are embedded and expressed in their cultural context can be captured with various methodologies.

Bottom-Up Approaches

As described earlier, Wright and Mischel (1988) used clustering techniques to identify different types of commonly used situational modifiers that the cultural experts in that context (the targets' peers and counselors) used to describe a particular cultural group. This is an example of a "bottom-up" strategy, in which the researcher recruits "experts" or informants in a given culture to provide the raw data for subsequent coding and clustering.

Top-Down Approaches

A second, "top-down" approach to assessment is one in which the researcher begins with a theory of the internal processing dynamics that may characterize a type, and is then able to hypothesize the distinctive *if . . . then . . .* profile for that type, as well as the psychological trigger features that define the profile (e.g., Downey & Feldman, 1996). A theory about a cultural group's distinctive processing dynamics can be derived from careful study about a group's history, or the social, environmental, and historical forces that have shaped its people. An excellent example of this approach is the careful analysis leading to the culture of honor research reviewed earlier. A hybrid approach, containing elements of both a top-down and a bottom-up approach, is seen in Mendoza-Denton et al. (2002), who not only hypothesized the dynamic of RS-race on the basis of historical and societal analysis but also interviewed people about the specific situations in which the dynamic would be played out.

Interpreting Cross-Cultural Differences in Global Traits

Researchers have shown quite convincingly that there are trait-level differences among cultural groups (Triandis & Suh, 2002). Again, the proposed approach is not incompatible: The C-CAPS predicts, and is able to account for, both *if . . . then . . .* patterns and broad differences between groups. In considering findings that two cultural groups differ—or do not—on a given trait, however, the C-CAPS approach uncovers alternative interpretations to a one-to-one correspondence between the trait and underlying dispositions.

Consider findings from Kammrath et al. (2005, Study 3), who presented people with several distinct *if . . . then . . .* patterns that were nevertheless identical in their overall interpersonal warmth. For example, one target was reliably friendlier toward authority figures than to peers, whereas a second target displayed precisely the opposite pattern. A third target was not differentially friendly toward authorities and peers. Participants rated their impressions of each target using Goldberg's transparent, bipolar Big Five scale (Golberg, 1992). From a global trait perspective, people should rate all targets equally on Agreeableness and Extraversion, given that all targets displayed the same overall level of interpersonal warmth. The results showed that although ratings of Extraversion did not differ across the three targets, the target that was warm toward authorities was seen as distinctly disagreeable, whereas the target that was friendly to peers was rated as quite agreeable (the third target was rated in the middle). These findings suggest caution in interpreting broad trait dimensions as indexes of overall behavior aggregates. In the research described here, the targets did *not* actually differ in their overall warmth, despite clear differences in perceivers' ratings of their Agreeableness.

A second caution in interpreting trait-level cultural differences too literally is seen in Shoda, Mischel, and Wright (1993), who also analyzed data from the boys' summer camp described earlier (Shoda et al., 1994; Wright & Mischel, 1988). For this analysis, the researchers analyzed the *if . . . then . . .* profile patterns of those boys who were collectively agreed to be prototypical exemplars of "friendly," "withdrawn," and "aggressive" children. Surprisingly, when looking at the children's physical aggression, it was not the prototypically "aggressive" children who displayed the most overall physical aggression—it was the campers labeled as "withdrawn." Evidently, even though the perceivers used the label "aggressive" to describe children and agreed as to which children could be described this way, the specific pattern to which the label referred did not necessarily correspond to the surface-level behavior. As another example, consider findings on gender stereotypes by Mendoza-Denton, Park, Kammrath, and Peake (2004). Despite the fact that men are stereotypically labeled as "assertive" and women as "passive," Mendoza-Denton et al. found that women are in fact expected to be more assertive than men in certain situations (e.g., those that have to do with home and hearth). The relevant point is that perceivers' labels do not necessarily correspond to the surface-level manifestations of behavior that the labels suggest.

As these examples suggest, the relationship between the trait terms people use to describe others and the behavior patterns to which they relate is not straightforward. People undeniably use traits, and the basic classification of these into five categories seems to have solid support, but their interpretation as reflecting biological dispositions of entire cultural groups (e.g., McCrae, 2004) seems premature. Having identified through careful, rigorous work that some groups of people differ from others in the traits ascribed to them, the logical next step seems not to look for biological differences, but rather to understand cultural variability in the lay theories associated with these traits.

CONCLUSIONS

In the seminal article "Cultural Psychology: What Is It?" Shweder (1990) refers to a song by Paul McCartney and Stevie Wonder, "Ebony and Ivory," with the lyric, "We all know that people are the same wherever you go." Shweder cites this lyric as an example of the intuitive lay notion, based on Platonic philosophy, of psychic unity—in other words, the idea that in spite of cultural superficialities, a basic humanity unites all of us (see Triandis, Chapter 3, this volume). In current cross-cultural conceptualizations, such psychic unity is claimed to be a universal personality trait structure that goes above and beyond cultural differences—with the strong implication that, indeed, people are the same wherever you go. Cultural psychology has suggested an alternative path to this approach, rejecting the notion of psychic unity and instead preferring to show that, by virtue of the fact that culture and psyche make each other up, people are just, irreducibly, not the same wherever you go.

And yet McCartney and Wonder do seem to have a fundamental point that cannot be easily dismissed. It stands to reason that, as a species, there should be a set of characteristics that unites all of us. Within the C-CAPS framework, the potential candidates for universality are the basic architecture of the system and its governing principles—availability, accessibility, applicability, and organization.

Despite calls not to equate personality exclusively with global traits, and warnings about the utility and comparability of broad constructs across cultures (Bock, 2000; Church, 2000; Kashima, 2001; Pervin, 1999), the tacit equation of consistency with "individual behavior dispositions that are expressed as consistent behavior across time and across situations" (Poortinga & Van Hemert, 2001, p. 1034) remains, in our reading, the default assumption among researchers interested in culture and personality. The cost of this assumption for the study of culture and personality is that it bypasses some of the most exciting advances in current personality science, and obscures opportunities for integration (Church, 2000; Mischel, 2004; Shoda & Mischel, 2000; Shoda et al., 2002; Triandis, 2000).

We have proposed here that a processing model that can account for person × situation interactions may be fruitfully applied to understanding how culture and person are mutually constitutive. This model departs from the classic notion of a bounded, causal entity called a "person" that exerts a unidirectional causal influence on behavior independent of situational or cultural forces. The framework offers a perspective that legitimizes cross-situational variability in behavior as the output of a culturally imbued, dynamic, meaning-making process (see Norenzayan et al., Chapter 23, this volume). It identifies an alternative set of mediating units—and their interrelationships—as the active ingredients of a cultural personality system. The cognitive–affective units and contextual variables outlined in Figure 7.3 are framed at a broad level, and require specification at the level of CAU contents and contextual variables to be able to offer prediction. In terms of the

contents and cultural manifestations of the C-CAPS, Shweder's (1991) description could not be more apt: "The mind, left to its own devices, is mindless" (p. 83).

Thus, rather than itself specifying a set of predictions, the C-CAPS framework offers a set of principles that researchers can use to guide their theory-building work. Such theory building, as we have reviewed, can occur in both a top-down or a bottom-up approach, but likely requires as a first step intimacy with a cultural group, through either observation or the insights of cultural informants (see also Cohen, Chapter 8, this volume). We have argued that insights in social cognition and personality science over the past two decades provide a set of principles for research that can lead to a cumulative science of culture–personality studies. A failure to take them into account risks falling prey to overgeneralizations and untenable stereotyping that in the past yielded studies of "national character" (Benedict, 1934) and "modal personality" (DuBois, 1944) ultimately untenable (see Triandis, Chapter 3, this volume).

REFERENCES

Allik, J., & McCrae, R. R. (2004). Toward a geography of personality traits: Patterns of profiles across 36 cultures. *Journal of Cross-Cultural Psychology*, *35*(1), 13–28.

Anderson, J. R. (1988). A spreading activation theory of memory. In A. Collins & E. E. Smith (Eds.), *Readings in cognitive science: A perspective from psychology and artificial intelligence* (pp. 138–154). San Mateo, CA: Kaufmann.

Ayduk, O., Downey, G., Testa, A., Yen, Y., & Shoda, Y. (1999). Does rejection elicit hostility in rejection sensitive women? *Social Cognition*, *17*, 245–271.

Barnouw, V. (1985). *Culture and personality*. Homewood, IL: Dorsey.

Bem, D. J., & Allen, A. (1974). On predicting some of the people some of the time: The search for cross-situational consistencies in behavior. *Psychological Review*, *81*, 506–520.

Benedict, R. (1934). *Patterns of culture*. Boston: Houghton Mifflin.

Betancourt, H., & López, S. R. (1993). The study of culture, ethnicity, and race in American psychology. *American Psychologist*, *48*(6), 629–637.

Bock, P. K. (2000). Culture and personality revisited. *American Behavioral Scientist*, *44*(1), 32–40.

Borkenau, P., Riemann, R, Spinath, F. M., & Angleitner, A (2006). Genetic and environmental influences on person × situation profiles. *Journal of Personality*, *74*, 1451–1479.

Bouchard, T. J., & Loehlin, J. C. (2001). Genes, evolution, and personality. *Behavior Genetics, 31,* 243–273.

Cantor, N., & Kihlstrom, J. F. (1989). Social intelligence and cognitive assessments of personality. In R. S. J. Wyer, & T. K. Srull (Eds.), *Advances in social cognition* (Vol. 2, pp. 1–59). Hillsdale, NJ: Erlbaum.

Cervone, D. (2004). The architecture of personality. *Psychological Review, 111*(1), 183–204.

Cervone, D. (2005). Personality architecture: Within-person structures and processes. *Annual Review of Psychology, 56,* 423–452.

Chan, W., & Mendoza-Denton, R. (2004, April). *Sensitivity to race-based rejection among Asian Americans.* Paper presented at the annual meeting of the Western Psychological Association, Phoenix, AZ.

Cheung, F. M., & Leung, K. (1998). Indigenous personality measures: Chinese examples. *Journal of Cross-Cultural Psychology, 29,* 233–248.

Church, A. T. (2000). Culture and personality: Toward an integrated cultural trait psychology. *Journal of Personality, 68*(4), 651–704.

Church, A. T., Katigbak, M. S., & Reyes, J. A. S. (1996). Toward a taxonomy of trait adjectives in Filipino: Comparing personality lexicons across cultures. *European Journal of Personality, 10,* 3–24.

Church, A. T., Katigbak, M. S., & Reyes, J. A. S. (1998). Further exploration of Filipino personality structure using the lexical approach: Do the big-five or big-seven dimensions emerge? *European Journal of Personality, 12,* 249–269.

CNN. (2005, January 14). Charleston again ranked best-mannered city. Available online at *www.CNN.com*

Cohen, D. (1997). Ifs and thens in cultural psychology. In R. S. J. Wyer (Ed.), *The automaticity of everyday life: Advances in social cognition* (Vol. 10, pp. 121–131). Mahwah, NJ: Erlbaum.

Cohen, D. (1998). Culture, social organization, and patterns of violence. *Journal of Personality and Social Psychology, 75*(2), 408–419.

Cohen, D., & Nisbett, R. E. (1994). Self-protection and the culture of honor: Explaining southern violence. *Personality and Social Psychology Bulletin, 20,* 551–567.

Cohen, D., & Nisbett, R. E. (1997). Field experiments examining the culture of honor: The role of institutions in perpetuating norms about violence. *Personality and Social Psychology Bulletin, 23*(11), 1188–1199.

Cohen, D., Nisbett, R. E., Bowdle, B. F., & Schwarz, N. (1996). Insult, aggression, and the Southern culture of honor: An "experimental ethnography." *Journal of Personality and Social Psychology, 70,* 945–960.

Cohen, D., Vandello, J., Puente, S., & Rantilla, A. (1999). "When you call me that, smile!": How norms for politeness, interaction styles, and aggression work together in southern culture. *Social Psychology Quarterly, 62,* 257–275.

Cole, M. (1996). *Cultural psychology: A once and future discipline.* Cambridge, MA: Harvard University Press.

Crocker, J., Major, B., & Steele, C. (1998). Social stigma. In D. T. Gilbert & S. T. Fiske (Eds.), *The handbook of social psychology* (4th ed., pp. 504–553). New York: McGraw-Hill.

Downey, G., & Feldman, S. I. (1996). Implications of rejection sensitivity for intimate relationships. *Journal of Personality and Social Psychology, 70,* 1327–1343.

DuBois, C. (1944). *The people of Alor: A socio-psychological study of an East Indian island.* Minneapolis: University of Minnesota Press.

Epstein, S. (1979). The stability of behavior: I. On predicting most of the people much of the time. *Journal of Personality and Social Psychology, 37,* 1097–1126.

Epstein, S. (1994). Trait theory as personality theory: Can a part be as great as a whole? *Psychological Inquiry, 5,* 120–122.

Epstein, S., & O'Brien, E. J. (1985). The person–situation debate in historical and current perspective. *Psychological Bulletin, 98,* 513–537.

Fiske, S. T. (2004). *Social beings: A core motives approach to social psychology.* Hoboken, NJ: Wiley.

Geertz, C. (1973). *The interpretation of cultures: Selected essays.* New York: Basic Books.

Gilbert, D. T., & Malone, P. S. (1995). The correspondence bias. *Psychological Bulletin, 117,* 21–38.

Goldberg, L. R. (1992). The development of markers for the Big-Five factor structure. *Psychological Assessment, 4,* 26–42.

Gosling, S. D., & John, O. P. (1999). Personality dimensions in non-human animals: A cross-species review. *Current Directions in Psychological Science, 8,* 69–73.

Gosling, S. D., Kwan, V. S. Y., & John, O. P. (2003). A dog's got personality: A cross-species comparative approach to personality judgments in dogs and humans. *Journal of Personality and Social Psychology, 85,* 1161–1169.

Hartshorne, H., & May, M. A. (1928). *Studies in deceit.* Oxford, UK: Macmillan.

Heine, S. J., Lehman, D. R., Markus, H. R., & Kitayama, S. (1999). Is there a universal need for positive self-regard? *Psychological Review, 106,* 766–794.

Higgins, E. T. (1996). Knowledge activation: Accessibility, applicability, and salience. In E. T. Higgins & A. W. Kruglanski (Eds.), *Social psychology: Handbook of basic principles* (pp. 133–168). New York: Guilford Press.

Hinton, G. E., McClelland, J. L., & Rumelhart, D. E. (1986). Distributed representations. In D. E. Rumelhart & J. L. McClelland (Eds.), *Parallel distributed processing: Explorations in the microstructures of cognition: Vol. I. Foundations* (pp. 77–109). Cambridge, MA: MIT Press/Bradford Books.

Hong, Y., Benet-Martinez, V., Chiu, C., & Morris, M.

W. (2003). Boundaries of cultural influence: Construct activation as a mechanism for cultural differences in social perception. *Journal of Cross-Cultural Psychology, 34,* 453–464.

Hong, Y., & Chiu, C. (2001). Toward a paradigm shift: From cross-cultural differences in social cognition to social-cognitive mediation of cultural differences. *Social Cognition, 19,* 181–196.

Hong, Y., & Mallorie, L. A. M. (2004). A dynamic constructivist approach to culture: Lessons learned from personality psychology. *Journal of Research in Personality, 38,* 59–67.

Hong, Y., Morris, M. W., Chiu, C., & Benet-Martinez, V. (2000). Multicultural minds: A dynamic constructivist approach to culture and cognition. *American Psychologist, 55*(7), 709–720.

Hoorens, V., & Poortinga, Y. H. (2000). Behavior in the social context. In K. Pawlik & M. R. Rosenzweig (Eds.), *International handbook of psychology* (pp. 40–53). London: Sage.

Humphreys, M. S., & Kashima, Y. (2002). Connectionism and self: Distributed representational systems and their implications for self and identity. In Y. Kashima, M. Foddy, & M. Platow (Eds.), *Self and identity: Personal, social, and symbolic* (pp. 27–54). Mahwah, NJ: Erlbaum.

Inkeles, A. (1996). *National character: A psycho-social study.* New Brunswick, NJ: Transaction.

Iyengar, S. S., & Lepper, M. R. (1999). Rethinking the value of choice: A cultural perspective on intrinsic motivation. *Journal of Personality and Social Psychology, 76,* 349–366.

Kammrath, L., Mendoza-Denton, R., & Mischel, W. (2005). Incorporating *if . . . then . . .* signatures in person perception: Beyond the person–situation dichotomy. *Journal of Personality and Social Psychology, 88,* 605–613.

Kaplan, B. (1954). *A study of Rorschach responses in four cultures.* Cambridge, MA: Harvard University Press.

Kashima, Y. (2001). Culture and social cognition: Toward a social psychology of cultural dynamics. In D. Matsumoto (Ed.), *The handbook of culture and psychology* (pp. 325–360). New York: Oxford University Press.

Kashima, Y. (2004). Person, symbol, sociality: Towards a social psychology of cultural dynamics. *Journal of Research in Personality, 38,* 52–58.

Kashima, Y., Kashima, E., Farsides, T., Kim, U., Strack, F., & Werth, L., et al. (2004). Culture and context-sensitive self: The amount and meaning of context-sensitivity of phenomenal self differ across cultures. *Self and Identity, 3,* 125–141.

Kitayama, S. (2002). Culture and basic psychological processes—toward a system view of culture: Comment on Oyserman et al. (2002). *Psychological Bulletin, 128,* 89–96.

Kitayama, S., & Markus, H. R. (1999). Yin and yang of the Japanese self: The cultural psychology of personality coherence. In D. Cervone & Y. Shoda (Eds.),

The coherence of personality: Social-cognitive bases of consistency, variability, and organization (pp. 242–302). New York: Guilford Press.

Kitayama, S., Markus, H. R., Matsumoto, H., & Norasakkunkit, V. (1997). Individual and collective processes in the construction of the self: Self-enhancement in the United States and self-criticism in Japan. *Journal of Personality and Social Psychology, 72,* 1245–1267.

Levy, S. R., Ayduk, O., & Downey, G. (2001). Rejection sensitivity: Implications for interpersonal and intergroup processes. In M. Leary (Ed.), *Interpersonal rejection* (pp. 251–289). New York: Oxford University Press.

Levy, S. R., West, T., Ramirez, L., & Karafantis, D. M. (2006). The Protestant work ethic: A lay theory with dual intergroup implications. *Group Processes and Intergroup Relations, 9,* 95–115.

Linton, R. (1936). *The study of man: An introduction.* New York: Appleton–Century.

Loehlin, J. C., McCrae, R. R., Costa, P. T. J., & John, O. P. (1998). Heritabilities of common and measure-specific components of the Big Five personality factors. *Journal of Research in Personality, 32*(4), 431–453.

Markus, H. R., & Kitayama, S. (1991). Culture and the self: Implications for cognition, emotion, and motivation. *Psychological Review, 98,* 224–253.

Markus, H. R., & Kitayama, S. (1998). The cultural psychology of personality. *Journal of Cross-Cultural Psychology, 29,* 63–87.

McAdams, D. P. (1999). Personal narratives and the life story. In L. A. Pervin & O. P. John (Eds.), *Handbook of personality: Theory and research* (2nd ed., pp. 478–500). New York: Guilford Press.

McCrae, R. R. (2000). Trait psychology and the revival of personality and culture studies. *American Behavioral Scientist, 44,* 10–31.

McCrae, R. R. (2004). Human nature and culture: A trait perspective. *Journal of Research in Personality, 38,* 3–14.

McCrae, R. R., & Allik, J. (2002). *The five-factor model of personality across cultures.* New York: Kluwer Academic/Plenum Press.

Mendoza-Denton, R. (1999). *Lay contextualism in stereotyping.* Unpublished dissertation, Columbia University, New York.

Mendoza-Denton, R., Ayduk, O. N., Shoda, Y., & Mischel, W. (1997). Cognitive–affective processing system analysis of reactions to the O. J. Simpson criminal trial verdict. *Journal of Social Issues, 53,* 563–581.

Mendoza-Denton, R., Downey, G., Purdie, V. J., Davis, A., & Pietrzak, J. (2002). Sensitivity to status-based rejection: Implications for African American students' college experience. *Journal of Personality and Social Psychology, 83,* 896–918.

Mendoza-Denton, R., Page-Gould, E., & Pietrzak, J. (2006). Mechanisms for coping with status-based rejection expectations. In S. Levin & C. Van Laar

(Eds.), *Stigma and group inequality: Social psychological approaches* (pp. 151–169). Mahwah, NJ: Erlbaum.

Mendoza-Denton, R., Park, S., Kammrath, L., & Peake, P. K. (2004, September). *Perceivers as social cognitive theorists: The case of gender stereotypes.* Paper presentation to the Psychology Department, Stanford University, Stanford, CA.

Mendoza-Denton, R., Shoda, Y., Ayduk, O., & Mischel, W. (1999). Applying cognitive-affective processing system (CAPS) theory to cultural differences in social behavior. In W. J. Lonner & D. L. Dinnel (Eds.), *Merging past, present, and future in cross-cultural psychology: Selected papers from the 14th international congress of the International Association for Cross-Cultural Psychology* (pp. 205–217). Lisse, The Netherlands: Swets & Zeitlinger.

Miller, J. G. (1997). Theoretical issues in cultural psychology. In J. W. Berry & Y. H. Poortinga (Eds.), *Handbook of cross-cultural psychology: Vol. 1. Theory and method* (pp. 85–128). Needham Heights, MA: Allyn & Bacon.

Miller, J. G. (1999). Cultural psychology: Implications for basic psychological theory. *Psychological Science, 10,* 85–91.

Mischel, W. (1968). *Personality and assessment.* New York: Wiley.

Mischel, W. (1973). Toward a cognitive social learning reconceptualization of personality. *Pyschological Review, 80,* 252–283.

Mischel, W. (2003). Challenging the traditional personality psychology paradigm. In R. J. Sternberg (Ed.), *Psychologists defying the crowd: Stories of those who battled the establishment and won* (pp. 139–156). Washington, DC: American Psychological Association.

Mischel, W. (2004). Toward an integrative science of the person. *Annual Review of Psychology, 55,* 1–22.

Mischel, W., & Morf, C. C. (2003). The self as a psycho-social dynamic processing system: A meta-perspective on a century of the self in psychology. In M. R. Leary & J. P. Tangney (Eds.), *Handbook of self and identity* (pp. 15–43). New York: Guilford Press.

Mischel, W., & Peake, P. K. (1982). Beyond *déjà vu* in the search for cross-situational consistency. *Psychological Review, 89,* 730–755.

Mischel, W., & Peake, P. K. (1983). Some facets of consistency: Replies to Epstein, Funder, and Bem. *Psychological Review, 90*(4), 394–402.

Mischel, W., & Shoda, Y. (1995). A cognitive-affective system theory of personality: Reconceptualizing situations, dispositions, dynamics, and invariance in personality structure. *Psychological Review, 102,* 246–268.

Mischel, W., & Shoda, Y. (1999). Integrating dispositions and processing dynamics within a unified theory of personality: The cognitive–affective personality system. In L. A. Pervin & O. P. John (Eds.), *Handbook of personality: Theory and research* (2nd ed., pp. 197–218). New York: Guilford Press.

Mischel, W., Shoda, Y., & Mendoza-Denton, R. (2002). Situation–behavior profiles as a locus of consistency in personality. *Current Directions in Psychological Science, 11,* 50–54.

Morris, M. W., Nisbett, R. E., & Peng, K. (1995). Causal attribution across domains and cultures. In D. Sperber & D. Premack (Eds.), *Causal cognition: A multidisciplinary debate* (pp. 577–614). New York: Clarendon Press/Oxford University Press.

Newcomb, T. M. (1929). *The consistency of certain extrovert–introvert behavior patterns in 51 problem boys.* New York: Columbia University, Teachers College Bureau of Publications.

Nisbett, R. E., & Cohen, D. (1996). *Culture of honor: The psychology of violence in the South.* Boulder, CO: Westview Press.

Obeyeskere, G. (1981). *Medusa's hair: An essay on personal symbols and religious experience.* Chicago: University of Chicago Press.

Peng, K., Nisbett, R. E., & Wong, N. Y. C. (1997). Validity problems comparing values across cultures and possible solutions. *Psychological Methods, 2*(4), 329–344.

Pervin, L. A. (1994). A critical analysis of current trait theory. *Psychological Inquiry, 5,* 103–113.

Pervin, L. A. (1999). The cross-cultural challenge to personality. In Y. Lee & C. R. McCauley (Eds.), *Personality and person perception across cultures* (pp. 23–41). Mahwah, NJ: Erlbaum.

Pervin, L. A. (2001). A dynamic systems approach to personality. *European Psychologist, 6*(3), 172–176.

Peterson, D. R. (1968). *The clinical study of social behavior.* New York: Appleton.

Piker, S. (1998). Contributions of psychological anthropology. *Journal of Cross-Cultural Psychology, 29,* 9–31.

Plaks, J. E., Shafer, J. L., & Shoda, Y. (2003). Perceiving individuals and groups as coherent: How do perceivers make sense of variable behavior? *Social Cognition, 21,* 26–60.

Poortinga, Y. H., & Hemert, D. A. (2001). Personality and culture: Demarcating between the common and the unique. *Journal of Personality, 69,* 1033–1060.

Pratto, F., Sidanius, J., Stallworth, L. M., & Malle, B. F. (1994). Social dominance orientation: A personality variable predicting social and political attitudes. *Journal of Personality and Social Psychology, 67,* 741–763.

Read, S. J., Jones, D. K., & Miller, L. C. (1990). Traits as goal-based categories—the importance of goals in the coherence of dispositional categories. *Journal of Personality and Social Psychology, 58,* 1048–1061.

Read, S. J., & Miller, L. C. (1998). *Connectionist models of social reasoning and social behavior.* Mahwah, NJ: Erlbaum.

Read, S. J., & Miller, L. C. (2002). Virtual personalities: A neural network model of personality. *Personality and Social Psychology Review, 6,* 357–369.

Ross, L., & Nisbett, R. E. (1991). *The person and the*

situation: Perspectives of social psychology. New York: McGraw-Hill.

Schwartz, S. H. (1992). Universals in the content and structure of values: Theoretical advances and empirical tests in 20 countries. In M. Zanna (Ed.), *Advances in experimental social psychology* (Vol. 25, pp. 1–66). New York: Academic Press.

Sellers, R. M., Caldwell, C. H., Schmeelk-Cone, K. H., & Zimmerman, M. A. (2003). Racial identity, racial discrimination, perceived stress, and psychological distress among African American young adults. *Journal of Health and Social Behavior, 44*(3), 302–317.

Shelton, J. N. (2000). A reconceptualization of how we study issues of racial prejudice. *Personality and Social Psychology Review, 4*(4), 374–390.

Shoda, Y. (1999). A unified framework for the study of behavioral consistency: Bridging person–situation interaction and the consistency paradox. *European Journal of Personality, 13,* 361–387.

Shoda, Y., LeeTiernan, S., & Mischel, W. (2002). Personality as a dynamical system: Emergency of stability and distinctiveness from intra- and interpersonal interactions. *Personality and Social Psychology Review, 6*(4), 316–325.

Shoda, Y., & Mischel, W. (1993). Cognitive social approach to dispositional inferences: What if the perceiver is a cognitive social theorist? *Personality and Social Psychology Bulletin, 19,* 574–585.

Shoda, Y., & Mischel, W. (1998). Personality as a stable cognitive–affective activation network: Characteristic patterns of behavior variation emerge from a stable personality structure. In S. J. Read & L. C. Miller (Eds.), *Connectionist models of social reasoning and social behavior* (pp. 175–208). Mahwah, NJ: Erlbaum.

Shoda, Y., & Mischel, W. (2000). Reconciling contextualism with the core assumptions of personality psychology. *European Journal of Personality, 14,* 407–428.

Shoda, Y., Mischel, W., & Wright, J. C. (1993). Links between personality judgments and contextualized behavior patterns: Situation–behavior profiles of personality prototypes. *Social Cognition, 4,* 399–429.

Shoda, Y., Mischel, W., & Wright, J. C. (1994). Intraindividual stability in the organization and patterning of behavior: Incorporating psychological situations into the idiographic analysis of personality. *Journal of Personality and Social Psychology, 67,* 674–687.

Shweder, R. A. (1990). Cultural psychology—What is it? In J. W. Stigler, R. A. Shweder, & G. Herdt (Eds.), *Cultural psychology: Essays on comparative human development* (pp. 1–43). Cambridge, UK: Cambridge University Press.

Shweder, R. A. (1991). *Thinking through cultures: Expeditions in cultural psychology.* Cambridge, MA: Harvard University Press.

Snyder, M., & Ickes, W. (1984): Personality and social behavior. In G. Lindzey & E. Aronson (Eds.), *Handbook of social psychology* (pp. 883–947). New York: Random House.

Steele, C. M. (1997). A threat in the air: How stereotypes shape intellectual identity and performance. *American Psychologist, 52,* 613–629.

Triandis, H. C. (1996). The psychological measurement of cultural syndromes. *American Psychologist, 51,* 407–415.

Triandis, H. C. (1997). Cross-cultural perspectives on personality. In R. Hogan, J. Johnson, & S. Briggs (Eds.), *Handbook of personality* (pp. 440–459). San Diego: Academic Press.

Triandis, H. C. (2000). Dialectics between cultural and cross-cultural psychology. *Asian Journal of Social Psychology, 3,* 185–195.

Triandis, H. C., Lambert, W. W., Berry, J. W., Lonner, W., Heron, A., Brislin, R. W., et al. (1980). *Handbook of cross-cultural psychology.* Boston: Allyn & Bacon.

Triandis, H. C., & Suh, E. M. (2002). Cultural influences on personality. *Annual Review of Psychology, 53*(1), 133–160.

Tylor, E. B. (1871). *The origins of culture.* Gloucester, MA: Peter Smith.

Vandello, J. A., & Cohen, D. (2004). When believing is seeing: Sustaining norms of violence in cultures of honor. In M. Schaller & C. S. Crandall (Eds.), *The psychological foundations of culture* (pp. 281–304). Mahwah, NJ: Erlbaum.

Vernon, P. E. (1964). *Personality assessment: A critical survey.* New York: Wiley.

Wallace, A. F. C. (1961). *Culture and personality.* New York: Random House.

Whiting, B. B., & Whiting, J. W. M. (1975). *Children of six cultures: A psycho-cultural analysis.* Cambridge, MA: Harvard University Press.

Whiting, J. W. M., & Child, I. L. (1953). *Child training and personality: A cross-cultural study.* New Haven, CT: Yale University Press.

Wright, J. C., & Mischel, W. (1988). Conditional hedges and the intuitive psychology of traits. *Journal of Personality and Social Psychology, 55,* 454–469.

Yeats, W. B. (1927). Among school children. In *The W. B. Yeats collection* [electronic resource; *www.collections.chadwyck.com*]. Alexandria, VA: Chadwyck-Healey.

CHAPTER 8

Methods in Cultural Psychology

DOV COHEN

Cultural psychologists who approach phenomena from, say, a social-psychological, developmental, or anthropological perspective not only inherit all the methodological problems and issues from their home disciplines, but also acquire many new ones. Studying a topic in more than one culture brings some special complexities. Furthermore, some standard methodological problems that are by and large ignored in one's home discipline (e.g., subject sampling) become major issues in cultural-psychological research. In contrast, very few (or perhaps no) methodological problems become easier when culture is added to the picture.

This chapter attempts to make explicit some of the methodological issues that pose extra challenges for cultural researchers. As with other research, the methodological challenges center around four themes: Causality, Operationalization, Sampling, and Interpretation (COSI). In brief, these four themes involve the questions: "Can I determine causality?", "What is my independent variable 'doing' to people, and/or what does my dependent variable actually measure?", "To what populations can I generalize my results?", and "Am I reading the data correctly?" (See summary in Table 8.1.)

This chapter is not an exhaustive list of issues cultural psychologists face, and it does not cover the methodological concerns of qualitative research. Rather, it starts exploring the four COSI questions by asking 10 subquestions. Richard Lewontin (1995) observed that scientists spend a great deal of time talking about methodological issues to which their field has cogent answers, and ignore those for which they do not have cogent answers. The list of subquestions below has some of both types of issues.

With respect to *causal* issues involving cultural differences, the subquestions we address have to do with determining (1) "What is the cultural dimension driving my differences?"; (2) "Are my cultural effects driven more by things that are 'in the head,' 'out in the world,' or some combination of both; and if so, how should I measure such effects?"; and (3) "What ecological, economic, or historical circumstances caused the cultural difference to emerge in the first place?"

With respect to the issue of participant *sampling*, the subquestions addressed are (1) "What population can I sensibly generalize about?" and (2) "How do I think about what is 'culture' and what is 'confound' when I pick my sample for study?"

TABLE 8.1. COSI: Four Questions Asked by a Young Field

Or, why is this discipline different from other disciplines in . . .

Causation

Cultural psychologists need to think in terms of multiple equilibria (rather than, or in addition to, straight correlational thinking). A cultural syndrome (e.g., collectivism) may be sensibly associated with one pattern of behavior in culture A (e.g., low emotional expressiveness, balanced affect) and the opposite sort of behavior in culture B (e.g., high emotional expressiveness, high positive affect). Multiple equilibria map onto multiple meaning systems that can be sensible, coherent, and follow their own cultural logics.

In understanding culture, we can locate causality inside the person (social-cognitive approaches, individual difference approaches), outside the person (situational–structural–practice approaches), and in the interaction between person and environment (culture X person X situation approaches, syndrome approaches).

Equilibrium does not equal adaptation, though functional explanations of cultural patterns may be a good place to start.

Operationalization

Cultural psychologists have to operationalize constructs in ways that are convincing and interpretable when seen through (at least) two different cultural lenses. Thus, they face the broad challenge of "translation" (of languages, situations, behaviors, reference groups, etc.) across cultures.

Cultural psychologists do have an advantage, though, in that the field's methodological pluralism gives researchers a full tool kit (e.g., surveys, laboratory experiments, field studies, analyses of cultural products, and more qualitative work) to produce convincing, convergent evidence, in which the strengths of one method offset the weaknesses of other methods.

Sampling

Cultural psychologists take the issue of participant sampling seriously. (That is the basis of our critique of mainstream psychology as primarily a psychology of the West). In the absence of probability sampling, however, how can one say something useful about either big-C Culture (American culture, Chinese culture, etc.) or little-c culture (the process by which people shape and are shaped by their world)? There are at least four different and contrasting sampling approaches to consider: typicality sampling versus just minimal difference sampling, and expert sampling versus inversion sampling. In thinking about which sampling approach to use, cultural psychologists need to think through some potentially thorny conceptual issues (e.g., what is culture, and what is confound?).

Interpretation

Cultural psychologists look at the "Necker cube" of culture, in which similarities are embedded within differences, and differences are embedded within similarities. Making the "familiar unfamiliar and the unfamiliar familiar" can reduce tendencies toward invidious comparisons with the Other. It softens comparisons and gets us out of our own frame of reference. Cultural psychology is about finding out how other ways of seeing the world (besides one's own) can be meaningful, sensible, and coherent.

The key to any convincing explanation is convergent evidence across methods. However, evidence that does not converge may also point to interesting cultural phenomena.

With respect to *operationalization*, the three subquestions are (1) "Am I 'translating' my variable correctly from one culture to another?"; (2) "What are the cost–benefit trade-offs of surveys versus experiments?"; and (3) "What other methods can provide convergent evidence?"

Finally, with respect to *interpretation*, the two subquestions are (1) "Am I really understanding what is similar and what is different in the cultures?" and (2) "Even if convergent evidence from multiple methods is the answer to most of my methodological problems, what happens if my evidence does not converge?"

The boundaries of the four elements of COSI can be quite fuzzy. However, for purposes of clarity in this chapter, the four elements are addressed in turn. The issues with causality are the most theoretical, the trickiest, and the ones that have the least cogent answers. The chapter begins with those as a starting point, because they lead into the sampling and operationalization issues. The O and S issues are more nuts-and-bolts and the answers to them are more (but not completely) cogent, with the ultimate answer lying in the need to collect converging evidence across a variety of methods. Finally, the chapter ends with interpretation issues, which are more abstract and have some larger implications for how we think about culture.

CAUSALITY

Leaving Terra Firma

Any study without a randomly assigned independent variable is by definition a correlational study and can therefore never prove causality. The vast majority of studies in cultural psychology fit into this correlational category, because culture is not a manipulated variable. We make statements such as "The Japanese were more likely to emphasize duties and the Americans, more likely to emphasize rights, *because* Japanese and American cultures differ in how they view the individual and the collectivity" or "Cultures A and B value harmony, *because* their agricultural practices require them to work together." These claims can be only suggested by our data. Nevertheless, a good portion of cultural studies make such causal claims (particularly of the first type); and using solid methodology often makes the difference between a strong suggestion of causality and a weak one.

Descriptive Studies

Studies in cultural psychology are often, but not always, of two different forms. One form is: Culture 1 has cultural syndrome X, whereas Culture 2 has syndrome Y. (Or sometimes, it is simply that Culture 1 has syndrome X, whereas Culture 2 does not). Examples of this sort of study are those showing that Eastern cultures tend to be more collectivistic, whereas Western cultures tend to be more individualistic, or that the South of the United States has a culture of honor, whereas the North of the United States does not (or has instead a culture of "dignity").

These studies may be purely descriptive, outlining the cultural patterns in one society versus another. The measured variables here tend to be face-valid representations of the cultural difference one is studying. So a researcher may offer evidence that Mexican culture is more collectivist than American culture by showing that they differ on an individualism–collectivism

scale, that they think about and behave toward ingroups and outgroups differently, or that they differ in how much they identify with their ingroups. Such evidence is descriptive because the measured (or "outcome") variable flows tautologically from the definition of individualism and collectivism. Furthermore, a researcher might conduct studies into the phenomenological experiences of people in a culture, explore a given cultural characteristic in depth, examine how this cultural characteristic manifests itself within a society or across societies, or study how cultural characteristic X is related to cultural characteristic Y (without worrying about causal direction; Asch, 1952/1987; D. Cohen, 2001; D. Cohen, Hoshino-Browne, & Leung, 2007; MacLeod, 1947; Rozin, 2001; Shweder, 1997). In such purely descriptive studies, no causal claims are made. As Rozin (2001) has pointed out, these studies are often a sensible place to start. More mature sciences (e.g., biology) began this way and still devote considerable attention to description. Rozin has argued that social psychologists, because of their status anxiety, have too quickly scanted important phenomena in need of basic descriptive work to build impressive formal models of less important phenomena. Cultural psychologists, too, may face the same temptation.

Causal Claims

Many studies attempt to be descriptive *and* make some form of causal claim. Obviously, in planning a study, it is extremely important first to think through what these causal claims might be. They often are of two kinds: (1) Culture 1 has syndrome X, whereas Culture 2 has syndrome Y because of reason R or (2) cultures differ in some local domain D, and these differences derive from some greater underlying difference in major cultural syndromes. Causal claim (1) tends to be more rare among cultural psychologists, so discussion of it is temporarily postponed.

Subquestion 1: "What Is the Cultural Dimension Driving My Differences?"

Claim: Differences in Local Domain D *Come from Deeper Differences in Underlying Syndromes* X *or* Y

This type of causal claim often gets made more or less implicitly. Examples of this type of claim might include the following: Japanese and

American conflict resolution styles derive from underlying differences in individualism versus collectivism; or East–West differences in approach versus avoidance motivation derive from more general differences in independence versus interdependence; or Korean versus Canadian differences in leadership style derive from underlying differences in holistic versus analytic thinking style; or Southern and Northern U.S. politeness patterns differ because of the presence or absence of a culture of honor; and so on. These studies are "causal" (rather than "merely" descriptive) in that the measured outcome variable does *not* tautologically derive from the definitions of the deeper cultural syndromes.

A crucial methodological issue involves the identification of the underlying dimension. At times, these claims can seem to derive from what Rosnow and Rosenthal (2002, p. 17) call the "principle of the drunkard's search." The name comes from an old joke about a man who has left the bar and is looking for his keys under the lamppost. He knows that the keys probably are not there, but that is where the light is good, so that is where he looks. A potential pitfall for cultural researchers is to look for the underlying causal dimension for a given phenomenon in a place where the light is already shining and the territory is well illuminated.

To continue the analogy, researchers such as Triandis, Hofstede, Markus, Kitayama, Bond, and others have shined a bright light on the cultural syndromes of independence versus interdependence or individualism versus collectivism. Thanks to their work, we know a great deal about these syndromes, and it has become a very salient way to describe cultures. However, there is a methodological problem if one relies too much on this salient individualism–collectivism difference for causal explanations. For example, one might make the following causal claims: Collectivist cultures tend to have inhibitory display rules, to downplay emotionality, to experience more negative affect, to have lower self-esteem and are more avoidance oriented than individualist cultures, which are more expressive, show higher positive affect and self-esteem, and are more approach oriented.

These may all be true, but two methodological issues should give us pause. The first is that cultures differ on any number of dimensions, in addition to the individualist–collectivist difference. China and the United States differ, for example, not just on individualism–collectivism but also on how tight versus loose they are, how fatalistic, how egalitarian, how religious, how ethnically homogenous, and so on (as well as on many "noncultural" demographic factors—a topic to be addressed later). A general readiness to attribute a difference between an Eastern and a Western culture to individualism–collectivism reflects a tendency to rely (and overrely) on this single well-explored dimension, instead of on many other underlying cultural dimensions that may be causally relevant.

Second, consider that much, though certainly not all, of the individualism–collectivism work has gone in the East–West direction, sampling countries from North America versus East or South Asia. Imagine instead what might have happened if the work had gone in the North–South direction, sampling countries from North America versus South and Central America. A number of our conclusions about the way collectivist cultures are and the way individualist cultures are might be reversed. We might conclude, for example, that collectivist cultures are happier (controlling for income effects), express more affect and assign greater significance to emotion, are more likely to think love should override pragmatic concerns in getting married, are more extroverted, and so on, compared to individualist cultures. The bias in how we have sampled individualist and collectivist cultures has led to certain conclusions about the way individualist and collectivist cultures "generally" are, and these conclusions might be reversed had researchers taken Latin American cultures as their collectivistic prototype rather than Asia.

There are at least two ways to think about what sorts of patterns different cultural syndromes give rise to, and these have very different implications for our methodologies. One way is to think in terms of "necessary" or "contingent" (probabilistic) facts (terms borrowed from the historian Fernand Braudel, 1980). In the search for necessary or contingent facts, we would look for the cultural syndromes that either necessarily or probably lead to certain types of behavior patterns. For example, individualist cultures tend to have more gender equality than collectivist cultures, because the sanctity of the person in such individualist cultures overrides his or her ascribed status or social roles. Or collectivist cultures use shame as a socializing tool, whereas individualist cultures are more likely to use guilt, because shame involves caring about others' approval, whereas guilt involves self-judgment and needs no audience. In research focused on necessary or probabilistic facts, a diverse sample of cultures is needed so that one can avoid the sampling biases of the type described earlier. In terms of methodology, one may have to sacrifice depth in the name of breadth, gathering data from as many cultures as is feasible, and glossing over the particularities of any one culture.

A second way to think about cultures is in terms of multiple equilibrium states. Although acknowledging that probabilistic facts exist, this way of thinking about culture would focus more on how the pieces of culture fit together in a rough equilibrium in a particular context. In this is also an implicit acknowledgment that many different equilibria might exist. People's behavior depends on the behavior of others around them, and as game theorists have noted, this mutual interdependence leads to multiple equilibria. Some cultures may be at one equilibrium point, others may be at another. (Research in this tradition would be the search for "conditioned facts" in Braudel's [1980] terms).

This statement of multiple equilibria recognizes the fact that there is more than one way to be a collectivist culture, and more than one way to be an individualist culture, for example. And an emphasis in this style of research, then, is to focus on meaning systems and the ways they make the parts of a given culture fit together. Breadth of cultures may be sacrificed for depth of understanding particular cultures. The research of Kitayama; Heine; and Markus and Hamedani (see Chapters 6, 29, and 1, respectively) is a classic example here. In an extensive series of experimental and questionnaires studies, they have elaborated on how the interdependent selfways of Japanese culture get manifested in phenomena such as the pursuit of interpersonal harmony; habits of self-criticism that produce a persistent drive for self-improvement, so that one can meet group standards; the giving of interpersonal sympathy and its role in supporting and enabling self-criticism; the *intra*personal realization of sympathy, so that one can also give sympathy to the self one is criticizing; and the treatment of the self as a social object whose actions, and even whose preferences, must situate oneself with

respect to the group. The point in this work is not necessarily to generalize the behavior patterns of North American and Japanese cultures to other cultures. Rather, the work is an exploration of different self-sustaining meaning systems, and this approach to research dictates a methodology that is more focused and less interested in how "probabilistic" facts play out across cultures.

One can imagine a different line of comparative research that examines Latin American and North American cultures, focusing on how interdependent Latino selfways get manifested in the normative expectation that one experience and express positive emotion (Diener & Suh, 2003; Diener & Tov, Chapter 28, this volume); the relational nature of this positive expression of emotion in conveying warmth; the way such emotionality suffuses both work and life (in contrast to the "Protestant relational ideology" that separates the "social–emotional" from the "task focus" relationship; Sanchez-Burks, 2002, 2004; Sanchez-Burks & Lee, Chapter 14, this volume); the cultural script of *simpatia* that promotes harmony through good feelings, congeniality, and charm (Triandis, Lisansky, & Betancourt, 1984); the faith in the most "irrational" of all positive emotions, romantic love (Levine, Sato, Hashimoto, & Verma, 1995; Franiuk, Cohen, & Pomerantz, 2002; cf. Hatfield, Rapson, & Martel, Chapter 31, this volume); and so on. Understanding the importance of harmony and the role of emotion is central in understanding both Asian and Latin American culture, but their roles seem to play out very differently in the two cultural contexts.

Subquestion 2: "Are My Cultural Effects Driven More by Things That Are 'in the Head,' by Things 'out in the World,' or by Some Combination of Both? If So, How Should I Measure Such Effects?"

Causality, Mind-Sets, Individual Differences, and Situations

One of the previously discussed methodological problems involves how one can impute causality (in the search for either "probabilistic facts" or "conditioned facts") and where one should locate it. Four approaches to this problem are discussed below, and as will be seen, conceptual and methodological issues tend to be tethered together here.

SOCIAL-COGNITIVE APPROACHES

One way to argue that a particular cultural "trait" leads to a particular behavior is to prime the mind-set that goes with that "trait" and examine its effect on the behavior of interest (Oyserman, Kemmelmeier, & Coon, 2002; Oyserman, Coon, & Kemmelmeier, 2002; Oyserman & Lee, Chapter 10, this volume).[1] In the area of individualism and collectivism, such work has been done through clever manipulations that ask respondents to think about the ways they are similar to family and friends (collectivist prime) versus different from them (individualist prime; Trafimow, Triandis, & Goto, 1991) or that prime the "we" concept (collectivist) versus the "I" concept (individualist) by having people circle the *we*'s or the *I*'s in a supposedly unrelated reading assignment (Gardner, Gabriel, & Lee, 1999). These priming exercises put people in a certain frame of mind, so that the experimental session simulates what it is like to have interdependent (or independent) thoughts either chronically accessible to an individual or chronically activated by different situations.

Work in this vein has suggested that priming social interdependence, for example, makes both Westerners and Asians more generous in their social comparisons (Stapel & Koomen, 2001; White, Lehman, & Cohen, 2006), more prevention focused in thinking about their goals (Lee, Aaker, & Gardner, 2000), and (for Westerners at least) more holistic in their thinking styles (Kuhnen, Hannover, & Schubert, 2001; Kuhnen & Oyserman, 2002). These findings parallel the same effects that are found when (unprimed) Asians and North Americans are compared, suggesting that social interdependence *can* produce such differences in principle and is a *plausible* explanation for why such differences arise in these cases.

The *manipulation* of the collectivist or individualist mind-set gives researchers tremendous help in establishing causality, because experimental manipulation is the only procedure that can indisputably establish cause. However, there are still some issues to sort through. First, such work does not establish that the chronic differences between cultures are in fact driven by the variable examined in the experiment, rather than by some other (unexamined) variable. To illustrate this point with an absurd example, Asian Americans have generally been found to be less emotionally expressive than European Americans. Imagine now that one might reverse this effect by giving Asian Americans an arousal-inducing hormone and giving European Americans an arousal-reducing hormone. Such hormones would probably override any culture main effect: The arousal-inducing hormone would lead both groups to be more expressive, whereas the arousal-reducing hormone would lead both groups to be less expressive. However, regardless of the manipulation's success, it obviously does *not* follow that chronic Asian American versus European American expressiveness differences are due to hormonal differences.

Second, this technique, by itself, cannot overcome the problems that come from sampling bias described earlier. For example, one may find that an interdependence prime makes Asian Americans less expressive of emotions. However, if one had drawn a sample of Latinos instead of Asian Americans, one might find that an interdependence prime makes them more expressive of emotions. The priming technique thus deals with causality *in a particular context*. One may be dealing with conditioned facts, such that what interdependence "causes" in one context may not be what it "causes" in another. Nevertheless, the manipulation of a mind-set through priming can make a powerful argument about causality in the groups under study, particularly when such priming evidence converges with evidence gained from one of the other approaches described below.

INDIVIDUAL DIFFERENCES

One can also study culture as a more traditional personality researcher might. Thus, a complementary method for dealing with issues of causation involves the statistical technique of mediation, using measurements that look for individual differences in how much people have internalized the cultural syndrome under study.[2] Respondents from Culture A and Culture B differ in their behavior in some domain D and one wants to attribute this to an underlying cultural syndrome X (and it is not simply a tautology to say that differences in domain D derive from differences in X). For example, Japanese and Canadian styles of handling conflict differ, and a researcher wants to attribute this difference to the greater individualism of Canadians. To use the individual-difference method, one would measure how individualistic or collectivistic a participant is, then use this individual-difference variable as a potential mediator of the cross-cultural difference. The usual testing of mediation is applied. First, one would demonstrate that the Japanese are, for example, more indirect in handling conflict than are Canadians. Second, one would show that (1) Japanese individuals have internalized collectivistic norms more than Canadians have, and (2) individual differences in this norm internalization predict individual differences in handling conflicts. At the third step, one enters both the dummy variable of culture (Japan vs. Canada) and the individual difference measure of internalized collectivism, and shows that whereas the individual-difference variable remains a significant predictor, the effect of the dummy variable is significantly lowered. Ideally, under this approach, the effect of the dummy variable would disappear completely to zero.[3]

Note again, however, that this does *not* solve the problem of biased sampling described earlier. Suppose, for example, that instead of Canadian and Japanese participants, the researcher had sampled, say, French and Israeli participants for the individualistic and collectivistic groups, respectively. Suppose further that the researcher found that Israelis were more direct in handling conflicts and were indeed more collectivistic. Suppose, finally, that among the French, and particularly among the Israelis, a blunt directness implied interpersonal engagement and respect, whereas indirectness implied a certain standoffishness or guardedness. One might then run the same mediation test and come to conclusions opposite those of the researcher who used the Canadian and Japanese sample and ran the same analysis.

Again, the technique also does not solve the problem of excluding other cultural syndromes. In the Canada–Japan study, for example, one might show that collectivism mediated an effect, but one could not rule out other variables that may have made Japanese participants prefer indirectness (a dialectic thinking style, a greater tolerance for ambiguity, greater deference to authority, etc.), unless one had also measured those other variables and shown they were unimportant. Every correlational analysis always has a third variable problem.

However, the mediational analysis does put the claim on firmer ground. Although it does not rule out the possibility that other variables may be important or that results would differ if

other cultures had been picked, it does make more *plausible* the claim that the difference between these two cultures is driven by differences in the internalization of an underlying collectivist or individualist orientation.

Furthermore, this method has the advantage of explicitly considering individual differences. Not all people are indoctrinated in a culture to the same degree. Not everyone believes or buys into the indoctrination to the same extent. Not everyone will be temperamentally suited to carry out cultural imperatives, even if they buy into them (Rozin, 2003). (Think of a temperamentally anxious person in a culture of honor, or a temperamentally introverted person in a culture whose practices, norms, and values require extraversion.) Additionally, not all subgroups within a culture adhere to the dominant culture's values, especially in ethnically and religiously heterogeneous countries. And even within ethnically or religiously homogenous societies, cultural knowledge is often distributed in a specialized fashion to some people who occupy certain roles and not others. Linton (1936, pp. 272–273) referred to cultural elements shared by only certain groups of people as "specialties" or "alternatives," as distinguished from "universals," which are known to all members of a culture. More recently Medin and Atran (2004) and others have explored the idea of distributed culture, with their work on environmental knowledge among the Maya, Q'eqchi', and Ladinos in Central America (Medin, Unsworth, & Hirschfield, Chapter 25, this volume).

INDIVIDUAL-DIFFERENCE MEDIATION ISSUES

Some additional major methodological issues arise, however, with this individual-differences approach—some of which are practical, whereas others are theoretical. These issues are not so much problems as they are challenges for developing a solid and more complete approach to the study of culture.

1. One of the practical issues is one that concerns all mediational analyses; that is, the mediator needs to be measured with some degree of reliability and validity. At present, mediators are usually measured with questionnaires (e.g., an individualism–collectivism scale; Smith & Bond, 2003). However, as is discussed in the section on operationalization, questionnaires are very often underwhelming

in their ability to detect cross-cultural differences. This is *not* per se an argument against mediational analyses. It is simply a reason why questionnaires may not be terribly useful as mediators.

In principle, there is no reason why mediators have to be measured via questionnaires. As long as they are valid, behavioral samples, performance on engaging tasks, or any other measure may serve as a mediator and stand in for the underlying construct. If researchers want to take the individual-difference perspective seriously, it will be useful to develop a repertoire of such nonquestionnaire measures that have demonstrated validity and *are practical to use* as mediating variables (Spencer, Zanna, & Fong, 2005).

2. The theoretical issues with the mediation method are different and quite interesting; by adopting the individual-difference mediation methodology, one is implicitly adopting a certain view of culture. This view locates culture within the individual. Beliefs are held by individuals. Behaviors are done by individuals. Affect is felt by individuals. Cognitions are thought by individuals (Bond, 2002). Whereas this is prima facie true, it does miss out on some things that some cultural psychologists would like to consider "cultural" and worthy of study (Fiske, 2002; Miller, 2002). More specifically, it can "reduce" culture to an individual-difference, inside-the-head variable that neglects how situations, practices, and institutional arrangements "afford" certain types of behavior, pulling for one pattern of thoughts and actions rather than another.

SITUATIONAL–STRUCTURAL APPROACH

A situational–structural approach that actually measures affordances that pull for a certain type of behavior—rather than merely asserting that such affordances exist—can require some creative thinking. However, such studies may help clarify why an individual-difference "reductionist" account will be necessarily incomplete. As one example of a interesting and creative situational approach, Kitayama, Markus, Matsumoto, and Norasakkunkit (1997; see also Morling, Kitayama, & Miyamoto, 2002) developed a method of "situation sampling" in which respondents were asked to generate as many situations as they could in which their own self-esteem either increased or decreased. Kitayama and colleagues

(1997) then sampled the situations generated by American and Japanese respondents, and presented them to others for ratings. American raters were more likely than Japanese raters to believe that their self-esteem would go up in the success situations and less likely to think their self-esteem would go down in the failure situations. But perhaps more importantly, the success situations generated by Americans were judged by both Japanese and Americans to be more affirming than the success situations generated by the Japanese, and the failure situations generated by the Japanese were judged to be more deflating than the failure situations generated by Americans. *If* one trusts the "situation sample" to reflect roughly the situations encountered in real life, then the argument can be made that American versus Japanese differences in self-enhancement (vs. self-criticism) at least partially derive from the differences in situations that Americans and Japanese encounter in day-to-day living. (The assumption of a perfect correspondence between the frequency of situations in "real life" and the frequency of situations generated and sampled in an experimental study is clearly untenable. However, it does *not* seem untenable that there is at least a positive correlation between the frequency of situations generated in the lab and situations encountered in real life.)

Another situational approach might drop the issue of "sampling" altogether and attempt to examine in the lab how "prototypical" situations from culture A and "prototypical" situations from culture B will each lead to different sorts of behavior. This too can be a useful way of demonstrating how situations from one culture or another afford different types of behavior. The predictions might involve (1) main effects (e.g., the "prototypical" situation of culture A leads to greater feelings of self-efficacy than that of culture B) and (2) interactions of the sort Morling et al. (2002) found (namely, routinely encountering the prototypical situation helps shape the person such that he or she becomes well-attuned to the affordances and practiced at the culturally appropriate ways of responding. Thus, there may be an interaction such that the prototypical situation of culture A leads to greater feelings of self-efficacy—and this is true *especially* for members of culture A). The disadvantages here are that (1) situations from one culture may not "translate" well to another culture (a point that is discussed later) and (2) the argument that a situation is prototypical in culture A must be asserted (rather than established through either observations or some technique similar to Kitayama's).[4]

"More" sociological forces also play a role in producing cultural differences (the word *more* is used here to indicate that there is no firm demarcation between where situations that are the purview of psychologists end and where structural forces that are the purview of sociologists begin). Yamagishi (1986, 1988; Yamagishi & Cook, 1993) and others, for example, have produced laboratory experiments that show in microcosm how "structural" factors—such as the presence or absence of a sanctioning system that punishes cheaters—shape people's behavior. In examining the "free rider" problem in which people do not contribute to public goods from which they benefit, Yamagishi (1988) contrasts two approaches: a cultural–individualistic approach and a cultural–institutional approach. The cultural–individualistic approach argues that behavior follows from internal values, such that collectivists do not free ride because they value contributing to the group. The cultural–institutional approach argues that behavior follows from the cultural institutions that have been established to create a certain type of behavior, such that collectivists do not free ride because systems of "mutual monitoring and sanctioning" are commonly established in collectivist cultures (more so than in individualist ones).

The explanations are not mutually exclusive. Thus, people with certain values are more likely to support certain types of institutions; conversely, certain institutions out in the world are more likely to socialize people to certain sorts of values. However, one of Yamagishi's contributions has been to take culture out of people's heads and show how important institutional forces are in this loop between individuals' values and the institutions that create (and are created by) them. More specifically, Yamagishi's experiments have (1) provided evidence for the cultural–institutional approach by showing how opportunities to develop sanctioning systems that punish cheaters and various systems of exchange affect people's decisions to cooperate or to free ride on the group; and (2) have provided evidence *against* the cultural–individualistic approach by showing that Japanese subjects are more likely than American subjects to exit from groups in which

there is no system to monitor and punish cheaters.

Finally, returning to the point that psychological and sociological approaches are intertwined, it is not always clear how one might draw a line between "situational" and "structural." Perhaps the most famous example of this is Milgram's (1974) 18 replications of the obedience experiment, which demonstrated the incredible power of situations and also served as an allegory for the structural forces in the modern state that enable genocides. The lessons of Milgram (make authority immediate and omnipresent, create distance between victim and victimizer, and allow people to shift responsibility for their actions elsewhere) are as much about macro-level sociological issues as they are about micro-level psychological forces in the immediate situation. Milgram himself viewed his obedience studies as preparation for a long-term project on "German character" (Blass, 2004, p. 65). The situational–structural variables were so important, however, that the cross-cultural project never made it out of New Haven, Connecticut.

The results of the studies discussed here suggest plausible arguments for ways in which cultural differences are not located solely within individuals but within practices, situations, collective representations, and institutional arrangements that afford certain types of behavior, enforce certain norms, or prime certain thoughts, and are more routinely encountered in one culture than another. Analyses that measures culture as an individual-difference variable "within the head" would be very usefully complemented by an approach "outside the head" that examined cultural practices, with the goal being a cultural psychology that investigates how culture and psyche "make each other up" or co-create each other (Kitayama & Markus, 1999; Markus & Hamedani, Chapter 1, this volume; Shweder, 1990; Adams & Markus, 2004).

Person × Situation × Culture Interactions/ Cultural Syndromes

A final note should be added about locating causation not just in persons or in situations but in person × situation interactions. Mischel, Mendoza-Denton, Shoda, and colleagues have discussed the notion of "behavioral signatures," or characteristic individual differences that emerge within particular situations (person × situation interactions; Mendoza-Denton & Mischel, Chapter 7, this volume; Mischel & Shoda, 1995). When one set of "behavioral signatures" characterizes many people within one culture but not another, it may then be helpful to think about Culture × Person × Situation interactions. This way of thinking is, in fact, consonant with Triandis's (1994) approach of discussing cultural syndromes. Such syndromes are not simple traits or behaviors, but are more like a *conglomeration* of traits and behaviors that cohere together meaningfully for people in a culture—even if they do not cohere together for people outside the culture (Cohen, 2001; Nisbett, 2005). Cultural syndromes and within-culture variability create the characteristic behavioral signatures of culture × person × situation interactions.

One example of this involves recent work on the cultural syndrome of honor. In some (though not all) honor groups, the syndrome of honor embraces (1) an ethic of bravery, in which one should be ready to commit violence to protect oneself if assaulted or one's reputation if insulted; and (2) an ethic of virtue, in which one is obliged to adhere to a moral code that demands prosocial reciprocity, trustworthiness, and so on. In most nonhonor cultures, virtue and violence do *not* go together; in fact, in most nonhonor cultures, a morally upright person would be both virtuous in his or her trustworthiness and altruism and slow to use violence. Experiments by Leung and Cohen (2007) with participants from two honor groups (U.S. Southerners and Latinos) and two nonhonor groups (Asian Americans and northern Anglo Americans) support this point. In brief, in Leung and Cohen (2007), it was those Asian Americans and northern Anglos who most eschewed honor-related violence who were (1) most helpful toward a confederate who had previously done them a favor and (2) least likely to cheat in an experimental task to win money. On the other hand, for those who came from a Southern U.S. or Latino culture of honor, it was those who *most* endorsed honor-related violence who also were the most helpful to a confederate and the least likely to cheat. Thus, among members of honor cultures, there was a characteristic "behavioral signature" defined by the syndrome of honor that demanded both a willingness to use violence to defend oneself and an altruistic desire to do good by being helpful and trustworthy. Among members of nonhonor cultures, a systematic but very different behavioral signature emerged, with the most pacifistic also being the most altruistic. A culture with a syndrome of honor creates one sort of person × situation interactions; one without such a syndrome creates a very different sort of person × situation interactions.

METHODS AND APPROACHES

Four approaches to culture have been noted thus far. An individual-differences approach may use experiments or, more commonly, questionnaires, but it will always include some measure of individual differences that is supposed to mediate the cultural effects. Social-cognitive approaches have thus far embraced the methodology of priming to simulate a certain cultural mind-set and then examine the consequences of holding that mind-set. Situation–structural approaches push this back one step further to look for the sorts of situations or structures that exist out in the world that channel or afford certain sorts of behavior; such an approach generally has pushed psychologists toward experimentation. A syndrome approach generally concentrates on the many ways a cultural theme manifests itself in a culture; such an approach favors an eclectic use of methods and may embrace both individual differences, situational–structural approaches, and their interaction.

In summary, although methodologies and theoretical approaches are not perfectly correlated, different methodologies seem generally to flow from different views of culture. And a researcher who unthinkingly adopts a certain methodology also is usually implicitly adopting a certain view of culture. The question is not which approach and method is better, but when should each approach be used. No matter what approach one starts with, it seems reasonable to assume that situations foster certain sorts of mind-sets, and certain mind-sets create certain situations (or make people construe situations a certain way). Situations and social structures create certain habits in people that shape their personalities; and people in turn create or re-create situations and structures that make sense to them. Furthermore, situations and persons interact in ways that may be defined by cultural syndromes, and these patterns of behavior or behavioral signatures may in turn reinforce (or sometimes change) the prevailing syndromes. And, within any culture, individual differences are guaranteed by differences in temperament, unique socialization experiences, and the existence of various "niches" within a culture that allow for various "types" of people to coexist within that cultural system (Cohen, 2001; Cooter, 1997; Konner, Chapter 4, this volume). The mix of persons within a system creates the niches, which in turn provide space for various "types" of people. Thus, taking a dynamic view of culture ultimately means we need to think from several approaches and, consequently, use a diverse set of methods.

If one were to attempt to build some grand model with individual differences, situations, institutional structures, social-cognitive construals, and cultural syndromes, the result almost surely would have causal arrows going in all directions. The trick is that (1) these arrows would not be equally strong, and (2) the strength of the arrows would probably vary across topics of study. We need to think about an issue from several different approaches, pick what we think is the most useful place to start, then see where to go from there.

Subquestion 3: "What Ecological, Economic, or Historical Circumstances Caused the Cultural Difference to Emerge in the First Place?"

The issue of causality also arises when we ask why the cultures under study are different in the first place. Obviously, part of the proximal answer has to do with the way individual psyches help co-create the culture through their behaviors, both individually and collectively (see Markus & Hamedani, Chapter 1, this volume). Understanding this process is one of the key goals of cultural psychology. However, sometimes we are also interested in the distal question of why certain cultural patterns arose in the first place. What were the ecological, economic, or historical factors that gave rise to the cultural pattern?

For example, Norenzayan, Choi, and Peng (Chapter 22, this volume; Nisbett, 2004; Nisbett, Chapter 35, this volume) have argued that a holistic thinking style developed in the East out of an environment and ecology that gave rise to large-scale agriculture, an endeavor that requires cooperation and interdependence. This social interdependence in turn gave rise to a holistic way of thinking, in which context and relationships took priority over individual objects and categories. In contrast, they theorized that an analytic thinking style arose in the West because the ecology of Greece encouraged herding and fishing rather than large-scale agriculture. Such ecological and economic circumstances meant that Greek society was less centralized and more fragmented than Chinese society. Greek social atomism in turn led to an atomistic, analytic mode of thought that concentrated on objects rather than relationships. Furthermore, Greece's place at the crossroads of the Mediterranean meant that there was a diverse "marketplace of ideas" and a need for formal systems of logic to sort out the good from the bad ideas.

Such ideas about social interdependence leading to more holistic thinking are given plausibility by laboratory experiments that set up these causal arguments in microcosm. For example, they are given plausibility by laboratory experiments showing that priming collectivism or priming individualism leads to more context-dependent or context-independent ways of thinking, respectively (Oyserman & Lee, Chapter 10, this volume; see also van Baaren, Horgan, Chartrand, & Dijkmans, 2004). These experiments make the causal argument somewhat more plausible, but to make a stronger statement about the links between ecology, economy, history, and culture, it is necessary to collect data on the actual ecological, economic, or historical circumstances themselves.

Ecology and Culture

The most famous contemporary example of this is Jared Diamond's (1999) *Guns, Germs, and Steel*, in which he traces the economic advancement and political dominance of cultures to early climatological and geographic factors that allowed for the domestication of plants and large animals. The development of agriculture in such societies led to surpluses that could sustain larger populations and occupational specialization. Thick population densities and the presence of domesticable animals in Eurasia also led to the development of certain crowd diseases. The germs of these diseases then became the most deadly forces as Eurasians spread across the globe. Diamond's book draws on the fields of anthropology, linguistics, genetics, and zoology to provide data for his argument.

Obviously, most of us have to be content with more humble undertakings than Diamond's. A few examples of such work empirically linking ecology to culture might include the following: Berry (1979) examined 17 cultures and showed that a culture's rate of conformity was highly correlated with whether its ecology encouraged cooperation (e.g., agricultural societies) or more individualistic activities (e.g., hunting and gathering societies); Henrich et al. (2001) examined 15 small-scale societies to see how fairly they would split a sizable amount of money provided by the experimenter, and they found that 50:50 splits were more likely to come from societies in which people (1) frequently engage in market transactions and (2) can realize big economic gains by cooperating with others outside the family; thus, a society in which the economic activity of whale hunting demands lots of cooperation tends to produce fairer offers than a society in which families are "almost entirely economically independent" of one another (Henrich et al., 2001, p. 76). Vandello and Cohen (1999) examined historical land use patterns of various U.S. states to see how 19th-century agricultural patterns predicted contemporary measures of individualism and collectivism, and so on.

Note that most of the examples above come from *cross-sectional* data. Thus, it is tempting to assume that ecological and economic factors preceded the development of cultural traits. However, without longitudinal data, one cannot rule out the possibility that the causation goes the other way. That is, one cannot rule out the possibility that more atomistic, less cooperative cultures gave rise to economies that did not require individual families to work with one another, whereas more cooperative cultures could take advantage of their synergy to create economic systems with more integration. To believe that ecology determines and *must necessarily* lead to certain economic and cultural arrangements is to assume that human cultures (1) do not alter their ecology, (2) do not move and self-select their ecological niches, and (3) always make the best use of their local ecology and thus inevitably end up at rational, adaptive economic and cultural arrangements. (If item 1, 2, or 3 is violated, then human choices and the cultural influences on them have entered the picture.) Assuming cultural arrangements are rational adaptations to the environment is a good place to start, but it is an assumption nonetheless.

ASSUMPTION NO. 1

In searching for a causal explanation, the usual assumption is that a cultural pattern is a certain way because it is functional or in some way adaptive for the culture. Again, this is probably a decent starting point in guiding research, but there are reasons to be wary. The first is that contemporary cultural patterns are not necessarily adapted to *current* environmental or ecological circumstances. Thus: the culture of honor may have arisen in the frontier South and West, but it may continue on long after the frontier has disappeared. High fertility rates that may have been adaptive in some agricultural settings persist after societies have become urbanized, child mortality rates have lessened, and children have become economic liabilities rather than assets (Triandis, 1994). Dysfunctional patterns of distrust, corruption, and "amoral familism" may persist even after autocratic governments have been displaced, and these patterns may undermine democracy and effective government (Putnam, 1993). And so on. Just as biological adaptations (e.g., a taste for fat and sugar) are no longer "adaptive" in places such as the United States, where people are surrounded by fat and sugar, so too are some cultural adaptations. A methodology that searches for the contemporary reasons why a cultural pattern is adaptive may come up empty-handed or worse; it may come up with a fallacious "just so" story for the current behavior.

There are at least some constraints in evolutionary psychology, because genes change only slowly (see also Atran, Chapter 17; Cole & Hatano, Chapter 5; Konner, Chapter 4; Li, Chapter 21; and Newson, Richerson, & Boyd, Chapter 18, all this volume). Think about the classic food preference example just given. People like McDonald's, but we know that a taste for McDonald's is not an adaptation, because McDonald's has only recently come into existence. Instead, our distant ancestors craved fats, sugars, and salts, and McDonald's has merely taken advantage of that ancestral adaptation (Symons, 1992). Cultural psychologists have a more difficult time than evolutionary psychologists, because cultures can change relatively rapidly (much more rapidly than genes); thus, cultural psychologists are not as constrained in their thinking about adaptations. It is possible to create many "just so" stories about why a given cultural pattern might be adaptive, because there is nothing that constrains our theorizing on *when*, *why*, and *in what circumstances* a cultural adaptation might have arisen.

Thus, a cultural pattern may in fact be adapted to current environmental circumstances. Or it may be adapted to any number of historical environmental circumstances. Or it may not be adaptive at all. A functionalist causal explanation may be false in some cases. Edgerton (1992) in particular has challenged what he calls "the myth of cultural adaptation." He asserts that cultural practices are rarely optimally functional, occasionally quite dysfunctional, and often unequal in the benefits they confer to different members of the society. Human culture may be as much a product of greed, xenophobia, sexism, shortsightedness, and irrationality, as our positive human qualities (see also Diamond, 2005). As much as possible, it makes sense to attempt to verify our general assumptions about adaptiveness and substantiate them in particular cases. Furthermore, we need to be precise about what *adaptive* means. Even when every individual is acting adaptively or rationally, that does not mean the overall cultural pattern is functional. An obvious example here is when the situation is structured as a "prisoner's dilemma" or a "tragedy of the commons." Every individual may behave rationally and adaptively, but the collective result is the worst possible, least functional outcome; and this worst possible outcome can also be a relatively stable equilibrium state.

Sources of Data

Researchers who study the links between ecologies, economies, history, and culture often need to work with archival data. Such data are abundant, though not always easy to find. Modern states are obsessive record keepers; however, depending on the topic, the records can vary in their quality and the amount of work needed to turn these records into manageable data. A great source for this data is data sets archived at the Inter-University Consortium for Political and Social Research (ICPSR; *www.icpsr.umich.edu/*). The Human Relations Area Files are available electronically and, as of 2004, had a searchable database with over 350,000 pages of information (*www.yale.edu/hraf*). Other databases, such as the Standard Cross-Cultural Sample of 186 so-

cieties (*eclectic.ss.uci.edu/~drwhite/worldcul/world.htm*), have been developed to avoid "Galton's problem" (the nonindependence of cultures due to either diffusion or a common history; Murdock & White, 2006). (Galton's "problem," of course, becomes an opportunity for researchers who study cultural diffusion and transmission; see Guglielmino, Viganotti, Hewlett, & Cavalli-Sforza, 1995; Pagel & Mace, 2004.) Still other collections should come online in the future.

Summary

In summary, not all cultural psychologists (particularly those doing the important basic work of description) need to worry about causality. But those who do need to think in terms of equilibriums (rather than, or in addition to, straight correlational thinking). Multiple ways of ordering the world can be meaningful, sensible, and coherent; discovering what these multiple cultural logics are is part of what cultural psychologists do.

Cultural psychologists also need to grapple with the question of where to begin: Social-cognitive, individual-difference, situational–structural, and cultural syndrome or culture × person × situation approaches all have something to contribute. Those doing more macro work also need to grapple with issues of gathering the sort of ecological, economic, and historical evidence that produces convincing arguments that go beyond just-so stories.

SAMPLING

The Causation section described how the sampling of cultures can drive our conclusions about what cultural syndrome gives rise to what patterns in particular domains. This section concentrates not on deciding which cultures to examine in our research, but on how we select participants once we have decided on the populations. As will be seen below, issues in sampling implicitly have views of culture built into them.

The issues to consider in thinking about sampling are as follows: What population are we hoping to generalize to, and what sorts of arguments are we trying to make? We first mention the relatively straightforward case of a researcher attempting to estimate a population parameter using a probability sample. We then deal with the more common case of researchers who do not use probability sampling.

Probability Sampling

In some cases the leap from sample to population can be made reasonably confidently—cases in which probability sampling is used and nonresponse rates are at an acceptably low level. From the populations, one develops a sampling frame (a list of all possible elements that could be included in the study). From the sample frame, one then draws the sample. Under probability sampling, all elements have a known and nonzero chance of being selected. Opinion surveys done with probability sampling are typically conducted by sociologists and political scientists or those working in collaboration with them. To get response rates at 80% or more, these usually have to be done by phone or in person, with multiple callbacks. There are various issues to consider with even very good probability samples (see Schuman & Kalton, 1985). But for the most part, one is on terra firma going from sample to population with most of these studies.

Studies using probability samples are often archived and available for secondary analysis by psychologists. This represents an excellent opportunity for those who study research questions related to the topics of such studies. However, because the secondary researcher was not the original investigator on the study, and the original investigator was probably not a cultural psychologist, one often has to make do with less than optimal questions. Large-scale surveys are extremely expensive, and the number of questions quite limited because time is at such a premium on them. Thus, psychologists going through survey archives may find that a typical survey does not cover a topic at the depths to which they are accustomed. However, the potential benefits of being able to find such data and use it in conjunction with data from a convenience sample (e.g., that gathered from the introductory psychology pool) are tremendous. Merely having a large N gathered from a convenience sample does not give generalizability; only a probability sample can give that. (This lesson was learned by the *Literary Digest* in the U.S. election of 1936. In a spectacularly wrong forecast, the *Digest* confidently predicted Landon would beat Roosevelt after getting 2.4 million survey respondents from across the country. Among other prob-

lems, however, the *Digest* constructed its sampling frame from sources such as telephone books, and car registration and country club membership lists. The problem was that in 1936, car ownership was not widespread, only one in four households had a telephone, and assuredly a smaller proportion than that belonged to country clubs. Of course, right now, a phone survey that uses random digit dialing (to get around the problem of unlisted phone numbers and cell phones) can get a pretty fair representation of the U.S. population. But that is *not* necessarily true in many countries, where telephones are far less common.

Good sources of large-scale survey data can be found at ICPSR, which houses data from sources such as World Values Surveys, National Opinion Research Center's General Social Survey (and its international counterparts), and the Institute for Social Research's National Election Study. Surveys such as these have a large N in any given year, and some of the same questions are asked from year to year. With such a large N, it is possible to investigate subcultures or systematic within-culture variation by socioeconomic status (SES), region, and so on; also, assuming one can reasonably aggregate across years, one can get a meaningful size N for small groups that do not show up in sufficient numbers in any given year. (For example, at 2% of the U.S. population, there will be 20 Muslims and 20 Jews in a survey of 1,000 respondents. Aggregating over, say, 10 years would give a more substantial 200 each.) Additionally, the repetition of questions in different years allows one to track changes over time, separate out generation effects from age effects, and, if the study is a panel study, follow the same people longitudinally over time.

Subquestions 1 and 2: "About What Population Can I Sensibly Generalize, and How Do I Think about What Is 'Culture' and What Is 'Confound' When I Pick My Sample?"

Nonprobability Sampling and Statements of Generalization: Too Big or Too Small?

For most cultural psychologists, secondary analysis of survey data will be used only as a complement to their main line of work. In the section on causation, the unavoidable problem was that no correlational study can prove causation. In the sampling section, the unavoidable problem is that no study without probability sampling can generate a safe generalization, because no one knows who exactly the study's sample represents.

Generalization is an inherent part of our work, however, as described in the following sections. How then do we deal with the unsolvable problem? Our sampling approaches are designed to be *suggestive* of some types of generalization, and a few imperfect approaches to sampling are described as a way to make studies more suggestive rather than less suggestive.

From Sample to Population and Vice Versa

In most noncultural psychology studies, the population is usually implicitly hypothesized to be all human beings, the sampling frame is the list of sophomores who have signed up for Psychology 1 this year, and the sample is the 80% of those who actually show up at the lab to participate in our study. In most culture studies, the population-to-sample link is only somewhat better. The population might implicitly be something like the 2.5 billion members of Eastern civilization and the billion members of Western civilization. The sampling frame is the Asian Americans and European Americans in the Psychology 1 pool, and the sample is those who show up. The absurdity of going "too big" in one's generalizations is obvious here.

Consider also the opposite problem of going "too small" and the paralysis it leads to in either selecting a sample or drawing conclusions. A researcher considers a study comparing the political cultures of Brazil and Argentina with the United States and Canada. The researcher wants to argue that some result illustrates a difference between the political cultures of Latin American and North American societies. A critic would correctly point out that Latin America is not "monolithic." The South American countries are different than the Central American countries. And within South America, the countries of Brazil and Argentina will be different from, say, Peru and Bolivia. Within Brazil, the states of northern Brazil will be much different than those of southern Brazil. And within southern Brazil, the state of São Paulo will be different from, say, the state of Santa Catarina. And within São Paulo state, the city of São Paulo will be different from those more inland. And within the city of São Paulo, . . . and the regression can go on ad infinitum, until one is thoroughly torn about

where to start the research and then afraid to make any homogenizing statement or generalize past the N specific subjects in the study once it has been completed.

For anyone not using a probability sample, the generalization problem is always there, whether or not it is acknowledged. For example, a researcher studying, say, parent–child socialization might sensibly say that she does not care if her results generalize to other Asian populations or to all Japanese. She may situate her research as examining processes and meanings within upper-middle-class Japanese and American parent–child interactions. That is, she may argue that her research concerns not the "grand" traditions (Eastern vs. Western culture, Buddhism, Confucian thought, etc.) but "local" traditions. (See also Glazer, 2000, on Redfield and Singer's notions of "great" and "little" traditions.) However, unless there was probability sampling, she has in fact no reason to believe her findings apply to other upper-middle-class Japanese and American parents, to other upper-middle-class Japanese and American parents from these particular towns, or even these particular neighborhoods, and so on.

If one wants to talk about one's findings as applicable to groups other than the specific subjects in the study, a generalization is being made. And perhaps more importantly, if one wants to talk about something as "cultural," then one is by definition talking about something shared among some group of people that is usually larger than the particular group of participants in this one study.

It is true that a researcher may not be interested in generalizing to estimate an exact population parameter (e.g., 57% of Japanese middle-class moms do it this way, whereas only 25% of American moms do). However, the researcher is implicitly generalizing whenever he or she describes something as "cultural," because he or she is usually referring to some set of practices and meanings that are either shared, acknowledged, or contested by some group of people (usually larger than the study N).

Sampling Approaches

The limitations of nonprobability samples lead to one of the fundamental paradoxes of cultural psychology. That is, part of cultural psychology's critique of mainstream psychology was that it was studying psychological principles that it claimed were universal, but that in fact were only tested on and perhaps true of only a small subsection of the population. Instead of a psychology of human nature, we essentially had a discipline that might have been what Shweder (1997, p. 155) would call "Anglo American cultural studies."

The work of cultural psychologists, however, has the same limitation in that it is similarly unclear how we can take findings from our sample and make them more broadly relevant to a study of culture. Given that any sample that is not a probability sample cannot pretend to know to whom the results generalize, how can one sample in a way that still allows one to say something useful about culture—either big-C Culture (Chinese culture, American culture, Mexican culture, etc.) or little-c culture (the process by which people make and are shaped by their world; Glazer, 2000)?

There are at least four approaches. They do not solve the problem that one cannot generalize past a sample without using probability sampling, and they all have different problems. However, they may all contribute something useful to understanding the way culture works. These four approaches might be called the typicality approach, the just minimal difference approach, the cultural experts approach, and the inversion approach.

TYPICALITY VERSUS THE JUST MINIMAL DIFFERENCE

A researcher is comparing cultures A and B. How should she draw her samples of people or families, or her sample of schools (or whatever her sampling unit is) from group A and B? One principle is to match on "typicality," so that one might compare "typical" groups in culture A with typical groups in culture B rather than having to compare typical groups in culture A with outlier groups in culture B. A competing way might be to match participants from the two cultures on the principle of the "just minimal difference." In the latter approach, one would try to match the samples as closely as possible on all variables, so that the only difference left is the difference in the cultural histories of the two groups. Practically speaking, the samples are made as similar as one can reasonably make them, so that exposure to culture A versus exposure to culture B becomes the *most*

obvious explanation when other obvious but "noncultural" factors have been equated.

The difficulty in the first approach is clear. How does one decide who is "typical"? It is far easier to decide who or what is *atypical* than to decide who is typical. For example, it is reasonably safe to say that a sample from the Upper West Side of Manhattan or Beverly Hills or northern Idaho may not be a "typical" American sample. But who would qualify as typical—a sample of people from Minnesota or Peoria, Illinois, or the ever-popular test market, Columbus, Ohio, with its location at the geographic and political center of the state that is "the epitome of American normalcy" (*Encyclopaedia Britannica*, 2004; Will, 2004a)? It is likely that by *typical* researchers probably mean *not atypical* in many obvious ways. Unless there is some well-established modal group that is statistically quite common or some culturally agreed on prototype, it is likely that *typicality* or not atypical is going to be a subjective call.

The latter approach—the just minimal difference—has an intuitive appeal to psychologists who primarily use controlled experiments. It is an attempt to mimic random assignment by keeping "everything else constant" and just concentrating on the cultural difference of interest. The problem is that there is no real random assignment, so there is no "everything else constant." However, there is also a deeper problem here: This approach implies that one is able to sort out what is the "cultural" factor from what is a confound or an extraneous factor. It is not clear that this is possible or even always desirable (see also Medin et al., Chapter 25, this volume).

One probably does not want to consider *all* differences between two cultural groups as a *cultural* difference (as opposed to an economic difference, ecological difference, demographic difference, etc.).[5] However, depending on the area of study, the line between what is cultural and what is, say, a confounding demographic factor can get quite blurry. For example, what does it mean for one to control for income when comparing cultural groups that renounce worldly success versus those that embrace it as a sign of the elect? Or what does it mean to control for education in comparing groups that emphasize formal schooling with those that do not? (See Glazer [2000, p. 226] also for similar discussions of preference for rural vs. urban living, or family size and structure as both a demographic variable and a "cultural feature par excellence," etc.). As Adams and Markus (2004) noted, one essential part of the "dynamic construction" approach to culture involves the blurring of the division between what is "culture" and what is "social structure," because both re-create each other. Some of that "everything else" that one is trying to get rid of may be a defining part of the cultural phenomena.

Then again, maybe not. Thinking about these issues forces a researcher to think about the nature of his or her study: (1) Is the aim to focus narrowly and analytically on a specific, circumscribed cultural practice, so that one can pinpoint its importance? (2) Is the goal to identify this difference as more "cultural," implying that it expresses some sort of chosen value for the group that will endure even if more "structural" or demographic changes occur? If either (1) or (2) is the aim of the study, that might push one toward a sample based on the "just minimal difference," so that one can focus in on the practice of interest, keeping at least *some* "other things equal." Or, for example, is the aim (3) to capture the "Gestalt" of the culture—to examine how the various aspects of the culture fit together and support one another (or clash)? If the latter is true, then that might push one more toward a sample based on some definition of "typicality," in which it does not make sense to "keep all else equal," because "all else" is part of what one is trying to study.

In some ways, the answer to the question of whether one wants to focus analytically or to capture a Gestalt is like the answer to the question of whether one wants vanilla or chocolate ice cream. The correct answer is, "Yes, both." In that case, within a given study one can sample not only widely but also strategically, selecting some of the sampling units based on the principle of "typicality," and others based on the principle of "just minimal difference." For example, if one is drawing a sample of, say, 10 schools, one can choose, say, five "typical" schools from each culture, then choose the other five schools with an eye toward matching them as closely as possible, so that one can isolate a particular characteristic of interest. Research budgets often do not allow for such sampling and, in that case, one simply has to determine the most important research goals for the study.

EXPERT SAMPLING VERSUS INVERSION SAMPLING

Expert sampling and inversion sampling represent two opposite approaches. One stacks the deck in favor of finding the cultural difference; the other stacks the deck against it. In expert sampling, one makes no pretense of studying the average group member. Instead, one tries to bring cultural systems into sharp relief by studying cultural "experts," where "experts" does not mean scholars but rather means the people most immersed in, most competent in, or who most embody a culture in its more "pure" form. Such a study with cultural experts may stand on its own, or it may be a prelude to future studies involving wider populations. For example, in studying reasoning about the natural world, Lopez, Atran, Coley, Medin, and Smith (1997) focused on Itza' Maya elders who spoke Itza'—clearly an exceptional group, because "the 'typical' Itza' speaks mainly Spanish" (Medin & Atran, 2004, p. 964). Then, once sharp cultural differences have been defined through studies that use expert sampling, subsequent research may go on to study the distribution and transmission of these "expert" ideas across networks within the community. The appeal of expert sampling is obvious and is quite consistent with Kurt Lewin's directive to "start strong." However, the drawbacks to this method are obvious as well: (1) It will not always be clear who the "experts" are, or who is most culturally competent (again, it is probably easier to identify who is not an expert or competent) and (2) depending on the size of the gulf between the experts and everybody else, the findings on the expert population may or may not prove useful in generating subsequent research with nonexpert populations.

A different possibility is to do the opposite of expert sampling and sample the subgroups that theoretically would be the *least* likely to produce a cultural difference. There are a few reasons one might do this type of inversion sampling. For example, one might want to strengthen the generalization inference by showing that the cultural difference exists even in extreme cases when the cards are stacked against it. Thus, in studying political culture, if one showed that even the most conservative Canadian province favored socialized medicine more than the most liberal U.S. state, one can make a stronger inference about a more general U.S.–Canada difference. A very different reason to engage in inversion sampling might be to test our understanding of a phenomena by "flipping it on its head," as Norbert Schwarz would say. Suppose, for example, one were studying differences in fatalism between Country A, which primarily grows a high volatility commodity a, and Country B, which primarily grows relatively stable commodity b. If one wanted to focus in on the connection between commodity volatility and fatalistic practices, it might be useful to include in one's sample some unusual regions from Country A that grew commodity b, and some unusual regions from Country B that grew commodity a.[6] In the typical regions of countries A and B, one might show how A's practices are more fatalistic than B's; but with the atypical regions, one might strengthen the argument about volatility and fatalism by showing that the effect flips on its head in these atypical regions. This type of sampling has an appeal to experimentally trained cultural psychologists. However, the same limits about claiming causality still apply, because the independent variable (in this case, commodity volatility) was still measured rather than manipulated.

College Student Sampling and Ethnic Group Sampling

Issues in college student sampling and ethnic group sampling are just special cases of the general issues discussed earlier. Nevertheless, they merit greater treatment, because practical considerations (ease of recruitment, ease of standardizing procedures, etc.) make using such samples quite popular.

College Student Samples

Given a desire to create the just minimal difference and the ready convenience of college samples, many researchers have opted (1) to find comparable colleges, then sample college students from various countries or (2) to study college students of different ethnic groups within a single country (see below for more on the latter). In psychology as a whole, somewhere around 80% of research on "normal" adults has used such college student samples (Rosnow & Rosenthal, 2002, p. 14). Within cultural psychology, no one has yet calculated a comparable estimate.

For cultural psychology, there are, of course, the usual hazards of using college student sam-

ples, then hoping to generalize beyond them. However, in cultural psychology, there are additional concerns as well. Within the United States, we have some suggestion of at least some of the ways college students differ from the rest of the population (see Sears, 1986), but such data may or may not be known for other countries. Furthermore, in almost every other place in the world, college students are likely to be an even more rarefied section of the population than they are in the United States, where approximately one in four persons ages 25 to 64 has a university education. By comparison, the number is only half that in places such as the progressive Scandinavian countries, the United Kingdom, and the other countries of the European Union (U.S. Bureau of the Census, 1999, p. 840). In most nations outside Europe, it will be lower still. The researcher trying to create the just minimal difference may wind up comparing a college student elite in the United States with a college student superelite elsewhere. This researcher may be equating on education, but he or she is not equating on social status or life chances. Whether there is an education effect or a social status effect—and on which one it might be more important to equate—is an issue that may vary depending on the research topic (see also Schooler, Chapter 15, this volume).

Many people's intuitions are that comparing a U.S. elite with a non-U.S. superelite will lessen the chance of finding cultural differences, because "cosmopolitan elites" share certain traits and values across the world (Shweder, 2000). For the researcher hoping to find a cultural difference, this is a good thing, because it means that the confounding factor usually works against the hypothesis rather than for it; thus, it cannot be a valid alternative explanation if differences are found.

However, in any given case, it is an open question whether cosmopolitan elites will be more like each other than are their respective populations. To the extent that one is comparing a Western culture with a non-Western culture *and* to the extent that elite status implies Westernization, the use of college student samples will probably work against the hypothesis. However, it is not clear that either modernization of a country or elite status within a country does actually lead to Westernization (Huntington, 1996). Probably in some countries and in some domains it does, and probably in some countries and in some domains it does not.

This is an empirical question, and we may or may not have the data to settle it for every particular domain of inquiry.

Comparisons between Ethnic Groups and between Countries

To create the "just minimal difference," some studies examine ethnic groups within a given country as opposed to between countries. For example, one might study Chinese Americans and European Americans rather than people in China and in the United States. There is much to be said for this approach, and, very practically, keeping the study at one location also helps to equate the operational details involved in actually running the study. For example, if one is running a study examining how European Americans and Chinese Americans respond to the loss of face, one can employ the same face-losing procedure with the same experimental confederates. And even when the study is not a high-impact (highly involving) laboratory experiment, a study that involves European Americans and Chinese Americans can use an English questionnaire to avoid translation ambiguities (discussed in the next section) or extraneous effects of language (discussed in Chiu, Leung, & Kwan, Chapter 27, this volume; Norenzayan, Choi, & Peng, Chapter 23, this volume; Perunovic, Ross, & Wilson, 2005; Wang & Ross, Chapter 26, this volume), if such effects are indeed extraneous.

However, if one wants to talk about Chinese culture and American culture, the comparison of European Americans with Chinese Americans minimizes some extraneous differences but creates others. For one thing, if one is using recent immigrants, a whole set of challenges accompanies trying to settle into a new culture. For another thing, even if one does not use recent immigrants, culture will be confounded with majority or minority status in most places in the United States. And as an entirely separate matter, immigrants are likely to be systematically different from their counterparts back home on at least some personality and demographic variables. In some cases, this is fine, because some preexisting differences and some challenges that new immigrants face may work against the hypothesis in question and so cannot be alternative explanations. However, in other cases, it will not always be clear that this is so. Thus, generalizing from Chinese immigrants to Chinese culture or generalizing from Chinese culture to Chinese immigrants is not a move that can be taken for granted (Glazer, 2000). Again, more abstractly, it may not be simple to go from the "local" traditions of a particular group in a particular place to the "grand" tradition (e.g., Eastern culture) from which it may have derived (and vice versa for the direction of inference).

A Novel Sample: Culture as an Experimentally Primed Variable

Samplings based on typicality, just minimal differences, expertise, and inversion are four of the multiple ways one might choose to sample. The just minimal difference approach and the inversion approach should be appealing to psychologists who come from an experimental background. However, the fundamental problem is that we cannot get rid of the third-variable problem, because we cannot randomly assign people to culture and consider it a manipulated variable.

There has been at least one ingenious sampling strategy for helping with this problem, though. Hong, Morris, Chiu, and Benet-Martínez (2000; Hong, Wan, Ching, No, & Chiu, Chapter 13, this volume) have done studies in which the sample is made up of bicultural individuals who have been socialized in two cultural traditions (in their research, they have used both residents of Hong Kong and Asian Americans). These bicultural individuals are then randomly assigned to receive an experimental manipulation in which they are primed with either Chinese icons (the Great Wall, a Chinese dragon) or American icons (Marilyn Monroe, the American flag).[7] In their research, they have, for example, shown that Chinese icons tend to push bicultural individuals toward Eastern, group-centered descriptions of events, whereas American icons tend to push them toward Western, individualistic descriptions. One does not get around the problem that bicultural individuals are a special subset of the population, but one does at least get around the problem of confounding culture with some of the other variables one would like to control. According to one way of thinking, bicultural individuals were a problem to be avoided—they were too tainted by culture A to be a "true" member of culture B, and vice versa. Hong et al.'s important move was to see working with such individuals as presenting an opportunity to manipulate (at least temporarily) cultural schemas. All sampling techniques are going to be flawed in some way, but as cultural psychology matures, it is likely that more of these clever sampling techniques will be developed as part of the discipline's repertoire.

Pragmatic Recruiting Concerns: Our Subjects Select Us

Whereas the previous sections have dealt mostly with how we select our subjects, a brief note should be added about how our subjects self-select into our studies. Two pragmatic recruiting concerns are (1) advertising culture in our studies and (2) paying participants. The effects of both are unclear, but the theoretical reasons why they may matter await further research.

The issue of how we advertise our studies is relevant both for studies that use community members and those that use psychology department participant pools and have to entice participants to sign up. Any researcher that uses sign-up methods faces the problem of participant self-selection. However, culture studies have an additional concern, in that they sometimes advertise for people of a particular ethnicity. At this point, I am unaware of any research that directly compares data from studies in which culture is explicitly advertised as a factor with those in which it is not. There may in fact be no differences, but it is possible that studies in which culture is advertised (1) are more likely to attract participants who are highly identified with their ethnicity; (2) may prime ethnicity for participants, thus making them more likely to follow cultural norms (Hong et al., 2000); (3) may produce "stereotype threat" effects (Steele, 1997, 1999); (4) may produce more "good subject" effects as participants try to give researchers the desired results; or (5) in an opposite fashion, may elicit more behavior that tries to disconfirm the stereotype, especially if that stereotype is negative. Four out of these five possibilities would exaggerate cultural differences. (Additionally, these effects may become even bigger when a large number of researchers use a participant pool with a small number of subjects who are, say, Asian American. Such a situation may produce "professional ethnics," with the same small

group of Asian Americans being used in culture study after culture study.) If advertising for culture does indeed affect the results, the researcher would probably want to know why, because some of these reasons (particularly items 3–5 from the preceding list) seem artifactual.

Finally, we know something about the distinguishing characteristics of volunteers for research in the United States: Volunteers tend to have higher SES, education, IQ scores, need for approval, are more likely to be female, and so on (Rosnow & Rosenthal, 2002). Much less is known about volunteers in other countries. Particularly when studies are conducted in poorer countries and "volunteers" are paid, one might expect that at least some of these volunteerism biases reverse (e.g., one may get "volunteers" lower in SES and education). How much of a concern this is will probably vary from study to study.

Sampling Technique(s) Appropriate to the Research Question

In summary, cultural psychologists need to take the issue of participant sampling seriously; that is the basis for the field's critique of mainstream psychology as a psychology of relatively elite Western populations. Rarely do cultural psychologists use probability sampling themselves, so it is definitionally unclear to whom our results generalize. Yet various sampling techniques may help us say something useful about either big-C Culture or little-c culture (e.g., typicality sampling vs. just minimal difference sampling, expert sampling vs. inversion sampling, bicultural sampling).

There are inevitably trade-offs in choosing one type of sample or another. Different sampling techniques have implicitly built into them different views of "what culture is." For example, as described earlier, questions of whether one is dealing with the grand traditions or local ones, of how best to keep "everything else equal," or whether one even wants to, are questions that are implicit in how the samples are selected. To make good decisions as researchers and good interpretations as readers, we need to define the research questions precisely, think through the sampling trade-offs we might make, and choose the sampling technique(s) most appropriate for our project.

OPERATIONALIZATION

Once one has thought through these issues, it is time to operationalize the hypothesis with measures of the dependent variable and measures or manipulations of the independent variable. Several excellent guides explore both the art and the science of operationalization (Berry, Poortinga, & Pandey, 1996; Gilbert, Fiske, & Lindzey, 1998; Schuman & Kalton, 1985; Schuman & Presser, 1981; Triandis & Berry, 1980; Triandis, 1994). This chapter can only briefly sketch out a few issues as they apply to culture. For all social scientists, the essential challenge of operationalization is to create variables that are convincing and interpretable. For cultural psychologists, these variables have to be convincing and interpretable when seen through (at least) two different cultural lenses.[8]

Subquestion 1: "Am I Translating My Variable Correctly from One Culture to Another?"

One of the big issues for cultural psychologists is that of "translation," which is loosely defined as making sure one's measures and manipulations are the same across cultures. The issue is obvious when it comes to language, but it also applies to translating situations and observations, as discussed later.

Linguistic Translation

If the study is to be conducted in two or more languages, one must have the materials translated and backtranslated. Thus, a first bilingual may translate materials from Vietnamese to Russian and a second bilingual will translate the materials back from Russian to Vietnamese. One can add a number of different protections, including having multiple bilinguals do the translation, the backtranslation, and reconcile any differences. Furthermore, one can conduct the process iteratively, subjecting the materials to multiple rounds of translation and backtranslation. It sounds straightforward enough, but anyone who has done it knows how difficult and tedious this can be.

A few examples illustrate the importance of slogging through what seem to be even the most tedious of issues. Monolingual English speakers probably think there could be nothing easier than translating the word *is*. But as President Bill Clinton observed in a very different context, "It depends on what the meaning of the word 'is' is."[9] In Spanish, the word *is* has two forms—*estar*, which is "generally used for temporary properties," and *ser*, which is generally used for permanent ones (Heyman & Diesendruck, 2002, p. 408; Sera et al., 1997). As Heyman and Diesendruck (2002) have shown, these two forms have consequences for attributions, such that Spanish-speaking children who hear a story about a girl who *es* shy are more likely to think the girl will be shy at other parties and 2 years in the future, as compared to those who heard that the girl *está* shy. A second example, the Twenty Statements Test, a common measure of self-construal, consists purely of 20 statements that begin "I am . . ." and ask the participant to complete the sentence. The usual findings are that Eastern respondents are more collectivistic, in that they more often give social role or category responses (e.g., "I am a man") compared to American respondents, who give more personality-oriented responses (e.g., "I am loud"). However, even the seemingly benign "I am" construction can be problematic, because the direct translation into Chinese is Wo *shi*—a construction "usually followed by a noun phrase and only occasionally an adjective" (Hong, Ip, Chiu, Morris, & Mennon, 2001). When Hong et al. dropped the *am* (or the *shi* in Chinese) from the Twenty Statements Test, Hong Kong and American participants gave very similar responses.

An issue of translation also seems to have partially led to the debate between Au (1983, 1984) and Bloom (1981, 1984) over the issue of Chinese speakers' inclination to engage in counterfactual thinking. Depending on how the stimulus materials are written and the subject population one uses, the number of counterfactual thoughts generated by Chinese (and English) speakers varied dramatically. Au argued that Bloom's materials were translated into "nonidiomatic" Chinese, and she argued that she could increase counterfactual reasoning when the materials were translated into a more idiomatic form. Ironically, Au claimed, Bloom's English-to-Chinese translators had rendered his materials less intelligible by translating the literal meaning instead of using forms more idiomatic to Chinese. Bloom (1984, p. 283) defended his translations (done by "native Chinese-speaking professors at the National Taiwan University") and in turn criticized Au's story materials. Translation, even when done by experts, is no simple matter.

Even within the English language, there can be a translation issue from region to region. Spanking, for example, means something different to Northerners and Southerners in the United States, because in the South, spanking is much more likely to be done with a paddle or a switch. Even with this difference in meaning, Southerners are more likely to favor a "good hard spanking." However, in analogous cases, one can imagine that differences in meaning could lead one to quite misleading conclusions. For example, if the word *argument* is taken to mean any sort of disagreement that involves raised eyebrows in culture A, whereas it means a shouting match that would drown out a rock concert in culture B, one might find that the frequency of "arguments" in culture A is startlingly high compared to that in culture B. In this case, the ambiguity in the word *argument* adds not only noise but also bias.

These differing definitions and standards can arise partly out of reference group effects that Heine and colleagues (2002) have explored. So, for example, when a respondent is asked whether she is "creative," she first needs to figure out what "creative" means ("Does it mean that I paint and write poetry? Or does it mean that I fire off snappy one-liners in the break room?"). Additionally, she needs to figure out what groups she should be comparing herself against ("Am I creative compared to chimpanzees? Compared to people my age? Compared to my fellow bank tellers? Compared to other Americans? Compared to other Americans *and* to the people in that other unknown culture that the researcher will be studying? Compared to all the humans in the world? Compared to some absolute standard that I have personally developed?"). People may not explicitly ask themselves these questions, but some definitions have to be implicitly constructed, and some comparison standard has to be set.[10] This is done with the aid of a reference group, implying, as Heine and colleagues (2002) have shown, that when a Japanese person answers a question such as "I have respect for the authority figures with whom I interact," he or she may be thinking of a very different comparison standard than that of an American (Singelis, 1994). In Heine et al.'s (2002) study, European Canadians' scores on an interdependence scale were equal to Japanese scores when no comparison group was given, were higher than Jap-

anese scores when members of each group were specifically told to compare themselves to people in their own culture, and were lower than Japanese scores when members of each group were specifically told to compare themselves to people in the other culture. (Obviously, people have to be knowledgeable about their own culture and other cultures to make these comparisons meaningful. But more generally, the point is that responses to Likert-scale attitude questions depend greatly on the reference group the respondent is using).

We can try to figure out the standards of comparison by asking respondents probing questions, or we may give respondents questions that ask specifically about the types of behaviors we are interested in. Furthermore, we can follow Schwartz's (1999) advice to avoid "vague quantifiers" such as *frequently*, *sometimes*, and so on, and instead ask for objective numbers. Thus, it is possible to turn some questions, such as "I frequently engage in violent pastimes" into "I go hunting ____ times per year," but it will not always be either possible to do so or meaningful to do so.

Translating Situations and Behaviors

By avoiding vague quantifiers and by asking more objective, behavioral questions, one generally lessens both the error and bias that results when participants from different cultures construe the question differently. High-impact lab experiments that call for specific behaviors go even further toward doing so. However, one still must be sure that the situations one constructs for a study and the behaviors observed translate from one culture to the next. The bargain one strikes for the sake of clarity is this: The more one specifies very particular situations, and the more narrowly one operationalizes a variable, the more one is implicitly pushed toward examining a phenomenon as an etic (universal) construct that is played out the same way across cultures—rather than as an emic or more culturally specific construct that is approached in a culture's own terms. Thus, the trade-off is that the more one is concrete, the less one will have error and bias about that particular set of behaviors; but also the more one is concrete, the greater the risk of missing emic phenomena or constructing what Triandis (1994, p. 69) called pseudoetics (false etics; see also LeVine, Chapter 2, and Triandis, Chapter 3, this volume).

This is essentially Cronbach's (1990) point about the fidelity-bandwidth trade-off, as applied to culture. Generally, there is a trade-off such that variables narrowly defined (low in bandwidth) can be measured with high fidelity (less noise), whereas those that are broadly defined across a range of observations (high in bandwidth) have lower fidelity (more noise). (*Note*: High bandwidth is *not* the same as simply being vague). Thus, one may measure, say, intelligence (Sternberg, Chapter 22, this volume), secure and insecure attachment (Morelli & Rothbaum, Chapter 20, this volume), reasoning ability (Norenzayan et al., Chapter 23, this volume), self-esteem (Kitayama et al., 1997), competitiveness, feelings of interdependence and connectedness (Brewer & Yuki, Chapter 12, this volume), religious behaviors, emotional expressions, passive–aggressive behaviors, mental health and illness (Marsella & Yamada, Chapter 33, this volume), patriotism, extroversion, love (Hatfield, Rapson, & Martel, Chapter 31, this volume), and so on. And the more concretely and precisely one measures these constructs, the less "noise" there will be. However, precision may also mean narrowness, and the narrower the construct is operationalized, the more likely it is to privilege one culture's definition of the construct over another's.

The coding of secure versus insecure behavior in the Strange Situation task is a possible illustration of the problem of narrow definitions (see Morelli & Rothbaum, Chapter 20, this volume). However, there are cases in which the problem is not simply the coding of behavior in a situation; rather, the problem is that *the entire situation* itself fails to translate. Shweder (1997, p. 155) provides a humorous example:

A team of psychologists from Scandinavia was doing comparative research [on] variations in the "universal" family meal. They wired ahead to a prominent local psychologist in this rural area of India and asked him to arrange for a family meal. . . . Being civil and polite, he did so, without ever telling them that in rural India there is no such thing as a family meal. The Scandinavian research team spent a few days in the area. The local psychologist convinced some family to sit down at a table together and food was served and they were filmed. But everyone was uncomfortable. Avoidance relationships were being violated. People kept getting up from the table and leaving. No one ever explained to the visitors that family meals should not be presumed to be part of some

universal grid. They returned home, coded the materials, and made some sort of inference about what was going on, without really ever understanding what was really going on.

Situations and behaviors—in both experimental paradigms and observational studies—can fail to "translate" across cultures. Ultimately, there is no substitute for background reading, having informants or collaborators familiar with the culture, pretesting measures, probing respondents for their understanding of concepts and behaviors, and using a combination of investigative techniques—some of which are "operant" methods, in that they are loosely controlled, exploratory, and driven primarily by the respondent, and others of which are "respondent" methods in that they are more tightly controlled, well-defined, and driven by specific hypotheses of the experimenter or interviewer (Triandis, 1994, p. 80).[11]

Subquestion 2: "What Are the Cost–Benefit Trade-Offs of Surveys versus Experiments?"

Strategies for Questionnaires and Experiments

Often, a research question can be plausibly answered by operationalizing the hypothesis in a naturalistic observational study, a questionnaire (open- or closed-ended), or a high-impact lab experiment. Again, the best answer about which one should do is: all of them. However, pragmatic concerns often dictate that one rather than the other needs to be done, or that one rather than the other at least needs to be done first. In nonqualitative cultural psychology research, this often comes down to the question of whether one should begin with questionnaires or experiments. There are two schools of thought on this issue. According to one school of thought, investigations need to start by casting the widest possible net to explore a phenomenon. The questionnaire (again either open- or closed-ended) is far more efficient for this purpose. Not only is it possible to run many, many participants at once, but it is also possible to ask about a wide array of situations and an extended history of behaviors. Say, for example, one is studying cultural differences in coping with stress across cultures. In a matter of a few pages, it is possible to ask about relationship stressors, academic stressors, work stressors, economic stressors, and so on. It is possible to ask about a history of situations that have happened in the past and to ask respondents to speculate on situations that might happen in the future. One can in this way get answers that cover a huge variety of situations.

The question, however, is whether and to what degree one should trust those answers. A mundane concern is that response set biases can potentially plague any sort of questionnaire research; however, what is particularly troublesome to cross-cultural researchers is the possibility that cultures are differentially susceptible to different response sets. For example, people from hierarchical cultures may be more likely to give extreme responses that use the end points of the scales; those from collectivistic cultures may be more likely to show the acquiescence bias (Johnson, Kulesa, Cho, & Shavitt, 2005; Lalwani, Shavitt, & Johnson, 2006; Triandis, 1994). Some protections can be put in place (e.g., having an equal number of reverse-scored and nonreverse-scored items can lessen problems created by the acquiescence bias), and one can do as much as possible to lessen the problem of social desirability biases (e.g., disguising the dependent variable, allowing participants to believe that their responses are anonymous, and truthfully assuring anonymity and confidentiality can reduce impression management effects).

However, there are deeper problems with any questionnaire data that can be very difficult to overcome. These involve problems in which the participant may not be able to correctly tell us about his or her behavior or attitudes, *even if he or she wants to*. Depending on the domain, people can have great difficulty identifying the reasons for their actions, articulating their preferences, predicting their future behavior, and predicting how they will feel about their future outcomes (Nisbett & Wilson, 1977; Gilbert & Wilson, 2000; Wilson & Dunn, 2004)—even when extremely important life events are involved (Pauker & Pauker, 1979). Of course, these points should not be pushed to the extreme (I can tell you that I prefer watching a movie to being hit with a hammer; I can tell you why I have that preference; and I can safely predict how I will feel after either experience). However, the difficulty in getting accurate self-reports is one reason some researchers prefer experiments and find that they produce bigger differences than do questionnaires.

The second school of thought on where to begin is to follow Kurt Lewin's advice and "start strong." In this case, one might look to a high-impact lab experiment to highlight a large effect. The following is very far from a perfect comparison, but consider a few examples. In national surveys, when asked whether they would approve of a man punching another man who "was drunk and bumped into the man and his wife on the street," around 7% of non-Southerners said "yes," whereas around 16% of Southerners did so (the effect size is small, r is approximately .15). In an experiment, when Northern and Southern university students were bumped into by a confederate and called an "asshole," 35% of Northerners responded with at least as much anger as amusement, whereas 85% of Southerners did so (the effect size is large, r is approximately .5; Cohen & Nisbett, 1994; Cohen, Nisbett, Bowdle, & Schwarz, 1996). On a questionnaire, when Northern and Southern students are asked how they would react to an annoying confederate who kept hitting them with paperwads, their predicted responses did not differ. However, when the experiment is actually run, differences do occur, with effect sizes in the medium and large range, depending on the specific behavioral measure (Cohen, Vandello, Puente, & Rantilla, 1999).

Effects from experiments have the potential to produce much bigger differences than questionnaires do, precisely because they are highly involving. Such highly involving studies are more likely to involve "online processing" compared to studies that do not psychologically engage a participant (Kitayama, 2002). This is likely to be particularly important for situations and behaviors that involve a lot of emotion. Emotions transform the way we experience the world, and in a "cool" state, it is not so easy to predict how one would behave in a "hot" state (Loewenstein & Schkade, 1999). Milgram (1974) provided a classic example. There is little chance that the behavior of subjects in Milgram's high-stakes, high-pressure experiment would have been predicted by anyone in a cold state filling out a questionnaire. In terms of more prosaic examples, anyone who has ever broken their diet after seeing a particularly delicious desert, said something in anger that they did not mean, or even bought too much at the grocery store because they were hungry, can attest to the simple truth that hot-state behavior is very different from, and cannot easily be predicted by, statements and behaviors made in a cold, detached state.

Even attitude questions that describe what might be a compelling scenario can only be so involving and even these often leave the situation underspecified. One can create the situation to be just right in the laboratory, but describing it on paper quickly becomes unwieldy. The bump and "asshole" experiment is an example:

"Imagine that you are in an unfamiliar building and you are walking along, minding your own business. You aren't in a hurry and no one is with you. Then someone who is about your size and who is wearing his baseball cap backwards starts to swagger down the hall, looking slightly miffed because you had earlier—through no fault of your own—interrupted his filing job. It's a tight hallway that you can both fit through if you each give a little, but as he walks down the hall, the man bumps into you firmly with his shoulder and calls you an "asshole" in a tone of voice that makes you think he isn't joking and he believes what he is saying. He definitely knows that he hit you, and though it's not clear if the bump was intentional, the "asshole" sure was. You know you weren't really at fault, and you may suspect that he knows this, too. Then he just keeps on walking without apologizing. He is neither stopping to directly confront you, nor is he running away. Rather, he intends to just walk on, like you're not going to do anything about it" [and so on].

In a live experiment, one can set up all the particulars to trigger the response in a way that is hard to do with underspecified questionnaire items.

Note here that the trade-offs between surveys and experiments perfectly complement each other. Surveys can ask about a wide array of situations but in a great many cases provide underwhelming evidence about differences in any particular situation. On the other hand, experiments can produce big differences in situations that we have constructed to be "just right." However, we cannot know whether the results from our "just right" situation generalize; and for that, questionnaires that allow us to ask about a variety of situations (without having to create them in the lab) can help a great deal.

Subquestion 3: "What Other Methods Can Provide Convergent Evidence?"

Beyond the Questionnaire and Lab Experiment

Cultural psychology is pluralistic in its methods, and it takes seriously the notion that converging evidence from diverse methodologies is the best type of support for an argument (Ellsworth & Gonzalez, 2003). A set of three attitude surveys will have weaknesses common to all attitude surveys; three lab experiments will have weaknesses common to all lab experiments; in general, three studies, all of the same methodology, are not as strong a support for a hypothesis as are three studies conducted with diverse methods. The weakness of any one methodology should be offset by the strengths of another.

As mentioned previously, cultural psychologists not only inherit all the weaknesses inherent in their home discipline but they also encounter new methodological problems that arise when they study a phenomenon across cultures. Hence, the standard appeal to all researchers to obtain converging evidence across methods is an even stronger imperative for cultural psychologists, who face extra methodological burdens. Thus, it is important to note that we are not and should not be restricting ourselves to operationalizing hypotheses using either paper-and-pencil questionnaires or experimental paradigms in traditional settings. Two additional techniques highlighted below are field "experiments" and the analyses of cultural products.

FIELD EXPERIMENTS

"Field experiments" is often used as a catch-all term for studies conducted outside the laboratory. Some of these are actually experiments in that they involve a manipulated variable (in addition to the nonmanipulated variable of culture). Others are more properly called "field studies," because there is no manipulated variable. These latter studies may involve experience sampling methods (in which participants are beeped at various intervals to complete questionnaires about their experiences as they go through the day; Diener & Tov, Chapter 28, this volume; Mesquita & Karasawa, 2002; Mesquita & Leu, Chapter 30, this volume) or they may involve (1) naturalistic observations in which the researcher has no role except to observe as discreetly as possible or (2) real-world reactions to events or stimuli that were actually created by the researcher (usually surreptitiously). An example of a naturalistic observation would be Levine and Norenzayan's (1999) study on the pace of life in different cultures, in which they measured the average walking speed in the business districts of various cities and also tracked the accuracy of public clocks. An example of a field study in which the researcher does surreptitiously provide a stimulus would be Levine, Martinez, Brase, and Sorensen's (1994) helping study, in which they had confederates in various downtown business districts pretend to be blind people needing help crossing the street, or had them walk along and drop their pens to see if passersby would pick them up, and so on. Such naturalistic and field observations have the advantage of capturing behavior outside the laboratory, where one can avoid artifacts that might result from impression management concerns, participant reactivity, stereotype threat, "good subject" effects, and so on. In addition, because they occur outside the confines of a university, such studies are likely to include samples broader than college student populations.

How much these studies mimic "typical" behavior in the real world often depends on how unusual a researcher's intervention is. For example, Feldman (1968) had researchers act as either natives or foreigners and (1) approach people in Boston, Paris, and Athens to ask them to mail a letter (relatively unusual); (2) take taxi rides to see whether the driver would cheat the passengers (normal); (3) ask for directions (normal), and so on. It is worth noting that the unusual task also had the most unusual results, being the only task in which Bostonians showed the greatest ingroup bias, preferentially mailing letters for fellow Americans rather than foreigners.

The field study can be conducted both with individuals as (unknowing) participants and also with organizations as unknowing participants. Salancik (1979) urged organizational researchers to conduct such experiments when he advocated "tickling" the organization to see how it responds and what this might reveal about the organization's true behavior as opposed to its stated mission. Putnam (1993) employed one such field study when he examined the effectiveness of various regional governments in Italy. A citizen (actually a confederate of the researcher) wrote to bureaucracies in each region with three requests. If no replies were received, follow-ups were made with phone calls and personal visits.

This "street-level" measure of responsiveness actually correlated reasonably well with other, very different measures of the regional governments' effectiveness; that is, bureaucratic performance in these field studies correlated significantly with the regional government's ability to pass budgets on time, enact reform legislation, and keep a stable cabinet. Because cultural psychologists can and should consider institutions, as well as individuals, as carriers and products of a culture, the field experiment that tickles an organization to investigate its goals (Salancik 1979), examines its responsiveness (Putnam, 1993), or finds out what is embraced versus what is stigmatized within that organization (Cohen & Nisbett, 1997) can be an important complement to traditional research paradigms that examine the individual as the unit of analysis.

Finally, there is an excellent opportunity to conduct field experiments as part of an intervention study. There are few researchers today who would re-create Sherif's (Sherif, Harvey, White, Wood, & Sherif, 1954) classic Robbers Cave experiments, setting up summer camps and introducing various manipulations. However, intervention programs—through public health campaigns, social work agencies, schools, political campaigns, and environmental programs—happen often in the world around us. These programs sometimes target a particular cultural group and other times focus on a general population, which may also have many cultural subgroups. The opportunity for cultural psychologists to propose some of these interventions, contribute to their design, or simply observe the results gives researchers a chance to study how different types of programs affect people from different cultures, how different chains of communication and influence get activated in different groups, how different cultural traditions either assimilate or accommodate new information and patterns of behavior, and so on. Such opportunities for field experiments (which use random assignment) or observational studies (which may have matched, if not randomly assigned, controls) give cultural psychologists an excellent chance to move into "the real world."

CULTURAL PRODUCTS

Cultural products exist out in the world. They are the laws that are passed, the advertising techniques that are used, the architectural

styles that are followed, the television programs that are made, the newspaper articles
that are written, the goods that are consumed,
the names that are given to people and places,
the words that are used, the dictionaries that
are compiled, the art that is produced, and so
on. All of these are within the purview of cultural psychologists. In fact, all of these have
been used by researchers investigating culture.
Morris and Peng (1994), and Lee, Hallahan,
and Herzog (1996) have analyzed Chinese and
American newspaper articles to examine the
causal explanations offered for various events.
To examine Asian versus U.S. differences in holistic versus analytic perception, Nisbett and
Masuda (2003) examined East Asian and
American artwork to show that background
rather than central figures were more emphasized in East Asian art; meanwhile, Miyamoto,
Nisbett, and Masuda (2006) photographed
and analyzed street scenes in Japanese and
American cities of various sizes to look at the
extent to which objects and buildings filled the
streetscapes and blended together or were
spaced apart so as to stand out and emphasize
their status as discrete entities. To examine the
extent to which regional cultures legitimated
violence, Baron and Straus (1989) examined
viewership of violent television shows, sub-
scription rates for violent magazines, per capita
production of college football players, and
state laws related to corporal and capital punishment. Similarly, Kelly (1999) examined
place and business names across the United
States and found that Southern states had more
violent names (e.g., Gun Point, FL; War, WV;
Battle Ax Church in Texas; or Gunsmoke Ken-
nels in Alabama). To examine persuasion in independent and interdependent cultures, Han
and Shavitt (1994) and Kim and Markus
(1999) examined Korean and American advertisements for their appeals (e.g., "The art of being unique" vs. "Sharing is beautiful"). To look
at the diminishing vocabulary of shame in
American culture, D. Cohen (2003) looked at
the prominence given to "shame" compared to
the prominence given to words such as *guilt*,
embarrassment, or *humiliation* in the dictionaries and thesauruses throughout various decades of the 19th and 20th centuries. Even the
many translations of the Bible reflected how
shame (relative to guilt) has been falling out of
religious vocabulary. The King James Bible
(1611) had a shame:guilt ratio of 5:1; at the
turn of the 20th century Bibles had a ratio of

3:1; and modern translations have now reduced the ratio to 1:1.

Some of these examples are aggregate behaviors; that is, they represent individual, "independent" decisions by people that are merely
summed together. Readership of violent magazines, for example, is an aggregate. Other such
products are more collective; that is, they require some form of collaboration to produce.
The streetscapes of Miyamoto et al. (2006) for
example, reflect the decisions of zoning boards;
architectural consultants; builders and business
owners who want to make their spaces appealing to customers, renters, landlords, and so on.
Such collective products are not the product of
any one person or group, but instead come out
of the push and pull of various forces within
the culture. (As is discussed in the "Interpretation" section, aggregates and collective
representations may differ in ways that can be
quite informative about the culture.)

Of course, the benefit that one gains examining a *collective* representation can also be a
drawback sometimes. With collective products,
for example, it can be difficult to determine
whether the product is created mostly as a
function of top-down choices made by the
elites of a culture or instead reflects a more
bottom-up process driven by preferences of the
mass public. One cannot pinpoint one particular causal agent, though one can potentially examine the processes by which such cultural
products are produced.

MORE QUALITATIVE METHODS

Research methods that are more qualitative are
not the subject of this chapter. However, such
methods can be a very valuable complement to
the more quantitative methods described here.
More qualitative studies can add richness,
depth, and vividness that more quantitative
studies cannot (LeVine, Chapter 2, this volume;
Miller, Fung, & Koven, Chapter 24, this volume). They add the *qualia* necessary for understanding what it is like to be an encultured human being (Shweder, 1997, Chapter 34, this
volume, and, in a different context, Nagel,
1974).

It should be noted that the distinction is really between studies that are "more qualitative" or "more quantitative." In qualitative
methods, there is usually some degree of
quantitativeness, because there is usually some
form of implicit counting. The statements that

"a few," "a minority of," "a majority of," "many," or "most" informants did a certain thing or felt a certain way reflects some sort of tally the researcher was making. Similarly, our quantitative methods require some sort of qualitative judgment whenever we, for example, analyze something a participant has written or said, in terms of the tone, degree of complexity, or affective content that it shows. (For that matter, on many self-report scales, we are asking participants to quantify their own judgment that they are, for example, feeling "mildly anxious" about something, "very satisfied with their life," "extremely in love" with their spouse, or "somewhat disgusted.")

In still other cases, we may quantitatively analyze data gleaned from the Standard Cross-Cultural Sample or Human Relations Area Files. Much of the research in these files was derived by anthropologists using qualitative methods or judgments. In this case, we are then using a quantitative method to aggregate qualitative data.

Summary

In summary, in addition to all the standard operationalization issues one must worry about, the cultural psychologist must construct variables that are interpretable and convincingly operationalize a construct when seen through (at least) two different cultural lenses. Thus, the cultural psychologist faces the additional problem of "translation," broadly defined to include language, behaviors, situations, reference groups, and so on. Cultural psychologists do have one advantage over their more discipline-bound colleagues, however. The field's youth and generally pluralistic outlook should foster a pluralism in methods as well. All methods have their individual weaknesses. However, with the field's pluralistic acceptance of diverse methodologies, cultural psychologists are given a full toolkit of techniques that can be used for both initial exploratory work and for producing the sort of convergent evidence across methodologies that makes for convincing social science arguments.

INTERPRETATION

Careful consideration of causal issues, sampling, and operationalization should lessen (but not eliminate) the difficulties of interpreta-

tion after the data are collected. There are certain inevitable problems that we encounter, and some of these were discussed earlier. However, there are other interpretational issues that arise, independent of the artifacts from any one study. Two issues considered below involve (1) how we interpret similarities and differences between cultures, and (2) how we interpret data that do not converge.

Subquestion 1: "Am I Really Understanding What Is Similar and What Is Different in the Cultures?"

"Quantifying" Similarities and Differences

The issue of similarities and differences between cultures occurs on multiple levels. At one level, the issue of heterogeneity within cultures can make differences between cultures look small in comparison. Various effect size measures can be employed to look at how "big" a cultural difference is; one of these, Cohen's d is the ratio of the difference in the means to the standard deviation (SD) within (pooled). This d can also be translated into an "intuitively compelling and meaningful" u_1, the percent of "the area covered by both populations combined that is not overlapped" (Cohen, 1988, p. 21). At a "small" d of .2, u_1 is 15%; at a "medium" d of .5 (which Cohen says may be "conceived of as one large enough to be visible to the naked eye"—that is, noticeable "in the course of normal experience"), u_1 is 33%; at a "large" d of .8, u_1 is 47% (pp. 22, 26).

Under this interpretation, d and u_1 may be considered as possible quantitative indices of similarities and differences between cultures. However, d (and u_1) are indicators of the size of the differences, *not* their importance. First, big differences can be trivial (as an absurd example, there is probably a culture effect such that Italians like eating pizza more than Saudi Arabians do, and the effect size is probably large here). Conversely, small and moderate effects may be quite important for any number of reasons: (1) Small differences at the center of the distribution can lead to large differences in the tails of the distributions (e.g., men may be somewhat more aggressive than women, on average, but men are tremendously more likely than women to be mass murderers); (2) small differences may have huge practical consequences. (For example, a shift of 5 percentage points would change who won the popular vote in many presidential elections, yet 5 percentage points translates to only one-tenth of a standard deviation for an evenly divided electorate. A 60-40 political "landslide" that might signal a major political realignment would translate to a difference of only four-tenths of a standard deviation; Ross & Nisbett, 1991); (3) small differences may become large differences when they accumulate over time. This is important when differences grow exponentially, as in compounding investments, in which total return is a function of initial investment multiplied by $(1 + r)^n$, where r is the rate of return and n is the number of compounding periods. And it is also true when accumulation involves only increasing the magnitude of the raw numbers involved, as in, for example, baseball. Following Abelson (1985), the correlation between a baseball player's batting average and success on any given trip to the plate is .05, equivalent to a d of .1. What separates Hall-of-Famers from benchwarmers is that differences accumulate over the course of a season or career; and (4) small and moderate differences *may* have important theoretical implications. (For example, the average effect size of the mere exposure effect is somewhere around a d of .4; the average effect for rewards undermining intrinsic motivation is around a d of .35; the average effect sizes for the relation between personality and various measures of heart functioning are in the $d = .2–.4$ range; Bornstein, 1989; Deci, Koestner, & Ryan, 1999; Lyness, 1993; Miller, Smith, Turner, Guijarro, & Hallet, 1996.) Similarities and differences between cultures may thus be quantified, but they cannot be interpreted without thinking about either practical or theoretical importance.

Controls and Boundaries

A second issue that arises in thinking about similarities and differences has to do with the importance of both boundary conditions and comparison conditions. Because of various response bias effects, a culture main effect may be difficult to interpret by itself. For example, in cases when one is measuring performance on some test, it is good to have definable parts of the test where one expects a cultural difference, and definable parts of the test where one either does not expect such a difference or expects a reversal. Thus, for example, if one expects culture A to show better memory than culture B for social stimuli, it is helpful to show that there are no differences (or a reversal) for

nonsocial stimuli. If culture A does better than culture B for social stimuli but there is no comparison condition of nonsocial stimuli, one cannot rule out the possibility that culture A simply took the task more seriously.

In this case, a comparison condition or comparison variable attempts to rule out the possibility of response biases that may create artifacts. In other cases, a comparison condition is theoretically meaningful because it puts boundary conditions on the phenomenon one is studying. Thus, for example, if a researcher wants to talk about culture A as a culture of honor, in which people are primed to be aggressive after being insulted, it is also helpful to have a control condition in which there is no affront and, hence, no greater readiness for aggression in culture A. The control condition aids in circumscribing the phenomena to honor-related infractions and helps rule out the explanation that culture A is simply a chronically aggressive culture across the board. Finally, some researchers may also choose to run control conditions that are expected to produce similarities that serve as an "anchor" in the way we think about the two cultures, preventing readers from drifting off into an extreme relativism.

Unfortunately, going for a culture × condition interaction (rather than simply a culture main effect) entails a large loss in power when one does not expect a crossover interaction. Think, for example, of a 2 (culture) × 2 (control vs. experimental condition) design in which one predicts a difference in the experimental condition and no difference in the control condition. Suppose that, as expected, there is a simple effect difference between the two cultural groups in the experimental condition ($t_1 = 2$, $p < .05$). Suppose further that, as expected, there is no simple effect difference between groups in the control condition ($t_2 = 0$, $p > .99$). *Assuming that the same pooled error term is used* across all of the t-tests, the t for the interaction term will be ($t_1 - t_2$) divided by the square root of 2. (In this case, where $t_1 = 2$ and $t_2 = 0$, the interaction $t = (2 - 0)/($square root of 2$) = 1.4$, $p > .15$) (Abelson, 1995). The control condition has already required the experimenter to double the n; but in addition, to make up for the loss in power, the experimenter will have to run many more participants than this to have a decent chance of detecting the interaction. (Of course, using Abelson's rule, if the control condition goes the *opposite* way to that of the experimental condition and the control condition difference is at least 42% as big as the experimental difference, there is a gain of power.) Designing studies in terms of interaction effects requires more thinking beforehand about appropriate comparison or boundary conditions, and it often requires more time and money to run more participants. However, the clarity such conditions can provide in interpretation can be well worth it.

The Necker Cube of Culture

A third issue about similarities and differences is more abstract, but it goes to the heart of what the cultural psychology field is or will become. That is, to the extent that cultural psychology can discuss both similarities and differences across cultures, it will be a richer field than if it can discuss only differences (see also Norenzayan & Heine, 2005; Konner, Chapter 4, this volume).

Cultural differences are embedded within similarities, and cultural similarities are embedded within differences. Depending on how we look at it, the similarities can look greater or the differences can look greater. A rich cultural psychology will force us to look at the "Necker Cube" of culture. Like the surfaces of the Necker cube, what pops out at us in our understanding of cultures will shift back and forth in terms of the ways the cultures are similar at one level and different at another. The implication is that cultural psychologists may design their research programs to be strong on both *integration* and *differentiation*. Phenomena that are different on the surface may have a similarity in terms of their deeper structure, and cultures that are similar on the surface may be quite different in their deeper structure. Two examples—one derived directly from empirical work, the other loosely derived from it—help to illustrate the point.

Starting in the 1990s, Heine and Lehman (1995, 1997a, 1997b, 1999; Heine, Takata, & Lehman, 2000; Heine, Kitayama, & Lehman, 2001; Heine, 2005, Chapter 29, this volume) began to publish an astonishing line of research, showing that some very robust self-enhancing biases did not seem to operate in Japan. One of their findings involved the "spread of alternatives" paradigm from cognitive dissonance research, in which participants make a choice and are then shown to rationalize that choice as a way to protect their self-esteem.

Heine and Lehman showed that this classic effect does not hold for the Japanese, presumably because dissonance effects, like other self-enhancing biases, did not operate in this population (Heine, Lehman, Markus, & Kitayama, 1999).

Two lines of research qualified Heine and Lehman's finding in important ways, however. In one, Hoshino-Browne et al. (2005) replicated the Heine and Lehman (1997a) result, showing that Asian Canadian participants (unlike their European Canadian counterparts) showed no rationalization effect when they made a choice for themselves. However, they also ran another condition in which participants were asked about a close friend's preferences, then had to choose a gift for this friend. In this condition, the findings reversed: The European Canadians showed no dissonance effect, whereas the Asian Canadians now began to rationalize their choice. Thus, it was not that dissonance phenomena existed in one culture but not another. Rather, both Asian Canadians and European Canadians rationalized to protect the self; however, the selves they were protecting were very different. The European Canadians were protecting the competent, rational, independent self that knows what it wants and goes out and gets it. The Asian Canadians were protecting the relational, interdependent self that is sensitive to other people and attends to their preferences. To make their point stronger, Hoshino-Browne et al. (2005) showed that a traditional self-affirmation task (which bolsters the self and typically wipes out the need to rationalize for European Americans) had no effect on Asian Canadians. Instead, they showed that only a new self-affirmation task that bolstered the interdependent self and shared values could wipe out dissonance effects for Asian Canadians.

In a separate but related line of work, Kitayama Snibbe, Markus, and Suzuki (2004; Kitayama, Duffy, & Uchida, Chapter 6, this volume) explored the idea that choices may threaten a person's self in very different ways in Japanese and American culture: A bad choice may threaten an American independent self, because it means that the self is not competent or efficacious. A bad choice may threaten a Japanese interdependent self, because others may then think of the person as foolish. Japanese may be relatively free of the independent threat when they make a choice but feel fully the interdependent threat when they make a decision. In several studies, Kitayama and colleagues (2004) replicated the Heine and Lehman (1997a) effect, showing no dissonance effects for Japanese. However, when Japanese participants were first forced to think about self-relevant others (e.g., by asking participants about what the average student's preferences would be), dissonance effects appeared in full force. Even putting participants in front of a poster that showed schematic line drawings of faces was enough to prime such interdependence concerns and produce dissonance effects for the Japanese. Like Hoshino-Browne et al. (2005), Kitayama et al. (2004) showed that dissonance occurred in the two cultures, but it was a very different kind of dissonance, invoking different threats to a different kind of self. Neither the Hoshino-Browne et al. (2005) nor the Kitayama et al. (2004) papers are a rejection of Heine and Lehman's (1997a) finding. They extended the finding by integrating (showing similar processes of rationalization following self-threat) and differentiating (showing how such threats and rationalizations were quite different for the two groups) to give a richer picture of self-threat, rationalization, and choice in the two cultures.

A different line of research pursued by Shweder, Rozin, Haidt, Miller and colleagues is not as tightly bound to particular studies, but provides another example of work that integrates and differentiates (Rozin, Lowery, Imada, & Haidt, 1999; Shweder, Much, Mahapatra, & Park, 1997). Shweder and colleagues developed a rich account of the "Big Three" of morality, showing how various ethical breaches cluster into events that violate principles of autonomy, community, or divinity (see also Haidt, Koller, & Dias, 1993; Miller, Chapter 19, this volume; Morelli & Rothbaum, Chapter 20, this volume; Rozin, Chapter 16, this volume). These three "ethical discourses" are found in the United States and India. However, the countries differ in which ones get foregrounded and which get backgrounded: In the United States, concerns with autonomy are foregrounded, whereas in India community and divinity are foregrounded.

Shweder and colleagues (1993) suggest *karma* as an "overarching moral metaphor" for South Asian morality, where karma is seen as a theory of personal responsibility. They then describe how the overarching concept of karma and the three subcategories of community, autonomy, and divinity also connect to American notions of personal responsibility,

communitarian concerns (e.g., secondhand smoke), the "moralization" of unhealthy behaviors as bad or disgusting, and an emergent American "neo-Puritanism" (Rozin, 1999; Shweder, 1993). The collective body of work is complex in the way it illuminates both the underlying similarities and differences in U.S. and Indian explanations of morality and suffering. As in the work by Hoshino et al. (2005) and Kitayama et al. (2004), the cultural analysis is like a Necker cube: Whether it is the differences or the similarities that strike us depends on the angle from which we are looking at the phenomena.

Subquestion 2: "What Happens If My Data Do Not Converge?"

The answer to methodological problems lies in thinking through our theories and collecting convergent evidence from multiple empirical methods. This answer is fine. However, what happens when the data do not converge? That is, what happens when the data from one methodology point to a different conclusion than the data from another methodology? We need to investigate whether this divergence is a result of artifacts or whether it is telling us something quite meaningful, and if so, what?

Artifacts

The first step involves thinking about and investigating possible methodological artifacts in our data and possible differences introduced by the use of different sampling techniques in different studies. In addition to any of the issues raised previously, culture researchers may have to watch out for other methodological artifacts because of the types of data with which we sometimes work. For example, statistical artifacts arise from working with aggregate data and grouped data. A standard example of *Simpson's paradox* is that shoe size is correlated with income. There may be no relationship between shoe size and income when considering just the men, and no relationship when considering just the women. However, when they are put together, there is a relationship between shoe size and income, because men, on average, have higher incomes and bigger feet. Consider a potential cultural example: There may be a negative relationship between an extended family support system and personal happiness. Within individualist cultures, more family support may mean more happiness; within collectivist cultures, the same may be true. However, when the cultures are put together, the relationship between support systems and happiness reverses, because collectivist cultures tend to have more family support and are on average less happy than individualist cultures.

When working with aggregate data, a researcher needs to be cautious of the *ecological fallacy*, in which one generalizes from aggregate-level data to individual processes. As a simple example, suppose that U.S. states with high numbers of educated people also had high rates of violent crime. The "generalization" from the aggregate level to the individual level would be that more education makes people more violent. The opposite is true, though: More education makes people less violent. It is just that states with higher numbers of educated people tend to have more urban areas, and more urban areas tend to have more violence.

Yet another problem arises when we try to extrapolate from within-group differences to between-group differences. This was famously on display in discussions of Herrnstein and Murray's (1994) *The Bell Curve*. In very rough form, the reasoning was as follows: We know that intelligence is highly heritable (i.e., genetic), and we know that there are differences on IQ tests between European Americans and African Americans. Therefore, the difference in IQ scores between European Americans and African Americans must be genetic. To illustrate the potential problems in going from a within-group explanation to a between-group explanation, Feldman (cited in Cavalli-Sforza and Cavalli-Sforza, 1995, p. 274) proposes this parallel example. Take two groups of 50 white Americans. We know that skin color is highly heritable, and this will be true within each of the two groups. Now send one group to a sunny place (Miami) and the other to a cloudy place (Champaign–Urbana) for the next year. Within each group, genetics will still predict skin tone, but the difference between groups is now the result of climate, not genetics. A cultural example follows: Suppose that more education predicts greater support for gender equality in both the United States and Denmark. One cannot then infer that Danes are more egalitarian because they tend to be better educated than Americans. In fact, Danes are not better educated; the powerful within-group

variable of education has no role in explaining the between-group difference.

These problems, which all stem from the "correlation is not causation" problem, are easy enough to spot when they are as obvious as the examples just given. However, many problems in research are much more subtle, and investigators need to be wary of these statistical artifacts in designing their studies and interpreting their data.

Does the Nonconvergence Represent a Real Cultural Phenomena?

Suppose, however, that no obvious methodological issues or statistical artifacts explain nonconvergent data. Obviously, we need to collect more data, but in what direction do we go? To decide this, we have two choices. We can believe either our data or our theory. (Here we run into an actor–observer problem. Einstein's dictum was that, as researchers, we tend to believe our theories more than our data. However, others tend to believe our data and not our theories: "No one but a theorist believes his theory; everyone puts faith in a laboratory result but the experimenter himself" [Galison, 2004, p. 69].) If one still believes the theory, then the next study should be designed to test the hypothesis in a new way and one hopes, provide clear results and also reconcile any conflicts.

Suppose, however, that one believes the data. There may be very good reasons for the conflicting results in studies, because the story may be more complex than originally thought. The conflicting results may, in fact, tell us something quite important about the cultural phenomena we are studying. Five very different examples hint at the wealth of possibilities:

1. A researcher finds that public behavior and cultural products tend to support a cultural norm *X*. However, in private attitude surveys, people do not seem to support norm *X*, and in fact support norm *Y*. It could be that for reasons previously discussed, attitude surveys just provide weaker results than analyses of behavior and collective representation. However, another possibility proposed by Miller and Prentice (1994) is that people may be in a state of "pluralistic ignorance." Everyone in a culture may be against norm *X* but may think that everyone else supports norm *X*. As a consequence, people behave in ways consistent

with the norm, even when no one privately believes it. Miller and Prentice (1994, Miller, 1999; see also Sears & Funk, 1990) have provided examples of this involving norms about drinking, racial attitudes, and other topics, and Kuran (1995) has proposed pluralistic ignorance as one of the forces that sustained communism in Eastern Europe, apartheid in South Africa, and the caste system in India for so long.

2. As a variation of this, a researcher finds that attitudinal and behavioral data both support norm X, but the behavioral data are much stronger. Again, this could be because our attitude measures are simply weaker. However, there could be another, more important reason, namely, that many behaviors are *social* behaviors. *They necessarily involve other people and require their participation*, meaning that there will not be a simple linear relationship between a person's internal predispositions and the actions he or she produces.

Take a hypothetical example of two cultures that differ in the proportion of people who have an aggressive mind-set. Suppose that in Culture A 6% of the people have such a mind-set, whereas culture B has 2% of such people. Suppose further that interpersonal interactions follow something like an "it takes two to tango" rule (Daly & Wilson, 1988). In culture B, for any single encounter, there is a .04% chance that aggressive people will randomly meet and a fight will ensue. For culture A, however, there is a .36% chance of such people meeting and fighting. The three to one difference in attitudes has become a 9 to 1 difference in behavior, because the "two to tango" rule means that differences in behavior go up as a function of the square of the difference in attitude.

This effect is magnified further for any behavior that requires the meeting of three like minds. In this case, the 3 to 1 difference in attitudes becomes a 27 to 1 difference in behavior. More generally, the difference in behavior will go up as a function of d^n, where d is the ratio of the difference in attitudes, and n is the number of people of similar mind-sets that need to meet to produce the behavior.

The odds become further altered if one makes two reasonable assumptions: (1) that in various population landscapes people interact with similar others at rates either greater or less than what would be expected by chance alone, and (2) that people are not single-minded in their approaches (e.g., "always act aggressively") but have a more complex set of decision rules that cover contingencies and give flexibility (e.g., "If I encounter a person of type X, then do A. If I encounter a person of type Y, then do B. If I encounter a person of type Z, then do C," and so on). In more complicated cases like these, game theoretical models and computer simulations can be of great help in thinking through how underlying distributions of attitudes in a population become translated into differences in behavior. The more general point for present purposes, however, is that differences between cultures in internal predispositions do not necessarily produce differences in behavior of the same magnitude, because social behaviors are some function of person A's disposition, person B's disposition, *and their interaction*.

3. A researcher conducts interviews and finds that all the people live in perpetual fear of their neighbors making violence against them. However, when she examines the public records, she finds that there has never been any violence in the community. This "paradox" is apparently not a terribly uncommon finding. The anthropologist Elizabeth Colson (1975, p. 37) writes:

> We listen to informants' fears and to their tales of violence . . . and we diagnose a world of warring factions, of feud, of frequent acts of aggression. . . . We look around us, however, and we find people apparently behaving with kindness, generosity, and forbearance, avoiding disputes and sharing resources, tolerant of each other's foibles. What we may miss is the connection between the two sets of social facts: the beliefs are related to the behavior. . . . It should therefore be no surprise to us if some people live in what appears to be a Rousseauian paradise because they take a Hobbesian view of their situation: they walk softly because they believe it necessary not to offend others whom they regard as dangerous. (See also Adams, 2005; D. Cohen et al., 1999; Knauft, 1985; Fiske, Kitayama, Markus, & Nisbett, 1998.)

If one had done only the analysis of records or observed only the quotidian practices in the community, one might conclude the culture was a Rousseauian paradise. If one had done only the interviews, one might conclude it was a Hobbesian battleground. Neither results of interviews nor analysis of records is completely true, and both are an essential part of the story.

4. A researcher finds large cultural differences when examining laws and other collective products. However, when he examines individual behavior and attitudes, he finds that the differences are far less extreme. Perhaps then the big differences in collective products result from polarization effects that occur when groups form. Groups may become more extreme than the individuals in them because, during collective decision making processes, (a) people may engage in posturing to line up with a perceived cultural ideal (see item 1); (b) a particularly persuasive argument may carry the day during group discussions (Brown, 1965); or (c) the shared information to which all group members have access gets discussed far more often and gets far more weight than idiosyncratic information that individuals may possess (Stasser & Titus, 1985).

5. A researcher employs three different measures of a cultural trait X. All measures are face valid, yet none of the measures correlate with each other. It is possible that at least one of the measures is not in fact valid, and it is possible that the underlying theme X lies more in the researcher's mind than in cultural "reality."

However, consider another way of thinking about the cultural phenomenon. One crude metaphor for culture is culture as "a bag of tricks," or less pejoratively, as a "tool kit." There is no reason that all the tools or all the tricks related to cultural theme X have to be distributed equally among all members of the population. Some members of the culture have tool A, some have tool B, and some have tool C. This parallels a distinction Linton (1936) made about "core" cultural elements distributed to all cultural members and "specialized" elements that are distributed to different subgroups of the population. It also parallels the distributional approach to culture that, for example, Medin and Atran (2004; Medin et al., Chapter 25, this volume) take when they look for patterns of agreement among members of a culture or subculture.

Glazer (1957) discussed a related point in talking about the Jewish religion as a religion of practices rather than a religion of dogma (see also Dimont, 1978). Judaism does not have a central, unifying dogma; it does not have a central authority, and it emphasizes behaviors rather than beliefs (A. Cohen, Siegel, & Rozin, 2003). Instead of a central doctrine, there are loosely related practices and traditions. In modern secular society, Jews pick and

choose from among these traditions and practices (Glazer, 1957; also D. Cohen, 2007). Some Jews derive religious meaning by keeping kosher; others are observant by sending their children to Hebrew School; still others observe by saying daily prayers, and so on. (In addition, Glazer [1957, p. 142] points out that some derive religious meaning from acts that may not be overtly religious, such as "liking Yiddish jokes, supporting Israel, raising money for North African Jews, and preferring certain kinds of food"). If one were to do a factor analysis of practices and behaviors that are valid reflections of people's various ways of being Jewish, there might not be a massively dominant, tightly clustered factor that one could call "Jewish observancy."

The above merely represent five examples that are nonartifactual explanations for results that do not converge. There are many others that point to potentially interesting cultural phenomena. A researcher interested in such phenomena can devise follow-up studies to test his or her post hoc explanation for the current pattern of divergent data.

Summary

In summary, the interpretational issues facing cultural psychologists are many. The use of multiple methods makes for a convincing argument when the data converge across them. However, the data do not always converge. At that point, the researcher needs to figure out whether this lack of convergence is artifactual, or whether it is a hint that will lead to real, interesting, and important phenomena yet to be discovered.

A coherent social science explanation will also be strong in the way it integrates and differentiates. The researcher staring at the Necker cube of culture will discover how similarities are embedded within differences, and how differences are embedded within similarities. This similarity–difference perspective makes our field richer scientifically.

On Science, Poetry, and Policy

The similarity–difference perspective is also important for a very different reason. T. S. Eliot (1998) once wrote that good poetry makes the unfamiliar familiar and the familiar unfamiliar.[12] Melford Spiro (1990) appropriated this observation to describe what anthropology was about. To make the unfamiliar familiar and the familiar unfamiliar by embedding differences within similarities and similarities within differences is good poetry. It is good science. And it is good policy. Ultimately, this familiar–unfamiliar, similarity–difference approach is what may prevent cultural psychology from degenerating into cultural stereotyping, or from being used as such. First, to the extent that we as a society come to see another group's practices as similar to our own, we lessen the distance between us and the Other.

Second, to the extent that cultural psychology encourages people to step outside their own frames of reference, we soften our judgments of the Other. Cultural differences are real, and they will be noticed. (J. Cohen, 1988, defines a medium effect size as "visible to the naked eye" and many of our effect sizes are much larger than this). Given then that the differences will be noticed, how does one interpret them?

One can either (1) view the differences in terms of the dominant discourse, in which case comparisons with the Other are likely to be invidious, or (2) one can approach the difference by assuming (at least initially) that the difference reflects some meaningful, coherent way of seeing the world that is different from one's own. Cultural psychology is about figuring out what those meaningful, coherent ways of seeing the world might be.

To deny that differences exist is to either assume that one's own cultural values are universal (or will be universal, as soon as those other people "come around"). And to deny that the differences will be noticed is to assume that the world's citizens are so dumb that they will never notice these differences that are "visible to the naked eye" in our increasingly pluralistic societies and interconnected world. Ultimately, one views differences through the prism of the dominant discourse, or one tries to study and understand the way other ways of seeing the world can be sensible, cogent, and meaningful. Cultural psychology does *not* imply a stance of moral relativism. (It does not imply that there are no moral standards; setting aside morality, it does not even imply that all cultural patterns are adaptive [see the section on Causation].) It does, however, imply a certain humility and urges us not to rush into either actions or judgments propelled by our own certitude (Fish, 2005; Shweder, 2003; Will, 2004b, 2005).

CONCLUSION

Researchers confront choices, because every method has its trade-offs. The methods themselves have assumptions built into them about what culture is. For example, they contain assumptions about how much we conceive of culture as being in the person versus "out there"; the methods contain assumptions about how readily cultural rules can be articulated, about what aggregates and collective products represent, and so on. Indeed, we make many assumptions by even thinking that a given cultural issue can be studied in some meaningful, tractable way.

As cultural researchers, we inherit all the problems of the disciplines in which we were trained, plus those that come with any attempt to understand, operationalize, sample, or interpret across cultures. We may face serious challenges, but working in our field also gives us some serious advantages. Cultural psychology is pluralistic in its methods, so its outlook is not limited by the use of a single paradigm or methodology. There is not yet, and I hope there never will be, a dogma to which cultural psychologists must adhere. And we are willing to listen to other fields, even if they are not (yet) willing to listen to us.

Finally, there is still plenty of "low-hanging fruit" for us to pick. Substantively, there are whole areas of the world yet to be explored by cultural psychologists, and a huge range of topics yet to be studied. Methodologically, the field is open for the discovery of new techniques and innovative ways of thinking about problems. The challenges we face and the opportunities we have are two sides of the same coin. If cultural psychologists have yet to find good answers to some of our methodological issues, it is because the field is still young. However, this same youth makes our field open, pluralistic, and full of opportunities.

NOTES

1. *Mind-sets* is used as a catch-all term: The prime may be doing a number of things, including activating scripts, making certain framings of a situation more accessible, activating different parts of the self-concept, and so on.

2. A mediational analysis does not have to involve a *chronic* individual difference; a mediation variable can also be a measurement of a temporary state or process (Smith & Bond, 2003). For an interesting and thought-

ful critique of mediation, see Spencer, Zanna, and Fong (2005), who advocate *manipulating* variables and finding moderators, rather than trying to measure mediators.

3. There is essentially a Zeno's paradox of mediation; that is, for any given causal connection, one can ask "What mediates this connection?" Thus, C may mediate the relation between A and B. One can then ask, "What mediates the connection between A and C (or B and C)?" If D mediates the connection between A and C, one can then ask "What mediates the connection between A and D (or between D and C)?" and so on. The example in the text assumes that this problem has been temporarily solved by temporarily accepting an individualistic or collectivistic orientation as being at an appropriate level of explanation.

4. More qualitative research would probably flesh out these prototypical situations, elaborate on scripts and rituals that accompany them, and describe them in terms of *practices*. Such work would likely take place outside the lab.

5. One might consider any difference between two cultural groups as definitionally a "cultural" difference. However, this chapter sticks with more conventional notions that there would be some differences that one would not want to call "cultural," and thus, there is a continuum of differences that run from "more cultural" to "less cultural."

6. If one were primarily focusing one's study on the relationship between crop volatility and fatalism, one might want to gather data from multiple countries that differed widely in the volatility of the crops they grew. However, for the sake of this example, pretend that for reasons discussed in the section on causation, the researcher wanted to focus in on these two cultures.

7. This sort of priming (the priming of cultural icons) and the priming described in the section on social cognitive approaches to culture are similar, in that they both demonstrate how flexible people can be in applying cultural schemas. However, the two types of priming lead to different sorts of inferences. Social cognitive priming is aimed at showing how a specific mind-set, implicit theory, or belief causes a behavior. In contrast, bicultural priming generally does *not* pinpoint a specific mind-set. Instead, bicultural priming tries to activate a very general mind-set—the worldview of "being Chinese" or "being American" for Chinese Americans, for example.

Social-cognitive priming and cultural icon priming may elicit either prime main effects or prime × culture of participant interactions. Such prime × culture interactions usually come in one of two forms. One might be called a *potentiating* prime and the other a *compensatory* prime. The logic behind a compensatory prime is that the prime will temporarily make accessible in culture A what is chronically accessible in culture B. Thus, for example, Heine et al. (2001) showed that priming European Americans with an incremental theory of ability makes them persist more on tasks, whereas it has no effect on Asians, who presumably already hold an incre-

mental theory as their default, chronically accessible theory. A *potentiating* prime, on the other hand, works on a very different principle, evoking a response from participants who are already "prepared" for the prime. Thus, Leung and Cohen (2007) found that an honor prime elicited the relevant honorable behaviors only among participants who were from cultures of honor (Southerners and Latinos). It did not have this effect for participants from other groups. The *potentiating* prime draws forth the prepared response from the honor group, but it has no effect on the other groups, because one cannot prime—or cannot *easily* prime—what is not there.

The cultural icon priming of Hong et al. (2000) follows the logic of a potentiating prime. A Chinese icon may draw forth a more "Chinese" response from a bicultural Asian American or Hong Kong resident, but it presumably would have little effect on a European American, who has no Asian identity to evoke (but cf. Bargh, Chen, & Burrows, 1996; Dijksterhuis & van Knippenberg, 1998; Kwan, 2007).

The compensatory versus potentiating prime distinction may be conceptually useful. However, some practical issues make the distinction blurry. Whether a prime potentiates a response depends not only on (1) how "prepared" the participants are with the accessible and relevant scripts and schemas but also on (2) how powerful the prime is. Thus, a relatively weak prime (e.g., a scrambled sentence task with words like *revenge* and *payback*) may act as a potentiating prime, calling forth a response only among those well prepared for a revenge mind-set. On the other hand, a 6-hour filmfest of revenge clips from John Wayne westerns, Charles Bronson *Death Wish* films, and the Arnold Schwarzenegger *Terminator* series may produce either a priming main effect (that shifts everyone) or a compensatory prime effect (if one group is already at ceiling). Because of cases like this, the logic of a potentiating prime ("One cannot prime what isn't there") might be modified to "One cannot easily prime what is not easily accessible."

8. For discussion of operationalization issues relevant to biological measures, see also Chiao and Ambady, Chapter 9; Levenson, Soto, and Pole, Chapter 32, both this volume; Tsai, Levenson, and McCoy, 2006.

9. Clinton explained the interpretation of "is" when talking about why he denied having sexual relations with a White House intern. "It depends on what the meaning of the word *is* is. . . . If *is* means is and never has been . . . that is one thing. . . . Now, if someone had asked me on that day, are you having any kind of sexual relations . . . that is, asked me a question in the present tense, I would have said no. And it would have been completely true" (Starr, 1998, footnote 1128). (Fortunately, the debate over whether Clinton lied never got to the point about whether *is* meant "Are you having sexual relations this very second?" However, further debate did center on the terms "sex" and "sexual relations," concerning what acts were covered under these expressions.)

10. The point can be taken too far. Sociologist Stanley Presser tells the story of his meetings with the famous survey sampling expert Leslie Kish. "How are you doing?" Presser would ask. "Compared to whom?" Kish would reply (MacFarquahar, 2004).

11. Thorough debriefings are especially important in culture research. Not only do some situations fail to translate but so also may the entire "frame" of the study—the conducting of a psychological experiment (Gintis, 2005). The "frame" of most laboratory psychology experiments is well understood by introductory psychology students: One goes to a room and performs some relatively innocuous task (possibly related to the experimental cover story, possibly not). In return, the experimenter gives you something of value that is relatively meaningless to him or her (either course credits or money from some deep pockets somewhere).

Henrich et al. (2001) found that this is not a universal script when they had members of various small-scale societies play economic games. (In one case, a respondent tried to attack the experimenter with a knife "because she thought he was an evil magician"; in another case, a rich herder in Mongolia refused to play because he did not want to take money away from the impoverished graduate student conducting the study; Gintis, 2005, personal communication, 2005).

12. Eliot's (1998, p. 108) exact quote was that good poetry makes "the familiar strange and the strange familiar," a notion he attributed to Coleridge.

REFERENCES

Abelson, R. (1985). A variance explanation paradox. *Psychological Bulletin, 97,* 128–132.

Abelson, R. (1995). *Statistics as principled argument.* Hillsdale, NJ: Erlbaum.

Adams, G. (2005). The cultural grounding of personal relationship: Enemyship in North American and West African worlds. *Journal of Personality and Social Psychology, 88,* 948–968.

Adams, G., & Markus, H. (2004). Toward a conception of culture suitable for a social psychology of culture. In M. Schaller & C. Crandall (Eds.), *The psychological foundations of culture* (pp. 335–360). Mahwah, NJ: Erlbaum.

Asch, S. (1987). *Social psychology.* New York: Oxford University Press. (Original work published in 1952)

Au, T. K. (1983). Chinese and English counterfactuals. *Cognition, 15,* 155–187.

Au, T. K. (1984). Counterfactuals: In reply to Alfred Bloom. *Cognition, 17,* 289–302.

Bargh, J., Chen, M., & Burrows, L. (1996). Automaticity of social behavior: Direct effects of trait construct and stereotype activation on action. *Journal of Personality and Social Psychology, 71,* 230–244.

Baron, L., & Straus, M. (1989). *Four theories of rape in American society.* New Haven, CT: Yale University Press.

Berry, J. (1979). A cultural ecology of social behavior. In L. Berkowitz (Ed.), *Advances in Experimental Social Psychology* (Vol. 12, pp. 177–206). New York: Academic Press.

Berry, J., Poortinga, Y., & Pandey, J. (1997). *Handbook of cross-cultural psychology.* Boston: Allyn & Bacon.

Blass, T. (2004). *The man who shocked the world.* New York: Basic Books.

Bloom, A. H. (1981). *The linguistic shaping of thought.* Hillsdale, NJ: Erlbaum.

Bloom, A. H. (1984). Caution—the words you use may affect what you say. *Cognition, 17,* 275–287.

Bond, M. H. (2002). Reclaiming the individual from Hofstede's ecological analysis—A 20-year odyssey: Comment on Oyserman et al. (2002). *Psychological Bulletin, 128,* 73–77.

Bornstein, R. (1989). Exposure and affect. *Psychological Bulletin, 106,* 265–289.

Braudel, F. (1980). *On history.* Chicago: University of Chicago Press.

Brown, R. (1965). *Social psychology.* New York: Free Press.

Cavalli-Sforza, L., & Cavalli-Sforza, F. (1995). *The great human diasporas.* Reading, MA: Perseus.

Cohen, A., Siegel, J., & Rozin, P. (2003). Faith versus practice. *European Journal of Social Psychology, 33,* 287–295.

Cohen, D. (2001). Cultural variation. *Psychological Bulletin, 127,* 451–471.

Cohen, D. (2003). The American national conversation about (everything but) shame. *Social Research, 70,* 1075–1108.

Cohen, D. (2005). *Tradition's thread.* Unpublished manuscript, University of Illinois, Urbana–Champaign.

Cohen, D., Hoshino-Browne, E., & Leung, A. (2007). Culture and the structure of personal experience: Insider and outsider phenomonologies of the self and social world. In M. Zanna (Ed.), *Advances in experimental social psychology* (pp. 1–67). San Diego: Academic Press.

Cohen, D., & Nisbett, R. E. (1994). Self-protection and the culture of honor. *Personality and Social Psychology Bulletin, 20,* 551–567.

Cohen, D., & Nisbett, R. E. (1997). Field experiments examining the culture of honor. *Personality and Social Psychology Bulletin, 23,* 1188–1199.

Cohen, D., Nisbett, R. E., Bowdle, B., & Schwarz, N. (1996). Insult, aggression, and the southern culture of honor. *Journal of Personality and Social Psychology, 70,* 945–960.

Cohen, D., Vandello, J., Puente, S., & Rantilla, A. (1999). When you call me that, smile! *Social Psychology Quarterly, 62,* 257–275.

Cohen, J. (1988). *Statistical power analysis for the behavioral sciences.* Hillsdale, NJ: Erlbaum.

Colson, E. (1975). *Tradition and contract.* Chicago: Aldine.

Cooter, R. (1997). Normative failure theory of law. *Cornell Law Review, 82,* 947–979.

Cronbach, L. (1990). *Essentials of psychological testing*. New York: HarperCollins.

Daly, M., & Wilson, M. (1988). *Homicide*. Hawthorne, New York: Aldine de Gruyter.

Deci, E., Koestner, R., & Ryan, R. (1999) A meta-analytic review of experiments examining the effects of extrinsic rewards on intrinsic motivation. *Psychological Bulletin, 125*, 627–668.

Diamond, J. (1999). *Guns, germs, and steel*. New York: Norton.

Diamond, J. (2005). The ends of the world as we know them. Retrieved on January 1, 2005, from *www.nytimes.com/2005/01/01/opinion/ 01diamond.html?incamp=article_popular_1&oref=login&pagewanted=print&position*

Diener, E., & Suh, E. (Eds.). (2003). *Culture and subjective well-being*. Boston: MIT Press.

Dijksterhuis, A., & van Knippenberg, A. (1998). The relation between perception and behavior, or how to win a game of Trivial Pursuit. *Journal of Personality and Social Psychology, 74*, 865–877.

Dimont, M. (1978). *The Jews in America*. New York: Simon & Schuster.

Edgerton, R. (1992). *Sick societies*. New York: Free Press.

Eliot, T. S. (1998). *The Sacred Wood and major early essays*. Mineola, NY: Dover.

Ellsworth, P., & Gonzalez, R. (2003). Questions and comparison. In M. Hogg & J. Cooper (Eds.), *The SAGE handbook of social psychology* (pp. 24–42). London: Sage.

Encyclopaedia Britannica. (2004). Retrieved November 2, 2004, from *www.britannica.com/ebi/article?tocId=9273747&query=christopher%20columbus&ct="ebi"*

Feldman, R. (1968). Response to compatriot and foreigner who seek assistance. *Journal of Personality and Social Psychology, 10*, 202–214.

Fish, S. (2005, December). Academic cross-dressing. *Harper's*, pp. 70–72.

Fiske, A. P. (2002). Using individualism and collectivism to compare cultures. *Psychological Bulletin, 128*, 78–88.

Fiske, A. P., Kitayama, S., Markus, H., & Nisbett, R. E. (1998). The cultural matrix of social psychology. In D. T. Gilbert, S. T. Fiske, & G. Linzey (Eds.), *Handbook of social psychology* (pp. 915–981). Boston: McGraw-Hill.

Franiuk, R., Cohen, D., & Pomerantz, E. (2002). Implicit theories of relationships. *Personal Relationships, 9*, 345–367.

Galison, P. (2004). Einstein's compass. *Scientific American, 291*, 67–69.

Gardner, W., Gabriel, S., & Lee, A. (1999). "I" value freedom, but "we" value relationships. *Psychological Science, 10*, 321–326.

Gilbert, D., Fiske, S., & Lindzey, G. (1998). *Handbook of social psychology*. New York: McGraw-Hill.

Gilbert, D., & Wilson, T. (2000). Miswanting. In J.

Forgas (Ed.), *Feeling and thinking* (pp. 178–197). New York: Cambridge University Press.

Gintis, H. (2006). *A framework for the unification of the behavioral sciences*. Retrieved October 25, 2006, from www.bbsonline.org/Preprints/Gintis-12052005/ Referees/Gintis-12052005_preprint.pdf

Glazer, N. (1957). *American Judaism*. Chicago: University of Chicago Press.

Glazer, N. (2000). Disaggregating culture. In L. Harrison & S. Huntington (Eds.), *Culture matters* (pp. 219–230). New York: Basic Books.

Guglielmino, C., Viganotti, C., Hewlett, B., & Cavalli-Sforza, L. (1995) Cultural variation in Africa. *Proceedings of the National Academy of Sciences, USA, 92*, 7585–7589.

Haidt, J., Koller, S., & Dias, M. (1993). Affect, culture, and morality, or is it wrong to eat your dog? *Journal of Personality and Social Psychology, 65*, 613–628.

Han, S., & Shavitt, S. (1994). Persuasion and culture. *Journal of Experimental Social Psychology, 30*, 326–350.

Heine, S. J. (2005). Constructing good selves in Japan and North America. In R. Sorrentino, D. Cohen, J. Olson, & M. Zanna (Eds.), *Culture and social behavior* (pp. 95–116). Mahwah, NJ: Erlbaum.

Heine, S. J., Kitayama, S., & Lehman, D. R. (2001). Cultural differences in self-evaluation. *Journal of Cross-Cultural Psychology, 32*, 434–443.

Heine, S. J., & Lehman, D. R. (1995). Cultural variation in unrealistic optimism. *Journal of Personality and Social Psychology, 68*, 595–607.

Heine, S. J., & Lehman, D. R. (1997a). Culture, dissonance, and self-affirmation. *Personality and Social Psychology Bulletin, 81*, 599–615.

Heine, S. J., & Lehman, D. R. (1997b). The cultural construction of self-enhancement. *Journal of Personality and Social Psychology, 72*, 1268–1283.

Heine, S. J., & Lehman, D. R. (1999). Culture, self-discrepancies, and self-satisfaction. *Personality and Social Psychology Bulletin, 25*, 915–925.

Heine, S., Lehman, D., Markus, H., & Kitayama, S. (1999). Is there a universal need for positive self-regard? *Psychological Review, 106*, 766–794.

Heine, S., Lehman, D. R., Peng, K., & Greenholtz, J. (2002). What's wrong with cross-cultural comparisons of subjective Likert scales? *Journal of Personality and Social Psychology, 82*, 903–918.

Heine, S. J., & Renshaw, K. (2002). Interjudge agreement, self-enhancement, and liking. *Personality and Social Psychology Bulletin, 28*, 442–451.

Heine, S. J., Takata, T., & Lehman, D. R. (2000). Beyond self-presentation. *Personality and Social Psychology Bulletin, 26*, 71–78.

Henrich, J., Boyd, R., Bowles, S., Camerer, C., Gintis, H., McElreath, R., et al. (2001). In search of *Homo economicus*: Experiments in 15 small-scale societies. *American Economic Review, 91*, 73–79.

Henrich, J., Boyd, R., Bowles, S., Gintis, H., Fehr, E., Camerer, C., et al. (2005). "Economic Man" in cross-cultural perspective. *Behavioral and Brain Sciences*, 28, 795–815.

Herrnstein, R., & Murray, C. (1994). *The bell curve.* New York: Free Press.

Heyman, G. D., & Diesendruck, G. (2002). The Spanish *ser/estar* distinction in bilingual children's reasoning about human psychological characteristics. *Developmental Psychology*, 38, 407–417.

Hong, Y., Ip, G., Chiu, C., Morris, M., & Menon, T. (2001). Construction of the self. *Social Cognition*, 19, 251–268.

Hong, Y., Morris, M., Chiu, C., & Benet-Martinez, V. (2000). Multicultural minds. *American Psychologist*, 55, 709–720.

Hoshino-Browne, E., Zanna, A. S., Spencer, S. J., Zanna, M. P., Kitayama, S., & Lackenbauer, S. (2005). On the cultural guises of cognitive dissonance. *Journal of Personality and Social Psychology*, 89, 294–310.

Huntington, S. P. (1996). *The clash of civilizations and the remaking of world order.* New York: Simon & Schuster.

Johnson, T., Kulesa, P., Cho, Y., & Shavitt, S. (2005). The relation between culture and response styles. *Journal of Cross-Cultural Psychology*, 36, 264–277.

Kelly, M. H. (1999). Regional naming patterns and the culture of honor. *Names*, 47, 3–20.

Kim, H., & Markus, H. (1999). Deviance or uniqueness, harmony or conformity? *Journal of Personality and Social Psychology*, 77, 785–800.

Kitayama, S. (2002). Culture and basic psychological processes—toward a system view of culture. *Psychological Bulletin*, 128, 89–96.

Kitayama, S., & Markus, H. (1999). Yin and yang of the Japanese self. In D. Cervone & Y. Shoda (Eds.), *The coherence of personality* (pp. 242–302). New York: Guilford Press.

Kitayama, S., Markus, H., Matsumoto, H., & Norasakkunkit, V. (1997). Individual and collective processes in the construction of the self. *Journal of Personality and Social Psychology*, 72, 1245–1267.

Kitayama, S., Snibbe, A. C., Markus, H. R., & Suzuki, T. (2004). Is there any "free" choice? *Psychological Science*, 15, 527–533.

Knauft, B. (1985). *Good company and violence.* Berkeley: University of California Press.

Kuhnen, U., Hannover, B., & Schubert, B. (2001). The semantic–procedural interface model of the self. *Journal of Personality and Social Psychology*, 80, 397–409.

Kuhnen, U., & Oyserman, D. (2002). Thinking about the self influences thinking in general. *Journal of Experimental Social Psychology*, 38, 492–499.

Kuran, T. (1995). *Private truths, public lies.* Cambridge, MA: Harvard University Press.

Kwan, V. (2007, January). *Imported cultural symbols affect everyday decisions.* Paper presented at cultural psychology preconference of the Society for Personality and Social Psychology annual meeting, Memphis, TN.

Lalwani, A. K., Shavitt, S., & Johnson, T. (2006). What is the relation between cultural orientation and socially desirable responding? *Journal of Personality and Social Psychology*, 90, 165–178.

Lee, A., Aaker, J., & Gardner, W. (2000). The pleasures and pains of distinct self-construals. *Journal of Personality and Social Psychology*, 78(6), 1122–1134.

Lee, F., Hallahan, M., & Herzog, T. (1996). Explaining real-life events: How culture and domain shape attributions. *Personality and Social Psychology Bulletin*, 22, 732–741.

Leung, A. K.-Y., & Cohen, D. (2007). *Within- and between-culture variation.* Urbana-Champaign: University of Illinois.

Levine, R., Martinez, T., Brase, G., & Sorenson, K. (1994). Helping in 36 U.S. cities. *Journal of Personality and Social Psychology*, 67(1), 69–82.

Levine, R., & Norenzayan, A. (1999). The pace of life in 31 countries. *Journal of Cross-Cultural Psychology*, 30(2), 178–205.

Levine, R., Sato, S., Hashimoto, T., & Verma, J. (1995). Love and marriage in eleven cultures. *Journal of Cross-Cultural Psychology*, 26(5), 554–571.

Lewontin, R. (1995). *Sex, lies, and social science.* Retrieved October 25, 2006, from *www.nybooks.com/contents/19950420*

Linton, R. (1936). *The study of man.* New York: Appleton–Century–Crofts.

Loewenstein, G., & Schkade, D. (1999). Wouldn't it be nice? In D. Kahneman, E. Diener, & N. Schwarz (Eds.), *Well-being* (pp. 85–105). New York: Russell Sage Foundation.

Lopez, A., Atran, S., Coley, J., Medin, D. L., & Smith, E. (1997). The tree of life. *Cognitive Psychology*, 32, 251–295.

Lyness, S. (1993). Predictors of differences between Type a and Type b individuals in heart rate and blood pressure reactivity. *Psychological Bulletin*, 114, 266–295.

MacFarquhar, L. (2004, October 18). The pollster. *The New Yorker*, pp. 85–94.

MacLeod, R. B. (1947). The phenomenological approach to social psychology. *Psychological Review*, 54, 193–210.

Medin, D. L., & Atran, S. (2004). The native mind: Biological categorization and reasoning in development and across cultures. *Psychological Review*, 111, 960–983.

Mesquita, B., & Karasawa, M. (2002). Different emotional lives. *Cognition and Emotion*, 16, 127–141.

Milgram, S. (1974). *Obedience to authority.* New York: Harper.

Miller, D. (1999). The norm of self-interest. *American Psychologist*, 54, 1053–1060.

Miller, D., & Prentice, D. (1994). Collective errors and errors about the collective. *Personality and Social Psychology Bulletin*, 20, 541–550.

Miller, J. (2002). Bringing culture to basic psychological theory—beyond individualism and collectivism. *Psychological Bulletin*, 128, 97–109.

Miller, T., Smith, T., Turner, C., Guijarro, M., & Hallet,

A. (1996). Meta-analytic review of research on hostility and physical health. *Psychological Bulletin*, *119*, 322–348.

Mischel, W., & Shoda, Y. (1995). A cognitive affective system theory of personality. *Psychological Review*, *102*, 246–268.

Miyamoto, Y., Nisbett, R. E., & Masuda, T. (2006). Culture and the physical environment: Holistic versus analytic perceptual affordances. *Psychological Science*, *17*, 113–119.

Morling, B., Kitayama, S., & Miyamoto, Y. (2002). Cultural practices emphasize influence in the United States and adjustment in Japan. *Personality and Social Psychology Bulletin*, *28*, 311–323.

Morris, M., & Peng, K. (1994). Culture and cause. *Journal of Personality and Social Psychology*, *67*, 949–971.

Murdock, G., & White, D. (2006). *Standard cross-cultural sample: On-line*. Retrieved October 24, 2006, from *eclectic.ss.uci.edu/~drwhite/worldcul/SCCS1969.pdf*

Nagel, T. (1974). What is it like to be a bat? *Philosophical Review*, *83*, 435–450.

Nisbett, R. (2004). *The geography of thought*. New York: Free Press.

Nisbett, R. (2005). The ghosts of cultural psychology. In R. Sorrentino, D. Cohen, J. Olson, & M. Zanna (Eds.), *Culture and social behavior* (pp. 251–258). Mahwah, NJ: Erlbaum.

Nisbett, R., & Masuda, T. (2003). Culture and point of view. *Proceedings of the National Academy of Sciences of the USA*, *100*, 11163–11170.

Nisbett, R., Peng, K., Choi, I., & Norenzayan, A. (2001). Culture and systems of thought. *Psychological Review*, *108*, 291–310.

Nisbett, R., & Wilson, T. (1977). Telling more than we can know. *Psychological Review*, *84*, 231–259.

Norenzayan, A., & Heine, S. (2005). Psychological universals: What are they and how can we know? *Psychological Bulletin*, *131*, 763–784.

Oyserman, D., Coon, H., & Kemmelmeier, M. (2002). Rethinking individualism and collectivism. *Psychological Bulletin*, *128*, 3–72.

Oyserman, D., Kemmelmeier, M., & Coon, H. (2002). Cultural psychology, a new look. *Psychological Bulletin*, *128*, 110–117.

Pagel, M., & Mace, R. (2004). The cultural wealth of nations. *Nature*, *428*, 275–278.

Pauker, S., & Pauker, S. (1979). The amniocentesis decision. *Birth Defects*, *15*, 289–324.

Perunovic, E., Ross, M., & Wilson, A. (2005). Language, culture and conceptions of the self. In R. Sorrentino, D. Cohen, J. Olson, & M. Zanna (Eds.), *Culture and social behavior* (pp. 165–180). Mahwah, NJ: Erlbaum.

Putnam, R. (1993). *Making democracy work*. Princeton, NJ: Princeton University Press.

Rosnow, R., & Rosenthal, R. (2002). *Beginning behavioral research*. Upper Saddle River, NJ: Prentice Hall.

Ross, L., & Nisbett, R. E. (1991). *The person and the situation*. New York: McGraw-Hill.

Rozin, P. (1999). The process of moralization. *Psychological Science*, *10*, 218–221.

Rozin, P. (2001). Social psychology and science. *Personality and Social Psychology Review*, *5*, 2–14.

Rozin, P. (2003). Five potential principles for understanding cultural differences in relation to individual differences. *Journal of Research in Personality*, *37*, 273–283.

Rozin, P., Lowery, L, Imada, S., & Haidt, J. (1999). The CAD triad hypothesis. *Journal of Personality and Social Psychology*, *76*, 574–586.

Salancik, G. (1979). Field stimulations for organizational behavior research. *Administrative Science Quarterly*, *24*, 638–650.

Sanchez-Burks, J. (2002). Protestant relational ideology and (in)attention to relational cues in work settings. *Journal of Personality and Social Psychology*, *83*, 919–929.

Sanchez-Burks, J. (2005). Protestant relational ideology. In R. Kramer & B. Staw (Eds.), *Research in organizational behavior* (pp. 267–308). New York: Elsevier.

Schuman, H., & Kalton, G. (1985). Survey methods. In G. Lindzey & A. Aronson (Eds.), *Handbook of social psychology* (pp. 635–697). New York: Random House.

Schuman, H., & Presser, S. (1981). *Questions and answers in attitude surveys*. New York: Academic Press.

Schwarz, N. (1999). Self-reports. *American Psychologist*, *54*, 93–105.

Sears, D. (1986). College sophomores in the laboratory. *Journal of Personality and Social Psychology*, *51*, 515–530.

Sears, D., & Funk, C. (1990). The limited effect of economic self-interest on the political attitudes of the mass public. *Journal of Behavioral Economics*, *19*, 247–271.

Sera, M. D., Bales, D. W., & del Castillo Pintado, J. (1997). *Ser* helps Spanish speakers identify "real" properties. *Child Development*, *68*, 820–831.

Sherif, M., Harvey, O., White, J., Hood, W., & Sherif, C. (1954). *Intergroup conflict and cooperation: The Robbers Cave experiment*. Norman: University of Oklahoma.

Shweder, R. (1990). Cultural psychology. In J. Stigler, R. Shweder, & G. Herdt (Eds.), *Cultural psychology* (pp. 1–43). Cambridge, UK: Cambridge University Press.

Shweder, R. (1993). "Why do men barbeque" and other postmodern ironies of growing up in the decade of ethnicity. *Daedalus*, *122*, 279–308.

Shweder, R. (1997). The surprise of ethnography. *Ethos*, *25*, 152–163.

Shweder, R. (2000). Moral maps, "first world" conceits, and the new evangelists. In L. Harrison & S. Huntington (Eds.), *Culture matters* (pp. 158–176). New York: Basic Books.

Shweder, R. (2003). *Why do men barbeque?* Cambridge, MA: Harvard University Press.

Shweder, R., Much, N., Mahapatra, M., & Park, L.

(1997). The "Big Three" of morality (autonomy, community, divinity) and the "Big Three" explanations of suffering. In A. Brandt & P. Rozin (Eds.), *Morality and health* (pp. 119–169). Florence, KY: Taylor & Frances/Routledge.

Singelis, T. (1994). The measurement of independent and interdependent self-construals. *Personality and Social Psychology Bulletin, 20*(5), 580–591.

Smith, P., & Bond, M. (2003). Honoring culture scientifically when doing social psychology. In M. Hogg & J. Cooper (Eds.), *The SAGE handbook of social psychology* (pp. 43–61). London: Sage.

Spencer, S. J., Zanna, M. P., & Fong, G. T. (2005). Establishing a causal chain: Why experiments are often more effective than mediational analyses in examining psychological processes. *Journal of Personality and Social Psychology, 89*, 845–851.

Spiro, M. (1990). On the strange and familiar in recent anthropological thought. In J. Stigler, R. Shweder, & G. Herdt (Eds.), *Cultural psychology* (pp. 47–61). Cambridge, UK: Cambridge University Press.

Stapel, D., & Koomen, W. (2001). I, we, and the effects of others on me. *Journal of Personality and Social Psychology, 80*, 766–781.

Starr, K. (1998). *Starr report.* Retrieved December 17, 2005, from *www.cnn.com/specials/multimedia/timeline/9809/starr.report/tab.html.*

Stasser, G., & Titus, W. (1985). Pooling of unshared information in group decision making. *Journal of Personality and Social Psychology, 48*, 1467–1478.

Steele, C. M. (1997). A threat in the air. *American Psychologist, 52*, 613–629.

Steele, C. M. (1999). Thin ice. *The Atlantic Monthly, 284*, 44–47, 50–54.

Symons, D. (1992). On the use and misuse of Darwinism in the study of human behavior. In J. Barkow, L. Cosmides, & J. Tooby (Eds.), *The adapted mind.* New York: Oxford University Press.

Trafimow, D., Triandis, H., & Goto, S. (1991) Some tests of the distinction between the private and the collective self. *Journal of Personality and Social Psychology, 60*, 649–655.

Triandis, H. (1994). *Culture and social behavior.* New York: McGraw-Hill.

Triandis, H., & Berry, J. (1980). *Handbook of cross-cultural psychology.* Boston: Allyn & Bacon.

Triandis, H. C., Marin, G., Lisansky, J., & Betancourt, H. (1984). *Simpatia* as a cultural script of Hispanics. *Journal of Personality and Social Psychology, 47*(6), 1363–1375.

Tsai, J., Levenson, R., & McLoy, K. (2006). Cultural and temperamental variation in emotional response. *Emotion, 6*, 484–497.

U.S. Bureau of the Census. (1999). *Statistical abstract of the United States.* Washington, DC: Author.

van Baaren, R. B., Horgan, T. G., Chartrand, T. L., & Dijkmans, M. (2004). The forest, the trees, and the chameleon: Context dependence and mimicry. *Journal of Personality and Social Psychology, 86*, 453–459.

Vandello, J., & Cohen, D. (1999). Patterns of individualism and collectivism in the United States. *Journal of Personality and Social Psychology, 77*, 279–292.

White, K., Lehman, D. R., & Cohen, D. (2006). Culture, self-construal, and affective reactions to successful and unsuccessful others. *Journal of Experimental Social Psychology, 45*, 582–592.

Will, G. (2004a, October 3). State and local disputes will drive the nation's choice. *Champaign-Urbana News-Gazette,* p. B2.

Will, G. (2004b, April 26). Shock and awe in Iraq. *Newsweek,* p. 64.

Will, G. (2005). The oddness of everything. Retrieved December 6, 2005, from *www.msnbc.msn.com/id/7856556/site/newsweek/page/2/.*

Wilson, T., & Dunn, E. (2004). Self-knowledge. *Annual Review of Psychology, 55*, 493–518.

Yamagishi, T. (1986). The provision of a sanctioning system as a public good. *Journal of Personality and Social Psychology, 51*, 110–116.

Yamagishi, T. (1988). Exit from the group as an individualistic solution to the free rider problem in the United States and Japan. *Journal of Experimental Social Psychology, 24*, 530–542.

Yamagishi, T., & Cook, K. (1993). Generalized exchange and social dilemmas. *Social Psychology Quarterly, 56*, 235–248.

CHAPTER 9

Cultural Neuroscience
Parsing Universality and Diversity across Levels of Analysis

JOAN Y. CHIAO
NALINI AMBADY

The existence of human diversity has been a source of contemplation and curiosity since the beginning of human history. In his encyclopedia *Etymologiae*, published in the seventh century, Isidori of Seville observed that diversity among humans existed not only in their appearance, such as color or body size, but also in the content of their minds (Jahoda, 2002). Philosophers, such as Descartes and Locke, continued speculation on the nature and origin of human diversity, introducing more formalized notions of culture and its relation to human nature into the lexicon. The study of culture and its role in humanity gained further prominence with the emergence of the field of anthropology in the late 19th century, which emphasized the study of cultural variation through observation of the customs, practices, values, and beliefs of different cultural groups, and later with the field of cultural psychology, which sought to apply the methodology of psychology and its emphasis on the individual mind to the study of cultural variation.

Contemporary cultural psychologists have made considerable progress in documenting cultural variation in human thought and action. The mutual constitution of culture and mind has been demonstrated in a variety of fundamental psychological processes, including the way people conceive of the self (Markus & Kitayama, 1991; Markus, Kitayama, & Heiman, 1996), how they make causal attributions (Morris & Peng, 1994), how they attend to and remember objects in their environment (Miyamoto & Kitayama, 2002; Kitayama, Duffy, Kawamura, & Larsen, 2003; Masuda & Nisbett, 2001), and how they perceive, experience, respond to, and predict their own and others' emotions (Elfenbein & Ambady, 2002; Lam, Buehler, McFarland, Ross, & Cheung, 2005; Mesquita & Frijda, 1992). A fundamental assumption of this research is that the human mind is intimately linked with its social world or cultural context, and that culture is continuously created through the actions and products of the individual minds that comprise it.

Cultural psychologists have been wary, however, about integrating biological perspectives into their research endeavors, perhaps because they assume that investigations into the biological bases of the mind reflect an empirical search for human universals rather than cultural differences (Norenzayan & Heine, 2005; Smedley & Smedley, 2005). Likewise, cognitive neuroscientists have viewed their discipline as a pursuit of universal truths rather than culturally specified instances about how the brain gives rise to the mind and vice versa (Kosslyn, 1999). Yet a growing number of studies show that both the structure and the function of the developing human brain is shaped both by the environment and by cultural experiences (Johnson & Munakata, 2005). Moreover, although recent advances in human genomics and molecular biology demonstrate that whereas the majority of the human genome is conserved across human cultures, variation in the frequency of different genes does exist between different human populations. This variation of genes between cultures suggests that cultural variation may emerge at multiple levels, possibly as a result of interactions between levels (e.g., gene–brain, culture–behavior, culture–gene, culture–brain–gene; Bonham, Warshauer-Baker, & Collins, 2005). Thus, we argue that cultural psychologists' notions of the "mutual constitution" of culture and mind needs to be broadened beyond interactions between culture and the mind, to interactions among culture, genes, and the brain.

Early articulations of this idea of bidirectional influences among culture, genes, mind, and the brain can be traced to the work of prominent developmental psychologists such as D'Arcy Thompson and C. Waddington, who laid down the original framework for what would later come to be known as *probabilistic epigenesis* (Johnson, 1997). According to this view, humans come into the world with sets of possible developmental trajectories (each with their own alternative end states, presumably described by the genome) that are then pursued, or not, over the course of development as a result of interactions with environmental input. The notion of *biocultural co-constructivism* was introduced more recently to account for the significance of plasticity across development in gene–environment interactions; humans may come into the world with a set of possible developmental trajectories, but once on a certain trajectory, plasticity may alter both the path and the end state (Li, 2003, Chapter 21, this volume). The empirical challenge brought on by both views is finding ways

to articulate precisely how neural mechanisms and psychological capacities emerge through complex, multilevel interactions between genetic forces and the cultural environment.

To designate an approach to meet this challenge, we introduce in this chapter the term "cultural neuroscience," which is a theoretical and empirical approach to investigate and characterize the mechanisms by which this hypothesized bidirectional, mutual constitution of culture, brain, and genes occurs. Specifically, we suggest that biological factors may lead to cultural variation at the neural and genetic levels, and that cultural factors may lead to variation in brain structure and function, as well as gene expression. To accomplish this, we first focus on identifying the conceptual landscape covered by the term "cultural neuroscience." Second, we describe the methodological tool box needed for accomplishing cultural neuroscience research. Third, we review recent progress in identifying cultural variation at the genetic and neural levels. Fourth, we discuss the nature and meaning of cultural variation across different levels of analyses. Finally, we identify important challenges and considerations that need to be addressed for cultural neuroscience to progress systematically and significantly.

CULTURAL NEUROSCIENCE: DEFINING THE LANDSCAPE

Cultural neuroscience is an area of research that investigates cultural variation in psychological, neural, and genomic processes as a means of articulating the interrelationship of these processes and their emergent properties (see Figure 9.1). A multilevel analytic approach to studying psychological phenomena and human behavior has become more popular, as demonstrated by the number of subfields that have proliferated in recent years, each incorporating neuroscience into a parent social science discipline; these include social neuroscience (Cacioppo, Lorig, Nusbaum, & Berntson, 2004), social-cognitive neuroscience (Ochsner & Lieberman, 2001), affective neuroscience (Davidson, 2003), and neuroeconomics (McCabe, 2003). Whereas cultural neuroscience shares the goal of these subfields to explain a given phenomenon in terms of an emergent property of interactions between mental and neural events, cultural neuroscience is distinctive in that it focuses squarely on examin-

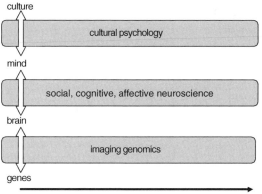

culture

cultural psychology

mind

social, cognitive, affective neuroscience

brain

imaging genomics

genes

ontogeny and phylogeny

FIGURE 9.1. Diagram of the cultural neuroscience framework.

ing psychological and neural processes that may vary across cultural groups in some meaningful way. Cultural neuroscience can be seen as a complementary endeavor to evolutionary psychology (see review by Cosmides, Tooby, & Barkow, 1992); however, whereas evolutionary psychology seeks to articulate the universal, evolved architecture of the mind shared by all humans, cultural neuroscience emphasizes cultural variation, specifically, investigating interactions between events at the psychological, neural, and genetic levels.

The Neuroscience of Culture versus Race

The goals and research questions of cultural neuroscience are to a certain extent similar to those driving the modern neuroscientific study of race. In recent years, the importance of social experience on brain function has been highlighted by studies showing that racial group membership affects neural processes underlying other basic aspects of social cognition, such as face perception and recognition, as well as social evaluation and bias (see Eberhardt, 2005, for a review). Work in this area has been groundbreaking in demonstrating how racial group membership (and racial experience more generally) can modulate the neural activity underlying basic perceptual and cognitive processes. Cultural neuroscience, however, is likely to illuminate how sociocultural and biological factors influence each other in ways not previously revealed by neuroscientific studies of race. Culture and race differ in a number of important respects (Betancourt & Lopez, 1993).

Culture refers to shared meaning systems, social practices, geographical space, social and religious values, language, ways of relating, diet, and ecology (Markus et al., 1996). In contrast, the concept of race, which typically refers to physical characteristics such as skin color, facial features, and hair type shared by people of a given ancestral origin, is shrouded in controversy about whether "race" refers solely to biological or socially constructed features that differentiate groups of people (Bonham et al., 2005; Smedley & Smedley, 2005). Individuals may belong to different races but may share the same culture. Whites, blacks, Hispanics, and Asians living in America, for example, share the same government structure and, to some extent, the same language, ecology, social values, and ways of relating, but are considered members of different racial groups. When neuroscience investigations of race and brain function include participants from the same culture (which, to date, all studies have), they do not capture how different meaning systems (e.g., collectivism and individualism), languages (e.g., Chinese and English), ways of reasoning (e.g., dialectism), and so on, may arise from, as well as alter, neural processing and genomic expression.

The suggestion that broad phenomena such as culture can be understood in terms of interactions between multilevel events (e.g., neural, situational, genetic) may be construed as a form of reductionism and may therefore be subject to criticisms typically associated with reductionist agendas. Philosophers of science and scientists of all kinds have long grappled with the problem of whether complex phenomena, such as consciousness, are truly reducible to their component parts (Dennett, 1995; Nagel, 1998). For instance, does reducing the phenomenon of consciousness into a description of neural events somehow fail to capture the context within which consciousness occurs, and do the phenomena that emerge from these neural events differ from the actual events themselves? The aim of cultural neuroscience *is not* to "reduce" culture into a description of genetic and neural processes at the expense of the characterization of emergent properties, nor is it intended to replace the language of culture with the language of neurons or molecules. The goal of a cultural neuroscience approach is empirically to shed light on the extent to which the cultural variation observable in human behavior and mental life is traceable to cultural variation at other levels of analysis and their interaction, including the biological and neural levels.

THE CULTURAL NEUROSCIENCE TOOL BOX: INTEGRATING METHODOLOGIES

What makes the study of cultural neuroscience a more viable empirical and theoretical proposition for modern scientists is the amalgamation of recent methodological advances in the fields of cultural psychology, cognitive neuroscience, and molecular biology. In recent years, cultural psychologists have made significant advances in articulating the criteria for creating culturally appropriate behavioral measures that ensure the psychological phenomenon of interest is testable in people of all cultures (Norenzayan & Heine, 2005). Cognitive neuroscience has revolutionized the study of the mind and brain by developing an arsenal of techniques for mapping neural structures to psychological functions at varying degrees of spatial and temporal resolution (Gazzaniga, Ivry, & Mangun, 2002; Handy, 2005; Heeger & Ress, 2002). Molecular biology has seen rapid transformation in recent years with the development of tools for enabling the efficient and economical translation of the human genome (Hariri & Weinberger, 2003). Taken together, the convergence of these tools enables the unprecedented ability to investigate the mutual constitution of genes, brain, behavior, mind, and culture (see Figure 9.2).

Behavioral Paradigms

The first important tool in the cultural neuroscience tool box is a compilation of *behavioral paradigms* appropriate for examining cognitive, perceptual, emotional, and social-cognitive phenomena in people of different cultures. The development of cross-culturally sensitive behavioral paradigms has proved challenging in several regards. The ways that tasks are created and administered may favor one cultural group over another in ease and intuitiveness; specifically, cultural differences may exist in response styles where people of certain cultures are more comfortable with completing questionnaires relative to others (Greenfield, 1997). Participants of certain cultures may be more likely to use the center rather than the extremities of a scale in a questionnaire (Chen, Lee, & Stevenson, 1995). Free-response formats requiring extensive translation may produce errors in meaning; such errors may also arise when translating the instructions of measures from one language to another (Brislin, 1970). Responses associated with demand characteristics may be more frequent when sampling from cultures that value "saving face" above accurate self-report (Heine, Takata, & Lehman, 2000), and culture may affect the different social referents used when providing self-reports (Heine, Lehman, Peng, & Greenholtz, 2002). Psychologists have created a number of solutions to these methodological worries, including back-translation (Brislin, 1970), incorporating different kinds of behavioral measures in a study (Nisbett & Cohen, 1996), and even using hidden behavioral measures (Heine et al., 2000).

Convergent Neuroscience Methods

The second component of the cultural neuroscience tool box is *convergent neuroscientific methods* for characterizing the neural processes underlying a given psychological function. There are several neuroscience tools available to psychologists interested in mapping neural structure to mental function, including functional MRI (fMRI), positron emission topography (PET), transcranial magnetic stimulation (TMS), magnetoencephalography (MEG), and event-related potentials (ERPs); each tool has its strengths and weaknesses (Gazzaniga et al., 2002). Imaging techniques, for example, such as fMRI and PET have very good spatial reso-

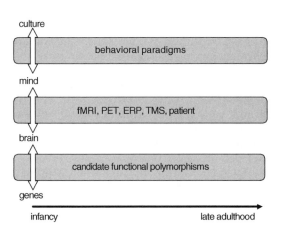

FIGURE 9.2. Diagram of the cultural neuroscience tool box.

lution (in cubic millimeters) and are crucial to identifying which brain regions are involved in different aspects of processing (Heeger & Ress, 2002). However, because they record differences in blood flow, which occurs on the level of seconds, and not neural activity directly, which occurs on the level of milliseconds, imaging techniques lack temporal precision. Cortical recording techniques, such as the ERP, are extremely temporally precise, because they directly record neural activity to the precision of milliseconds and are therefore good for determining when a process is occurring or when a difference in neural processing emerges (Handy, 2005). Unlike fMRI and PET, the ERP lacks spatial precision, because it records electrical signals only from cortical regions directly under the scalp. This is particularly problematic for the study of subcortical areas, such as the amygdala, that have been strongly implicated in the processing of emotions. MEG, a methodology with both the advantages of brain imaging techniques and ERPs directly records electrical activity from the brain, thus having extremely high temporal resolution. MEG also has good spatial resolution due to the high number (e.g., approximately 300 channels) and sensitivity of the channels used to record electrical activity.

TMS and studies of patients with brain lesions are currently the only way of discerning which regions in a normal brain are *necessary* for performing a certain function, such as recognizing faces or emotional expressions. TMS uses rapidly changing magnetic fields to induce electric fields in a specific brain region and can be applied repetitively (Paulus, Hallett, Rossini, & Rothwell, 1999). In a typical TMS experiment, a powerful magnet that is held over a cortical region of the brain (e.g., the motor cortex or frontal gyri) delivers magnetic pulses for a few minutes. The application of these magnetic pulses affects electrical and biochemical activity in the directed brain region and in interconnected brain regions. Typically, the region in which TMS is applied undergoes suppression of activity or temporary dysfunction, creating a "temporary functional lesion." If this neural dysfunction is accompanied by behavioral decline, one can infer that a given brain regions is *necessary* for a particular mental function. Similarly, by testing a given behavioral paradigm in patients with discrete brain lesions, one can infer whether or not a brain region is *necessary* to produce a certain behavior.

Disadvantages of patient studies are that lesion sites rarely completely overlap nor is severity of brain damage identical across patients. Such heterogeneity in location and severity of brain lesions may affect the degree to which one can infer that a specific area of the brain is critical. Thus, the advantage of TMS is that one can examine the necessity of a given neural structure within the same location across several normal brains.

Given their different strengths and weaknesses, no individual neuroscientific method can independently capture the rich complexity with which the brain processes cognitive and emotional information. Rather, it is the convergence of findings from multiple techniques that enables us to make sound inferences about neural structures and their psychological function. ERPs tell us when neural processes are occurring. MRI and fMRI provide information about the structure and function of the human brain. TMS and patient populations provide information about whether a given brain region is necessary for a given psychological function.

Genes and Their Functional Polymorphisms

Genes, the fundamental physical and functional unit of heredity, substantially influence every level of human biology, including neural function and mental processes. Genes are thought to account for a majority of psychiatric illnesses, prompting many studies that attempt to map specific genes onto various cognitive, emotional, and personality styles and disorders (Hariri & Weinberger, 2003). The entire human genome comprises a relatively small number of unique genes, approximately 20,000 to 30,000, many of which are found in the genomes of other species, from simple organisms, such as bacteria and fruit flies, to more complex ones, such as sheep and monkeys (Cavalli-Sforza, 2005). Although the actual number of genes is small, individual genes can take on various forms, known as polymorphisms, that result from evolutionary "mistakes" whereby the original genetic structure is modified in small but significant ways: through snips, repeats, and deletions of base pairs. There are approximately 3 million polymorphic variation sites in the human genome, and it is the variation in these sites across populations and subpopulations that has yielded surprising and potent insights into the possible origins of psychological and neural differences across individuals and cultures (Cavalli-Sforza, 1998, 2005).

Hence, the third part of the cultural neuroscience tool box is a means of determining the presence or absence of functional polymorphisms and their variants in an individual. Identifying functional polymorphisms is important to designing experiments that test whether a given neural or mental process is influenced by one's genome. Blood samples and cheek swabs are the primary ways of obtaining DNA from individuals; body samples are then amplified through polymerase chain reactions (PCRs) tailored to isolate specific functional polymorphisms (Gelernter, Kranzler, & Cubells, 1997). Once the variants of a given polymorphism in an individual is identified (e.g., short or long allele carrier), they can then be separated into different groups and the participant's neural and psychological responses can be compared in light of his or her genomic profile.

These three basic components of the cultural neuroscience tool box—(1) culturally appropriate behavioral paradigms, (2) neuroscience tools, and (3) functional polymorphisms—offer an unprecedented amount of experimental power for cross-level analyses of cultural variation. These tools allow the measurement of individual mental, neural, and genomic information, and comparisons of individuals from different cultures at every level. A multilevel analysis has long been considered necessary for a full articulation of the mutual constitution of culture and the mind; the unification of novel experimental techniques in the cultural neuroscience tool box described earlier provides the means to achieve this. As existing tools improve and new tools are introduced, the tool box will need to be updated and refined.

CULTURAL VARIATION IN BEHAVIOR

Numerous behavioral studies, mostly comparing Easterners (e.g., Chinese, Japanese) and Westerners (e.g., Western Europeans, European Americans), suggest that there is significant cultural variation in basic psychological processes, including mathematical thinking, reasoning style, memory, emotion, and the self (see review, in Markus & Kitayama, 1991; Nisbett & Norenzayan, 2002). For example, Mandarin speakers talk about time as if it were vertical,

whereas English speakers refer to it as horizontal (Boroditsky, 2001). Easterners tend to attend to the background or situation, whereas Westerners focus on the object within a scene (Masuda & Nisbett, 2001). Furthermore, Easterners tend to perceive objects and people, and the situation in which they are embedded as mutually interdependent; thus, they may use holistic strategies for perceiving people and scenes. Westerners, however, who are more likely to perceive objects and people as independent from the situation, apply a more analytic strategy for perceiving entities in their environment (Nisbett & Norenzayan, 2002). These examples provide a window into the degree to which culture shapes basic psychological processing and serve as a foundation for research that examines cultural variation at other levels of analysis, including genes and the brain. Because behavioral findings that document cultural variation in mind and behavior are well represented in other chapters, we focus our discussion on cultural variation beyond behavior.

CULTURAL VARIATION IN THE BRAIN

The vast majority of cognitive neuroscience research has focused on elucidating functional relationships among brain, mind, and behavior, which are presumed invariant across cultures (Plomin & Kosslyn, 2001). However, there are several reasons to suspect meaningful cultural variation in brain structure and function. First, as discussed earlier, there seems to be significant cultural variation in functional polymorphisms associated with primary cognitive and affective capacities. Furthermore, approximately 70% of genes are expressed in the brain. Thus, cultural variation in brain function is possible to the extent that these functional polymorphisms affect efficiency and capacity of neurotransmission (Hariri & Weinberger, 2003). Second, experience, particularly perceptual or social experience during certain periods of development, can play a definitive and shaping role in the acquisition and maturation of neural mechanisms underlying a wide range of fundamental skills, including language (Neville & Bavelier, 1998), music comprehension (Janata & Grafton, 2003), face processing (Gauthier & Nelson, 2001), and spatial navigation (Wolbers, Weiller, & Buchel,

2004; Maguire et al., 2000). To the extent that cultural rules, values, beliefs, and practices shape perceptual and social experience, and to the extent that experience differs between cultures, cultural differences in neural responses underlying cognitive and affective processes are likely to exist (Park & Gutchess, 2002). Third, behavioral research suggests significant cultural variation, particularly between Westerners and East Asians, in their basic perceptual, cognitive, and affective strategies, that may have emerged as a result of divergent philosophical and reasoning traditions (e.g., holistic vs. analytic) between the East and West (Nisbett, Peng, Choi, & Norenzayan, 2001). To the extent that neural mechanisms underlie psychological ones, we would expect to find differences in neural activity for psychological functions where notable behavioral differences exist between cultures. Finally, the neural bases of a given mental function may vary across cultural groups either in terms of structures and circuitry recruited to perform a given task (e.g., to recognize emotions or colors) or the degree to which these structures are activated during the task, even in absence of observable behavioral or genetic differences. Thus, investigating cultural variation in brain structure and function is both a viable and necessary endeavor for fulfilling the goals of both cultural psychology (e.g., to articulate meaningful cultural differences) and cognitive neuroscience (e.g., to identify and explain brain structure and function).

Despite notable progress in describing cultural variation at the behavioral and genetic levels in recent years, still relatively little is known about the ways the structure and function of the human brain vary across different cultures. To date, the lion's share of empirical research on cross-cultural differences in the brain has been in the domain of language (e.g., the neural bases for cross-linguistic differences and multilingualism; Paulesu et al., 2000; Bolger, Perfetti, & Schneider, 2005; Xue, Chen, Jun, & Dong, 2006). Empirical progress in investigation of cross-cultural differences in neural activity for a broader range of psychological phenomena, from object perception (Ketay, Hedden, Aron, Markus, & Gabrieli, 2005) and theory of mind (Kobayashi & Temple, 2004) to music (Morrison, Demorest, Aylward, Cramer, & Maravilla, 2003) and taste perception (McClure et al., 2004), is also growing rapidly.

CULTURAL VARIATION IN THE HUMAN GENOME

Incredible controversy has ensued in recent years over the question of whether racial or cultural differences exist at the level of the human genome and if it even makes sense to apply concepts such as race and culture to the genome (Sankar & Cho, 2002; Wang & Sue, 2005). Such controversy is not without merits. The human genome is incredibly conserved, with only approximately 0.2% to 0.4% of the genome varying across individuals (Tishkoff & Kidd, 2004). Mutation, migration, genetic drift, and selection are all sources of normal genetic variation in cultures (Cavalli-Sforza, 1998, 2005). Individual genomic variation accounts for approximately 90% of total genomic variation. There also exists variation in genes at the population level, but on a much smaller scale, because people are more likely to mate with others who live close to them, and to share the same language and phenotypic qualities (e.g., assortative mating; Tishkoff & Kidd, 2004; Wang & Sue, 2005). Given that the majority of the genome does not appear to vary across cultural groups or populations, does it even make sense to pay attention to cultural variation in genomic frequencies?

We argue that although it occurs on a much smaller scale relative to individual genetic variation, genomic variation at the population level should not be ignored; instead, it should be considered seriously, with scientific rigor and ethical care. We prefer to discuss population variation in the genome in terms of culture rather than race, because culture refers not only to ethnic heritages and phenotypic similarities between individuals but, perhaps more importantly, also to shared lifestyles, diet, geographical region, and other environmental aspects that likely have a significant interaction with brain function, gene expression, and selection. Both the sheer range of genomic frequency variation in the number of genes that demonstrate group frequency variation and the number of cultural groups for which frequency distribution differs are impressive, posing a formidable challenge for molecular biology research (Cheung et al., 2000). Indeed, molecular biologists have designed online databases (e.g., ALFRED[1]) on the Web to facilitate public dissemination of catalogues documenting variation in genomic frequencies for populations all over the world: from the Khung San tribe in Africa to the Yemenites in Eastern Europe (Osier et al., 2002). Although it is possible that cultural variation in allelic frequency for many genes will not have direct functional consequences on the mind or brain, there is growing evidence to the contrary. Here, we highlight two functional polymorphisms, *DRD4* and *5-HTT*, with significant cultural variation in genomic frequencies that has already been demonstrated to influence psychological and neural mechanism substantially.

DRD4: Dopamine Regulator Gene

The dopamine receptor gene, *DRD4*, is one of the most polymorphic genes. Variants of the *DRD4* vary in the number of imperfect 48 base pair (bp) tandem repeats, ranging from 2 to 11 repeat units, but most commonly 4 to 7 repeats. The number of repeat units on the *DRD4* affects the size of the dopamine receptor and its ability to bind to dopamine-like molecules (Benjamin et al., 1996). Variation of the *DRD4* gene has been linked to novelty-seeking behavior and psychiatric disorders (Gelernter, Kranzler, Coccaro, et al., 1997). Considerable evidence suggests that the seven-repeat *DRD4* variant is involved with increased novelty-seeking, risk-taking behavior and hyperactivity (see review by Munafo et al., 2003). The frequency of long versus short-allele carriers of the *DRD4* gene varies significantly across cultures. A low proportion of the East Asian population carries the long-allele variant of *DRD4* (e.g., 1% carry seven repeats), whereas an extremely high proportion of the South American Indian population carries the long-allele version (e.g., 78% carry seven repeats; Chen, Burton, Greenberger, & Dmitrieva, 1999).

There are several possible explanations for this cultural variation in the genome. One is the *founder's effect*, whereby a higher proportion of long alleles within a migratory population may be due to the fact that founders of that population migrated as a behavioral consequence of carrying the long allele of the *DRD4*, which promoted exploratory behavior. A second possibility is *natural selection*, whereby South Americans carrying the long allele had an advantage relative to their short-allele-carrying counterparts, thus providing them with a reproductive/survival advantage. A third hypothesis is *random mutation*, whereby frequency differences in long- versus short-allele versions of *DRD4* within a small population

result from spontaneous mutation, such that over each successive generation, by chance, long-allele individuals leave more descendants relative to short-allele individuals, which then leads to a reduction in heterogeneous genetic variation within that population over time.

Chen and colleagues (1999) conducted regression analyses to determine the factor(s) driving the variation of *DRD4* between East Asians and South American Indians. In particular, they compiled existing data on *DRD4* allele frequencies of 2,320 individuals from 39 populations, and on the long-term migration pattern (e.g., 1,000 to 30,000 years ago) for these populations. They found that populations known to migrate had a significantly larger proportion of individuals with the long allele of the *DRD4* relative to nonmigratory populations. Chen and colleagues speculate that this association is not due to founder's effects, because the rate of long alleles of *DRD4* is identical for immigrants (e.g., Chinese and Japanese immigrants in the United States) and their respective comparison group (e.g., Chinese in China and Japanese in Japan). This suggests that the increased rate of long alleles among migratory groups more likely resulted from adaptation to the challenges of migration rather than to a particular subset of individuals who founded the migratory groups. Future research is needed to determine whether the striking cultural variation in *DRD4* allele frequency between East Asian and South American populations corresponds with cultural variation in neural mechanisms underlying novelty-seeking behavior, risk taking, or hyperactivity.

5-HTT: Serotonin Regulator Gene

The serotonergic uptake transporter gene, *5-HTT*, is another polymorphism known for cultural variation. *5-HTT* codes for proteins that regulate the reuptake of serotonin at brain synapses and plays a critical role in the regulation of emotional processes. Similar to variants of the *DRD4* gene that differ in length, the two main variants of the *5-HTT* gene, short (s/s) and long (l/l), differ in the length of the promoter region that subsequently affects when, where, and how much protein is made. The long allele of the *5-HTT* is associated with higher transcription efficiency relative to the short allele, ultimately promoting higher levels of serotonin in the synapse.

Behavioral genetics studies examining the functional role of *5-HTT* in emotion have found that individuals carrying the short allele were slightly more prone to abnormal levels of anxiety relative to long-allele carriers (Lesch et al., 1996), a finding later corroborated by others (Katsuragi et al., 1999; see review by Sen, Burmeister, & Ghosh, 2004). People with the short allele were also found to acquire conditioned fear responses more readily than those without this allele (Garpenstrand, Annas, Ekblom, Oreland, & Fredrikson, 2001). Finally, a study by Caspi and colleagues (2003) showed that individuals with the short allele for this gene were more susceptible to stressful life events and twice as likely to suffer from depressive symptoms, diagnosable depression, and suicidality compared to individuals with the long allele.

Further evidence for a critical role of *5-HTT* in emotion processing comes from imaging genomics research examining the relationship between *5-HTT* and brain function. In particular, recent work has linked the *5-HTT* serotonin uptake gene to amygdalar function. A recent imaging genomics study by Hariri and colleagues (2002) demonstrated that individuals with the short allele showed greater amygdalar activation during an emotion-matching task relative to individuals with the long allele. Another imaging study by Furmark and colleagues (2004) found enhanced right amygdalar response in social phobics with one or two copies of the short allele compared to social phobics who were homozygous for the long allele during anxiety provocation. Greater amygdalar reactivity in response to emotional stimuli in short-allele carriers relative to long-allele carriers may underlie their heightened sensitivity or arousal to emotional stimuli, ultimately leading to higher rates of anxiety and depression disorders. These findings, though preliminary, are groundbreaking, because they show a direct relationship between genes and brain function, whereas previously researchers had only been able to study the relationship between genes and behavior. Moreover, examining the link between genes and brain function may prove more fruitful than studying the link between genes and behavior, because genetic variation in both studies accounted for more than 20% of variance in brain function even though no differences in behavioral measures (e.g., emotion matching task) emerged between the short- and long-allele groups in these particular studies.

Critically, Japanese and Caucasians from Western Europe and the United States significantly differ in the number of individuals within the cultural group that carry the short versus long allele of the *5-HTT* genotype. Several behavioral genetics studies have reported that in a typical Japanese sample, 70–80% of individuals carry the short allele (s/s or s/l) compared to 20–30% of individuals carrying the long allele. In a typical Caucasian sample, 55–60% of individuals carry the long allele and only 40–45% of individuals are short-allele carriers of the *5-HTT* genotype (Gelernter, Kranzler, & Cubells, 1997; Gelernter, Kranzler, Coccaro, et al., 1997; Hariri & Weinberger, 2003). Several behavioral genetics research groups have also reported this cultural difference among independent samples of Japanese and Caucasians, further validating this potentially important finding (Kumakiri et al., 1999). A critical research direction for the future is to investigate the relationship between this cultural difference in frequency of short- versus long-allele carriers of *5-HTT* and cultural differences in behavioral performance on anxiety, personality or emotion measures, as well as brain functioning, such as in amygdalar reactivity to emotional stimuli (Chiao et al., 2004).

To the extent that *5-HTT* is relevant to normal and abnormal emotion processing, it is important to consider how and why Japanese and European populations differ so dramatically in their ratio of short- versus long-allele carriers and what implications this has for cultural differences in emotion at the neural and behavioral level.[2] Behavioral geneticists speculate that the population differences may reflect a combination of varying behavioral adaptation in different populations, adaptation related to other phenotypes, and genetic drift of another important but neutral polymorphism (Gelernter, Kranzler, & Cubells, 1997; Gelernter, Kranzler, Coccaro, Siever, & New, 1998). Whether this difference in frequency of short- versus long-allele carriers between Japanese and Caucasian populations drives the cultural variation in cognition and emotion observed at behavioral and neural levels is an intriguing question for future research.

Despite growing evidence that substantial variation in genomic frequencies exists across cultures, we are only beginning to understand its functional scope and the broader implications for explaining cultural variation in psychological processes, brain structure, and function. Enthusiasm for this endeavor is to be met with caution, because scholars need not look too far back in history for examples of arguments whereby genomic differences across the races were documented as a means of justifying a racial hierarchy (Eberhardt, 2005; Fraser, 1995). As Gould (1981) and others have aptly cautioned, science does not operate solely in an objective vacuum but in the mosh pit of social, political, and historical ideologies and environments. Scientists should be aware of the moral issues at stake when conducting cultural neuroscience research and take responsibility to protect against potential misuse or misinterpretation of their findings by the lay public, media or naïve scholars.

Correspondence of Culture Variation across Levels of Analysis

One way that investigations of cultural differences in brain function may prove useful is to provide converging evidence that extends behavioral research to demonstrate cultural differences in cognitive, emotional, or perceptual abilities. A recent fMRI study comparing neural activity during the Framed Line Test (FLT) between East Asians living in the United States for less than 7 years and European Americans provides a compelling example (Ketay et al., 2005). Originally created by Kitayama and colleagues (2003), the FLT assesses one's capacity both to incorporate and to ignore contextual information in a nonsocial domain. In the original version of the FLT, participants are presented with a square frame with a vertical line embedded within it and are then shown another square frame of the same or different size. They are asked to draw a line that is either identical to the first line in the first square frame in absolute length (absolute condition) or proportionate to the height of the surrounding frame (relative condition). The absolute condition requires one to ignore the context (both the first and second frame) when reproducing the line, whereas the relative condition requires one to incorporate context when reproducing the line. Results from a previous behavioral study of the FLT showed that Asians were more accurate in the relative condition, whereas European Americans were more accurate in the absolute condition (Kitayama et al., 2003).

In the recent neuroimaging study of the FLT, participants performing a modified version of

the task viewed a series of stimuli, each comprising a line inside a square, both of which varied systematically in size across trials. Specifically, participants judged whether either (1) the proportional size of the line relative to the square was the same as the stimuli just seen in the previous trial (relative condition) or (2) the absolute length of the line, regardless of the square size, was the same (absolute condition). Results from this study revealed cultural variation in neural responses to the extent that certain brain regions were recruited to perform the relative and absolute line judgment tasks. East Asians demonstrated greater recruitment of the dorsolateral prefrontal cortex (DLPFC), a brain region important in working memory tasks, for absolute versus relative line judgments, whereas European Americans showed more engagement of the anterior cingulate cortex (ACC), a brain region typically engaged during cognitive conflict, for relative versus absolute line judgments. These fMRI results extend previous behavioral results showing that East Asians and European Americans use different cognitive strategies to perceive objects embedded within a background by demonstrating differential recruitment of neural circuitry during such perceptual judgments between cultural groups.

Culture Variation in Neural Systems

Cultural differences may also exist at the neural level, even in the absence of cultural differences in the behavioral level. For example, an fMRI study by Gutchess, Welsh, Boduroglu, and Park (2006) compared neural activation between East Asian Americans and European Americans as they performed unintentional encoding of a series of pictures of objects (e.g., elephant), backgrounds (e.g., beach) and objects embedded in meaningful backgrounds (e.g., elephant on a beach), and rated how pleasant they found the pictures (e.g., *pleasant*, *neutral*, or *unpleasant*). After scanning, participants were given a surprise recognition test. Ratings of pleasantness did not interact with the culture of participants. Moreover, East Asian Americans and European Americans performed equally well, suggesting that task difficulty was equivalent across the two groups of participants, but significant group differences emerged in recruitment of distinct brain regions. Specifically, European Americans activated more regions implicated in object processing, including the bilateral middle temporal gyrus, left superior parietal/angular gyrus, and right superior temporal/supramarginal gyrus. These results suggest that people of different cultural groups may use different encoding strategies and recruit different neural systems, even though both groups perform on object recognition tasks with equivalent behavioral competence.

In a cross-cultural fMRI study conducted in our laboratory on the neural bases of emotion recognition, Japanese participants, living in Japan, and European American participants, living in the United States, were scanned while explicitly recognizing Japanese and European American happy, neutral, fearful, and angry facial expressions (Chiao et al., 2004). Behavioral results indicated that all participants recognized facial expressions in Japanese and European American faces equally well. However, neuroimaging results showed that more Japanese than European American participants recruited distinct neural networks while judging ingroup versus outgroup emotional expressions. Hence, cultural variation in how the brain processes information may exist even when cultural variation is not observable in behavior; thus, inquiry into cultural variation at the neural level has the serious potential to provide novel insight into the universality and cultural specificity of neural processing.

Culture as Experience

Another way that cultural differences at the neural level may emerge is in brain regions that are experience-dependent or experience-sensitive. Modulation in these regions reflects the degree of familiarity or exposure to a given type of stimulus or task and may be accompanied by heightened skill or proficiency in a given behavioral task. One example of this kind of cultural difference at the neural level comes from fMRI and ERP face recognition studies in adults, showing that activity in the fusiform gyrus differs for faces of different racial or cultural groups and may be moderated by degree of interracial exposure (Golby, Gabrieli, Chiao, & Eberhardt, 2001). Another example of the influence of musical expertise or familiarity on neural responses comes from studies comparing neural responses to music in professional musicians and in novices. Recent ERP research suggests that familiarity with a given musical instrument alters neural re-

sponses to that instrument's sound. In particular, Turkish listeners showed a greater P3 amplitude response to hearing music from a familiar instrument (e.g., *ney*) relative to an unfamiliar instrument (e.g., cello), suggesting that hearing familiar music increases the allocation of attentional resources during memory (Arikan et al., 1999). Moreover, Morrison and colleagues (2003) used fMRI to compare neural activity in professional musicians (expert) and novices (control) while they listened to music of their own (Western-familiar) versus other culture (Chinese-unfamiliar). They found no difference in neural responses during listening to Western versus Chinese music in either music experts or novices, supporting the view that differences in cultural content (e.g., genre of music) do not necessarily affect brain responses. However, professional musicians demonstrated greater activity in the right superior temporal gyrus in response to both music genres, and in the right midfrontal region for Western music and the left midfrontal region for Chinese music. This latter finding indicates that expertise or training in a given skill, namely, listening to music, enhances activity in brain regions underlying that capacity. Moreover, the rostromedial prefrontal cortex in Western music experts demonstrates sensitivity to Western tonal structure, such that different voxels within this region activate for different tonal keys (Janata et al., 2002). Taken together, these studies illustrate how cortical responses may be shaped by cultural experience.

Culture as a Perceptual Filter

Culture may influence cortical responses not only through the shaping of perceptual experience but also by providing a body of semantic knowledge with which to filter and interpret perceptual experiences. In an interesting attempt to examine whether cultural knowledge influences perceptual experience and its neural correlates, McClure and colleagues (2004) compared neural activity while drinking either Coke or Pepsi. Double-blind behavioral tests indicated that people demonstrate strong preferences for either Coke or Pepsi. Moreover, regression analyses comparing behavioral and neural data revealed that activity in the ventromedial prefrontal cortex (VMPFC) was positively correlated with these behavioral preferences for anonymously delivered Coke and Pepsi. Moreover, when delivery of Coke or

Pepsi was preceded by cultural information (e.g., picture of a Coke or Pepsi can), a broader range of brain regions was recruited, including bilateral hippocampus and DLPFC, relative to when delivery was preceded by a simple light. These results suggest that taste preferences are shaped by at least two kinds of neural response: (1) in the VMPFC, associated primarily with the chemical composition of the drink; and (2) in the bilateral hippocampus and DLPFC, associated with cultural knowledge of the drink. Thus, cultural associations to drinks built up over time through exposure to advertisements, can influence neural activity during gustatory perception and significantly shape gustatory preferences.

FURTHER METHODOLOGICAL CONSIDERATIONS FOR CULTURAL NEUROSCIENCE RESEARCH

The growing number of cultural neuroscience investigations demonstrates the viability of a cultural neuroscience approach. However, just as early cross-cultural behavioral research was hampered by methodological problems, it is important to address methodological issues that hinder the progress of cultural neuroscience research on questions of interest.

Inclusion of Participants from All Cultures

The first issue involves participant sampling and access to necessary equipment. Currently, neuroscience research is conducted on expensive, stationary, and high-maintenance equipment (e.g., fMRI, ERP) available predominantly in rich, industrialized regions within North America, Japan, and Western Europe. Successful application of neuroscience methods to psychology questions requires extensive user training and technical support. This situation severely limits this research to these geographical regions or countries, therefore limiting the groups of participants studied. Evidence of a sampling bias is evident, because over 96% of imaging sites where basic cognitive and affective neuroimaging research is conducted are based in Western Europe or the United States (Raichle, 2003). Thus, one methodological problem that needs to be resolved is how to facilitate neuroscience research for scientists and participants in cultures where the technology and scientific instrumentation necessary to conduct these experiments is absent or difficult

to access. A possible solution is to develop and use neuroscience methods that are transportable to countries where the cultural group of interest resides. The solution to the problem of how to facilitate neuroscience research in regions of the world where the necessary technology does not exist or is difficult to access is likely to require international cooperation and support from governments and private institutions in countries where the necessary scientific technology and infrastructure is already available. Although this is a challenging problem, finding ways to include diverse populations in neuroscience research is crucial to characterize fully mechanisms and structures in the human brain.

Testing within a Culture or between Cultures?

To sidestep this participant sampling problem, most cross-cultural neuroscience investigations to date have been conducted at one scanner site, using recent immigrants or bilingual speakers as participants, rather that multiple scanner sites, so that participants may be tested in their native environment (Gutchess et al., in press; Ketay et al., 2005; Kobayashi & Temple, 2004). Although this strategy has the benefit of eliminating the possibility of introducing noise due to testing environment alone, it may lack some ecological validity because recent immigrants or bilinguals, through acculturation, may identify more with their current culture during testing and adopt strategies optimal for that cultural environment, thereby reducing the probability of finding cultural variation at the neural level. An alternative strategy is to test participants across multiple scanner sites located in each cultural group's native environment (Chiao et al., 2004). This strategy optimizes ecological validity, because the researchers are also likely to belong to the same culture, enhancing the probability that participants' frame of mind while performing the task strictly relates to their own culture. It is possible that this strategy also introduces another potential confound of variance, namely, differences in signal attributable solely to differences in scanner sites. However, previous neuroimaging studies to examine reliability of fMRI and PET results acquired in different testing sites have found that minimal differences in the data were attributable solely to scanner environment, suggesting that comparing imaging results collected from two different scanner sites is appropriate and potentially a more advantageous strategy for conducting cultural neuroscience research (Casey et al., 1998; Ojemann et al., 1998).

Culturally Appropriate Brain Templates

Another pressing methodological issue involves the creation of culturally appropriate brain templates for spatial normalization of imaging data and brain atlases used for structure–function mapping. For neuroimaging studies, it is necessary to normalize the images of individual brains to a standard spatial template. Some scientists have argued that brain size and shape significantly vary across different racial groups (Park & Gutchess, 2002). Because the spatial normalization templates and brain atlas used currently (e.g., Montreal Neurological Institute [MNI] space and Talairach Daemon) were created by averaging brain images of predominantly white individuals, it is plausible that these templates are inadequate for capturing subtle but significant variation in brain structure that may subsequently affect where differences in brain function are mapped and observed (Evans et al., 1992; Mazziotta, Toga, Evans, Fox, & Lancaster, 1995; Talairach & Tournoux, 1988). Such considerations may be especially important when studying phenomena that reveal themselves in small areas of brain tissue, such as subnuclei within the amygdala.

Selection of Experimental Measures

A third methodological issue concerns the experimental materials used (e.g., stimuli, task, and procedure). As reviewed earlier in this chapter, cultural psychologists faced many problems in developing sound cross-cultural behavioral measures. In adapting these behavioral paradigms to neuroscience research, several considerations emerge (Aguirre & D'Esposito, 1999). First of all, neuroimaging and electrophysiological experiments typically require many trials depending on the type of design. Because some scientists may want to examine cultural variation in neural responses for tasks in which a behavioral difference has already been demonstrated, an event-related design would be most appropriate so that behavioral responses for each trial can be recorded and mapped onto individual physiological events. In particular, event-related fMRI

designs, which involve recording of behavioral and neural responses on a trial-by-trial basis, typically require more power than block or parametric designs; thus it will be important to include a sufficient number of trials per relevant condition (Buckner & Braver, 1999). Furthermore, tasks, instructions and stimulus displays need to be modified, so that they have equivalent meaning across cultures. When designing neuroimaging studies based on prior cross-cultural behavioral work, special consideration may be given to selecting paradigms that yield a large effect because of the typical smaller sample size in neuroimaging studies relative to cultural psychology behavioral studies. Finally, whereas some of the most effective cultural psychology behavioral paradigms involve tasks that require participants to provide responses beyond a button press (e.g., drawing a line or describing an event), behavioral responses in a majority of current neuroimaging environments are restricted to button presses or vocal responses to minimize potential face and body movement, which can create a significant artifact in the neuroimaging data. Although cultural psychology and neuroscience methods bring unique issues to the experimental design table, each of these issues is resolvable, as suggested by recent progress in cultural neuroscience research.

Genotyping Participants

A fourth methodological concern involves integrating cross-cultural genomic data with neuroimaging. Finding an adequate number of participants (e.g., 15–20) who carry the short- and long-allele version of a given functional polymorphism may require genotyping three times the number of desired participants—particularly for polymorphisms that include a rare version. Once preliminary genotyping has identified an adequate number of participants in both cultures, other neural and behavioral testing can be administered. Integrating genotyping with neural and behavioral assays may have profound explanatory power in explaining cultural differences in neural responses and behavior. For example, significant variation may exist in behavior and/or neural activity between cultural groups; however, further inspection may show that these cultural differences are really driven by differences in ratio of short- to long-allele carriers between cultural groups. Although the pragmatic difficulties of conducting such research are likely to be great, the potential for discovering new ways of explaining cultural variation across all levels of analysis is tremendous.

IMPLICATIONS OF CULTURAL NEUROSCIENCE FOR BASIC AND APPLIED RESEARCH

The ability for a cultural neuroscience framework to provide novel links between sociocultural and biological phenomenon is unprecedented. The development of paradigms and tools with the three fields of cultural psychology, social–cognitive–affective neuroscience, and imaging genomics make this endeavor possible in ways never previously imagined. We do not expect that the study of all psychological and biological phenomena will necessitate a cultural neuroscience approach. Rather, the goal and challenge for cultural neuroscience is to identify the phenomena that *can* be readily mapped within and across levels. It is these phenomena that hold the promise to provide a window into our understanding of the interplay of sociocultural and biological forces.

There are at least two foreseeable benefits of a cultural neuroscience approach for basic and applied research: the merging of natural and social sciences, and the enhancement in the condition; and care of human health across different cultural groups.

Merging the Scientific Study of Culture and Biology

The study of culture and biology has long been stratified within universities and academic subfields, creating a deep conceptual and methodological schism between these different communities of researchers. Snow (1959) once hypothesized that molecular biology could serve as a bridge between the two areas of thought. However, only modest progress has been made so far, because genetic–behavior association studies have only been mildly successful. We hypothesize that cultural neuroscience stands in an even greater position to bridge the culture–biology gap by pulling perspectives and methodologies from every area of psychology (from evolutionary and cognitive to cultural and developmental psychology), as well as from the fields of anthropology, molecular biology, and neuroscience. The tools needed to investigate the links between multiple levels of analysis are available in ways not previously imaginable, and the results of utilizing these tools to investigate phenomena using a cultural neuroscience approach are likely to enable us to articulate with greater specification our conceptions of culture and its mutually influential relationship with biology. The cultural neuroscience framework aims to reshape the trend to specialize and stay within the confines of one's academic subfield toward a transdisciplinary integration of theoretical knowledge and methodological expertise across the social and natural sciences.

Implications for Population Health

The important interplay of culture and genes in the study of population health has long been appreciated (Shields et al., 2005). This belief stems from the fact that significant differences exist in the frequency with which certain health conditions occur across cultural groups. For example, because of "founder effects," Ashkenazi Jewish people have a greater prevalence of Tay–Sachs disease, and cystic fibrosis is more common among people from Northern Europe (Exner, Dries, Domanski, & Cohen, 2001; Wang & Sue, 2005). Another example is population differences in allelic frequency of the gene *CYP2A6*, which affects the likelihood of nicotine addiction (Shields et al., 2005). Protective forms of the *CYP2A6* are very rare in people who self-identify as European or African (less than 3%), but they are more prevalent in people who self-identify as Japanese or Korean (as great as 24%; Shields et al., 2005). How do differences in genetic frequencies affect brain systems and behavior underlying physical and mental health conditions? How do cultural forces affect the expression and function of these genes, and their effect on brain and behavior?

The answers to these intriguing questions are finally within our empirical grasp. Our hope is that the cultural neuroscience framework may be used effectively to identify and investigate candidate phenomena using the prescribed, multiple levels of analytic approach. By integrating across disciplines and methodologies from cultural to biological levels of analysis, we will meaningfully enhance our chances of understanding of how sociocultural and biological forces interact and shape each other, and finding potential ways to direct this knowledge toward timely issues in population health.

ACKNOWLEDGMENTS

We would like to thank Angela Gutchess, Kristin Bellanca, Nicholas Rule, Jan Leu and participants of the 2002 Harvard Culture, Emotion and the Brain workshop for their helpful comments. This work was supported by a National Science Foundation Graduate Research Fellowship to Joan Y. Chiao and by National Institutes of Health Grant No. R01 MH070833-01A1 to Nalini Ambady.

NOTES

1. *alfred.med.yale.edu/alfred/aboutalfred.asp*
2. This cultural difference at the level of genes is not in the actual makeup of the *5-HTT* functional polymorphism, or in how the gene expresses itself, but in the frequency of carriers of the gene or the ratio of people carrying the short- or long-allele version of the gene in the entire population.

REFERENCES

Aguirre, G. K., & D'Esposito, M. (1999). Experimental design for brain FMRI. In A. L. Baert, K. Sartor, & J. E. Youker (Eds.), *Functional MRI* (pp. 369–380). New York: Springer.

Arikan, M. K., Venrim, M., Oran, O., Inan, S., Elhih, M., & Demiralp, T. (1999). Music effects on event-related potentials of humans on the basis of cultural environment. *Neuroscience Letters, 268*(1), 21–24.

Benjamin J., Li, L., Patterson, C., Greenberg, B. D., Murphy, D. L., & Hamer, D. H. (1996). Population and familial association between the D4 dopamine receptor gene and measures of novelty seeking. *Nature Genetics, 2*, 81–84.

Betancourt, H., & Lopez, S. R. (1993). The study of culture, ethnicity, and race in American psychology. *American Psychologist, 48*, 629–637.

Bolger, D. J., Perfetti, C. A., & Schneider, W. (2005). Cross-cultural effect on the brain revisited: Universal structures plus writing system variation. *Human Brain Mapping, 25*(1), 92–104.

Bonham, V. L., Warshauer-Baker, E., & Collins, F. S. (2005). Race and ethnicity in the genome era: The complexity of the constructs. *American Psychologist, 60*(1), 9–15.

Boroditsky, L. (2001). Does language shape thought?: English and Mandarin speakers' conceptions of time. *Cognitive Psychology, 43*(1), 1–22.

Boroditsky, L. (in press). Linguistic relativity. In *Encyclopedia of cognitive science*. MacMillan.

Brislin, R. (1970). Back-translation for cross-cultural research. *Journal of Cross-Cultural Psychology, 1*(3), 185–216.

Buckner, R. L., & Braver, T. S. (1999). Event-related functional MRI. In A. L. Baert, K. Sartor, & J. E. Youker (Eds.), *Functional MRI* (pp. 441–450). New York: Springer.

Cacioppo, J. T., Lorig, T. S., Nusbaum, H. C., & Berntson, G. G. (2004). Social neuroscience: Bridging social and biological systems. In C. Sansone, C. C. Morf, & A. T. Panter (Eds.), *The Sage handbook of methods in social psychology* (pp. 383–404). Thousand Oaks, CA: Sage.

Casey, B. J., Cohen, J. D., O'Craven, K., Davidson, R. J., Irwin, W., Nelson, C. A., et al. (1998). Reproducibility of fMRI results across four institutions using a spatial working memory task. *NeuroImage, 8*(3), 249–261.

Caspi, A., Sugden, K. Moffitt, T. E., Taylor, A., Criag, I. W., Harrington, H., et al. (2003). Influence of life stress on depression: Moderation by a polymorphism in the 5-HTT gene. *Science, 301*, 386–389.

Cavalli-Sforza, L. L. (1998). The DNA revolution in populations. *Trends in Genetics, 14*(2), 60–65.

Cavalli-Sforza, L. L. (2005). The human genome diversity project: Past, present and future. *Nature Reviews: Genetics, 6*(4), 333–340.

Chen, C., Burton, M. L., Greenberger, E., & Dmitrieva, J. (1999). Population migration and the variation of dopamine (DRD4) allele frequencies around the globe. *Evolution and Human Behavior, 20*, 309–324.

Chen, C., Lee, S. Y., & Stevenson, H. W. (1995). Response style and cross-cultural comparison. *Psychological Science, 6*, 170–175.

Cheung, K. H., Osier, M. V., Kidd, J. R., Pakstis, A. J., Miller, P. L., & Kidd, K. K. (2000). ALFRED: An allele frequency database for diverse populations and DNA polymorphisms. *Nucleic Acids Research, 28*(1), 361–363.

Chiao, J. Y., Iidaka, T., Bar, M., Aminoff, E., Nogawa, J., & Ambady, N. (2004). *Culture influences neural responses during emotion recognition.* Poster presented at the 34th Annual Society for Neuroscience meeting, San Diego.

Cosmides, L., Tooby, J., & Barkow, J. (1992). Evolutionary psychology and conceptual integration. In *The adapted mind: Evolutionary psychology and the generation of culture* (pp. 3–18). New York: Oxford University Press.

Davidson, R. J. (2003). Affective neuroscience and psychophysiology: Toward a synthesis. *Psychophysiology, 40*, 655–665.

Dennett, D. (1995). *Darwin's dangerous idea: Evolution and the meanings of life.* New York: Simon & Schuster.

Eberhardt, J. L. (2005). Imaging race. *American Psychologist, 60*, 181–190.

Elfenbein, H. A., & Ambady, N. (2002). On the universality and cultural specificity of emotion recognition: A meta-analysis. *Psychological Bulletin, 128*, 203–235.

Evans, A. C., Marrett, S., Neelin, P., Collins, L., Worsley, K., Dai, W., et al. (1992). Anatomical mapping of functional activation in stereotactic coordinate space. *NeuroImage, 1*(1), 43–53.

Exner, D. V., Dries, D. L., Domanski, M. J., & Cohen, J. N. (2001). Lesser response of angiotensin-converting-enzyme inhibitor therapy in black as compared with white patients with left ventricular dysfunction. *New England Journal of Medicine, 344,* 1351–1377.

Fraser, S. (1995). *The bell curve wars.* New York: Basic Books.

Furmark, T., Tillfords, M., Garpenstrand, H., Marteinsdottir, I., Langstrom, B., Oreland, L., & Fredrikson, M. (2004). Serotonin transporter polymorphism related to amygdala excitability and symptom severity in patients with social phobia. *Neuroscience Letters, 362*(3), 189–192.

Garpenstrand, H., Annas, P., Ekblom, J., Oreland, L., & Fredrikson, M. (2001). Human fear conditioning is related to dopaminergic and serotonergic biological markers. *Behavioral Neuroscience, 115*(2), 358–364.

Gauthier, I., & Nelson, C. (2001). The development of face expertise. *Current Opinion in Neurobiology, 11,* 219–224.

Gazzaniga, M. S., Ivry, R., & Mangun, G. R. (2002). *Cognitive neuroscience: The biology of the mind.* New York: Norton.

Gelernter, J., Kranzler, H., Coccaro, E. F., Siever, L. J., & New, A. S. (1998). Serotonin transporter protein gene polymorphism and personality measures in African American and European American subjects. *American Journal of Psychiatry, 155*(10), 1332–1338.

Gelernter, J., Kranzler, H., Coccaro, E., Siever, L., New, A., & Mulgrew, C. L. (1997). D4 dopamine-reception (DRD4) alleles and novelty seeking in substance-dependent, personality-disorder, and control subjects. *American Journal of Human Genetics, 61*(5), 1144–1152.

Gelernter, J., Kranzler, H., & Cubells, J.F. (1997). Serotonin transporter protein (SLC6A4) allele and haplotype frequencies and linkage disequilibria in African- and European-American and Japanese populations and in alcohol-dependent subjects. *Human Genetics, 101*(2), 243–246.

Golby, A. J., Gabrieli, J. D. E., Chiao, J. Y., & Eberhardt, J. L. (2001). Differential fusiform responses to same- and other-race faces. *Nature Neuroscience, 4*(8), 845–850.

Gould, S. J. (1981). *The mismeasure of man.* New York: Norton.

Greenfield, P. (1997). Culture as process: Empirical methods for cultural psychology. In J. W. Berry, Y. H. Poortinga, & J. Pandey (Eds.), *Handbook of cross-cultural psychology* (Vol. 1, pp. 301–346). Boston: Allyn & Bacon.

Gutchess, A., Welsh, R. C., Boduroglu, A., & Park, D. C. (2006). Cultural differences in neural function associated with object processing. *Cognitive, Affective and Behavioral Neuroscience, 6*(2), 102–109.

Handy, T. C. (2005). *Event-related potentials: A methods handbook.* Cambridge, MA: MIT Press.

Hariri, A. R., Mattay, V. S., Tessitore, A., Kolachana, B., Fera, F., Goldman, D., et al. (2002). Serotonin transporter genetic variation and the response of the human amygdala. *Science, 297,* 400–404.

Hariri, A. R., & Weinberger, D. (2003). Imaging genomics. *British Medical Bulletin, 65,* 237–248.

Heeger, D. J., & Ress, D. (2002). What does fMRI tell us about neuronal activity? *Nature Reviews: Neuroscience, 3,* 142–151.

Heine, S. J., Lehman, D. R., Peng, K., & Greenholtz, J. (2002). What's wrong with cross-culural comparisons of subjective Likert scales? The reference group effect. *Journal of Personality and Social Psychology, 82*(6), 903–918.

Heine, S. J., Takata, T., & Lehman, D. R. (2000). Beyond self-presentation: Evidence for Japanese self-criticism. *Personality and Social Psychology Bulletin, 26,* 71–78.

Jahoda, G. (2002). Culture, biology and development across history. In H. Keller, Y. H. Poortinga, & A. Schoemerich (Eds.), *Between culture and biology: Perspectives on ontogenetic development* (pp. 13–29). Cambridge, UK: Cambridge University Press.

Janata, P., Birk, J. L., Van Horn, J. D., Leman, M., Tillmann, B., & Bharucha, J. J. (2002). The cortical topography of tonal structures underlying Western music. *Science, 298,* 2167–2170.

Janata, P., & Grafton, S. T. (2003). Swinging in the brain: Shared neural substrates for behaviors related to sequencing and music. *Nature Neuroscience, 6*(7), 682–687.

Johnson, M. H. (1997). *Developmental cognitive neuroscience: An introduction.* Oxford, UK: Blackwell.

Johnson, M. H., & Munakata, Y. (2005). Processes of change in brain and cognitive development. *Trends in Cognitive Science, 9*(3), 152–158.

Katsuragi, S., Kunugi, H., Sano, A., Tsutsumi, T., Isogawa, K., Nanko, S., et al. (1999). Association between serotonin transporter gene polymorphism and anxiety-related traits. *Biological Psychiatry, 45*(3), 368–370.

Ketay, S., Hedden, T., Aron, A., Markus, H., & Gabrieli, J. D. E. (2005). Cultural differences in neural activation during relative versus absolutely perceptual judgments (Program No. 409.24). *2005 Abstract Viewer/Itinerary Planner.* Washington, DC: Society for Neuroscience.

Kitayama, S., Duffy, S., Kawamura, R., & Larsen, J. T. (2003). Perceiving an object and its context in different cultures: A cultural look at new look. *Psychological Science, 14,* 201–206.

Kobayashi, C., & Temple, E. (2004). *Neural basis of Japanese theory of mind is different from English one?* Paper presented at the 34th Annual Society for Neuroscience meeting, San Diego.

Kosslyn, S. M. (1999). If neuroimaging is the answer, what is the question? *Philosophical Transactions of the Royal Society of London B, 354*(1387), 1283–1294.

Kumakiri, C., Kodama, K., Shimizu, E., Yamanouchi, N., Okada, S., Noda, S., et al. (1999). Study of the association between the serotonin transporter gene regulatory region polymorphism and personality traits in a Japanese population. *Neuroscience Letters*, 263, 205–207.

Lam, K. C., Buehler, R., McFarland, C., Ross, M., & Cheung, I. (2005). Cultural differences in affective forecasting: the role of focalism. *Personality and Social Psychological Bulletin*, 31(9), 1296–1309.

Lesch, K. P., Bengel, D., Heils, A., Sabol, S. Z., Greenberg, B. D., Petri, S., et al. (1996). Association of anxiety-related traits with a polymorphism in the serotonin transporter gene regulatory region. *Science*, 274(5292), 1527–1531.

Li, S.-C. (2003). Biocultural orchestration of developmental plasticity across levels: The interplay of biology and culture in shaping the mind and behavior across the life span. *Psychological Bulletin*, 129(2), 171–194.

Maguire, E. A., Gadian, D. G., Johnsrude, I. S., Good, C. D., Ashburner, J., Frackowiak, R. S. J., et al. (2000). Navigation-related structural change in the hippocampi of taxi drivers. *Proceedings of the National Academy of Sciences USA*, 97(8), 4398–4403.

Markus, H., & Kitayama, S. (1991). Culture and the self: Implications for cognition, emotion and motivation. *Psychological Review*, 98, 224–253.

Markus, H., Kitayama, S., & Heiman, R. (1996). Culture and "basic" psychological principles. In E. T. Higgins & A. W. Kruglanski (Eds.), *Social psychology: Handbook of basic principles* (pp. 857–913). New York: Guilford Press.

Masuda, T., & Nisbett, R. E. (2001). Attending holistically vs. analytically: Comparing the context sensitivity of Japanese and Americans. *Journal of Personality and Social Psychology*, 81, 922–934.

Mazziotta, J. C., Toga, A. W., Evans, A., Fox, P., & Lancaster, J. (1995). A probabilistic atlas of the human brain: Theory and rationale for its development. *NeuroImage*, 2, 89–101.

McCabe, K. (2003). Neuroeconomics. In L. Nadel (Ed.), *Encyclopedia of cognitive science* (pp. 294–298). New York: Macmillan.

McClure, S., Li, J., Tomlin, D., Cypert, K. S., Montague, L. M., & Montague, P. R. (2004). Neural correlates of behavioral preference for culturally familiar drinks. *Neuron*, 44, 379–387.

Mesquita, B., & Frijda, N. H. (1992). Cultural variations in emotions: A review. *Psychological Bulletin*, 112, 179–204.

Miyamoto, Y., & Kitayama, S. (2002). Cultural variation in correspondence bias: The critical role of attitude diagnosticity of socially constrained behavior. *Journal of Personality and Social Psychology*, 83, 1239–1248.

Miyamoto, Y., Nisbett, R. E., & Masuda, T. (2006). Culture and the physical environment: Holistic versus analytic perceptual affordances. *Psychological Science*, 17(2), 113–119.

Morris, M., & Peng, K. (1994). Culture and cause: American and Chinese attributions for social and physical events. *Journal of Personality and Social Psychology*, 67, 949–971.

Morrison, S. J., Demorest, S. M., Aylward, E. H., Cramer, S. C., & Maravilla, K. R. (2003). FMRI investigation of cross-cultural music comprehension. *NeuroImage*, 20(1), 378–384.

Munafo, M. R., Clark, T. G., Moore, L. R., Payne, E., Walton, R., & Flint, J. (2003). Genetic polymorphisms and personality in healthy adults: A systematic review and meta-analysis. *Molecular Psychiatry*, 8(5), 471–484.

Nagel, T. (1998). Conceiving the impossible and the mind–body problem. *Philosophy*, 73(285), 337–352.

Neville, H. J., & Bavelier, D. (1998). Neural organization and plasticity of language. *Current Opinion in Neurobiology*, 8(2), 254–258.

Nisbett, R. E., & Cohen, D. (1996). *Culture of honor: The psychology of violence in the South*. Boulder, CO: Westview Press.

Nisbett, R. E., & Norenzayan, A. (2002). Culture and cognition. In H. Pashler & D. L. Medin (Eds.), *Stevens handbook of experimental psychology: Cognition* (3rd ed., Vol. 2, pp. 561–597). New York: Wiley.

Nisbett, R. E., Peng, K., Choi, I., & Norenzayan, A. (2001). Culture and systems of thought: Holistic vs. analytic cognition. *Psychological Review*, 108, 291–310.

Norenzayan, A., & Heine, S. J. (2005). Psychological universals: What are they and how can we know? *Psychological Bulletin*, 135, 763–784.

Ochsner, K., & Lieberman, M. (2001). The emergence of social cognitive neuroscience. *American Psychologist*, 56, 717–734.

Ojemann, J. G., Buckner, R. L., Akbudak, E., Snyder, A. Z., Ollinger, J. M., McKinstry, R. C., et al. (1998). Functional MRI studies of word-stem completion: Reliability across laboratories and comparison to blood flow imaging with PET. *Human Brain Mapping*, 6(4), 203–215.

Osier, M. V., Cheung, K. H., Rajeevan, H., Pakstis, A. J., Kidd, J. R., Miller, P. L., et al. (2002). ALFRED (ALlele FREquency Database): A resource for genetic anthropology and human population genetics. *Human Origins and Disease: CSHL Meeting Abstracts of Papers*, 43.

Park, D. C., & Gutchess, A. H. (2002). Aging, cognition and culture: A neuroscientific perspective. *Neuroscience and Biobehavioral Reviews*, 26(7), 859–867.

Paulesu, E., McCrory, E., Fazio, F., Menoncello, L., Brunswick, N., Cappa, S. F., et al. (2000). A cultural effect on brain function. *Nature Neuroscience*, 3(1), 91–96.

Paulus, W., Hallett, M., Rossini, P. M., & Rothwell, J. C. (1998). Transcranial magnetic stimulation. In *Proceedings of the International Symposium on Transcranial Stimulation*. Gottingen: Elsevier.

Peng, K., Nisbett, R., & Wong, N. Y. C. (1997). Validity problems comparing value across cultures and possible solutions. *Psychological Methods, 2,* 329–344.

Plomin, R., & Kosslyn, S. M. (2001). Genes, brain and cognition. *Nature Neuroscience, 4,* 1153–1155.

Raichle, M. E. (2003). Functional brain imaging and the human brain. *Journal of Neuroscience, 23*(10), 3959–3962.

Sankar, P., & Cho, M. K. (2002). Toward a new vocabulary of human genetic variation. *Science, 298*(5597), 1337–1338.

Sen, S., Burmeiter, M., & Ghosh, D. (2004). Meta-analysis of the association between a serotonin transporter promoter polymorphism (5-HTTLPR) and anxiety-related personality traits. *American Journal of Medical Genetics B, 127*(1), 85–89.

Shields, A. E., Fortun, M., Hammonds, E. M., King, P. A., Lerman, C., Rapp, R., et al. (2005). The use of race variables in genetic studies of complex traits and the goal of reducing health disparities: A transdisciplinary perspective. *American Psychologist, 60*(10), 77–103.

Smedley, A., & Smedley, B. (2005). Race as biology is fiction, racism as a social problem is real: Anthropological and historical perspectives on the social construction of race. *American Psychologist, 60*(1), 16–26.

Snow, C. P. (1959). *The two cultures and the scientific revolution.* New York: Cambridge University Press.

Talairach, J., & Tournoux, P. (1988). Co-planar stereotaxic atlas of the human brain: 3-dimensional proportional system—an approach to cerebral imaging. New York: Theime.

Tishkoff, S. A., & Kidd, K. K. (2004). Implications of biogeography of human populations for "race" and medicine. *Nature Genetics, 36*(11), S21–S27.

Umekage, T., Tochigi, M., Marui, T., Kato, C., Hibino, H., Otani, T., et al. (2003). Serotonin transporter-linked promoter region polymorphism and personality traits in a Japanese population. *Neuroscience Letters, 337,* 13–16.

Wolbers, T., Weiller, C., & Buchel, C. (2004). Neural foundations of emerging route knowledge in complex spatial environments. *Cognitive Brain Research, 21,* 401–411.

Wang, V. O., & Sue, S. (2005). In the eye of the storm: Race and genomics in research and practice. *American Psychologist, 60*(1), 37–45.

Xue, G., Chen, C., Jin, Z., & Dong, Q. (2006). Cerebral asymmetry in the fusiform areas predicted the efficiency of learning a new writing system. *Journal of Cognitive Neuroscience, 18,* 923–931.

CHAPTER 10

Priming "Culture"
Culture as Situated Cognition

DAPHNA OYSERMAN
SPIKE WING-SING LEE

Culture can be operationalized as a set of structures and institutions, values, traditions, and ways of engaging with the social and nonsocial world that are transmitted across generations in a certain time and place (e.g., Shweder & LeVine, 1984); that is, culture is both temporally continuous and specific. It is located in a time and situated in a geographic and social place. Because of its situated character, culture is neither perfectly transmitted to all members of a cultural group nor is it perfectly uniform across all members of a culture. In other words, though cultures are shared, they are not fully "in the head" of any particular member of a culture (e.g., Mendoza-Denton & Mishel, Chapter 7, this volume). A number of theorists have described the variability in cultural knowledge spread or dissemination within a population (Atran, Medin, & Ross, 2005; Sperber, 2001). These authors all note that because culture is situated, one's place within a society and the social networks within which one is embedded should influence the aspects of "culture" to which one has access. Both context and change in context (e.g., through immigration) may (Kitayama, Ishii, Imada,

Takemura, & Ramaswamy, 2006) or may not (Atran et al., 2005) carry with it cultural change depending in part on features of the social networks in which one is embedded before and after contextual change.

Situated variability *within* cultural groups is of course not the whole story. The nature and meaning of subtle and not-so-subtle historical and current differences and similarities *between* cultural groups is a main interest of cultural and cross-cultural psychology. Felt difference can be large. Travelogues, comedy routines, diversity training, and business guides all attempt to illuminate (and bridge) differences in how time is understood, what appropriate norms for politeness are, and why other elements of everyday life seem opaque to outside observers coming from different racial/ethnic, religious, or other groups, different societies, nation-states, or regions of the world. Everyday situations, such as how winning or losing in sports is communicated (Markus, Uchida, & Omoregie, 2006); everyday language use such as whether or not personal pronouns can be omitted (E. Kashima & Y. Kashima, 1998); and the everyday assumptions

255

that make up organizational structures, documents, and mission statements (e.g., Rokeach & Ball-Rokeach, 1989) reflect these differences. Defined in this way, culture is clearly important. As a construct, it captures the breadth and diversity of humanness.

Unfortunately, this very breadth makes it difficult to systematically model "culture" to make predictions about when and how cultures systematically influence cognition, affect, motivation, and behavior. Although understanding a specific culture or a certain group within a culture at a certain time and place may be interesting, parsimonious and predictive rather than detailed and descriptive modeling is the central goal of cultural and cross-cultural psychology. Cultural and cross-cultural psychologists do not simply want to understand the ways that Americans and Japanese differ, or the ways that Germans and Chinese differ. Rather, the essential goal is to understand the ways that culture influences how the mind works and to identify cultural contingencies that moderate general processes of human cognition.

To take on this challenge, cultural psychologists must posit general processes that both differ in their average or likely occurrence across cultures and provide systematic prediction about the what (content) and how (process) of cognition. A number of potentially useful basic organizing constructs (e.g., "tight" vs. "loose" cultures—Triandis, 1995; "masculine" vs. "feminine" cultures—Hofstede, 1980; survival vs. self-expression—Inglehart, 1997; honor–modesty vs. shame—Gregg, 2005; see also Cohen, 2001), and frameworks (e.g., the ecocultural model—Berry, 1976, 1994; Georgas, 1988; 1993) have been proposed to address the basic process question. To date the two constructs that have most captured popular appeal are individualism and collectivism (e.g., Hofstede, 1980, 2001; Kagitçibasi, 1997; Kashima, Kashima, & Aldridge, 2001; Oyserman, Coon, & Kemmelmeier, 2002; Triandis, 1995).

Individualism, as described by Triandis (Chapter 3, this volume), characterizes a cultural syndrome in which the individual is the basic unit of analyses and societal structures are assumed to be of value to the extent that they support individual happiness. Collectivism, on the other hand, describes a cultural syndrome in which the group is the basic unit of analyses and societal structures are assumed

to be of value to the extent that they support preservation and enhancement of group resources. As reviewed by Oyserman, Coon, et al. (2002), plausible consequences of individualism and collectivism for basic concerns of psychology—how we make sense of ourselves and others (self-concept, relationality) and how we think more generally (cognition)—are easily discerned. These are outlined below.

Individualism implies that a basic self-goal is to feel good about oneself as a unique and distinctive person, and to define these unique features in terms of abstract traits. As a cultural syndrome it also implies that relationships are likely to feel chosen and voluntary rather than permanent and fixed; relationships thus construed can be worked on and improved or left when costs and benefits are imbalanced following equity norms. With regard to cognition, judgment, reasoning, and causal inference, individualism as a cultural syndrome implies that focus is generally oriented toward the person rather than the situation or social context, because the decontextualized self is assumed to be a stable, causal nexus (Choi, Nisbett, & Norenzayan, 1999; Miller, 1984; Morris & Peng, 1994; Newman, 1993). Thus, individualism promotes a decontextualized, as opposed to a situation-specific, reasoning style that assumes social information is not bound to social context. Oyserman and colleagues have described this style as a "separate and pull apart" style as opposed to a situation-specific, relational "embed and connect" style (Markus & Oyserman, 1989; Oyserman, Kemmelmeier, & Coon, 2002).

Collectivism implies that a basic self-goal is to attain and maintain group membership, so that the self is defined in terms of both group memberships and the traits and abilities relevant for maintaining these (e.g., loyalty, perseverance). As a cultural syndrome collectivism also implies that important group memberships are ascribed and fixed, viewed as "facts of life" to which people must accommodate; that boundaries between ingroups and outgroups are stable, relatively impermeable, and important; therefore, ingroup exchanges are based on equality or even generosity principles (Morris & Leung, 2000; Sayle, 1998; Triandis, 1995). With regard to cognition, judgment, reasoning, and causal inference, collectivism as a cultural syndrome implies that social context, situational constraints, and social roles figure prominently in person perception and causal reasoning (Miller, 1984; Morris & Peng, 1994), and that meaning is contextualized and memory is likely to contain richly embedded detail.

Indeed, a key strength of the individualism–collectivism operationalization of culture is that it sets the stage for specific and testable predictive models. Its parsimony has facilitated use of standard social-psychological priming methods to study effects of making salient features of individualism (or collectivism) on individual-level psychological processes. This narrowed focus of inquiry into culture as operationalized by the individualism and collectivism axes has been helpful in that it has led to specific and novel predictions about how cultural influence works and its impact on basic psychological processes.

For example, E. Kashima and Y. Kashima (1998; Y. Kashima & E. Kashima, 2003) use the individualism and collectivism frame to posit difference by culture group on whether language structure emphasizes or deemphasizes individual actors via pronoun dropping. Dropped pronouns allows the self to be in the background, to introduce one's spouse by saying "wife" rather than "my wife," to describe one's action by saying "going" rather than "I am going." Similarly, Markus and her colleagues (e.g., Markus & Kitayama, 1991; Markus & Oyserman, 1989; Oyserman, 1993) use the individualism and collectivism frame to posit difference by culture group on whether basic self-schemas are separate or connected, resulting in a chronic independent or interdependent way of making sense of the self. Perhaps most intriguingly, the individualism and collectivism frame is being used to posit difference by culture in both content and process of cognition—what and how we think (for earlier reviews, see Oyserman, Coon, et al., 2002; Oyserman, Kemmelmeier, et al., 2002).

In this chapter we provide a brief summary of the mostly correlational evidence suggesting that a focus on individualism and collectivism captures at least some important aspects of culture and cross-cultural difference, highlighting what appear to be systematic differences between Western European and especially Anglo-Saxon–based and other cultures. We then examine gaps in causality that correlational evidence cannot address and propose that to understand the processes underlying how individualism and collectivism influence motivation, cognition, and behavior, more systematic experimental approaches are needed. We high-

light the efficacy of a particular experimental paradigm that involves priming or bringing to mind particular content or cognitive processes. We outline what the priming literature can tell us about the effects of culture (both as operationalized by individualism and collectivism, and as operationalized by other relevant axes, such as high power–low power and equality) on content and process of cognition. We suggest a situated cognition approach to culture and outline what the cultural syndrome priming literature tells us about how culture influences what we think and how we process information about ourselves and the world.

INDIVIDUALISM AND COLLECTIVISM: OPERATIONALIZING, ASSESSING, AND EXAMINING CONSEQUENCES

Operationalization

Individualism is most commonly operationalized as personal independence, and collectivism is most commonly operationalized as obligation and duty to the ingroup, according to Oyserman, Coon, et al. (2002), who examined how individualism and collectivism were assessed in the 20 years after Hofstede (1980) introduced the terms to cross-cultural psychology. Whereas they found 27 distinct scales and noted that no single scale was dominant, they also noted that scale items tended to be modified across studies, so that a subset of items was relatively commonly used. They content-coded scale items, identifying 15 core constructs, seven describing individualism and eight describing collectivism, that together accounted for almost 90% of items across each of the scales.

With regard to collectivism scales, over 85% of scales had at least one item focused on "sense of duty to group," with about 75% having at least one item focused on "relatedness to others." Other identified constructs, in descending order, were "seeking others' advice," "harmony" and "working in groups," "sense of belonging to a group," "contextualized self," and "valuing hierarchy." With regard to individualism scales, almost all scales included at least one item focused on "valuing personal independence." There was less of a consensus on other items, with one-third or fewer of the scales including items focused on "personal achievement," "self-knowledge," "uniqueness," "privacy," "clear communication," and "competition."[1]

Assessment

As reviewed in this volume by Triandis (Chapter 3) and in a recent thorough review and meta-analytic synthesis (Oyserman, Coon, et al., 2002), there is consistent evidence of the effectiveness of modeling cultural difference in terms of individualism and collectivism. The meta-analytic synthesis compared the United States (European Americans) with other countries, and European Americans with other Americans, on individualism and/or collectivism using all English language studies published between 1980 and 2000 and any unpublished data provided after listserve requests. Cross-national comparisons included 50 studies comparing the United States and at least one other country. Although 64 different countries were represented in the comparisons, almost half of all studies focused on comparisons between East Asian regions and America as befits

the focus on U.S.–Asian comparison in the cultural literature. Within-U.S. comparisons included 35 studies yielding 68 comparisons of European Americans with African Americans, Asian Americans, or Latino Americans. Results provide evidence of average cross-national difference in individualism and collectivism that broadly map onto East and West difference, with some exceptions (Oyserman, Coon, et al., 2002).

With regard to cultural differences in basic values, the meta-analysis shows significant differences in endorsement of individualism values (e.g., personal independence and uniqueness) and collectivism values (e.g., group membership and group processes). Although relying on responses to attitude scales has limitations (see Uskul & Oyserman, 2006, for a review), the overall picture across studies is that on average European Americans are higher in self-rated individualism and lower in self-rated collectivism than Africans, Eastern Europeans, and Asians. This is graphically presented in Figure 10.1. All data points are located in the

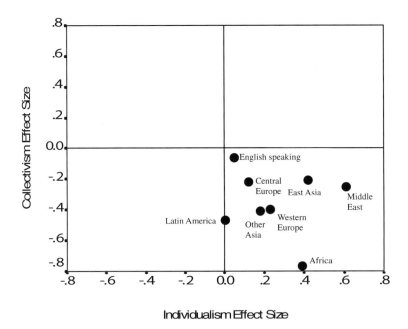

FIGURE 10.1. Are Americans more individualistic and less collectivistic than others? Simultaneous mapping of effects sizes of comparisons between the United States and other regions of the world on individualism and collectivism. Positive effect sizes reflect higher European American individualism and collectivism; negative effect sizes reflect lower European American individualism and collectivism. Adapted from Oyserman, Coon, and Kemmelmeier (2002). Copyright 2002 by the American Psychological Association. Adapted by permission.

lower right quadrant, reflecting higher U.S. individualism and lower U.S. collectivism. Differences are not significant with other English-speaking countries (e.g., Australia, Canada, Great Britain, and New Zealand), suggesting a common cultural core of high individualism and low collectivism. Latin Americans are overall higher in collectivism but not lower in individualism—a cultural syndrome that fits the twin ideas of *machismo* and *simpatico*. Combined effect sizes for comparisons with East Asia were moderate,[2] as were combined effect sizes for Africa and the Middle East. Taken together, these findings corroborate conventional expectations of cultural theorists.

In addition to this generally confirming picture, Oyserman, Coon, et al. (2002) reported some interesting caveats. First, the meta-analysis suggests that although European American and individuals from other English-speaking countries do not differ in individualism and collectivism, they differ from Western Europeans. European Americans are *lower* in collectivism than Europeans, suggesting a uniquely Anglo-American way of being (high individualism and low collectivism) but challenging the notion of a single "Western" culture.

Second, although the data support the general assertion that European Americans are higher in individualism and lower in collectivism than Asians, effect sizes for Asian regions are similar to those for European regions, with large effects only for U.S.–Africa comparisons. The Asian and European findings challenge the notion of a general "East" versus "West" cultural syndrome and suggest that a more nuanced approach is needed to understand individualism and collectivism within, as well as between, societies. Indeed, Oyserman, Coon, et al. (2002) report large internal heterogeneity within East Asian countries. Consistent with the assumption of high American individualism and low American collectivism, U.S.–China comparisons yield moderate to large effects and do not vary by scale content. But U.S.–Korea and U.S.–Japan comparisons yield small effects for individualism, and collectivism and differences are contingent on scale. No U.S.–Korean difference is found unless collectivism scales include relatedness; if included, Koreans are higher in collectivism. Japanese are lower in collectivism when collectivism scales include

seeking group harmony, defining the self in context, sense of belonging to groups, and acceptance of hierarchy. Japan–U.S. collectivism comparison is in the expected direction (though still small) only when scales include working in a group and exclude seeking harmony.

Third, although two of three within-U.S. comparisons parallel international comparisons, the within-U.S. comparison of African Americans and European Americans shows a stark difference from the U.S.–Africa comparison. European Americans exhibit higher individualism and lower collectivism than Asian Americans, and lower collectivism than Latino Americans (but are indistinguishable on individualism from Latino Americans). However, African Americans exhibit higher individualism and are indistinguishable in collectivism compared to European Americans. These findings (presented graphically in Figure 10.2) challenge the assumption that high individualism and low collectivism is part of a European tradition brought to America and most accessible to European Americans, and suggest that African Americans are in some important ways quintessential Americans.

Moreover, effects for comparisons with Asian Americans and African Americans (though not for comparisons with Latino Americans) are influenced by individualism scale content. Including personal uniqueness items in individualism scales increases the difference between Asian Americans and European American and the difference between African Americans and European Americans. Asian American individualism scores decrease and African American scores increase compared to those of European Americans. Including personal competition items in individualism scales increases the individualism scores of both Asian Americans and African Americans, but not of European Americans. Thus, when individualism scales include personal competition, Asian Americans and European Americans no longer differ in individualism, whereas the difference between African Americans and European Americans increases—with the difference favoring African Americans. Taken together, results suggest first that general assumptions about cross-group differences in individualism and collectivism have some empirical support; second, that future research should not assume that any pair of between-

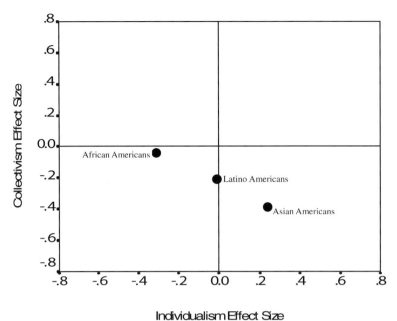

FIGURE 10.2. Are European Americans higher in individualism and collectivism than African Americans, Asian Americans or Latino Americans? Simultaneous mapping of effects sizes of comparisons between European Americans and other Americans on individualism and collectivism. Positive effect sizes reflect higher European American individualism and collectivism; negative effect sizes reflect lower European American individualism and collectivism. Adapted from Oyserman, Coon, and Kemmelmeier (2002). Copyright 2002 by the American Psychological Association. Adapted by permission.

group difference is due to individualism–collectivism difference; and third, that how individualism and collectivism are operationally defined does matter.

Consequences of Individualism and Collectivism

Taken as a whole, the meta-analytic review suggests that the individualism and collectivism value axes do provide a reasonable organizing structure. If individualism and collectivism differ in meaningful ways cross-culturally, the next question to be answered is the extent that these differences in values matter for how individuals make sense of themselves, how they connect and relate to others, and what and how they think about the world—the plausible consequences of individualism and collectivism described in the opening sections of this chapter. Here, too, we base our conclusions on the review of Oyserman, Coon, et al. (2002), who analyzed the associations of individualism and collectivism with self-concept, relationality, and cognition based on all retrievable English language studies published between 1980 and 2000 (and unpublished data).

Self-Concept

Oyserman, Coon, et al. (2002) reviewed 30 studies that assessed self-esteem, self-concept, or personality, and associated these with individualism and/or collectivism. They found that research typically compared groups within the United States or two countries and assumed differences in chronic cultural syndrome rather than assessed individualism and/or collectivism. If the assumption that cross-group difference is due to difference in individualism and/or collectivism is valid, then an argument can be made that individualism is associated with more optimism or higher self-esteem, whereas collectivism is associated with a more interpersonal and social self-concept. According to this review, effect sizes for self-concept differences are variable. Large effects occur especially when the researcher examined collective or ingroup-focused content and directly assessed individualism and/or collectivism. Because research is either correlational or lacks direct assessment or manipulation of salience of cultural syndrome, research in this domain remains open to criticism and more critical assessment of the culture → self causal claim.

Relationality

We reviewed 71 studies that assessed close relationships (family, intimate relationships), ingroup–outgroup interactions (social behavior, communication style, conflict resolution style), and work or organizational contexts (working in groups, organizational conflict management). Broadly speaking, these studies suggest that individualism and collectivism as cultural syndromes are associated with differences in relationality and group relations: Individualism is associated with ease of interaction with strangers, preference for direct rather than indirect communication style; collectivism is associated with ingroup preference in relationships and different forms of face saving. Effect sizes are often moderate to large, though highly variable. Effects for conflict management are heterogeneous. Work and organizational research allows for stronger conclusions than close relationship and ingroup–outgroup relations studies, because the former research almost always included both direct assessment of individualism and collectivism, experimental manipulation, and cross-national rather than within-U.S.-only comparison.

Cognition

Whereas research on content of self-concept and relationality supports the notion that individualism and collectivism as cultural syndromes matter in everyday life, potential impact of culture on cognitive process is particularly intriguing, as noted by Norenzayan, Choi, and Peng in Chapter 23, this volume. Oyserman, Coon, et al. (2002) reviewed 39 studies examining cultural and cross-cultural aspects of attribution style, explanations, and persuasion. Americans were consistently more likely to focus on dispositions rather than situations in providing rationales for behavior or explaining causality than were participants from non-Western countries. Where measured, individualism and collectivism appeared to mediate this effect, and where calculable, effect sizes tended to be moderate to large, with separate orthogonal effects for individualism and collectivism.

Whereas the research reviewed by Oyserman, Coon, et al. (2002) focused predominantly on social cognition, in the past few years, evidence of cross-national differences between the United States, China (Nisbett, 2003) and Japan (Kitayama, Duffy, Kawamura, & Larsen, 2003) in non-social-cognitive processes has emerged as well. This emerging research suggests that Americans are faster and more accurate in recall of abstract and central information, Chinese are more accurate with details and elements of the whole (including the background), and Japanese are more accurate with proportions between elements. Researchers studying cultural and cross-cultural differences in cognition nowadays use experimental methods and diverse participants, providing a strong basis for assertions that individualism and collectivism are associated with differences in cognitive style and attribution processes (for a review, see Norenzayan et al., Chapter 23, this volume).

CULTURE AS SITUATED COGNITION: INTERPRETING THE MEANING OF ASSOCIATIONS BETWEEN CULTURAL SYNDROME AND COGNITIVE CONTENT AND PROCESS

How are these findings to be interpreted? Most provocative is the possibility that culture influences not only the content but also the nature of our thinking. One possible model is that distal differences—in philosophy, religion, language, history—create proximal differences in how we think (Nisbett, 2003; see also Norenzayan et al., Chapter 23, this volume). This perspective, with its focus on distal cultural difference, implies that cultural differences in cognition require socialization in the traditions of one's culture and are hence relatively fixed and difficult to change.

A number of studies suggests otherwise. For example, among immigrants to the United States, Marian and Kaushanskaya (2004) demonstrate that when randomly assigned to use English rather than Russian, participants describe memories that focus on the self significantly more than when these memories are retrieved in Russian. Ross, Xun, and Wilson (2002) demonstrate that when randomly assigned to describe themselves in English rather than Chinese, Chinese students studying in Canada give responses that do not differ significantly from European-heritage Canadians. Among Hong Kong Chinese students filling out questionnaires while Hong Kong was still under British rule, endorsement of Chinese cultural values *increased* when participants were randomly assigned to fill out the questionnaire in English rather than Chinese (Bond & Yang, 1982; Yang & Bond, 1980). These results suggest that cultural values are complex, can be situationally primed in the moment, and that what comes to mind in the moment is the working subset that is relevant to the task at hand (see also Oyserman, Kemmelmeier, et al., 2002).

Cultures Vary in the Salience of Individualism and Collectivism in Various Situations

What then would be the process by which distal differences influence current meaning making? A possible process model is that various distal differences influence social structures and situations to increase or decrease likelihood of experiencing the self (and the social world) as separate or connected, but that all cultures provide sufficient experience of individualism and collectivism to allow either to be primed when situationally relevant, because all cultures are rooted in evolutionary and natural

selection with the same adaptive needs (see Cohen, 2001; Oyserman, Kemmelmeier, et al., 2002). A society that did not have the potential to invoke group loyalty would not be likely to survive to benefit individual members over time, nor would a society that did not provide spaces for individual choice when group needs were met. Following this reasoning, Figure 10.3 presents a process model linking these distal and proximal features.

The notion that societies include both individualism and collectivism in various ways seems at first glance novel. However, quite a large number of social scientists endorse the perspective that individualism and collectivism are not opposing ends of the same dimension but are rather domain-specific, orthogonal constructs differentially elicited by current contextual and social cues (e.g., Bontempo, 1993; Kagitçibasi, 1987; Lehman, Chiu, & Schaller, 2004; Oyserman, 1993; Rhee et al., 1996; Singelis, 1994; Sinha & Tripathi, 1994; Triandis, Bontempo, Villareal, Asai, & Lucca, 1988). As we outline below, thinking about both individualism and collectivism as situationally cued opens the possibility of addressing basic questions about whether and

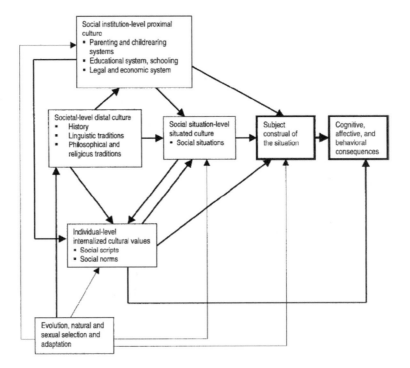

FIGURE 10.3. A socially contextualized model of cultural influences. Adapted from Oyserman, Kemmelmeier, and Coon (2002). Copyright 2002 by the American Psychological Association. Adapted by permission.

how culture might influence content of thoughts (e.g., what comes to mind when one thinks of oneself, which values feel most central, how close one feels to others), and social and nonsocial cognition (e.g., what content and which cognitive procedures comes to mind).

Priming Individualism and Collectivism

Why Use Priming?

Cross-national comparisons and studies using bilingual participants "feel" ecologically valid: They use real differences in terms of where one lives and the language one speaks, and document an association between these differences and how individuals make sense of themselves and their social worlds, and how they think more generally. However, these comparisons make it difficult to answer questions about psychological processing; that is, they are mute as to whether individualism and collectivism are the active ingredients in observed differences, and if so, which aspects of individualism and collectivism make a difference. To answer these process questions, it is necessary to manipulate experimentally the salience of individualism and collectivism as syndromes and to compare results when different facets of these syndromes are brought to mind. Indeed, an emerging experimental technique based in social cognition research involves efforts to prime individualism or collectivism and in this way isolate effects on a dependent measure.

Priming involves making content and/or procedures temporarily accessible. The influence of construct accessibility on social perception is well documented (Higgins & Bargh, 1987). Accessibility can be the temporary result of priming (Srull & Wyer, 1978, 1979) or a more chronic result of routine or habitual activation of a construct in one's everyday environment (Bargh, 1984; Higgins, 1989, 1996). Temporary and chronic accessibility effects are similar (thus, comparable) and independent (thus, additive) in influencing in social judgments (Bargh, Bond, Lombardi, & Tota, 1986; Rudman & Borgida, 1995). Recent priming and chronic activation are both predictive of construct accessibility.

In the laboratory, priming typically involves presenting participants with a series of ostensibly unrelated tasks. When participants are not made aware of a connection between tasks (i.e., of researcher intent to influence them), semantic content and procedural knowledge

cued by the first task "spill over" into subsequent tasks. By studying this spillover effect (e.g., comparing group differences between priming tasks) and comparing spillover effects to cross-national differences, it is possible to test models of cultural influence on content and process of cognition.

Priming as a technique holds promise of creating an experimental analogue of chronic differences between cultural groups by temporarily focusing participants' attention on different culture-relevant content or mind-set. Primes can cue semantic or content knowledge, as well as procedural or mind-set knowledge; culture-relevant values, norms, goals, beliefs, and attitudes can be cued automatically, without participants' awareness. For culture, priming most commonly involves making active ingredients of either individualism or collectivism salient and assessing effect of priming as a between-participant variable.

Of course, priming can only make accessible that which is there. Like all priming methods, the culture-priming tasks can only be effective if semantic content and procedural mind-set knowledge relevant to each construct are available to be primed. Thus, relevant content and procedural knowledge already has to be in memory. One cannot be individualism-primed if one has available in memory only collectivism-relevant semantic and procedural knowledge; similarly one cannot be collectivism-primed if one has available in memory only individualism-relevant semantic and procedural knowledge.

Thus, a basic assumption in priming literature must be that across societies and cultures, individuals are capable of thinking about themselves and the world as both separate and independent, and as connected and interdependent, even if they are typically likely to focus on one or the other. Given universality of both a basic sense of bodily and spatial-symbolic separateness (Burris & Rempel, 2004) and a sense of social connectedness and need to belong (Baumeister & Leary, 1995), this assumption seems warranted. It is not plausible that human minds are structured only to see separation or only connection (see Cohen, 2001; Oyserman, Kemmelmeier, et al., 2002).

CONCEPTUAL PRIMING

The literature on priming has distinguished between conceptual priming and mind-set priming (Bargh & Chartrand, 2000; Galinsky, Gruenfeld, & Magee, 2003). Conceptual priming, also termed "semantic priming," involves activation of specific mental representations such as traits, values, norms, or goals that then serve as interpretive frames in the processing of subsequent information (Higgins, 1996). Once a concept is primed, concepts associated with it in memory are also activated through spreading activation (Neely, 1977).

Following the auto-motives model (e.g., Bargh, 1990), goal constructs are stored in memory and can be conceptually primed. Once stored, goals for achievement, for power, for remembering, for impression formation, and other pursuits can be primed without explicit, conscious intention formation (Chartrand & Bargh, 1996). For example, Bargh, Raymond, Pryor, and Strack (1995) and Chen, Lee-Chai, and Bargh (2001) exposed participants to words associated with possession of power in the lab and showed priming effects; that is, bringing to mind words associated with power also activated specific, individualized goals associated with power, and these influenced participant perception and behavior. Priming power makes salient sexualized images of women among men already likely to sexually harass (Bargh et al., 1995). Priming power can make salient self-interest or social responsibility goals, depending on individual differences in agentic self-interest versus communal orientation (Chen et al., 2001).

Priming power turned on a semantic network of associated meanings. The result of priming power depended on what participants associated with power. Following this line of reasoning, average between-society or between racial/ethnic group differences attributed to differences in cultural syndrome may be due to differences in the semantic networks primed in everyday situations. Objects and practices continually activate corresponding culturally meaningful concepts and thoughts; that is, cultures may prime different cognitive content by creating differing semantic, associative, and content networks that together influence what we think about ourselves, others, and the world, what feels persuasive, and so on.

MIND-SET PRIMING

Whereas conceptual priming activates a concept or meaning structure, mind-set priming activates procedural knowledge, a way of thinking (Bargh & Chartrand, 2000). Just as conceptual priming cannot prime novel meaning, but only meaning that has been stored in memory, mind-set priming cannot prime procedural knowledge that does not exist in memory. Mind-set priming involves the nonconscious carryover of a previously stored mental procedure or way of making sense of the world. For example, when primed to think about either whether to engage in a goal (deliberate goal pros and cons) or how to engage in a goal (implement strategies to attain the goal), participants later use this same thinking style in a second, unrelated task (e.g., Gollwitzer, Heckhausen, & Steller, 1990).

Mind-set priming is consistent with a general assumption that processing strategies are situated and tuned to meet current situational requirements (for a review, see Schwarz, 2002, 2006). These processing strategies or procedures can be thought of as part of a procedural tool kit used to structure thinking. When cued, they provide ways of reasoning about the world and have been also termed heuristics or naive theories. For example, experiencing ease might mean that the task was simple or that one is talented. Interpretation depends in part on the naive theory brought to mind to make sense of experience (Schwarz, 2006). Procedural priming cues a procedure, thus allowing it to be set into motion and studied separately from its everyday context.

Social cognition research has suggested a number of likely chronic or easily cued procedures. For example, Schwarz and colleagues (e.g., Schwarz & Bless, 1992; Strack, Schwarz, & Gschneidinger, 1985), in their assimilation–contrast model, describe assimilation as the more chronic cognitive procedure style and contrast as the cue-able alternative cognitive procedure; that is, individuals automatically assimilate and integrate new information with already present information, unless they are cued to use a contrasting procedure. When contrasting is cued, they automatically separate new from already present information. Cues to use a contrasting procedural style include everyday differences triggers such as belonging to a different time, place, or group.

More generally, mood, perceived distance, and perceived power have been studied as procedural triggers. Schwarz and Clore (1996, 2007) describe mood as providing procedural cues: Positive mood cues less effortful, heuristic processing and negative mood cues more effortful, systematic processing. Trope and Liberman (2003) describe distance and anything that cues distance (including temporal distance) as providing procedural cues (see also Boroditsky, 2000). Distal objects and events are processed abstractly, in terms of core, gist, and superordinate structure; proximal objects and events are processed concretely, in terms of detail, particulars, and subordinate structure. Mood (Gasper & Clore, 2002), power (Smith & Trope, 2006), and self-regulatory focus (Förster & Higgins, 2005) have also been studied as mind-set primes for local versus global processing style. Bad mood, low power, and a caution-oriented prevention self-regulatory focus trigger local processing, whereas good mood, high power, and success-oriented promotion self-regulatory focus trigger global processing.

With regard to cultural and cross-cultural psychology, some of these procedures have been linked to particular gender and cultural groups. Thus, for example, Markus and Oyserman (1989) proposed that women and individuals from non-Western societies are more likely to view themselves as importantly connected. They contrasted women and non-Westerners with men and individuals from Western societies, who are more likely to view themselves as importantly separate from others, and argued that basic cognitive procedures connected with these divergent basic self-schemas cue different cognitive procedures— connect, integrate versus separate, and distinguish. These arguments were refined by Markus and Kitayama (1991) in their follow-up review, in which connected self-schemas were termed interdependent self-construals and separate self-schemas were termed independent self-construals, with the proposal that this difference in self-concept is true of average differences between Eastern and Western ways of self-construal. Cross and Madson (1997) made the same argument for gender (for a different perspective on gender and culture see Kashima et al., 1995).

Following these initial reviews of the literature, empirical work demonstrating the association of "separate" and "connected" self-schemas with preference for "separating" and "connecting" cognitive processes was carried out by Woike (1994). Woike and her colleagues describe connected self-schemas as communion self-concepts and separate self-schemas as agency self-concepts (following Bakan, 1966),

and term the relevant preferred cognitive processes integration and distinction respectively (Woike, 1994; Woike, Lavezzary, Barksy, 2001). They find that the cognitive procedure chronically preferred by those with an agentic self-schema is to distinguish or separate, whereas the cognitive procedure chronically preferred by those with a communal or connected self-schema is to connect and integrate. Following from the separated and connected self-schema models, this difference in basic cognitive procedures has also been corroborated in more explicitly culture-focused research (Hannover & Kühnen, 2004; Kühnen, Hannover, & Schubert, 2001; Kühnen & Oyserman, 2002).

SUMMARY

Priming studies artificially prime or cue certain procedures in a controlled environment. The same outcomes are likely to be cued in everyday situations as well. Both conceptual and mind-set priming processes are likely to occur, and both are likely to be important for researchers seeking to understand the process by which distal differences in societies (their histories, philosophical and religious traditions, and ecological niches) influence "online" differences in the sense individuals make of their social and nonsocial world and how they go about thinking—cognitive content and structure. By focusing attention on likely differences in content and procedures cued in the moment, our goal in this chapter is to provide a causal model of proximal cultural difference rather than a model outlining potential distal cultural difference. We now turn to evidence that culture may influence cognitive content and process either by nonconscious or conscious activation of cognitive content or procedures.

What Is the Evidence That Accessible Cultural Syndromes Influence What and How We Think?

By providing an experimental manipulation, conceptual and mind-set priming techniques hold promise of clarifying at least some of the active ingredients of chronic cross-national differences. However, to demonstrate that priming techniques evoke what is understood to be culture rather than some other semantic and procedural knowledge, the first task is to demonstrate that priming does in fact evoke *culturally relevant* semantic knowledge—values, content of self-concept, and ways of interacting with others (relationality). That is, priming collectivism (individualism) should make collective (individualistic) values more salient and likely to be endorsed, render relational and group membership (individual traits, unique self-features) content of self-concept more accessible and likely to be recalled, and increase felt closeness to ingroup members. Once this impact of priming on conceptual knowledge has been demonstrated, the impact of priming on culturally relevant procedural knowledge can be examined.

Types of Primes

Because primes are tools or means of evoking semantic and procedural knowledge, causal inference from priming results is strengthened if results are consistent across different types of primes. Consistent effects across differing prime types provide convergent evidence that the latent constructs of individualism and collectivism are being evoked. Similarly, causal inference is strengthened if priming individualism and collectivism works in both Eastern and Western countries, because this will constitute evidence that both Eastern and Western countries socialize for both individualism and collectivism. Before turning to evidence that priming results can be observed using different methods and among members of different cultures, we outline briefly each of the various individualism and collectivism primes used in the field.

Oyserman and Lee (2007) have conducted an extensive review of the culture priming literature. They find that primes are diverse in content, in type of task used, and in their transparency to the participant. This diversity is helpful, if meta-analytic results from priming studies are consistent across these different levels of collectivism primes, this will constitute evidence that the underlying process of collectivism is the same across different levels of groups (relational vs. collective)—an issue unresolved by the cross-cultural, cross-national comparative literature.

With regard to priming individualism, tasks typically focus on the individual self (using "I" as a prime), on the self as different or unique, and on difference and separateness more generally. With regard to priming collectivism, tasks focus not only on connection, using "we" as a prime, but also on similarity or obligation to

family, as well as larger groups, such as teams. That is, collectivism primes focus on what has been termed "relational," as well as "collective," identities: friends, family, others with whom one is likely to have a close and personal bond, as well tribal affiliation or membership in larger groups where a close and personal bond with all group members is unlikely (for distinction between relational and collective identities, see Brewer & Gardner, 1996; Roccas & Brewer, 2002).

As detailed below, each of the priming tasks can clearly be viewed as a conceptual prime. Words related to individualism and collectivism are primed and likely to bring to mind relevant values, ways of being a self, ways of engaging with others, and ways of making sense of the world. A question to be explored is whether it can also be shown that these tasks prime procedural knowledge—activating cognitive procedures of separating out and focusing on a main object, the figure versus connecting, integrating, and focusing on the whole. Thus, the question is when words like *separate*, *different*, and *dissociate* or words like *similar*, *connect*, and *together* are used in instructions or in the task itself, do they prime mind-sets rather than simply content knowledge?

Priming Individualism and Relationally Focused Collectivism

While collectivism has mostly been described in terms of focus on group membership, much of the cross-national research has focused on within-group contexts, examining more relational rather than group-level processes. Not surprisingly then, two of the common primes also focused on priming a relational level of "we." As outlined below, these are the Similarities and Differences with Family and Friends task (SDFF) and the Pronoun Circling task. One or the other of these primes is used in almost half of all culture-priming studies (Oyserman & Lee, 2007).

SIMILARITIES AND DIFFERENCES WITH FAMILY AND FRIENDS TASK (SDFF)

Trafimow, Triandis, and Goto (1991, Study 1) developed this task. To prime individualism or "I" the instructions are as follows: "For the next 2 minutes, you will not need to write anything. Please think of what makes you different from your *family and friends*. What do you expect yourself to do?" To prime collectivism (in this case a "relational we") the instructions are as follows: "For the next 2 minutes, you will not need to write anything. Please think of what you have in common with your *family and friends*. What do they expect you to do?" (p. 651; italics added). As noted in the italicized text, the focus is on others with whom one has a close relation. The SDFF may be assumed to prime conceptual knowledge: Activating concepts of one's similarities to (differences from) close others should activate relevant values, ways of describing oneself, and engagement with others.

PRONOUN CIRCLING TASK

Brewer and Gardner (1996) developed an initial version of this task that contrasted "we" with "they." This work was refined by Gardner, Gabriel, and Lee (1999), who developed the initial form of the pronoun circling task comparing a focus on "I" (as well as "me" and "my"), with a focus on "we," where "we" refers to friends who go together into the city. Specifically the task is to circle personal singular and plural pronouns in a paragraph. Following the initial work of Brewer and Gardner, a number of different paragraphs have been used. The original paragraph was: *We* go to the city often. *Our* anticipation fills *us* as *we* see the skyscrapers come into view. *We* allow *ourselves* to explore every corner, never letting an attraction escape *us*. *Our* voice fills the air and street. *We* see all the sights, *we* window shop, and everywhere *we* go *we* see *our* reflection looking back at *us* in the glass of a hundred windows. At nightfall *we* linger, *our* time in the city almost over. When finally *we* must leave, *we* do so knowing that *we* will soon return. The city belongs to *us* (italics added to show relational collective prime). Because the concepts "I" and "we" are primed, the pronoun circling task may be assumed to prime conceptual knowledge: Activating concepts "I" and "we" should activate relevant values, ways of describing oneself, and engagement with others.

Priming Individualism and Collectivism That Is Both Relationally and Collective Group-Focused

Three collectivism primes did focus on the collective level, in conjunction with a more relational level. Two of these primes, scrambled sentence tasks and subliminal priming, are standard in the priming literature. Scrambled

sentences and subliminal prime can in principle use collective or relational words, and indeed, current usage has words such as *team* and *group*, which are likely to be more collective than relational. The third prime has participants imagine themselves in the shoes of a Sumerian warrior, making choices in part due to group (tribe) membership, as well as family concerns; this common prime is similar to the SDFF prime in that instructions simply ask participants to imagine the situation. These primes are also often used, constituting almost 40% of published culture-priming research (Oyserman & Lee, 2007).

SCRAMBLED SENTENCE TASK

The scrambled sentence task (Srull & Wyer, 1979) is one of the standard tools for priming. According to Oyserman and Lee's (2007) review, the following words have been used to prime individualism, the words *I, me, mine, distinct, different, competitive, own, free, unique, dissociate, assertive, unusual, autonomy, alone, apart, autonomous, detached, different, dissimilar, distinct, diverge, independence, individual, isolate, separate, solitude, split, unique,* and *self-contained* are included. To prime collectivism, the words *we, us, ours, join, similar, alike, share, cooperative, agreeable, help, group, respect, partnership, together, team, support, others, attached, alliance, closeness, cohesive, connection, inseparable, interdependence, intimate, joint, merged, overlap, similar, shared, together, union,* and *friendships* were used. Given the concepts primed, the scrambled sentence task may be assumed to prime cultural-syndrome-relevant conceptual knowledge.

SUBLIMINAL PRIMING

Subliminal methods are also standard priming techniques. Subliminal priming involves presentation of target words or pictures at a speed too fast (e.g., 35 ms) for conscious processing. Only one published use can be located in the culture priming literature. Oishi, Wyer, and Colcombe (2000, Study 3) included in their priming task the following words: *own, mine, compete, 1, me, individual, distinct,* and *free* (vs. *share, ours, cooperate, us, we, group, same,* and *team*). Subliminally primed concepts may be assumed to prime cultural-syndrome-relevant conceptual knowledge.

SUMERIAN WARRIOR STORY

Trafimow et al. (1991, Study 2) developed this task. The instructions read, "We would like you to read a couple of paragraphs on the following page. After reading these paragraphs, you will be asked to make a judgment about the main character" (p. 652). The participant is then given a lengthy text to read that either focuses attention on individual-talent or tribe-membership and family considerations as rationale for the choice. Because concepts related to individual choice versus focus on tribe and family are primed, the task may be assumed to prime conceptual knowledge.

Priming Individualism and Group-Focused Collectivism

Two other primes attempted to evoke group focus explicitly in their collectivism primes. Group focus was prime by either instantiating a group in the lab or by having participants imagine that they were part of a team or alone, or by having participants imagine themselves or their family consuming grape juice. While quite different from the other primes, this kind of minimal group fits with classic social identity research (e.g., Tajfel, 1982, 2001; Tajfel & Forgas, 2000; Tajfel & Turner, 2004). It could be argued to be relevant to the cross-national literature examining collectivism via preference for working in groups (see Oyserman, Coon, et al., 2002), as well as to Hofstede's (1980) workplace-based focus in the initial cross-culture research comparing countries on individualism. To the extent that work group concepts prime relevant cultural syndrome constructs, the tasks may be assumed to prime conceptual knowledge.

GROUP INSTANTIATION AND GROUP IMAGINATION

Three studies used a "group instantiation prime" (Briley & Wyer, 2002, Studies 1–3). Individualism priming involved individual conditions (performing the task individually, being seated at single-person desks separated by partitions). Collectivism priming involved group formation and intergroup competition (being seated at five-person tables, working as a group, giving the group a name, being told that points were rewarded to the group and competing against other groups).

Seven studies used a "group imagination" prime (Aaker & Lee, 2001, Study 2 Pretest, Studies 2–4; Lee, Aaker, & Gardner, 2000, Studies 2–4). Individualism priming involved imagining oneself competing in a singles' tennis match or consuming grape juice. Collectivism priming involved imagining oneself competing on a tennis team or one's family consuming grape juice.

Language as Prime

Oyserman and Lee (2006) were able to locate 10 studies (Bond & Yang, 1982; Kemmelmeier & Cheng, 2004; Marian & Kaushanskaya, 2004; Ralston, Cunniff, & Gustafson, 1995; Ross et al., 2002; Tavassoli, 2002; Trafimow, Silverman, Fan, & Law, 1997; Watkins & Gerong, 1999; Watkins & Regmi, 2002; Yang & Bond, 1980) that used language as their priming method. The assumption is that English carries with it knowledge about American or Anglo-Saxon culture and therefore evokes individualism, whereas other non-Western languages carry with them knowledge about a home culture that is assumed to be more collectivist. This prime can only be used with participants who are fluent in both English and another language. Although in principle any two languages can be used, Oyserman and Lee (2007) found studies comparing responses in English to those in Chinese, Cebuano, Nepali, and Russian—languages rooted in cultures assumed higher in collectivism.

Although researchers clearly assume that English is a prime for individualism, and this may be so, it is not entirely clear what exactly is being evoked by use of English. It may be a foreign language (e.g., Kemmelmeier & Cheng, 2004), the language of the colonizer (e.g., Yang & Bond, 1980), or a second home language (e.g., Ross et al., 2002) depending on social-historical backgrounds and social cues, in the experimental situation. Likewise, although researchers clearly assume that use of native language primes some form of collectivism—whether feelings of interdependence, or more general collective focus, it is not entirely clear what is being evoked. Using a non-native language may suggest that one is to communicate with an outsider; therefore, one may need to take the other's likely frame of reference into account. Thus, the larger context and the context primed by the experiment are both likely to matter. For example, using one's native tongue in one's home country with a native-language-speaking researcher may have different effects than if one does so in another country, say, as a student in the United States or Canada. For a Hong Kong Chinese student, the meaning of using English in Hong Kong (e.g., Bond & Yang, 1982) may differ from the meaning of using English in Canada (Ross et al., 2002). These distinctions highlight both the situated nature of language use and its effects on cognition and the need for further work to better understand these situated effects. If language priming shows effects on values, self-concept, and relationality, it can be assumed that language is a conceptual prime. If language priming also shows effects on cognitive processes, then it can be assumed that language is a procedural prime as well.

WHAT DOES THE PRIMING LITERATURE REVEAL?

Priming is a relatively new entry into the cultural and cross-cultural literature. But cultural and cross-cultural psychologists have adopted the primes we introduced earlier to evoke individualism and collectivism, and to examine their effects on a number of dependent measures among various cultural groups. In this section we review the empirical findings of this body of research.

The Nature of the Literature

Oyserman and Lee (2007) conducted a search of the English-language published literature and found 67 studies with 5,818 participants that primed both individualism and collectivism. These priming studies examined effects on values (typically items from Schwartz, 1992; Triandis, 1995; Triandis, McCusker, & Hui, 1990), relationality (e.g., social obligation), self-concept (typically coding from the Twenty Statements Test [TST; Kuhn & McPartland, 1954]), well-being (e.g., life satisfaction), and cognition. Priming studies were conducted in English, German, Dutch, and Chinese. Studies were conducted in four regions and eight countries: North America (the United States and Canada), East Asia (Hong Kong and Singapore), Western Europe (Germany and the Netherlands), and Other Asia (Nepal and the Philippines).

Seven studies presented a cross-national replication of priming effects (Aaker & Lee, 2001,

Study 2 Pretest & Study 2; Briley & Wyer, 2001, Study 4; Gardner et al., 1999, Study 2; Lee et al., 2000, Studies 3–5) and one study presented priming as a replication of cross-national difference (Haberstroh, Oyserman, Schwarz, Kühnen, & Ji, 2002, Study 2). Even though these studies provided information on Hong Kong and China, the bulk of studies ($n = 36$) were conducted in the United States and, whether in the United States or not, most studies were conducted in English ($n = 44$). Studies not conducted in English were conducted in Germany, the Netherlands, and Hong Kong, or used language as a prime. Most studies did not provide explicit information about racial/national heritage of participants. It is unclear whether studies did not provide the information because they did not include racial/ethnic majority participants or whether race/ethnicity was not reported because sample sizes were too small for subgroup analyses. Only about one-third of studies included gender in the design.

Hypothesized Effects

Following the cultural syndrome model described previously, the expected impact of priming on values, self-concept, relationality, and cognition can be outlined as follows: With regard to values compared to when collectivism is primed, when individualism is primed, endorsement of relational or collective values would be lower and endorsement of individualistic values would be higher. With regard to self-concept, compared to when collectivism is primed, when individualism is primed, unique traits and attributes related to self-concept should be more accessible, and social or relational aspects of self-concept should be less accessible. With regard to relationality, compared to when collectivism is primed, when individualism is primed, we expected less accessibility of feelings of social obligation and closeness to ingroup others. With regard to cognition, compared to when collectivism is primed, when individualism is primed, we expected more accessibility of context-independent cognitive processing and less accessibility of context-dependent cognitive processing.

Overall Priming Main Effects

Culture priming had a significant and small-to-moderate effect (mean weighted $d = 0.34$, mean unweighted $d = 0.45$) that did not differ significantly when Asian or Asian American compared to European or European American participants were included. Overall, results suggest that priming does influence culture-relevant content (values, self-concept, and relationality) and process (cognition). Effects are relatively robust to prime with some exceptions as noted below. By unpacking the main effect of priming to ask how priming influences each of these culture-relevant constructs and processes, and whether effects are consistent across prime and sample, Oyserman and Lee (2007) provide evidence that at least part of the process by which culture has its effects is via priming of knowledge (semantic priming) and mind-set (procedural priming).

Moderator Analyses

Effect of Prime Type

The majority of studies primed cultural syndrome by using language and six of the seven tasks (with the exception of subliminal priming) described in the prior section. A few studies used various tertiary unclassified primes. The most common priming tasks were Pronoun Circling ($n = 15$), Sumerian Warrior ($n = 12$), SDFF ($n = 10$), and using language as a prime ($n = 10$). Mean weighted effect sizes were moderate for Sumerian Warrior and SDFF primes, and small for Pronoun Circling, scrambled sentence ($n = 7$), group imagination ($n = 8$), and group instantiation ($n = 3$) tasks. Reflecting perhaps the ambiguity of what exactly is being primed, especially small effects (weighted $d = 0.10$) were found for language primes. Estimating effects sizes by whether the collectivism primed was relational, collective, or both, Oyserman and Lee (2007) report moderate effects when collective primes included both relational and collective group levels, but small effects when only the relational or collective level was primed. This increased effect size of the mixed primes may reflect the fact that they were better able to cue cultural-syndrome-relevant content in working memory. Alternatively, these differences may be an artifact of differential use of the primes for different dependent variables. While the most common priming task, the Pronoun Circling task, has been used with a variety of dependent variables (self-concept, cognition, values), other tasks, such as the SDFF, have been used mostly with a single dependent variable.

Effect of Dependent Variable

Significantly different effects of culture syndrome priming were found depending on the culture-relevant construct assessed. Culture syndrome priming had significant but small effects on values (based on $n = 15$ studies) and self-concept (based on $n = 21$ studies), but moderate-to-large effects on relationality (based on $n = 13$ studies) and cognition (based on $n = 28$ studies). To understand the nature of these effects, each culture-relevant construct was assessed separately.

VALUES

Studies examining the effect of priming on values could be divided into those using known individualism and collectivism value scales (as reported earlier, those of Triandis and Schwartz) and those using other value items (e.g., "Chineseness," Bond & Yang, 1982; Ross et al., 2002; Yang & Bond, 1980; emotional connectedness, self-sacrifice, and individuality, Briley & Wyer, 2001, Study 4; equality proverbs, Briley & Wyer, 2002, Study 3; justice values, Kemmelmeier, Wieczorkowska, Erb, & Burstein, 2002, Study 3). Because effect of cultural syndrome priming on responses to known individualism and collectivism value scales is a plausible validity check of the priming manipulation itself, Oyserman and Lee (2006) examined effect size for these studies separately and found effects in the moderate range. This is an important validity check for the priming procedure.

Further analyses reported by Oyserman and Lee (2007) suggest some difference in effect size by prime. Whereas the Sumerian Warrior task, the SDFF, and the scrambled sentence tasks have on average a moderate impact on accessibility of cultural values, the Pronoun Circling task, the group imagination task, and the group instantiation task have only a small effect on accessibility of cultural values. No effect of language priming was found.

SELF-CONCEPT

Among the 21 studies examining the effect of cultural syndrome priming on self-concept, most operationalized it with content coding of variants of the TST (Kuhn & McPartland, 1954). Other studies used items from either Singelis's (1994) or Leung and Kim's (1997)

Self-Construal Scales or created their own items. Small effects were found whether researchers content-coded for number of personal traits or number of collective identities generated in the TST. No effect of cultural syndrome priming was found for number of relational identities generated. It is possible that a more complex relationship exists between cultural syndrome priming and self-concept than can be captured by content-coding TST responses; that is, current research is based on categorizing responses as social or personal self-focused. When a social self is cued, however, it seems likely that it will cue how one is that self—for example, thinking of oneself as a daughter or as a Muslim will cue the relevant traits associated with this identity (e.g., willful or obedient). If each word is coded separately, then the latter descriptors will be coded as private selves, yet this may not be how they are intended (for further discussion of this issue see, e.g., Oyserman, 2007).

It is also possible that effects are dependent on prime type. When language was used as a prime with English as the individualism prime, and Chinese (Ross et al., 2002), Cebuano (Watkins & Gerong, 1999), or Nepali (Watkins & Regmi, 2002) as the collectivism primes, participants referred more to others in Chinese than in English, and described more relational but fewer collective selves in Cebuano and Nepali than in English. However, they also used more trait self-descriptors in Cebuano. Further analyses reported by Oyserman and Lee (2007) suggest that the Sumerian Warrior, the Pronoun Circling, the group imagination, and the language priming tasks all have on average a small effect on accessible content of self-concept, whereas the SDFF task has on average a moderate effect. The SDFF task involves bringing to mind similarities to (or differences from) family and friends, suggesting that the effect of priming on self-concept content may be particularly clear when the prime brings to mind semantic content that is very close to the task at hand.

RELATIONALITY

Average effects of priming cultural syndrome on relationality are moderate. Some studies show effects on reported social obligation (e.g., Gardner, Gabriel, & Dean, 2004). Other studies show effects on behavioral measures of psychological closeness (Holland, Roeder, van Baaren, Brandt, & Hannover, 2004, Study 2); that is, relative to when individualism was primed, when collectivism was primed, participants sat closer to a confederate.

Size of effect appears to be dependent on the type of prime used (Oyserman & Lee, 2007). Further analyses reported by Oyserman and Lee suggest that language priming has a small effect on accessible knowledge about relationality; the Sumerian Warrior task and the Pronoun Circling task have, on average, a moderate effect, and the SDFF and the scrambled sentence tasks have on average a large effect. Whereas the SDFF explicitly focuses on relationships, scramble sentence tasks do not, so the larger effect in the latter two prime conditions is unlikely to be solely due to bringing to mind family and friends.

COGNITION

Taken together, studies priming cultural syndrome and then assessing accessibility of individualism and collectivism values, relationality, and relevant self-concept content provide assurance that priming cultural syndrome using the kinds of primes described previously does seem to activate relevant constructs and make accessible the values, and ways of thinking about oneself and relating to others described in the cross-cultural literature. These results suggest that at least in part, culture's impact is via priming of semantic knowledge and networks.

Social cognition studies support this claim, showing effects of priming on conceptual knowledge. For example, Haberstroh et al. (2002, Study 1) find that semantic priming of cultural syndrome shifts sensitivity to conversational norms, making collectivism-primed German participants as sensitive as nonprimed Chinese participants. Taken as a whole, the results of cultural-syndrome-priming studies not only provide a "live" process model but also highlight that cultural impact is indeed situated in the immediate context. Contexts are cultural because they evoke certain values, ways of being a self, ways of engaging others, relevant attitudes, and sensitivities to others.

Although a process model that focuses on conceptual priming effects is interesting, as we noted at the outset of this chapter, cultural psychologists have argued for an even deeper impact of culture. Cultural psychologists have argued that culture influences not only what we think but also how we think. The studies priming cultural syndrome, then assessing accessibility of relevant cognitive procedural knowledge provide insight into this latter claim. Thus, for example, Stapel and Koomen (2001, Study 1) primed cultural syndrome, then presented participants with social comparison information. They found that participants were more likely to contrast their self-description with the other after individualism priming and more likely to assimilate information about the other into their self-description after collectivism priming. These effects suggest effects of priming on mind-set, in this case, use of a contrast or exclusion-focused cognitive mind-set procedure rather than an assimilation or inclusion-focused cognitive mind-set procedure.

In the cognitive domain across studies, effect size was moderate whether the cognitive construct assessed was an attitude, judgment, or social cognition (and the prime activated conceptual knowledge), or a nonsocial cognitive process was assessed (and the prime activated procedural knowledge). In an example of procedural priming, Kühnen and Oyserman (2002) showed that priming cultural syndrome influenced speed with which respondents recognized letters in an embedded letters task (Study 1) and accuracy of recall of figures embedded in context (Study 2). More recently in our lab we have demonstrated that priming cultural syndrome influences Stroop color-naming latency effects. Because the Stroop task requires participants to separate and pull apart features of the stimuli, both Americans and Koreans showed effects such that relative to collectivism priming, individualism priming speeds latency of accurate Stroop color response on difficult trials (those in which color and word are incongruent; Cha, 2006; Oyserman, Sorensen, & Reber, 2006).

The procedural knowledge that appears to be primed by the cultural syndrome tasks focuses on separate versus connected reasoning. This distinction is similar to the one made by Nisbett and his colleagues (see Norenzayan, Choi, & Peng, Chapter 23, this volume) but does not require that the cultural syndrome itself be set by distal cultural features such as Eastern versus Western cultural and philosophic and religious traditions. Further analyses reported by Oyserman and Lee (2007) suggest that effects of priming cultural syndrome on cognition are relatively robust to the specific

prime used. The Sumerian Warrior task, the Pronoun Circling task, the SDFF, the scrambled sentence task, group imagination, and language as prime all have on average a moderate effect on both cognition content and process (though effects for the group instantiation task are small[3]). Taken as a whole, the cultural syndrome priming studies suggest that there is a procedure relevant to the individualism syndrome and a procedure relevant to the collectivism syndrome.

Comparison of Priming Cultural Syndrome with a Control Comparison Condition

Although most studies did not provide a control condition, those that did use a control comparison show a small effect size for both the comparison between individualism prime and control and the comparison between collectivism prime and control. In these control comparison studies, effects for individualism priming did not depend on which dependent variables were assessed, whereas for collectivism priming, effects were moderate for relationality and cognition, and extremely small for self-concept and values. Relative to control conditions, on average, individualism priming produced greater shift than collectivism priming, with two caveats. First, studies using the scrambled sentence task produced equal shift from comparison whether individualism or collectivism was primed. Second, when collectivism priming included both relational and group-level collective focus, a larger shift from comparison for collectivism priming than for individualism priming was observed. Taken as a whole, no single priming task can be considered the gold standard for future work. However, the mixed-level collectivism primes and the scrambled sentence primes seem to provide a mix of ecological validity (taking into account multiple levels) and maximal control (content of sentences can be tailored to enhance results).

SUMMARY AND CONCLUSIONS

Cross-cultural comparisons suggest that culture matters, influencing how the self is defined, how relationships with others are imagined, what is of value and worth, and how the mind works. Cross-national comparisons can be high in ecological validity: They demonstrate real differences between real groups. A meta-analytic review suggests that cross-national variability in culture is patterned, that assumed value differences can be assessed through survey response. However, these studies are limited. Reliance on survey response leaves open questions about interpretability of comparisons, and studies that lack experimental manipulation cannot illuminate the process by which culture matters, leaving as a black box the mechanism through which culture influences individuals. To address these problems, social cognition research provides semantic and procedural priming as tools to assess the impact of some key aspects of cultural syndromes on content and process of thinking.

To answer these process questions, it is necessary to experimentally manipulate the salience of individualism and collectivism as syndromes and to compare results when different facets of these syndromes are brought to mind. A recent comprehensive review of the cultural-syndrome-priming literature supports the cross-cultural psychological contention that culture matters; that is, priming some culture-relevant content shows a clear impact on accessible cultural knowledge, resulting in shifting values, altered descriptions of content of self-concept, and differences in understanding about one's social obligations and relations with others. These findings suggest that culture is a conceptual prime, activating relevant knowledge. Perhaps most importantly and fundamentally, priming influences situated cognitive process in culturally meaningful ways; that is, priming individualism and collectivism cultural syndromes made accessible different procedural knowledge. The mind-set of individualism is to pull apart and separate, to contrast figure from ground, self from other. The mind-set of collectivism is to connect and integrate, to assimilate figure with ground, self with other. These findings suggest that culture is also a procedural prime, activating relevant naïve theories as to how to make meaning.

Cultural-syndrome-priming literature does not simply support prior suppositions about the influence of culture. It also provides new information suggesting that individualism and collectivism do influence how we think, the cognitive procedures evoked. Moreover, far from being immutable, cultural differences are malleable in the moment. Because cultural syndrome priming can be understood as setting up a situation that cues or makes subjectively sa-

lient isolated active ingredients of culture, the evidence that cultural syndrome priming is effective suggests that such malleability is also plausible in everyday life. Subtle priming evoked subjective construals that afford and elicit culturally meaningful and relevant thoughts, feelings, and behaviors. Thus, although they feel natural, real, and immutable, cultural meanings and cultural differences are likely fluid. Like any other reasoning, culturally situated reasoning is action-based; the situation cues what is relevant to making meaning and taking action in the moment. The finding that cultural syndrome priming influences both content and process is particularly important, because procedural knowledge or naive theories about how to process information and make meaning of meta-cognitive experience matter for the sense we make of not only ourselves and others, motivation, goal pursuit, and goal persistence but also for intergroup dialogue.

Clearly there is much to be done. Priming research does not yet include regions of the world such as Latin America, Africa, and the Middle East. To understand more about the underlying process, to make predictions with regard to differences in real groups other than college students, it will be necessary to conduct priming research off college campuses. Good cultural syndrome primes should provide the ability to test effects within and across countries, and to test effects with non-college-student participants. Use of varied primes is recommended because no prime alone should be assumed to embody fully the latent construct of "culture" or even its active ingredients.

Moreover, cultural-syndrome-priming research to date has focused on the procedural knowledge likely to be linked with individualism and collectivism, and has not yet begun to examine the procedural knowledge associated with other cultural axes. Culture itself is not just individualism and collectivism, and the priming literature should not be confined to this particular domain. A likely future focus is Hofstede's (1980) power distance construct.

Thus, Shavitt et al. (2006) have provided evidence that, taking hierarchy into account (what they have termed "horizontal" and "vertical" individualism and collectivism) adds to predictions based solely on individualism and collectivism. Disentangling power and individualism–collectivism may be an important step toward utilizing priming techniques to study this syndrome. For example, Oyserman (2006) has proposed that the relevant cultural axis may focus on responses to high power, low power, and equality, separate from individualism and collectivism. Fiske (1991) and others have suggested that priming to have power is likely to cue global processing, and priming not have power is likely to cue local processing.

Culture-based power researchers will also want to know what happens when equality is cued. Whether equality cues high-power or low-power cognitive procedures is likely to depend on whether equality is synonymous with lack of power within a culture. Much like individualism and collectivism, cultural-syndrome-priming research can begin to provide information about both the content and the procedures that these cultural syndromes bring to mind. Future high- and low-power cultural syndrome researchers will need to examine impact on both content and procedures, as well as to ask whether power, once primed, has the same effect on mind-set or procedural knowledge cross-culturally and whether equality, once primed, carries with it high or low power-linked procedures.

Articulating effects of power separate from as well as in conjunction with individualism and collectivism may increase clarity of prediction. Priming individualism and collectivism could have very different effects on values in contexts that are simultaneously high or low in power. For example, using Triandis's articulation of horizontal and vertical individualism and collectivism, it is possible that in a vertical, individualist culture, priming individualism should lead to endorsement of inequality or competition, whereas in a horizontal, individualist culture, priming individualism should lead to endorsement of equality.

Finally, future research is also needed to untangle language and other features of priming. As noted in this volume (e.g., Chiu, Leung, & Kwan, Chapter 27; Norenzayan et al., Chapter 23; Wang & Ross, Chapter 26; all this volume), language itself is related to culture, memory, and cognition. Although studies using language are limited to participants who are bi- or multilingual, potential effects of language can be operationalized and studied with other primes, thus disentangling language from other culture-relevant factors. To date average effects for language prime studies are very small. This may be due to the necessity of using populations that

know two or more languages well. These bilingual or multilingual people are likely also to be to some extent bicultural or multicultural. Regardless of the type of prime used, populations that chronically move back and forth between cultural frames may be different from other populations.

Indeed, one form of priming research has focused explicitly on bicultural or multicultural individuals (Hong, Morris, Chiu, & Benet-Martínez, 2000). This work uses icons (e.g., the Great Wall of China, the Statue of Liberty) to cue one cultural syndrome or another. Because of this focus on individuals with detailed knowledge of multiple cultures, this work is somewhat different in focus from the research we have reviewed. Like the language priming requirement that participants know two or more languages well, this form of priming requires that participants know more than one culture well. Rather than assuming that all societies include both individualism and collectivism, this body of work assumes that some individuals experience both individualism and collectivism due to immigration or globalization of American cultural influence. Because of this focus, icon priming research can be seen as rooted in research focused on immigration, acculturation, and acculturative stress. However, in principle, icon-based priming should be able to show effects for both semantic and procedural knowledge.

Current research evidence does not include replication of effects with biculturals using language and icon priming, and with others using other priming tasks. Therefore, we cannot yet tell whether effects are the same or different between these populations, and if there are differences whether these are in quantity (i.e., effect size), quality (e.g., whether both content and procedural knowledge can be primed), or in both quantity and quality of effects. We speculate that effects will not differ in quality but may differ in quantity across groups more or less exposed to cultural shifts. Following our model of culture as situated cognition, it is likely that neither language alone nor biculturalism alone explains differences across postmodern societies. Rather, effects are due to situated meaning. Language and icons matter to the extent that they carry meaning in context. Meanings in situation matter, because culture from our perspective is a form of situated cognition; it provides cues as to who one is, what is meaningful, and how to process information about the world.

ACKNOWLEDGMENTS

We thank Ayse Uskul for her comments on an earlier draft of this chapter and Jill Fortain for her assistance with references and figures.

NOTES

1. Whereas the bulk of research on culture focuses on these two loosely defined cultural syndromes, a number of related constructs are not fully integrated into this body of work. Oyserman, Coon, et al. (2002) note that authors disagree as to whether familialism (relatedness to family, seeking harmony with family members, supporting and seeking advice from family) is *separate* from collectivism (Gaines et al., 1997), the *essential core* of collectivism (Lay et al., 1998), or an important *element* of collectivism, distinct from a nonkin-focused type of collectivism (Rhee, Uleman, & Lee, 1996). Similarly, the place of hierarchy and competition within an individualism and collectivism framework is not fully articulated. Hofstede (1980) originally proposed individualism and power, or as he termed it, "power distance," as separate cultural factors, a view paralleled in Fiske's (1991) taxonomy of basic social relationships, and more recently advocated by Triandis and his colleagues, who proposed including hierarchical or egalitarian aspects of social relationships in analyses of individualism–collectivism (cf. Singelis, Triandis, Bhawuk, & Gelfand, 1995; Triandis & Gelfand, 1998). By including a horizontal–vertical dimension to discussion of cultural differences, different dimensions of individualism and collectivism can be distinguished depending on whether they presume equal or different status between individuals, namely, "horizontal individualism," "horizontal collectivism," "vertical individualism," and "vertical collectivism." According to this framework, cultures high in horizontal individualism tend to be egalitarian, with individuals being independent and of comparable power and status. Countries identified as having this pattern are the Scandinavian countries (Singelis et al., 1995; Shavitt, Lalwani, Zhang, & Torelli, 2006; Triandis & Gelfand, 1998). Cultures high in horizontal collectivism tend to be egalitarian, with individuals committed to the good of the group; only Israeli kibbutzim are identified with this pattern (Shavitt et al., 2006). Most high individualism cultures tend to champion competition between individuals, resulting in acceptable inequality between individuals; most high collectivism cultures also include both clear hierarchies and acceptance of differential outcomes given one's place in the hierarchy. Thus, although equality is thus possible, most cultures are "vertical" to some degree (Shavitt et al., 2006). Triandis's work does raise the question of whether cultures differ in how high and low power influence the sense individual members make of themselves and their world—what and how they think. This is explored further in a later section.

2. Effect sizes are reported following the recommendations of J. Cohen (1992) in interpreting the meaning of the observed effect sizes: Effect sizes of less than $d = 0.2$ are described as "small"; those of $d = 0.5$–0.7 are described as "moderate"; and those above $d = 0.8$, as "large."

3. Small effects were also found for studies that pursued a more complex interaction effect. Lee, Aaker, and Gardner (2000, Studies 2–4, Aaker & Lee, 2001, Studies 1–4), Briley and Wyer (2002, Study 3), and Mandel (2003, Study 1) all examined the hypothesis that priming individualism and collectivism is potentiated when matched with primed or chronic self-regulatory focus (individualism matched with promotion focus, collectivism matched with prevention focus). Across these studies, a small effect was found for match.

REFERENCES

Aaker, J. L., & Lee, A. Y. (2001). "I" seek pleasures and "we" avoid pains: The role of self-regulatory goals in information processing and persuasion. *Journal of Consumer Research, 28,* 33–49.

Atran, S., Medin, D. L., & Ross, N. O. (2005). The cultural mind: Environmental decision making and cultural modeling within and across populations. *Psychological Review, 112,* 744–776.

Bakan, D. (1966). *The duality of human existence.* Chicago: Rand McNally.

Bargh, J. A. (1984). Automatic and conscious processing of social information. In R S. Wyer, Jr. & T. K. Srull (Eds.), *Handbook of social cognition* (Vol. 3, pp. 1–43). New York: Erlbaum.

Bargh, J. A. (1990). Auto-motives: Preconscious determinants of social interaction. In E. T. Higgins & R. M. Sorrentino (Eds.), *Handbook of motivation and cognition* (Vol. 2, pp. 93–130). New York: Guilford Press.

Bargh, J. A., Bond, R. N., Lombardi, W. J., & Tota, M. E. (1986). The additive nature of chronic and temporary sources of construct accessibility. *Journal of Personality and Social Psychology, 50,* 869–878.

Bargh, J. A., & Chartrand, T. L. (2000). The mind in the middle: A practical guide to priming and automaticity research. In H. T. Reis & C. M. Judd (Eds.), *Handbook of research methods in social and personality psychology* (pp. 253–285). Cambridge, UK: Cambridge University Press.

Bargh, J. A., Raymond, P., Pryor, J. B., & Strack, F. (1995). Attractiveness of the underling: An automatic power → sex association and its consequences for sexual harassment and aggression. *Journal of Personality and Social Psychology, 68,* 768–781.

Baumeister, R. F., & Leary, M. R. (1995). The need to belong: Desire for interpersonal attachments as a fundamental human motivation. *Psychological Bulletin, 117,* 497–529.

Berry, J. W. (1976). *Cross-cultural research and methodology series: III. Human ecology and cognitive style: Comparative studies in cultural and psychological adaptation.* Oxford, UK: Sage.

Berry, J. W. (1994). An ecological perspective on cultural and ethnic psychology. In E. J. Trickett, R. J. Watts, & D. Birman (Eds.), *Human diversity: Perspectives on people in context* (pp. 115–141). San Francisco, CA: Jossey-Bass.

Bond, M. H., & Yang, K. S. (1982). Ethnic affirmation versus cross-cultural accommodation: The variable impact of questionnaire language on Chinese bilinguals from Hong Kong. *Journal of Cross-Cultural Psychology, 13,* 169–185.

Bontempo, R. (1993). Translation fidelity of psychological scales: An item response theory analysis of an individualism–collectivism scale. *Journal of Cross-Cultural Psychology, 24,* 149–166.

Boroditsky, L. (2000). Metaphoric structuring: Understanding time through spatial metaphors. *Cognition, 75,* 1–28.

Brewer, M. B., & Gardner, W. L. (1996). Who is this "we"?: Levels of collective identity and self-representations. *Journal of Personality and Social Psychology, 71,* 83–93.

Briley, D. A., & Wyer, R. S. (2001). Transitory determinants of values and decisions: The utility (or nonutility) of individualism and collectivism in understanding cultural differences. *Social Cognition, 19,* 197–227.

Briley, D. A., & Wyer, R. S. (2002). The effect of group membership salience on the avoidance of negative outcomes: Implications for social and consumer decisions. *Journal of Consumer Research, 29,* 400–415.

Burris, C. T., & Rempel, J. K. (2004). "It's the end of the world as we know it": Threat and the spatial-symbolic self. *Journal of Personality and Social Psychology, 86,* 19–42.

Cha, O. (2006). *"I" see trees, "We" see forest: Cognitive consequences of independence vs. interdependence.* Unpublished doctoral dissertation, University of Michigan, Ann Arbor, MI.

Chartrand, T. L., & Bargh, J. A. (1996). Automatic activation of impression formation: Nonconscious goal priming reproduces effects of explicit task instructions. *Journal of Personality and Social Psychology, 71,* 464–478.

Chen, S., Lee-Chai, A. Y., & Bargh, J. A. (2001). Relationship orientation as a moderator of the effects of social power. *Journal of Personality and Social Psychology, 80,* 173–187.

Choi, I., Nisbett, R. E., & Norenzayan, A. (1999). Causal attribution across cultures: Variation and universality. *Psychological Bulletin, 125,* 47–63.

Cohen, D. (2001). Cultural variation: Considerations and implications. *Psychological Bulletin, 127,* 451–471.

Cohen, J. (1992). A power primer. *Psychological Bulletin, 112,* 155–159.

Cross, S. E., & Madson, L. (1997). Models of the self: Self-construals and gender. *Psychological Bulletin, 122,* 5–37.

Fiske, A. P. (1991). *Structures of social life: The four elementary forms of human relations.* New York: Free Press.

Förster, J., & Higgins, E. T. (2005). How global versus local perception fits regulatory focus. *Psychological Science, 16,* 631–636.

Gaines, S. O., Jr., Marelich, W. D., Bledsoe, K. L., Steers, W. N., Henderson, M. C., Granrose, C. S., et al. (1997). Links between race/ethnicity and cultural values as mediated by racial/ethnic identity and moderated by gender. *Journal of Personality and Social Psychology, 72,* 1460–1476.

Galinsky, A. D., Gruenfeld, D. H., & Magee, J. C. (2003). From power to action. *Journal of Personality and Social Psychology, 85,* 453–466.

Gardner, W. L., Gabriel, S., & Dean, K. K. (2004). The individual as "melting pot": The flexibility of bicultural self-construals. *Cahiers de Psychologie Cognitive* [Current Psychology of Cognition], 22, 181–201.

Gardner, W. L., Gabriel, S., & Lee, A. Y. (1999). "I" value freedom, but "we" value relationships: Self-construal priming mirrors cultural differences in judgment. *Psychological Science, 10,* 321–326.

Gasper, K., & Clore, G. L. (2002). Attending to the big picture: Mood and global versus local processing of visual information. *Psychological Science, 13,* 34–40.

Georgas, J. (1988). An ecological and social cross-cultural model: The case of Greece. In J. W. Berry, S. H. Irvine, & E. B. Hunt (Eds.), *Indigenous cognition: Functioning in cultural context* (pp. 105–123). Dordrecht, the Netherlands: Martinus Nijhoff.

Georgas, J. (1993). Ecological–social model of Greek psychology. In U. Kim & J. W. Berry (Eds.), *Indiginous psychologies: Research and experience in cultural context* (pp. 56–78). Thousand Oaks, CA: Sage.

Gollwitzer, P. M., Heckhausen, H., & Steller, B. (1990). Deliberative and implemental mind-sets: Cognitive tuning toward congruous thoughts and information. *Journal of Personality and Social Psychology, 59,* 1119–1127.

Gregg, G. (2005). *The Middle East: A cultural psychology.* New York: Oxford University Press.

Haberstroh, S., Oyserman, D., Schwarz, N., Kühnen, U., & Ji, L. J. (2002). Is the interdependent self more sensitive to question context than the independent self?: Self-construal and the observation of conversational norms. *Journal of Experimental Social Psychology, 38,* 323–329.

Hannover, B., & Kühnen, U. (2004). Culture, context, and cognition: The Semantic Procedural Interface model of the self. In W. Stroebe & M. Hewstone (Eds.), *European review of social psychology* (Vol. 15, pp. 297–333). Hove, UK: Psychology Press/Taylor & Francis (UK).

Higgins, E. T. (1989). Knowledge accessibility and activation: Subjectivity and suffering from unconscious sources. In J. S. Uleman & J. A. Bargh (Eds.), *Unintended thought* (pp. 75–123). New York: Guilford Press.

Higgins, E. T. (1996). Knowledge activation: Accessibility, applicability, and salience. In E. T. Higgins & A.

W. Kruglanski (Eds.), *Social psychology: Handbook of basic principles* (pp. 133–168). New York: Guilford Press.

Higgins, E. T., & Bargh, J. A. (1987). Social cognition and social perception. *Annual Review of Psychology, 38,* 379–426.

Hofstede, G. (1980). *Culture's consequences.* Thousand Oaks, CA: Sage.

Hofstede, G. (2001). *Culture's consequences: Comparing values, behaviors, institutions and organizations across nations* (2nd ed.). Thousand Oaks, CA: Sage.

Holland, R. W., Roeder, U. R., van Baaren, R. B., Brandt, A. C., & Hannover, B. (2004). Don't stand so close to me: The effects of self-construal on interpersonal closeness. *Psychological Science, 15,* 237–242.

Hong, Y. Morris, M., Chiu, C., & Benet-Martínez, V. (2000). Multicultural minds: A dynamic constructivist approach to culture and cognition. *American Psychologist, 55,* 709–720.

Inglehart, R. (1997). *Modernization and postmodernization: Cultural, economic, and political change in 43 societies.* Princeton, NJ: Princeton University Press.

Kağitçibaşi, Ç. (1987). *Growth and progress in cross-cultural psychology.* Berwyn, PA: Swets North America.

Kağitçibaşi, Ç. (1997). Wither multiculturalism? *Applied Psychology: An International Review, 46,* 44–49.

Kashima, E. S., & Kashima, Y. (1998). Culture and language: The case of cultural dimensions and personal pronoun use. *Journal of Cross-Cultural Psychology, 29,* 461–486.

Kashima, Y., & Kashima, E. S. (2003). Individualism, GNP, climate, and pronoun drop: Is individualism determined by affluence and climate, or does language use play a role? *Journal of Cross-Cultural Psychology, 34,* 125–134.

Kashima, Y., Kashima, E., & Aldridge, J. (2001). Toward cultural dynamics and self-conceptions. In S. Constantine & M. B. Brewer (Eds.), *Individual self, relational self, collective self* (pp. 277–298). New York: Psychology Press.

Kashima, Y., Yamaguchi, S., Kim, U., Choi, S. C., Gelfand, M. J., & Yuki, M. (1995). Culture, gender, and self: A perspective from individualism–collectivism research. *Journal of Personality and Social Psychology, 69,* 925–937.

Kemmelmeier, M., & Cheng, B. Y. M. (2004). Language and self-construal priming: A replication and extension in a Hong Kong sample. *Journal of Cross-Cultural Psychology, 35,* 705–712.

Kemmelmeier, M., Wieczorkowska, G., Erb, H. P., & Burstein, E. (2002). Individualism, authoritarianism, and attitudes toward assisted death: Cross-cultural, cross-regional, and experimental evidence. *Journal of Applied Social Psychology, 32,* 60–85.

Kitayama, S., Duffy, S., Kawamura, T., & Larsen, J. (2003). Perceiving an object and its context in different cultures. *Psychological Science, 14,* 201–206.

Kitayama, S., Ishii, K., Imada, T., Takemura, K., & Ramaswamy, J. (2006). Voluntary settlement and the spirit of independence: Evidence from Japan's "northern frontier." *Journal of Personality and Social Psychology, 91,* 369–384.

Kuhn, M. H., & McPartland, T. S. (1954). An empirical investigation of self-attitudes. *American Sociological Review, 19,* 68–76.

Kühnen, U., Hannover, B., & Schubert, B. (2001). The semantic-procedural interface model of the self: The role of self-knowledge for context-dependent versus context-independent modes of thinking. *Journal of Personality and Social Psychology, 80,* 397–409.

Kühnen, U., & Oyserman, D. (2002) Thinking about the self influences thinking in general: Cognitive consequences of salient self-concept. *Journal of Experimental Social Psychology, 38,* 492–499.

Lay, C., Fairlie, P., Jackson, S., Ricci, T., Eisenberg, J., Sato, T., et al. (1998). Domain-specific allocentrism–idiocentrism: A measure of family connectedness. *Journal of Cross-Cultural Psychology, 29,* 434–460.

Lee, A. Y., Aaker, J. L., & Gardner, W. L. (2000). The pleasures and pains of distinct self-construals: The role of interdependence in regulatory focus. *Journal of Personality and Social Psychology, 78,* 1122–1134.

Lehman, D. R., Chiu, C. Y., & Schaller, M. (2004). Psychology and culture. *Annual Review of Psychology, 55,* 689–714.

Leung, T., & Kim, M. S. (1997). *A revised self-construal scale.* Honolulu: University of Hawaii at Manoa.

Mandel, N. (2003). Shifting selves and decision making: The effects of self-construal priming on consumer risk-taking. *Journal of Consumer Research, 30,* 30–40.

Marian, V., & Kaushanskaya, M. (2004). Self-construal and emotion in bicultural bilinguals. *Journal of Memory and Language, 51,* 190–201.

Markus, H., Uchida, Y., & Omoregie, H. (2006). Going for the gold: Models of agency in Japanese and American contexts. *Psychological Science, 17,* 103–112.

Markus, H. R., & Kitayama, S. (1991). Culture and the self: Implications for cognition, emotion, and motivation. *Psychological Review, 98,* 224–253.

Markus, H. R., & Oyserman, D. (1989). Gender and thought: The role of the self-concept. In M. Crawford & M. Gentry (Eds.), *Gender and thought: Psychological perspectives* (pp. 100–127). New York: Springer-Verlag.

Miller, J. G. (1984). Culture and the development of everyday social explanation. *Journal of Personality and Social Psychology, 46,* 961–978.

Morris, M. W., & Leung, K. (2000). Justice for all?: Progress in research on cultural variation in the psychology of distributive and procedural justice. *Applied Psychology: An International Review, 49,* 100–132.

Morris, M. W., & Peng, K. (1994). Culture and cause: American and Chinese attributions for social and physical events. *Journal of Personality and Social Psychology, 67,* 949–971.

Neely, J. H. (1977). Semantic priming and retrieval from lexical memory: Roles of inhibitionless spreading activation and limited-capacity attention. *Journal of Experimental Psychology: General, 106,* 226–254.

Newman, L. S. (1993). How individualists interpret behavior: Idiocentrism and spontaneous trait inference. *Social Cognition, 11,* 243–269.

Nisbett, R. E. (2003). *The geography of thought: How Asians and Westerners think differently . . . and why.* New York: Free Press.

Oishi, S., Wyer, R. S., & Colcombe, S. J. (2000). Cultural variation in the use of current life satisfaction to predict the future. *Journal of Personality and Social Psychology, 78,* 434–445.

Oyserman, D. (1993). The lens of personhood: Viewing the self and others in a multicultural society. *Journal of Personality and Social Psychology, 65,* 993–1009.

Oyserman, D. (2006). High power, lower power and equality: Culture beyond individualism and collectivism. *Journal of Consumer Psychology, 16,* 352–356.

Oyserman, D. (2007). Social identity and self-regulation. In A. W. Kruglanski & E. T. Higgins (Eds.), *Social psychology: Handbook of basic principles* (2nd ed.). New York: Guilford Press.

Oyserman, D., Coon, H. M., & Kemmelmeier, M. (2002). Rethinking individualism and collectivism: Evaluation of theoretical assumptions and meta-analyses. *Psychological Bulletin, 128,* 3–72.

Oyserman, D., Kemmelmeier, M., & Coon, H. M. (2002). Cultural psychology, a new look: Reply to Bond (2002), Fiske (2002), Kitayama (2002), and Miller (2002). *Psychological Bulletin, 128,* 110–117.

Oyserman, D., & Lee, W. S. (2007). *Cultural syndromes influence what and how we think: Effects of priming individualism and collectivism.* Manuscript under review.

Oyserman, D., Sorensen, N., Cha, O., & Schwarz, S. (2006). *Thinking about "Me" or "Us" in East and West: Priming independence and interdependence and Stroop performance.* Manuscript under review.

Oyserman, D., Sorensen, N., & Reber, R. (2006). *What did you say? Priming cultural syndrome, verbal fluency and auditory accuracy.* Manuscript under review.

Ralston, D. A., Cunniff, M. K., & Gustafson, D. J. (1995). Cultural accommodation: The effect of language on the responses of bilingual Hong Kong Chinese managers. *Journal of Cross-Cultural Psychology, 26,* 714–727.

Rhee, E., Uleman, J. S., & Lee, H. K. (1996). Variations in collectivism and individualism by ingroup and culture: Confirmatory factor analyses. *Journal of Personality and Social Psychology, 71,* 1037–1054.

Roccas, S., & Brewer, M. B. (2002). Social identity complexity. *Personality and Social Psychology Review, 6,* 88–106.

Rokeach, M., & Ball-Rokeach, S. J. (1989). Stability and change in American value priorities, 1968–1981. *American Psychologist, 44,* 775–784.

Ross, M., Xun, W. Q. E., & Wilson, A. E. (2002). Language and the bicultural self. *Personality and Social Psychology Bulletin, 28,* 1040–1050.

Rudman, L. A., & Borgida, E. (1995). The afterglow of construct accessibility: The behavioral consequences of priming men to view women as sexual objects. *Journal of Experimental Social Psychology, 31,* 493–517.

Sayle, M. (1998). The social contradictions of Japanese capitalism. *Atlantic Monthly, 281,* 84–94.

Schwartz, S. H. (1992). Universals in the content and structure of values: Theoretical advances and empirical tests in 20 countries. In M. P. Zanna (Ed.), *Advances in experimental social psychology* (Vol. 25, pp. 1–65). New York: Academic Press.

Schwarz, N. (2002). Situated cognition and the wisdom of feelings: Cognitive tuning. In L. F. Barrett & P. Salovey (Eds.), *The wisdom in feelings: Psychological processes in emotional intelligence* (pp. 144–166). New York: Guilford Press.

Schwarz, N. (2006). Individualism and collectivism. *Journal of Consumer Psychology, 16,* 324.

Schwarz, N., & Bless, H. (1992). Constructing reality and its alternatives: An inclusion/exclusion model of assimilation and contrast effects in social judgment. In L. L. Martin & A. Tesser (Eds.), *The construction of social judgments* (pp. 217–245). Hillsdale, NJ: Erlbaum.

Schwarz, N., & Clore, G. L. (1996). Feelings and phenomenal experiences. In E. T. Higgins & A. W. Kruglanski (Eds.), *Social psychology: Handbook of basic principles* (pp. 433–465). New York: Guilford Press.

Schwarz, N., & Clore, G. L. (2007). Feelings and phenomenal experiences. In A. W. Kruglanski & E. T. Higgins (Eds.), *Social psychology: Handbook of basic principles* (2nd ed.). New York: Guilford Press.

Shavitt, S., Lalwani, A. K., Zhang, & Torrelli, ? (2006). The horizontal/vertical distinction in cross-cultural consumer research. *Journal of Consumer Psychology, 16,* 352–356.

Shweder, R. A., & LeVine, R. A. (Eds.). (1984). *Culture theory: Essays on mind, self, and emotion.* New York: Cambridge University Press.

Singelis, T. M. (1994). The measurement of independent and interdependent self-construals. *Personality and Social Psychology Bulletin, 20,* 580–591.

Singelis, T. M., Triandis, H. C., Bhawuk, D., & Gelfand, M. J. (1995). Horizontal and vertical dimensions of individualism and collectivism: A theoretical and measurement refinement. *Cross-Cultural Research: The Journal of Comparative Social Science, 29,* 240–275.

Sinha, D., & Tripathi, R. C. (1994). Individualism in a collectivist culture: A case of coexistence of opposites. In U. Kim, H. C. Triandis, Ç. Kağitçibaşi, S. C. Choi, & G. Yoon (Eds.), *Individualism and collectiv-*

ism: Theory, method, and applications (pp. 123–136). Thousand Oaks, CA: Sage.

Smith, P. K., & Trope, Y. (2006). You focus on the forest when you're in charge of the trees: Power priming and abstract information processing. *Journal of Personality and Social Psychology, 90,* 578–596.

Sperber, D. (2001). Mental modularity and cultural diversity. In H. Whitehouse (Ed.), *The debated mind: Evolutionary psychology versus ethnography* (pp. 23–56). New York: Berg.

Srull, T. K., & Wyer, R. S., Jr. (1978). Category accessibility and social perception. *Journal of Personality and Social Psychology, 37,* 841–856.

Srull, T. K., & Wyer, R. S., Jr. (1979). The role of category accessibility in the interpretation of information about persons: Some determinants and implications. *Journal of Personality and Social Psychology, 37,* 1660–1672.

Stapel, D. A., & Koomen, W. (2001). I, we, and the effects of others on me: How self-construal level moderates social comparison effects. *Journal of Personality and Social Psychology, 80,* 766–781.

Strack, F., Schwarz, N., Bless, H., Kübler, A., & Wänke, M. (1993). Awareness of the influence as a determinant of assimilation versus contrast. *European Journal of Social Psychology, 23,* 53–62.

Strack, F., Schwarz, N., & Gschneidinger, E. (1985). Happiness and reminiscing: The role of time perspective, affect, and mode of thinking. *Journal of Personality and Social Psychology, 49,* 1460–1469.

Tajfel, H. (1982). Social psychology of intergroup relations. *Annual Review of Psychology, 33,* 1–39.

Tajfel, H. (2001). Social stereotypes and social groups. In. M. A. Hogg & D. Abrams (Eds.), *Intergroup relations: Essential readings* (pp. 132–145). New York: Psychology Press.

Tajfel, H., & Forgas, J. P. (2000). Social categorization: Cognitions, values and groups. In C. Strangor (Ed.), *Stereotypes and prejudice: Essential readings* (pp. 49–63). New York: Psychology Press.

Tajfel, H., & Turner, J. C. (2004). The social identity theory of intergroup behavior. In J. T. Jost & J. Sidanius (Eds.), *Political psychology: Key readings* (pp. 276–293). New York: Psychology Press.

Tavassoli, N. T. (2002). Spatial memory for Chinese and English. *Journal of Cross-Cultural Psychology, 33,* 415–431.

Trafimow, D., Silverman, E. S., Fan, R. M. T., & Law, J. S. F. (1997). The effects of language and priming on the relative accessibility of the private self and the collective self. *Journal of Cross-Cultural Psychology, 28,* 107–123.

Trafimow, D., Triandis, H. C., & Goto, S. G. (1991). Some tests of the distinction between the private self and the collective self. *Journal of Personality and Social Psychology, 60,* 649–655.

Triandis, H. C. (1995). *Individualism and collectivism.* Boulder, CO: Westview.

Triandis, H. C., Bontempo, R., Villareal, M. J., Asai, M., & Lucca, B. (1988). Individualism and collectivism: Cross-cultural perspectives on self-ingroup relationships. *Journal of Personality and Social Psychology, 54,* 323–338.

Triandis, H. C., & Gelfand, M. J. (1998). Converging measurement of horizontal and vertical individualism and collectivism. *Journal of Personality and Social Psychology, 74,* 118–128.

Triandis, H. C., McCusker, C., & Hui, C. H. (1990). Multimethod probes of individualism and collectivism. *Journal of Personality and Social Psychology, 59,* 1006–1020.

Trope, Y., & Liberman, N. (2003). Temporal construal. *Psychological Review, 110,* 403–421.

Uskul, A., & Oyserman, D. (2006). Question comprehension and response: Implications of individualism and collectivism. In B. Mannix, M. Neale, & Y. Chen (Eds.), *Research on managing groups and teams: Vol. 9. National culture and groups* (pp. 173–201). Oxford, UK: JAI Press.

Watkins, D., & Gerong, A. (1999). Language of response and the spontaneous self-concept: A test of the cultural accommodation hypothesis. *Journal of Cross-Cultural Psychology, 30,* 115–121.

Watkins, D., & Regmi, M. (2002). Does the language of response influence self-presentation?: A Nepalese test of the cultural accommodation hypothesis. *Psychologia: An International Journal of Psychology in the Orient, 45,* 98–103.

Woike, B. A. (1994). The use of differentiation and integration processes: Empirical studies of "separate" and "connected" ways of thinking. *Journal of Personality and Social Psychology, 67,* 142–150.

Woike, B. A., Lavezzary, E., & Barksy, J. (2001). The influence of implicit motives on memory processes. *Journal of Personality and Social Psychology, 81,* 935–945.

Yang, K. S., & Bond, M. H. (1980). Ethnic affirmation by Chinese bilinguals. *Journal of Cross-Cultural Psychology, 11,* 411–425.

PART III

IDENTITY AND SOCIAL RELATIONS

CHAPTER 11

Social Relationships
in Our Species and Cultures

ALAN P. FISKE
SUSAN T. FISKE

Social relationships are the primary channel through which cultures are transmitted, and conversely, culture informs social relationships. This occurs because culture is what organisms acquire by interacting in a community or social network; that is, culture includes those aspects of organisms' capacities, motives, ideas, biology, practices, institutions, artifacts, and landscapes that result from engaging in social relationships. Humans have exceptional specializations for learning from others, including a sophisticated capacity for imitating purposeful action. Humans also have proclivities to modify their innate social–relational dispositions in accord with the precedents, principles, and prototypes provided by the communities in which they participate. Thus, culture is transmitted through culturally informed social relationships.

But how does this work? How does the human psyche enable people to bootstrap their social relations, using universal mechanisms to develop culturally particular forms of sociality? To answer this fundamental question for cultural psychology, we need to know what aspects of human social relations are endogenous

(intrinsic to humans), and how these universal aspects give rise to cultural variation. At the same time, we need to know how people recognize and deploy the actions that create and modulate social relationships. Finally, we need both to identify the core motives that drive sociality and to determine how culture shapes their intensity and orientation. These are the questions we explore in this chapter.

This chapter first presents some perspectives on culture and social relationships. The first perspective considers five *core social motives* that motivate people to relate to others in the first place. Then we describe 15 highly salient human relationships, the *roles* most often culturally elaborated, socially institutionalized, cognitively schematized, and emotionally motivated. Cultural and social psychologists have generally ignored most relationships that are phenomenologically salient around the world. A third perspective analyzes four *relational models* that people use to coordinate with each other; these are the elementary building blocks that people implement in culturally distinctive ways and combine to construct complex social systems. The fourth perspective focuses on how people perceive outsiders and strangers in a two-dimensional *framework of warmth and competence*, based on intent and status. Finally, we tie together the third and fourth perspectives for a more general take on *how people respond to each other*. All these perspectives explain ways that universal social-psychological adaptations give rise to culturally particular social-psychological processes.

CORE SOCIAL MOTIVES

Over the last century, psychologists have repeatedly identified a limited set of core social motives that underlie human behavior (S. Fiske, 2004; Stevens & Fiske, 1995). An essential foundation of the human adaptive niche is other people—the social groups, networks, and relationships in which humans participate (Caporael, 1997; A. Fiske, 2000; S. Fiske, 2004). Most important, people seek *social belonging* with their own kind, the most basic social motive of all (S. Fiske, 2004; Baumeister & Leary, 1995). Belonging enables people to survive and thrive (e.g., Berkman, Glass, Brissette, & Seeman, 2000; House, Landis, & Umberson, 1988; Stansfield, Bosma, Hemingway, & Marmot, 1998). People's core social motive to belong with others ensures their attempts to gain acceptance and avoid rejection (S. Fiske, 2004). From these attempts follow the remaining core social motives: to maintain socially shared *understanding*, a sense of *control* over outcomes, a special sympathy for the *self*, and *trust* in certain ingroup others. The core social motives provide a potentially universal perspective on human sociality, as we shall see.

Belonging

The importance of belonging is a cultural constant. To illustrate the complementarity of our species' evolved proclivities and their cultural variations, consider this core social motive of belonging. Although people are attracted to others everywhere and form relationships everywhere, the mechanisms differ slightly. For example, similarity predicts attraction, at least across wealthy, educated cultural samples that have been studied (Bond & Smith, 1996; Rai & Rathore, 1988), and this makes adaptational sense. Similarity correlates with ingroup membership, suggesting more trust and control than

outgroup members probably afford, especially given that their goals may differ from those of the ingroup (S. Fiske & Ruscher, 1993). Similarity also functions to affirm mutual group membership by indicating that the people involved represent variations on the group's shared prototype or image of itself (e.g., Abrams, Marques, Bown, & Dougill, 2002; Hogg, 2001). Familiarity, often correlated with similarity, also encourages friendship (a type of ingroup formation) in both American and Japanese samples, for example (Heine & Renshaw, 2002).

However, cultures may vary in the extent to which people value similarity in relationships, with Americans valuing similarity more (Heine & Renshaw, 2002). Of course, Americans might define "similarity" as having a single, shared attribute or interest, whereas Japanese might require more shared attributes to feel similar.

Relatedly, cultures may combine universal principles with culture-specific enactments in other domains that encourage relationship. On the one hand, cultures tend to agree about what is physically attractive (Berry, 2000). For both men and women, young, symmetrical, and prototypical features are good. Some features obviously depend on gender; for example, in women (Cunningham, 1986; Cunningham, Roberts, Barbee, Druen, & Wu, 1995), childlike features (large eyes spaced far apart, small nose, small chin), some mature features that might also indicate being slender (narrow face, prominent cheekbones), expressive features (high eyebrows, large smile), and sexual cues (larger lower lip as in a sexual pout, well-groomed, full hair) are favored. What is attractive in men is less often studied, but high cheekbones and rugged jaws appear to be favored (Berry, 2000).

On the other hand, although physical attractiveness predicts interpersonal attraction in many cultures, cultures vary in what they infer from beauty. Western samples report that beautiful people are socially warm and skilled (Feingold, 1992). Several East Asian samples appear to link attractiveness to a cultural ideal distinct from Western ones (Chen, Shaffer, & Wu, 1997; Dion, Pak, & Dion, 1990; Shaffer, Crepaz, & Sun, 2000; Wheeler & Kim, 1997). Chinese immigrants to Canada, those most involved in their Chinese community, do not display the American attractiveness stereotype (Dion et al., 1990). A physical attractiveness stereotype, however, does emerge in some Asian cultures (Korea and Taiwan), but the content differs. Unlike people in the United States, attractive people in Korea are not presumed to be more powerful but are instead presumed to show more concern for others and more integrity. American and Korean views of social potency apparently differ (Wheeler & Kim, 1997). For Taiwanese participants, cultural context also mattered: Taiwanese who endorsed Western values showed the stereotype most on individualist traits (Shaffer et al., 2000), whereas those who most accepted Chinese traditions showed the stereotype on the most extreme (positive and negative) traits but not more moderates ones, presumably less important (Chen et al., 1997). In each case, although certain aspects appear universal (the importance of belonging, responding to similarity, and attractiveness), the culture shapes the specific manifestations.

Belonging Securely versus Widely

Belonging, the most central core motive, is posited to be universal, but it is enacted differently depending on culture. Several theories contrast Eastern and Western views, with relevance for belonging. Cultural self theory (Markus & Kitayama, 1991) contrasts Japanese interdependent selves, focused on relational motives to maintain harmony, with American independent selves, focused on self-enhancing motives to keep autonomy. Basic trust theory (Yamagishi & Yamagishi, 1994) contrasts Japanese caution with American trust, respectively requiring a long confirmation and preference for well-known associates versus a short confirmation and openness to strangers.

Different enactments of belonging motives fit several cultural observations. Individualists have more relationships, but collectivists appear to have closer, more sensitive, and fewer relationships, with more rules (Verkuyten & Masson, 1996). Americans feel a moral duty to help a relative, depending on how much one likes the relative, whereas Indians find it is a moral duty to help a relative regardless of individual liking (Miller & Bersoff, 1998). East Asian close relationships are more often involuntary, stable, and good enough (Ho, 1998). People are often closer to their families of birth in East Asia than in Western settings (Takahashi, Ohara, Antonucci, & Akiyama, 2002). For example, spousal relationships are

secondary to father–son relationships in Confucian hierarchies. Cultures do differ dramatically in their expectations about marriage (Bond & Smith, 1996; Smith & Bond, 1994). One broad-brush contrast would be marriages arranged to reinforce social networks versus individual romantic choice. Attachment processes may respectively emphasize symbiotic harmony or generative tension between individuals and relationships (Rothbaum, Weisz, Pott, Miyake, & Morelli, 2000). But in many settings, people perceive their own relationships as better than other people's (Endo, Heine, & Lehman, 2000).

Broadly, though, the theme of wide versus secure belonging captures some cultural variations (S. Fiske & Yamamoto, 2005). These cultural variations in belonging underlie variations in the other core social motives that operate in the service of this fundamental, universal motive for belonging as noted earlier: shared understanding, effective control, self enhancement, and trust.

Understanding

To belong, people seek a *socially shared understanding*; this proves to be a core social motive (Augoustinos & Innes, 1990; S. Fiske, 2002a, 2004; Hardin & Higgins, 1996). If you are the only one who thinks that every glacial granite boulder can potentially crush you, you will not travel easy in Vermont, and locals will think you are nuts; conversely, if you do not believe in witches and sorcery, you will not understand events in Burkina Faso, and locals will think you are nuts. People are demonstrably motivated to develop a socially shared understanding of each other and their environment. A shared information framework allows people to function in groups and in any kind of relationship. It informs their assessment of their own rejection and acceptance. This understanding is likely to operate along particular dimensions that facilitate belonging, and these dimensions are, we suggest, pancultural.

Understanding Relationships versus Persons

Although socially shared understanding appears universal, people's strategies for understanding also show some cultural variation, consistent with emphasis on autonomy and unvarnished honesty, or emphasis on interdependence and social harmony. For example, in Anglo American culture, people focus on understanding individuals, but in more interdependent cultures, people may well focus more on understanding networks of relationships among people.

Controlling as a Group or Individual

People are highly motivated to know the contingencies between their own actions and outcomes (S. Fiske, 2002a, 2004). Feelings of control reflect feeling effective in one's environment. Attributional processes operate in the service of perceived intentional control, another core social motive (S. Fiske, 2004; Pittman, 1998). Feeling efficacious promotes both individual health and group life, so people try to restore lost control, but cultures and individuals vary on this motive. Exactly how people imagine another's intentions depends on cultural factors (A. Fiske, Kitayama, Markus, & Nisbett, 1998).

Previous research on interdependence shows that American students do attend to persons who control their outcomes, and this effect correlates with measures reflecting a basic motive for a sense of personal control (Dépret & Fiske, 1999; Erber & Fiske, 1984; Neuberg & Fiske, 1987; Ruscher & Fiske, 1990; Stevens & Fiske, 2000). Americans, at least, search for information that will restore a sense of personal prediction and control when their outcomes depend on another person. Similarly, when their sense of control is threatened generally, they search for information about others in their environment (Pittman & Pittman, 1980).

Cultural differences in control (A. Fiske et al., 1998) reflect varying emphases on social harmony: the extent to which the individual cedes control to ingroup others, seeking to create and maintain collective compatibility. For example, a scale of harmony control (Morling & Fiske, 1999) includes items such as feeling secure in accepting the care of friends, getting one's own needs met by meeting the needs of others, and going along with intangible forces larger than the self. As one cultural contrast, for example, Texan Latinos score higher than Texan Anglos. As another example, independent Americans achieve control by influencing the world, whereas interdependent Japanese achieve control by mature adjustment and compromise to circumstances and relationships. American women with normal pregnancies coped best by individual acceptance, whereas Japanese women coped best by social assurance (Morling, Kitayama, & Miyamoto, 2003). In general, Americans specialize in primary control, whereas Japanese and other East Asians may specialize more in cooperation-based secondary control (Morling & Evered, 2006).

Self-Enhancement

Maintaining a *special status for the self* appears to be yet another core social motive (S. Fiske, 2004). This special status (whether inflated self-esteem, self-improvement, or self-sympathy) depends on culture but seems to engage self-protection, self-improvement, and self-maintenance.

Enhancing Relationship versus Self

The self plays a special role in people's lives. In a wide-ranging literature review, many Western samples tend to enhance the self relative to other people, or relative to other people's view of them (Kwan, John, Kenny, Bond, & Robins, 2004). But the Japanese, for instance, tend to be more modest and view the self more in the context of group memberships (Markus & Kitayama, 1991). Some have posited that East Asians view the self with a special sympathy, despite its admitted flaws (Heine, Lehman, Markus, & Kitayama, 1999). This self may be improved, although the task is difficult and success is not guaranteed. Sympathy in relationships balances against self-criticism, each enabling the other (Kitayama & Markus, 1999).

Trusting

Jointly meaningful normative models for relationships direct sociality at interpersonal and intergroup levels, reflecting people's need to know whom to trust and more specific rules for interaction depending on culture; *trusting at least some close others* serves as another core social motive (S. Fiske, 2004; Gurtman, 1992; Yamagishi, 2002).

Trusting Selectively versus Widely

Americans generally have positive expectations about other people, as a baseline (S. Fiske, 2002, 2004). They trust other people in general not to create unprovoked negative outcomes for themselves. In Japan, trust operates more narrowly, within the ingroup, and only then based on the assurance of knowing the other person's incentive contingencies (Yamagishi, 1998). As a result of the more narrow trusting motive and the embedding of self in a network, caution should be more evident in Japanese data on belonging and rejection.

Our initial cultural comparisons between one East Asian setting (Japan) and an American setting (Yamamoto et al., 2004) entail five kinds of preliminary comparative data: (1) societal stereotypes reflecting rejection between groups, (2) reported norms about rejection among friends, (3) a scenario study about potential rejection, (4) a study of expected interaction and potential rejection, and (5) a study of actual interaction and actual rejection. In each case, we find both cultural similarities and differences reflecting the motive to belong more securely or more loosely (S. Fiske & Yamamoto, 2005). Our initial data suggest that people in the two cultures sometimes have different motives and metaexpectations about interpersonal relationships, although all are highly motivated to belong in relationships and show hurt at interpersonal rejection. Americans' sense of wide, loose belonging apparently fits autonomous understanding, with people being direct and speaking what they view as the truth. They view relationships as a matter of individual choice and control, show self-confidence and self-enhancement, and trust optimistically until their trust is violated.

The Japanese apparently have slightly different motives and metaexpectations. They prioritize social harmony, relation-oriented motives, and do not mind saying different things in different situations. Thus, they do not think feedback is necessarily true, even if their partner evaluates them positively. To the Japanese, one makes positive or flattering statement about another to reinforce solidarity, show respect, and protect the other's "face."

Conclusion Regarding Core Social Motives

Regardless of culture, belonging, understanding, controlling, self-enhancing, and trusting all operate in the context of interpersonal compatibility, with implications for people's well-being in the face of acceptance and rejection. Each culture interprets and transmits ways of enacting these motives in characteristic ways. One venue for enacting these abstract, universal core social motives is culturally institutionalized relationships, namely social roles.

PEOPLE'S EXPERIENCE OF SOCIAL ROLES: AN ETHNOLOGICAL PHENOMENOLOGY OF INSTITUTIONALIZED RELATIONSHIPS

People often organize their interactions according to institutionalized sets of cultural roles. These roles are explicitly schematized, motivationally salient, culturally elaborated frameworks for social relationships. Anthropologists and sociologists have extensively studied these institutionalized relationships for two reasons. First, these relationships organize everyday intentions and present important constraints, so that people explicitly interpret others' action and justify their own action in terms of these roles. Institutionalized relationships comprise much of the texture of life as experienced—they are among the most salient aspects of the phenomenology, experience, or natural history of sociality. Second, some institutionalized relationships are more or less universal, whereas many others are widespread, so they permit meaningful cross-cultural comparison and analysis. To understand the psychology of everyday social relations, cultural and social psychologists need to recognize these institutionalized relationships and connect their theories to them.

As the second of three ways to describe specific patterns of human relationships, we want to go beyond the range typically considered by social and cultural psychologists to illustrate the varieties of widespread kinds of relationships, none of which is universal, but none is completely particular, either. These 15 types are among those most often culturally elaborated, socially institutionalized, cognitively schematized, and emotionally motivated; thus, they are salient ways of organizing social cognition, motivation, emotion, and evaluation in large subsets of the world's cultures. Surprisingly, no established list or taxonomy enumerates them, but the following are most of the important ones:

• *Marriage*: Close economic coordination and sharing of many significant resources; constitutive of parental relations and often the offsprings' group membership; usually involving coresidence and nearly always some kind of exclusivity in sexual rights. Marriage is virtually universal, although specific features vary dramatically, notably, how marriages connect groups and create networks, how they are arranged and dissolved, and whether multiple concurrent or successive spouses, or other sexual partners, are permissible for husbands, wives, or both.

• *In-lawship*: Structured, often obligatory relationships with in-laws. In many traditional societies, each kin group "gives" brides to specific kin groups, which entails myriad special norms and practices. These relations are typically asymmetrical: The husband and his kin have economic or labor obligations to the wife's kin and must be circumspect or avoidant. Conversely, often there is a joking relationship (see the next type of relationship) with the spouse's younger siblings. (See references below.)

• *Joking and funerary relationships*: A relationship in which the parties are required to tease, insult, roughhouse, and act rudely to each other, usually including sexual jokes or advances. Sometimes participants may freely appropriate each other's possessions. Partners typically attend each other's funeral, where they make a mockery of the ritual proceedings and may have responsibilities as executor. Joking partners commonly are defined by kinship roles (e.g., between grandchild and grandparent, or with the spouse's younger siblings), or relations between pairs of communities or ethnic groups. Widespread across Africa and many other regions, joking relationships are often complemented by avoidance in other relationships in which extreme circumspection is required (typically, especially with one's mother-in-law) (e.g., Labouret, 1929; Paulme, 1939; Radcliffe-Brown, 1940/1965a, 1949/1965b).

• *Compadrazgo*: The relationship between a person and his or her godchild's parents. A close, trusting relationship entails lifelong hospitality, aid, and cooperation and precludes sexual relations with the compadre's spouse. Traditionally, this relationship is universal in the Catholic societies north of the Mediterranean and in many neighboring societies, along with Latin America (e.g., Lynch, 1986; Mintz & Wolf, 1950; Nutini & Bell, 1980; Nutini, 1984).

• *Agemates*: A relationship among men initiated in a particular span of years (typically not at the same event), entailing mutual aid in warfare and raiding, pooling of resources to pay fines, fellowship, and feasting. This usually requires permissive access to each other's wives. This relationship, which is present in nearly all the pastoral societies of east and northeast sub-Saharan Africa, is also present in variations elsewhere (e.g., Baxter & Almagor, 1978; Hollis, 1905; Llewelyn-Davies, 1981; Spencer, 1988).

• *Kinship*: Complex constellation of relationships and group membership involving close cooperation and core social identities. Kin usually perceive that they share some essential corporeal essence. Children may belong to the father's group, the mother's group, or both. Kinship is important in virtually all cultures and usually is by far the most important organizing framework for sociality. (Some classics include Ember & Ember, 1983; Evans-Pritchard, 1951; Fox, 1967; Lévi-Strauss, 1949/1969; Needham, 1971; Radcliffe-Brown & Forde, 1960.)

• *Milk-kinship*: Close bond between a woman and someone else's child she has suckled, creating a relationship closely resembling that resulting from birth. This extends to milk-kinship of both parties' kin. It is important in all Islamic societies, and many other cultures in Africa north of the equator, and the Balkans (e.g., Altorki, 1980; Dettwyler, 1988; Khatib-Chahidi, 1992).

• *Ritual covenant* ("blood brotherhood"): Strong bond of reciprocal altruism, trust, and aid in many cultures created by ingesting or absorbing each other's blood. This covenant is often formed across ethnic groups, usually between men. Traditionally widespread in Africa and present in many other parts of the world, it usually involves sexual taboos and expectations of partners' bestowal of a bride (e.g., Beidelman, 1963; Evans-Pritchard, 1933; Tegnaeus, 1952).

• *Reciprocal exchange of prestige goods*: Either simultaneously or alternately, partners give presents to each other, sometimes ritually valuable objects with little or no use value. The standard for the exchange is even matching, but partners may compete to overmatch each other. This custom is famous in Melanesia (e.g., Leach & Leach, 1983; Macintyre, 1983; Malinowski, 1922/1961).

• *Rotating credit associations*: A defined group of people meet at regular intervals. At each meeting, each participant makes an equal contribution to a pool of money, and one person takes the entire pool. The order of turn-taking among the participants may be decided ahead of time, or by lot on each occasion. The practice is widespread (e.g., Ardner, 1964; Geertz, 1962; Hart, 1977; Vélez-Ibañez, 1983).

• *Sodalities and secret societies*: Ritually constituted voluntary groups that engage in joint activities such as political action, enforcement of morals in the community, or collective ritual or religious responsibilities. This widespread practice is especially common in Africa and Melanesia (e.g., Boas, 1970; Fortune, 1932; Gregor, 1979; MacKenzie, 1996; Mak, 1981; Murphy, 1980; Tuzin, 1984).

• *Castes*: Social categories defined by birth that restrict intermarriage, sexual relations, eating together, or other social contact with lower castes. They are often associated with occupation and nearly always form a status hierarchy. (There is a fuzzy taxonomic boundary between castes and ethnic groups.) Caste systems are widespread (e.g., Bynum, 1992; Camara, 1976; Höffer, 1979; Khare, 1976; Marriott, 1976; Orenstein, 1968; Paulme, 1968; Powdermaker, 1939/1993; Yalman, 1963; Wyatt-Brown, 1982).

• *Slavery*: A relationship in which one person or group owns another, with rights to the product of that person's labor and children, and other controls; usually includes rights to sell the other. The practice has been widespread (including, notably, in classical Greece) (e.g., Kopytoff, 1982; Lovejoy, 1981; Rubin & Tuden, 1977).

• *Prostitution and concubinage*: Sexual acts in return for material considerations. The practice is universal. (For a subtle analysis of these practices in classical Greece, see Davidson, 1998.)

• *Totemic relations*: A group's or an individual's identification with a species of animal (or occasionally a plant species or other natural phenomenon). Totemic groups usually are exogamous (do not marry within the group) and are typically defined by common descent, often putatively from the totem animal. Totemism nearly always entails a taboo against eating the totem, and/or killing it, but sometimes with important ritual exceptions. The practice is widespread; in attenuated form, it is evident in team names and mascots (e.g., Douglas, 1966; Durkheim, 1912/1915; Fortes, 1945, 1966/1987; Frazer, 1910/1968; Goldenweiser, 1910/1963; Tambiah, 1969).

This cannot be an exhaustive list of the most widespread, highly structured, culturally im-

portant types of institutionalized relationships, but it is a start.[1] There are many other widespread types of institutionalized social relationships, most notably, relationships with gods, but most other institutionalized relationships are more variable and culture-specific in form and are therefore less amenable to cross-cultural comparison. To our knowledge, aside from the very different sociological typology of Simmel (1971), there have been no previous attempts to lists the most widespread types of institutionalized relationships. In any case, these are many of the major relational schemas for which anthropologists keep an eye out, and whose local nuances are the focus of a lot of fieldwork. At the very least, psychologists may find it a useful glossary for conversations with anthropological colleagues, microsociologists, and informants in other cultures. Moreover, powerful and pervasive social motives, emotions, evaluations, sanctions, cognitive schemas and processes, and much of social action in general are oriented to these institutionalized social relationships. Unless researchers are aware of these institutionalized relationships, they will not understand most of their informants' intentions, evaluations, or obligations.

Theorists have explored factors that may explain the institutionalization of many of these relationship types (see their respective references). But no general theory explains why this set of particular social relationships is institutionalized in a great many cultures. Why do *these* particular 15 role sets tend to diffuse, endure, and become elaborated and institutionalized, in contrast to the innumerable rarer ones that are not often institutionalized? With regard to relational models theory (RMT, covered in the next section), it is intriguing to note that the greatest number of these are primarily communal sharing (CS) relationships; many of the others are predominantly authority ranking (AR) relationships, or ones that combine aspects of CS and AR. In a very few, equality matching (EM) or market pricing (MP) predominate. RMT posits that, in general, the primary intrinsic motivations for relationships differ in typical intensity, with CS > AR > EM > MP. This is one plausible, partial basis for the prevalence of these institutionalized relationships: They meet basic psychosocial needs. For example, the trusting and intimate relationships among agemates, compadres, and ritual covenants are pleasant and rewarding. Joking partners enjoy the teasing and banter. In addition, it seems likely that many of these institutionalized relationships comprise combinations of relational models that are functionally complementary in some way, at one or more levels. Marriage and kinship effectively organize subsistence activities and material resources, as well as provide necessary frameworks for child-rearing and socialization. Another factor in their prevalence and persistence may have to do with the ways they combine with other relationships. For example, prostitution is clearly related to occupational opportunities for women, together with marriage practices such as male age of marriage, spousal roles, and taboos on sexual relations before marriage, or during pregnancy or lactation. Anthropologists have repeatedly demonstrated how joking partners, ritual covenants, in-laws, and compadres provide crucial alternative economic and political alliances that complement relations to spouses and kin. More generally, to account for the distribution of these institutionalized relationships across and within cultures, we might begin by looking at the manner in which these institutionalized relationships combine with each other, and with more culture-specific relationships. Can we identify a combinatorial syntax of social relationships?

But these are speculations, and cultural psychologists have a virtually open field for exploring the psychological sources of these institutionalized relationships and the psychological consequences of participating in each. The study of institutionalized relationships is an excellent starting point for cultural social psychology, with the notable advantage that they are readily apparent to the observer and well represented in the explicit, reflective, semantic awareness of informants. Moreover, studying them would join cultural and social psychology to their sister disciplines, psychological and social anthropology.

However, there are certain disadvantages of using roles or institutionalized relationships to analyze cultures. Some of these institutionalized relationships are not present in all cultures, and many social interactions in any culture are not shaped by any of them. As we indicated, no theoretical framework encompasses them all, let alone explains them. Nor are they elementary—they are not the basic constituents of sociality. Having considered broad social motives and more specific types of social roles, we now turn to elementary social relationships.

RELATIONAL MODELS

Theory

Relational models theory (RMT) posits that people rely on four elementary models to generate, understand, coordinate, evaluate, and sanction most aspects of nearly all social interaction in all cultures (A. Fiske, 2001, 2002, 2004a). These relational models (RMs) are the basis for most social motives, moral emotions, and evaluative judgments (A. Fiske, 2002). People tend to seek and sustain these four types of relationships largely for their own sake; these relationships are all intrinsically meaningful to varying degrees depending on the RM, culture, gender, age, and individual personality.

Communal sharing (CS) is the organization of interaction according to something socially meaningful that participants have in common (and that differentiates them from outsiders). CS operates when people take joint responsibility for something such as raising a child, when they share resources such as an ocean or food, or when they act with compassion because they identify with another's suffering. CS also underlies the killing of women who besmirch the family's collective honor and the ethnic cleansing of people who pollute the communal purity of the nation. It also operates in collective responsibility, so that an attack on any member of the group motivates other group members to attack any member of the attacking group indiscriminately. CS can be as deep as intense love, or as superficial as sharing access to a drinking fountain or a highway. In abstract terms, CS is a relational structure called an "equivalence group," resembling a categorical scale. With respect to a given interaction, a set of people are either socially equivalent or they are categorically different.

The most intense CS relationships are formed metonymically, when participants' sharing of some aspect of their bodies, or the acknowledgment of something their bodies share in common, creates a categorical bond among the social persons. The process is *consubstantial assimilation* (making their substances similar). In CS, people perceive that their bodies are the same in some way: sharing some essential substance such as "blood" or "genes"; having some crucial surface feature such as (a particular type of) circumcision or skin color; or even moving rhythmically in unison (A. Fiske, 2004b). CS is created and sustained by giving birth, nursing, partaking in each other's blood in bonding rites, and commensal eating and drinking—especially partaking in religious sacrifice. Skin-to-skin contact also promotes CS. Undergoing extreme physical deprivation and peril together likewise creates CS bonds. Prolonged military drill and dancing also tend to have this effect.

Semiotically analyzed, the constitution of CS through consubstantial assimilation is indexical, because the sharing of bodily or comestible substances is a material sign of the social relationship: Sharing materializes social cohesion and identification in concrete biologically significant form. For example, people perceive giving birth to a child to cause the CS relationship between mother and child; people perceive blood-bonding covenants to create mutual obligations, because the partners incorporate each other's blood, which binds them morally by connecting their material substance. This constitutive indexicality is congruent with people's communication and cognitive representations of CS as bodily equivalence—that is, people represent the CS connection as same substance, same surface, or synchronous motion. Thus, people *express* CS in the same ways they *create* it, corresponding to the ways they *think* of it. Probably, children also *seek to identify* their CS groups in this way: for example, by attending to who nurses, shares food, holds, and sleeps with them. Conversely, these proclivities for recognizing CS filter its *cultural transmission*. Only those cultural implementations that resonate with these prepared expectations of CS will be readily diffused and repeatedly transmitted. Moreover, whereas any aspect of persons can be equivalent, consubstantial assimilation is uniquely evocative; it motivates and commits people, binding them emotionally.

Authority ranking (AR) structures social interaction in an ordinal hierarchy of asymmetrical relationships. Higher ranking people are entitled to deference and respect from subordinates; subordinates are entitled to pastoral protection from leaders who should stand up for them in dealings with outsiders or higher superiors. AR manifests in status differentiation, privilege, and chain of command. AR includes awe and obedience to superior beings, morality based on the commandments or will of gods and elders, seniority systems, and ranking of people according to achievement or ascription. AR underlies violent contests for dominance

and punishment for disloyalty. Formally, AR is a linear ordering whose meaningful relations and operations correspond to those of a linear scale. Inequality is directional and transitive.

AR is constituted via *social physics*: through space, time, and magnitude (A. Fiske, 2004b). People assume their rank and display it by arranging themselves above and below, or in front and behind; that is, people are ranked as "superiors" and "inferiors," as "leaders" and "followers." Higher ranking people come first, or have seniority by being first. Those "higher" in rank are entitled to bigger abodes, bigger shares, and more personal space; they are "greater" than the "little" people who are ranked "lower." In many unrelated languages, rank is marked by plural linguistic forms, such as the royal "we" or the respectful *vous*.

This social use of space, time, and magnitude is iconic and metaphoric: Relations in space, time, and magnitude are maps of social relations. The linear ordering of positions in any of these physical dimensions corresponds to a linear social rank ordering. This iconic constitution of AR relations reflects a corresponding cognitive representation of AR: People think of rank as position, magnitude, and temporal precedence. Likewise, children anticipate this, searching for these signs of ranking in order to participate in local AR relations. Furthermore, this social physics uniquely evokes the emotions and motives that sustain AR. And communication about AR relies primarily on spatial, temporal, and magnitude representations: The chief is higher, in front of, and bigger than his "subordinates," and precedes them (he is superior, leads his followers, has precedence, may be addressed in the plural, occupies a greater social and architectural space, etc.). People occasionally invent and impose other media for constituting and conveying hierarchy, but the filter of innate cognitive expectations and affective responses makes space, time, and magnitude the predominant medium of AR in all cultures.

Equality matching (EM) is coordination in which people attend to additive differences, anchored with reference to even balance. In EM, people keep track of whether they are equal, or what needs to be done to make them equal. Examples include taking turns; in-kind reciprocity, such as favors or dinner invitations; tit-for-tat revenge; equal distributions or contributions; and decisions by vote or lottery. In CS, some aspect or resource of the participants is the same, undifferentiated—"What's mine is yours." In EM, participants are separate but equal; you and I are different but on a par, evenly matched: One person, one vote, and every vote counts, but my vote is not your vote. The relations and operations that are socially meaningful in EM correspond to those defined in an interval scale (formally known as an ordered Abelian group).

People constitute EM with *concrete operations* that *operationally define* even balance (cf. Piaget, 1932, 1952). People are made equal by procedures such as taking turns, drawing straws, or flipping a coin; casting a ballot; lining up on a starting line and commencing simultaneously; beginning and ending work at the same time; counting out shares in rounds of one-to-one correspondence; or comparing shares by aligning them or weighing them in a pan balance. Legitimately conducted, these operations create equality, ostensibly demonstrate it, invoke binding norms, and evoke emotions motivating compliance. Again, the constitutive, communicative, and cognitive systems for EM are congruent with each other and with the processes that mediate children's discovery of the local implementations of EM relations and, hence, their cultural transmission.

Market pricing (MP) structures interaction according to ratios or rates, where all socially relevant aspects of a situation reduce to a common metric. Aspects of an MP interaction frame by proportionality: for example, when morality is framed as justice in due proportion to what each person deserves. Examples include cost/benefit calculations, judgments based on utilitarian rationality, distributions proportional to contributions, and, of course, prices, wages, rents, interest, taxes, and tithes. In MP, multiplication, division, and the distributive law are meaningful because they are in a ratio scale (formally, an Archimedean ordered field).

Abstract, *arbitrary symbols* are the primary medium for constituting and communicating MP. Indeed, cognizing MP proportions, ratios, and rates essentially requires symbolic representation. Displaying a price, making a bid, signing a check, or assenting to a written contract necessarily depend on symbols whose meaning is arbitrarily created by convention. The calculus of cost/benefit analysis and utilitarian morality depends on reducing all values to an abstract numerical metric. The quintessential medium of MP is price (including

wages, rents, interest, fines, etc.), which represents the exchange ratio for a quantity of a commodity against all other commodities in the economy; all features of the object blend into this one number (Simmel, 1900/1990). The reification of prices is the symbol representing prices: money. Contemporary representations of money exhibit its purely abstract, conventional quality: digitally symbolized accounts and transfers that are embodied in no particular material object or place.

Thus people typically constitute, cognize, and communicate each RM in its own, distinctive medium. Children are prepared to discover their community's implementation of the RMs by attending to and trying out these RM-specific media; conversely, these are the channels through which these implementations are culturally transmitted.

To simplify, so that we do not have to refer to all five of the aspects of this constitution–communication–cognition–cultural learning–cultural transmission system every time, we can call this the *conformation system* of the RM: consubstantial assimilation for CS, social physics for AR, concrete operations for EM, and abstract symbolism for MP.

Research

People use these four relational models to make moral judgments, to generate ideologies and political platforms, to give social meaning to land and objects, to exchange objects, to make contributions or distributions, to organize labor, to make group decisions, and to construct social identities. Complex social relationships, groups, activities, institutions, and communities combine models that are sequentially linked, hierarchically embedded, or otherwise concatenated. Every use of any model must be culturally informed, because the models are incomplete: They do not specify with whom, where, when, or how they are to be implemented—or which model is to be used in which aspects of an interaction. Culture provides prototypes and precedents that guide people in applying the models in mutually congruent implementations that permit coordinated action (A. Fiske, 2000).

Wide-ranging research using a wide variety of methods (see Haslam's, 2004, review; A. Fiske & Haslam, 2005) shows that RMs organize three types of naturally occurring social errors in five cultures; people confuse persons with whom they interact in the same RM. Also, when people intentionally select a substitute for their original partner in an activity, they pick someone with whom they relate according to the same RM. When people list all their acquaintances, they produce runs (clusters) of acquaintances with whom they have the same RM—even though this cannot be a conscious strategy. When asked to sort their acquaintances freely into categories according to how they relate to them, they tend to place people according to the RM that governs their interactions with them. When people judge the similarity of their relationships with others, similarity is a function of whether they use the same or a different RM to relate to the persons. Taxometric studies that use a variety of methods all show that, as theorized, the RMs are psychologically distinct categories, not continuous dimensions. Individual differences in specific patterns of aberrant RM implementations correspond to specific personality disorders. Aberrant implementations of RMs are associated with vulnerability to depression, bipolar disorder, and psychosis. RMT also illuminates organizational behavior and management, political psychology, and the anthropology of the family (reviewed in Haslam, 2004). People detest and derogate explicit framing of trade-offs that apply an illegitimate RM (A. Fiske & Tetlock 1997). The endowment effect results largely from the meaning of objects as mediators of RMs, and the value people place on objects depends on the RMs that the objects are tokens of; that is, the price (if any) at which people are willing to sell an object depends on the social relationship in which they received an object, and the price people are willing to pay for an object depends on the relationship that the object represents for them (McGraw & Tetlock, 2005; McGraw, Tetlock, & Kristel, 2003). The implementation of EM predicts self-enhancement, whereas five measures of individualism do not (Thomsen, Sidanius, & Fiske, 2006). Families and groups get along when they coordinate using the same RM but are frustrated and angry when they attempt to interact using different RMs, or the same RM implemented in different ways (Sondak, 1998; Vodosek, 2003; Goodnow, 2004). (For additional studies and theoretical applications of RMT, see the bibliography at *www.rmt.ucla.edu.*)

RMs are innate and universal, but their application to organize concrete interactions is necessarily cultural. According to RMT, cultural variation is the corollary of the indeterminacy of *mods*, the elementary relational structures. For example, children have an innate intuitive understanding of linear ordering in sociality, the AR mod; they cannot innately know who occupies what position in each hierarchy in their community, or in what contexts people are ranked with respect to what aspects of an interaction. Children depend on their culture to provide prototypes and precedents to guide them in implementing AR. To participate in meaningful, coordinated interaction, children have to implement each RM in accord with the specific cultural prototypes and precedents that others in their community are using. Relational mods cannot be implemented in their abstract, indeterminate, innate form: They must be implemented in specific, culturally informed coordination systems. Culture provides *preos* (precepts, principles, precedents, and prototypes) that complement and complete innate but indeterminate relational mods. Children learn these preos through the conformation system in which they are culturally transmitted, mentally cognized, and communicated in everyday representations.

RMT posits that humans are innately sociable: They seek to form and sustain relationships largely as intrinsic ends in themselves. Children and adults have innately structured motives specific to each RM. People need CS relationships especially, but also AR and EM relationships. To a lesser degree, they may also sometimes need MP relationships. Of course, individuals differ in the strength of these motives, and cultures differ in which motives they recognize, legitimate, foster, suppress, or redirect; cultures also differ in where they orient each motive. In an African village, people meet most of their CS motives within permanent kin relationships and some enduring friendships; in an American city, the middle-class seeks to meet its CS needs in (often impermanent) romantic dyads, as well as friendships and associations.

RMT posits that RMs coordinate most mutually meaningful social relationships. Of course, people do not have meaningful social relationships with most other people. Indeed, people may be present in the same space, or causally affect each other, without participating in a meaningfully coordinated relationship. If they simply ignore each other's sociality, ignoring each other's existence or treating each other like nonsocial objects, then we say they have a *null* relationship. For example, a forager gathers the fruit from a tree without concerning herself about any other person's potential rights to that fruit, so she has a null relationship with those others. Likewise, if bullets are flying, I seek cover behind a log or a body; I treat the body as merely a shield like the log, having a null relationship with the log and—in the moment, at least—with the person whose body it is, even if the person later turns out to be alive.

If a person attends to the other's sociality but is not guided, motivated, or obligated by any RM—although aware that the other's cognition and motivation *is* socially organized—that person's orientation can be characterized as *asocial*; that is, the orientation is asocial if the other person is nothing but a means to nonsocial ends—if a relationship with the other is neither intrinsically motivated nor felt to be morally binding. Psychopaths are asocial, and pure Machiavellianism is asocial.[2]

RMT is a comprehensive synthesis of major theories of sociality, but it differs from other theories in several respects. First, several other major theories, such as Tönies's contrast of *Gemeinschaft* and *Gesellschaft*, or Durkheim's mechanical versus organic solidarity, have described a subset of the four basic types of relationships but left out one or two of the basic forms. Although a few other theories have recognized all four basic forms of sociality in one particular domain of social life, RMT is the only theory that encompass all domains of social coordination and shows how the same RMs operate across domains. No other approach provides a unified theory of interpersonal, intergroup, organizational/institutional, and international coordination. RMT connects ideology, economy, and polity to social psychology and to many forms of psychopathology. RMT also uniquely integrates social cognition, communication, constitution, cultural transmission, and children's social development, along with social emotions, motives, moral judgments and values, sanctions, and the maintenance, redress and repair, and termination of social relations. No other general theory of sociality incorporates into the same framework universals, individual differences, and variation across cultures. Moreover, RMT aims, at least, to formulate an integrative understanding of the mechanisms and processes of natural selection, neuroanatomy, neuro-

physiology, ontogeny, and culture that shape social relations—and are in turn shaped by social relations. Also, RMT is one of the few theories that recognizes that humans have evolved to be intrinsically social. Moreover, RMT sees children as sophisticated, active culture seekers. The development of sociality is not just socialization or internalization, it is a process of externalization in which children strive to connect their innate social proclivities—the four mods—with the local cultural implementations—preos. Cultural prototypes and precedents complement and complete children's innate relational proclivities, coming together to form definite models for social coordination.

Nevertheless, RMT has some major limitations. As currently formulated, RMT does not address the long-term ecological, societal, and functional factors that affect which RM coordinates which domains in which cultures and *how* RMs are implemented; nor does is explain how implementations change historically. Nor does RMT address the situational, demographic, and strategic factors that affect people's choice of RMs and their implementations when they have a cultural choice, at the margins. Furthermore, RMT does not explain what goes on outside the framework of RMs, or before people adopt an RM; that is, it does not encompass cognition, motives, or emotions in either null or asocial relations. This is just what the social-cognitive content model (SCCM) covers—including the ways that people cognize persons as potential relational partners. Both RMT and SCCM posit that humans are fundamentally social beings with strong relational needs; SCCM addresses the ways in which cognition about persons serves core social motives.

SOCIAL-COGNITIVE CONTENT MODEL: AN EXPANSION OF THE STEREOTYPE CONTENT MODEL

Theory

When people respond to another social entity, whether a group or an individual, they do so in the service of core social motives. The motive to belong is central; it is the motive for seeking to form or join CS relationships (A. Fiske, 2002b; S. Fiske, 2004; Leary & Baumeister, 2000). People want to connect with other people in their own group, arguably, to survive and thrive. The core motive to belong defines ingroup (own group) and outgroup (all other groups). Ingroup *belonging* matters because the ingroup by definition shares one's goals, which facilitates other core social motives, as described earlier—socially shared *understanding*, a sense of *controlling* one's outcomes, *enhancing* the self, and *trusting* close others (S. Fiske, 2004). The outgroup by definition does not share the ingroup's goals, and is at worst indifferent and at best hostile, so the outgroup is viewed as threatening and elicits negative affect (S. Fiske & Ruscher, 1993). This approach to social behavior highlights the importance of knowing who is with "us" and who is against "us," in the service of furthering shared goals. The approach has elements in common with other emphatically social adaptational perspectives on social cognition (e.g., Kurzban & Leary, 2001; Neuberg, Smith, & Asher, 2000), but it focuses less specifically on reproductive strategies and more on social surviving and thriving within a group. People are demonstrably healthier if they are not socially isolated. This approach also fits a pragmatic, goal-based analysis of social behavior (S. Fiske, 1992). In this view, social perception provides the foundation for social survival within one's group. Some principles are universal, although their instantiations vary by culture, as we will see.

If the core motive of ingroup belonging matters so much, then people's central concern when encountering another person or group will be the other's group membership; that is, in RM terms, the CS group(s) to which the other belongs. Previous theoretical work and research on the continuum model show that such social category–based responses are rapid and primary, coming before more individuated, person-specific responses (e.g., S. Fiske & Neuberg, 1990; S. Fiske, Lin, & Neuberg, 1999). Our subsequent and current work more closely examines the nature of these social categories. We proceed from the premise that the crucial categories essentially answer: friend or foe? And then: able or unable? That is, when people encounter strangers, they first want to know the strangers' intentions (good or ill) and their ability to enact them (capability). If the intentions are good, then the social other's goals are at least compatible, and the other is ingroup or a close ally. Otherwise, the other is threatening. And whether the goals are compatible or not, people want to know whether the other actually matters (if capable) or not (if incapable).

The stereotype content model (SCM; S. Fiske, Xu, Cuddy, & Glick, 1999; S. Fiske, Cuddy, Glick, & Xu, 2002) proposes that soci-

etal groups are universally perceived along two primary dimensions, warmth and competence. These are the two primary dimensions of general stereotype content. *Warmth* is anchored at the positive end by characteristics such as friendly, good-natured, warm, and sincere: Is the other friend or foe? *Competence* is anchored by characteristics such as capable, confident, competent, and skillful: Is the other able or unable? Perceived warmth occurs in relation to society in general (Group X is or is not nice people in general) but also in interpersonal relationships (Person X is always nice or not nice to me). Perceived competence occurs in relation not only to society in general (valued skills) but also to specific relationships contexts (relevant skills). People tend to conflate these two levels, believing that their experience, or their group's experience, represents the true nature of those other social entities.

Related Research

The two dimensions have received copious support from several areas of psychology. These dimensions emerge in classic American person perception studies (S. Fiske, Cuddy, & Glick, 2007). And in more recent Western person perception research, these two dimensions account for more than 80% of the variance in global impressions of individuals. Similar twin dimensions appear in European work on social value orientations, in construals of others' behaviors, and in voters' ratings of political candidates in the United States and Poland. Related dimensions also describe Western national stereotypes (e.g., competence and morality); and emerge in analyses of prejudices toward many specific social groups in the United States and Europe (e.g., S. Fiske et al., 2007).

These two dimensions differ from two other broad frameworks that might at first seem similar. First, the semantic differential dimensions of evaluation, potency, and activity (Osgood, Suci, & Tannenbaum, 1957) do not correspond, because both warmth and competence entail evaluation (better to be high on both); moreover, both vary in the potency and activity of their expression. Second, the perceived warmth and competence dimensions correspond to people's impressions of others, whereas the Big Five personality traits (Extraversion, Agreeableness, Conscientiousness, Openness to Experience, and Neuroticism) correspond to measured consistency in behavior (Wiggins & Trapnell, 1997). People do not necessarily perceive each other along five dimensions, but may opt for a more pragmatic sense of their social relationship, based on intent (warmth) and ability to enact it (competence).

Evidence from the United States

The SCM proposes that stereotype contents respond to fixed principles that apply across varied perceivers and groups. In the United States, stereotype content and its social structural correlates are systematic, generating three fundamental hypotheses (S. Fiske et al., 1999, 2002). First, across groups, *stereotypes share common dimensions of content: warmth and competence*. Second, *many outgroups receive evaluatively mixed stereotypes*: more positive on one dimension and less positive on another. Third, locations of groups along *these dimensions of stereotype content follow from social structural variables:* Perceived status predicts stereotypical competence, and perceived competitiveness predicts stereotypical (lack of) warmth. The SCM maps stereotypes, and a group's location on the map results from its place in the social structure.

Previous U.S. datasets (S. Fiske et al., 1999, 2002), including a representative sample survey (Cuddy, Fiske, & Glick, in press-b), have mapped several dozen American groups (e.g., poor people, rich people, old people, middle-class people, disabled people, Asians, Jews). The groups reliably differentiate in this two-dimensional space of liking (warmth) and respecting (competence); that is, they spread out in all quadrants of the space, and cluster analyses typically identify clusters in each quadrant of the space. These findings support the first hypothesis, common dimensions.

To investigate the second hypothesis, that many stereotypes rate differently on warmth and competence, we examined the distribution of the groups in the map of outgroups. Only a few groups land in the most obvious, unmixed combinations of liking and respect (pride-inspiring groups such as Christians and the middle class) or disliking and disrespect (contempt-inspiring groups such as the homeless and poor). The interesting combinations are mixed and elicit ambivalence: Liked but disrespected, the pitied groups are high on perceived warmth but low on perceived competence (e.g., older, disabled). Conversely, the envied, disliked but respected groups are low on perceived warmth but high on perceived competence (e.g., rich, Asian, Jewish). Many of the groups, often the majority, land in the mixed competence × warmth quadrants, high on one and low on the other, as predicted.

Much additional support for the mixed stereotypes hypothesis—that many groups are perceived as high on one dimension but low on the other—stems from research on stereotypes of specific social groups. Two types of stereotyped groups materialize in this literature: those viewed as kind but helpless, and those viewed as skillful but cunning. Envious prejudice is directed at the latter groups, who are seen as threateningly competent and untrustworthy (Cuddy, Fiske, & Glick, in press-a; in press-b). For example, "nontraditional" women, such as career women and feminists, are perceived to possess agentic but not communal traits, and are respected but disliked— the embodiment of envious prejudice. Envious prejudice also targets Asian Americans, who are characterized by stereotypes such as excessive competence (too ambitious, too hardworking) and lack of sociability. Similarly, stereotypes of Jews combine business acumen with interpersonal self-interest. Viewed grudgingly as worthy of respect, such groups are not well liked, and they elicit envy, a loaded emotion that involves both hostility and depression. Envy tends to be directed toward higher-status people when their standing is seen as unjustly gained.

Groups seen as benevolent but incapable of competing in mainstream society sit in the opposite corner of the map. This type of prejudice reflects liking but disrespect and often targets traditional women and elderly people, both perceived as high communal but low agentic (Cuddy et al., in press-a, in press-b). Viewed as harmless but pathetic, they typically elicit pity, a paternalistic response. Pity goes to individuals whose stigmas are viewed as uncontrollable and to lower-status people (Cuddy et al., in press-a, in press-b).

Still, some groups receive evaluatively consistent stereotypes. Groups whose members are perceived as both hostile and indolent are most susceptible to the traditional form of antipathy normally associated with derogated groups. These groups elicit contempt (S. Fiske et al., 2002) that tends to be directed toward stigmatized people whose negative outcomes are perceived by others as avoidable. For example, homelessness, obesity, and AIDS all elicit anger, but only when attributed to individual weaknesses or moral shortcomings. Welfare recipients and poor people of any race also elicit disgust and contempt more than any other quadrant's groups (S. Fiske, Cuddy, & Glick, 2002).

Conversely, ingroups and mainstream social groups are favored as both warm and competent. These groups typically elicit pride and admiration (S. Fiske, Cuddy, & Glick, 2002), apparently because of their valued attributes that reflect on but do not detract from the self. All four of these patterns—for ingroups, extremely negative outgroups, and the two mixed types of groups—support the frequency of evaluatively mixed stereotypes, the SCM's second hypothesis.

In keeping with the SCM's third major hypothesis, different locations in the social structure—high or low status, more or less competition—predict intergroup stereotypes, emotions, and behaviors. Status and competition both operationalize relative to society in general. People report how groups are viewed by society, and their own relative position does not much affect their knowledge of where groups stand relative to each other. People respond in much the same ways to individuals of higher and lower status who compete or not with them as individuals (Caprariello, Cuddy, & Fiske, 2004; DiChiara & Fiske, 2004).

Focusing on the friend–foe dimension, competition reliably predicts a perceived lack of warmth. Groups perceived to compete with the ingroup or with society in general (e.g., by being exploitative) are seen as unfriendly. The evidence reviewed in the next section shows that this effect is reliable, though moderate in size.

Also, status reliably predicts perceived competence. People apparently endorse meritocracy more than sour grapes: Groups get what they deserve. The research reviewed in the next section shows that this status–competence effect is large and robust.

Evidence from Europe and from East Asia

The SCM previously had been tested only in U.S. samples. If the SCM describes universal human principles, then they should not be limited to American perceivers or other culturally related contexts. Although it proposes systematic principles of societal stereotypes and their relation to social structure, some aspects should be culturally variable. In this research (Cuddy, Fiske, Kwan, et al., in press), the SCM revealed theoretically grounded cross-cultural, cross-group similarities and differences across 10 nations. Student samples ($N = 1,028$) from seven European and three East Asian samples (Japan, South Korea, and Hong Kong) supported three hypothesized cross-cultural similarities: (1) Perceived warmth and competence reliably differentiate societal group stereotypes; (2) many outgroups receive evaluatively mixed stereotypes; and (3) high-status groups stereotypically are competent, and competitive groups stereotypically lack warmth.

Our comparative data uncovered one consequential cross-cultural difference: The three East Asian cultures did not locate their own reference groups (ingroups and societal prototype groups) in the most positive cluster (high-competence/high-warmth). Most discussions of prejudice (e.g., Brewer & Brown, 1998; S. Fiske, 1998) hold that outgroup derogation requires obvious reference-group favoritism. But although the East Asian samples showed less self-enhancement and diminished reference-group favoritism, they apparently did so without eliminating outgroup derogation. This, on a societal level, is analogous to modesty with regard to the self, a phenomenon frequently observed in East Asian samples compared to Western ones (Markus & Kitayama, 1991).

The different SCM quadrants elicit not only different stereotypic traits and distinct emotional prejudices but also specific patterns of discriminatory behavior, resulting in the Behaviors from Intergroup Affect and Stereotyping (BIAS) map (Fiske, Cuddy, & Glick, 2002). As noted earlier, people are proud of or admire high-competence, high-warmth ingroups and reference groups; this elicits helping and association. Low-competence, low-warmth outgroups receive contempt and disgust, which elicits both active harm (attack, fight) and passive harm (exclude, demean).

Two evaluatively mixed clusters receive ambivalent emotions and behavior: People report envy and jealousy of high-competence but low-warmth groups, which elicits both active harm (sparked by dislike) and passive association (because of their high status). Low-competence but high-warmth groups receive pity and sympathy, which elicits both passive harm (sparked by disrespect) and active help (because they pose no threat). These behavior predictions are supported in the U.S. national survey data, as well as student samples (Cuddy et al., in press-b), but they await cross-cultural comparison.

The SCM applies to the perception of individuals as much as groups, and even to the perception of individuals not perceived as group members per se; that is, the same structural features (status and competition) that predict impressions of groups (stereotypes and emotional prejudices) should predict impressions of individuals. In recognition of this prediction and of its origins in person perception research, we refer to the overarching principle as the SCCM. We would expect the general principles of the SCCM to be culturally universal. For example, in the American case, the self and close friends (allies) would appear as warm and competent. Across many cultures, people prefer friends and mates with a few specific traits that fit the generality of this prediction, namely, kindness and intelligence (Buss, 1989; Buss & Barnes, 1986). Various SCCM aspects, but especially those involving self, might again show cultural variability, as has been demonstrated for the SCM.

The Social-Cognitive Content Model

The expanded SCM, termed the SCCM, suggests that for adaptive purposes, people need to know immediately whether other social entities (individuals, groups) are with them or against them, as in the sentry's call, "Who goes there? Friend or foe?" Upon knowing the other's intent, a secondary question is the other's competence to enact that intent (the sentry wants to know whether the other is armed). The SCCM emphasizes dimensions that indicate the nature of the perceiver's interdependence with others. But cultural enactments of belonging in relationships differ, for example, along dimensions of belonging securely to a few, stable, long-term relationships or many, unstable, shorter-term relationships. The core motives approach that emerges in the SCCM demonstrates again that universals and cultural particulars are products of the same adaptive system by which people survive and thrive within social relationships.

RSVP: RELATIONAL STRUCTURE, VALENCE, AND PULL

Relating SCCM and RMT

SCCM is a theory of the perception and evaluation of persons and groups, especially when no concrete relationship has (yet) been established between the perceiver and the target persons. It describes structural relations between groups in society, and the members of these groups, on the basis of relative status/power and their competition or cooperation. RMT is a theory of structures for coordinating and evaluating interactions, when such normative coordination occurs. Processes at the SCCM and RMT levels are connected, because the perception of strangers, distant acquaintances, and groups is predominantly oriented toward anticipating the nature of the potential relationship that might be formed with them. People need to know how they are going to coordinate if they start to interact with the person(s) they are perceiving; moreover, they want to decide whether to engage or to avoid engagement. So people think about others primarily as potential relational partners (A. Fiske & Haslam, 1996). Conversely, based on their experience in relationships they do form, people engaged in any RM evaluate their existing and former partners on dimensions of warm to hostile, and competent to incapable.

Furthermore, RMT and SCCM readily connect, first because they each address both individual and group levels of analysis. RMT posits that the four RMs organize relations among groups and relationships of persons to groups, as well as among individuals (A. Fiske, 1991, 2004a). Similarly, SCCM posits that the dimensions that underlie perception of groups also underlie perception of individuals in status and competition structures.

Second, the two models cover a range of intensity, defined here as "pull." Pull is related to attractiveness, or rather, motivation to relate to the other. Pull is the *desired amount* of relationship: the depth, breadth, and duration of sociality that people seek with a given individual or group. RMT posits that any of the four RMs can be implemented at any intensity; a relationship can have any level of *pull*; that is, any type of relationship can encompass any extent, frequency, duration, and range of interactive domains, and can involve any level of motivation and normative obligation.[3] The limiting case, where pull is zero, is a null relationship, in which people do not use any RM to evaluate or sanction any aspect of their interactions (A. Fiske, 1991). Lacking any impetus to engage in a coordinated relationship, people respond to others primarily according to their perceived warmth and competence, the SCCM dimensions.

Relationship Priorities

People usually prefer warm relationships to hostile relationships. Furthermore, competent people are able to make things happen, and are hence attractive relationship partners—people want to connect with them—provided they are not perceived as likely to be hostile. So the greater the competence and the warmth of each potential participant in a prospective relationship, the greater the disposition of other potential participants to form a relationship with them, and then to extend, intensify, and deepen the relationship; that is, warmth and competence predict pull (attraction). The other's competence and warmth relevant to self interact in their positive effects on relationship pull, because the greater someone's competence, the more the person can do for and with you, if so inclined. Conversely, hostility and competence interact in their negative effects on relationship pull: A competent person can do you a lot of harm, if so inclined. So, overall, we predict the following ordinal scale of relationship pull (the motivation to relate intensely):

Competent + Warm > Incompetent + Warm > Incompetent + Hostile > Competent + Hostile

Although warmth enhances all relationships, making them function better, warmth is not equally important in all four RMs; for different relationships, the consequences of warmth differ. Note that we do not equate warmth with CS; any relationship can be warm (friendly, nice, sincere, and trustworthy), and CS relationships need not *necessarily* be warm; people may share a public park or a highway without being warm. Nevertheless, warmth is most crucial to CS relationships, important in AR (both up and down), variably but generally less crucial in EM, and an important basis for trust in MP, but not essential so long as there are external enforcement mechanisms. Conversely, it seems likely that the intrinsic rewards of the RMs vary considerably, so that people find some types of relationships more satisfying than others, and hence warmer. The order of intrinsic reward is also CS > AR > EM > MP.

Likewise, although competence has an impact on all relationships, the consequences of competence differ for different RMs. Competence is crucial to MP and also fairly important in EM. Competence is less important in CS—people love babies and may loyally tend to totally incapacitated sick and elderly partners. In AR, there is an asymmetry: People demand high competence in their superiors but tolerate lesser competence in their subordinates. Indeed, when status is achieved (vs. ascribed), rel-

evant kinds of competence *result* in higher status. The effects on pull can be summarized as follows:

Importance of Warmth: CS > AR > EM > MP

Importance of Competence: MP > EM > CS

Higher AR > Lower AR

But the causal processes operate not only from valence (warmth, competence) and pull (attractiveness) to RM but also in the other direction. SCCM theorizes that people perceive social superiors as competent; in an AR relationship, people perceive those above them as competent and those below them as incapable. In 13 worldwide student and adult samples, the status–competence correlation averages .89 (Cuddy, Fiske, Kwan, et al., in press). Putting SCCM and RMT together leads to the prediction, as yet untested, that status will be most highly correlated with perceptions of competence in just the domains where AR operates in a given culture; that is, people are ranked in some social domains but not others, so they will perceive the greatest competence differences in abilities that operate in those domains compared to abilities related to cultural domains in which AR does not operate.

SCCM also theorizes that people perceive competitors as hostile (correlation averages .25). Competitors are people whose goals or interests are mutually exclusive with self, putting them at odds with each other. Competition divides people, precluding CS relationships. The opposite of competition is having a shared interest in attaining mutually interdependent aims, where each person can only get what he or she seeks if the other person does too. This means that they have important outcomes in common—they have some kind of CS relationship. For this reason, and because of the intrinsically rewarding nature of CS, we posit that CS relationships generate warmth. However, violation of a CS or AR relationship often instantly transforms warmth into extreme hostility. To summarize:

AR → Competence differentiation:
    Higher status → higher perceived competence
        in abilities related to the
        ranked domain,
    Lower status → lower perceived competence
        in abilities related to the
        ranked domain.
CS → Warmth, but
    Violation of CS or AR → Hostility.

What about EM and MP? Do they affect perceptions of competence and warmth? Both can be implemented as frameworks for competitiveness, that is, as the starting point for comparative AR. Indeed, competitiveness may even enhance performance in EM and MP: Games, sports, or election contests and other rivalries are structured by EM, whereas competition among buyers and among sellers makes MP systems efficient. Sometimes this competitiveness develops into hostility, but excessive hostility is not conducive to functional EM or MP. On the contrary, a background presupposition of a sufficient level of warmth, or at least trust based on shared interests in sustaining functional cooperation, facilitates both EM and MP.

MP tends somewhat to enhance perceptions of competence. MP is linked to division of labor and consequent specialization, resulting in specialized competence, such that each party is uniquely competent in its own specialty. EM can work either way. When implemented as the framework of rules that establishes the conditions for a contest, EM often results in an assessment of relative competence that enhances perceptions of the competence of the victorious competitor and diminishes the perceived competence of the loser. When each side attempts to humiliate the other side by outdoing it, even turn-taking can be a contest with this effect. But when implemented as balanced equality in performance, EM tends to result in a leveling sense of evenly matched competence—provided all parties adequately carry out their turns. In short, when acting within an EM framework, failing to match others results in evaluative derogation and attribution of incompetence.

In short, dynamics go from not only valence (warmth, competency) to pull (attraction) and type of relationship but also in the other direction, from RM to valence and pull. Integrating RMT with SCCM produces a theory that we call *relational structure, valence, and pull. Répondez s'il vous plaît* means "please respond," so RSVP is an apt name for a theory that highlights how people respond to each other. RSVP posits that valence (warmth and competence together) strongly affects pull—people's desire to form and intensify relationships. Conversely, relationships structured according to each of the four RMs have distinctive effects on perception of the warmth and competence of relational partners, and the pull to intensify or withdraw from the relationship.

RSVP also goes beyond either SCCM or RMT, because it extends both and connects them, providing a more comprehensive characterization of the aspects of sociality that determine action and affect. RMT has nothing to say about how people cognize or evaluate others before they form a relationship, but SCCM characterizes the fundamental dimensions of cognizing and evaluating others in this presocial state. SCCM has nothing to say about how interpersonal relationships are structured, whereas RMT characterizes the fundamental structures for coordination.

When people relate to each other, there is more to the interaction than can be captured by the quantitative warmth and competence dimensions. But there is also more to a relationship than can be captured by its relational structure alone. RSVP posits that the key attributes that determine the nature of a social relationship are the *relational structure, its valence, and its pull.*

Metatheoretical and Methodological Issues in Cultural Comparisons

For more than two decades, cultural psychologists have relied on a comparative schema based on the constructs of individualism and collectivism or independence and interdependence (A. Fiske et al., 1998). Indeed, this contrast goes back to the foundation of social science in the work of Tönnies (1887/1988) and Durkheim (1893/1933). However, recent work questions these constructs, so we do not use them here. Different measures of each construct neither correlate with each other nor yield the same classification of cultures (A. Fiske, 2002). Although individualism and collectivism were originally theorized to be polar opposites (Hofstede, 2001), measures of the two constructs are generally orthogonal (Oyserman, Coon, & Kemmelmeier, 2002). Measures of individualism do not correlate with the key constructs they were theorized to be functionally tied to, such as self-enhancement (Thomsen et al., 2006). Moreover, both constructs lump all social relationships together, positing that their motivational and cognitive importance covary: Either all relationships are more important than "individual" goals, or all are less important than individual goals. The ethnographic evidence indicates, on the contrary, that social relationships are crucial in all cultures, but that *different* relationships are salient in different cultures—and that elementary relational models are implemented differently according to cultural prototypes. The construct of "individualism" bundles together a disparate set of features that happen to be historically prominent in contemporary Western ideological construals of modern Western society, contrasting them with the supposed "collectivism" of societies whose only common feature is that they are not modern and Western.

Perspectives

Cultural psychology has focused on cognitive differences between cultures, because it arose largely from the realization that cognitive processes previously thought to be universal in fact vary as a function of culture. We need to pay more attention to explaining *why* this variation exists at all—why are human sociality and cognition so diverse? What is it about the human psyche that makes it depend on culture? The uniquely human adaptive advantage consists of linked capacities to learn from others and to flexibly and rapidly adapt social relations to utilize diverse and changing ecological niches. This social learning and relational flexibility result in cultural diversity. Yet we still know little about how this cultural transmission occurs.

To be cultural, psychology has to explain how people become proficient, motivated participants in the particular social networks into which they are born or later enter; that is, cultural psychology must explain how people develop into culturally informed beings and continue to acculturate. In this chapter we have described a wide range of institutionalized relationships, as well as four types of RMs. We have posited that children are intrinsically motivated to form relationships, and that they expect to find the cultural cues for these social relationships in distinct media corresponding to the type of relationship: bodily assimilation for CS; above, in front, earlier, greater, or stronger for AR; concrete operations that are ostensive procedural definitions for EM; and abstract conventional symbols, such as money and utility, for MP. These are the media in which humans are prepared to constitute and communicate social relationships, and in which they cognize them. These are the channels through which cultures transmit their prototypes and

precedents for implementing RMs. Moreover, these are the modes of action that evoke relational motives and invoke normatively binding social commitments.

Children also learn to relate to different kinds of strangers and evaluate ingroup members based on perceived intent (cooperative–competitive) and status, inferring respectively the others' warmth and competence. The pull (attraction) of a relationship depends on warmth–competence combinations and on whether it is a null relationship or a developed RM. Each RM can be implemented in different ways, resulting in distinctive evaluations of relational partners as warm or hostile, capable or incompetent. Social relationships are intrinsically motivated, fulfilling basic relational and other needs; the intensity, form, and orientation of these needs are inevitably shaped by the prevalent social experiences in each culture, but all humans are fundamentally relational animals. Yet every human is necessarily social in a distinctive, culturally informed manner.

NOTES

1. We thank Nancy Levine for her comments and a couple of additions to this list.

2. Cultures, types of relationships, specific relationships, and individuals seem to vary in the degree to which the identity of the particular partner is important to the relationship. Parsons described aspects of this issue in terms of his universalism versus particularism pattern variable (Parsons & Shils, 1951; Parsons & Bales, 1955). Americans regard the identity of their spouses as fundamental to their marriages; on the other hand, one customer can substitute for another pretty easily, or one grocer for another, without much consequence. However, some American MP relationships are very dependent on the particular identities of the partners; there are no good substitutes. Levy (1973) discovered that, compared to people in many cultures, Tahitians were much less concerned about the identity of the children in their home; people often request and grant fostering rights to others. Likewise, although not indifferent, Tahitians are comparatively unconcerned about *who* their lover or spouse is; what is important is to have one, and whereas some are better than others and one gets used to a particular person, it does not have to be anyone in particular. Pham (2006) showed that cultures differ in whether they focus on sustaining existing relationships or forming new ones.

3. These components of pull appear to be analytically distinct, but at this point we think that parsimony is more important than conceptual discrimination, so for now we collapse them into one dimension, pull.

REFERENCES

Abrams, D., Marques, J., Bown, N., & Dougill, M. (2002). Anti-norm and pro-norm deviance in the bank and on the campus: Two experiments on subjective group dynamics. *Group Processes and Intergroup Relations, 5,* 163–182.

Altorki, S. (1980). Milk-kinship in Arab Society: An unexplored problem in the ethnography of marriage. *Ethnology, 19,* 283–244.

Ardner, S. (1964). The comparative study of rotating credit associations. *Journal of the Royal Anthropological Institute, 94,* 201–209.

Augoustinos, M., & Innes, J. M. (1990). Towards an integration of social representations and social schema theory. *British Journal of Social Psychology, 29,* 213–231.

Baumeister, R. F., & Leary, M. R. (1995). The need to belong: Desire for interpersonal attachments as a fundamental human motivation. *Psychological Bulletin, 117,* 497–529.

Baxter, P. T. W., & Almagor, U. (Eds.). (1978). *Age, generation and time: Some features of East African age organizations.* New York: St. Martin's Press.

Beidelman, T. O. (1963). The blood covenant and the concept of blood in Ukaguru. *Africa, 33,* 321–342.

Berkman, L. F., Glass, T., Brissette, I., & Seeman, T. E. (2000). From social integration to health: Durkheim in the new millennium. *Social Science and Medicine, 51,* 843–857.

Berry, D. S. (2000). Attractiveness, attraction, and sexual selection: Evolutionary perspectives on the form and function of physical attractiveness. In M. P. Zanna (Ed.), *Advances in experimental social psychology* (Vol. 32, pp. 273–342). New York: Academic Press.

Boas, F. (1970). *The social organization and the secret societies of the Kwakiutl Indians.* New York, Johnson Reprint Corporation.

Bond, M. H., & Smith, P. B. (1996). Cross-cultural social and organizational psychology. In J. T. Spence, J. M. Darley, & D. J. Foss (Eds.), *Annual review of psychology* (Vol. 47, pp. 205–235). Palo Alto, CA: Annual Reviews.

Brewer, M. B., & Brown, R. J. (1998). Intergroup relations. In D. T. Gilbert, S. T. Fiske, & G. Lindzey (Eds.), *Handbook of social psychology* (4th ed., Vol. 2, pp. 554–594). New York: McGraw-Hill.

Buss, D. M. (1989). Sex differences in human mate preferences: Evolutionary hypothesis tested in 37 cultures. *Behavioral and Brain Sciences, 12,* 1–49.

Buss, D. M., & Barnes, M. (1986). Preferences in human mate selection. *Journal of Personality and Social Psychology, 50,* 559–570.

Bynum, V. E. (1992). *Unruly women: The politics of social and sexual control in the Old South.* Chapel Hill and London: University of North Carolina Press.

Camara, S. (1976). *Gens de la parole: Essai sur la condition et le rôle des griots dans la société Malinké.* Paris: Mouton.

Caporael, L. R. (1997). The evolution of truly social cognition: The core configurations model. *Review of Personality and Social Psychology, 1,* 276–298.

Capriello, P., Cuddy, A. J. C., & Fiske, S. T. (2004). *Social structure beliefs alter stereotypes.* Unpublished manuscript, Princeton University, Princeton, NJ.

Chen, N. Y., Shaffer, D. R., & Wu, C. (1997). On physical attractiveness stereotyping in Taiwan: A revised sociocultural perspective. *Journal of Social Psychology, 137,* 117–124.

Cuddy, A. J. C., Fiske, S. T., & Glick, P. (in press-a). Competence and warmth as universal trait dimensions of interpersonal and intergroup perception: The Stereotype Content Model and the BIAS map. In M. P. Zanna (Ed.), *Advances in experimental social psychology.* New York: Academic Press.

Cuddy, A. J. C., Fiske, S. T., & Glick, P. (in press-b). The BIAS map: Behaviors from intergroup affect and stereotypes. *Journal of Personality and Social Psychology.*

Cuddy, A. J. C., Fiske, S. T., Kwan, V. S. Y., Glick, P., Demoulin, S., Leyens, J.-P., et al. (in press). Is the stereotype content model culture-bound?: A crosscultural comparison reveals systematic similarities and differences. *British Journal of Social Psychology.*

Cunningham, M. R. (1986). Measuring the physical in physical attractiveness: Quasi-experiments on the sociobiology of female facial beauty. *Journal of Personality and Social Psychology, 50,* 925–935.

Cunningham, M. R., Roberts, A. R., Barbee, A. P., Druen, P. B., & Wu, C. (1995). "Their ideas of beauty are, on the whole, the same as ours": Consistency and variability in the crosscultural perception of female physical attractiveness. *Journal of Personality and Social Psychology, 68,* 261–279.

Davidson, J. N. (1998). *Courtesans and fishcakes: The consuming passions of classical Athens.* New York: St. Martins.

Dépret, E. F., & Fiske, S. T. (1999). Perceiving the powerful: Intriguing individuals versus threatening groups. *Journal of Experimental Social Psychology, 35,* 461–480.

Dettwyler, K. A. (1988). More that nutrition: Breast-feeding in urban Mali. *Medical Anthropology Quarterly, 2,* 172–183.

DiChiara, J., & Fiske, S. T. (2004). *Status competition and interpersonal perception.* Unpublished raw data, Princeton University, Princeton, NJ.

Dion, K. K., Pak, A. W., & Dion, K. L. (1990). Stereotyping physical attractiveness: A sociocultural perspective. *Journal of Cross-Cultural Psychology, 21,* 158–179.

Douglas, M. (1966). *Purity and danger: An analysis of concepts of pollution and taboo.* London: Routledge & Kegan Paul.

Durkheim, É. (1933). *The division of labour in society* (G. Simpson, trans.). New York: Free Press. (Original work published 1893)

Durkheim, É. (1915). *The elementary forms of the religious life* (J. W. Swain, trans.). New York: Free Press. (Original work published 1912)

Ember, M., & Ember, C. (1983). *Marriage, family, and*

kinship: Comparative studies of social organization. New Haven, CT: Human Relations Area Files Press.

Endo, Y., Heine, S., & Lehman, D. R. (2000). Culture and positive illusions in close relationships: How my relationships are better than yours. *Personality and Social Psychology Bulletin , 26,* 1571–1586.

Erber, R., & Fiske, S. T. (1984). Outcome dependency and attention to inconsistent information. *Journal of Personality and Social Psychology, 47,* 709–726.

Evans-Pritchard, E. E. (1933). Zande blood-brotherhood. *Africa, 6,* 369–401.

Evans-Pritchard, E. E. (1951). *Kinship and marriage among the Nuer.* Oxford, UK: Clarendon Press.

Feingold, A. (1992). Good-looking people are not what we think. *Psychological Bulletin, 111,* 304–341.

Fiske, A. P. (1991). *Structures of social life: The four elementary forms of human relations.* New York: Free Press.

Fiske, A. P. (2000). Complementarity theory: Why human social capacities evolved to require cultural complements. *Personality and Social Psychology Review, 4,* 74–94.

Fiske, A. P. (2002a). Using individualism and collectivism to compare cultures: A critique of the validity and measurement of the constructs: Comment on Oyserman et al. *Psychological Bulletin, 128,* 78–88.

Fiske, A. P. (2002b). Moral emotions provide the self-control needed to sustain social relationships. *Self and Identity, 1,* 169–175.

Fiske, A. P. (2004a). Four modes of constituting relationships: Consubstantial assimilation; space, magnitude, time, and force; concrete procedures; abstract symbolism. In N. Haslam (Ed.), *Relational models theory: A contemporary overview* (pp. 61–146). Mahwah, NJ: Erlbaum.

Fiske, A. P. (2004b). Relational models theory 2.0. In N. Haslam (Ed.), *Relational models theory: A contemporary overview* (pp. 3–25). Mahwah, NJ: Erlbaum.

Fiske, A. P., & Haslam, N. (1996). Social cognition is thinking about relationships. *Current Directions in Psychological Science, 5,* 143–148.

Fiske, A. P., & Haslam, N. (2005). The four basic social bonds: Structures for coordinating interaction. In M. Baldwin (Ed.), *Interpersonal cognition* (pp. 267–298). New York: Guilford Press.

Fiske, A. P., Kitayama, S., Markus, H. R., & Nisbett, R. E. (1998). The cultural matrix of social psychology. In D. T. Gilbert, S. T. Fiske, & G. Lindzey (Eds.), *Handbook of social psychology* (4th ed., Vol. 2, pp. 915–981). New York: McGraw-Hill.

Fiske, A. P., & Tetlock, P. (1997). Taboo tradeoffs: Reactions to transactions that transgress spheres of exchange. *Political Psychology, 17,* 255–294

Fiske, S. T. (1992). Thinking is for doing: Portraits of social cognition from daguerreotype to laserphoto. *Journal of Personality and Social Psychology, 63,* 877–889.

Fiske, S. T. (1998). Stereotyping, prejudice, and discrimination. In D. T. Gilbert, S. T. Fiske, & G. Lindzey (Eds.), *Handbook of social psychology* (4th ed., Vol. 2, pp. 357–411). New York: McGraw-Hill.

Fiske, S. T. (2002a). Five core social motives, plus or minus five. In S. J. Spencer, S. Fein, M. P. Zanna, & J. Olson (Eds.), *Motivated social perception: The Ontario Symposium* (Vol. 9, pp. 223–246). Mahwah, NJ: Erlbaum.

Fiske, S. T. (2002b). What we know now about bias and intergroup conflict: Problem of the century. *Current Directions in Psychological Science, 11,* 123–128.

Fiske, S. T. (2004). *Social beings: A core motives approach to social psychology.* New York: Wiley.

Fiske, S. T., Cuddy, A. J. C., & Glick, P. (2002). Emotions up and down: Intergroup emotions result from perceived status and competition. In D. M. Mackie & E. R. Smith (Eds.), *From prejudice to intergroup emotions: Differentiated reactions to social groups* (pp. 247–264). Philadelphia: Psychology Press.

Fiske, S. T., Cuddy, A. J. C., & Glick, P. (2007). Universal dimensions of social perception: Warmth and competence. *Trends in Cognitive Science, 11,* 77–83.

Fiske, S. T., Cuddy, A. J., Glick, P., & Xu, J. (2002). A model of (often mixed) stereotype content: Competence and warmth respectively follow from perceived status and competition. *Journal of Personality and Social Psychology, 82,* 878–902.

Fiske, S. T., Lin, M. H., & Neuberg, S. L. (1999). The continuium model: Ten years later. In S. Chaiken & Y. Trope (Eds.), *Dual process theories in social psychology* (pp. 231–254). New York: Guilford Press.

Fiske, S. T., & Neuberg, S. L. (1990). A continuum model of impression formation, from category-based to individuating processes: Influence of information and motivation on attention and interpretation. In M. P. Zanna (Ed.), *Advances in experimental social psychology* (Vol. 23, pp. 1–74). New York: Academic Press.

Fiske, S. T., & Ruscher, J. B. (1993). Negative interdependence and prejudice: Whence the affect? In D. M. Mackie & D. L. Hamilton (Eds.), *Affect, cognition and stereotyping: Interactive processes in group perception* (pp. 239–268). San Diego: Academic Press.

Fiske, S. T., Xu, J., Cuddy, A. C., & Glick, P. (1999). (Dis)respecting versus (dis)liking: Status and interdependence predict ambivalent stereotypes of competence and warmth. *Journal of Social Issues, 55,* 473–491.

Fiske, S. T., & Yamamoto, M. (2005). Coping with rejection: Core social motives, across cultures. In K. D. Williams, J. P. Forgas, & W. von Hippel (Eds.), *The social outcast: Ostracism, social exclusion, rejection, and bullying* (pp. 185–198). New York: Psychology Press.

Fortes, M. (1945). *The dynamics of clanship among the Tallensi: Being the first part of an analysis of the social structure of a Trans-Volta tribe.* Oxford, UK: Oxford University Press.

Fortes, M. (1987). Totem and taboo. In M. Fortes, *Religion, morality and the person: Essays on Tallensi religion* (pp. 110–142). Cambridge, UK: Cambridge University Press. (Original work published 1966)

Fortune, R. (1932). *Omaha secret societies* (Columbia

University Contributions to Anthropology, Vol. 14.). New York: Columbia University Press.

Fox, R. (1967). *Kinship and marriage: An anthropological perspective.* Cambridge, UK: Cambridge University Press.

Frazer, J. G. (1968). *Totemism and exogamy: A treatise on certain early forms of superstition and society.* London: Dawsons of Pall Mall. (Original work published 1910)

Geertz, C. (1962). The rotating credit association: A "middle rung" in development. *Economic Development and Cultural Change, 10,* 241–263.

Goldenweiser, A. A. (1963). Totemism, an analytical study. *Journal of American Folk-lore, 23,* 179–293. (Original work published 1910)

Goodnow, J. J. (2004). The domain of work in households: A relational models approach. In N. Haslam (Ed.), *Relational models theory: A contemporary overview* (pp. 167–196). Mahwah, NJ: Erlbaum.

Gregor, T. A. (1979). Secrets, exclusion, and the dramatization of men's roles. In M. L. Margolis & W. E. Carter, (Eds.), *Brazil, anthropological perspectives: Essays in honor of Charles Wagley* (pp. 250–269). New York: Columbia University Press.

Gurtman, M. B. (1992). Trust, distrust, and interpersonal problems: A circumplex analysis. *Journal of Personality and Social Psychology, 62,* 989–1002.

Hardin, C. D., & Higgins, E. T. (1996). Shared reality: How social verification makes the subjective objective. In R. M. Sorrentino & E. T. Higgins (Eds.), *Handbook of motivation and cognition* (Vol. 3, pp. 28–34). New York: Guilford Press.

Hart, D. V. (1977). *Compadrinazgo: Ritual kinship in the Philippines.* DeKalb: Northern Illinois University Press.

Haslam, N. (2004). Research on the relational models: An overview. In N. Haslam (Ed.), *Relational models theory: A contemporary overview* (pp. 27–57). Mahwah, NJ: Erlbaum.

Heine, S. J., Lehman, D. R., Markus, H. R., & Kitayama, S. (1999). Is there a universal need for positive self-regard? *Psychological Review, 106,* 766–794.

Heine, S. J., & Renshaw, K. (2002). Interjudge agreement, self-enhancement, and liking: Cross-cultural divergences. *Personality and Social Psychology Bulletin, 28,* 578–587.

Ho, D. Y. F. (1998). Interpersonal relationships and relationship dominance: An analysis based on methodological relationism. *Asian Journal of Social Psychology, 1,* 1–16.

Höffer, A. (1979). *The caste hierarchy and the state in Nepal: A study of the Muluki Ain of 1854.* Innsbruck: Universitätsverlag Wagner.

Hofstede, G. H. (2001). *Culture's consequences: Comparing values, behaviors, institutions, and organizations across nations* (2nd ed.). Thousand Oaks, CA: Sage.

Hogg, M. A. (2001). A social identity theory of leadership. *Personality and Social Psychology Review, 5,* 184–200.

Hollis, A. C. (1905). *The Masai: Their language and folklore.* Oxford, UK: Clarendon Press.

House, J. S., Landis, K. R., & Umberson, D. (1988). Social relationships and health. *Science, 241,* 540–545.

Khare, R. S. (1976). *The Hindu hearth and home.* Durham, NC: Carolina Academic Press.

Khatib-Chahidi, J. (1992). Milk kinship in Shi'ite Islamic Iran. In V. Maher (Ed.), *The anthropology of breast feeding: Natural law or social construct* (pp. 109–132). New York: St. Martin's Press.

Kitayama, S., & Markus, H. R. (1999). Yin and yang of the Japanese self: The cultural psychology of personality coherence. In D. Cervone & Y. Shoda (Eds.), *The coherence of personality: Social cognitive bases of personality consistency, variability, and organization* (pp. 242–302). New York: Guilford Press.

Kopytoff, I. (1982). Slavery. *Annual Review of Anthropology, 11,* 207–230.

Kopytoff, I. (1988). The cultural context of African abolition. In S. Miers & R. Roberts, (Eds.), *The end of slavery in Africa* (pp. 115–138). Madison: University of Wisconsin Press.

Kurzban, R., & Leary, M. R. (2001). Evolutionary origins of stigmatization: The functions of social exclusion. *Psychological Bulletin, , 127,* 187–208.

Kwan, V. S. Y., John, O. P., Kenny, D. A., Bond, M. H., & Robins, R. W. (2004). Reconceptualizing individual differences in self-enhancement bias: An interpersonal approach. *Psychological Review, 111,* 94–110.

Labouret, H. (1929). La parenté à plaisanteries en Afrique Occidentale. *Africa, 2,* 244–254.

Leach, J. W., & Leach, E. (Eds.). (1983). *The Kula: New perspectives on Massim exchange.* Cambridge, UK: Cambridge University Press.

Leary, M. R., & Baumeister, R. F. (2000). The nature and function of self-esteem: Sociometer theory. In M. P. Zanna (Ed.), *Advances in experimental social psychology* (Vol. 32, pp. 1–62). New York: Academic Press.

Lévi-Strauss, C. (1969). *The elementary structures of kinship* (Rev. ed., J. H. Bell Trans.; J. R. von Sturmer & R. Needham (Eds.). Boston: Beacon Press. (Original work published 1949)

Levy, R. I. (1973). *Tahitians.* Chicago: University of Chicago Press.

Llewelyn-Davies, M. (1981). Women, warriors, and patriarchs. In S. B. Ortner & H. Whitehead (Eds.), *Sexual meanings: The cultural construction of gender and sexuality* (pp. 330–358). New York: Cambridge University Press.

Lovejoy, P. E. (Ed.). (1981). *The ideology of slavery in Africa.* Beverly Hills, CA: Sage.

Lynch, J. H. (1986). Godparents and kinship in early medieval Europe. Princeton, NJ: Princeton University Press.

Macintyre, M. (1983). *The Kula: A bibliography.* Cambridge, UK: Cambridge University Press.

MacKenzie, D. (1996). *Violent solutions: Revolutions, nationalism, and secret societies in Europe to 1918.* Lanham, MD: University Press of America.

Mak, L.-F. (1981). *The sociology of secret societies: A study of Chinese secret societies in Singapore and peninsular Malaysia*. Kuala Lumpur: Oxford University Press.

Malinowski, B. (1961). *Argonauts of the Western Pacific: An account of native enterprise and adventure in the archipelagoes of Melanesian New Guinea*. New York: Dutton. (Original work published 1922)

Markus, H. R., & Kitayama, S. (1991). Culture and the self: Implications for cognition, emotion, and motivation. *Psychological Review, 98*, 224–253.

Marriott, M. (1976). Hindu transactions: Diversity without dualism. In B. Kapferer (Ed.), *Transaction and meaning: Directions in the anthropology of exchange and symbolic behavior* (pp. 109–142). Philadelphia: Institute for the Study of Human Issues.

McGraw, A. P., & Tetlock, P. E. (2005). Taboo trade-offs, relational framing and the acceptability of exchange. *Journal of Consumer Psychology, 15*, 2–15.

McGraw, A. P., Tetlock, P. E. A., & Kristel, O. V. (2003). The limits of fungibility: Relational schemata and the value of things. *Journal of Consumer Research, 30*, 219–229.

Miller, J. G., & Bersoff, D. M. (1998). The role of liking in perceptions of the moral responsibility to help: A cultural perspective. *Journal of Experimental Social Psychology, 34*, 443–469.

Mintz, S. W., & Wolf, E. R. (1950). An analysis of ritual co-parenthood (*compadrazgo*). *Southwestern Journal of Anthropology, 6*, 341–368.

Morling, B., & Evered, S. (2006). Secondary control reviewed and defined. *Psychological Bulletin, 132*, 269–296.

Morling, B., & Fiske, S. T. (1999). Defining and measuring harmony control. *Journal of Research in Personality, 33*, 379–414.

Morling, B., Kitayama, S., & Miyamoto, Y. (2003). American and Japanese women use different coping strategies during normal pregnancy. *Personality and Social Psychology Bulletin, 29*, 1533–1546.

Murphy, W. P. (1980). Secret knowledge as property and power in Kpelle society: Elders versus youth. *Africa, 50*, 193–207.

Needham, R. (Ed.). (1971). *Rethinking kinship and marriage*. London: Tavistock.

Neuberg, S. L., & Fiske, S. T. (1987). Motivational influences on impression formation: Outcome dependency, accuracy-driven attention, and individuating processes. *Journal of Personality and Social Psychology, 53*, 431–444.

Neuberg, S. L., Smith, D. M., & Asher, T. (2000). Why people stigmatize: Toward a biocultural framework. In T. F. Heatherton, R. E. Kleck, M. R. Hebl, & J. G. Hull (Eds.), *The social psychology of stigma* (pp. 31–61). New York: Guilford Press.

Nutini, H. (1984). *Ritual kinship: Ideological and structural integration of the compadrazgo system in rural Tlaxcala* (Vol. 2). Princeton, NJ: Princeton University Press.

Nutini, H., & Bell, B. (1980). *Ritual kinship: The structure and historical development of the compadrazgo system in rural Tlaxcala* (Vol. 1). Princeton, NJ: Princeton University Press.

Orenstein, H. (1968). Toward a grammar of defilement in Hindu sacred law. In M. Singer & B. S. Cohen (Eds.), *Structure and change in Indian society* (pp. 115–131). New York: Wenner-Gren Foundation.

Osgood, C. E., Suci, G. J., & Tannenbaum, P. H. (1957). *The measurement of meaning*. Urbana: University of Illinois Press.

Oyserman, D., Coon, H. M., & Kemmelmeier, M. (2002). Rethinking individualism and collectivism: Evaluation of theoretical assumptions and meta-analysis. *Psychological Bulletin, 178*, 3–72.

Parsons, T., & Bales, R. F. (1955). *Family, socialization and interaction process*. Glencoe, IL: Free Press.

Parsons, T., & Shils, E. A. (Eds.). (1951). *Toward a general theory of action*. Cambridge, MA: Harvard University Press.

Paulme, D. (1939). Parenté à plaisanteries et alliance par le sang en Afrique Occidentale. *Africa, 12*, 433–444.

Paulme, D. (1968). Pacte de sang, classes d'âge et castes en Afrique noir. *Archives Européenes de Sociologie, 9*, 12–33.

Pham, L. B. (2006). Social relationship practices: An alternative account of cultural differences in mentalities. Manuscript under review.

Piaget, J. (1932). *The language and thought of the child*. 2nd ed. New York: Harcourt, Brace.

Piaget, J. (1952). *The child's conception of number*. New York: Humanities Press. (Original work published 1932)

Piaget, J. (1965). *The moral judgment of the child* (M. Gabain, Trans.). New York: Free Press. (Original work published 1932)

Pittman, T. S. (1998). Motivation. In D. T. Gilbert, S. T. Fiske, & G. Lindzey (Eds.), *Handbook of social psychology* (4th ed., Vol. 1, pp. 549–590). New York: McGraw-Hill.

Powdermaker, H. (1993). *After freedom: A cultural study in the deep south*. Madison: University of Wisconsin Press. (Original work published 1939)

Radcliffe-Brown, A. R. (1965a). On joking relationships. In *Structure and function in primitive society: Essays and addresses* (pp. 90–104). New York: Free Press. (Original work published 1940)

Radcliffe-Brown, A. R. (1965b). A further note on joking relationships. In *Structure and function in primitive society: Essays and addresses* (pp. 105–116). New York: Free Press. (Original work published 1949)

Radcliffe-Brown, A. R., & Forde, D. (Eds.). (1960). *African systems of kinship and marriage* [Published for the International African Institute]. New York: Oxford University Press.

Rai, S. N., & Rathmore, J. (1988). Attraction as a function of cultural similarity and proportion of similar attitudes related to different areas of life. *Psycholingua, 29*, 123–131.

Rothbaum, F., Pott, M., Azuma, H., Miyake, K., & Weisz, J. (2000). The development of close relationships in Japan and the United States: Paths of symbiotic harmony and generative tension. *Child Development, 71*, 1121–1142.

Rothbaum, F., Weisz, J., Pott, M., Miyake, K., & Morelli, G. (2000). Attachment and culture: Security in the United States and Japan. *American Psychologist*, *55*, 1093–1104.

Rubin, V., & Tuden, A. (Eds.). (1977). Comparative perspectives on slavery in New World plantation societies. *Annals of the New York Academy of Sciences*, *292*, whole volume.

Ruscher, J. B., & Fiske, S. T. (1990). Interpersonal competition can cause individuating processes. *Journal of Personality and Social Psychology*, *58*, 832–843.

Shaffer, D. R., Crepaz, N., & Sun, C. R. (2000). Physical attractiveness stereotyping in cross-cultural perspective: Similarities and differences between Americans and Taiwanese. *Journal of Cross-Cultural Psychology*, *31*, 557–582.

Simmel, G. (1971). *On individuality and social forms: Selected writings* [Edited and with an Introduction by D. N. Levine]. Chicago: University of Chicago Press.

Simmel, G. (1990). *The philosophy of money* D. Frisby (Ed.), T. Bottomore & D. Frisby (Trans., 2nd ed.). London: Routledge. (Original work published 1900)

Smith, P. B., & Bond, M. H. (1994). *Social psychology across cultures: Analysis and perspective*. Needham Heights, MA: Allyn & Bacon.

Sondak, H. (1998). Relational models and organizational studies: Applications to resource allocation and group process. In C. L. Cooper & D. M. Rousseau (Eds.), *Trends in organizational behavior* (Vol. 5, pp. 83–102). Chichester, UK: Wiley.

Spencer, P. (1988). *The Maasai of Matapato: A study of rituals of rebellion*. Bloomington: Indiana University Press, in association with the International African Institute.

Stansfield, S. A., Bosma, H., Hemingway, H., & Marmot, M. G. (1998). Psychosocial work characteristics and social support as predictors of SF-36 health functioning: The Whitehall II study. *Psychosomatic Medicine*, *60*, 247–255.

Stevens, L. E., & Fiske, S. T. (1995). Motivation and cognition in social life: A social survival perspective, *Social Cognition*, *13*, 189–214.

Stevens, L. E., & Fiske, S. T. (2000). Motivated impressions of a powerholder: Accuracy under task dependency and misperception under evaluation dependency. *Personality and Social Psychology Bulletin*, *26*, 907–922.

Takahashi, K., Ohara, N., Antonucci, T. C., & Akiyama, H. (2002). Commonalities and differences in close relationships among the Americans and Japanese: A comparison by the individualism/collectivism concept. *International Journal of Behavioral Development*, *26*, 453–465.

Tambiah, S. J. (1969). Animals are good to think and good to prohibit. *Ethnology*, *8*, 423–459.

Tegnaeus, H. (1952). *Blood brothers: An ethnosociological study of the institutions of blood-brotherhood with special reference to Africa*. New York: Philosophical Library.

Thomsen, L., Sidanius, J., & Fiske, A. P. (2006). Interpersonal leveling, independence, and self-enhancement: A comparison between Denmark and the US, and a relational practice framework for cultural psychology. *European Journal of Social Psychology*, *36*, 1–25.

Tönnies, F. (1988). *Community and society [Gemeinschaft und Gesellschaft]* (C. P. Loomis, Trans., with an Introduction by John Samples). New Brunswick, NJ: Transaction. (Original work published 1887)

Tuzin, D. (1984). Miraculous voices: The auditory experience of numinous objects. *Current Anthropology*, *25*, 579–596.

Vélez-Ibañez, C. (1983). *Bonds of mutual trust: The cultural systems of rotating credit associations among urban Mexicans and Chicanos*. New Brunswick, NJ: Rutgers University Press.

Verkuyten, M., & Masson, K. (1996). Culture and gender differences in the perception of friendship by adolescents. *International Journal of Psychology*, *31*, 207–217.

Vodosek, M. (2003). *Finding the right chemistry: Relational models and relationship, process, and task conflict in culturally diverse research groups*. Unpublished doctoral dissertation, University of Michigan, Ann Arbor.

Whalen, P. J. (1998). Fear, vigilance, and ambiguity: Initial neuroimaging studies of the human amygdala. *Current Directions in Psychological Science*, *7*, 177–188.

Wheeler, L., & Kim, Y. (1997). What is beautiful is culturally good: The physical attractiveness stereotype has different content in collectivistic cultures. *Personality and Social Psychology Bulletin*, *23*, 795–800.

Wiggins, J. S., & Trapnell, P. D. (1997). Personality structure: The return of the Big Five. In R. Hogan, J. Johnson, & S. Briggs (Eds.), *Handbook of personality psychology* (pp. 737–765). New York: Academic Press.

Wyatt-Brown, B. (1982). *Southern honor: Ethics and behavior in the Old South*. New York: Oxford University Press.

Yalman, N. (1963). On the purity of women in the castes of Ceylon and Malabar. *Journal of the Royal Anthropological Institute*, *93*, 25–58.

Yamagishi, T. (1998). *The structure of trust: An evolutionary game of mind and society*. Tokyo: Tokyo University Press.

Yamagishi, T. (2002). The structure of trust: An evolutionary game of mind and society. *Hokkaido Behavioral Science Report*, No. SP-13.

Yamagishi, T., & Yamagishi, M. (1994). Trust and commitment in the United States and Japan. *Motivation and Emotion*, *18*, 129–166.

Yamamoto, M., Miyamoto, S., Fiske, S. T., Miki, H., Okiebisu, et al. (2004). *Comparative data on friendship*. Unpublished raw data, University of Tsukuba, Japan.

CHAPTER 12

Culture and Social Identity

MARILYNN B. BREWER
MASAKI YUKI

The concept of "social identity" has been invoked throughout the human sciences whenever there is need for a conceptual bridge between individual and group levels of analysis. Social identity provides a link between the psychology of the individual—the representation of self—and the structure and process of social groups within which the self is embedded. As a consequence, the social identity concept has been invented and reinvented in a wide variety of theoretical frameworks, and across all the social and behavioral science disciplines (Brewer, 2001; Stryker, 1987; Thoits & Virshup, 1997).

The ubiquity of social identity theory and research throughout the social sciences reflects some universal features of human society that derive from the profoundly social nature of human beings as a species. Group living is part of human evolutionary history, inherited from our primate ancestors but evolved to a level of interdependence beyond that of any other social primate (Brewer & Caporael, 2006; Caporael, 1997). With coordinated group living as the primary survival strategy of the species, the social group in effect provided a buffer between the individual organism and the exigencies of the physical environment. Given the morphology and ecology of evolving hominids, the in-

terface between hominids and their habitat must have been a group process. Finding food, defending against predation, moving across a landscape—these matters of coping with the physical habitat—are largely group processes. Over time, if exploiting a habitat is more successful as a collective group process than as an individual process, then not only would more successful groups persist, but so also would individuals who were better adapted to group living. Thus, we would expect that the basic elements of human psychology—cognition, motivation, and emotion—would be attuned to the structural requirements of social groups and social coordination.

The capacity for social identification—considering the self as a part of a larger social unit—is one feature of human psychology that serves to regulate and maintain the essential relationship between individuals and their social groups. In all societies, individuals view themselves as part of defined social groupings (*ingroups*) characterized by mutual cooperation and reciprocal obligation (Levine & Campbell, 1972; Sumner, 1906). Although the capacity for social identity is postulated to be universal, the locus and content of social identities are clearly culturally defined and regulated. Thus, social identity provides a rich area for study of the interface between individual psychology and systems of cultural practices and meaning.

The study of cultural differences in social identification is most often couched in terms of the distinction between *individualism* and *collectivism* as one basic dimension of cultural norms and values (Hofstede, 1980; Triandis, 1989; 1995). As it is most generally understood, individualistic cultures are characterized by an emphasis on autonomy and differentiation of the individual self from others, whereas collectivist societies are characterized by social embeddeness and interdependence (Oyserman, Coon, & Kemmelmeier, 2002). In terms of self-definition, individualists are assumed to focus primarily on the distinction between self and others (me vs. not me) and collectivists on the distinction between ingroup (us) and outgroup (them), with little differentiation of the individual self within the ingroup. As a consequence, collectivists are expected to show high levels of ingroup–outgroup discrimination in their social behavior, whereas individualists are expected to be more universalistic and nondiscriminatory. In terms of goals and values, individualists give priority to personal goals over the goals of collectives, whereas collectivists either make no distinction between personal and collective goals, or if they do, they subordinate their personal goals to collective goals (Triandis, 1989). With regard to ingroup identity, the central theme of individualism is the conception of individuals as autonomous beings who are separate from groups; the central theme of collectivism is the conception of individuals as aspects of groups or collectives (Triandis, Chan, Bhawuk, Iwao, & Sinha, 1995).

Given the universal requirements of group living and social interdependence, we believe that this bipolar characterization of culture anchored by individualism at one end of a dimension and collectivism on the other is too simplistic. And, indeed, the representation of individualistic societies described earlier is inconsistent with decades of research on social identity and ingroup bias that has been conducted almost exclusively in highly individualistic Western societies (cf. Brewer, 1979; Tajfel & Turner, 1979; Abrams & Hogg, 2001). Furthermore, a recent comprehensive review of cross-national studies of individualism and collectivism (Oyserman et al., 2002) indicates that Americans (who generally score high on measures of individualism) are found to be no less collectivistic than East Asians (particularly Japanese and Korean) on several components of collectivist values and attitudes.

We do not doubt that societies differ in terms of degree of individualism, specifically, the extent to which a culture emphasizes independence and autonomy over interdependence and harmony (Markus & Kitayama, 1991; Oyserman et al., 2002; Schimmack, Oishi, & Diener, 2005). What we challenge is the notion that individualism precludes social identification with social groups and collectives. In our view, a more complete understanding of cultural differences in social identity will start from the recognition that *all* societies must meet primary needs for both individual and social identity, and provide for an effective interface between individual self-interest and collective interests and welfare. What differs across cultures is *how* social identification processes are represented and channeled to regulate social cooperation and achieve a balance between expression of individuality and social conformity (Brewer & Roccas, 2001). We present a thesis that complements previous work on individualism and collectivism by showing how societies that are traditionally classified as collectivistic differ from more individualistic societies in the nature and structure of social identities. In this chapter we hope to elucidate the role of culture in shaping (1) the meaning of ingroups, (2) the relationship between group identity and trust, and (3) the nature of ingroup–outgroup biases.

SOCIAL IDENTITY THEORY: BASES OF INGROUP IDENTIFICATION

Within social psychology, the most elaborated theory of social identity and ingroup bias is social identity theory (SIT), as developed by Tajfel and Turner (1979), and the related self-categorization theory (SCT), developed by Turner and colleagues in subsequent years (Turner, Hogg, Oakes, Reicher, & Wetherell, 1987). Thus, we begin our review with a synopsis of SIT and related research, then show how the introduction of a cultural perspective leads to qualification and modification of the theory.

Social identity is defined as "that part of an individual's self-concept which derives from his knowledge of his membership of a social group ... together with the value and emotional significance attached to that membership" (Tajfel, 1981, p. 255). SCT extended this definition to include the idea that social identities are *depersonalized* representations of the self, entailing "a shift towards the perception of self as an interchangeable exemplar of some social category and away from the perception of self as a unique person" (Turner et al., 1987, p. 50). SIT, as articulated by Tajfel (1978) and Turner (1975, 1985), represents the convergence of two traditions in the study of intergroup attitudes and behavior—social categorization (as represented in the work by Doise [1978], Tajfel [1969], and Wilder [1986]) and social comparison (as exemplified by Lemaine [1974] and Vanneman and Pettigrew [1972]). The theoretical perspective rests on two basic premises:

1. Individuals organize their understanding of the social world on the basis of categorical distinctions that transform continuous variables into discrete classes; categorization has the effect of minimizing perceived differences *within* categories and accentuating intercategory differences.
2. Because individual persons are themselves members of some social categories and not others, social categorization carries with it implicit *ingroup–outgroup* (we–they) distinctions; because of the self-relevance of social categories, the ingroup–outgroup classification is a superimposed category distinction with affective and emotional significance.

These two premises provide a framework for conceptualizing any social situation in which a particular ingroup–outgroup categorization is made salient. In effect, the theory posits a basic *intergroup schema* with the following characteristic features: (1) assimilation within category boundaries and contrast between categories such that all members of the ingroup are perceived to be more similar to the self than members of the outgroup (the *intergroup accentuation* principle); (2) positive affect (trust, liking) selectively generalized to fellow ingroup members but not to outgroup members (the *ingroup favoritism* principle); and (3) intergroup social comparison associated with perceived negative interdependence between ingroup and outgroup (the *social competition* principle).

SIT in conjunction with SCT provides a single comprehensive theory of group behavior and the cognitive processes that underlie a range of intergroup and group phenomena. The basic tenet of these theories is that group behaviors derive from cognitive representations of the self in terms of a shared social category membership, in which there is effectively no psychological separation between the self and the group as a whole. This phenomenon is referred to as *depersonalization of self-representation*, whereby the cognitive representation of the self shifts from *personal self* to *collective self* (Hogg & Abrams, 1988; Hogg & Turner 1987).

SIT articulates how cognitive representations of self and a relevant ingroup correspond when ingroup identification (social identity) is psychologically salient. When individuals categorize the self and view themselves as indistinguishable from the ingroup, they also view other ingroup members as interchangeable with one another. The representation of the ingroup is embodied in a "prototype," defined by features shared by group members. Such prototypical features capture ingroup similarities and intergroup differences that distinguish the ingroup from comparison outgroups. Perceptions of the self and other ingroup members are then assimilated to this ingroup prototype. When a shared social identity is salient, ingroup members are perceived as similar to one another, and the ingroup as a whole is perceived to be a homogeneous unit (Doosje, Ellemers, & Spears 1995; Haslam, Oakes, Turner, & McGarty, 1996; Simon & Hamilton, 1994). The affective and behavioral consequences of social identity lead to intergroup situations characterized by preferential treatment of ingroup members, mutual distrust between ingroup and outgroup, and intergroup competition.

Culture and Meaning of Social Identity

Parallel to individualism and collectivism, SIT/SCT postulate a continuum anchored by personal (individuated) identity at one end and social (collective) identity at the other. The shift between personal and social identities is presumed to lie in universal cognitive processes associated with social categorization and category salience. Against this view of a single continuum, Brewer and Gardner (1996) postulated that there are three different levels of the "social self"—the *individual, relational,* and *collective*—as distinct self-representations with different structural properties, bases of self-evaluation, and motivational concerns (see also

Kashima & Hardie, 2000; Gabriel & Gardner, 1999; Sedikides & Brewer, 2001). The individual self is the representation of self as a unique person, differentiated from other individuals. The relational self is the self defined in terms of connections and role relationships with significant others (Aron, Aron, Tudor, & Nelson, 1991; Cross & Madson, 1997; Gilligan, 1982; Markus & Kitayama, 1991). The collective self is the social identity of SCT, defined in terms of prototypical properties shared among members of a common ingroup (Turner et al., 1987).

The relational and collective levels of self postulated by Brewer and Gardner (1996) represent two different forms of social identification (i.e., processes by which the individual self is extended to include others as integral to the self-concept). The critical distinction between these is that relational selves are *personalized*, incorporating dyadic relationships between the self and specific close others, and the extension of these relationships in the form of networks of interpersonal connections. By contrast, collective selves involve *depersonalized* connections with others by virtue of common membership in a symbolic group. Collective identities do not require interpersonal knowledge or coordination, but rely on shared symbols and cognitive representations of the group as a unit independent of personal relationships within the group.

Drawing on this distinction between relational and collective social selves, Yuki (2003) suggested that the predominant characteristics of group cognition and behavior may differ across certain cultural contexts. According to this framework, processes consistent with SIT and SCT are most applicable to intergroup situations involving people from Western cultures. The typical characteristics of group cognition and behavior for East Asians, however, may be qualitatively different from those of Westerners. Whereas people in Western cultures tend to emphasize the categorical distinctions between ingroups and outgroups, East

Asians may have a stronger tendency to think about groups as predominantly *relationship-based*. In group contexts, East Asians tend to perceive themselves as a "node" embedded within a network of shared relationship connections (i.e., family members, friends, colleagues, acquaintances, friends of friends, etc.) rather than within strict, bounded groups per se. Within this framework, the ingroup for East Asians is cognitively represented as a relatively stable and structured network of relationships among group members.

Whereas SIT implicates intergroup comparison as a key source of ingroup identification and cooperation, Yuki's framework proposes that East Asian collectivism is based largely on the promotion of cooperative behaviors and maintenance of relational harmony *within* ingroups. It is important to note that this framework does not suggest that East Asians ignore the ingroup as a meaningful social unit, and research indeed suggests that they do impose boundaries between ingroups and outgroups (Gudykunst, 1988; Smith & Bond, 1999). However, East Asians tend not to depict their ingroups as depersonalized entities (as conceptualized in SIT), but as complex networks of interrelated individual members (Chang, Lee, & Koh, 1996; Hamaguchi, 1977; Ho, 1993; Hwang, 1999; King & Bond, 1985; Kim & Lee, 1994; Lebra, 1976; Munro, 1985). This type of group representation is consistent with research demonstrating that there are different bases for group entitativity and group attraction, with some groups emphasizing their categorical, depersonalized nature, and others emphasizing the structured relational networks and interpersonal bonds among members (Hamilton, Sherman, & Lickel, 1998; Prentice, Miller, & Lightdale, 1994; Seeley, Gardner, Pennington, & Gabriel, 2003).

A summary representation of the postulated differences between relational and collective bases of social identity is provided in the Table 12.1.

TABLE 12.1. Comparing Relational and Collective Social Identity

	Relational	Collective
Self-concept	Individuated/connected directly or indirectly with others	Depersonalized/defined in terms of prototypicality
Motivation	Reciprocity	Intergroup status/competition
Group representation	Interpersonal network	Depersonalized entity

Rather than thinking about groups as categories of depersonalized members, East Asians are especially concerned about maintaining a high level of knowledge about the complex relational structure within the ingroup. According to Yuki (2003), East Asian group members chronically perceive themselves to be personalized from and connected with other members, and they are aware of the exact location of the self within the group represented as a network. Furthermore, some theorists have suggested that it is this relational knowledge that allows East Asians to strategically promote self-interests within the complex relational structure in a group (Yamagishi, Jin, & Miller, 1998). Relational knowledge determines the expected behavior of individuals within the group and serves to maintain mutually beneficial relationships among group members (Aoki, 2001; Hwang, 1999; Nakane, 1970).

Experimental findings from a study by Yamagishi and Kosugi (1999) provide indirect evidence for this view. These researchers found that their Japanese participants who had high external locus of control and low generalized trust (characteristics typical in collectivistic societies) were in fact better at judging good and bad relationships among classmates than were participants who were high in internal locus of control and generalized trust.

Overall, then, the conceptualization of ingroups and group behavior in East Asia tends to place less emphasis on categorization, intergroup comparison, and depersonalization of the self, and places more emphasis on maintaining harmony within groups, being sensitive to the needs and feelings of others, and being aware of the relationship structure within the group (Yuki, 2003). In a collectivist society, where awareness of interdependence and status relationships is high, relational ties are the key to social identification with ingroups.

Two Bases of Social Identity

Although Yuki's (2003) theory was developed specifically in the context of comparisons between Western cultures (particularly Western Europe and the United Sates) and East Asian cultures (particularly Japan), we believe that the distinction between relationship-based and category-based social identities provides a useful framework for viewing cultural effects on social identity processes more broadly. In fact, many East Asian cultures other than Japan appear to emphasize relationship-based social identity, although specific forms do vary from culture to culture. Pye (2000) argues that Chinese social identities are based on particularistic relationships that radiate out from immediate family to extended kin to shared identities based on hometown or university attendance, whereas Japanese social bonds are more subjective and based on personal relationships of indebtedness and obligation (p. 126). Relationship-based social identity is also prevalent in Africa. For instance, Adams and Dzokoto (2003) suggest that social identity in West Africa is best characterized as "relational individualism," in that individuals make case-by-case decisions as to whether to trust others by taking into account the relational connections to them (Shaw, 2000). This ethos is very different from the depersonalized collective self of SIT. Many Africanists, in fact, have argued that larger, more depersonalized collective identities, such as ethnicity and nationality, are the product of social constructions that emerged only after European colonization (e.g., Nagel, 1994; Yeros, 1999).

Across all societies, individuals maintain close personal relationships, small-group interpersonal networks, and membership in large, symbolic groups (Brewer & Caporael, 2006; Caporael, 1997). But cultural systems rely more or less heavily on these different forms of social connection as the primary locus for defining the social self and exercising social control over individual behavior. It is primarily Western European and North American individualistic cultures that rely heavily on abstract, categorical group memberships in constructing social identities. Other cultures appear to rely more on relational networks to do so. Two theoretical perspectives can be brought to bear to help account for this broad cross-cultural variation of the basis of social identity.

According to Berry's (1979) ecological model of culture, cultural differences in social relationships emerge in part from socio-ecological factors such as geography, social structure, and mobility. Drawing on this model, Oishi (2005) has argued that social mobility plays an especially important role in determining salient aspects of self and ingroups. In a low-mobility society, group membership is generally ascribed and predetermined. People cannot escape from the group even if they find that their own attitudes, goals, and so on, are not fully compatible with those of fellow group members. What they have to do is to maintain good relationships with others, by recognizing and accommodating individual differences in attitudes, goals, and so on, within the group. Thus, relationships rather than similarity or homogeneity define group boundaries.

By contrast, in a society where individuals move frequently, group memberships do not last as long as in a society where individuals live in the same community for a long period of time. To the extent that social aspects of the self (e.g., relationships, roles, group membership) change more frequently in a highly mobile society than they do in a nonmobile society, collective selves should be less consistent across time in the former society than in the latter. Instead, groups are formed around similarities and common interests, with symbols to demarcate group membership and coordinated action. Given the association between mobility and individualism (Triandis, 1995), this ecological model provides an explanation for why individualism is associated with depersonalized, symbolic collective identities, whereas less mobile, collectivistic societies are characterized by stable, relationship-based social identities.

A second, related, explanation for the observation that individualism is associated with category-based social identity comes from Brewer and Roccas (2001), who contend that the nature of collective selves is shaped and constrained by the relative importance placed on values of independence (individual autonomy) versus interdependence in relations between the self and others in a society. With emphasis on obligation, mutual interdependence, and responsibility to ingroup others in societies with relational collectivistic values, social identification with groups is a high-investment commitment. This means that the benefits of group inclusion are high, in that groups provide security and guaranteed mutual aid. Yet it also implies that the costs of inclusion are also high in terms of obligations and duties to fellow group members that demand time and resources. When intragroup obligations are strong and underwritten by group norms and sanctions, the benefits of group inclusion can best be met within relatively small, stable, and exclusive social units. Accordingly, in collectivist cultures, relationship-based ingroups are optimal.

Individualistic value orientations, with a strong emphasis on individual autonomy and social mobility, have very different implications for the demands and level of investment associated with group memberships. At first glance, it may appear that individualistic values are incompatible with the very notion of collective social selves. To the contrary, we believe that individualism has very direct effects on the need for inclusion in larger social units, such that individual autonomy and collective identity with large, depersonalized groups are quite compatible. Because individualism gives greater weight to personal interests and preferences in resolving potentially conflicting demands of individual achievement and the welfare of others, obligations to groups and fellow group members are neither absolute nor highly reliable. Thus, the potential benefits of ingroup inclusion are diffused and probabilistic, and individuals need to be part of larger and more inclusive social units to reap the benefits of security and mutual aid associated with group membership. In effect, the attachment to large, depersonalized groups, such as nation, ethnicity, and religion, is a function of the loss of the tightly interdependent community associated with social mobility and individualism.

Cultural values and practices that embody implicit rules of social exchange, expectations of mutual obligation, and sources of social approval all shape where individuals invest their self-definition, affective attachments, and, most important, social identities. These cultural effects on which social identities matter in turn determine the role that social identification plays in interpersonal and intergroup behavior.

Bases of Ingroup Identity: Some Empirical Findings

The distinction between relationship-based and category-based social identities helps to make sense of some otherwise anomalous findings in the literature on the relationship between individualism–collectivism and self-concept. The simple assumption has been that the self-concepts of persons in individualistic cultures consist primarily of idiocentric traits and attributes, whereas members of collectivist cultures incorporate more social references, including allocentric, relational constructs and group memberships, in their salient self-representations (Triandis, 1989). But comparative research on the spontaneous self-concept of respondents in different cultures has not consistently supported this simple relationship between culture and content of representations of the self. Some studies comparing self-descriptions of participants from individualistic and collectivist societies (including Kenya, Malaysia, India, Japan, China, and Korea), and individualistic societies (U.S., Britain, and Australia) have found support for the contention that collectivists generate a larger proportion of social identity references (Bochner, 1994; Dhawan, Rosemen, Naidu, Thapa, & Rettek, 1995; Kashima et al., 1995; Ma & Schoeneman, 1997; Ross, Xun, & Wilson, 2002; Trafimow, Triandis, & Goto, 1991; Triandis, McCusker, & Hui, 1990). On the other hand, some studies have found that U.S. respondents used an equal, or sometimes even greater, proportion of social descriptors in their spontaneous self-concepts than respondents from Japan, China, or Korea (Bond & Cheung, 1983; Cousins, 1989; Ip & Bond, 1995; Rhee, Uleman, Lee, & Roman, 1995).

The picture becomes a bit clearer when one looks more closely at different types of social identity responses in these studies. In general, participants from collectivist cultures generate more references to social relationships and role identities in their spontaneous self-descriptions, but respondents in individualistic cultures generate an equal or greater number of references to social group or social category memberships. Furthermore, in their meta-analysis of cross-cultural comparisons of individualism and collectivism, Oyserman et al. (2002) found that Americans score high on collectivism when measures include items tapping a "sense of group belonging" as an aspect of collectivist orientation.

In a particularly comprehensive cross-cultural test using sentence completion responses to the Twenty Statements Test (TST; Kuhn & McPartland, 1954) as a measure of salient self-concept, Watkins et al. (1998) obtained responses from a large number of university students from four different individualistic cultures (Australia, Canada, New Zealand, and whites in South Africa) and five collectivist cultures (China, Ethiopia, Philippines, Turkey, and blacks in South Africa). Self-descriptions were classified as idiocentric (e.g., personal qualities, traits, attitudes), allocentric (relational constructs: sociable, good friend, etc.), small-group memberships (e.g., family relationships), and large group memberships ("I am a student," "I am Chinese," etc.). The re-

sults indicated a great deal of variability across the nine cultures in the percentage of responses of each type. Overall, however, members of individualistic cultures and of collectivist cultures generated approximately the same proportion (65–70%) of idiocentric self-descriptions. What differed was not the total proportion of social self-descriptions but rather the *type* of social reference that appeared most frequently. On average, respondents from countries classified as collectivistic generated more responses categorized as *allocentric* or *small-group* memberships, whereas respondents from individualistic countries generated more references to *large-group* memberships.

In an experimental study, Brewer and Gardner (1996) found that the frequency of relational terms or references to large-group memberships in TST self-descriptions could be influenced by a priming manipulation that induced participants to think about either small-group relations or large collectives. When the meaning of *we* was contextualized to refer to interpersonal relationships, responses to the Who Am I? test included a larger proportion of relationship identities (e.g., "I am a daughter," "I am a good friend") compared to a control condition in which no *we* priming was given. On the other hand, when the *we* prime was presented in the context of a large collective group, responses to the TST included a larger proportion of category memberships (e.g., "I am an American," "I am a woman"). These experimental findings confirm that relational and collective responses to the TST are sensitive to the activation of different types of social identities.

Overall, then, findings from a variety of studies regarding the presence of social identifiers in spontaneous self-concept are consistent with the idea that cultures do not differ in *whether* social identities are important aspects of the self-concept but in *what type* of social identity is more salient.

In a more direct test of cultural differences in the meaning of ingroup social identities, Yuki (2003) conducted a comparative study between Japan and the United States on predictors of the strength of ingroup identity and loyalty. He asked both American and Japanese university students to report how they perceived two kinds of ingroups of different sizes—their nation and a small social group to which they belonged (e.g., club or activity group). One set of measures involved perceived relational connections with the groups, such as knowledge about individual differences and relationships among group members, and the sense of interconnectedness between the self and other group members. Another set of measures pertained to features of the ingroup as a social category, such as perceived intragroup homogeneity and status relative to outgroups. Yuki found that for Japanese students, ingroup identification and loyalty were determined solely by the relational factors, with no significant correlation with the categorical factors. In contrast, among American students, identity and loyalty were associated significantly with both the relational and the categorical factors. This pattern of findings is consistent with our model of cultural difference in the meaning and cognitive representation of social ingroups.

SOCIAL IDENTITY AND SOURCES OF SELF-WORTH

Understanding the bases on which individuals in different cultures define ingroups and social identities takes on added significance when one considers the relationship between social identity and psychological functioning. Cultural values and practices influence which social units have the most impact on members' self-representations and what qualities contribute most to positive psychological well-being (Deaux, 1993). One line of research on social identity effects investigates the extent to which individuals derive their sense of self-worth and well-being from their social group memberships or social relationships. In cultures where depersonalized, symbolic, or categorical group identities are most prominent, collective self-enhancement may be an important source of self-worth. In cultures where ingroups are defined primarily as relational networks, well-being and self-esteem may be more closely associated with enhancement of the quality of relationships and relationship partners. This hypothesis helps us integrate some divergent sets of findings from the cross-cultural literature.

In the United States, the self-enhancing function of group identity has been studied primarily in relation to the concept of "collective self-esteem" (Luhtanen & Crocker, 1992), which refers to individuals' evaluations of their social identities and the role of their group memberships in contributing to their personal self-worth. Measurement of collective self-esteem

has identified four related but distinct components (subscales)—*identity importance* (how important group memberships are to the individuals' self-concept), *member esteem* (individuals' assessment of their value as group members), *private esteem* (individuals' personal evaluation of their membership groups), and *public esteem* (individuals' assessment of how others evaluate their membership groups). In initial studies of the collective self-esteem scale, each of these components was found to correlate to some degree with personal self-esteem (Luhtanen & Crocker, 1992). However, consistent with Yuki's (2003) findings regarding the importance of intergroup comparison and status on ingroup identity and loyalty among white college students in the United States, public collective self-esteem is a significant contributor to personal self-esteem (Crocker, Luhtanen, Blaine, & Broadnax, 1994; Luhtanen & Crocker, 1992). Even among low-status minority groups, strength of ethnic identification and collective self-esteem is positively related to measures of self-worth and well-being (Branch, Tayal, & Triplett, 2000; Crocker et al., 1994; Verkuyten & Lay, 1998), suggesting that group identification serves to buffer self-worth from the effects of social discrimination (Branscombe, Schmitt, & Harvey, 1999).

By contrast, evidence suggests that for East Asians, collective ingroup enhancement is not a significant basis of personal self-esteem (Heine, 2003). This seems particularly true when the target ingroup is a large categorical collective, such as national or university identities. Hewstone and Ward (1985), for instance, obtained evidence of group-effacing attributional biases among Chinese in reference to their ethnic group. Bond and Hewstone (1988) found that British high school students in Hong Kong had more positive images of the ingroup than did Chinese students. Similarly, Rose's (1985) cross-national study found that Americans had more positive views of their country than did Japanese, and Heine and Lehman (1997) found that Japanese students' ratings of their own universities were worse than ratings by students from rival universities. Finally, Snibbe, Kitayama, Markus, and Suzuki (2003) found significantly less ingroup favoritism among Japanese football fans compared with their American counterparts. In contrast to American students, who clearly showed intergroup bias, their Japanese counterparts, although equally identified with their university and the sports team, did not show any evidence of intergroup bias.

Importantly, although East Asians rarely enhance their collective self-esteem, they do exhibit significant relationship-enhancing bias, as indicated by the difference between evaluations of their own relationships and of "average" relationships (Endo, Heine, & Lehman, 2000; see also Sedikides, Gaertner, & Toguchi, 2003). Even the absence of self-enhancement and the emphasis on self-critical attitudes have been interpreted as being designed to maintain good relationships with others (Heine & Lehman, 1997; Kitayama, Markus, Matsumoto, & Norasakkunkit, 1997). The motivational significance of relationship enhancement for Asians is further suggested by the finding that relationship harmony is more strongly associated with subjective well-being in Hong Kong than in the United States (Kwan, Bond, & Singelis, 1997; Kurman & Sriram, 1997).

CONSEQUENCES OF SOCIAL IDENTITY FOR INTRAGROUP AND INTERGROUP PROCESSES

Considering social identity from a cultural perspective has implications for understanding group-level phenomena, as well as individual self-concepts. Our general point is that different bases for social identity have different implications for how social identity regulates intragroup and intergroup processes and outcomes (see Hong, Wan, No, & Chiu, Chapter 13, this volume). By considering how culture shapes the meaning of ingroups, we can shed some light on apparent anomalies in the cross-cultural literature on trust and intergroup behavior.

Intragroup Processes: Trust and Cooperation

In the social science literature, there has been a recent resurgence of interest in trust as a central psychological construct (Buchan, Croson, & Dawes, 2002; Foddy, Platow, & Yamagishi, 2003; Kramer, 1999; Yamagishi, Foddy, Makimura, Matsuda, & Platow, 2003). For our purposes, "trust" is defined as an expectation of beneficent treatment from others in uncertain or risky situations (Foddy et al., 2003). In general, the concept of trust reflects a belief that others will act in a way that will benefit (or not harm) oneself, *before* one knows the outcome of other's behaviors (Dasgupta, 1988).

Trust is typically called for in situations where another person has the potential to gain at one's expense but can choose *not* to do so (Yamagishi & Yamagishi, 1994).

Of particular interest is the role of trust in contexts and institutions where participants must decide whether to rely on others without personal knowledge about them or history of an interpersonal relationship (Cook, 2001; Foddy et al., 2003; Kramer, 1999; Ostrom, 1998; Tyler, 2001; Yamagishi et al., 2003; Yamagishi & Yamagishi, 1994). Although it is generally difficult to establish trust in a person whom one does not know personally, such impersonal trust is essential for the creation and maintenance of many forms of economic exchange, organizations, and social and political institutions.

Macy and Skvoretz (1998) state that the "earliest trust rule is based on social distance—trust neighbors, but not outsiders" (p. 651). Individuals may trust others if they know (or believe) that they and others are directly or indirectly connected through mutual friendships or acquaintances (Coleman, 1990). A shared network of interpersonal relationships provides a mechanism for extending *personalized* trust to unknown others who are part of the social network. On the other hand, shared category membership (a common ingroup) may be a basis for *depersonalized* trust (Brewer, 1981; Buchan et al., 2002; Macy & Skvoretz, 1998; Yamagishi & Kiyonari, 2000). As a consequence of shifting psychologically from the personal to the collective level of identity, one may be less likely to distinguish the interests of other ingroup members from those of oneself, leading to increasing trust toward fellow ingroup members whether personally known or not. Research on the consequences of social identity has demonstrated that mere shared ingroup membership is sufficient to engender trust and cooperation. When a shared social categorization has been made salient, individuals are more likely to trust that an allocator will share resources fairly (Foddy et al., 2003), to cooperate to conserve group resources (e.g., Brewer & Kramer, 1986; DeCremer & van Vugt, 1999), and to contribute to a public good without knowing whether others are also contributing their share (Wit & Kerr, 2002).

But recent research shows that this tendency to trust ingroup members is qualified by cultural differences. Interestingly, evidence indicates that this ingroup bias in trust is actually larger for those who have an individualistic cultural orientation or people from individualistic cultures, rather than for collectivists and people from collectivistic cultures. Buchan et al. (2002), for instance, tested individuals' willingness to trust others in an investment game involving an indirect exchange situation. They found that participants with an individualistic cultural orientation increased their levels of trust in unknown others (in terms of amount of monetary investment) when an arbitrary category boundary was introduced to provide exchange participants with a common social group identity. Participants with a collectivist orientation, however, did not alter their level of trust, whether a category identity had been made salient or not. Using a similar procedure in a subsequent study, Buchan, Croson, and Johnson (2003) found that U.S. participants showed a clear ingroup bias in trust, whereas Chinese participants did not show such a tendency at all. Likewise, Yamagishi et al. (2003) found that sharing group membership (e.g., same country, same university) was sufficient to generate higher trust in ingroup members for Australians, but not for Japanese.

These counterintuitive findings regarding the relationship between collectivist cultural values and intragroup trust can be explained (at least in part) by recognizing the difference between relationship-based and category-based ingroups. As we have been arguing, East Asians' group behaviors are predominantly intragroup- and relationship-based. Groups are constructed so that members can monitor each other's behavior, and high visibility of individual members may serve as a mechanism for inhibiting potential freeriding (Miller & Kanazawa, 2000; Yamagishi et al., 1998). In fact, Yamagishi's cross-cultural experiments showed that Japanese became less cooperative and less trusting toward the ingroup when there was no system of ingroup monitoring and sanctioning, whereas Americans did not change their level of cooperation and trust as a function of the presence or absence of a monitoring and sanctioning system (Yamagishi, 1988a, 1988b). In contrast to a mechanism of cooperation based on depersonalized shared group membership, relationship-based trust and cooperation are dependent on interpersonal connections and reciprocal obligations (Yamagishi et al., 1998).

This evidence of cultural differences led Yuki, Maddux, Brewer, and Takemura (2005) to speculate that differences in the meaning of ingroups (and corresponding social identities) are associated with different bases of ingroup trust and cooperation across cultures. More specifically, they hypothesized that Americans' group behavior is based on the categorical distinctions between ingroups and outgroups, and depersonalized trust is based on knowledge that self and other share membership in a bounded social category. By contrast, if Japanese group behavior is driven more by the importance of relationship networks, trust should be highest toward individuals who are presumed to share a direct or indirect network of relationships with the self, regardless of category boundaries. Shared ingroup membership may provide one basis for inferring relational connections to an unknown other, but potential network ties across category boundaries should be equally likely to elicit trust. In other words, it was predicted that if an unknown outgroup member shares an indirect interpersonal connection with the self (through a personal acquaintance), this cross-group relationship link should generate trust for an outgroup member in Japan but not in the United States.

Results from two experiments supported the hypothesis that the bases of ingroup trust differ across cultures. Across both studies, Americans tended to trust strangers based on the categorical differentiation between those who share the same group memberships and those who do not, and having an acquaintance in the outgroup had no effect on levels of trust. This pattern demonstrates that trust is depersonalized for Americans, consistent with the social identity model in which group behavior and cognition are based primarily on categorical differentiation between ingroup and outgroups. In contrast, trust for Japanese participants depended more on the likelihood that targets shared direct or indirect relationship links. In particular, the presence of a potential cross-group relationship had a strong effect on outgroup trust for Japanese. The results from our Japanese samples are congruent with the hypothesis that Japanese group behavior and cognition are relationship-based (Yuki, 2003), with Japanese trusting those who most likely shared direct and indirect interpersonal relationships, as exemplified by the high levels of trust toward both ingroup members and outgroup members with potential relationship connections. Overall, then, these experiments on trust support our general theoretical framework that representations of ingroups and bases of social identity differ across cultural context.

Intergroup Processes:
Ingroup–Outgroup Discrimination

In addition to intragroup behavior, the cultural basis of ingroup identity has important implications for *intergroup* relations. Ingroup–outgroup discrimination refers to differences in behavior directed toward members of ingroups in comparison to outgroup members, particularly behaviors that benefit ingroup members and/or disadvantage outgroupers. The question here is whether ingroups based on relational interdependence and ingroups based on symbolic categories have similar effects on attitudes and behavior toward outgroup members.

In the literature on individualism–collectivism, the claim has been made that members of collectivist cultures make sharper distinctions between ingroup behavior and outgroup behavior than do members of individualistic cultures (Triandis, 1995). As Iyengar, Lepper, and Ross (1999) put it, "As the self-other boundary becomes less distinct, the distinction between ingroup members and outgroups members assumes greater significance. . . . Assimilating ingroup members to self may lead individuals to contrast ingroup and outgroup members more sharply, making them relatively more susceptible to different cognitive, perceptual, and motivational biases" (p. 279).

A number of comparative studies have supported this idea that collectivist values are associated with greater ingroup–outgroup differentiation. For example, Leung (1988) found that in responses to conflict scenarios between two disputants, Hong Kong Chinese college students were less likely to pursue a conflict with an ingroup disputant (close friends) and more likely to pursue a conflict with an outgroup disputant (strangers) than were American students. Similarly, studies on distributive justice have shown that people from collectivist cultures apply different reward allocation norms to ingroup and outgroup. Leung and Bond (1984), for instance, found that Chinese participants shared the rewards more equally with the friends, but with an outgroup stranger they adhered to the equity norm more closely than did the Americans. Likewise, Mahler, Greenberg, and Hayashi (1981) asked students in Japan and in the United States how rewards should be divided in a set of stories describing two workers. American participants tended to favor an equity allocation based on relative contribution of the two workers, regardless of whether the workers were friends. Japanese participants, on the other hand, favored an equality allocation when the two workers were described as strongly connected, though their allocation preferences were the same as Americans when the story implied that the two workers were not strongly connected.

In contrast to these findings that indicate that East Asians discriminate between ingroup and outgroup situations more than Americans do, the implications from research by Yuki (2003), cited previously, indicate that intergroup comparisons between social categories are more important to Americans than to Japanese. In the European and American literature on social identity, the role of category salience in ingroup–outgroup discrimination has been well documented in experimental research using the minimal intergroup paradigm (Tajfel, 1970; Tajfel, Billig, Bundy, & Flament, 1971; Brewer, 1979; Turner, 1981; Diehl, 1990).

"Minimal groups" are depersonalized social categories based on arbitrary category distinctions between ingroup and outgroup. Indeed, there is evidence to suggest that ingroup bias based on such categorical distinctions may in fact be more pronounced in Western than in Asian cultures. Wetherell (1982) conducted a study to test cross-cultural robustness of ingroup favoritism in minimal groups in New Zealand. She found that children with a Polynesian background showed weaker ingroup bias than did those with European background, and they instead attempted to benefit both ingroup and outgroup members. In the previously cited study by Buchan et al. (2003), half of the participants played the role of "responders," who were asked to decide whether they should return a portion of the money received (with trust) from the "senders," who were either in the (minimal) ingroup or outgroup. The results showed that American participants exhibited significant ingroup bias, returning a greater amount of money to the ingroup than to outgroup senders, whereas Chinese showed the opposite tendency. Furthermore, this cultural difference was mediated by cultural orientation of individualism–collectivism (i.e., the effect of culture disappeared when individual difference in individualism–collectivism was statistically controlled), with individualists showing more ingroup bias than collectivists within both countries. Other evidence suggests that East Asians do not readily engage in outgroup discrimination in minimal group settings when discrimination does not indirectly benefit the self (Yamagishi, Jin, & Kiyonari, 1999).

The apparent contradiction in conclusions drawn in the literature about the relative ingroup–outgroup discrimination of collectivistic and individualistic societies can be resolved when one looks more closely at how ingroups are defined in different studies and what types of intergroup discrimination are being assessed. In the typical minimal group studies, ingroups are defined as genuinely categorical, in the sense that they are determined based on arbitrary bases, such as by lottery, dot estimation tendency (overestimator vs. underestimator), and artistic preference, and, more importantly, there is no substantial interdependence among members. However, as discussed earlier, ingroups for collectivists are more relationship-based networks, where interdependence within ingroup is of crucial importance. In contrast to the positive intergroup distinctiveness principle governing intergroup behaviors, as depicted by SIT, East Asian intergroup behaviors can be characterized as strategies that maximize one's own personal interest by maintaining mutually beneficial relationships with fellow ingroup members (Hamaguchi, 1977; Yamagishi et al., 1998).

In East Asian cultures, the obligation to cooperate is applicable primarily in interaction with friends rather than with strangers. In a recent experiment on the effects of cultural cues on social behavior, subsequent to being primed with Chinese (vs. American or culture-neutral) symbols, Chinese American biculturals were more cooperative when they played the prisoner's dilemma game with their friends. However, culture priming did not affect these biculturals' cooperative or competitive choices when they played the game with strangers (Wong & Hong, 2005).

Congruent with this reasoning, a series of studies by Yamagishi and colleagues (Jin, Yamagishi, & Kiyonari, 1996; Karp, Jin, Yamagishi, & Shinotsuka, 1993) showed that Japanese engage in ingroup favoritism in a minimal group situation when an apparent cue of intragroup interdependence is provided. In a condition where participants were each told that he or she was the only person within the ingroup who was given the reward allocation task, they did not show ingroup favoritism. They did, however, favor the ingroup when it was emphasized clearly that everyone in the experiment was performing the reward allocation task, which supposedly made them think about interdependence (and reciprocity) within their group. These findings are consistent with Benedict's (1946) suggestion that the source of Japanese ingroup loyalty is the maintenance of strictly reciprocal relationships with fellow ingroup members. In contrast, participants in minimal group experiments in North America and Australia show significant ingroup discrimination even when reciprocal interdependence within groups has been eliminated (e.g., Perreault & Bourhis, 1998; Platow, McClintock, & Liebrand, 1990), suggesting that ingroup favoritism in these cultures is based on desire to benefit the ingroup as a whole rather than on expectation of reciprocal favors.

SUMMARY AND CONCLUSIONS

Our thesis throughout this chapter has been based on the idea that all cultures rely on social identification and ingroup loyalty, trust, and cooperation as an essential mechanism of social coordination and social control. The nature of social identities, however, is embedded in cultural values and practices, with the consequence that ingroup boundaries and ingroup–outgroup distinctions may be culture-specific. Although the nature of these differences in defining ingroups and social identity may vary along a number of dimensions, we have emphasized one important distinction, namely, the difference between social identities based on networks of interpersonal relationships and social identities based on shared membership in depersonalized collectives. We have reviewed research showing that this distinction is consistent with findings from cross-cultural comparisons of bases of self-esteem, intragroup trust, and intergroup discrimination. A great deal of the empirical research conducted in this area involves comparison between individualistic cultures, represented by the United States, Europe, and Australia, and collectivistic cultures, represented by East Asia. We are convinced, however, that this distinction can be used more broadly in future research on the role of culture in shaping and defining social identity and its consequences for individual, group, and intergroup processes.

REFERENCES

Abrams, D., & Hogg, M. A. (2001). Collective identity: Group membership and self-conception. In M. Hogg & R. Tindale (Eds.), *Blackwell handbook of social psychology: Group processes* (pp. 425–460). Oxford, UK: Blackwell.

Adams, G., & Dzokoto, V. A. (2003). Self and identity in African studies. *Self and Identity*, 2, 345–359.

Aoki, M. (2001). *Toward a comparative institutional analysis*. Cambridge, MA: MIT Press.

Aron, A., Aron, E. N., Tudor, M., & Nelson, G. (1991). Close relationships as including other in the self. *Journal of Personality and Social Psychology*, 60, 241–253.

Benedict, R. (1946). *The chrysanthemum and the sword: Patterns of Japanese culture*. Boston: Houghton Mifflin.

Berry, J. W. (1979). A cultural ecology of social behavior. *Advances in Experimental Social Psychology*, 12, 177–206.

Bochner, S. (1994). Cross-cultural differences in the self concept: A test of Hofstede's individualism/collectivism distinction. *Journal of Cross-Cultural Psychology*, 25, 273–283.

Bond, M. H., & Cheung, T. (1983). College students' spontaneous self-concept: The effect of culture among respondents in Hong Kong, Japan, and the United States. *Journal of Cross-Cultural Psychology*, 13, 186–200.

Bond, M. H., & Hewstone, M. (1988). Social identity theory and the perception of intergroup relations in Hong Kong. *International Journal of Intercultural Relations*, 12, 153–170.

Branch, C. W., Tayal, P., & Triplett, C. (2000). The relationship of ethnic identity and ego identity status among adolescents and young adults. *International Journal of Intercultural Relations*, 24, 777–790.

Branscombe, N. R., Schmitt, M. T., & Harvey, R. D. (1999). Perceiving pervasive discrimination among African Americans: Implications for group identification and well-being. *Journal of Personality and Social Psychology*, 77, 135–149.

Brewer, M. B. (1979). Ingroup bias in the minimal intergroup situation: A cognitive–motivational analysis. *Psychological Bulletin*, 86, 307–324.

Brewer, M. B. (1981). Ethnocentrism and its role in interpersonal trust. In M. Brewer & B. Collins (Eds.), *Scientific inquiry and the social sciences* (pp. 345–360). San Francisco: Jossey-Bass.

Brewer, M. B. (2001). The many faces of social identity: Implications for political psychology. *Political Psychology*, 22, 115–125.

Brewer, M. B., & Caporael, L. R. (2006). An evolutionary perspective on social identity: Revisiting groups. In M. Schaller, J. Simpson, & D. Kenrick (Eds.), *Evolution and social psychology* (pp. 143–161). Philadelphia: Psychology Press.

Brewer, M. B., & Gardner, W. (1996). Who is this "we"?: Levels of collective identity and self representation. *Journal of Personality and Social Psychology*, 71, 83–93.

Brewer, M. B., & Kramer, R. D. (1986). Choice behavior in social dilemmas: Effects of social identity, group size, and decision framing. *Journal of Personality and Social Psychology*, 50, 543–549.

Brewer, M. B., & Roccas, S. (2001). Individual values, social identity, and optimal distinctiveness. In C.

Sedikides & M. Brewer (Eds.), *Individual self, relational self, collective self* (pp. 219–237). Philadelphia: Psychology Press.

Buchan, N. R., Croson, R., & Dawes, R. M. (2002). Swift neighbors and persistent strangers: A cross-cultural investigation of trust and reciprocity in social exchange. *American Journal of Sociology*, 108, 168–206.

Buchan, N. R., Croson, R., & Johnson, E. J. (2003). *Let's get personal: An international examination of the influence of communication, culture, and social distance on trust and trustworthiness* (Working paper). University of Wisconsin, Madison.

Caporael, L. R. (1997). The evolution of truly social cognition: The core configurations model. *Personality and Social Psychology Review*, 1, 276–298.

Chang, W. C., Lee, L., & Koh, S. (1996, June). *The concept of self in a modern Chinese context*. Paper presented at the 50th Anniversary Conference of the Korean Psychological Association, Seoul, Korea.

Coleman, J. S. (1990). *Foundations of social theory*. Cambridge, MA: Harvard University Press.

Cook, K. S. (Ed.). (2001). *Trust in society*. New York: Russell Sage Foundation.

Cousins, S. D. (1989). Culture and self-perception in Japan and the United States. *Journal of Personality and Social Psychology*, 56, 124–131.

Crocker, J., Luhtanen, R., Blaine, B., & Broadnax, S. (1994). Collective self-esteem and psychological well-being among White, Black, and Asian college students. *Personality and Social Psychology Bulletin*, 20, 503–513.

Cross, S. E., & Madson, L. (1997). Models of the self: Self-construals and gender. *Psychological Bulletin*, 122, 5–37.

Dasgupta, P. S. (1988). Trust as commodity. In D. Gambetta (Ed.), *Trust: Making and breaking cooperative relations* (pp. 49–72). Oxford, UK: Blackwell.

Deaux, K. (1993). Reconstructing social identity. *Personality and Social Psychology Bulletin*, 19, 4–12.

DeCremer, D., & van Vugt, M. (1999). Social identification effects in social dilemmas: A transformation of motives. *European Journal of Social Psychology*, 29, 871–893.

Dhawan, N., Rosemen, I., Naidu, R., Thapa, K., & Rettek, S. (1995). Self-concepts across two cultures: India and the United States. *Journal of Cross-Cultural Psychology*, 26, 606–621.

Diehl, M. (1990). The minimal group paradigm: Theoretical explanations and empirical findings. In W. Stroebe & M. Hewstone (Eds.), *European review of social psychology* (Vol. 1, pp. 263–292). Chichester, UK: Wiley.

Doise, W. (1978). Groups *and individuals: Explanations in social psychology*. Cambridge, UK: Cambridge University Press.

Doosje, B., Ellemers, N., & Spears, R. (1995). Perceived intragroup variability as a function of group status and identification. *Journal of Experimental Social Psychology*, 31, 410–436.

Endo, Y., Heine, S. J., & Lehman, D. R. (2000). Culture

and positive illusions in close relationships: How my relationships are better than your relationships. *Personality and Social Psychology Bulletin, 26*, 1571–1586.

Foddy, M., Platow, M., & Yamagishi, T. (2003). *Group-based trust in strangers: Evaluations or expectations?* Unpublished manuscript, La Trobe University, Melbourne, Australia.

Gabriel, S., & Gardner, W. L. (1999). Are there "his"and "hers" types of interdependence?: The implications of gender differences in collective versus relational interdependence for affect, behavior, and cognition. *Journal of Personality and Social Psychology, 77*, 642–655.

Gilligan, C. (1982). *In a different voice: Psychological theory and women's development.* Cambridge, MA: Harvard University Press.

Gudykunst, W. B. (1988). Culture and intergroup processes. In M.H. Bond (Ed.), *The cross-cultural challenge to social psychology* (pp. 165–181). Thousand Oaks, CA: Sage.

Hamaguchi, E. (1977). *"Nihon rashisa" no saihakken* [The rediscovery of "Japaneseness"]. Tokyo: Nihon Keizai Shinbunsha.

Hamilton, D. L., Sherman, S. J., & Lickel, B. (1998). Perceiving social groups: The importance of the entitativity continuum. In C. Sedikides, J. Schopler, & C. A. Insko (Eds.), *Intergroup cognition and intergroup behavior* (pp. 47–74). Mahwah, NJ: Erlbaum.

Haslam, S. A., Oakes, P. J., Turner, J. C., & McGarty, C. (1996). Social identity, self-categorization, and the perceived homogeneity of ingroups and outgroups: The interaction between social motivation and cognition. In R. M. Sorrentino & E. T. Higgins (Eds.), *Handbook of motivation and cognition: Vol. 3. The interpersonal context* (pp. 182–222). New York: Guilford Press.

Heine, S. J. (2003). An exchange between Heine and Brown & Kobayashi regarding Brown & Kobayashi (2002): Self-enhancement in Japan?: A reply to Brown & Kobayashi. *Asian Journal of Social Psychology, 6*, 75–84.

Heine, S. J., & Lehman, D. R. (1997). The cultural construction of self-enhancement: An examination of group-serving biases. *Journal of Personality and Social Psychology, 72*, 1268–1283.

Hewstone, M., & Ward, C. (1985). Ethnocentrism and causal attribution in Southeast Asia. *Journal of Personality and Social Psychology, 48*, 614–623

Ho, D. F. Y. (1993). Relational orientation in Asian social psychology. In U. Kim & J. W. Berry (Ed.), *Indigenous psychologies: Research and experience in cultural context* (pp. 240–259). Newbury Park, CA: Sage.

Hofstede, G. (1980). *Culture's consequences: International differences in work-related values,* Beverly Hills, CA: Sage.

Hogg, M. A., & Abrams, D. (1988). *Social identifications: A social psychology of intergroup relations and group processes.* London: Routledge.

Hogg, M. A., & Turner, J. C. (1987). Intergroup behaviour, self-stereotyping, and the salience of social cate-

gories. *British Journal of Social Psychology, 26*, 325–340.

Hwang, K. K. (1999). Filial piety and loyalty: Two types of social identification in Confucianism. *Asian Journal of Social Psychology, 2*, 163–183.

Ip, G. W. M., & Bond, M. H. (1995). Culture, values, and the spontaneous self-concept. *Asian Journal of Psychology, 1*, 29–35.

Iyengar, S. S., Lepper, M. R., & Ross, L. (1999). Independence from whom? Interdependence with whom?: Cultural perspectives on ingroups versus outgroups. In D. Prentice & D. Miller (Eds.), *Cultural divides: Understanding and overcoming group conflict* (pp. 273–301). New York: Russell Sage Foundation.

Jin, N., Yamagishi, T., & Kiyonari, T. (1996). Bilateral dependency and the minimal group paradigm. *Japanese Journal of Psychology, 67*, 77–85. (in Japanese)

Karp, D. R., Jin, N., Yamagishi, T., & Shinotsuka, H. (1993). Raising the minimum in the minimal group paradigm. *Japanese Journal of Experimental Social Psychology, 32*, 231–240.

Kashima, E., & Hardie, E. A. (2000). The development and validation of the Relational, Individual, and Collective Self-Aspects (RIC) Scale. *Asian Journal of Social Psychology, 3*, 19–48.

Kashima, Y., Yamaguchi, S., Kim, U., Choi, S., Gelfand, M., & Yuki, M. (1995). Culture, gender, and self: A perspective from individualism-collectivism research. *Journal of Personality and Social Psychology, 69*, 925–937.

Kim, U., & Lee, S.H. (1994, June). *The Confucian model of morality, justice, selfhood and society: Implications for modern society.* Paper presented at the Eighth International Conference on Korean Studies, Seoul.

King, A. Y. C., & Bond, M. H. (1985). The Confucian paradigm of man: A sociological view. In W. T. Tseng & D. Wu (Eds.), *Chinese culture and mental health* (pp. 29–46). New York: Academic Press.

Kitayama, S., Markus, H. R., Matsumoto, H., & Norasakkunkit, V. (1997.) Individual and collective processes in the construction of the self: Self enhancement in the United States and self-criticism in Japan. *Journal of Personality and Social Psychology, 72*, 1245–1267.

Kramer, R. M. (1999). Trust and distrust in organizations: Emerging perspectives, enduring questions. *Annual Review of Psychology, 50*, 569–598.

Kuhn, M. H., & McPartland, T. S. (1954). An empirical investigation of self-attitudes. *American Sociological Review, 19*, 68–76.

Kurman, J., & Sriram, N. (1997). Self-enhancement, generality of self-evaluation, and affectivity in Israel and Singapore. *Journal of Cross-Cultural Psychology, 28*, 421–441.

Kwan, V., Bond, M. H., & Singelis, R. M. (1997). Pancultural explanations for life satisfaction: Adding relationship harmony to self-esteem. *Journal of Personality and Social Psychology, 73*, 1038–1051.

Lebra, T. S. (1976). *Japanese patterns of behavior.* Honolulu: University of Hawaii Press.

Lemaine, G. (1974). Social differentiation and social originality. *European Journal of Social Psychology*, 4, 17–52.

Leung, K. (1988). Some determinants of conflict avoidance. *Journal of Cross-Cultural Psychology*, 19, 125–136.

Leung, K., & Bond, M. H. (1984). The impact of cultural collectivism on reward allocation. *Journal of Personality and Social Psychology*, 47, 793–804.

Levine, R. A., & Campbell, D. T. (1972). *Ethnocentrism: Theories of conflict, ethnic attitudes and group behavior*. New York: Wiley.

Luhtanen, R., & Crocker, J. (1992). A collective self-esteem scale: Self-evaluations of one's social identity. *Personality and Social Psychology Bulletin*, 18, 302–318.

Ma, V., & Schoeneman, T. (1997). Individualism versus collectivism: A comparison of Kenyan and American self-concepts. *Basic and Applied Social Psychology*, 19, 261–273.

Macy, M. W., & Skvoretz, J. (1998). The evolution of trust and cooperation between strangers: A computational model. *American Sociological Review*, 63, 638–660.

Mahler, I., Greenberg, L., & Hayashi, H. (1981). A comparative study of rules of justice: Japanese versus American. *Psychologia*, 24, 1–8.

Markus, H. R., & Kitayama, S. (1991). Culture and the self: Implications for cognition, emotion, and motivation. *Psychological Review*, 98, 224–253.

Miller, A. S., & Kanazawa, S. (2000). *Order by accident: The origin and consequences of conformity in contemporary Japan*. Boulder, CO: Westview.

Munro, D. J. (1985). Introduction. In D. J. Munro (Ed.), *Individualism and holism: Studies in Confucian and Taoist value* (pp. 1–34). Ann Arbor: University of Michigan Press.

Nagel, J. (1994). Constructing ethnicity: Creating and recreating ethnic identity and culture. *Social Problems*, 41, 152–176.

Nakane, C. (1970). *Japanese society*. Berkeley: University of California Press.

Oishi, S. (2005). *The flexible inclusion and exclusion of others in self-concept*. Unpublished manuscript, University of Virginia, Charlottesville.

Ostrom, E. (1998). A behavioral approach to the rational choice theory of collective action. *American Political Science Review*, 92, 1–22.

Oyserman, D., Coon, H. M., & Kemmelmeier, M. (2002). Rethinking individualism and collectivism: Evaluation of theoretical assumptions and meta-analyses. *Psychological Bulletin*, 128, 3–72.

Perreault, S., & Bourhis, R. Y. (1998). Social identification, interdependence and discrimination. *Group Processes and Intergroup Relations*, 1, 49–66.

Platow, M., McClintock, C., & Liebrand, W. (1990). Predicting intergroup fairness and ingroup bias in the minimal group paradigm. *European Journal of Social Psychology*, 20, 221–240.

Prentice, D., Miller, D., & Lightdale, J. (1994). Asymmetries in attachments to groups and to their members: Distinguishing between common-identity and common-bond groups. *Personality and Social Psychology Bulletin*, 20, 484–493.

Pye, L. (2000). Traumatized political cultures: The after effects of totalitarianism in China and Russia. *Japanese Journal of Political Science*, 1, 113–128.

Rhee, E., Uleman, J., Lee, H. K., & Roman, R. J. (1995). Spontaneous self-descriptions and ethnic identities in individualistic and collectivistic cultures. *Journal of Personality and Social Psychology*, 69, 142–152.

Rose, R. (1985). National pride in cross-national perspective. *International Social Science Journal*, 103, 85–96.

Ross, M., Xun, W. Q. E., & Wilson, A. E. (2002). Language and the bicultural self. *Personality and Social Psychology Bulletin*, 28, 1040–1050.

Schimmack, U., Oishi, S., & Diener, E. (2005). Individualism: A valid and important dimension of cultural differences between nations. *Personality and Social Psychology Review*, 9, 17–31.

Sedikides, C., & Brewer, M. B. (Eds.). (2001). *Individual self, relational self, collective self*. Philadelphia: Psychology Press.

Sedikides, C., Gaertner, L., & Toguchi, Y. (2003). Pancultural self-enhancement. *Journal of Personality and Social Psychology*, 84, 60–79.

Seeley, E., Gardner, W., Pennington, G., & Gabriel, S. (2003). Circle of friends or members of a group? Sex differences in relational and collective attachment to groups. *Group Processes and Intergroup Relations*, 6, 251–263.

Shaw, R. (2000). "Tok af, lef af": A political economy of Temne techniques of secrecy and self. In I. Karp & D. Masolo (Eds.), *African philosophy as cultural inquiry* (pp. 25–49). Bloomington: Indiana University Press.

Simon, B., & Hamilton, D. L. (1994). Self-stereotyping and social context: The effects of relative in-group size and in-group status. *Journal of Personality and Social Psychology*, 66, 699–711.

Smith, P. B., & Bond, M. H. (1999). *Social psychology across cultures* (2nd ed.). Boston, MA: Allyn & Bacon.

Snibbe, A. C., Kitayama S., Markus H. R., & Suzuki T. (2003). They saw a game: A Japanese and American (football) field study. *Journal of Cross-Cultural Psychology*, 34, 581–595.

Stryker, S. (1987). Identity theory: Developments and extensions. In K. Yardley & T. Honess (Eds.), *Self and identity* (pp. 89–104). New York: Wiley.

Sumner, W. G. (1906). *Folkways*. New York: Ginn.

Tajfel, H. (1969). Cognitive aspects of prejudice. *Journal of Social Issues*, 25, 79–97.

Tajfel, H. (1970). Experiments in intergroup discrimination. *Scientific American*, 223(2), 96–102.

Tajfel, H. (1978). Social categorization, social identity and social comparison. In H. Tajfel (Ed.), *Differentiation between social groups* (pp. 61–76). London: Academic Press.

Tajfel, H. (1981). *Human groups and social categories*. Cambridge, UK: Cambridge University Press.

Tajfel, H., Billig, M., Bundy, R., & Flament, C. (1971). Social categorization and intergroup behaviour. *European Journal of Social Psychology*, *1*, 149–178.

Tajfel, H., & Turner. J. C. (1979). An integrative theory of intergroup conflict. In W. Austin & S. Worchel (Eds.), *Social psychology of intergroup relations* (pp. 33–47). Chicago: Nelson.

Thoits, P. A., & Virshup, L. V. (1997). Me's and we's: Forms and functions of social identities. In R. Ashmore & Lee Jussim (Eds.), *Self and identity: Fundamental issues* (Vol. 1, pp. 106–133). New York: Oxford University Press.

Trafimow, D., Triandis, H. C., & Goto, S. G. (1991). Some tests of the distinction between the private self and the collective self. *Journal of Personality and Social Psychology*, *60*, 649–655.

Triandis, H. C. (1989). The self and social behavior in differing cultural contexts. *Psychological Review*, *96*, 506–520.

Triandis, H. C. (1995). *Individualism and collectivism*, Boulder, CO: Westview.

Triandis, H. C., Chan D., Bhawuk, D., Iwao, S., & Sinha, J. (1995). Multimethod probes of allocentrism and idiocentrism. *International Journal of Psychology*, *30*, 461–480.

Triandis, H. C., McCusker, C., & Hui, C. H. (1990). Multimethod probes of individualism and collectivism. *Journal of Personality and Social Psychology*, *59*, 1006–1020.

Turner, J. C. (1975). Social comparison and social identity: Some prospects for intergroup behaviour. *European Journal of Social Psychology*, *5*, 5–34.

Turner, J. C. (1981). The experimental social psychology of intergroup behaviour. In J. Turner & H. Giles (Eds.), *Intergroup behaviour* (pp. 66–101). Oxford, UK: Blackwell.

Turner, J. C. (1985). Social categorization and the self-concept: A social cognitive theory of group behavior. In E. Lawler (Ed.), *Advances in group processes* (Vol. 2, pp. 77–122). Greenwich, CT: JAI Press.

Turner, J. C., Hogg, M., Oakes, P., Reicher, S., & Wetherell, M. (1987). *Rediscovering the social group: A self-categorization theory*. Oxford, UK: Blackwell.

Tyler, T. R. (2001). Why do people rely on others?: Social identity and the social aspects of trust. In K. S. Cook (Ed.), *Trust in society* (pp. 285–306). New York: Russell Sage Foundation.

Vanneman, R. D., & Pettigrew, T. F. (1972). Race and relative deprivation in the urban United States. *Race*, *13*, 461–486.

Verkuyten, M., & Lay, C. (1998). Ethnic minority identity and psychological well-being: The mediating role of collective self-esteem. *Journal of Applied Social Psychology*, *28*, 1969–1986.

Watkins, D., Adair, J., Akande, A., Gerong, A., McInerney, D., Sunar, D., et al. (1998). Individualism–collectivism, gender and the self-concept: A nine culture investigation. *Psychologia*, *41*, 259–271.

Wetherell, M. (1982). Cross-cultural studies of minimal groups: Implications for the social identity theory of intergroup relations. In H. Tajfel (Ed.), *Social identity and intergroup relations* (pp. 207–240). Cambridge, UK: Cambridge University Press.

Wilder, D. A. (1986). Social categorization: Implications for creation and reduction of intergoup bias. In L. Berkowitz (Ed.), *Advances in experimental social psychology* (Vol. 19, pp. 291–355). New York: Academic Press.

Wit, A. P., & Kerr, N. L. (2002). Me versus just us versus us all: Categorization and cooperation in nested social dilemmas. *Journal of Personality and Social Psychology*, *83*, 616–637.

Wong, R. Y., & Hong, Y (2005). Dynamic influences of culture on cooperation in the Prisoner's Dilemma. *Psychological Science*, *16*, 429–434.

Yamagishi, T. (1988a). Exit from the group as an individualistic solution to the free rider problem in the United States and Japan. *Journal of Experimental Social Psychology*, *24*, 530–542.

Yamagishi, T. (1988b). The provision of a sanctioning system in the United States and Japan. *Social Psychology Quarterly*, *51*, 265–271.

Yamagishi, T., Foddy, M., Makimura, Y., Matsuda, M., & Platow, M. (2003). *Contextualized and decontextualized use of social categories: Comparisons of Australians and Japanese on group-based trust and cooperation* (Working Paper Series No. 7). Sapporo, Japan: Hokkaido University, Department of Behavioral Science.

Yamagishi, T., Jin, N., & Kiyonari, T. (1999). Bounded generalized reciprocity: Ingroup boasting and ingroup favoritism. *Advances in Group Processes*, *16*, 161–197.

Yamagishi, T., Jin, N., & Miller, A. S. (1998). Collectivism and in-group bias. *Asian Journal of Social Psychology*, *1*, 315–328.

Yamagishi, T., & Kiyonari, T. (2000). The group as the container of generalized reciprocity. *Social Psychology Quarterly*, *63*, 116–132.

Yamagishi, T., & Kosugi, M. (1999). Character detection in social exchange. *Cognitive Studies*, *6*, 179–190. (in Japanese)

Yamagishi, T., & Yamagishi, M. (1994). Trust and commitment in the United States and Japan. *Motivation and Emotion*, *18*, 129–166.

Yeros, P. (Ed.). (1999). *Ethnicity and nationalism in Africa: Constructivist reflections and contemporary politics*. London: Macmillan.

Yuki, M. (2003). Intergroup comparison versus intragroup cooperation: A cross-cultural examination of social identity theory in North American and East Asian cultural contexts. *Social Psychology Quarterly*, *66*, 166–183.

Yuki, M., Maddux, W. W., Brewer, M. B., & Takemura, K. (2005). Cross-cultural differences in relationship- and group-based trust. *Personality and Social Psychology Bulletin*, *31*, 48–62.

CHAPTER 13

Multicultural Identities

YING-YI HONG
CHING WAN
SUN NO
CHI-YUE CHIU

The new millennium has started off in the direction of increased global connectivity and intercultural migration. According to the United Nations' 2002 report, at least 185 million people worldwide currently reside outside the country of their birth, and the number of immigrants has more than doubled since 1975, excluding tourism or other kinds of short-term entries. In general, developed countries received more migrants from undeveloped countries than the other way round. As a result, one of every 10 persons living in the more developed regions is a migrant. Although the United States and Germany are the two countries with the largest number of migrants, many other countries around the globe have comparably large immigrant populations as well. For example, more than 17% of the Canadian population and more than 21% of the Australian population are foreign born. In addition to migration, rapid growth in international travel and telecommunication has increased people's exposure to foreign cultures.

Critical analyses have effectively dispelled the early naive enthusiasm that the world is becoming a global village and that all regional differences will be resolved through multilateral cultural hegemony (cf. Parameswaran, 2002; van Strien, 1997). In fact, despite the rhetoric of the global village, to many people living in multicultural societies, increased intercultural connectivity has heated up the fields in which the meanings of "the self" are contested. What does it mean to be a multicultural being? What does it mean to have a multicultural self? Such questions pertain to the nature of the multicultural mind and multicultural identities, and deserve serious attention from cultural psychologists. Our primary goal in this chapter is to draw attention to these important questions and to set up a tentative agenda for further discussion on these topics.

CONCEPTUAL DISTINCTIONS

Cultural Identity and Collective Identity

Before we start, it is worth discussing our definition of "multicultural identities" and how it is related to other types of self-representations. Brewer and Gardner (1996; see also Sedikides & Brewer, 2001) have delineated three ways to represent the self, namely, the individual self (which is characterized by an individual's personal attributes), the relational self (which is characterized by personal relationships with significant others), and the collective self (which is characterized by memberships in social groups or categories). These three self-representations allow people to define the self in three ways—individual (personal) identity, relational (social) identity, and collective identity. We add another identity, cultural identity, by which we refer to self-definition with reference to a *knowledge tradition* (Barth, 2002), or a collection of ideas and practices shared or widely distributed in a delineated population.[1]

On the surface, the construct of cultural identity may seem redundant with that of collective identity. However, this would be the case only when we equate a knowledge tradition (or culture) with a designated group, a practice with which many psychologists and anthropologists have taken issue (Appadurai, 1996; Friedman, 1994). Treating culture as a group is defensible only when a particular knowledge tradition is completely shared in the designated group. To be sure, there are cases where a particular knowledge tradition is widely distributed in a collective. However, even the most widely distributed knowledge tradition is seldom shared completely among all members of a group. For example, Christianity is widely distributed among Norwegians. About 90% of Norwegians are Christians, but a sizable percentage (10%) of them are not. Therefore, the Norwegian collective identity does not overlap completely with a Christian identity. Conversely, there are also instances in which people who identify with a particular knowledge tradition are geographically dispersed and do not belong to a well-defined collective (e.g., environmentalists around the world).

Furthermore, a collective identity may be conferred on people even when they do not necessarily identify with the knowledge tradition widely shared in the group. This is the case particularly for ascribed collective identities or identities conferred on an individual without the individual's prior consent (e.g., racial identity, gender identity, or the religious identity of Catholic babies who were baptized at birth). In short, collective identity and cultural identity are distinct constructs.

That said, we must acknowledge that although cultural identity and collective identity are distinct constructs, cultural *identification* and collective *identification* are intimately related. Level of identification refers to the degree to which one forms a unit relation between the self and the pertinent identity. Individuals who have strong identification with a knowledge tradition believe that this cultural identity is an integral part of their self-definition. Conversely, individuals who have weak identification with a knowledge tradition view this cultural identity as being tangential to their self-definition. Similarly, identification with a collective refers to the extent to which group membership of the collective is central to a person's self-definition.

When individuals (e.g., Chinese) identify strongly with a widely believed knowledge tradition (e.g., Confucianism) to define a collective (e.g., ethnic Chinese), they may also identify strongly with the collective. Likewise, when identification with a collective is strong, identification with the knowledge tradition widely believed to characterize the collective may be strong too (Jetten, Postmes, & McAuliffe, 2002; McAuliffe, Jetten, Hornsey, & Hogg, 2003).

Multicultural Mind and Multicultural Self

Cultural learning directly through personal experiences with the practices in a culture, or indirectly through observations of how the knowledge tradition is institutionalized in a society or implemented in practices, is the process whereby a knowledge tradition is acquired. A knowledge tradition available to an individual increases in cognitive accessibility as it is repeatedly called out and applied to understand one's experiences and to coordinate social actions. However, it would be a mistake to assume that individuals who possess knowledge of a particular cultural tradition will necessarily identify with it (Jetten et al., 2002). We emphasize that learning and acquiring a certain knowledge tradition does not entail identification with it. Experiences of short-term cultural travelers provide a good illustration of this point. Tourists, international students, or expatriate workers may be able to acquire the knowledge traditions in a foreign society and apply the newly acquired knowledge to guide their practices in the foreign land, without identifying with these knowledge traditions (Chiu & Chen, 2004).

By extension, individuals who have been exposed extensively to two (or more) knowledge traditions may have developed some degree of fluency in both. The increased frequency and intensity of intercultural contacts described at the beginning of this chapter has greatly facilitated multicultural learning. Admittedly, the acquisition of a knowledge tradition that is radically different from the one that is most familiar may initially create a "shocking" experience (Ward, Bochner, & Furnham, 2001). However, when individuals have acquired a knowledge tradition that is sufficiently different from their native one, they may choose to apply the native or new knowledge tradition in a given concrete situation, cognitively place them in juxtaposition, and attempt to integrate the knowledge from different cultural sources to foster a creative synthesis (Chiu & Hong, 2005). In this sense, the meeting of more than one knowledge tradition in a person can increase flexibility in cognitive and behavioral responding, and bring forth a stream of cultural innovations and creativity.

Individuals who are fluent in more than one cultural tradition can identify with one, all, or some cultural traditions. The issue of managing dual or multiple cultural identities does not emerge until bicultural or multicultural individuals are confronted with the task of defining the self with reference to certain knowledge tradition(s). We illustrate our arguments with bicultural identities, assuming that the same arguments apply equally well to multicultural identities. When bicultural individuals manage and negotiate their dual cultural identities, they may need to consider the affective, social, and political implications of the identity options available to them. This may be accompanied by feelings of confusion and ambivalence, as well as intrapsychic conflicts, particularly when the issue of divided allegiance is made salient, such as when new immigrants in some countries are expected to assimilate into the mainstream culture. Some bicultural individuals may construct an integral bicultural identity by synthesizing their dual identities. Such creative synthesis has been a topic of focal attention in cultural psychology. There is also an extant literature on the implications of various multiple-identities management strategies for psychological adjustment and well-being.

Making a distinction between multicultural knowledge (mind) and multicultural identification (self) also allows us to discuss the possible interactions between these two constructs. For example, given that knowledge tradition is the object of cultural identification, it is inconceivable that a person would identify with a culture without having at least some vague ideas of what constitutes the culture's knowledge tradition. In some situations, individuals may express and affirm their cultural identity by applying the pertinent cultural knowledge, although the application of cultural knowledge does not always entail cultural identification.

The distinction between acquiring cultural knowledge and cultural identification is therefore a theoretically important one. This distinction has offered us a refreshing perspective to reorganize the rapidly expanding literature on multicultural mind and multicultural self. To exploit the theoretical utility of this distinction, we have organized this chapter into four major sections: We (1) describe the psychological principles that underlie application of multicultural knowledge, (2) review the psychological processes involved in the management and expression of multicultural identities, (3) discuss the possible interactions of multicultural knowledge and multicultural identities, and finally (4) situate the microscopic psychological processes reviewed thus far in the global, sociopolitical contexts where the dynamic interactions of the multicultural mind and the multicultural self unfold *in vivo*.

In summary, by bringing a sharper focus to the seemingly blurry distinction between the multicultural mind and the multicultural self, we seek to shed some light on the dynamic processes whereby multicultural individuals choose between different cultural lenses to construct the reality, depending on the changing needs of the moment. We also strive to illuminate how multicultural individuals construct a self-identity that fits their experiences in an evolving multicultural environment.

MANAGEMENT AND APPLICATION OF BICULTURAL KNOWLEDGE

When individuals become experts in more than one culture, they may switch cultural frames in response to cues of changing cultural demands in the environment. Specifically, their social information processing is channeled through the lenses of more than one culture, and their interpretive biases could be pushed in the direction of one or the other culture by the presence of cultural cues in the immediate environment, a process we call "cultural frame switching." Such dynamic and flexible application of cultural knowledge results in adaptive responses to the shifting bicultural milieus. In this section, we introduce the basic cognitive principles that mediate cultural frame switching, and discuss its implications for adaptive and competent intercultural behaviors.

Principles of Knowledge Activation

The term "culture" is used here to designate a coalescence of loosely organized knowledge (or learned routines) that is produced, distributed, and reproduced among a collection of interconnected individuals. To the extent that culture consists of a network of distributed knowledge, application of cultural knowledge should follow the basic principles that govern knowledge activation in specific situations: the principles of availability, accessibility, and applicability (Higgins, 1996; Wyer & Srull, 1986).

Availability of Bicultural Knowledge

Some knowledge items are more widely distributed in one culture than in others. Individuals must be aware of the relative distribution of knowledge across cultures before they can apply knowledge discriminatively and appropriately in different cultural contexts.

Extensive experiences with several different cultures may increase people's awareness of the uneven distribution of various knowledge items in these cultures. There is some evidence for the idea that extensive bicultural experiences produce calibrated representations of the second culture. Although both Hong Kong and New York City are cosmopolitan cities, Hong Kong people arguably have more exposure to New York culture than do New Yorkers to Hong Kong culture. Given such asymmetry in the direction of cultural contacts, Lee (2002) found that Hong Kong undergraduates are more accurate in estimating the distribution of knowledge (e.g., general knowledge about flowers and landmarks) among New York undergraduates than are New York undergraduates in estimating the distribution of knowledge among Hong Kong undergraduates.

Other researchers have obtained similar findings in the estimations of subjective psychological knowledge. American undergradu-

ates are *slightly* more proud of their personal history of fulfilling personal aspirations (promotion pride) than of their personal success in meeting parental expectations (prevention pride; see Higgins et al., 2001, for discussions of these constructs). American undergraduates tend to be very accurate when they estimate the relative strength of promotion and prevention pride in American college student culture. Chinese undergraduates in Beijing have relatively limited experiences with American culture. When asked to estimate the relative strength of promotion pride and prevention pride among American college students, they overestimated the difference of American students' endorsement of promotion pride and prevention pride by three times. By comparison, Hong Kong undergraduates have more exposure to American culture than do students in Beijing. Although Hong Kong undergraduates also overestimated the difference of American students' endorsement of promotion pride and prevention pride, the magnitude of overestimation was much smaller (Ip, Chen, & Chiu, 2003). In short, with frequent contacts with a second culture, refined cultural knowledge about that culture is acquired. Availability of such knowledge leads to sensitivity to the distribution of different knowledge items in this culture.

Chronic Accessibility

Chronic accessibility of a knowledge item is a product of frequent use of that item (Higgins, 1996). Knowledge items that are frequently used in a cultural group are usually widely shared (Lau, Chiu, & Lee, 2001; Lau, Lee, & Chiu, 2004; Sechrist & Stangor, 2001), frequently reproduced in communication (Lyons & Kashima, 2001), widely represented in external or public carriers of culture (Menon & Morris, 2001), and cognitively accessible to members of the group (Hong, Morris, Chiu, & Benet-Martinez, 2000).

For example, in Asian cultures, group agency and aspects of the interdependent self are relatively well represented in commercial advertisements (Han & Shavitt, 1994; Kim & Markus, 1999), newspaper articles (Menon, Morris, Chiu, & Hong, 1999) and the languages (Kashima & Kashima, 1998). By contrast, in Western cultures, direct personal agency and aspects of the independent self are relatively well represented in these media. In addition, when asked to describe themselves,

Asians spontaneously mention more interdependent or group-related self-statements, and fewer independent self-statements than do Westerners, indicating that the interdependent or group-related self is more chronically accessible to Asians than to Westerners (Rhee, Uleman, Lee, & Roman, 1995; Wang, 2001). As such, cultures may differ in the chronic accessibility of ideas and practices.

Temporary Accessibility

Temporary accessibility refers to the heightened activation of a representation evoked by cues in the immediate context, which may remind individuals of an idea that is not chronically accessible. For example, although among American undergraduates the independent self has high chronic accessibility, American undergraduates mention more group attributes and fewer personal attributes when their collective self ("we") is primed than when their individual self ("I") is primed. This finding indicates that both individual and collective self-construals are available to some American undergraduates, and contextual priming calls out one or the other kind of self-construals (Gardner, Gabriel, & Lee, 1999; Trafimow, Triandis, & Goto, 1991). Similar findings have been obtained among Chinese students (Trafimow, Silverman, Fan, & Law, 1997; Gardner et al., 1999).

The principle of temporary accessibility may explain the phenomenon of cultural frame switching that many biculturals have experienced. Some individuals who have become enmeshed in more than one culture navigate situations in the second culture as experts. These biculturals may switch their mode of interpretation: In one situation everything is filtered through one cultural lens; in the next, through another one. Hong and her associates (Hong, Chiu, & Kung, 1997; Hong et al., 2000; Hong, Benet-Martinez, Chiu, & Morris, 2003) proposed that this occurs through spontaneous activation of cultural frames, which are interconnected knowledge structures, in response to cues of the cultural requirements of a situation. In one experiment that tested this idea, Chinese American biculturals (Hong Kong Chinese, Chinese Americans) were primed with either Chinese cultural icons (e.g., the Chinese dragon) or American cultural icons (e.g., Mickey Mouse). When primed with Chinese (vs. American) cultural icons, these biculturals were more inclined to use a group agency model to interpret an ambiguous event; they made more group attributions and fewer individual attributions. Analogous culture priming effects have been found on spontaneous self-construal (Ross, Xun, & Wilson, 2002) and cooperative behaviors (Wong & Hong, 2005). In addition, the culture priming effect has also been replicated in studies that used different bicultural samples (Chinese Canadians, Dutch Greek bicultural children), and a variety of cultural primes (e.g., language, experimenter's cultural identity; Ross et al., 2002; Verkuyten & Pouliasi, 2002).

Applicability of Cultural Knowledge

Cultural frame switching is not a knee-jerk response to situational cues. The evoked cultural frame is appraised for its applicability to the judgment context before it is applied; an accessible cultural idea does not impact judgments or behaviors unless it is applicable to the task at hand. As noted, Chinese-American biculturals would more likely apply a group (vs. individual) agency perspective to interpret a stimulus event when primed with Chinese cultural icons than when they are primed with American cultural icons. However, this occurs only when the group (vs. individual) agency perspective is applicable in the judgment context, such as when the tension between group agency and individual agency is highlighted (Hong et al., 2003).

Similarly, in Chinese cultural contexts, a cooperative (vs. competitive) script is applicable only in interaction with friends, not in interactions with strangers. Thus, subsequent to being primed with Chinese (vs. American or culture-neutral) primes, Chinese American biculturals are more cooperative when they play the prisoner's dilemma game with their friends. However, culture priming does not impact these biculturals' cooperative or competitive choices when they play the game with strangers (Wong & Hong, 2005).

Summary

Culture, like other knowledge, impacts judgments and behaviors when it is activated. Activation of cultural knowledge follows the general principles of availability, chronic accessibility, temporary accessibility, and applicability. As the foregoing analysis illustrates, retrieval of a specific cultural knowledge item is a probabilistic (as opposed to deterministic) process contingent upon the individual's chronic cultural experiences, the unfolding cultural milieu, and the situation-appropriateness of cultural knowledge. Thus, culture does not rigidly determine human behaviors. Instead, like other knowledge, culture is a cognitive resource for grasping experiences and pursuing life goals.

Bicultural Knowledge and Cultural Competence

Individuals with bicultural knowledge have more than one set of cultural tools to interpret the world (cf. DiMaggio, 1997; Shore, 1996). These tools may foster competent behaviors in at least three ways.

First, when people generate creative exemplars in a conceptual domain (e.g., animals on the planet Mars), even their most creative exemplars resemble the highly accessible exemplars in a related domain (e.g., animals on Earth, with eyes and legs). Apparently, a major constraint on creative conceptual expansion is the influence of the highly accessible exemplars (T. Ward, Patterson, Sifonis, Dodds, & Saunders, 2002). Normative, conventional views and ideas in a culture are frequently used to interpret and understand the world. If a cultural lens is used frequently enough to make sense of the environment, it becomes a learned routine, and a part of "routinized" culture (Ng & Bradac, 1993). Thus, although culture provides conventional tools for sense making and problem solving, it also impedes creativity (T. Ward et al., 2002).

If the categorical accessibility norms in a culture result from chronic cultural experiences, bicultural experiences may help to foster creative expansion of ideas. To elaborate, Idea A may have high categorical accessibility in Culture I and low categorical accessibility in Culture II. Conversely, Idea B may have high categorical accessibility in Culture II and low categorical accessibility in Culture I. An individual who has extensive experiences in Cultures I and II may be able to retrieve Ideas A and B spontaneously, place the two ideas in juxtaposition and through creative insights integrate the two ideas into a novel idea. This process, often referred to as "novel conceptual combination," has been shown to have beneficial effects on creative conceptual expansion (Hampton, 1997; Simonton, 1997, 2000; W.

Wan & Chiu, 2002). Indeed, many examples of creative conceptual expansion in daily life result from integrating indigenous cultural exemplars from diverse cultures. For example, furnishing a New York apartment with traditional Ming Dynasty furniture may give a creative postmodern feel to this home. Consistent with this idea, we found in a recent study that among European American university students, those who have more experiences with other cultures have a greater tendency to sample ideas from other cultures (Middle Eastern and Far Eastern cultures) and integrate them in a creative conceptual expansion task (Leung, Chiu, & Hong, 2003).

Second, in intercultural communication, bicultural experiences allow individuals to discover, adjust, and integrate new attitudes and values from the second culture (Casmir, 1992). As such, knowledge of other cultures may help to establish the common ground in intercultural interactions, such as international business negotiation or management of culturally heterogeneous work teams (e.g., Earley, 2002; Earley & Ang, 2003; Pinkley & Northcraft, 1994). Consistent with this idea, Chinese Americans, who are familiar with both Chinese and American cultures, are likely to know that Americans have higher promotion pride than do Chinese. Therefore, when Chinese Americans try to persuade a Chinese or American to purchase an insurance policy, they use more promotion-focused arguments for an American target than for a Chinese target (Leung et al., 2003).

Third, accurate knowledge of another culture is linked to better intercultural interaction quality. For example, among Mainland Chinese university students in Hong Kong, some have more accurate knowledge of the values of their host culture (Hong Kong culture) than others. Those who have more accurate knowledge have more satisfactory interactions with the local students and the university staff than do those who have less accurate knowledge (Li & Hong, 2001).

In summary, as bicultural experiences accumulate, so does bicultural knowledge. Bicultural knowledge can foster culturally competent behaviors and creative endeavors. However, as noted, individuals who have acquired knowledge from a second culture may or may not identify with the second culture. If that is the case, how do biculturals negotiate cultural identity?

MANAGEMENT OF MULTICULTURAL IDENTITIES

Cultural identities may be uniquely represented within each multicultural individual (Roccas & Brewer, 2002). Based on how multiple cultures are structurally represented, there may be little competition for psychological resources among cultural identities. However, even though there may be little internal conflict *within* multicultural individuals, the differing demands and expectations placed on members of each cultural group—to be culturally authentic, to be loyal to the group, speak the language, and follow the norms, along with numerous others— necessitate management of situation-appropriate responses.

Successful management of multicultural identities thus involves resolution of conflicts arising from these manifold internal and external demands. Thus, management of multiple identities requires both overt and conscious flexibility (Birman, 1998; Phinney & Devich-Navarro, 1997), along with more subtle adaptability to the cultural requirements of the situation (e.g., changes in field dependence [Kitayama, Duffy, Kawamura, & Larsen, 2003]; self-esteem levels [Hetts, Sakuma, & Pelham, 1999]). Additionally, it entails increased proficiency in choosing among identity options to emphasize the desirable aspects of the self in context (Sprott, 1994; Waters, 1990). Although numerous means of managing multiple cultural identities are available to multiculturals, possible limitations exist as to the scope of management strategies employed. Depending on prescribed social policies within a society (e.g., Berry, 2001), attitudes toward multiculturalism held by the majority or dominant group (e.g., LaFromboise, Coleman, & Gerton, 1993; Montreuil & Bourhis, 2001), or available personal resources (e.g., Camilleri & Malewska-Peyre, 1997), individuals may negotiate their multiple identities through integration, alternation, or synergy strategies. Although engagement in multicultural identity negotiation may yield overt behaviors in tune with changing cultural environments, management processes may also generate internal ambivalence regarding identity loyalties and cultural affiliation.

Multicultural Identities and Their Development

Recent acculturation models (e.g., Lee, Sobal, & Frongillo, 2003; Ryder, Alden, & Paulhus, 2000; Tsai, Ying, & Lee, 2000) have emphasized the multidimensionality of cultural selves: As individuals acquire knowledge and practices of a new culture, knowledge and practices of heritage cultures are retained. Moreover, these cultural identities can coexist within any given individual without adverse psychological consequences.

Furthermore, individuals may strategically evoke cultural identities to enhance their consonance with changing environments. As Padilla and Perez (2003) point out, in adapting to a new cultural context, newcomers may engage different identity strategies depending on contextual factors such as the cultural and racial diversity of the place of settlement, the dominant group's assignment of value to the identities brought by newcomers from their prior experiences, or the extant relations among dominant and nondominant groups prior to their arrival. Importantly, these contextual factors contribute to newcomers' motivations to acculturate to the mainstream culture.

The foregoing analysis implies that multiculturals may *develop* and *adjust* their multicultural identities in response to changing circumstances to increase the alignment of the identities with individuals' prior experiences, and current goals and affordances. This developmental perspective to multicultural identities has two major advantages. First, many writers have focused on the hypothesized negative consequences of identity shifts. Terms such as "culture shock," "acculturative stress," and "identity confusion" are illustrative of the negative slant with which multicultural identity management has been addressed. From the developmental perspective, these seemingly negative experiences grow out of the awareness of cultural differences and the deliberate effort to retain or reformulate the current identity in light of new cultural experiences. These "negative experiences" surface only at certain transitional stages of multicultural identity development.

Second, a developmental perspective demands attention to identify and analyze the processes involved in the construction and management of multicultural identity. Recent studies have captured a few snapshots of these processes. Coming in contact with different cultural traditions increases self-awareness of one's own cultural embeddedness (Sussman, 2000; Zaharna, 1989). This heightened awareness then allows one to make comparisons, to distance oneself, or to choose from among available cultural identity options (Camilleri & Malewska-Peyre, 1997; Verkuyten & de Wolf, 2002). With prolonged contact, individuals may develop adjustment repertoires that in turn lead to sustained identity shifts or the internalization of new cultural identities. Once multiple identities are internalized, proficient management of multiple identity demands requires that complex knowledge structures associated with each cultural identity—episodic memories and meaning systems composed of values, beliefs, behaviors, practices; significant others and acquaintances—be appropriately accessed in changing contexts, while new cultural knowledge is concurrently encoded into memory. Smooth management of such complex multicultural identity processes may be facilitated by increased sociopolitical support for multicultural societies (Berry, 2001) in which individuals would have ready access to many different ways of negotiating multicultural identities. As individuals gain greater access to multicultural-oriented life experiences, different identity-management strategies, which were initially intentionally and effortfully controlled, may be practiced at a relatively automatic or nonconscious level.

Strategies of Multicultural Identity Negotiation

Every multicultural identity may have a unique developmental history and a distinct developmental trajectory. Nonetheless, existing research and theory on multicultural identity negotiation may be organized into three broad categories of identity negotiation strategies: integration, alternation, and synergy. Preference for identity negotiation strategies may change over the life course, and any given individual may synchronously utilize all or a combination of these three distinct modes of identity negotiation.

In one class of identity negotiation models, *integration*, identities become blended and merged into one coherent identity (LaFromboise et al., 1993; Sprott, 1994). Integration models assume that elements from multiple cultures fuse into a unitary (multicultural) identity. As such, integration models view the development of multicultural identities as additive, in that new cultural identities are "added to" existing cultural identities. However, elements from one culture may be cued in differ-

ent circumstances, bringing to the fore, relative to other internalized cultures, aspects of the self associated with the cued culture. Integration models often describe multiculturals as having highly developed identities in each culture, which are utilized in culturally appropriate ways in different contexts (e.g., Oyserman, 1993; Oyserman, Sakamoto, & Lauffer, 1998; Suinn, Ahuna, & Khoo, 1992; Yamada & Singelis, 1999).

The second class of negotiation models, *alternation*, involves switching back and forth among cultural identities depending on the fit of the identity with the immediate context. Ross et al. (2002) showed that when responding in Cantonese or Mandarin, bilingual–bicultural Chinese Canadians shifted their self-descriptions toward a pattern typical of Chinese than when responding in English. Hong and her colleagues have also demonstrated that biculturals readily shift cultural interpretive frames based on available cultural cues (Hong et al., 1997, 2000, 2003; No & Hong, 2004a). Although cultural knowledge is indeed distinct from cultural identity, it would not be a stretch to assume that aspects of the self are also accessed and applied in response to cultural cues.

In the third class of negotiation strategies, *synergy*, entirely new identities are forged as a result of contact with different cultural models (Anthias, 2001). In contrast to integration or alternation, synergy posits that new identities emerge which cannot be reduced to the sum of their parts (e.g., Benet-Martinez, Leu, Lee, & Morris's [2002] notion of a "third culture"). As an example, in our new line of research on cultural hybridization (No, Wan, & Chiu, 2005), we posit that Korean American culture (or Chinese American culture, etc.) is not a direct summation of components from Korean culture (i.e., the culture of Korea) and American culture (i.e., the culture of the United States), but rather is a unique cultural configuration that results from a transformation of the components themselves when they interact with one another. As such, an individual who identifies as Korean American embodies an entirely new set of knowledge traditions, one that arises and unfolds in a specific historical context of ethnic Koreans residing in an American landscape. In the domain of language, synergy is best encapsulated in the process of creolization, in which a new grammar is constructed out of the continued interaction of groups speaking two or more distinct languages. In this respect,

Grosjean (1989) notes that it may be inaccurate to transport paradigms of neurolinguistic research developed from monolingual speakers to that of bilingual speakers. Bilinguals must instead be approached as a person with a "unique and specific linguistic configuration . . . and not the sum of two monolinguals" (p. 6). By acknowledging the unique and specific effects of bilingualism, linguistic research has been extended to examine phenomena such as code switching and language borrowing. Furthermore, Grosjean argues that the synergistic effects of bilingualism do not entail a loss of competency in the original languages—an idea that resonates with research on cultural hybridization (e.g., Korean Americans are to some extent culturally competent in Korean culture and in American culture).

Identity Ambivalence, Marginalization, and Alienation

In an early analysis of migration and identity, Park (1928) approached the internal conflict and ambivalence arising from identification with multiple cultural groups through the notion of "marginal man," a person who feels simultaneous detachment and involvement with multiple cultural groups. Identification with multiple cultural groups engenders psychological conflict when values and practices of heritage and mainstream cultural groups are perceived to be too distant or in opposition (Benet-Martinez et al., 2002). Identity ambivalence may also result from the fluctuating responses of others to multiculturals, depending on the salient identity features of a context (Turner, Hogg, Oakes, Reicher, & Wetherell, 1987), such as when multiculturals are approached with intimacy and familiarity in one context and responded to with fear and distance by the same individuals in another context (Zaharna, 1989). Additionally, identity conflict may arise due to exclusion or rejection by desired cultural groups. Exclusion is then turned inward and attributed to lack of cultural knowledge or language fluency (Kanno, 2003; Pang, 2000).

Identity ambivalence, marginalization, and alienation may also result from intragroup conflicts among newly arrived and established cultural groups who settle within the same geographical area. Feeling excluded by the established group increases the likelihood that migrants develop ambivalent or marginal identities. Niemann, Romero, Arredono, and Ro-

driguez (1999) found that U.S. Mexicans perceived more rejection and discrimination from Chicanas/Chicanos (U.S.-born Mexican Americans) than from Anglo Americans. Japanese Peruvians and Japanese Brazilians who traveled to Japan as migrant workers during the late 1980s and throughout the 1990s were treated as Peruvians/Brazilians by the Japanese, but as Japanese in their respective countries of Peru and Brazil, although of mixed blood and being of second- or third-generation status (Tsuda, 2003; Takenaka, 1999).

Psychological Adjustment to Bicultural Experiences

Berry and his colleagues (Berry, Poortinga, Segall, & Dasen, 1992; Berry & Sam, 1997) have put forth an influential model of acculturative strategies. As individuals come in contact with multiple cultural groups, they may accommodate their identity to the mainstream culture (*assimilate*); simultaneously retain their heritage cultural identity, while developing the mainstream cultural identity (*integrate*); reject the mainstream cultural identity, opting instead for their heritage cultural identity (*separate*); or reject both mainstream and heritage cultural identifications (*marginalize*). Berry hypothesizes that integration is most conducive to psychological well-being, although the evidence for this hypothesis is inconclusive (Rogler, Cortes, & Malgady, 1991; Rudmin, 2003).

A key issue seems to be the generation cohort of the immigrants. For instance, Furnham and Li (1993) found that second-generation Chinese in Britain, who were more likely to report feeling that they were part of the host community, were significantly more likely than those who did not feel part of the host community to report greater psychological symptoms. Similarly, Robins and Regier (1991) found that the lifetime prevalence of mental illness of U.S.-born Mexican Americans was much higher than that of first-generation Mexican American immigrants. Organista, Organista, and Kurasaki (2002) thus suggested that the poorer mental health of native-born Mexican Americans, despite their greater assimilation into the U.S. culture than first-generation Mexican Americans, "has to do with their especially stressful experience in America as a devalued and discriminated ethnic minority group" (p. 154).

Aside from focusing on the acculturation strategy per se, some researchers have examined the cognitive factors that underlie vulnerability in adjusting to bicultural experience. For one, Benet-Martinez and Haritatos (2005) found that Asian Americans who view their Asian identity and American identity as conflicting showed greater depression and anxiety than do those who view their two identities as less conflicting. In other research, Hong and her associates (Chao, Chen, Roisman, & Hong, in press; No & Hong, 2004a, 2004b; cf. Hong, Roisman, & Chen, 2006) proposed that biculturals' beliefs about race—whether race is an essentialist entity (reflecting biological essence, unalterable, and indicative of abilities and traits) or a socially constructed, dynamic construct—predict the extent to which they can successfully achieve psychological adaptation to both cultures. The researchers argued that an essentialist race belief would give rise to perception of less permeability between racial group boundaries. Therefore, ethnic minorities holding an essentialist race theory would have a harder time integrating experiences with both their ethnic and host cultures. Consistent with this idea, Chao et al. (in press) found that the stronger the Chinese Americans participants endorse an essentialist race theory, the higher their skin conductance reactivity (sweating more compared to the rest period) when talking about their own bicultural experiences, suggesting that an essentialist race theory is associated with more effortful defense.

Summary

When multiculturals negotiate cultural identity, they do not just retrieve their knowledge of the pertinent cultures. They turn cultural traditions into objects of reflection; they cognitively juxtapose these traditions and evaluate their significance with references to prior cultural experiences and current intercultural relations. Whereas the multicultural mind grows out of multicultural experiences, multicultural identity is both a product of deliberate reflectiveness and an ongoing personal project.

INTERACTION OF MULTICULTURAL KNOWLEDGE AND MULTICULTURAL IDENTITIES

Multicultural mind and multicultural identity are distinct constructs, but they do work to-

gether. This section explicates how cultural representations support a variety of cultural identification processes, including categorical perception, cultural identification, and affirmation of cultural identity. Next, we discuss how identification influences application of knowledge in specific multicultural contexts.

The Role of Cultural Representations in Cultural Identification

Cultural Prototypes and Categorical Perceptions

As noted, cultural identification involves defining the self with reference to one or more cultural traditions. Once cultural identification occurs, a person's perceptual focus shifts from the idiosyncratic characteristics of the self to the prototypical features of the culture (cf. Hogg, 2001, 2003). Prototypical features of a culture consist of symbolic elements (e.g., beliefs, values) and behaviors that epitomize the culture and maximally distinguish it from other cultures. In short, they are normatively agreed upon ideological and behavioral characteristics that define the culture. When identification with a culture is strong, or when cultural identity is made salient, perceptions of the social world are filtered through the lens of culture; thoughts and behaviors are not seen as signatures of individual personality, but are interpreted in terms of their consonance with cultural prototypes.

Thus, the varying degrees to which people's thoughts and behaviors adhere to cultural prototypes provide a gradient for differentiating and evaluating people (e.g., Haslam, Oakes, McGarty, Turner, & Onorato, 1995). Individuals who exhibit culture-prototypical thoughts and behaviors are perceived by other members of the culture to be good representatives of the culture, and are evaluated favorably. Conversely, those who exhibit culture-atypical thoughts and behaviors are often marginalized and evaluated negatively (Marques & Paez, 1994; Marques, Abrams, Paez, & Martinez-Taboada, 1998).

Cultural prototypes become a major criterion for interpersonal perception when cultural identification is strong, or when cultural identity is made salient. For example, in an organizational role-play experiment (McAuliffe et al., 2003), an employee showing collectivist behavior is perceived more positively than an employee showing individualist behaviors, when the organization has a collectivist organization culture. This effect is particularly pronounced among those who strongly identify with the organization.

C. Wan, Chiu, Tam, et al. (2007) have proposed an intersubjective consensus approach to identifying culture-prototypical values. This approach involves assessment of the general consensus among people in the culture on the distributions of different values in the culture. Through their experiences in a culture, people learn about and even participate in the construction of the common beliefs and values that are important to the culture. Such collective representations do not necessarily correspond to most cultural members' private personal values (cf. Miller & Prentice, 1994). Yet when people in the same culture agree that certain values are widely shared in the culture, these values are likely to be culture-prototypical values. C. Wan and Chiu (2003) applied the intersubjective consensus approach to identify culture-prototypical values in an American undergraduate student culture and replicated the findings from the McAuliffe et al. (2003) study. Specifically, when their university student identity is made salient, student participants perceive a target student who endorses culture-prototypical values (values generally believed to be widely distributed in the student culture) to be friendlier, kinder, and more sincere than a target student who is not known to have these values (C. Wan & Chiu, 2003).

Cultural Prototypes and Cultural Identification

People may perceive others based on whether they display culture-prototypical values. They may also construct their own cultural identity based on how much they personally endorse culture-prototypical values: Individuals who endorse these values tend to identify with the culture, and those who do not have relatively weak cultural identification. Consistent with this idea, C. Wan, Chiu, Tam, et al. (2007, Study 1) found that university undergraduate students' identification with the undergraduate student culture is positively related to endorsement of culture-prototypical values identified through the intersubjective consensus approach. Analogous findings have been obtained in identification with other culturally constructed categories (e.g., gender [C. Wan &

Chiu, 2005]; political identification [C. Wan, Chiu, & Tam, 2005]).

Prototypical representations are also involved in identification with more than one culture. Consider the following two hypothetical cultures. Some values are prototypical features in Cultures A and B, but some are prototypical features only in Culture A, and others are prototypical features only in Culture B. Bicultural individuals know what values fall into each category. In addition, their relative strength of identification with the two cultures may be reflected in their relative endorsement of the different categories of values. Using the intersubjective consensus approach, researchers have been able to identify values that are prototypical features in Culture A but not in Culture B, and vice versa. In addition, it has also been shown that biculturals who identify strongly with Culture A (rather than with Culture B) tend to endorse values that are prototypical features of Culture A (C. Wan, Chiu, Peng, et al., in press).

Affirmation of Cultural Identity

When people identify with a culture, that culture heavily impacts their behaviors. Thus, people who identify strongly (vs. weakly) with a culture are more likely to follow cultural norms (Jetten et al., 2002, Study 1). For example, North Americans who strongly identify with North American culture are more individualist than are the weak identifiers. Similarly, Indonesians who strongly identify with Indonesian culture are more collectivist than individuals who weakly identify with the culture. Furthermore, when identification with a cultural group is strong, norms (shared attitudes) have greater impact on behavioral intentions than do personal attitudes, and the reverse is true when cultural identification is weak (Terry & Hogg, 1996; Terry, Hogg, & White, 1999).

When their cultural identity is threatened, people may attempt to affirm their cultural identity, often by asserting their adherence to cultural tradition. For example, research has examined how people respond to cultural identity threat. In this situation, high identifiers rate themselves as more collectivist when the cultural norm is collectivist than when it is individualist. Additionally, their behavioral intentions are more consistent with collectivist norms than are those of low identifiers (Jetten et al., 2002, Study 3).

Aside from identity threat, mortality salience may also increase the need to affirm one's cultural identity. Research has shown that when the terror of death is made salient, people manage their existential terror by asserting their membership in a valued cultural group, thereby endorsing the prototypical cultural values (Halloran & Kashima, 2004; Kashima, Halloran, Yuki, & Kashima, 2004; see review by Greenberg, Solomon, and Pyszczynski, 1997).

In summary, cultural prototypes as special kinds of cultural representations play an important part in a broad range of cultural identification processes, including categorical perceptions, cultural identification, and cultural identity affirmation.

Management of Multicultural Identities and Application of Multicultural Knowledge

The interaction between multicultural knowledge and multicultural identities has been most extensively studied in culture priming experiments. As mentioned, in culture priming, specific features of a social context activate certain piece of cultural knowledge, which is then applied in the specific situation. The presence of a cultural priming effect depends on the presence of knowledge about the culture being primed. Furthermore, how a piece of cultural knowledge is related to people's specific responses to cultural cues depends on their identity management concerns in that situation (Chiu & Chen, 2004). Specifically, multicultural individuals, in any given context, may show an assimilation or a contrast response to the cued culture. When knowledge of both cued cultures is available, contextual cues can push biculturals' responses in the direction of the cued culture, producing an assimilation effect (Hong et al., 2000; Wong & Hong, 2005). However, when cultural identity is made salient, or when one's cultural identity is under threat, the motivation to affirm one's cultural identity may drive a contrast effect. Under this circumstance, contextual cues may push biculturals' responses away from the cued culture. For example, presenting highly Welsh-identified Welsh speakers with speech samples of British Standard English may lead these speakers to exaggerate their Welsh accent when their minority status is also made salient in the situation (Bourhis & Giles, 1977).

The likelihood of displaying an assimilation or contrast effect is also related to how biculturals cognitively represent the pertinent cultures. Biculturals may perceive their two cultural identities as compatible and integrated, or as conflicting and separate (Benet-Martinez et al., 2002). Chinese American biculturals who perceive their Chinese and American identities as compatible tend to show an assimilation effect, whereas those who perceive their Chinese and American identities as conflicting tend to show a contrast effect. Apparently, when two cultural identities are perceived to be compatible, cultural cues do not evoke strong reactance, and biculturals display responses consistent with the activated cultural frames. However, when biculturals feel that they are torn between two conflicting cultures, cultural cues may elicit psychological reactance and produce a contrast effect.

According to Benet-Martinez et al. (2002) the perceived compatibility between two cultures is an important determining factor in whether biculturals integrate the two cultural identities into one, combined, emerging identity. Consistent with this proposal, research has suggested that the bigger the perceived distance between two cultures, the more difficult it is for cultural travelers to acculturate into the second culture (e.g., Dunbar, 1994; C. Ward & Searle, 1991).

Another factor that predicts the tendency to display assimilation or contrast effects is the extent to which biculturals believe that "race" is an essentialist entity, which we already discussed briefly (No & Hong, 2004a, 2004b). When Korean Americans hold an essentialist belief about race, they tend to view the boundary between their own ethnocultural group and the mainstream group as impermeable. The mainstream American icons remind them of their minority status (i.e., "I am a Korean") and the Korean cultural values associated with their minority identity (No & Hong, 2004b). Therefore, instead of displaying an American response pattern, they show a response pattern that is consistent with the highly accessible Korean identity. For example, North Americans are more likely to show egocentric projection of emotion (e.g., "Others must feel sad too when I am sad") than are East Asians, who in turn are more likely than North Americans to show relational projection of emotion (e.g., "Others must feel sympathetic when I am sad"; Cohen & Gunz, 2002). Korean Americans who believe in an essentialist race theory show an increased tendency to make relational projection subsequent to being primed with American cultural icons, an indication of contrast effect (No & Hong, 2004a).

To summarize, when identity issues are not involved, culture priming produces an assimilation effect. However, when identity issues are brought into the scene, more complicated response patterns emerge, suggesting that culture primes do not just call out the corresponding cultural knowledge. Instead, they increase awareness of the intercultural relations in the society, activate perceptions of the identity compatibility and malleability, and evoke feelings and values attached to one's cultural identities. All these effects take place within an intercultural context, embedded within a broader network of power relations in the society.

GLOBALIZATION AND THE REMAKE OF THE CULTURAL LANDSCAPE

Thus far, our discussion has focused on the basic principles of multicultural psychology, which explain the molecular processes in multicultural psychology. However, a complete analysis of multicultural psychology demands attention to a critical analysis of the embeddedness of individual psychology in a rich historical and political multicultural context. Cultural psychology has barely set foot on this intellectual territory. Yet this may be the territory where theories of multicultural psychology will meet new challenges.

With the rapid growth of global linkages and consciousness, social life is increasingly organized on a global scale. Human beings have entered the era of globalization. Both the referential and connotative meanings of *globalization* may vary, depending on the context in which the term is used. However, most writers agree that globalization involves "the compression of the world and the intensification of consciousness of the world as a whole" (Robertson, 1992, p. 8).

As globalization proceeds, more previously isolated economies are integrated into the world economy via international trade and investment. Some countries, such as China, have benefited enormously through this process of integration and have enjoyed rapid growth in gross domestic product (GDP). However, there is also ample evidence that the gap between the richest and poorest countries, and that between the richest and poorest groups of individuals in many nations (including the most industrialized states; e.g., the United States and Western European countries) have increased (Alderson & Nielsen, 2002). For instance, within an industrialized country, the problem of income inequality has been aggravated by direct investment outflow, import of cheaper consumer goods and, to a lesser extent, inflow of international labor through migration (Alderson & Nielsen, 2002). These developments make it necessary to conceptualize negotiation of cultural identities within the confines of power relations in both local and global contexts.

At the same time, the rapid speed of air transportation, and the instantaneous electronic transfer of information and capital, have led to what Anthony Giddens (1985) refers to as time–space distanciation, or the experiential compression of time and space. A postmodern, global culture is often characterized as one "of virtuality in the global flows which transcend time and space" (Castells, 1998, p. 350). Increasingly, the forces that have grounded different knowledge traditions to a confined space have disintegrated.

As the pace of globalization accelerates, so does population movement across national borders. At the beginning of this chapter, we presented some statistics on migration. Migration influences the ethnic composition of both the sending and receiving countries. Many migrants are *temporary* international workers (e.g., Filipino domestic helpers in Hong Kong, seasonal farm laborers) who move from one country to another and back again. Business travel and tourism are two other major components of population movements. For example, Canada has a population of about 31 million people but has close to 50 million entries by nonresident travelers annually. Similarly, the United States receives approximately 97 million international travelers annually by air alone (Richmond, 2002).

The demographic changes accompanying globalization have important implications for the coordination of knowledge and negotiation of identities in cosmopolitan cities. To begin, globalization requires integration of local economies into the global market, which is grounded in the capitalist logic. The capitalist logic is grounded in "instrumental rationality," a kind of rationality defined in terms of efficiency and feasibility of achieving goals via calculative strategization of the means (Weber,

1904/1958). Instrumental rationality flourished in Europe during the Enlightenment period, when a coalescence of individualist ideas became popular. These ideas include religious individualism (the emphasis on the individual's personal relationship with God, and the belief that salvation is contingent on personal faith and needs no intermediaries), economic individualism (the belief that rewards depend on individual performance), political individualism (the belief that political systems are set up to satisfy individual needs, and that individual rights are protected by law), methodological individualism (the belief that all social phenomena should be understood as resulting from the psychological processes of individuals), and psychological individualism (the belief in the value of the individual, self-actualization, individual uniqueness, and individual identity; Ho & Chiu, 1994; Lukes, 1973). This collection of ideas constitutes the major contents of the mainstream knowledge tradition in most industrialized countries, consisting of the United States and most Western European countries. The question is: Will globalization ultimately lead to homogenization of cultures via *global hegemony*?

Globalization and Homogenization of Cultures

At first glance, the global hegemony project is destined to succeed. The Western economic powers, representatives of the global market force, may have a dominating influence over other, non-Western (local) nations not only in the economic sphere but also in the direction of cultural restructuring. Globalization has been labeled as new, modern, scientific and results-oriented. The global culture embraces consumerism, individualism, competition, and efficiency. These cultural ideals could be falsely established as universal, overriding local traditions. The hegemonic influence seldom takes the form of enforced domination. Instead, it often assumes the form of voluntary submission to the reference culture (van Strien, 1997). In addition, the capitalist logic in the global market demands strict adherence to the same collection of efficient economic and social practices that turn out controllable, predictable results. Furthermore, an expanding consumerist culture, with its attendant global marketing strategies, tends to exploit similar, basic material desires and create similar lifestyles (Parameswaran, 2002).

There is some evidence that globalization may lead to the demise of local cultures. First, a defining feature of globalization is the continuing transformation of the society via science and technology (Fischer, 1999). Penetration of science and technology education, which supports and is in turn supported by instrumental rationality, is a hallmark of globalization in a country. In a comparative study of 20 nations that differ widely in the extent of globalization (e.g., from Sweden to Romania, Brazil, Mexico, and Thailand), Tzeng and Henderson (1999) reported that the best country-level predictor of the level of globalization is the country's level of involvement in science education. Countries with more mature global economies have greater educational expenditures per capita, a higher percentage of the adult population with college-level education, a greater number of university professors per capita, a greater number of foreign students in national universities, and a greater number of students attending institutions of higher learning abroad. In addition, people in countries with more mature global economies have stronger identification with the value of scientific education.

There is some tentative evidence that exposure to the global culture, directly via exposure to global industries such as tourism, or indirectly through participation in a science and technology educational institution, may lead to the demise of indigenous knowledge traditions. In one study, participants from Kenya and the United States responded to the TST, which requires the participant to generate 20 self-descriptive statements. Among pastoral nomads in Kenya, only 18% of their spontaneous self-descriptions referenced personal attributes. The remaining 82% of their self-descriptions referenced memberships in social categories. By comparison, the percentage of self-descriptions that referenced personal attributes was 42% for hotel workers and university staff in Kenya, 83% for university students in Kenya, and 87% for American undergraduates (Ma & Schoeneman, 1997). There is also evidence that, compared to Japanese students who have never been abroad, students who have visited a Western country report higher self-esteem (Heine, Lehman, Markus, & Kitayama, 1999).

However, findings from the kind of comparative studies described in the previous paragraph are difficult to interpret because of self-selection bias. For example, in the study conducted in Kenya, it is possible that college students, as well as workers in hotels and universities, belonged to a self-selected sample with a strong preference for the global knowledge tradition or a cosmopolitan (vs. tribal) identity. Thus, their American-like responses to the TST could be expressions of their identity choice rather than indentations caused by globalization's inevitable erosive effects.

Globalization and Cultural Diversity

Some writers contend that globalization will not result in homogenization of culture. Lal (2000) offers a distinction between material and cosmological beliefs in a culture. "Material" beliefs pertain to ways of making a living or beliefs about the material world, particularly the economy. By contrast, "cosmological" beliefs are related to the definition of humankind's place in the world. More specifically, cosmological beliefs define the purpose and meaning of life, and an individual's relationship to others. Whereas the material beliefs in the global culture increase in popularity as a country is integrated into the global market, cosmological beliefs in local knowledge traditions are relatively resistant to the influence of globalization.

There is some evidence for this hypothesis. Based on data from the three waves of the World Values Surveys, which include 65 societies, Inglehart and Baker (2000) found that economic development is associated with increased endorsement of values that emphasize secularism, rationality, and self-expression. However, the broad knowledge tradition of a society (e.g., Protestantism, Confucianism) leaves an imprint on work-related values (e.g., importance of good pay, job security, work pressure, trade union, working with pleasant people) that endures despite the erosive effects of globalization.

Fu and Chiu (2003) also found that among Hong Kong undergraduates, with globalization, Western values compatible with instrumental rationality (e.g., creativity) have high cognitive accessibility. By comparison, Western moral values rooted in political individualism (e.g., liberty and human rights) are less accessible. In the moral domain, Confucian values of interpersonal mutuality continue to enjoy high cognitive accessibility. In short, instead of homogenizing culture, globalization may lead to *pluralization* of cultures via the meeting of global and local cultures in one locality.

The presence of plural cultures may result in internal *differentiation*, with one segment of the population favoring the traditional culture and others favoring the emerging new cultural modes and lifestyles. For example, globalization has brought about contested views about females in India. On the one hand, in Hindu patriarchal beliefs, the female gender is essential and primordial (Mahalingam, 2003). In one study, American and Indian participants were asked to imagine that a man's brain was transplanted to a woman's head, and vice versa. Most American participants believed that a brain transplant would change the gender behaviors of both a man and a woman. By contrast, most Indian participants, particularly Brahmin males, believed that a brain transplant would change the gender behaviors of men only, and that women are biologically predisposed to behave in a feminine manner; they would exhibit feminine qualities that even the most radical medical intervention could not have altered (Mahalingam & Rodriguez, 2003).

On the other hand, globalization has brought new educational and employment opportunities to women in India, reducing their reliance on husbands and fathers. In addition, as documented in an in-depth ethnographic study in West Bengal, India (Ganguly-Scrase, 2003), in promoting a consumerist ideology, the mass media have created a new consumerist subject—a glamorous "liberated" woman that epitomizes independent mobility through shopping. In Bengal, whereas older women favor the traditional Indian view of womanhood, many younger women use images of the new consumerist subject to construct new models of womanhood that stand in opposition to the traditional patriarchal gender norms and challenge the gender ideologies in Bengali culture.

Globalization has been characterized as a process that generates contradictory spaces (Sassen, 1998), because the spread of the global culture may provoke resistance and reactions from local cultures. The *contestation* of global and local cultures could range from out-and-out rebellions against globalization (e.g., the antiglobalization demonstration that took place in Seattle during the World Trade Organization Conference in 1999) to engagement in practices that embody oppositional local cultural meanings. For example, Thompson and Arsel (2004) studied local coffee shops in Chicago as the embodiment of such oppositional cultural meanings in stark contrast to global cultural meanings that Starbucks represents. Some of these local coffee shops are decorated with countercultural symbols and bohemian atmospherics, whereas others exhibit a more polished, bourgeois ambiance. Some regular patrons of these coffee shops denounce Starbucks for crowding out all the local coffee shops, and view local coffee shops as exuding an alternative, antiestablishment aura, and as outposts for like-minded activists to challenge prevailing corporate power structures.

Contestation of global and local cultures may also result in adaptation of norms or practices to local traditions, a process often referred to as *glocalization*. In the marketplace, the globalized capital seeks complete domination (Parameswaran, 2002). The shopping mall is an outpost of the globalized economy. Because a high percentage of malls are planned and built by no more than 10 transnational architectural firms, malls throughout the world share common features of aesthetics, architecture, and design. For this reason, the shopping mall is also an architectural symbol of globalization. However, as Salcedo (2003) noted, even in the shopping mall, which has been assumed to be an archetypical globalized space, aspects of the local culture are co-opted into the world of consumption. For example, in the Phillipines' Megamall, there is a church constructed for Catholic masses. In Saudi Arabia, there is a mall where foreign women perform the sales work and men are prohibited to enter.

In summary, although there have been some concerns that globalization might undermine cultural diversity through the processes of pluralization, contestation, and glocalization, there are also reasons to believe that globalization will foster cultural diversity.

The Political Context of Identity Negotiation

Identity negotiation is a historically constituted process. Processes such as colonization, globalization, and racial tensions are integral parts of the context of identity negotiation. Take colonization as an example: By the time of World War I, the European powers ruled over 85% of the rest of the globe. The world map has changed drastically since then, as the world order is reconstituted in response to the aftermath of the world wars, the civil and ethnic wars following them, and the collapse of the Communist Bloc. Many former colonies have

established national independence. However, the impact of colonization on cultural identity negotiation can still be felt in some neo-Colonial regions.

For example, Réunion, an island in the Indian Ocean, was uninhabited when the Portuguese discovered it in 1513. From the 17th to the 19th centuries, French immigration supplemented by Africans, Chinese, Malays, and Malabar Indians gave the island its ethnic mix. The plantation workers, many of whom were slaves, spoke different languages and were obliged to communicate through Creole, a linguistic intermediary easily understood by all. Gradually, Creole cemented relations between different ethnic components in the slave society; the Creole identity became a common identity built around the Creole language and bound together heterogeneous cultures. Today, "creolization" is used in cultural discourse to refer to the process whereby a human group attempts "to create a new local culture from the whole range of cultural resources available to the different components that together constitute a creolized society" (Medea, 2002, p. 127).

In 1946, Réunion entered the neo-Colonial era when the island became a French départment. Since then, the French government has implemented a series of assimilation policies emphasizing French culture and denying the worth of the Réunionese people's language, values, and culture. The cultural assimilation process was accompanied by the imposition of a globalized economy, dominated by the service sector, with its consequent focus on consumption, international finance, banks, and multinational corporations. These changes have rejuvenated the identity negotiation process on the island. For example, cultural movements to assert a distinctive Creole identity emerged (Medea, 2002), bringing around a continuous contestation of the global French culture and the local Creole culture.

In a multicultural environment, cultural clashes may lead to adoption of separatist strategies in identity management, whereas countries in the wake of severe racial antagonism may seek to replace exclusionist identities with an inclusive one. South Africa's social history provides a good illustration of both processes. After the South African government publicly admitted the failure of apartheid policies in 1989, an immediate issue was how to find a cultural identity that would promise unity and reconciliation after decades of racial tension and cultural clashes. Against this historical backdrop, South Africans rediscovered the biblical symbol of the rainbow to represent peaceful harmonization of different racial and cultural traditions. In 1994, Archbishop Desmond Tutu proclaimed proudly in a televised Thanksgiving service: "We are the rainbow people of God. We are free—all of us, black and white together!"

The rainbow people identity is both an inclusive identity and a political symbol, consciously crafted to achieve a political purpose. It is an identity defined by a peaceful union of diverse cultural and racial traditions. Survey research in South Africa revealed initial strong support for the rainbow people identity. In 1994, 65% of South Africans favored the rainbow people identity, but the percentage of supporters dropped to 48% in 1999. In 1996, 17% of South Africans considered the rainbow people identity a source of national pride, but the percentage dropped to 11% in 1999 (Dickow & Moller, 2002). The waning appeal of the rainbow people identity casts doubt on the efficacy of using an inclusive identity to manage diverse cultural groups in a multicultural nation.

Compared to the ethnic relations in South Africa, ethnic relations in the United States, albeit more subtle, are by no means less influential in shaping the course of multicultural identities negotiation. On the one hand, the widely held ideology of American culture being a "melting pot" has exerted pressure on ethnic minorities to assimilate into the American mainstream culture (see Hirschman, 1983). On the other hand, research has shown that ethnic/minority Americans are less likely than white Americans to be seen as full-fledged members of the society. For example, Devos and Banaji (2005) found that the category "American" is associated with being white for most white respondents. Similarly, Cheryan and Monin (2005) found that white American perceivers consider Asian American faces less American than white American faces. More important, the Asian Americans, made aware of this perception, may react to it by asserting their American identity. For instance, in one experiment (Cheryan & Monin, 2005, Study 5), a white experimenter subtly denied Asian American participants' American identity by telling them at the beginning of the experiment, "Actually, you have to be an American to be in this study." This manipulation led Asian American participants to exhibit behaviors that affirmed their American identity.

Many minority group members in the United States are sensitive to both the differentness and the disadvantageousness of their ethnic cultural tradition. Here is how a Vietnamese American informant in an ethnographic study expressed her frustration: "I have been here 18 years and if somebody had been to Viet Nam and spoke the language would think they knew that country well . . . [but] Americans still think of me as a foreigner" (Sparrow, 2000, p. 188). With the awareness of their differentness and disadvantageousness, some minority group members have sought to fit into the mainstream culture by developing a secondary cultural identity, as revealed in the report of another informant in the same ethnographic study: "As a result of all these differences and having been forced to adapt to this new culture, I have developed another cultural identity which is capable of surviving in this new environment. . . . This identity functions like a second personality that appears when it is necessary to adopt a culturally appropriate behavior in the new culture" (p. 192). The same themes of ethnocultural discrimination, the desire to preserve the heritage cultural tradition, consciousness of the benefits of biculturalism, and motivation for bicultural identity development also emerged in an ethnographic study of a Chinese community in Chicago (Lu, 2001).

For Japanese in Brazil, the turns of events in the global context changed their social status in Brazil and the way they managed their multicultural identities (Tsuda, 2001). Japanese migration to Brazil began at the beginning of the 20th century, when the Brazilian government decided that Japanese workers were technologically minded enough to work in Brazil's expanding coffee plantations. Encounters with the ethnically and culturally different Brazilians heightened the salience of the imported workers' Japanese identity.

The rise of Japan as a global imperial power in the 1930s fueled an anti-Japanese movement in Brazil. The tide of anti-Japanese sentiment rose as Japan entered World War II. In response to their negative minority status, some Japanese in Brazil began to adopt the majority cultural patterns in exchange for better acceptance into majority society. As a result, a synthetic bicultural identity known as Japanese Brazilian emerged and gained popularity among the Brazilian-born Japanese.

After World War II, Japan rapidly rose to the top of the global order to become the second largest economy in the world, thereby reversing the hierarchical relationship between Brazil and Japan on the global scale. As Japan rose in global prominence and prestige, Japanese Brazilians started to embrace their Japanese cultural heritage and distance themselves from the undesirable, underdeveloped aspects of Brazil's culture. The result has been a reaffirmation of their Japanese identity after decades of assimilative attempts to become more Brazilian.

Ironically, when the Brazilian economy crumbled in the 1980s, some Japanese Brazilians, attracted by the abundance of job opportunities, migrated to Japan, only to discover that they would be treated as "foreigners" in their "homeland." They were seen to have been "Brazilianized," and were socially and culturally marginalized. By immigrating to Japan, these Japanese Brazilians had subjected themselves to a new set of power relations and were obliged to participate in a new round of cultural identity negotiation (Tsuda, 2001).

In short, the cases described here illustrate the historical constitution of cultural identity. Each country or group has its unique social and political history, and has therefore followed a distinctive course of cultural identity development. The goal of the review in this section is not to delineate the universal principles that govern negotiation of cultural identities. On the contrary, our goal is to highlight the complexity of such negotiation processes, and how such processes may change course in response to the changing power relations in the society. Nonetheless, the examples reviewed here illustrate the multiplicity of cultural traditions represented in the mind of individuals in a globalized world, and the sociopolitical dimensions that underlie negotiations of multicultural identities. These are the two recurrent themes that have emerged from the rapidly expanding empirical literature we reviewed in previous sections.

CONCLUDING REMARKS

Hong et al. (2000) have proposed a dynamic constructivist approach to studying the influences of multiple cultures on individuals. At the heart of this approach is the idea that all individuals are capable of representing multiple cultures in their minds and switching between representations of cultures. As such, culture should not be seen as a static, monolithic entity. Instead, it should be understood as a collection of variably shared knowledge representations that people use to navigate the social world. Accordingly, culture should not be treated as synonymous with a demarcated population defined with respect to certain demographic, geographic, national, or ethnic characteristics. We acknowledge that meanings are unevenly distributed in different cultural groups, and that such uneven distribution of meanings may give rise to stable, meaningful, between-group differences (see review by Lehman, Chiu, & Schaller, 2004). However, the presence of such differences does not justify a reified and essentialist view of culture.

The dynamic constructivist approach conceptualizes the multicultural mind and multicultural identity as distinct but interrelated theoretical constructs. Acquisition of knowledge from a new culture does not always produce identification of that culture. Accordingly, although the global culture is spreading rapidly around the world, homogenization of cultures is not an inevitable outcome of globalization. Indeed, multiculturalism and globalization are likely to coexist.

The increased frequency and intensity of intercultural contacts will inevitably change the agenda of cultural-psychological research. On the one hand, knowledge of multiple cultures can be a valuable resource; individuals with a multicultural mind are equipped with several sets of interpretive tools to grasp experiences. We have reviewed how exposure to other cultures is linked to increased creativity and competence in intercultural interactions.

On the other hand, experiences with multiple cultures can also raise identity concerns, particularly in situations where individuals need to pledge their allegiance to one or the other cultures. The identity negotiation processes often take place amid the power relations in the society. There is a pressing need for cultural psychologists to address these processes as they redefine the intercultural and intergroup landscape in the coming decades.

NOTE

1. We endorse the view that culture consists of a network of loosely organized knowledge that is produced,

distributed, and reproduced among a collection of inter-connected individuals (Chiu & Chen, 2004; Shore, 1996; Sperber, 1996). According to Barth (2002), knowledge constitutes "all the ways of understanding that we use to make up our experienced, grasped reality" (p. 2), and includes all learned routines of thinking, feeling, and interacting with people.

REFERENCES

Alderson, A. S., & Nielsen, F. (2002). Globalization and the great U-turn: Income inequality trends in 16 OECD countries. *American Journal of Sociology, 107*, 1244–1299.

Anthias, F. (2001). New hybridities, old concepts: The limits of "culture." *Ethnic and Racial Studies, 24*, 619–641.

Appadurai, A. (1996). *Modernity at large: Cultural dimensions of globalization.* Minneapolis: University of Minnesota Press.

Barth, F. (2002). An anthropology of knowledge. *Current Anthropology, 43*, 1–18.

Benet-Martinez, V., & Haritatos, J. (2005). Bicultural Identity Integration (BII): Components and psychosocial antecedents. *Journal of Personality, 73*, 1015–1050.

Benet-Martinez, V., Leu, J., Lee, F., & Morris, M. W. (2002). Negotiating biculturalism: Cultural frame switching in biculturals with oppositional versus compatible cultural identities. *Journal of Cross-Cultural Psychology, 33*, 492–516.

Berry, J. W. (2001). A psychology of immigration. *Journal of Social Issues, 57*, 615–631.

Berry, J. W., & Sam, D. L. (1997). Acculturation and adaptation. In J. W. Berry, M. H. Segall, & C. Kağitçibaşi (Eds.), *Handbook of cross-cultural psychology: Vol. 3. Social behavior and applications* (2nd ed., pp. 291– 326). Boston: Allyn & Bacon.

Berry, J. W., Poortinga, Y. H., Segall, M. H., & Dasen, P. R. (1992). *Cross-cultural psychology: Research and applications.* Cambridge, UK: Cambridge University Press.

Birman, D. (1998). Biculturalism and perceived competence of Latino immigrant adolescents. *American Journal of Community Psychology, 26*, 335–354.

Bourhis, R. Y., & Giles, H. (1977). The language of intergroup distinctiveness. In H. Giles (Ed.), *Language, ethnicity and intergroup relations* (pp. 119–135). London: Academic Press.

Brewer, M. B., & Gardner, W. (1996). Who is this "we"?: Levels of collective identity and self representations. *Journal of Personality and Social Psychology, 71*, 83–93.

Camilleri, C., & Malewska-Peyre, H. (1997). Socialization and identity strategies. In J. W. Berry, P. R. Dasen, & T. S. Saraswathi (Eds.), *Handbook of cross-cultural psychology: Vol. 2. Basic processes and human development* (2nd ed., pp. 41–67). Boston: Allyn & Bacon.

Casmir, F. L. (1992). Third-culture building: A paradigm shift for international and intercultural communication. *Comunnication Yearbook, 16*, 407–428.

Castells, M. (1998). *The end of millennium.* Oxford, UK: Blackwell.

Chao, M., Chen, J., Roisman, G. I., & Hong, Y. (in press). Essentializing race: Implications for bicultural individuals' cognition and physiological reactivity. *Psychological Science.*

Cheryan, S., & Monin, B. (2005). "Where are you really from?": Asian Americans and identity denial. *Journal of Personality and Social Psychology, 89*, 717–730.

Chiu, C., & Chen, J. (2004). Symbols and interactions: Application of the CCC model to culture, language, and social identity. In S. H. Ng, C. Candlin, & C. Chiu (Eds.), *Proceedings of ICLASP8.* Hong Kong: City University of Hong Kong Press.

Chiu, C., & Hong, Y. (2005). Culture: Dynamic processes. In A. J. Elliot & C. S. Dweck (Eds.), *Handbook of competence and motivation* (pp. 489–505). New York: Guilford Press.

Cohen, D., & Gunz, A. (2002). As seen by the other . . . : Perspectives on the self in the memories and emotional perceptions of Easterners and Westerners. *Psychological Science, 13*, 55–59.

Devos, T., & Banaji, M. (2005). American = white? *Journal of Personality and Social Psychology, 88*(3), 447–466.

Dickow, H., & Moller, V. (2002). South Africa's "rainbow people," national pride and optimism: A trend study. *Social Indicators Research, 59*, 175–202.

DiMaggio, D. (1997). Culture cognition. *Annual Review of Sociology, 23*, 263–287.

Dunbar, E. (1994). The German executive in the U.S. work and social environment: Exploring role demands. *International Journal of Intercultural Relations, 18*, 277–291.

Earley, P. C. (2002). Redefining interactions across cultures and organizations: Moving forward with cultural intelligence. *Research in Organizational Behavior, 24*, 271–299.

Earley, P. C., & Ang, S. (2003). *Cultural intelligence: Individual interactions across cultures.* Stanford, CA: Stanford University Press.

Fischer, M. M. J. (1999). Emergent forms of life: Anthropologies of late or postmodernities. *Annual Review of Anthropology, 28*, 455–478.

Friedman, J. (1994). *Cultural identity and global process.* London: Sage.

Fu, J. H., & Chiu, C. (2003). *Studying cultures from a shorter distance: Change and maintenance of cultural values in multicultural environment.* Manuscript under review

Furnham, A., & Li, Y. H. (1993). The psychological adjustment of the Chinese community in Britain: A study of two generations. *British Journal of Psychiatry, 162*, 109–113.

Ganguly-Scrase, R. (2003). Paradoxes of globalization, liberalization, and gender equality: The worldviews of the lower middle class in West Bengal, India. *Gender and Society, 17,* 544–566.

Gardner, W. L., Gabriel, S., & Lee, A. (1999). "I" value freedom, but "we" value relationships: Self-construal priming mirrors cultural differences in judgment. *Psychological Science, 10,* 321–326.

Giddens, A. (1985). *The nation–state and violence.* Cambridge, UK: Polity Press.

Greenberg, J., Solomon, S., & Pyszczynski, T. (1997). Terror management theory of self-esteem and cultural worldview: Empirical assessments and conceptual refinements. In P. M. Zanna (Ed.), *Advances in experimental social psychology* (Vol. 29, pp. 61–141). San Diego: Academic Press.

Grosjean, F. (1989). Neurolinguists, beware!: The bilingual is not two monolinguals in one person. *Brain and Language, 36,* 3–15.

Halloran, M. J., & Kashima, E. S. (2004). Social identity and worldview validation: The effects of ingroup identity primes and mortality salience on value endorsement. *Personality and Social Psychology Bulletin, 30,* 915–925.

Hampton, J. A. (1997). Emergent attributes in combined concepts. In T. B. Ward, S. M. Smith, & J. Vaid (Eds.), *Creative thought: An investigation of conceptual structures and processes* (pp. 83–110). Washington, DC: American Psychological Association.

Han, S., & Shavitt, S. (1994). Persuasion and culture: Advertising appeals in individualistic and collectivistic societies. *Journal of Experimental Social Psychology, 30,* 326–350.

Haslam, S., Oakes, P. J., McGarty, C., Turner, J. C., & Onorato, R. S. (1995). Contextual changes in the prototypicality of extreme and moderate outgroup members. *European Journal of Social Psychology, 25,* 509–530.

Heine, S. J., Lehman, D. R., Markus, H., & Kitayama, S. (1999). Is there a universal need for positive self-regard? *Psychological Review, 106,* 766–794.

Hetts, J. J., Sakuma, M., & Pelham, B. W. (1999). Two roads to positive regard: Implicit and explicit self-evaluation and culture. *Journal of Experimental Social Psychology, 35,* 512–559.

Higgins, E. T. (1996). Knowledge activation: Accessibility, applicability and salience. In E. T. Higgins & A. E. Kruglanski (Eds.), *Social psychology: Handbook of basic principles* (pp. 133–168). New York: Guilford Press.

Higgins, E. T., Friedman, R. S., Harlow, R. E., Idson, L. C., Ayduk, O. N., & Taylor, A. (2001). Achievement orientations from subjective histories of success: Promotion pride versus prevention pride. *European Journal of Social Psychology, 31,* 3–23.

Hirschman, C. (1983). America's melting pot reconsidered. *Annual Review of Sociology, 9,* 397–423.

Ho, D. Y. F., & Chiu, C. (1994). Component ideas of individualism, collectivism, and social organization: An application in the study of Chinese culture. In U. Kim, H. C. Triandis, C. Kağitçibaşi, G. Choi, & G. Yoon (Eds.), *Individualism and collectivism: Theory,*

method and applications (pp. 137–156). Thousand Oaks, CA: Sage.

Hogg, M. A. (2001). A social identity theory of leadership. *Personality and Social Psychology Review, 5,* 184–200.

Hogg, M. A. (2003). Social identity. In M. R. Leary & J. P. Tangney (Eds.), *Handbook of self and identity* (pp. 462–479). New York: Guilford Press.

Hong, Y., Benet-Martinez, V., Chiu, C., & Morris, M. W. (2003). Boundaries of cultural influence: Construct activation as a mechanism for cultural differences in social perception. *Journal of Cross-Cultural Psychology, 34,* 453–464.

Hong, Y., Chiu, C., & Kung, T. M. (1997). Bringing culture out in front: Effects of cultural meaning system activation on social cognition. In K. Leung, Y. Kashima, U. Kim, & S. Yamaguchi (Eds.), *Progress in Asian social psychology* (Vol. 1, pp. 135–146). Singapore: Wiley.

Hong, Y., Morris, M. W., Chiu, C., & Benet-Martinez, V. (2000). Multicultural minds: A dynamic constructivist approach to culture and cognition. *American Psychologist, 55,* 709–720.

Hong, Y., Roisman, G. I., & Chen, J. (2006). A model of cultural attachment: A new approach for studying bicultural experience. In M. H. Bornstein & L. Cote (Eds.), *Acculturation and parent child relationships: Measurement and development* (pp. 135–170). Mahwah, NJ: Erlbaum.

Inglehart, R., & Baker, W. E. (2000). Modernization, cultural change, and the persistence of traditional values. *American Sociological Review, 65,* 19–51.

Ip, Y., Chen, J., & Chiu, C. (2003). *Intersubjective consensus on regulatory focus.* Unpublished raw data, University of Illinois, Urbana–Champaign.

Jetten, J., Postmes, T., & McAuliffe, B. (2002). "We're all individuals": Group norms of individualism and collectivism, levels of identification and identity threat. *European Journal of Social Psychology, 32,* 189–207.

Kanno, Y. (2003). *Negotiating bilingual and bicultural identities: Japanese returnees betwixt two worlds.* Mahwah, NJ: Erlbaum.

Kashima, E. S., Halloran, M. J., Yuki, M., & Kashima, Y. (2004). The effects of personal and collective mortality salience on individualism: Comparing Australians and Japanese with higher and lower self-esteem. *Journal of Experimental Social Psychology, 40,* 384–392.

Kashima, E. S., & Kashima, Y. (1998). Culture and language: The case of cultural dimensions and personal pronoun use. *Journal of Cross-Cultural Psychology, 29,* 461–486.

Kim, H. S., & Markus, H. R. (1999). Deviance or uniqueness, Harmony or conformity?: A cultural analysis. *Journal of Personality and Social Psychology, 77,* 785–800.

Kitayama, S., Duffy, S., Kawamura, T., & Larsen, J. T. (2003). Perceiving an object and its context in different cultures: A cultural look at New Look. *Psychological Science, 14,* 201–206.

LaFromboise, T., Coleman, H. L., & Gerton, J. (1993). Psychological impact of biculturalism: Evidence and theory. *Psychological Bulletin, 114*, 395–412.

Lal, D. (2000). Does modernization require Westernization? *Independent Review, 5*, 5–24.

Lau, I. Y., Chiu, C., & Lee, S.-L. (2001). Communication and shared reality: Implications for the psychological foundations of culture. *Social Cognition, 19*, 350–371.

Lau, I. Y., Lee, S.-L., & Chiu, C. (2004). Language, cognition and reality: Constructing shared meanings through communication. In M. Schaller & C. Crandall (Eds.), *The psychological foundations of culture* (pp. 77–100). Mahway, NJ: Erlbaum.

Lee, S.-L. (2002). *Communication and shared representation: The role of knowledge estimation.* Unpublished doctoral dissertation, University of Hong Kong, Hong Kong.

Lee, S., Sobal, J., & Frongillo, E. A. (2003). Comparison of models of acculturation: The case of Korean Americans. *Journal of Cross-Cultural Psychology, 34*, 282–296.

Lehman, D., Chiu, C., & Schaller, M. (2004). Culture and psychology. *Annual review of psychology.* Palo Alto, CA: Annual Reviews.

Leung, K. A., Chiu, C., & Hong, Y. (2003). *Communication and regulatory focus.* Unpublished raw data, University of Illinois, Urbana–Champaign.

Li, Q., & Hong, Y. (2001). Intergroup perceptual accuracy predicts real-life intergroup interactions. *Group Processes and Intergroup Relations, 4*, 341–354.

Lu, X. (2001). Bicultural identity development and Chinese community formation: An ethnographic study of Chinese schools in Chicago. *Howard Journal of Communications, 12*, 203–220.

Lukes, S. (1973). *Individualism.* Oxford, UK: Blackwell.

Lyons, A., & Kashima, Y. (2001). The reproduction of culture: Communication processes tend to maintain cultural stereotypes. *Social Cognition, 19*, 372–394.

Ma, V., & Schoeneman, T. J. (1997). Individualism versus collectivism: A comparison of Kenyan and American self-concepts. *Basic and Applied Social Psychology, 19*, 261–273.

Mahalingam, R. (2003). Essentialism, culture, and beliefs about gender among the Aravanis of Tamil Nadu, India. *Sex Roles, 49*, 489–496.

Mahalingam, R., & Rodriguez, J. (2003). Essentialism, power and cultural psychology of gender. *Journal of Cognition and Culture, 3*, 157–174.

Marques, J., Abrams, D., Paez, D., & Martinez-Taboada, C. (1998). The role of categorization and in-group norms in judgments of groups and their members. *Journal of Personality and Social Psychology, 75*, 976–988.

Marques, J., & Paez, D. (1994). The black sheep effect: Social categorization, rejection of ingroup deviates, and perception of group variability. In W. Stroebe & M. Hewstone (Eds.), *European review of psychology* (Vol. 5, pp. 37–68). New York: Wiley.

McAuliffe, B. J., Jetten, J., Hornsey, M., & Hogg, M. A. (2003). Individualist and collectivist norms: When it's ok to go your own way. *European Journal of Social Psychology, 33*, 57–70.

Medea, L. (2002). Creolisation and globalization in a neo-Colonial context: The case of reunion. *Social Identities, 8*, 125–141.

Menon, T., & Morris, M. W. (2001). Social structure in North American and Chinese cultures: Reciprocal influence between objective and subjective structures. *Journal of Psychology in Chinese Societies, 2*, 27–50.

Menon, T., Morris, M. W., Chiu, C., & Hong, Y. (1999). Culture and the construal of agency: Attribution to individual versus group dispositions. *Journal of Personality and Social Psychology, 76*, 701–717.

Miller, D. T., & Prentice, D. A. (1994). Collective errors and errors about the collective. *Journal of Personality and Social Psychology, 20*, 541–550.

Montreuil, A., & Bourhis, R. Y. (2001). Majority acculturation orientations toward "valued" and "devalued" immigrants. *Journal of Cross-Cultural Psychology, 32*, 698–719.

Ng, S. H., & Bradac, J. (1993). *Power is language: Vernal communication and social influence.* Newbury Park, CA: Sage.

Niemann, Y. F., Romero, A. J., Arredondo, J., & Rodriguez, V. (1999). What does it mean to be "Mexican"?: Social construction of an ethnic identity. *Hispanic Journal of Behavioral Sciences, 21*, 47–60.

No, S., & Hong, Y. (2004a, January). *Negotiating bicultural identity: Contrast and assimilation effects in cultural frame switching.* Poster presented at the annual conference of the Society for Personality and Social Psychology, Austin, TX.

No, S., & Hong, Y. (2004b, January). *Bicultural frame switching: Belief in race as fixed moderates minority reactivity toward cultural primes.* Poster presented at the annual conference of the American Psychological Society, Chicago, IL.

No, S., Wan, C., & Chiu, C. (2005). *Cultural hybridization among Chinese and Korean ethnics residing in the United States.* Unpublished raw data, University of Illinois, Urbana–Champaign.

Organista, P. B., Organista, K. C., & Kurasaki, K. (2002). The relationship between acculturation and ethnic minority mental health. In K. M. Chun, P. B. Organista, & G. Marin (Eds.), *Acculturation: Advances in theory, measurement, and applied research* (pp. 139–162). Washington, DC: American Psychological Association.

Oyserman, D. (1993). The lens of personhood: Viewing the self and others in a multicultural society. *Journal of Personality and Social Psychology, 65*, 993–1009.

Oyserman, D., Sakamoto, I., & Lauffer, A. (1998). Cultural accommodation: Hybridity and the framing of social obligation. *Journal of Personality and Social Psychology, 74*, 1606–1618.

Padilla, A. M., & Perez, W. (2003). Acculturation, social identity, and social cognition: A new perspective. *Hispanic Journal of Behavioral Sciences, 25*, 35–55.

Pang, C. L. (2000). *Negotiating identity in contemporary Japan: The case of Kikokushijo*. London: Kegan Paul.

Parameswaran, R. (2002). Local culture in global media: Excavating colonial and material discourses in National Geographic. *Communication Theory, 12,* 287–315.

Park, R. E. (1928). Human migration and the marginal man. *American Journal of Sociology, 33,* 881–893.

Phinney, J. S., & Devich-Navarro, M. (1997). Variations in bicultural identification among African American and Mexican American adolescents. *Journal of Research on Adolescence, 7,* 3–32.

Pinkley, R. L., & Northcraft, G. B. (1994). Conflict frames of reference: Implications for dispute processes and outcomes. *Academy of Management Journal, 37,* 193–205.

Rhee, E., Uleman, J. S., Lee, H. K., & Roman, R. J. (1995). Spontaneous self-descriptions and ethnic identities in individualistic and collectivistic cultures. *Journal of Personality and Social Psychology, 69,* 142–152.

Richmond, A. H. (2002). Globalization: Implications for immigrants and refugees. *Ethnic and Racial Studies, 25,* 707–727.

Robertson, R. (1992). *Globalization: Social theory and global culture*. London: Sage.

Robins, L. N., & Regier, D. A. (Eds.). (1991). *Psychiatric disorders in America: The epidemiologic catchment areas study*. New York: Free Press.

Roccas, S., & Brewer, M. (2002). Social identity complexity. *Personality and Social Psychology Review, 6,* 88–106.

Rogler, L. H., Cortes, D. E., & Malgady, R. G. (1991). Acculturation and mental health status among Hispanics: Convergence and new directions for research. *American Psychologist, 46,* 585–597.

Ross, M., Xun, W. Q. E., & Wilson, A. E. (2002). Language and the bicultural self. *Personality and Social Psychology Bulletin, 28,* 1040–1050.

Rudmin, F. W. (2003). Critical history of the acculturation psychology of assimilation, separation, integration, and marginalization. *Review of General Psychology, 7,* 3–37.

Ryder, A. G., Alden, L. E., & Paulhus, D. L. (2000). Is acculturation unidimensional or bidimensional?: A head-to-head comparison in the prediction of personality, self-identity, and adjustment. *Journal of Personality and Social Psychology, 79,* 49–65.

Salcedo, R, (2003). When the global meets the local at the mall. *American Behavioral Scientist, 46,* 1084–1103.

Sassen, S. (1998). *Globalization and its discontents: Essays on the new mobility of people and money*. New York: New Press.

Sechrist, G. B., & Stangor, C. (2001). Perceived consensus influences intergroup behavior and stereotype accessibility. *Journal of Personality & Social Psychology, 80,* 645–654.

Sedikides, C., & Brewer, M. B. (2001). Individual self, relational self, and collective self: Partner, opponents, or strangers? In C. Sedikides & M. B. Brewer (Eds.), *Individual self, relational self, collective self* (pp. 1–4). Ann Arbor, MI: Psychology Press.

Shore, B. (1996). *Culture in mind: Cognition, culture, and the problem of meaning*. New York: Oxford University Press.

Simonton, D. K. (1997). Foreign influence and national development: The impact of open milieus on Japanese civilization. *Journal of Personality and Social Psychology, 72,* 86–94.

Simonton, D. K. (2000). Creativity: Cognitive, personal, developmental, and social aspects. *American Psychologist, 55,* 151–158.

Sparrow, L. M. (2000). Beyond multicultural man: Complexities of identity. *International Journal of Intercultural Relations, 24,* 173–201.

Sperber, D. (1996). *Explaining culture: A naturalistic approach*. Cambridge, MA: Blackwell.

Sprott, J. E. (1994). "Symbolic ethnicity" and Alaska natives of mixed ancestry living in Anchorage: Enduring group or a sign of impending assimilation? *Human Organization, 53,* 311–322.

Suinn, R. M., Ahuna, C., & Khoo, G. (1992). The Suinn–Lew Asian Self-Identity Acculturation Scale: Concurrent and factorial validation. *Educational and Psychological Measurement, 52,* 1041–1046.

Sussman, N. M. (2000). The dynamic nature of cultural identity throughout cultural transitions: Why home is not so sweet. *Personality and Social Psychology Review, 4,* 355–373.

Takenaka, A. (1999). Transnational community and its ethnic consequences: The return migration and the transformation of ethnicity of Japanese Peruvians. *American Behavioral Scientist, 42,* 1459–1474.

Terry, D. J., & Hogg, M. J. (1996). Group norms and the attitude-behavior relationship: A role for group identification. *Personality and Social Psychology Bulletin, 22,* 776–793.

Terry, D. J., Hogg, M. A., & White, K. M. (1999). The theory of planned behaviour: Self-identity, social identity and group norms. *British Journal of Social Psychology, 38,* 225–244.

Thompson, C. J., & Arsel, Z. (2004). The Starbucks brandscape and consumers' (anticorporate) experiences of glocalization. *Journal of Consumer Research, 31,* 632–642.

Trafimow, D., Silverman, E. S., Fan, R. M.-T., & Law, J. S. F. (1997). The effects of language and priming on the relative accessibility of the private self and the collective self. *Journal of Cross-Cultural Psychology, 28,* 107–123.

Trafimow, D., Triandis, H. C., & Goto, S. G. (1991). Some tests of the distinction between the private self and the collective self. *Journal of Personality and Social Psychology, 60,* 649–655.

Tsai, J. L., Ying, Y., & Lee, P. A. (2000). The meaning of "being Chinese" and "being American: Variation among Chinese American young adults." *Journal of Cross-Cultural Psychology, 31,* 302–332.

Tsuda, T. (2001). When identities become modern: Japanese emigration to Brazil and the global contextualization of identity. *Ethnic and Racial Studies, 24,* 412–432.

Tsuda, T. (2003). *Strangers in the ethnic homeland: Japanese Brazilian return migration in transnational perspective.* New York: Columbia University Press.

Turner, J. C., Hogg, M., Oakes, P., Reicher, S., & Wetherell, M. (1987). *Rediscovering the social group: A self-categorization theory.* Oxford, UK: Blackwell.

Tzeng, O. C. S., & Henderson, M. M. (1999). Objective and subjective cultural relationships related to industrial modernization and social progress. *International Journal of Intercultural Relations, 23,* 411–445.

van Strien, P. J. (1997). The American "colonization" of northwest European social psychology after World War II. *Journal of the History of the Behavioral Sciences, 33,* 349–363.

Verkuyten, M., & de Wolf, A. (2002). Being, feeling and doing: Discourses and ethnic self-definitions among minority group members. *Culture and Psychology, 8,* 371–399.

Verkuyten, M., & Pouliasi, K. (2002). Biculturalism among older children: Cultural frame switching, attributions, self-identification, and attitudes. *Journal of Cross-Cultural Psychology, 33,* 596–609.

Wan, C., & Chiu, C. (2003). *Intersubjective consensus and person perception.* Unpublished raw data, University of Illinois, Urbana–Champaign.

Wan, C., & Chiu, C. (2005, January). *They think men and women are different, and I agree! The role of intersubjective consensus in gender identification.* Poster presented at the 6th annual meeting of the Society of Personality and Social Psychology, New Orleans, LA.

Wan, C., Chiu, C., Peng, S., & Tam, K. (in press). Measuring cultures through intersubjective norms: Implications for predicting relative identification with two or more cultures. *Journal of Cross-Cultural Psychology.*

Wan, C., Chiu, C., & Tam, K. (2005, May). *Who voted for Bush?: Intersubjective representations of what Republicans and Democrats like and dislike.* Hot Topic Talk at the 17th Annual Convention of American Psychological Society, Los Angeles, CA.

Wan, C., Chiu, C., Tam, K., Lee, S., Lau, I. Y., & Peng, S. (2007). Perceived cultural importance and actual self-importance of values in cultural identification. *Journal of Personality and Social Psychology, 92,* 337–354.

Wan, W. W., & Chiu, C. (2002). Effects of novel conceptual combination on creativity. *Journal of Creative Behavior, 36,* 227–240.

Wang, Q. (2001). Culture effects on adults' earliest childhood recollection and self-description: Implications for the relation between memory and the self. *Journal of Personality and Social Psychology, 81,* 220–233.

Ward, C., Bochner, S., & Furnham, A. (2001). *The psychology of culture shock* (2nd ed.). Philadelphia: Routledge.

Ward, C., & Searle, W. (1991). The impact of value discrepancies and cultural identity on psychological and sociocultural adjustment of sojourners. *International Journal of Intercultural Relations, 15,* 209–225.

Ward, T. B., Patterson, M. J., Sifonis, C. M., Dodds, R. A., & Saunders, K. N. (2002). The role of graded category structure in imaginative thought. *Memory and Cognition, 30,* 199–216.

Waters, M. C. (1990). *Ethnic options: Choosing identities in America.* Berkeley: University of California Press.

Weber, M. (1958). The Protestant ethic and the spirit of capitalism (T. Parsons, Trans.). New York: Scribner's. (Original work published 1904)

Wong, R. Y., & Hong, Y. (2005). Dynamic influences of culture on cooperation in the prisoner's dilemma. *Psychological Science, 16,* 429–434.

Wyer, R. S., & Srull, T. K. (1986). Human cognition in its social context. *Psychological Review, 93,* 322–359.

Yamada, A., & Singelis, T. M. (1999). Biculturalism and self-construal. *International Journal of Intercultural Relations, 23,* 697–709.

Zaharna, R. S. (1989). Self-shock: The double-binding challenge of identity. *International Journal of Intercultural Relations, 13,* 501–525.

CHAPTER 14

Cultural Psychology of Workways

JEFFREY SANCHEZ-BURKS
FIONA LEE

The domain of work constitutes a major portion of our lives. A study conducted by the Economic Policy Institute found that the average worker in the United States spends 1,900 hours a year, roughly a third of one's total waking hours, at work. Furthermore, the number of hours individuals spend at work has steadily increased in the United States (e.g., a typical person works 20 days more a year than 25 years ago; Linstedt, 2002; Wessel, 2003). This trend of increasing hours at work is also documented in the European Union, despite social and political efforts to resist such trends (Frost, 2005). These figures do not take into account working hours outside the office; with the proliferation of telecommunication technologies, it is not uncommon for people to handle work-related e-mails, paperwork, and phone calls at home, during their commute, or while on vacation (Barker, 1998). Given work's dominant claim on people's daily lives, understanding the cultural psychology of *workways* is critical to understanding the cultural psychology of social life. Workways describe a culture's signature pattern of workplace beliefs, mental models, and practices that embody a society's ideas about what is true, good, and efficient within the domain of work.

How much cultural variability is there in workways? Some have suggested that trends in business globalization may have reduced cross-cultural differences in workways; as a result of efforts by multinational corporations to standardize structures and tasks, as well as the large percentage of managers getting their training from U.S. business schools, or programs modeled after U.S. business schools (Hébert, 2005), cultural variance in workways in contemporary organizations is minimized and subsumed by the larger "business" culture. According to this view, the world of work increasingly serves as a "culture free or culture neutral zone" (Birnbaum-More & Wong, 1995).

However, these claims about the cultural universality of workways are not supported by recent empirical evidence showing that cultural differences are amplified rather than diminished in work contexts (e.g., Sanchez-Burks, 2002). As we describe later in this chapter, several studies have shown that East–West differences in relational attunement— sensitivity to social, emotional, and relational cues—are more prominent in work than in nonwork settings (Sanchez-Burks et al., 2003). Far from being culture neutral, workways remain deeply colored by the palette of historical, ideological, and sociocultural influences that operate in the larger societal context, and may well be a domain that amplifies these dynamics.

Research showing that cultural divides widen within the workplace can be problematic from a practical standpoint. Intercultural contact is often necessary at work, where fluent communication and coordination must occur in the face of deep-seated cultural differences. Within major U.S. cities, for instance, about one-fourth of the population was born in a foreign country (e.g., 36%, Los Angeles; 25%, Boston; 21%, Chicago, and about 11% of the U.S. population, or 26 million individuals; U.S. Bureau of the Census, 2000), such that most individuals have little choice but to interact with colleagues, suppliers, and customers of different cultural and ethnic backgrounds. Increases in cross-cultural contact at work also stem from the recent increase of multinational corporations; many large corporate mergers have united companies from different cultures (e.g., Daimler–Chrysler, Ericsson–GTE, Hitachi–GE), creating an environment where people from different cultures have to cooperate, communicate, and coordinate closely and effectively.

Indeed, there is general recognition by business researchers and practitioners that cultural differences in workways can create problems in job performance, that cultural differences are not well understood, and that they are difficult to manage. For example, the business press is rife with stories of successful managers assigned to an international post and failing spectacularly to replicate their success at home. Approximately 15–50% of managers assigned to work with colleagues abroad curtail their assignments because of an inability to manage cultural differences in interpersonal behaviors, such as receiving and giving feedback, communicating criticisms and differences in opinion, and expressing emotions at work (Bird, Heinbuch, Dunbar, & McNulty, 1993; Copeland & Griggs, 1985; Deshpande & Visweswaran, 1992; Eschbach, Parker, & Stoeberl, 2001; Tung, 1987). These failures of intercultural work directly affect businesses' bottom lines, with each failure costing an estimated $50,000 to $350,000 (Copeland & Griggs, 1985). From an applied perspective, there is tremendous interest in understanding how cross-cultural differences and dynamics

affect interpersonal processes in the workplace, as well as specific interventions organizations can enact to diminish problems and misunderstandings that arise from such differences.

In this chapter, we lay an initial groundwork for a cultural psychology of workways. In doing so, we draw from a variety of research in social, organizational, and cultural psychology—for example, studies examining workplace relational styles, dynamics of intercultural contact, managerial and organizational perceptions, and social networks—to discuss how these dynamics reflect on cultural theory and research. Attention is given to how work affects cross-cultural dynamics, as well as how cross-cultural dynamics affect work. To the extent that both culture and work are important sources of context for individuals, this chapter also has broader implications for understanding the relationship between the individual and the context.

The reviews included in this chapter are not exhaustive but are intended to highlight emerging characteristics of the cultural psychology of workways. These characteristics include (1) greater attention to historical, ideological, and sociocultural influences that create, maintain, and transform approaches to work; (2) a focus on the specific cognitive and behavioral mechanisms that produce cultural variation at work; and (3) increased emphasis on research that produces rich accounts of culture-specific workways. We begin by tracing historical accounts of culture and work.

LOOKING BACK: HISTORICAL PERSPECTIVE ON CULTURE AND WORK

The domain of culture and work is not a new to scholarly inquiry. The earliest written accounts of cultural variation, dating around the 6th century B.C., describe the unique social patterns of merchants as they traded along the shores of the Black Sea, and how the diversity of cultural practices affected this work (Ascherson, 1996; Herodotus, 2003). Similarly, the emergence of unique workways was one of the defining features of early America (Crèvecoeur, 1782/1981; de Tocqueville, 1840/1990). Historically, accounts of culture and work have been characterized by two constant and defining themes that remain central to the cultural psychology of workways: attempts to understand how cultural beliefs shape the context of work, and how the context of work influences cultural beliefs (Fiske, Kitayama, Markus, & Nisbett, 1998).

Debates over Influence of Structure versus Beliefs

Work played a dominant role in the 19th-century debates about the influence of "macro" social–organizational structures on beliefs (Marx, 1873/1992) versus the influence of "micro" beliefs on social–organizational structures (Weber, 1904/1930). For Karl Marx, the structural conditions of the workplace produced particular psychological states (e.g., alienation) that form the basis of sociocultural worldviews and workways. Although Max Weber did not directly disagree with this perspective, he argued that prevailing cultural ideologies played a key role in creating culturally unique workways. For example, he argued that the early (17th and 18th centuries) Calvinists believed that work was part of a religious calling and was valuable in its own right, that idle talk and sociability was distracting to one's work duties, and that individuals ought to maintain an unsentimental impersonality at work (Bendix, 1977; Fischer, 1989; Landes, 2000). In cultures influenced by this theology, such as the United States, these beliefs about work were secularized and incorporated in the contemporary culture, so that attitudes such as valuing work in and of itself, relying on the self, and limiting personal indulgences are not merely representative of Calvinist Protestants but largely descriptive of Americans as a whole (Furnham, 1990; Lenski, 1961).

Causal evidence of this mutual constitution of context and mind was convincingly provided through a series of influential studies carried out a century later by sociologists Kohn and Schooler (1983). Supporting the influence of social structure on psychology (e.g., Marx, 1873/1992; Whyte, 1956), their studies showed that features of one's occupational context (e.g., the relative complexity of one's job and the degree of self-direction in organizing tasks) have a direct influence on people's beliefs and behaviors that extends beyond the closing workday's whistle. Moreover, they provided evidence of a reverse causal path whereby individual-level cognitions and personality characteristics shape the conditions of work (particularly over extended periods of time), suggesting that psychology also influences social structures (e.g., Bellah, Madsen, Sullivan,

Swidler, & Tipton, 1996; McClelland, 1961; Weber, 1904/1930).

Sociocultural History in Cultural Theory

Early studies on culture and work typically focused on a society's social history, describing how historical practices and ideologies sowed the seeds for contemporary cultural patterns. Similar to the notion of path-dependence used by economists (e.g., Arthur, 1994), the origins of contemporary cultural workways were traced to prior social-historical events or conditions rather than to factors in the immediate, current environment (for reviews see Arthur, 1994). This, of course, was central to Weber's (1904/1930) thesis on the Protestant work ethic (PWE); as mentioned earlier, Weber traced beliefs in the United States about the value of work, limits to self-indulgences, and self-reliance to the ideologies of the founding Calvinist communities in 17th-century New England. Other studies showed how sociocultural practices perpetuated these culturally unique belief systems through the generations. For example, Winterbottom (1953) compared the child-rearing practices of Protestant and Catholic mothers in the United States and found that Protestant mothers spent more time communicating PWE values and motivations (cf. McClelland, 1961), and introduced them at earlier ages in their child's development.

As a matter of historical coincidence, a different movement around the same period introduced a similar notion of hard work as moral imperative in Japan. Robert Bellah (1957) argued that early religious beliefs during the Tokugawa period (1600–1868) in Japan left a lasting imprint on contemporary Japanese workways. Particularly, Bellah showed that early doctrines of Buddhism, Confucianism, and Shintoism encouraged ways of thinking that underlie Japan's contemporary economic and industrial development. For instance, early cultural emphasis on the family fostered the emergence of many small, family-owned enterprises. Similar to development of the PWE in the United States, secular and religious beliefs mutually influenced each other. On the one hand, religious values that placed political and family leaders in the realm of the "divine" encouraged compliance to government policies and interventions directed to spur industrialization. On the other hand, hard work and self-sacrifice were viewed as ways to achieve religious enlightenment. As Bellah (1985) argued, the central value system that developed in the Tokugawa period remains influential in contemporary secular Japanese culture, perhaps in a more intense form.

The lasting effects of social history on culturally unique workways extend beyond moral imperatives toward hard work and self-sacrifice. For example, Schooler (1976) found that cultural variations in self-direction and authority orientation in the workplace could be predicted by when a cultural group's ancestral country abolished serfdom and hence changed the "macro" work context (e.g., England in 1603, German states in 1815, Poland in 1861). This trend was observed after controlling for social class, occupation, and religion. In other words, contemporary cultural differences in workways reflected sociocultural conditions generations ago. These studies demonstrate the importance of investigating the influence of a group's prior social-historical conditions on the development and availability of specific psychological beliefs and attitudes.

The Study That Spawned a Movement: Hofstede at IBM

The spark that ignited a widespread interest in culture and work was a multinational survey study of IBM employees (Hofstede, 1980). By focusing on self-reported preferences for work-related characteristics, Hofstede sidestepped complex issues regarding the role of social-historical conditions, ideology, or the mutual influence of context and mind in constituting cultural workways. Hofstede proposed that national cultures vary along four dimensions: (1) *power distance*, or an individual's preference for equality–inequality between individuals in a group; (2) *uncertainty avoidance*, or an individual's preference for structure; (3) *masculinity/femininity*, or an individual's prevalence for assertiveness, performance, success, and competition (masculinity) versus quality of life, warm personal relations, service, care for the weak, and solidarity (femininity); and (4) *individualism versus collectivism*, or an individual's preference for acting as an individual or acting in a group.

Of course, these dimensions did not originate with the publication of Hofstede's *culture's consequences*; themes about individual versus community or equality versus inequality

were discussed much earlier by many social scientists (e.g., Durkheim, 1933; Mead, 1967; Parsons, Bales, & Shils, 1953; Reisman, 1961; Whyte, 1956; Tönnies, 1887/2002; Kluckhohn & Strodtbeck, 1961). Hofstede's study, however, launched a widespread research interest in cross-cultural industrial–organizational psychology (for excellent reviews, see Hui & Luk; 1997; Earley & Gibson, 1998). Furthermore, despite the study's exclusive focus on work settings, Hofstede's dimensions of culture became a dominant framework for understanding cross-cultural differences across virtually all settings, work and nonwork alike.

(Back) Toward a Cultural Psychology of Workways

Despite decades of research focusing on cultural variation along broad value dimensions such as individualism–collectivism or power distance, there is a paucity of valid, reliable evidence that these dimensions can explain (i.e., mediate or moderate) distinct psychological or behavioral outcomes (Briley & Wyer, 2001; Earley & Mosakowski, 2002; Heine, Lehman, Peng, & Greenholtz, 2002; Takano & Osaka, 1999; but see Earley, 1989, for an exception). More recently, cultural scholars have focused on the specific cognitive structures and processes that guide behavior (Morris & Young, 2002), and linking these cognitions to social-historical and contextual features unique to a cultural group (Sanchez-Burks, 2002). This strategy of combining methodological advances in social-cognitive psychology with the rich social-historical approach of earlier cultural psychology has developed more precise, richer models of cultural workways. Specifically, this involves taking into account the role of context, as well as specific mental schemas, and mapping out the conditions under which one expects both cultural differences and similarities. We review examples of this work in subsequent sections of this chapter.

WORKPLACE RELATIONAL STYLES

Culturally Specific Workplace Relational Styles

Although the majority of cross-cultural psychology emphasizes cultural comparisons, examining how two or more cultures differ along any number of variables, one prevailing stream of research in cross-cultural psychology of work has examined culturally indigenous or culturally unique workplace relational styles. "Workplace relational styles" refer to people's beliefs about the function of relationships in the workplace, as well as relational behaviors at work (e.g., communicating with others, attending to another person's needs). This more anthropological approach of examining, in depth, unique patterns of interpersonal relating within a single culture has identified a number of culturally specific workplace relational styles that reflect deep-seated ideologies about the nature of social–emotional ties within and across work domains (e.g., Ayman & Chemers, 1983; Diaz-Guerrero, 1967; Earley, 1997; Markus & Kitayama, 1991; Triandis, Marin, Liansky, & Betancourt, 1984).

Chaebol

Organizational research within South Korea suggests that work relations are modeled after the tradition of *chaebol*, or "company familism" (Kim, 1988). Here, work relationships are not unlike family relationships. Managers or work supervisors play a paternal role in relation to their subordinates (Hui & Luk, 1997). In this way, work organizations are typically a network of tight-knit, highly personal relationships. Variations of *chaebol* can be found in other Asian cultures, such as Japan and India (Hui, Eastman, & Yee, 1995; Kanungo, 1990; Kool & Saksena, 1988; Sinha, 1980). Managers in these cultures take care to learn about the personal lives of their subordinates; attend the "personal" events of employees, such as a relative's funeral; and actively intervene on behalf of their employees in personal affairs, such as marital problems or family finances (Triandis, Dunnette, & Hough, 1994). Similarly, an employee's sense of obligation to his or her boss extends beyond the boundaries of the office or workday. Subordinates are expected to assist their bosses at work, but the boss should expect the subordinate similarly to provide assistance outside of work, and for non-work-related tasks such as household chores or assisting in family events (Hampden-Turner & Trompenaars, 1993).

Guanxi

In Chinese organizations, business relations are characterized by a distinct emphasis on building dense networks of personal relationships.

Entrepreneurs conduct their business by developing *you-yi*, or deep friendships based on mutual obligation in which business people make connections in their social networks available to one another (Solomon, 1999; Wall, 1990). This Chinese system of dense networks, or *guanxi*, differs from networking in Western businesses because of its transitive nature (Cai, 2001; Farh, Tsui, Xin, & Cheng, 1998; Li, Tsui, & Weldon, 2000). Whereas a French businessperson interested in connecting with a target person in a fellow French colleague's network might typically ask the colleague to facilitate such a connection, a Chinese operating under the principle of *guanxi* would assume that he or she has direct access to any person in the colleague's network. Thus, more than using common network ties as a way to create familiarity and a base for generating goodwill, *guanxi* describes the transitive nature of obligations in Chinese business practices.

Guanxi also influences preferences for business partners. For example, rather than making business decisions based on "objective" measures, such as price, product quality, or technical skills, it would not be uncommon for a Chinese businessperson to do business with another person more because he or she comes from the same village or has a mutual acquaintance. These social "contracts" are seen as reassurances that a business partner will indeed be reliable and trustworthy (Sanchez-Burks, 2005). For many Asians, establishing *guanxi* is an essential condition to an effective working relationship (Hampden-Turner & Trompenaars, 1993).

Simpatía

Like most other relationships, work relations in Latin cultures are guided by the relational script of *simpatía* (Diaz-Guerrero, 1967; Triandis et al., 1984). Similar to many East Asian cultures, *simpatía* emphasizes social harmony, such that respecting and understanding others' feelings is valued above all, and conflict is minimized (Markus & Lin, 1999). Unlike many East Asian cultures, *simpatía* also emphasizes the expressive displays of personal charm, graciousness, and hospitality—even to those outside one's personal networks (Diaz-Guerrero, 1967; Lindsley & Braithwaite, 1996; Sanchez-Burks, Nisbett, & Ybarra, 2000). *Simpatía* is a valued characteristic in many Latin cultures, even within the workplace. For example, within Italy, it is has been found to be a necessary (though not sufficient) prerequisite to leadership (Dechert, 1961).

Protestant Relational Ideology

Although the culture-specific relational styles reviewed thus far—*chaebol*, *guanxi*, and *simpatía*—all suggest a heightened emphasis on relationships at the workplace, research on American workways shows a different pattern. Specifically, American workways are guided by *Protestant relational ideology* (PRI), an ideology that combines Lutheran teachings about the importance of work with Calvinist imperatives for restricting relational, social–emotional concerns while working (Sanchez-Burks, 2002). As put in practice by the early Calvinists, these restrictions were relaxed outside of work such that paying attention to others' social–emotional cues was considered entirely appropriate at play and leisure (Daniels, 1995; Fischer, 1989). Thus, PRI is characterized by a divide in relational attunement, or attention to affective issues and relational concerns, between work and nonwork contexts (Bendix, 1977; Lenski, 1961). Specifically, relational attunement among Americans is reduced in work settings compared to social, nonwork settings (Sanchez-Burks, 2005).

The social-historical origins of PRI were demonstrated in an experiment comparing levels of relational attunement in work versus nonwork settings between two American samples with highly similar demographic profiles (socioeconomic background, educational background, religiosity) but differed in whether their religious upbringing was connected to PRI (Protestant) or not (non-Protestant) (Sanchez-Burks, 2002, Study 1). Participants were primed for either a work context or a nonwork context, then performed an "emotional Stroop test" in which they heard positively or negatively valenced words read in an affect-appropriate tone (e.g., a sad voice for funeral) or an affect-inappropriate tone (e.g., a sad voice for wedding). Participants had to identify the semantic valence (good–bad) of each word and ignore the emotional tone of the spoken word. When primed for the nonwork context, emotional tone of voice equally confused both Protestant and non-Protestant groups (i.e., when the tone was affect-inappropriate, participants took longer to identify the semantic valence of the word). How-

ever, when primed for the work context, emotional tone of voice had significantly less effect for the Protestants compared to the non-Protestant participants; the Protestant participants were better at blocking out emotional content, but only in the work context. It appears that Protestant and non-Protestant Americans had different workplace relational styles: Whereas the non-Protestants attended to emotional content in both work and nonwork contexts, Protestants limited their processing of emotional cues in the work context only.

This pattern was replicated in a study that examined levels of nonconscious behavioral mirroring, a behavior that reflects attention to another person in the relationship (Sanchez-Burks, 2002, Study 2). Participants with a Calvinist religious upbringing did not engage in nonconscious mirroring of another person when primed with a work context. However, non-Calvinist participants in work and nonwork contexts, as well as Calvinist participants in nonwork contexts, all showed higher levels of mirroring. Again, being at work or in a work relationship appears to reduce relational attunement and sensitivity for Americans raised in a Calvinist tradition. Though secular American culture in general is strongly affected by Calvinistic teachings (Bendix, 1977; Daniels, 1995; Fischer, 1989; Lenski, 1961), these studies show that the influence of PRI on workways seems particularly pronounced for those raised in this religious tradition.

Culturally Indigenous Workplace Relational Styles: A Summary

Taken together, research on workplace relational styles shows tremendous diversity in the mental models people use to navigate and manage relationships in the workplace. Some workplace relational styles, such as *chaebol*, *guanxi*, or *simpatía*, rely on a heightened sensitivity to interpersonal relationships in the workplace. In cultures where these workplace relational styles are dominant, being at work often may require attention on two foci—the task at hand (e.g., the budgetary implications of a proposal being presented by a coworker) and the relational dimension of the social interaction (e.g., coworkers' nonverbal gestures that unfold while they describe the proposal). Of course, this heightened relational attunement serves only as a basic building block upon which such diverse forms of workways as *chaebol* or *simpatía* are possible.

In contrast to these work patterns based on heightened relational attunement, American workways appear as an exception, characterized in part by a relational style in which affective and relational concerns are less carefully monitored and are given diminished importance. As we describe in the next section, this pattern of behavior is specific to work. Outside work, Americans are just as attentive to social–emotional cues as East Asians. This moderating role of context highlights both cultural differences and cultural similarities in workways.

It is important to note that workplace relational patterns are reflected in variables across multiple levels of analysis, from cognitions to behaviors to social network structures. For example, *chaebol* describes family-like relationships in the workplace, *guanxi* is about the use of informal relationships at work, *simpatía* emphasizes display of and attention to subtle relational and social–emotional cues at work, and PRI is about the separation of work and nonwork relationships. In the next section, we turn to research describing workplace communication and feedback, dynamics that further reflect cultural workways in general, and cultural variation in workplace relational attunement in particular.

Relational Attunement and Indirectness in Workplace Communication

"Relational attunement," or attention to affective issues and relational concerns, is often examined in the context of communication. Specifically, people's awareness and comprehension of subtle or indirect cues in interpersonal communication are often used as an indicator of relational attunement (Earley, 1997; Holtgraves & Yang, 1992; Ting-Toomey, 1988). Grice (1968) differentiated between "sentence meaning," which refers to the literal or semantic meaning of an utterance, and "speaker meaning," which refers to what the speaker intends to accomplish with the remark. Relational attunement can be seen as sensitivity to discrepancies between sentence and speaker meaning.

From the speaker's point of view, relational attunement can be defined as the speaker's intention to do more than merely transmit the literal or sentence meaning of the words exchanged (Grice, 1968). Indeed, speakers can use a wide variety of subtle communication cues to transmit indirect meaning (Brown & Levinson, 1987; Goffman, 1959). For example, one can convey criticism of a colleague's work by avoiding eye contact (nonverbal), offering faint praise (verbal indirect meaning), or using a critical tone of voice (verbal emotion; Ambady, Koo, Lee, & Rosenthal, 1996; Lee, 1993; Goffman, 1967). Similarly, relational attunement can be used by speakers with more malevolent or devious intentions, for example, in the form of subtle sarcasms that protect one from accountability for negative remarks (DePaulo & Kashy, 1998).

From the listener's point of view, relational attunement can be understood as the listener's awareness of and attention to subtle communication cues to infer speaker meaning. Imagine a man talking to a colleague about his new supervisor. He mentions that she seems nice and fair. His colleague laughs, shrugs his shoulders, and says, "Well, yes, I suppose she *is* nice and fair. Best of luck to you." If the listener is relationally attuned, he or she will be able to "read between the lines" and likely conclude from the colleague's verbal tone and gestures that the new supervisor is probably a very difficult boss. In contrast, if the listener is not relationally attuned, he is less likely to use and attend to subtle communication cues, more likely to expect themselves and others to communicate more directly or "say it as it is," and only attend to the explicit meaning of what is said (Holtgraves, 1997). Using this example, the listener is likely to infer from the colleague's statement that the new supervisor is indeed a nice and fair person.

Avoiding misunderstanding therefore requires that communicators have similar levels of relational attunement. For example, if the colleague is using indirect cues and nonverbal gestures to convey his message that the new supervisor is a difficult boss, but the listener assumes that the comments can be interpreted literally, misunderstandings can occur (Brown & Levinson, 1987; Earley, 1997; Lee, 1993; Prentice & Miller, 1999). We next describe cultural research on relational attunement, focusing on studies of indirect communication and nonverbal communication at work.

Indirectness

One common assumption is that East Asians are more indirect in their communication than

Westerners. Because East Asians are presumably more attentive to maintaining face for others, they are more likely to "couch" the meanings of their words with subtle verbal and nonverbal cues, and to pay attention to these cues in interpreting others' speech (Earley, 1997; Lee, 1993, 1999; Ting-Toomey, 1988). However, recent studies on indirectness suggest this may not always be the case. Sanchez-Burks et al. (2003) used self-report and implicit measures of indirectness to compare managers in the United States, China, Korea, and Singapore. The self-report measure was a modified version of Holtgrave's (1997) indirectness questionnaire, in which respondents indicated their use of indirect cues in communication within work and outside of work. The behavioral measure of indirectness asked respondents to interpret the meaning of a message communicated between either two friends or two coworkers; here, indirectness refers to going beyond sentence meaning to infer speaker meaning.

The study found the expected cultural difference in indirectness in work settings; Chinese and Koreans managers were more indirect (both as speakers and as listeners) than their American counterparts at work. For example, when asked to interpret the performance feedback, "There is room for improvement but overall this is good," East Asian managers were more likely to infer that this message was feedback given for relatively poor performance, whereas American managers did not go beyond the explicit meaning of the message and inferred that this message conveyed a relatively positive assessment. However, no reliable cultural differences in indirectness were found outside work settings. For example, when asked to interpret the same message framed as a discussion between two friends about a personality test, American managers were just as indirect as East Asian managers (see Figure 14.1).

According to the dynamic constructivist perspective of culture (Hong, Morris, Chiu, & Benet-Martinez, 2000), cultural interpretive frames or schemas guide behaviors only when they come to the foreground (i.e., become available, salient, and applicable) in the individual's mind. In this sense, cultural differences are dynamic and context-dependent. Consistent with this perspective, cultural differences in indirectness vary depending on the contextual cues that make different relational styles

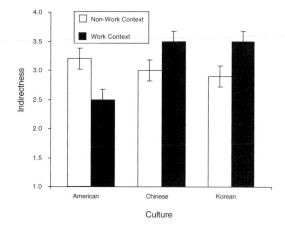

FIGURE 14.1. Indirectness as a function of context and participant's culture. Adapted from Sanchez-Burks et al. (2003). Copyright 2003 by the American Psychological Association. Adapted by permission.

more or less accessible. Within the context of work, American managers activate a particular relational schema that diverges from that of their East Asian counterparts. However, outside the context of work, American and East Asian managers adopt similar relational schemas in their use of indirectness.

Nonlinguistic Cues

We found similar moderating effects of context in research on nonverbal communication at work. Ambady et al. (1996) compared how Korean and American managers use nonlinguistic cues in their workplace communications. American and Korean managers were videotaped communicating good news (getting an unexpected bonus) or bad news (losing an expected bonus) to either a boss, a peer, or a subordinate. Content-filtered versions of these videos were rated by Korean or American coders for use of nonlinguistic cues.

The results showed that, compared to Americans, Korean managers were more sensitive to the hierarchical nature of the relationship and modified their use of nonlinguistic cues as a function of this relationship. For example, Korean managers were rated as using more nonlinguistic cues when the listener was higher in status; they were more likely to exhibit nonlinguistic cues that communicated other-enhancement, affiliation, and self-deference when communicating to a boss than to a peer or a subordinate. In contrast, American managers did not vary their use of nonlinguistic cues to bosses, peers, or subordinates. However, American managers were influenced by the content of the message, using more nonlinguistic cues when communicating bad news than good news. Korean managers, on the other hand, did not vary their use of nonlinguistic cues based on the content of the message. Overall, the results demonstrated that Korean managers showed higher levels of relational attunement than American managers in hierarchical situations, whereas the reverse was true when the content of the message was particularly negative.

Although this study only examined within-culture communication (the raters of nonlinguistic cues were from the same culture as the managers who produced the cues), the observed cultural difference can be a source of misunderstanding and misinterpretation in the workplace. For example, when Korean speakers use a lot of nonlinguistic cues to signal the higher status of the listener, American listeners might mistakenly interpret these cues to mean the content of the message is extremely negative. Or when American speakers use a lot of nonlinguistic cues to signal extreme criticism, the Korean listener might mistakenly interpret these cues to reflect merely the listener's relative status, rather than as a signal for the severity of the situation.

Relational Attunement at Work: A Summary

Relational attunement is of critical concern in the multicultural workplace. As mentioned, when speakers and listeners have different norms of relational attunement, misunderstandings and misinterpretations of information can easily occur. The research evidence we have reviewed shows that cultural influences in relational attunement are complex; specifically, culture interacts with context in different ways to influence relational attunement. Cultural differences in relational attunement can be more apparent in some situations than in others (e.g., in work vs. nonwork contexts, or when transmitting good vs. bad news), or more apparent in some relationships than in others (e.g., in hierarchical relationships).

This raises several implications. First, though cultural *differences* have been the focus of much cultural theory and research, these studies also highlight cultural *similarities*, describing contexts and situations in which people from different cultures do not behave differently from one another. These complex interaction effects between culture and context are all too often overlooked in efforts to array cultures along broad value dimensions. Second, the nature of these cultural patterns and interactions appears better explained by specific psychological mechanisms—deep-seated beliefs and cognitive processes—that are not always accessible to participants. This idea that internal cognitive or affective systems are differentially brought to the fore as situational cues change is similar to other conceptions of how personality differences are moderated by context (Mischel & Shoda, 1995). Third, this work has particular relevance for practice. To the extent that work often requires effective communication between people of different cultural backgrounds, it is critical to understand the conditions in which discrepancies in relational attunement are especially large. This concern with managing and minimizing problems in intercultural interpersonal contact is particularly salient when considering issues of diversity, to which we turn our attention next.

MANAGING DEMOGRAPHIC AND CULTURAL DIVERSITY

Diversity is a large topic of research in the organizational and management literature (for a review, see Williams & O'Reilly, 1998). Diversity, as it has been studied, relates to issues around the management of demographic differences—to what happens when people of different gender, nationality, age, functional expertise, education, tenure, religion, and ethnicity relate to one another in the context of work. Although psychologists have long tackled this problem by focusing on issues such as prejudice, stereotyping, and discrimination, organizational researchers also are interested in the question of whether demographic diversity leads to better outcomes (Chatman, Polzer, Barsade, & Neale, 1998).

There are many reasons why a demographically diverse workforce might enhance work-related effectiveness and productivity. Given the increasingly diverse marketplace—both globally and locally—firms must be able to sell to different types of customers and work with different types of vendors to remain competitive in the long run. Firms that have a diverse workforce are presumably better able to take advantage of the opportunities of the global marketplace and thrive (Williams & O'Reilly, 1998). A related argument suggests that work units—firms or teams—that bring together different opinions, perspectives, backgrounds, and expertise are more likely to generate creative and innovative ideas, which are critical for long-term survival and success of the firm (e.g., Jehn, Northcraft, & Neale, 1999; Lau & Murninghan, 1998).

However, the evidence that demographic diversity leads to more effective work performance has been, at best, mixed. Though demographic diversity can enhance task effectiveness in complex environments—as diversity brings about more approaches, perspectives, and opinions—it also increases emotional conflict within the work unit (Brief, 2000). Indeed, extensive research on intergroup dynamics suggests that mere contact between groups often gives rise to adverse dynamics such as implicit and explicit ethnocentrism, outgroup stereotyping, and intergroup hostility (R. Brown, 1986). The increase in interpersonal and social conflict that results from demographic diversity tends to undermine task effectiveness (Jehn, 1995), and this does not abate until the minority group reaches a critical mass (e.g., in traditionally male professions when women represent close to 50% of the work unit; Allmendinger & Hackman, 1995). Although the potential promise of demographic diversity has not been borne out by research, several streams of research on cultural workways suggest a new approach to defining and theorizing about diversity.

Demographic and Work Styles Diversity

The research literature on diversity most commonly focuses on the demographic features of individuals (e.g., ethnicity, nationality, age, gender) as the source of interpersonal difference and, therefore, conflict. An implicit assumption in this literature is that people's category membership is the primary form of diversity at the workplace. This focus, unfortunately, overlooks another potentially more important form of difference, namely, cultural variations in the mental models and relational styles people bring to the workplace. Organizational researchers have focused on differences in observable demographic characteristics, with little attention to the substantive differ-

ences that lie underneath them, whereas cultural psychologists have generated rich theory and empirical data on cultural variations that could make a difference in the workplace.

Work Team and Coworker Preferences

Recent research on work team preferences has taken initial steps to bridge these streams of work. Social and organizational psychologists have argued that ingroup biases stemming from a social categorization process create a preference, when given the choice, to work with others who have similar category membership (e.g., functional background, age group, nationality, gender, ethnicity; Pelled, 1996; Chatman et al., 1998; Williams & O'Reilly, 1998). For example, provided the opportunity to choose between an Anglo or a Latino workgroup, an Anglo worker is more likely to choose the Anglo workgroup.

However, surface-level demographic characteristics are confounded with culturally specific relational schemas; for example, people's cognitions and behaviors about appropriate relational behaviors at work tend to reflect their cultural or ethnic group memberships. In a study that disentangled these relative influence, Sanchez-Burks et al. (2000) asked participants to choose between two groups—an ethnic ingroup that exhibited a work style of an ethnic outgroup, and an ethnic outgroup that exhibited a work style of an ethnic ingroup. The results showed that 85% of participants showed a preference for the ethnic outgroup. In other words, similarity in working style was far more important than similarity in ethnicity per se in choosing teams and coworkers.

This finding suggests that preference for one's own ethnicity actually might reflect a preference for a certain culturally bound work style. It may be difficult to assess in actual work settings, however, whether a discriminatory action against an outgroup member reflects an ethnic bias or a working style bias. Nonetheless, to the extent people automatically infer a particular working style (or any other characteristic) simply based on another person's ethnicity, the consequences of both types of prejudice are similarly insidious.

The idea that working style, rather than ethnicity, is a more powerful shaper of people's decisions about what team to join or with whom to work can offer a different approach to reducing prejudice and discrimination. Focusing too narrowly on demographic characteristics as the source of minority disadvantage runs the risk of missing the underlying mechanism of the prejudicial behavior (i.e., working style incongruence). If given substantive information about other people's work styles, observers may be less likely to rely on demographic categories such as ethnicity as a heuristic to infer work styles, and thus less likely to rely on these demographic categories to guide their preferences and choices of teams and colleagues (e.g., Sanchez-Burks et al., 2000).

Implications for Mentor–Protégé Relationships

In addition to work team and coworker preference, diversity also has implications for mentor–protégé relationships. According to research on leader–member exchange theory (Graen, Novak, & Sommerkamp, 1982; Paglis & Green, 2002; Sherony & Green, 2002), superiors rather quickly identify subordinates with whom they will form informal mentoring relationships. Demographic biases have been shown to have an important role in these decisions, often to the detriment of minority demographic groups (e.g., Pelled & Xin, 1997). In the United States, for example, male managers tend to form mentoring relationships with male rather than female protégés, or white managers tend to form mentoring relationships with white rather than nonwhite protégés (Thomas, 1993). Given that mentoring relationships are considered an essential resource for climbing the corporate ladder, many scholars and practitioners have suggested that women and ethnic minorities are inherently at a disadvantage because of this type of prejudice and discrimination in the corporate world.

However, supervisors' early preferences for subordinates actually might reflect preferences for work style similarity rather than demographic similarity. Lacking other information about these relatively new employees who are potential protégés, it is not unreasonable for supervisors to infer working styles based on demographic characteristics such as ethnicity— particularly given the substantive overlap between working styles and membership in different cultural demographic groups. However, as actual working styles of protégés' become developed and apparent over time, mentors might seek out mentoring relationships with people who share their own working styles regardless of demographic congruence. Similar to

work group or coworker preferences, it might be the case that given substantive information about working styles, mentors will pick protégés not primarily based on demographic congruence, but rather on congruence in working styles. Nonetheless, the implication of this shift in preference from ethnicity to relational work style does not necessarily alleviate problems of intergroup bias. To the extent that relational styles of the dominant group remains favored over those more common among underrepresented cultural groups, this cultural-psychological perspective on workways suggests the possibility of an overlooked, nuanced form of institutional discrimination.

Extreme Diversity and Hybrid Cultures

Further evidence that diversity can be conceptualized as managing differences in work styles (rather than demographic group membership) comes from an innovative study by Earley and Mosakowski (2000). In a series of experiments with four-person managerial teams that worked within a large multinational firm headquartered in Bangkok, they varied the level of cultural diversity represented in the teams. The results replicated an expected effect in which split teams (two members from one country, and two members from another country) experienced more negative dynamics and performed worse compared to homogeneous teams (all members sharing a common nationality). But they also formed teams that had "extreme" levels of diversity—in which each member came from a different country—such that no two members held a common cultural background. These teams with extreme levels of diversity performed better than split teams and did just as well as the homogenous teams. As Earley and Mosakowski observed, in the absence of any common cultural work styles or schemas, these highly diverse teams created a hybrid culture in which team-specific norms, rules, and expectations emerged. In short, extreme levels of demographic differences allowed these teams, over time, to develop a new and shared work style, and this similarity of work style was a positive predictor of performance.

Interethnic Interviews

The consequences and implications of diversity are perhaps most controversial when one considers minorities' access to jobs and career mobility. Overt and aversive racism continue to be a factor in hiring and promotion decisions within organizations today (Brief, 2000; Murrell, Dietz-Uhler, Dovidio, & Drout, 1994). An interviewer's ethnic biases can create a disadvantage for minority job candidates, even if these biases are not conscious or intentionally applied (Dovidio & Gaertner, 2000). A classic experiment on interethnic interviews conducted by Word, Zanna, and Cooper (1974) showed that nonconscious ethnic biases can be manifested in multiple ways; for example, white interviewers asked fewer questions, remained more physically distant, and made less eye contact during interviews with black candidates compared to white candidates. These differences create a self-fulfilling prophecy whereby the interviewer's ethnic biases negatively and nonconsciously affect the performance of the candidate.

However, perceived incompatibilities in the working styles of two cultural groups also can create disadvantages for minority targets or job candidates, creating conditions for what might be referred to as a *cultural incongruence prophecy* (Sanchez-Burks, 2005), which suggests that a target's behavior can be influenced by differences between the evaluator's and the target's culturally related cognitions. Evidence for this idea comes from a study examining nonconscious behavioral mirroring in the context of an interethnic job interview (Sanchez-Burks, Blount, & Bartel, 2007). Prior research shows that people have a nonconscious tendency to mirror others' behavior in social interactions, and that people have more positive subjective experiences of rapport as a result of mirroring exhibited by interaction partners (Chartrand & Bargh, 1999; Cheng & Chartrand, 2003; LaFrance, 1979). Both mirroring and its effect on perceived rapport are moderated by attentiveness to relational cues (van Baaren, Maddux, Chartrand, de Bouter, & Van Knippenberg, 2003).

Given that cultural groups differ in relational attunement (Sanchez-Burks, 2002), there should be cultural differences in the display and sensitivity to the effects of mirroring. Empirical evidence indeed shows that mirroring is more common within more relationally attuned, interdependent cultures compared to more independent cultures (van Baaren et al., 2003; van Baaren, Horgan, Chartrand, & Dijkmans, 2004), and these differences in the enactment of mirroring become pronounced

within work settings (Sanchez-Burks, 2002). More recently, Sanchez-Burks, Blount, and Bartel (2007) reasoned that Latinos' greater attentiveness to relational cues should increase their susceptibility to the negative effects of not receiving mirroring in a social interaction, whereas Anglo Americans' inattentiveness to relational cues at work would reduce their vulnerability to the negative experience of not receiving behavioral mirroring. They examined the implications of these differences in a field experiment in which Anglo American and Latino midlevel employees of a U.S. Fortune 500 company participated in a mock interview in a headquarters' office suite. Participants were randomly assigned to an Anglo American interviewer who mirrored, or did not mirror, the gestures, mannerisms, and postures of the applicants (while maintaining similar levels of propinquity and positivity, such as amount of smiling, across both conditions). The interviews were videotaped, and later an independent panel of professional recruiters and interview coaches, blind to the experimental conditions, evaluated participants' performances using these videos. The results showed that, overall, the absence of interviewer mirroring negatively affected all participants. More important, the performance of Latinos was more affected by mimicry than that of Anglo Americans; compared to those in the mirroring condition, Latino interviewees in the nonmirroring condition performed more poorly, and reported higher levels of anxiety and lower levels of self-esteem.

Although the mirroring of the interviewer in this study was experimentally manipulated, prior research showed that Anglo Americans are generally less likely to mirror or exhibit behavioral mirroring overall (van Baaran et al., 2003), and particularly in work settings (Sanchez-Burks, 2002). To the extent that most interviewers in corporate America tend to be Anglo Americans, this creates a naturally occurring environment in which Latinos would underperform in interview situations. These results suggest that differences in behavioral mirroring in the workplace, even in the absence of any overt or implicit racism against ethnic/minority groups, can result in outcomes that disadvantage the minority group. Adding to earlier themes of how a cultural perspective provides unique insights into intergroup biases, this research reveals how the workways of a dominant group operate as an institutionalized form of discrimination, such that it does not re-quire malevolent individual biases to create an inhospitable environment for minorities. In this way, even subtle differences in cultural workways can provide difficult challenges for facilitating diversity in organizations.

Managing Diversity: A Summary

In this section, we argue that marrying cultural psychology with diversity research is a fruitful endeavor. Although diversity has been typically examined in organizational research as differences in observable or surface characteristics (e.g., gender, race, or age), differences in less observable characteristics such as belief systems, preferences, work styles, and mental models also can be important factors that undermine intercultural contact. From a practical standpoint, interventions to increase diversity in the workplace can benefit from an increased focus on helping individuals to develop shared workways and workplace relational schemas across racial and ethnic lines.

As mentioned, the preference for and perpetuation of a dominant, culturally unique workway can be just as insidious as the preference for a dominant ethnic group. Organizational structures and practices, such as selection and attrition (Schneider, 1987), can reproduce and sustain a singular work style, mental model, or cultural ideology that undermines diversity in workways. For example, in a study of corporate recruiters of U.S.-based Fortune 500 firms, Heaphy, Sanchez-Burks, and Ashford (2007) found that job candidates who built rapport with an interviewer by blurring the work and nonwork divide (e.g., by mentioning a girlfriend or commenting on family pictures of the interviewer) were less likely to be granted a second interview. In other words, job candidates who do not conform to the uniquely American workway of restricting personal issues at work are less likely to be recruited. These institutional practices that reinforce homogeneity in workways do little to help business organizations reap the advantages of an ethnically diverse workforce. Of greater concern, given that workways are often culture-bound, organizations that pursue homogeneity of workways are also likely to bring about homogeneity of cultures and ethnicities. Indeed, organizations may justify or couch racially discriminatory hiring practices behind the more "politically correct" motivation of preserving a singular workplace relational style.

On a more optimistic note, organizational change can play a role in facilitating larger cultural change. For example, in the dot-com boom of the 1990s, there are many examples of companies bucking normative traditions by embracing nonwork activities in the workplace—employees playing ping-pong during breaks at work, or going on whitewater rafting trips as a company. Or, as mentioned, as the marketplace becomes more global and companies become more multinational, it is increasingly a fact of life that employees have to adapt to and work with people with dramatically different workways. Echoing the ideas of Marx (1873/1992), individuals exposed to these different institutional environments are likely to develop different ways of working (e.g., different norms of blending work and nonwork activities) and may in turn be catalysts for bringing about larger changes in cultural ideology.

ORGANIZATIONAL AND MANAGERIAL PERCEPTIONS AND EXPECTATIONS

Cultural research in the organizational and managerial literature has focused on a plethora of managerial practices that differ across cultures. Many of these more applied findings have important contributions to psychological theory and research. In the next section, we highlight several key findings in this area, including cross-cultural research on attributions in the workplace, expectations of conflict, and beliefs about professionalism.

Cross-Cultural Attributions for Performance

Work is a domain where performance—success or failure—is of important consequence for both the individual and the organization, and attributions or explanations of performance have been a topic of extensive research in cultural workways. In this section we review three lines of research that have particular bearing on cultural psychology—positivity attributional biases, attributions to individuals versus groups, and organizational attributions.

Positivity Biases

How managers make attributions about positive and negative events such as success and failure has important implications for the future performance of employees and the organization at large. For example, the propensity to make dispositional attributions to explain performance can lead managers to overlook important structural causes of failure (in the case of poor outcomes), or misappropriate resources to a few undeserving employees (in the case of good outcomes). The latter phenomenon was eloquently described by Malcolm Gladwell (2002) in his analysis of the downfall of the now infamous Enron Corporation. According to Gladwell, no expenses were spared to hire the best and brightest individuals from elite business schools during the heyday of Enron. These employees were fast-tracked and given huge financial and strategic responsibilities, even though they were underqualified, undertrained, and inexperienced. When these individuals failed, they were given more, rather than less, responsibility and control. Enron's culture of identifying a few winners, then maintaining their "star" status by consistently making dispositional attributions for their successes, while making situational attributions for their failures, contributed to the ultimate downfall of the entire company.

This propensity to focus on dispositional attributions of winners is consistent with cultural research on the positivity bias, or the propensity to make internal attributions for others' successes and external attributions for others' failures (the positivity bias is similar to the self-serving bias, except that the attributions are directed toward others; Sears, 1983). The Hallahan, Lee, and Herzog (1997) content analysis of how sports journalists make attributions about winners and losers found cultural variation in how the positivity attributional bias is expressed. Specifically, journalists from Western cultures predominantly focused on winners, making internal attributions for their successes, and praising their abilities to the sky. This results in a "star" culture in Western societies, where disproportionate attention is paid to the winners, and extraordinary and outstanding abilities and talents are attributed to them. Journalists from Eastern cultures, in contrast, predominantly focused on losers, making external attributions for their losses. In Eastern cultures, effort is expended on equalizing winners and losers, so that no one stands out—journalists spent more time making excuses for the losers, so that they did not appear below average or subpar.

Group versus Individual

Research has shown cultural differences in how individuals versus social collectives are held accountable for outcomes. Zemba, Young, and Morris (2005) found that Japanese were more likely than Americans to attribute organizational outcomes to a single leader (e.g., CEO). Specifically, they found that Japanese attributed blame to a business leader for harms caused by the organization (e.g., environmental accident), whereas Americans were reluctant to do so unless there was a clear connection between the action and the individual. Relatedly, Japanese leaders were more likely to take the blame and resign for organizational failure, it was not caused directly by their own actions and even if the cause originated before the leader became a member of the organization. Individual representatives of the group—such as the CEO or the leader—are viewed as the proxy of the group and have to assume blame for organizational level failures.

The notion that cultural differences exist in the status of groups and individuals also is salient in the literature on motivation. How to motivate workers to perform well or to exhibit other behaviors that the organization finds desirable is of great interest to business scholars and practitioners. The early work of William Ouchi (1981) showed that, in contrast to American managers, Japanese managers used the work team as the source for motivation for individual workers. Similarly, DeVoe and Iyengar (2004) showed that whereas American managers tend to attribute their subordinates' motivation exclusively to work-related incentives (e.g., salary), Latin American and Chinese managers are more likely to believe that social incentives (e.g., belonging to a group, building harmonious relationships) are more important sources of motivation for their subordinates. Like other research on cultural psychology, an individual's inextricable embeddedness within the social collective appears to be much more salient in Eastern than in Western cultures (Sagiv & Schwartz, 2000a).

Organizational Attributions

Besides individuals, social collectives such as organizations also make attributions. For example, several studies examined the attributions business organizations make for their performance by content analyzing the text in their annual reports to shareholders (Bettman & Weitz, 1983; Lee, Peterson, & Tiedens, 2004; Salancik & Meindl, 1984; Staw, McKechenie, & Puffer, 1983). Ambady, Shih, Hallahan, and Lee (2005) have used this technique to examine attributions across cultures. Specifically, they content-analyzed the attributions contained in the annual reports of publicly traded companies in four countries—India, Hong Kong, Singapore, and the United States. Results showed that Indian companies changed from a prototypical Eastern attributional style (more external attributions, or attributing performance to competitors, government policy, or economic conditions) before 1991—the year India experienced a large-scale economic restructuring to allow more Western capital—to a prototypical Western attributional style (more internal attributions, or attributing performance to managerial decisions or internal strategy) after 1991. During the same time period, attributions made by Singapore and U.S. companies (countries with no large-scale economic or political change during the 1991 time frame) showed no changes in their attributions. Also, attributions in Hong Kong companies changed from a prototypical Western attributional style before 1997—the year when Hong Kong was handed over to China from British rule—to a prototypical Eastern attributional style. Again, Singapore and U.S. companies showed no changes in attribution styles during the same time.

These results have several implications. First, they show that cultural differences in attribution styles are reflected in not only individual-level inferences of causality but also the publicly communicated inferences of social collectives. Although annual reports are written by individuals, they nevertheless represent the views of the business organization as a collective. The results show that, like individuals, organizational attributions reflect East–West differences in preference for internal versus external attributions. Second, cultural differences in organizational attributions are sensitive to larger cultural, political, and economic influences. Whether the observed attributional shifts in Indian and Hong Kong firms reflect changes in how the executives or employees of the organizations actually thought about their performance, or the organization's attempts at appealing to different audiences over time, they changed in predictable ways with larger "macro" forces in the economic and political environment, and the change occurred quite

quickly (a year after the seminal event). It appears that the cultural differences in organizational attributions are highly transitory and sensitive to the larger context.

Expectations about Conflict across Cultures

Research on conflict at work has most commonly focused on how different types of conflict affect individual and team performance. Although the data are somewhat equivocal, there is some evidence (primarily from U.S. and Northern European samples) that task conflict—disagreements about the work itself—can facilitate team performance and creativity through constructive debate (Jehn & Bendersky, 2003; DeDreu & Weingart, 2003). In contrast, relationship conflict—disagreements and dynamics unrelated to the task, which involve interpersonal tensions and personality clashes—is a robust and reliable predictor of team underperformance and dissatisfaction (DeDreu & Weingart, 2003).

However, expectations of and reactions to conflict do not mirror the empirical findings and further exhibit cultural differences. Neuman, Sanchez-Burks, Ybarra, and Goh (2005) conducted two studies comparing perceptions of task and relationship conflict among Americans, Koreans, Chinese, and Japanese managers. The results showed that both Americans and East Asians believed task conflict was a roadblock to success. Though East Asians also believed relationship conflict was detrimental to task performance, Americans did not believe that relationship conflict necessarily affected team performance. In fact, when given the opportunity to join a talented team that would likely experience relationship conflict, Americans were twice as likely as East Asians to state that they would join such a team.

Thus, there are both cultural differences and cultural similarities regarding beliefs about conflict: Americans share with other cultures the belief that task conflict limits team performance, but differ from other cultures in beliefs about the detrimental effects of relationship conflict on team performance. These findings are consistent with PRI, the uniquely American workway that minimizes the importance of social and emotional concerns at work; Americans expected work-related conflict to exact a toll on work performance but did not expect personal or social conflict to play a role at work. This suggests that "conflict frames," or subjective construals of conflict that influence decisions and behaviors (Gelfand et al., 2001, 2002; Pinkley, 1990), are more strongly shaped by prevailing cultural ideologies than by the actual relationship between conflict and performance.

Culturally Bound Beliefs about Professionalism

"Being professional," in the vernacular of Western business speak, is an often-used standard invoked by organizations to regulate behavior of its members, or by individuals to manage others' impressions using culturally and organizationally relevant cues such as décor or dress (Elsbach, 2003, 2004; Rafaeli & Dutton, 1997). Yet exactly what "being professional" means is rarely explicitly defined. Although idiosyncrasies may exist between industries, organizations, and even roles within a firm, notions such as professionalism can provide a window into culturally implicit meanings about how to behave appropriately while at work.

Recent research suggests that perceptions of professionalism are indeed culturally bound. Heaphy et al. (2007) assessed people's schema of professionalism by having managers from multiple cultures affix images of work-related items (e.g., a stapler, file folder, or an award certificate) and non-work-related items (e.g., a family photo or a child's drawing) to an image of an empty office cubicle of a person described as having either a "professional" or an "unprofessional" reputation. Results showed that perceptions of professionalism entailed restricting the amount of nonwork symbols to fewer than 20%. Interestingly, far from a cultural universal, this perception of professionalism was moderated by the amount of experience managers had working in the United States. Specifically, the more time managers had lived and worked in the United States, the more likely they were to perceive restriction of personal content displayed in the office as an indicator of high professionalism. Of course, all societies have beliefs about appropriate behavior at work. Though translations of professionalism appear in many cultures—*puro* in Japan, *epangelmatismos* in Greece, *profesionalismo* in Mexico—this research suggests that its particular connotations within American business are far from universal and, instead, are deeply imbued with tacit cultural meanings.

FUTURE DIRECTIONS

In this section, we highlight streams of research that may be particularly fruitful for the study of cultural workways in particular, and cultural psychology more generally. Particularly, we highlight theories, variables, and methodological approaches that are less common in psychological research but potentially provide a rich perspective for cultural psychology research in the future.

Social Networks

Cultural psychology of workways is not limited to a study of people's minds or social contexts. Social networks, or the pattern of interconnections between individuals, play an important role in the mutual constitution of individuals and institutions within cultures (Morris, Poldony, & Ariel, 2000). Social network research examines actual patterns of social behavior—who talks with whom, whom people go to for task and personal advice, to whom people hand off their work—and the consequences of these various network strategies for individual, team, and organizational outcomes and behaviors.

Social network analysis offers much potential for future research in cultural psychology. For instance, multiplexity, or the degree of overlap in a social network, is a particularly interesting variable in that it taps both the content and the structure of the interconnecting web of people's social relations. The level of multiplexity in individuals' networks indicate the extent to which the same set of people serve multiple roles (e.g., the same person has the roles of confidant, coworker, and cousin simultaneously). For example, given the central PRI tenet of separating work and nonwork domains, the social networks of individuals in cultures influenced by PRI should have lower levels of multiplexity (Kacperczyk, Sanchez-Burks, & Baker, 2005).

Recent cross-cultural evidence supports this notion. Ariel et al. (2000) compared social networks among employees of a multinational bank in Spain, Germany, and the United States. They found that despite organizational attempts at standardization across its branches, there remained substantial cultural variations in actual patterns of social relations. For example, in Spain, employees' networks showed greater multiplexity, that is, more overlap between advice and personal networks, such that the same person would be sought out for both work and personal advice. In contrast, American employee networks showed significantly lower multiplexity, indicating two nonoverlapping networks, one for work-related issues and one for personal issues.

Transitivity is another network characteristic that may be an important predictor for success within some Asian cultures (Gelfand & Cai, 2004). As mentioned, professional networks in China are fashioned in a way that is consistent with the broader notion of *guanxi*, in which two people who are connected based on mutual obligations can expect people in each other's networks to respond in kind despite being one step removed in the social network. For example, imagine Kaiping wishes a favor from a potential business associate, Chi-Ying, someone he does not know personally. Both Kaiping and Chi-Ying, however, are connected to a mutual friend Lijun. It is acceptable under the principle of *guanxi* for Kaiping to approach Chi-Ying directly, without going through Lijun. Kaiping can further expect Chi-Ying to offer him the same favors and special treatment she would offer to Lijun (Gelfand & Cai, 2004).

Understanding and adapting to social network characteristics such as mutiplexity or transitivity may be a particularly critical skills for operating effectively in today's global marketplace. For example, having a network with a lot of multiplexity may be advantageous for a businessperson generating new business in Spain. Or having a highly transitive social network may benefit an entrepreneur who wishes to expand her business into China. In short, having network characteristics that fit in with another culture might facilitate one's success in operating within that culture.

The ability to alternate between multiple network strategies to "fit in" across multiple cultures may be an additional skill that predicts success in the global marketplace. For instance, businesspeople who have to work within multiple cultures might have to switch back and forth between a high-transitive and a low-transitive network, or a high-multiplex or a low-multiplex network, depending on their colleagues' cultural background. In this way, achieving "cultural fluency" may entail understanding and evoking different network structures across cultural divides.

Besides examining the relationship between various network characteristics and perfor-

mance across cultures, future research might also examine antecedents to culturally adaptive network structures and skills. For instance, prior exposure to different cultures might create more flexibility in network structures and strategies, such that multicultural individuals (who identify with different cultures) may have more facility in switching back and forth between different types of networks. Furthermore, network structures might powerfully affect individual belief systems. For example, the American entrepreneur who participates (willingly or not) in the Spanish business world and develops higher multiplexity in her social networks as a result might begin to attenuate her own beliefs about separation of work and nonwork life.

Organizational Culture

Cross-cultural research typically examines culture at the level of a nation (e.g., Japan vs. the United States) or the level of ethnic groups (e.g., Asian Americans vs. Latinos). Yet cross-cultural research also can be conducted at the level of the work group or work organization. "Organizational culture" refers to the observable values and norms that characterize an organization (Schein, 1996) or to commonly held schemas (ways of thinking about and doing things) that individuals within an organization might share. Organizational culture has been called a variety of terms, such as "organizational personality" (Barnard, 1968), corporate climate, corporate soul, or organizational psychounity (Denison, 1996).

In one sense, organizational culture is analogous to national or ethnic cultures (Alutto, 2002). Both types of "cultures" entail shared beliefs, values, and norms of a particular social system, be it a business organization or an entire society. One can think of organizations as nested in nations, where a country might have numerous organizations within it, and organizational cultures are influenced by the larger national culture in which they operate. Likewise, one can think of nations as nested in organizations—where multiple national units exist within a single organization (e.g., Hofstede's [1980] multinational study of IBM), and differences between national units are influenced by the larger organizational or firm culture.

Comparing these two research streams—organizational culture and national cultures—

side by side, it is evident that dimensions and concepts used to describe national cultures have been used to describe cultures within organizations or firms. For example, the concept of individualism–collectivism (INDCOL), originally used in cross-national comparisons, has been used to examine cultural differences between business firms, functional departments, or work teams within the same country (Lee, 1997, 1999). Particularly, multiple studies have examined how creating a more collectivistic versus individualistic orientation within a work group (via experimental manipulations) affects group and organizational dynamics (Chatman & Barsade, 1995; Lee, 1997, 1999).

Despite this limited cross-fertilization of the two literatures, little theory or research has explored the similarities and differences of cultures at these various levels of analysis. In an exception, Earley and Mosakowski (2002) suggest that, compared to organizations, national cultures are less transient and less affected by the entry and exit of any single individual. However, these differences have blurred as organizations have grown increasingly large, diverse, and global, whereas national values have been shown to be much more susceptible to environmental jolts and changes (Ambady et al., 2005).

Thus, one important direction for future research is examining the relationship between national cultures, organizational cultures, and individual psychology. One possible proposition is that organizational cultures may reflect the larger national culture in which they operate. For example, value differences that exist between cultures (i.e., autonomy–embeddedness, hierarchy–egalitarianism, mastery–harmony) may affect organizational cultures (Sagiv & Schwartz, 2000b). For example, organizations in autonomous cultures may be relatively open to change and diversity, but organizations in embedded cultures function as extended families, taking responsibility for organizational members in all domains of life. Organizations in hierarchical cultures may emphasize the chain of authority, assigning well-defined roles and goals to individual members, whereas organizations in egalitarian cultures may be more flexible in allowing individuals to decide how they will enhance organizational goals. Organizations in mastery cultures may be dynamic, competitive, and strongly oriented to achievement and success, whereas organizations in harmony cultures may be more concerned with the organization's integration and impact on the larger society and environment.

Another possible proposition may focus on the interface between organizational and national cultures. Specifically, the fit between organizational and national culture may predict organizational performance. One may argue that organizations with cultures that fit in with the prevailing values of the larger national culture might be more successful, or more favorably perceived by shareholders and the general public. To the extent that organizations exhibit cultural values that are inconsistent with the larger culture, they may violate expectations held by the general public about what is generally good and desirable, leading to unfavorable impressions and lower stock prices (Lee et al., 2004). Alternatively, one may argue that organizations with cultures that differ from the prevailing values of the larger national culture will be viewed as more innovative and cutting edge.

Cultural Intelligence

Thinking is for doing and, within the domain of work, learning about culture is critical for successfully navigating cultural differences. The recent construct of cultural intelligence offers one such mechanism through which people can manage cross-cultural differences. Earley and Ang (2003) wondered why some people operate well in new cultures, while others have difficulty fully understanding or practicing new cultural values and behaviors. They suggested that this ability cannot be fully explained by social or emotional intelligence, empathy, or other individual differences. They coined the term "cultural intelligence" (or CQ) to describe an individual's ability to adapt to new and unfamiliar cultures. CQ has cognitive components (grasping culture-specific knowledge, as well as metacognitive skills such as self-awareness and ability to create new categories), motivational components (willingness to adapt and change oneself as the cultural context changes), and behavioral components (ability to generate new behaviors within a new cultural context).

As mentioned earlier, difficulty in managing cross-cultural business relationships is both common and costly (Copeland & Griggs, 1985), and many of these failures may be attributed to insufficient levels of CQ (Earley & Ang, 2003). CQ, though an individual difference, can indeed be developed. For example, cognitions such as culture-specific knowledge—how to conduct a meeting in Japan or how to exchange gifts in China—can be learned, as can metacognitive skills relevant to CQ, such as social perception, reasoning, or self-monitoring. Similarly, motivation can be increased through goal-setting exercises to change individual attitudes. Behavioral change can be instilled through behavioral modification techniques.

CQ is a promising individual-level variable that directly addresses the concept of cultural fluency in intercultural interactions. Although CQ is applicable to most, if not all, dimensions along which cultures vary, future research may find that the usefulness of CQ is moderated by the nature of cross-cultural differences. For example, when individuals have to negotiate between cultural phenomena about which they do not have clear or intuitive understanding—for example, differences between high- and low-context cultures—CQ might prove especially helpful. Or when individuals are reluctant to admit to certain culturally ingrained behaviors due to self-presentation concerns, such as being less relationally attuned in certain settings, having high CQ or being trained in CQ might have a strong effect on improving the quality and effectiveness of intercultural contact.

Examining Cultures by Using Dilemmas

Dilemmas are an underutilized methodology for examining cultural differences. This approach is exemplified in the research of Hampden-Turner and Trompenaars (1993), who presented to respondents in multiple cultures a series of work-related dilemmas and asked them to make a choice between two extreme positions. For example, managers were asked to choose between the following descriptions of a company:

1. As a system designed to perform functions and tasks in an efficient way. People are hired to fulfill these functions with the help of machines and other equipment. They are paid for the tasks they perform.
2. As a group of people working together. The people have social relations with other people and with the organization. The functioning is dependent on these relations.

Using this approach, they found important cultural differences and similarities specific to work, but with clear implications for broader contexts. For instance, in the aforementioned dilemma, only 36% of the managers from Japan chose (1), whereas this option was favored by 70% or more of the managers in the United States, with Sweden and Italy somewhere in between (56% and 46%, respectively). Hampden-Turner and Trompenaars argued that managers' decisions in such dilemmas reflect and express the national culture in which they operate—dimensions such as universalism, collectivism, and achievement.

Though some researchers (Oyserman, Coon, & Kemmelmeier, 2002) have questioned the validity of value dimensions such as INDCOL as a useful way to understand cultural differences, this criticism may reflect the problems with using scales as a way to measure values, rather than the concept of values per se. Indeed, Hampden-Turner and Trompenaars (1993) found that theoretically grounded dilemmas based on individualism and collectivism show consistent and theoretically explainable cross-cultural variation. This, together with the consensus with which other cultural theorists have described constructs analogous to INDCOL (e.g., Durkheim, 1933; Kluckhohn & Strodtbeck, 1961; Parsons et al., 1951; Reisman, 1961; Tönnies, 1887/2002), suggests that broad value dimensions could be usefully reexamined with the dilemma methodology in future research. Specifically, when the validity of self-reported values cannot be established (see Heine et al., 2002; Peng, Nisbett, & Wong, 1997), or when experimental methodologies are not viable (as in many applied field settings), the dilemma methodology exemplified in the research by Hampden-Turner and Trompenaars (1993) offers much promise.

CONCLUSION

The emerging research on cultural psychology and workways offers a unique perspective that is relevant for theory and research in cultural psychology. The interplay between the micro, psychological processes and the macro, structural processes that characterize the research on cultural workways provides critical insights for understanding how and why cross-cultural differences and similarities emerge, as well as when they may be particularly problematic for intercultural relations.

In understanding what constitutes a psychology of workways, it should be noted that much of experimental psychology may have unintentionally been studies on work. The most commonly used methodological paradigm in psychology experiments engages participants in a task-oriented "work" setting. For example, participants often come to an office and are asked to perform in some sort of problem-solving, decision-making, perceptual, or interpersonal task. Participants are typically given a set of instructions, and asked to follow them and perform accordingly within a given time frame. Also, participants typically receive some sort of compensation—money or course credit—for the "work" they perform.

Although participating in a short psychological experiment is clearly different than long-term employment within an organization or work group, participants in a typical psychology experiment are more likely to have a "working" mind-set than "playing" or social, nonworking mind-set, unless such a context is explicitly primed or created (e.g., studies of romantic partners). Findings from the experimental literature may therefore largely be studies of work-related cognitions, feelings, and behaviors. To the extent that a large part of cultural psychology employs this experimental paradigm, this may contribute to a cultural literature that overestimates the prevalence of certain types of cultural differences and underestimates other types of cultural differences. In this way, research on cultural workways provides a contextual anchor for assessing the cultural psychology of social life.

REFERENCES

Allmendinger, J., & Hackman, J. R. (1995). The more, the better?: A four-nation study of the inclusion of women in symphony orchestras. *Social Forces, 74*(2), 423–460.

Alutto, J. (2002). Culture, levels of analysis, and cultural transition. In F. Yammarino & F. Dansereau (Eds.), *The many faces of multi-level issues* (pp. 321–326). San Francisco: JAI Press.

Ambady, N., Koo, J., Lee, F., & Rosenthal, R. (1996). More than words: Linguistic and nonlinguistic politeness in two cultures. *Journal of Personality and Social Psychology, 70*(5), 996–1011.

Ambady, N., Shih, M., Hallahan, M., & Lee, F. (2005). *Stock explanations: Culture and causal attributions in letters to shareholders.* Unpublished manuscript, Tufts University, Medford, MA.

Arthur, W. B. (1994). *Increasing returns and path dependence in the economy.* Ann Arbor: University of Michigan Press.

Ascherson, N. (1996). *Black Sea.* New York: Hill & Wang.

Ayman, R., & Chemers, M. M. (1983). Relationship of supervisory behavior ratings to work group effectiveness and subordinate satisfaction among Iranian managers. *Journal of Applied Psychology, 68,* 338–341.

Barker, R. (1998, October 12). So your workers want to telecommute. *BusinessWeek.* Available at *www.businessweek.com*

Barnard, C. (1968). *The functions of the executive.* Cambridge, MA: Harvard University Press.

Bellah, R. N. (1957). *Tokugawa religion.* New York: Free Press.

Bellah, R. N. (1985). *Tokugawa religion: The cultural roots of modern Japan.* New York: Free Press.

Bellah, R. N., Madsen, R., Sullivan, W. M., Swidler, A., & Tipton, S. M. (1996). *Habits of the heart: Individualism and commitment in American life.* Berkeley: University of California Press.

Bendix, R. (1977). *Max Weber: An intellectual portrait.* Berkeley: University of California Press.

Bettman, J., & Weitz, B. (1983). Attributions in the boardroom: Causal reasoning in corporate annual reports. *Administrative Science Quarterly, 28,* 165–183.

Bird, A., Heinbuch, S., Dunbar, R., & McNulty, M. (1993). A conceptual model of the effects of area studies training programs and a preliminary investigation of the model's hypothesized relationships. *International Journal of Intercultural Relations, 17*(4), 415–435.

Birnbaum-More, P., & Wong, G. (1995). Acquisition of managerial values in the People's Republic of China and Hong Kong. *Journal of Cross-Cultural Psychology, 26*(3), 255–275.

Brief, A. P. (2000). Just doing business: Modern racism and obedience to authority as explanations for employment discrimination. *Organizational Behavior and Human Decision Processes, 81*(1), 72–97.

Briley, D. A., & Wyer, R. S. (2001). Transitory determinants of values and decisions: The utility (or nonutility) of individualism and collectivism in understanding cultural differences. *Social Cognition, 19,* 197–227.

Brown, P., & Levinson, S. (1987). *Politeness: Some universals in language usage.* Cambridge, UK: Cambridge University Press.

Brown, R. (1986). *Social psychology* (2nd ed.). New York: Free Press.

Cai, D. A. (2001). Looking below the surface: Comparing subtleties of U.S. and Chinese culture in negotiation. In J. Weiss (Ed.), *Tigers roar: Asia's recovery and its impact* (pp. 217–237). New York: Sharpe.

Chartrand, T. L., & Bargh, J. (1999). The chameleon effect: The perception–behavior link and social interaction. *Journal of Personality and Social Psychology, 76*(6), 893–910.

Chatman, J. A., & Barsade, S. G. (1995). Personality, organizational culture, and cooperation: Evidence from a business simulation. *Administrative Science Quarterly, 40*(3), 423–443.

Chatman, J. A., Polzer, J. T., Barsade, S. G., & Neale, M. A. (1998). Being different yet feeling similar: The influence of demographic composition and organizational culture on work processes and outcomes. *Administrative Science Quarterly, 43*(4), 749–780.

Cheng, C. M., & Chartrand, T. L. (2003). Self-monitoring without awareness: Using mimicry as a nonconscious affiliation strategy. *Journal of Personality and Social Psychology, 85*(6), 1170–1179.

Copeland, L., & Griggs, L. (1985). *Going international: How to make friends and deal effectively in the global marketplace.* New York: Random House.

Crèvecoeur, J. (1981). *Letters from an American farmer.* New York: Penguin Books. (Original work published 1782)

Daniels, B. C. (1995). *Puritans at play.* New York: St. Martin's Press.

Dechert, C. R. (1961). "Simpatía" and leadership: A study of group relations among Italian government employees. *Bolletino di Psicologia Applicata, 43–44,* 1–9.

De Dreu, C. K. W., & Weingart, L. R. (2003). Task versus relationship conflict, team performance, and team member satisfaction: A meta-analysis. *Journal of Applied Psychology, 88*(4), 741–749.

Denison, D. (1996). What IS the difference between organizational culture and organizational climate?: A native's point of view on a decade of paradigm wars. *Academy of Management Review, 21*(3), 619–654.

DePaulo, B. M., & Kashy, D. A. (1998). Everyday lies in close and casual relationships. *Journal of Personality and Social Psychology, 74*(1), 63–79.

Deshpande, S., & Viswesvaran, C. (1992). Is cross-cultural training of expatriate managers effective: A meta analysis. *International Journal of Intercultural Relations, 16,* 295–310.

de Tocqueville, A. (1990). *Democracy in America.* New York: Vintage Books. (Original work published 1840)

DeVoe, S. E., & Iyengar, S. S. (2004). Managers' theories of subordinates: A cross-cultural examination of manager perceptions of motivation and appraisal of performance. *Organizational Behavior and Human Decision Processes, 93*(1), 47–61.

Diaz-Guerrero, R. (1967). *Psychology of the Mexican.* Austin: University of Texas Press.

Dovidio, J. F., & Gaertner, S. L. (2000). Aversive racism and selection decisions: 1989 and 1999. *Psychological Science, 11*(4), 315–320.

Durkheim, É. (1933). *The division of labor in society* New York: Free Press.

Earley, P. C. (1989). Social loafing and collectivism: A comparison of United States and the People's Republic of China. *Administrative Science Quarterly, 34,* 565–581.

Earley, P. C. (1997). *Face, harmony, and social structure: An analysis of organizational behavior across cultures.* New York: Oxford University Press.

Earley, P. C., & Ang, S. (2003). *Cultural intelligence: An analysis of individual interactions across cultures.* Palo Alto, CA: Stanford University Press.

Earley, P. C., & Gibson, C. B. (1998). Taking stock in our process on individualism–collectivism: 100 years of solidarity and community. *Journal of Management Special Issue: Yearly Review of Management, 24*(3), 265–304.

Earley, P. C., & Mosakowski, E. (2000). Creating hybrid team cultures: An empirical test of transnational team functioning. *Academy of Management Journal, 43*(1), 26–49.

Earley, P. C., & Mosakowski, E. (2002). Linking culture and behavior in organizations: Suggestions for theory development and research methodology. In F. Yammarino & F. Dansereau (Eds.), *Research in multi-level issues* (Vol. 1, pp. 297–319). Newbury Park, CA: JAI Press.

Elsbach, K. D. (2003). Organizational perception management. *Research in Organizational Behavior, 25,* 297–332.

Elsbach, K. D. (2004). Interpreting workplace identities: The role of office décor. *Journal of Organizational Behavior, 25*(1), 99–128.

Eschbach, D. M., Parker, G. E., & Stoeberl, P. A. (2001). American repatriate employees' retrospective assessments of the effects of the cross-cultural training on their adaptation to international assignments. *International Journal of Human Resource Management, 12,* 270–287.

Farh, J.-L., Tsui, A., Xin, K., & Cheng, B.-S. (1998). The influence of relational demography and *guanxi*: The Chinese case. *Organizational Science, 9,* 471–488.

Fischer, D. (1989). *Albion's seed: Four British folkways in America.* New York: Oxford University Press.

Fiske, A. P., Kitayama, S., Markus, H. R., & Nisbett, R. E. (1998). The cultural matrix of social psychology. In D. Gilbert, S. Fiske, & G. Lindzey (Eds.), *Handbook of social psychology* (Vol. 2, pp. 915–981). San Francisco: McGraw-Hill.

Frost, L. (2005, March 23). France's assembly lengthens 35-hour workweek. *The Associated Press.* Retrieved October 10, 2006, from www.postgazette.com/pg/05082/476118.stm

Furnham, A. (1990). *The Protestant work ethic: The psychology of work related beliefs and behaviours.* New York: Routledge.

Gelfand, M., & Cai, D. A. (2004). Cultural structuring of the social context of negotiation. In M. J. Gelfand & J. M. Brett (Eds.), *The handbook of negotiation and culture.* Palo Alto, CA: Stanford University Press.

Gelfand,, M. J., Higgins, M., Mishii, L. H., Raver, J. L., Dominguez, A., Murakami, F., et al. (2002). Culture and egocentric perceptions of fairness in conflict and negotiation. *Journal of Applied Psychology, 87*(5), 833–845.

Gelfand, M. J., Nishii, L. H., Holcombe, K. M., Dyer, N., Ohbuchi, K., & Fukuno, M. (2001). Cultural influences on cognitive representations of conflict: Interpretations of conflict episodes in the United States and Japan. *Journal of Applied Psychology*, 86(6), 1059–1074.

Gladwell, M. (2002, July 22). The talent myth: Are smart people overrated? *The New Yorker Magazine*, pp. 100–105.

Graen, G., Novak, M., & Sommerkamp, P. (1982). The effects of leader-member exchange and job design on productivity and satisfaction: Testing a dual attachment model. *Organizational Behavior and Human Performance*, 30, 191–231.

Grice, H. P. (1968). Utterer's meaning, sentence-meaning and word-meaning. *Foundations of Language*, 4, 225–242.

Goffman, E. (1959). *The presentation of self in everyday life*. Garden City, NY: Doubleday.

Goffman, E. (1967). *Interaction ritual: Essays in face-to-face behavior*. New York: Pantheon Books.

Hallahan, M., Lee, F., & Herzog, T. (1997). It's not just whether you win or lose it is also where you play the game: Cross-cultural differences in the positivity bias. *Journal of Cross-Cultural Psychology*, 28, 768–778.

Hampden-Turner, C., & Trompenaars, A. (1993). *The seven cultures of capitalism: Value systems for creating wealth in the United States, Japan, Germany, France, Britain, Sweden, and the Netherlands*. New York: Doubleday.

Heaphy, E., Sanchez-Burks, J., & Ashford, S. (2007). *American professionalism: Contents and consequences of an organizational role schema*. Unpublished manuscript, University of Michigan, Ann Arbor.

Hébert, R. (2005). A world of difference. *APS Observer*, 18(4), 24–25.

Heine, S., Lehman, D., Peng, K., & Greenholtz, J. (2002). What's wrong with cross-cultural comparisons of subjective Likert scales?: The reference-group effect. *Journal of Personality and Social Psychology*, 82(6), 903–918.

Herodotus. (2003). *The histories* [Penguin classics]. New York: Penguin.

Hofstede, G. (1980). *Culture's consequences*. Beverly Hills, CA: Sage.

Holtgraves, T. (1997). Styles of language use: Individual and cultural variability in conversational indirectness. *Journal of Personality and Social Psychology*, 73(3), 624–637.

Holtgraves, T., & Yang, J. (1992). The interpersonal underpinnings of request strategies: General principles and differences due to culture and gender. *Journal of Personality and Social Psychology*, 62, 246–256.

Hong, Y., Morris, M., Chiu, C., & Benet-Martinez, V. (2000). Multicultural minds: A dynamic constructivist approach to culture and cognition. *American Psychologist*, 55, 709–720.

Hui, C., Eastman, K., & Yee, C. (1995). The relationship between individualism–collectivism and satisfaction at the workplace. *Applied Psychology: An International Review*, 44, 276–282.

Hui, C., & Luk, C. (1997). Industrial/organizational psychology. In J. Berry, M. Segall, & C. Kağitçibaşi (Eds.), *Handbook of cross-cultural psychology* (Vol. 3, pp. 371–412). Needham Heights, MA: Allyn & Bacon.

Jehn, K. A. (1995). A multimethod examination of the benefits and detriments of intragroup conflict. *Administrative Science Quarterly*, 40(2), 256–282.

Jehn, K. A., & Bendersky, C. (2003). Intragroup conflict in organizations: A contingency perspective on the conflict outcome relationship. *Research in Organizational Behavior*, 25, 187–242.

Jehn, K. A., Northcraft, G. B., & Neale, M. A. (1999). Why differences make a difference: A field study of diversity, conflict, and performance in workgroups. *Administrative Science Quarterly*, 44(4), 741–763.

Kacperczyk, A., Sanchez-Burks, J., & Baker, W. (2005). *Chameleon social networks patterns and cross-cultural fluency*. Unpublished manuscript, University of Michigan, Ann Arbor.

Kanungo, R. (1990). Culture and work alienation: Western models and Eastern realities. *International Journal of Psychology*, 25, 795–812.

Kim, S. U. (1988). The role of social values and competitiveness in economic growth: With special reference to Korea. In D. Sinha & H. S. R. Kao (Eds.), *Social values and development: Asian perspectives* (pp. 76–92). New Delhi: Sage.

Kluckhohn, F., & Strodtbeck, F. L. (1961). *Variations in value orientations*. Evanston, IL: Row, Peterson.

Kohn, M. L., & Schooler, C. (1983). *Work and personality: An inquiry into the impact of social stratification*. Norwood, NJ: Ablex.

Kool, R., & Saksena, N. K. (1988). Leadership styles and its effectiveness among Indian executives. *Indian Journal of Applied Psychology*, 26(1), 9–15.

LaFrance, M. (1979). Nonverbal synchrony and rapport: Analysis by the cross-lag panel of technique. *Social Psychology Quarterly*, 42(1), 66–70.

Landes, D. (2000). Culture makes almost all the difference. In S. P. Huntington & L. E. Harrison (Eds.), *Culture matters: How values shape human progress* (pp. 2–14). New York: Basic Books.

Lau, D. C., & Murnighan, J. K. (1998). Demographic diversity and faultlines: The compositional dynamics of organizational groups. *Academy of Management Review*, 23(2), 325–340.

Lee, F. (1993). Being polite and keeping mum: How bad news is communicated in organizational hierarchies. *Journal of Applied Social Psychology*, 23(14), 1124–1149.

Lee, F. (1997). When the going gets tough, do the tough ask for help?: Help seeking and power motivation in organizations. *Organizational Behavior and Human Decision Processes*, 72(3), 336–363.

Lee, F. (1999). Verbal strategies for seeking help in organizations. *Journal of Applied Social Psychology*, 29(7), 1472–1496.

Lee, F., Peterson, C., & Tiedens, L. (2004). *Mea culpa*: Predicting stock prices from organizational attributions. *Personality and Social Psychology Bulletin*, *30*(12), 1–14.

Lenski, G. (1963). *The religious factor*. New York: Anchor Books.

Li, J., Tsui, A., & Weldon, E. (2000). *Management and organization in the Chinese context*. New York: Macmillan.

Lindsley, S. L., & Braithwaite, C. A. (1996). You should "wear a mask": Facework norms in cultural and intercultural conflict in maquiladoras. *International Journal of Intercultural Relations*, *20*(2), 199–225.

Linstedt, S. (2002, October 14). Wonder where your time goes?: You probably spent it at work. *Buffalo News*, p. B7.

Markus, H., & Kitayama, S. (1991). Culture and the self: Implications for cognition, emotion, and motivation. *Psychological Review*, *98*(2), 224–253.

Markus, H. R., & Lin, L. R. (1999). Conflictways: Cultural diversity in the meanings and practices of conflict. In D. A. Prentice & D. R. Miller (Eds.), *Cultural divides: Understanding and overcoming group conflict* (pp. 302–333). New York: Russell Sage Foundation.

Marx, K. (1992). *Capital: A critique of political economy*., New York: Penguin Books. (Original work published 1873)

McClelland, D. (1961). *The achieving society*. New York: Van Nostrand.

Mead, M. (1967). *Male and female*. New York: HarperCollins.

Mischel, W., & Shoda, Y. (1995). A cognitive-affective system theory of personality: Reconceptualizing situations, dispositions, dynamics, and invariance in personality structures. *Psychological Review*, *102*(2), 246–268.

Morris, M. W., Poldony, J. M., & Ariel, S. (2000). Missing relations: Incorporating relational constructs into models of culture. In P. C. Earley & H. Singh (Eds.), *Innovations in international and cross-cultural management* (pp. 52–90). Thousand Oaks, CA: Sage.

Morris, M. W., & Young, M. J. (2002). Linking culture to behavior: Focusing on more proximate cognitive mechanisms. In F. Yammarino & F. Dansereau (Eds.), *Research in multi-level issues: Vol. 1. The many faces of multi-level issues* (pp. 327–341). New York: Elsevier.

Murrell, A. J., Dietz-Uhler, B. L., Dovidio, J. F., & Drout, C. (1994). Aversive racism and resistance to affirmative action: Perception of justice are not necessarily color blind. *Basic and Applied Social Psychology*, *15*(1/2), 71–86.

Neuman, E., Sanchez-Burks, J., Ybarra, O., & Goh, K. (2005). *American optimism about the consequences of workgroup conflict*. Unpublished manuscript, University of Michigan, Ann Arbor.

Ouchi, W. (1981). *Theory Z*. Reading, MA: Addison-Wesley.

Oyserman, D., Coon, H. M., & Kemmelmeier, M. (2002). Rethinking individualism and collectivism: Evaluation of theoretical assumptions and meta-analyses. *Psychological Bulletin*, *128*(1), 3–72.

Paglis, L. L., & Green, S. G. (2002). Both sides now: Supervisor and subordinate perspectives on relationship quality. *Journal of Applied Social Psychology*, *32*(2), 250–277.

Parsons, T., Bales, R. F., & Shils, E. (1953). *Working papers in the theory of action*. New York: Free Press.

Pelled, L. H. (1996). Demographic diversity, conflict, and work group outcomes: An intervening process theory. *Organizational Science*, *7*, 615–631.

Pelled, L. H., & Xin, K. R. (1997). Birds of a feather: Leader–member demographic similarity and organizational attachment in Mexico. *Leadership Quarterly*, *8*(4), 433–450.

Peng, K., Nisbett, R. E., & Wong, N. (1997). Validity problems comparing values across cultures and possible solutions. *Psychological Methods*, *2*(4) 329–344.

Pinkley, R. L. (1990). Dimensions of conflict frame: Disputant interpretations of conflict. *Journal of Applied Psychology*, *75*(2), 117–126.

Prentice, D., & Miller, D. (1999). *Cultural Divides: Understanding and overcoming group conflict*. New York: Russell Sage Foundation.

Rafaeli, A., & Dutton, J. (1997). Navigating by attire: The use of dress by female administrative employees. *Academy of Management Journal*, *40*(1), 9–45.

Riesman, D. (1961). *The lonely crowd*. New Haven, CT: Yale University Press.

Sagiv, L., & Schwartz, S. H. (2000a). Value priorities and subjective well-being: Direct relations and congruity effects. *European Journal of Social Psychology*, *30*, 177–198.

Sagiv, L., & Schwartz, S. H. (2000b). A new look at national culture: Illustrative applications to role stress and managerial behavior conference presentations. In N. Ashkenasy, M. Peterson, & C. Wilderom (Eds.), *Handbook of organizational culture and climate* (pp. 417–436). Thousand Oaks, CA: Sage.

Salancik, G., & Meindl, J. (1984). Corporate attributions and strategic illusions of management control. *Administrative Science Quarterly*, *29*, 238–254.

Sanchez-Burks, J. (2002). Protestant relational ideology and (in)attention to relational cues in work settings. *Journal of Personality and Social Psychology*, *83*(4), 919–929.

Sanchez-Burks, J. (2005). Protestant relational ideology: The cognitive underpinnings and organizational implications of an American anomaly. In R. Kramer & B. Staw (Eds.), *Research in organizational behavior* (Vol. 26, pp. 265–305). New York: Elsevier.

Sanchez-Burks, J., Blount, S., & Bartel, C. (2007). *The role of behavioral mirroring and relational attunement in intercultural workplace interactions*. Unpublished manuscript, University of Michigan, Ann Arbor.

Sanchez-Burks, J., Lee, F., Choi, I., Nisbett, R. E., Zhao, S., & Koo, J. (2003). Conversing across cultures: East–West communication styles in work and nonwork contexts. *Journal of Personality and Social Psychology, 85*(2), 363–372.

Sanchez-Burks, J., Nisbett, R. E., & Ybarra, O. (2000). Cultural styles, relational schemas, and prejudice against out-groups. *Journal of Personality and Social Psychology, 79*(2), 174–189.

Schein, E. (1996). Culture: The missing concept in organization studies. *Administrative Science Quarterly, 41,* 229–240.

Schneider, B. (1987). The people make the place. *Personnel Psychology, 40,* 437–453.

Schooler, C. (1976). Serfdom's legacy: An ethnic continuum. *American Journal of Sociology, 81*(6), 1265–1286.

Sears, D. (1983). The person-positivity bias. *Journal of Personality and Social Psychology, 44*(2), 233–250.

Sherony, K. M., & Green, S. G. (2002). Coworker exchange: Relationships between coworkers, leader-member exchange, and attitudes. *Journal of Applied Psychology, 87*(3), 542–549.

Sinha, J. B. (1980). *Nurturant task leader.* New Delhi: Concept.

Staw, B., McKechenie, P., & Puffer, S. (1983). The justification of organizational performance. *Administrative Science Quarterly, 28,* 582–600.

Takano, Y., & Osaka, E., (1999). An unsupported common view: Comparing Japan and the U.S. on individualism/collectivism. *Asian Journal of Social Psychology, 2*(3), 311–341.

Thomas, D. (1993). Racial dynamics in cross-race developmental relationships. *Administrative Science Quarterly, 38,* 169–194.

Ting-Toomey, S. (1988). Intercultural conflict styles: A face-negotiation theory. In Y. Y. Kim & W. B. Gudykunst (Eds.), *Theories in intercultural communication* (pp. 213–238). Newbury Park, CA: Sage.

Tönnies, F. (2002). *Community and society.* Piscataway, NJ: Transaction Publishers. (Original work published 1887)

Triandis, H. C., Dunnette, M. D., & Hough, L. M. (1994). *Handbook of industrial and organizational psychology.* Palo Alto, CA: Consulting Psychology Press.

Triandis, H. C., Marin, G., Lisansky, J., & Betancourt, H. (1984). *Simpatía* as a cultural script of Hispanics.

Journal of Personality and Social Psychology, 47, 1363–1375.

Tung, R. L. (1987). Expatriate assignments: Enhancing success and minimizing failure. *Academy of Management Review, 1*(2), 117–125.

U.S. Bureau of the Census. (2000). *Nativity, citizenship, year of entry, and region of birth.* Retrieved October 10, 2006, from *www.census.gov*

van Baaren, R., Horgan, T., Chartrand, T., & Dijkmans, M. (2004). The forest, the trees, and the chameleon: Context dependence and mimicry. *Journal of Personality and Social Psychology, 86,* 453–459.

van Baaren, R. B., Maddux, W. M., Chartrand, T. L., de Bouter, C., & Van Knippenberg, A. (2003). It takes two to mimic: Behavioral consequences of self construals. *Journal of Personality and Social Psychology, 84,* 1093–1102.

Wall, J. A., Jr. (1990). Managers in the People's Republic of China. *Academy of Management Executive, 4*(2), 19–32.

Weber, M. (1930). *Protestant ethic and the spirit of capitalism.* Winchester, MA: Allen & Unwin. (Original work published 1904)

Wessel, H. (2003, November 16). A 40-hour workweek just a dream to many. *Houston Chronicle.* Retrieved October 10, 2006, from www.chron.com/CDA/archives/archive.mp/?id=2003-37-8256

Williams, K. Y., & O' Reilly, C. A., III. (1998). Demography and diversity in organizations: A review of 40 years of research. *Research in Organizational Behavior, 20,* 77–141.

Word, C. O., Zanna, M. P., & Cooper, J. (1974). The nonverbal mediation of self- fulfilling prophecies in interracial interaction. *Journal of Experimental Social Psychology, 10,* 109–120.

Whyte, W. H. (1956). *Organization man.* New York: Simon & Schuster.

Winterbottom, M. R. (1953). *The relation of childhood training in independence to achievement motivation.* Unpublished doctoral dissertation, University of Michigan, Ann Arbor.

Zartman, W., & Berman, M. (1982). *The practical negotiator.* New Haven, CT: Yale University Press.

Zemba, Y., Young, M., & Morris, M. W. (2005). *Blaming executives for organizational harms: How intuitive logics of Japanese and Americans differ.* Unpublished manuscript, Tokyo University, Tokyo, Japan.

CHAPTER 15

Culture and Social Structure

The Relevance of Social Structure to Cultural Psychology

CARMI SCHOOLER

This chapter is written from the perspective of someone who functions professionally as not only a psychologist but also a sociologist. In fact, much of the chapter is written from a sociological perspective. This perspective is particularly germane for understanding the relevance of social structure—in brief, the arrangement of roles within a social system—to the concerns of cultural psychologists. Cultural psychology focuses on how one level of suprapersonal social phenomena—culture—affects the psychological functioning of the individual. It shares with much of psychology a distinct tendency to neglect the psychological effects of social structure. In doing so, cultural psychologists tend to treat all individuals in a culture as being subject to the same socioenvironmental influences. This is definitely not the case. Dissimilarities in social–structural position, almost by definition, result in differences in the nature of the environment to which the individual is exposed.

The issue is not merely one of "independent" social–structural and cultural effects on psychological function. There is also the distinct possibility that culture and social structure may interact in affecting psychological functioning. Not only may cultural effects on psychological functioning vary among individuals in different social–structural positions, but the same social–structural position may also have different effects in different cultures.

In examining potential interactions between culture and social structure we should also consider the possible "reverse" effects of the psychological functioning of individual members of a society on its culture. As Cohen (2001) has noted, "Environmental circumstances lead to different cultural 'traits'. Different ecologies . . . predispose a culture to different social structures" (p. 452). Particularly relevant to the question of the effects of social structure are cases in which psychological changes among individuals in various social–structural positions in a society—changes resulting from changes in that society's socioeconomic structure (e.g., modes of production and distribution)—end up affecting its culture. Such effects of modes of production on the psychological functioning and values of individuals in different social–structural positions within a society are among the principal social mechanisms underlying the hypotheses cited by Cohen (2001) as leading to differences in cultural values both across different societies and historically within a given society.

SOME DEFINITIONS

Before providing specific examples of these potential causal interconnections among culture, social structure, and psychological functioning, it is heuristically useful to define "culture" and "social structure," as well as a series of related terms that help explicate their potential relationships. The definitions I present are adaptations and modifications of the general view of noted sociologist Robert Merton (1957a, 1957b) and well within the mainstream of sociological thought (for an extended discussion and elaboration of this theoretical framework, see Schooler, 1994).

- *Status:* A position in a social system occupied by designated actors (i.e., individuals or social organizations) that comprises a set of roles that define the incumbents' expected patterns of interrelationships with incumbents of related statuses. Statuses may be ranked hierarchically in terms of the interrelated concepts of (1) prestige, (2) unequal distribution of relatively scarce social resources and unequal opportunity for acquiring them, and (3) power—the ability to induce others to fulfill one's goals. When statuses are considered in terms of such a hierarchical perspective, the term "social status" is frequently used.
- *Social class:* The term "social class" is often used almost interchangeably with the term "social status." Most sociologists who deal with stratification, however, distinguish between the two. They reserve use of the term "social class" to reflect the types of societal divisions envisaged by Marx. Thus, Kohn and Slomczynski (1990) describe social classes as "groups defined in terms of their relationship to ownership and control over the means of production, and their control over the labor power of others" (p. 2). I would amend this definition to include also ownership and control over the means of distribution. The focus of this review is on the more general concept—status.

- *Social structure:* The patterned interrelationships among a set of individual and organizational statuses, as defined by the nature of their interacting roles.
- *Culture:* A historically determined set of denotative (what is), normative (what should be), and stylistic (how done) beliefs shared by a group of individuals who have undergone a common historical experience and participate in an interrelated set of social structures. In a more expansive form, the definition could include the institutional, instrumental, and material embodiments of these beliefs.
- *Society or sociocultural system:* A set of persons and social positions that possesses both a culture and a social structure.
- *Caste,* the final term whose definition I present, is particularly germane to the issue of the relationship of social structure and culture, because it combines facets of both. In 1930, Kroeber defined a caste as "an endogenous and hereditary subdivision of an ethnic unit occupying a position of superior or inferior rank or social esteem in comparison with other such subdivisions" (p. 254). I would only add that castes "restrict the occupation of their members and their association with members of other castes . . . through social barriers sanctioned by custom, law or religion" (Lowe, McHenry, & Pease, 1985).

It should be noted that the definition of "culture" posits subordinate social structures. In turn, social structure is, by definition, posited to be superordinate to individual psychological functioning. These definitions thus presuppose that culture, social structure, and psychological functioning, although causally and ontologically related, represent different levels of phenomena (for a full discussion of emergent levels of reality based on the work and conceptualizations of the comparative animal psychologist T. Christian Schnierla [1951], see Schooler, 1994). Nevertheless, subordinate and superordinate levels of phenomena can affect each other. Thus, just as the characteristics of the superordinate cultural level may affect the characteristics of the subordinate social–structural level, the characteristics of the subordinate social–structural level can affect the superordinate cultural level.

Much more speculative is the possibility that among these levels of phenomena, superordinate levels tend to affect subordinate levels more quickly than the other way around. If so, then psychological phenomena would more quickly be affected by social–structural phenomena than the reverse; in turn, social–structural phenomena, would be affected more quickly by cultural phenomena than the reverse. Empirically, such a possibility is suggested by a series of findings (e.g., Schooler, 1976; Kohn & Schooler, 1983; Schooler & Naoi, 1988; M. Naoi & Schooler, 1990) in which the effects of superordinate-level phenomena on subordinate-level phenomena are contemporaneous, whereas the effects of subordinate-level phenomena on superordinate-level phenomena are lagged (i.e., they occur over a longer period of time).[1]

As elaborated by Schooler (1994), a possible theoretical explanation for such a temporal ordering starts with the truism:

> Everything that exists has not been dysfunctional long enough or severely enough to cease being able to exist. From this perspective, the hypothesis about the different speeds at which things change can be reframed in terms of how long an element in a particular system can be dysfunctional before it ceases to exist, possibly by leading to the destruction of the system (e.g., organism, social structure, sociocultural system) of which it is a part. Thus, perhaps, because less redundancy is likely to exist at subordinate than at superordinate levels, the lower the level of phenomena, the shorter the period for which it can tolerate dysfunctional elements. . . . If more complex levels tend to have a greater degree of redundancy, a greater number of dysfunctional elements would be necessary to disrupt them. . . . Dysfunctional elements in a person's thought processes are likely to threaten the thinker's existence more quickly than dysfunctional elements in a social structure are likely to lead to the end of the social structure. In a similar manner, cultural level phenomena may be more resistant to change than social structural level phenomena because phenomena at the sociocultural system level are superordinate to those at the social structural level: not only are social structures elements of cultural level phenomena, but cultural beliefs affect the role expectations that pattern social structures. (p. 268; Schooler, 1994, contains a more extended discussion of the theory)

Leaving aside the question of the exact mechanisms through which such effects occur, social structures are obviously affected by what happened in their past. Thus, social structures are influenced by past history, just as are cultures. For out present purposes, the important

distinction, is that, as noted earlier, a society's culture seems apt to change more slowly than its social structure. Cultures tend to remain affected by events in the relatively distant past, including such specific ones as which side holding which ideology won what battle, or which unusual person with what abilities and beliefs appeared when. A society's social structure, on the other hand, is affected by not only its historically determined culture but also by relatively immediate exigencies such as its socioeconomic processes of production and distribution (Schooler, 1996). It is at least in part to take into account this possibility that, as a matter of emphasis, the term "historically determined" is included in the definition of culture, but not in the definition of social structure.

Whether or not there actually is a consistent difference between the speeds with which culture, social structure, and individual psychological functioning generally affect each other, it is clear that these three levels of phenomena do affect each other. In the next several sections I provide examples of such effects that are pertinent to the issue of the relevance of social structure to cultural psychology. I begin by supplying evidence of the direct relevance of social structure to the study of the psychology of the individual by presenting three illustrative examples in which social structure directly affects psychological functioning: (1) the psychological effects of occupational conditions; (2) the interconnections of social structure, stress, and mental and physical health; and (3) the effects of social structure on the psychological determinants of educational outcomes.

Because this cultural psychology handbook is replete with instances in which culture affects individual psychological functioning, I omit parallel examples demonstrating such cultural effects. Instead, I devote the bulk of the review to illustrating and discussing how the effects of culture and social structure often interact in affecting psychological functioning. As a consequence of such interactions, it is often necessary to take into account culture and social structure simultaneously if we are to understand the effects of each. I conclude my literature review by discussing several examples of how cultural and social–structural factors interrelate in affecting how caste membership influences psychological functioning—with caste itself representing a dense interweaving of cultural and social–structural elements.

EFFECTS OF SOCIAL STRUCTURE ON PSYCHOLOGICAL FUNCTIONING

Central to my discussion of the effects of social structure on psychological functioning is the hypothesis that social–structural differences in the complexity of the environments, particularly work environments, faced by individuals in different positions in a society's social structure play an important part in accounting for social status differences in levels of intellectual functioning and self-directed orientations and values in that society. My reasoning centers on a rough-hewn theory of the psychological processes through which complex environments have their effects (Schooler, 1984, 1990a). According to this theory, the complexity of an individual's environment is defined by its stimulus and demand characteristics. The more diverse the stimuli, the greater the number of decisions required, the greater the number of considerations to be taken into account in making these decisions, and the more ill defined and apparently contradictory the contingencies, the more complex the environment. Such environments put a premium on intellectual flexibility—the ability to use an assortment of approaches and vantage points in confronting cognitive problems in a nonstereotypical way. To the degree that such an environment rewards cognitive effort, individuals should be motivated to develop their intellectual capacities and to generalize the resulting cognitive processes to other situations. Conversely, continued exposure to relatively simple environments may have the opposite effects. The theory is consistent with findings of a large body of research from a wide range of disciplines, including animal-based neurobiology (e.g., Kempermann, Kuhn, & Gage, 1997; Greenough, Cohen, & Juraska, 1999), indicating that exposure to complex environments increases intellectual functioning throughout the life course and across species (Schooler, 1984, 1990a, 2007). I define intellectual functioning by the level of complexity of the problems that the individual is currently able to solve.

Nonintellective aspects of psychological functioning should also be affected by environmental complexity. To the extent that complex environments reward initiative and independent judgment, such environments should foster a generalized orientation to self-directedness rather than conformity to external authority. It is also plausible that experience in complex environments leads to the development of a kind of subjectivism deriving from both the feeling that locus of control is and should be within oneself and the importance given to mental processes by the emphasis placed on effective cognitive functioning (Schooler, 1972).

The hypothesis about the positive effects of doing self-directed substantively complex work on intellectual functioning provides a clue to, at least, a partial explanation of what has been termed the "Flynn effect" (Neisser, 1998)—the trend in industrial societies, ever since testing began, for scores over a wide range of intelligence tests to rise by about 3 IQ points per decade (Flynn, 1987). If technical and economic development leads to more complex environments and to more intellectually demanding work conditions, such increased environmental complexity should result in higher levels of intellectual functioning. Such an increase in environmental complexity almost certainly occurred in the move from rural to urban settings, and from premodern agricultural to commercial and manufacturing occupations. There is also evidence that the substantive complexity of work continues to increase at later levels of development (Attwell, 1987; Dickens & Flynn, 2001; Form, 1987; Penn, Michael, Rose, & Rubery, 1994). Given this increasing complexity of work demands and other aspects of life, and the causal link between levels of environmental complexity and intellectual functioning, the ongoing gains in intelligence test performance that Flynn (1987) found can be seen as due, in some large part, to the way the world has become more complex. For a full discussion of the plausibility of this view of the Flynn effect, see Schooler (1998).

More generally, the complexity of the intellectual demands made by modern occupational and other social conditions can also be seen as contributing to what have been described as the psychological consequences of modernization. The pioneer quantitative, cross-national study examining the psychological correlates of modernization was the Project on the Sociocultural Aspects of Development. Led by Alex Inkeles, its goal was to test his hypothesis "that the standardized institutional environments of modern society induce standard patterns of response, despite the countervailing randomizing effects of persisting traditional patterns of culture" (Inkeles, 1960, p. 1). It did so by examining the degree to which individuals "incorporate as personal attributes qualities which are analogous to or derive from the organizational properties of the institutions and roles in which ... [they] are regularly and deeply involved" (Inkeles, 1983, p. 8). Tying this question specifically to modern experience, Inkeles and Smith (1974) selected the factory as an embodiment of many aspects of such experience. From an analysis of factory characteristics they derived a set of qualities that they assumed would be learned and incorporated as personal attributes by men who experienced extended factory employment after growing up in a premodern rural village. This set of qualities, which they called *individual modernity*, consisted of openness to new experience, independence from traditional authority, belief in science and medicine for solving human problems, educational and occupational ambition, punctuality and orderliness, and interest in civic affairs (Inkeles, 1969).

The research was conducted in six industrializing nations—Argentina, Bangladesh, Chile, India, Israel and Nigeria; almost 6,000 men served as survey respondents. Analyses of the data indicated that the various hypothesized aspects of modernity, do, in fact, co-occur in a syndrome of individual modernity. Furthermore, the findings demonstrated robust cross-national empirical relationships between the various psychological aspects of individual modernity and work in industrial settings, as well as exposure to such other concomitants of modernization as urbanization, education and mass media. In each of the countries studied, exposure to social-structural conditions associated with industrialization was generally shown to be empirically correlated with the psychological characteristics predicted by the Project's theory.

Despite the strength of its empirical findings, the Project has been criticized for a variety of ideological reasons. For example, from the neo-Marxist perspective, Wallerstein (1974) has characterized it as an apologia for the capitalistic, imperialistic status quo. Somewhat similarly, from the postmodernist perspective, Luke (1991) sees the modernity thesis as a "dehistoricized, desocialized and de-culturalized-social theory" (p. 284) that the power elite uses as a legitimating ideology to control the masses socially.

Despite these ideological complaints, there does not seem to have been any major study that refutes the original Inkeles and Smith (1974) empirical conclusions. In fact, Inglehart and Baker's (2000) reanalysis of an extensive series of cross-national surveys in terms of traditional values versus secular–rational values and survival versus self-expression values strongly attests to the general validity of Inkeles et al.'s general findings about the psychological effects of modernization. Thus, Inglehart and Baker conclude that although "the broad cultural heritage of a society— Protestant, Roman Catholic, Orthodox, Confucian or Communist—leaves an imprint on values that endures despite modernization ... economic development is associated with shifts away from absolute norms and values towards values that are increasingly rationale, tolerant, trusting and participatory" (p. 19). A complaint that can be legitimately raised about Inkeles and his colleagues is their conceptual and empirical ambiguity about how the socioenvironmental conditions and psychological characteristics they associate with modernity relate to each other. Although Inkeles and his associates (Inkeles, 1983; Inkeles & Smith, 1974) described several mechanisms through which such changes may take place (i.e., reward and punishment, modeling, exemplification, and generalization), they never empirically isolate which aspects of the modernization experience have these effects.

Psychological Effects of Occupational Conditions

The attempt to specify how the social-structurally determined environmental conditions that individuals face in modern societies affect their psychological functioning was an underlying aim of the project on the psychological effects of occupational conditions that Melvin Kohn and I originally conceived in the early 1960s. The initial impetus of the study was to test the hypothesis that social status differences in occupational conditions were the cause of the social status differences in parental values that Kohn (1959) had previously found. In the course of developing our research protocol, our goals expanded greatly. The general purpose of the study became to test the hypothesis that social status differences in people's orientations toward themselves and their environments, in the values they hold for themselves and their children, and even in the ways that they think, are a function of the nature and conditions of their work.

To delineate the exact linkages between individuals' conditions of work and their psychological characteristics, we did not compare specific jobs; rather, we conceived of a job in terms of a series of dimensions. Among these were substantive complexity, closeness of supervision, routinization (seen as indicative of occupational self-direction), ownership, bureaucratization, position in the hierarchy, and time pressure. Substantive complexity was the keystone concept in regard to occupational self-direction, in terms of both our theoretical perspective and empirical findings. We defined "substantively complex work" as work that in its very substance requires thought and independent judgment (Kohn & Schooler, 1983, p. 106). Indices for the latent concept of substantive complexity of work are derived from detailed open- and closed-ended questions about the participants' work with things, data (or ideas), and people. The questions provide the basis for seven ratings: appraisals of the complexity of each respondent's reported work with things, with data, and with people based on those of the *Dictionary of Occupational Titles* (U.S. Department of Labor, 1965), as well as respondents' estimates of the amount of time they spent working at each type of activity.

The original sample of 3,101 men interviewed in 1964 was representative of all men in the United States employed in civilian occupations. In a 1974 follow-up, a representative subsample of those men, who were then under 65 years old, was reinterviewed, and their wives and children were interviewed for the first time. Analyzing the men's longitudinal data with the then newly developed technique of structural equation modeling (SEM; (Joreskog, 1973), we found that jobs that facilitate occupational self-direction, increase intellectual functioning, and promote a self-directed orientation to self and to society (Kohn & Schooler, 1983).[2] Further findings demonstrated that opportunities for exercising occupational self-direction are to a large extent determined by a job's location in the social structure of society. Other results indicated that oppressive working conditions produce a sense of distress. In all of these findings there is the consistent implication that the principal process by which occupations affect personality is generalization from the lessons of the job to life off the job. Interviews with the male respondents' wives revealed a similar pattern of psychological effects of occupational conditions among employed women (J. Miller, Schooler, Kohn, & Miller, 1979).

In 1994, I and my colleagues in the National Institute of Mental Health (NIMH) Section on Socioenvironmental Studies carried out a 20-year follow-up survey on the surviving members of the adult 1974 sample. Our findings, (Schooler, Mulatu, & Oates, 1999, 2004) are based on the 166 men and 78 women who were working when interviewed, both times that they were surveyed. These findings replicate and extend the earlier Kohn and Schooler (1983) findings about the effects of substantively complex self-directed work on intellectual functioning, and self-directed values and orientations when the sample was 20 years younger. Our new findings provide consistent, credibly strong evidence that even in old age, carrying out self-directed, complex tasks on the job has a positive effect on intellectual processes and also increases self-directed orientations. Because each of these general psychological characteristics is both caused by and causes high social status, our findings also confirm and elucidate the complex causal patterns through which social status, occupational conditions, and psychological functioning affect each other (Schooler et al., 2004).

From the very beginning, Kohn and I realized that cross-national replication represented one of the best ways to test the generalizability of our hypotheses. In fact, the first cross-national attempt to test these hypotheses (Pearlin & Kohn, 1966) was actually carried out in Turin well before the analysis of the data from the original 1964 U.S. survey was completed. Consequently, its indices, particularly for occupational self-direction, are only approximate. Still, the Turin study was the first to provide evidence that the relationship between social stratification and fathers' valuation of self-direction for children is substantially attributable to occupational self-direction. The study even provided evidence that the relationship between the men's social stratification position and their wives' values is in part attributable to the men's job conditions.

The cross-national replications methodologically closest to the Kohn–Schooler U.S. NIMH studies were carried in Poland and Japan, in direct collaboration with the NIMH investigators. The major purpose of these collaborations was to ascertain whether social–structural position has similar psychological effects in a Western and a non-Western, and in a capitalist and a noncapitalist, society. Finding similarities among these three countries in the psychological effects of being in an advantageous social–structural position and in the importance of occupational self-direction in explaining these effects, would provide considerable evidence that our findings have cross-cultural generality.

The Polish survey, directed by Kazimierz Slomczynski, was conducted in 1978 with the collaboration of Melvin Kohn (see Kohn & Slomczynski, 1990, for the most complete English description). The probability sample of 1,557 men was representative of men living in urban areas and employed full time in civilian occupations. The study was designed to be an exact replication of the main parts of the Kohn–Schooler study. Questions about occupational self-direction and psychological functioning were adopted from the Kohn–Schooler interview schedule. Overall, the Polish replication provided very strong confirmation of the Kohn–Schooler hypotheses. The findings

> demonstrate that occupational self-direction plays the pivotal role in explaining both the effects of social structure on personality and the effects of personality on achieved position in the social structure. Position in the class structure and in the stratification order affect men's values, intellectual flexibility and self-directedness of orientation primarily *because* they affect occupational self-direction; occupational self-direction, in turn, affects these facets of psychological functioning. These facets of psychological functioning affect men's positions in the social structure mainly *because* they affect occupational self-direction, which then affects class placement and status achievement. (Kohn & Slomczynski, 1990, p. 170)

Analyses of a replication carried out in Poland in 1992 and a companion study carried out in the Ukraine in 1993 (Kohn et al., 1995) indicate that radical social change does not change the pattern of relationships between social structure and personality found under stable social conditions. Instead, radical social change transforms social structures. In the process of transformation, the social structures of Poland and Ukraine increasingly resembled the social structures of the more capitalist types of society. By late 1992, Poland exhibited the capitalist pattern and early in 1993, Ukraine was not far behind (Kohn et al., 1997). The individuals in these societies changed as their social statuses changed—evidence that the psychological functioning of the individual is quite sensitive to social–structural change.

The Japanese replication was carried out by researchers at Tokyo and Osaka Universities under the direction of Atsushi Naoi, with my collaboration. The interview consisted primarily of questions translated from the original Kohn–Schooler U.S. survey. The 629 male respondents were drawn from a random probability sample of employed males, 26–65 years old. The results indicated that advantageous social–structural positions are related to parental valuation of self-direction, to intellectual flexibility, and to self-directedness of orientation for Japan very much as they are for the United States and Poland. Occupational self-direction has the same psychological effects and plays precisely the same role in explaining the relationships of social–structural position and personality for Japan as it does for the United States and Poland (A. Naoi & Schooler, 1985). These findings hold true even when traditionality of job settings and economic centrality of industry are statistically controlled (Schooler & Naoi, 1988).

As was the case in the United States, a similar pattern of psychological effects of occupational self-direction was found when the employed wives ($N = 246$) of the sampled Japanese men were interviewed (M. Naoi & Schooler, 1990). Because one of the most consistent themes in accounts of Japanese culture is the deemphasis of individualism and the importance placed on psychological interdependence (A. Naoi & Schooler, 1985), finding that occupational self-direction has the same effects in Japan as in the more individualistically oriented United States represents a very real increase in the generalizability of our hypotheses about the effects of occupational conditions.

Social Structure, Stress, and Mental and Physical Health

There is an extensive literature examining the interrelationships among social structure, stress, and mental and physical health. The most general findings are that relatively poor social–structural position is related to relatively high levels of stress (e.g., McLeod & Kessler, 1990; Stansfield, Head, & Marmot, 1998) and relatively poor mental health (Marmot, Ryff, Bumpass, Shipley, & Marks, 1997) and physical health (Adler, Marmot, McEwan, & Stewart, 1999). Intriguingly, the impact of social structure on health is not merely at the poverty line. The relationship is so regularly linear that it has been described as a gradient in which health status apparently improves with every increment of socioeconomic status (SES; Adler & Ostrove, 1999; Marmot, 1999). SEM analyses of the data from our 1974–1994 longitudinal survey confirmed that "a notable part of the effect of SES on health is due to psychological distress" (Mulatu & Schooler, 2002, p. 22).

Gallo and Matthews (2003) provide a full and excellent review of the relevant research literature on the role of negative emotions in the association between SES and health. They conclude by presenting "a general framework for understanding the roles of cognitive emotional factors, suggesting that low SES environments are stressful and reduce individuals' reserve capacity to manage stress, thereby increasing vulnerability to negative emotions and cognitions" (p. 10). As this framework implies, "studies that account for initial differences in stress exposure suggest that at every level of stress, individuals with low SES report more emotional distress than those with higher SES" (p. 34). Thus, social–structural position affects not only the amount of stress to which an individual is exposed but also the ability of that individual to deal with the resultant stress level.

Social Structure and Educational Outcomes

There is ample evidence that social structure affects educational outcomes. From kindergarten on, those from families relatively high in social status do better in school and go further up the educational ladder than those from less privileged social origins. The social–structural differences in level of schooling are not merely reflections of possible differences in mental ability that may derive from some combination of genetic and environmental factors. Also involved are social–structurally based differences in self-directedness and self-regulation, aspirations, perceptions of others' views of oneself, and actual and perceived resources.

Much of the best research in this area has been carried out by the Wisconsin Longitudinal Study of Social and Psychological Factors in Aspirations and Achievements (for a summary, see Sewell, Hauser, Springer, & Hauser 2001). The original data collection for this study was based on a 1957 survey of the postsecondary educational plans of all high school seniors in the public, private, and parochial schools of Wisconsin. Follow-up surveys that included not only a representative subsample of the original respondents but also their siblings and spouses were carried out in 1975–1977, 1992–1994, and 2002–2003. Throughout, the analyses have been carried out by some of the most sophisticated data analysts in the social sciences. In terms of educational aspirations, the Wisconsin researchers found that "for each gender, socioeconomic status is a powerful determinant of who will plan on college—even when intelligence measured is controlled" (Sewell et al., 2001, p. 8). Furthermore, it is the children's "perceptions of their parents' intent to encourage their educational aspirations that is crucial to the development and maintenance of those aspirations. . . . The educational attainments of both parents has strong positive effects on the aspirations of their children" (Sewell et al., 2001, p. 9).

In terms of actual academic attainment, Sewell et al. (2001) report that "when academic ability was controlled by dividing the sample into quarters according to the students' measured cognitive ability, we still found that higher socioeconomic status students attained substantially higher educations than did lower status student" (p. 13). A high-ability student coming from a family of high SES was approximately 3.5 times more likely to obtain a graduate degree or professional education than a student with similar cognitive ability who came from a family with low SES.

Sewell et al. (2001) concluded that "perhaps the most interesting finding was that educational aspiration strongly affected educational attainment, independent of its relationship to measured intelligence and socioeconomic status" (p. 14). Thus, educational attainment was strongly affected by a psychological characteristic—individuals' educational aspirations—that had been strongly affected by their perceptions of their parents' educational expectations for them. These perceptions were in turn affected by their families' positions in the social structures of their societies. This pattern of findings provides an example of how psychological characteristics, even noncognitive ones that are affected by a family's position in the social structure of its society, may decrease the likelihood of intergenerational mobility and thus increase the likelihood of reproduction of social status across generations.

The consequences for school performance of the effects of social structure on children's psychological functioning manifest themselves at the very beginning of the school career. Here too, such social structural differences are not limited to possible differences in intellectual functioning. As we have seen, the original impetus of the Kohn–Schooler occupation studies was to substantiate earlier findings that higher status parents were more likely than lower status parents to have values for their children that emphasized self-directedness rather than conformity, and to link these differences to disparities in the job demands of high- and low-status occupations (Kohn & Schooler, 1983).

Whether or not the SES differences in parental values are responsible for SES differences in childrens' self-regulation, such differences in self-regulation appear to exist and appear to predict school adjustment. Convincing evidence that this is the case is provided by Miech, Essex, and Goldsmith (2001) in a study using longitudinal data from 451 mothers in the Wisconsin Study of Family and Work. The mothers' survey included questions assessing their children's levels of self-regulation before they entered kindergarten. The kindergarten teachers assessed the children's: (1) overall problems in interpersonal relationships in school, (2) hyperactivity–attention deficiency, and (3) present and future academic ability. Miech et al. found that "self-regulation served as a mediator of the association between children's SES and both interpersonal problems at school and teachers' expectations" (p. 102). For example, after the influence of self-regulation was controlled, "the association between SES and relationship difficulties was diminished by 39 percent and was not statistically significant" (p. 108).

A source of unease among educators is the possibility that students may lose some of the skills and knowledge that they have acquired during the school year over summer vacation. Of particular concern has been the possibility raised by evidence collected in past decades that such loss was greater among children coming from lower SES families (e.g., Heyns, 1978; Entwisle, Alexander, & Olsen, 1997). These earlier studies did not take into account the timing of the pre- and postvacation tests during the school year. By not doing so, they left open the possibility that at least part of the differences found were due to social background differences in rates of learning while schools are in session. Recent analyses of data from a nationally representative U.S. sample (Burkam, Ready, Lee, & LoGerfo, 2004) have found that

even when time of testing is taken into account, students from different SES levels differ in what happens to their skills during the period between kindergarten and first grade. When the students are divided into quintiles in terms of their family SES, those from higher SES backgrounds continue to learn during the summer, whereas those from lower SES backgrounds lose some of the knowledge and abilities that they have learned. For reading, these differences follow a linear trend across SES quintiles. For mathematics and general knowledge the differences are not strictly linear: The lowest SES quintile loses knowledge and ability during vacation; the upper SES quintile gains knowledge, whereas the knowledge levels of the middle three quintiles remain the same.

There has been a strong suspicion (e.g., Entwisle et al., 1997) that such SES differences in the cognitive effects of vacations may be due to SES differences in the intellectual content and stimulation of the environments to which children are exposed when they are not in school. Burkam et al.'s (2004) analyses do not provide strong support for such a contention. They admit, however, that their measures may not adequately assess the relevant environmental characteristics. Nevertheless, whatever the exact causal mechanisms, Burkam et al.'s analyses provide a compelling example of the psychological effects of individuals' positions in the social structure of their societies—effects that influence individuals' abilities to take full advantage of the opportunities that their societies provide.

The Importance of Social Structure

In this section I have provided evidence that individuals' positions in the social structures of their societies can vitally affect them. We have seen how social–structural position can affect intellectual functioning and orientations to oneself and to others. We have seen how it can affect health, the level of stress to which individuals are exposed, their ability to cope with this stress, and their physical and mental health. The presented evidence shows that the effects of social–structural position extend beyond individuals to their families. This evidence demonstrates that parents' social–structural positions affect the school performance and educational attainment of their children—not only in terms of intellectual functioning but even when the level of their children's intellectual functioning is controlled.

The evidence that I have presented is only a selection from the vast amount of evidence that attests to the importance to individuals of their positions in the social structures of their societies. Underlying all of this evidence is the general principle that advantaged position in the social structure of, at least modern industrial and postindustrial societies, does not merely result in economic advantage (financial capital). Such favored positions also result in gains in human capital (peoples' skills and abilities as used in employment), social capital (the social network of the individual's family, friends, acquaintances, and contacts), and cultural capital (social status-linked cultural tastes, knowledge, and abilities). These forms of capital, although different, have the distinct possibility of converting into each other, so that a gain (or loss) in one form of capital can result in gains (or losses) in the others. It is just such ramifications of the effects of social status that make it so important for cultural, and other, psychologists to keep social structure in mind as they pursue their research and develop their theories.

SOME EXAMPLES OF THE INTERACTION OF SOCIAL STRUCTURE AND CULTURE IN AFFECTING PSYCHOLOGICAL FUNCTIONING

Cross-national studies testing hypotheses about the psychological effects of occupational conditions have come up with a variety of findings that involve interactions between a society's cultural characteristics and the ways that society's social structure affects the psychological functioning of its members. Thus, although both the Polish and the Japanese replications confirmed the cross-national generalizability of the Kohn–Schooler hypotheses, both studies provided intriguing evidence of how a nation's culture can also affect the ways conditions of work affect the individual psychologically.

The cross-national discrepancies between Polish and U.S. findings tend to center around cultural differences in attitudes toward authority (Kohn & Slomczynski, 1990). Thus, in the United States, the substantive complexity of work is generally the most important aspect of occupational self-direction for explaining the impact of social structure. In Poland, closeness of supervision is relatively more important and has its primary psychological impact through its effect on authoritarianism–conservatism. The positive correlation of closeness of supervision with authoritarianism–conservatism is notably higher there than in the United States. Kohn and Slomczynki see this higher correlation "as reflecting the greater saliency of authority in Polish than in American society. . . . It was in the self-interest of both the state bureaucracy and the church to support those elements of traditional Polish culture that encourage people to obey all forms of authority" (p. 207).

Another cross-national difference that Kohn and Slomczynski (1990) see as reflecting the greater cultural acceptance of traditional modes of authority in Poland compared to the United States is in the relative roles of fathers and mothers in the intergenerational transmission of values. In the United States, fathers tend to play a relatively important role; in Poland, mothers play the predominant role. Kohn and Slomczynski (1990) do not attribute this cross-national discrepancy to differing economic and political systems in the two countries. Rather they "think it is a historically rooted cultural contrast: Polish fathers play a more traditional role than do US fathers in the division of labor within the family and in the socialization of children. . . . The traditional Polish pattern where mothers have primary responsibility for child rearing and fathers' roles in the socialization of children focus on control and punishment, still obtains in many families" (p. 208).

When we examine Japan, we find that most of the cross-national differences relate to the nature and pervasiveness of the psychological effects of organizational position. The pattern of findings provides support for those who emphasize the general psychological importance of the group to the individual in Japanese culture and the specific importance to the Japanese worker of the organization for which he or she works (A. Naoi & Schooler, 1985), as well as for those who stress the cultural importance of hierarchical position (Nakane, 1970). In Japan, ownership and high position in the work hierarchy increase self-confidence and decrease self-deprecation. These job characteristics have no such effects in the United States (Kohn & Schooler, 1983) and may actually have had the opposite effects in socialist Poland (Kohn & Slomczynski, 1990). In Japan, as opposed to the United States and Poland, ownership and high hierarchical position at work lead to greater authoritarian–conservatism.

High hierarchical level at work also leads to more idea conformity and less personally responsible standards of morality. The scale measuring authoritarian-conservatism in Japan is actually marked by a higher degree of obeisance and respect for authority than its counterpart in the United States. The greater authoritarian-conservatism of Japanese in favorable organizational positions may reflect culturally embedded attitudes. Because of the "strong tendency for consequential human relations to have a vertical structure" in accord with Japanese cultural values (Caudill, 1973, p. 249; Nakane, 1970), Japanese in authority may tend to believe that such obeisance is appropriate, that moral principles can be bent to their needs, and that others share these beliefs.

Japan also provides an example of how cultural inertia may slow down social–structural and, consequently, psychological change. The evidence is strong that self-directedness is valued even less for women than for men in Japanese culture (Lebra, 1984; Schooler & Smith, 1978). It is highly plausible that this difference fosters the social–structural differences we find when we compare job roles of Japanese men and their wives (M. Naoi & Schooler, 1990). The wives' jobs are significantly lower in every component of occupational self-direction. Thus, Japanese cultural norms increase the likelihood that women will work in generally subservient, non-self-directed, low-prestige positions. As we have seen, occupying such positions reduces the self-directedness of their orientations. This would increase the likelihood that they will remain amenable to the cultural norms disvaluing women's autonomy (which, of course, played a part in their original discriminatory occupational placement) and decrease their motivation to organize in defense of women's rights. It will be interesting to see what may happen as a result of the recent trend for Japanese women to attain higher status jobs. There is evidence (Faiola, 2004) that this trend may result in a lesser willingness to get involved in "traditional" marriages with Japanese men—marriages that even a quarter of a century ago were often characterized by a psychological disengagement of Japanese wives from their husbands (Schooler & Smith, 1978).

Individuals' orientations toward themselves and others are affected by not only interactions between culture and social structure, as reflected by occupational position but also by interactions between culture and social–structural position, as embodied in education. Authoritarianism represents a striking example of such an interaction between culture and education. A substantial body of research links relatively favorable social–structural position with nonauthoritarian, generally self-directed orientations (for a review of the literature, see Farnen & Meleon, 2002). As indicated by the studies of the psychological effects of occupational conditions described above, much of this relationship may be due to the greater level of occupational self-direction that generally characterizes occupations well situated within the social structures of the relevant societies. Nevertheless, as we have seen in the case of Japan, a society's cultural values may influence the strength of the relationship between favorable social–structural occupational positions and self-directed orientations, sometimes doing so to the extent that it is reversed. Similarly, although there is a general tendency for education, which is typically an important indicator of both adult social status and social status of origin, to be linked to nonauthoritarian, self-directed orientations, there are a more than a few instances in which cultural values affect the strength of the relationship.

Simpson (1972) examined the relationship between education and authoritarianism in four societies. In the United States and Finland, he found the strong, expected relationship. In Costa Rica, education reduced authoritarianism only after the eighth grade. In Mexico, education had little effect on authoritarianism. Simpson hypothesized that "education will reduce authoritarianism only when the educational system emphasizes cognitive rather than rote learning or is manned by nonauthoritarian teachers" (p. 223). Duckitt (1992), who retested this hypothesis in a study that dealt with several potential concerns about the Simpson study, used an established measure of authoritarianism (Ray, 1979) whose items were balanced in terms of whether agreement or disagreement was indicative of authoritarianism. He dealt with the issue of whether Simpson's findings might result from noneducational socioeconomic differences between the countries by comparing English- and Afrikaans-speaking white South Africans; although the two groups are generally matched on socioeconomic dimensions, Afrikaans culture is generally viewed as more authoritarian. Duckitt concluded that the findings for English speaking White South Africans were consistent with a considerable amount of research indicating that increasing levels of formal education are associated with lower levels of authoritarianism . . . but the findings for Afrikaans speakers were not. The results of this study support Simpson's (1972) earlier observation that the relationship between education and authoritarianism may not be invariant and that, in certain sociocultural contexts, it will be severely attenuated or even absent. (p. 706)

In further support of this conclusion it is worth noting that Kohn and Slomczynski (1990) found no direct relationship between levels of authoritarianism and years of schooling in the Polish educational system—a system that may well have been characterized by authoritarian teachers and curricula.

In a more wide-ranging analysis based on representative data from over 40 countries, Farnen and Meleon (2002) found that the correlation between education and authoritarianism was substantially lower among states that had a history of totalitarian rule compared to those who had no history (−.22 vs. −.30). A similar pattern of correlations was found when states that were rated high on a state authoritarianism scale were compared to those rated medium and low on that scale (−.33 vs. −26 vs. −.17.). Interestingly, when Farnen and Meleon compared the correlation between education and authoritarianism among economically developed, developing, and undeveloped countries, the size of the negative correlation decreased as the level of economic development decreased (−.33 vs. −.25 vs. −15). Unfortunately, Farnen and Meleon did not carry out any analyses that simultaneously examined the effects of a history of totalitarian rule, high state authoritarianism, and economic development, so that we cannot know how much each of these cultural and socioeconomic factors independently affected the correlation, or whether they may have interacted in doing so.

It is also the case that what may initially appear to be culturally determined cross-national differences in interactions between cultural and social–structural variables may be the result of cross-national economic differences. Kunovich (2004) used hierarchical linear modeling to analyze multilevel data from 17 East and West European countries. He found that at the overall individual level, education and income reduced prejudice, and that prejudice increased when the individual occupied a labor market position likely to involve direct competition with immigrants. When, however, he compared the magnitude of these effects in the different countries, he found that these effects "are weaker in Eastern Europe compared to Western Europe, largely because of poor economic conditions. . . . Countries with poor economic conditions have weaker relationships between the social structural variables and prejudice" (p. 20).

CASTE: CULTURE AND SOCIAL STRUCTURE COMMINGLED

As described earlier, "castes" are the defining units of a system of rigid social stratification, sanctioned by custom, law, or religion. Caste systems are characterized by hereditary status, endogamy, and caste-based restrictions on occupation and social contact. As such, caste systems represent a true meld of culture and social structure, so that almost all effects of caste membership can be seen as an interaction between the two. Although the social science conceptualization of caste was originally developed on the basis of the Hindu system, castes exist in many countries and cultures. Examples in West Africa are *forgerons* (ironworkers) and *griots* (oral historians, praisers of famous men). Examples in Europe are tinkers and gypsies. An example in modern-day Japan is the Burakumin—descendents of a caste that worked in occupations associated with death. Burakumin were considered to be below the lowest rung of the traditional Tokugawa Japanese caste system. In that system, the Samurai were officially on the highest rung, followed by farmers, craftspeople, and merchants. It is also the case that the Japanese nobility, based on relationship to the Emperor, could then, and now, be considered a distinct caste, as might also past, and possibly present, European nobles.

A particular complication of caste systems that may affect individuals' attitudes and psychological functioning is that the culturally ascribed social status of the members of particular castes may not be mirrored in their socioeconomic position. An example of this is reported by Biswas and Pandey (1996) in a study of individual mobility and perception of social status among Indian tribal and caste groups. They found an interaction between caste and mobility in the perception of both status and relative poverty. In the perception of status

> mobile scheduled [i.e. very low status] caste . . . groups, even if they perceive their economic conditions as better . . . perceive their social status as lower. . . . The upper class immobile group perceived their social status as higher even though their socioeconomic condition was lower. . . . In the case of the perception of relative poverty, the immobile upper caste people perceived more relative poverty than did the immobile scheduled caste . . . People. (p. 209)

Biswas and Pandey concluded that

> in Indian society the upper caste feel entitled to and are expected to have an economically privileged range. . . . That is why the upper caste immobile respondents feel more deprived and relatively poorer than do their immobile counterparts in the scheduled caste . . . groups. The scheduled caste people may have accepted their ascribed low social position and may not feel entitled to greater economic facilities and thus do not perceive themselves as relatively more deprived; they therefore perceive less relative poverty. (p. 210)

Another interaction between caste and social structure occurs when values and modes of thinking that might be predicted as arising from the relative complexity and intellectual demandingness of caste members' educational and occupational experiences are counteracted by values deriving from these caste members' felt needs to preserve the caste's status in society.

An example of this can be seen in a study of the correlates of individualism and collectivism in Sri Lanka (Freeman, 1997). According to Freeman, "In Sri Lanka . . . occupational status is an index of one's rank within a traditional caste hierarchy . . . (homemakers, wage laborer, unskilled . . . professional with advanced degree; senior government or military official)" (p. 327). He predicted that those in high-status occupations would tend to hold idiocentric values stressing individualism and disvaluing collectivism. Freeman did so on the basis of reasoning analogous to that underlying the Kohn and Schooler (1983) and the Schooler et al. (1999, 2004) studies on the psychological effects of occupational conditions. "Post hoc analyses revealed that, quite opposite to prediction, a group of highly educated individuals, also high in occupational status, received some of the lowest idiocentrism scores in the entire

sample. These are the high caste, 'traditional elite' of the country" (p. 333). Freeman explained this unexpected finding by noting that

> [a] traditional system of caste by definition is opposed to the idiocentrist values of independence and self-determination. These values would understandably be rejected by the traditional elite, because they represent a threat to the social system that supports the high status of this group. By the same token, by endorsing idiocentrist values, educated lower- and middle-caste respondents may be expressing a rejection of the traditional status quo, and also expressing their aspirations beyond a low or intermediate status in the caste system. (p. 333)

Freeman notes that it is pertinent "that other social change theorists have observed similar patterns in other traditional cultures, such that the middle classes are most receptive to the processes of change in the status quo, whereas, the traditional elites and uneducated lower classes, albeit for different reasons, tend to be more resistant to change" (p. 333).

CONCLUSIONS

I hope that these theoretical discussions and empirical examples of the interconnections of social structure and culture have succeeded both in raising the methodological concern and piquing the theoretical interests of cultural psychologists. In terms of cultural psychologists' methodological approaches, given the above examples of how individuals' positions in the social structures of their societies can notably affect their psychological functioning, it is important that cultural psychologists pay attention to social–structural issues in designing their research. The importance of their doing so is increased by the possibility, illustrated by these examples, that cultural and social–structural factors may interact so that the effects of culture on psychological functioning may be dependent on the social–structural statuses of the individuals being investigated while, conversely, the effects of social–structural position may be affected by culture.

It would seem to sometimes be the case that when the "expected" psychological outcomes of being in a particular social–structural position challenge the traditional values and self-views of those in that position, the length of time that it takes for such effects to occur is extended, if they occur at all. Among examples of this tendancy that I have discussed are (1) the unexpectedly high levels of authoritarianism–conservatism among Japanese managers, (2) the more positive than might be expected self-views of relatively upper status castes that have had recent histories of downward economic mobility, (3) the less positive than might be expected self-views of low-status castes that have histories of recent upward mobility, (4) the relatively socially conservative authoritarian views of high-caste, elite Sri Lankans. What social scientists cannot say, or even hypothesize, at the present time is under what conditions such, or other, interactions between culture and social structure are likely to occur.

Given the demonstrated effects of social status on psychological functioning among individuals in the same society, and the evidence that these effects may be affected by interactions with culture, it is probably best that general conclusions about cultural differences between societies be based on samples that include a wide range of the statuses in the societies being compared. It is probably not sufficient to limit comparisons across cultures to individuals in the same social–structural position or positions, although, in many instances, doing so provides some level of control.

Unfortunately, the proviso about the dangers of basing conclusions about cross-cultural differences on studies of individuals in a single social–structural position applies to college students, who occupy a status that has been the focus of a large proportion of the research, particularly experimental research, in cultural psychology. Reason for concern about the general dependence on college students as experimental subjects in psychology experiments was provided over a decade and half ago in a review by Sears (1987; see also Schooler, 1989). Sears showed that the great majority of social-psychological studies conducted from the early 1960s until the time of his article had relied almost exclusively on college students tested in the laboratory. The most prestigious research was, if anything, more likely to have done so. These trends seem to have continued until the present. Sears also presented evidence suggesting the possibility that such subjects are likely to have less crystallized attitudes, less formulated senses of self, stronger cognitive skills, stronger tendencies to comply with authority, and more unstable peer group relationships than do older adults. He concludes that these

peculiarities of social psychology's predominant database may have unwittingly, and perhaps misleadingly, contributed to such major substantive conclusions: that people are easily influenced, behave inconsistently with their attitudes, do not rest their self-perceptions on introspection, and are highly egocentric. Sears also raised the possibility that this database may have contributed to the strong emphasis in contemporary social psychology upon cognitive processes. In terms of cultural psychology research, it is also quite plausible that the selection processes that affect the level and nature of an individual's education may differ across countries, resulting in psychological differences among individuals of nominally equivalent educational levels. Similarly, as seen in the case of authoritarianism, there is evidence that systematic cross-national differences, such as those in educational processes, may also lead to theoretically important differences in the psychological characteristics of individuals at nominally equivalent educational levels (e.g., college sophomores). Given these trends and possibilities, it is incumbent on cultural psychologists to base their conclusions on individuals from a range of educational levels. More generally, given the possibility of interactions such as those found between culture and social structure, it would seem to be important when describing the psychological effects of a society's culture, that cultural psychologists specify the segments of society to which they believe their conclusions apply.

The importance of taking social structure into account when considering the psychological effects of culture goes beyond a concern for placing appropriate limits on the extent of the empirical claims one makes. Paying attention to social structure is also important for understanding how culture and social structure function, how each affects the other, and how they may interact in having their psychological effects. An example of how social structure and culture may affect each other can be seen in the ramifications of the findings described earlier, that across a number of industrialized cultures, intellectually demanding work on the job increases intellectual functioning and individualistic self-directed orientations to self and others. These findings strongly raise the possibility that changes in a society's modes of production and distribution may affect the cognitive functioning, orientations, and values of its members. As noted earlier, it is just such societal differences in modes of production and distribution that the various theories reviewed by Cohen (2001) hypothesize to underlie the cultural dissimilarities and consequent psychological differences that are of central concern to cultural psychologists. One example of such concern with the effects of modes of production is Nisbett and Cohen's (1996) theoretical explanation of how a history derived from herding-based economy led the Southern United States to develop a culture of honor, with its psychological and behavioral consequences. Another example is Nisbett's (2003) tracing of Asian versus Western psychological differences to differences between cultures deriving from societies originally based on the large-scale, cooperative agriculture that was predominant in Asia as opposed to the subsistence, small-scale agriculture that characterized much of ancient Europe.

In terms of social–structural effects, it is important to note that not all social statuses within a given society may be similarly affected by a particular set of societal changes. Nor may all social statuses within a society be in similar positions to affect that society's cultural values. Given these possibilities, changes in a society's culture may come to be affected by not only the number of individuals whose psychological functioning and beliefs are affected by changes in a society's production or distribution of its "goods" but also the social–structural positions of the individuals whose psychological functioning and beliefs are so changed—hence, the theoretical importance of examining not only overall changes in socioenvironmental factors such as the nature of work and its consequent psychological effects in a given society but also the distribution of such changes within that society's social structure.

The possibility also exists of the development over time of a feedback loop between a society's socioeconomic functioning and the intellectual functioning of some of its members. Such a feedback loop might involve several stages: (1) Changes in modes of production and distribution within a particular society lead to increases in levels of occupational self-direction, and hence to increases in intellectual functioning; (2) these increases in intellectual functioning occur among individuals whose positions within that society's social structure lead to the development of new, more effective modes of that society's economic functioning; (3) these new modes of economic functioning

similarly involve increases in the intellectual demands placed on individuals in social–structural positions that permit them to affect their society's productiveness; (4) the resultant increases in level of individual intellectual functioning in such social–structural positions lead to still more effective and plausibly more complex intellectually demanding modes of production. Of course, it is equally plausible that if changes in a particular society's modes of production and distribution lead to a decrease in levels of occupational self-direction among individuals who are in social–structural positions that permit them to affect their society's productiveness, then the result might be a feedback loop that would eventually lead to less effective modes of production, distribution, and intellectual functioning.

The finding that occupational self-direction leads to self-directed orientations to self and society raises the possibility that the degree to which the modes of production within a society promote occupational self-direction may come to affect the level of individualism of that society's cultural norms. Here, too, there may develop over time a feedback loop between the individualistic values of those in particular locations in a given society's social structure and that society's modes of production and socioeconomic operation.

There has been a wide range of sociological theorizing that individualism, through one process or another, encourages economic development. Such a possibility is one of the foundations of Weber's argument in the debate about the importance of the Protestant ethic for the growth of Western capitalism (Tawney, 1963; Weber, 1958). Goldstone's (1987) argument that technical and economic progress is dependent on individuals' being open to innovation, pluralism, and the taking risks also suggests ways in which a self-directed individualistic orientation may encourage technical and economic development. Goldstone attributed the historical economic stagnation of a wide range of countries to the intolerance of innovation resulting from a "suppression of alternatives and emphasis on internal cultural orthodoxy" (p. 132) . To the degree that self-directed orientations loosen one's ties to and concerns about the social groups to which one belongs (Macfarlane, 1986; Schooler, 1990b), individuals strongly interested in their own success may also be more willing to engage in risky ventures than would those constrained by concerns over the repercussions of their actions to the social groups with which they identify. In addition, individuals with self-directed orientations may be freer to act without concern for the constraints that such group ties impose, providing for greater flexibility in both the geographical movement and occupational behavior of workers.

Although there may often be a link between individualistic values and economic development, the existence of individualistic, self-directed cultural norms does not guarantee economic development. Such cultural norms apparently characterize both preliterate, immediate-return hunter-gatherer societies (Woodburn, 1982) and subarctic hunting societies (Ridington, 1988). In neither case did self-directed individualistic orientations lead to economic development. Nor do the orientations and values that individuals within a society derive from their work experiences necessarily have a relatively immediate effect on their society's norms. Many factors, including the effectiveness of the institutions shielding a given society's established norms from change, can affect the degree to which, and the speed with which, the society's cultural norms are affected by the psychological consequences of its members' occupational conditions. Nevertheless, it remains distinctly plausible that such effects can and have occurred. For more elaborated discussions of these issues, see Schooler (1990b, 1994, 1996, 1998).

I began this review by noting the general lack of attention that psychologists pay to social structure as a variable that may potentially affect the psychological functioning of the individual. I hope that in the course of the review I have convinced those interested in cultural psychology of the importance of paying attention to the nature of the social structures of the societies whose cultures' psychological effects they are investigating. Of at least equal importance is that cultural psychologists take into account the social–structural positions of the individuals they are studying within the societies whose cultural effects they are investigating. As we have seen, cultures and social structures can interact both in terms of how they affect each other and how they affect the individual. Consequently, a full understanding of culture, of social structure, and of individual psychological functioning can only be truly achieved if attention is paid to each of these facets of reality and none is neglected.

NOTES

1. Cultural lag—the continuing psychological effects of cultural beliefs and practices in the face of material and social–structural change—has long been noted by sociologists (e.g., Ogburn [1950, 1964]). Evidence for the persistent long-term effects of culture on social structure and psychological functioning is presented by the finding (Schooler, 1976) that, compared to men from ethnic groups whose home countries abolished serfdom relatively early, American men from ethnic groups with a relatively recent and pervasive history of serfdom tend to show the nonindividualistic, conformist orientation, and intellectual inflexibility of men working under environmental conditions characteristic of serfdom. This pattern of findings strongly suggests that the restrictive social and occupational conditions that prevailed within feudal European societies seem to have affected those societies' cultures in a manner analogous to the way the lack of occupational self-direction affects an individual's intellectual functioning and orientations to self and others. The resultant pattern of persistent ethnic cultural differences has continued to affect both individuals' positions in the social structures of their society and their psychological functioning across generations and across the changes represented by industrialization and immigration the United States.

Evidence of the relatively more rapid effect of social structure on psychological functioning than of psychological functioning on social structure can be found in the Kohn and Schooler (1983) findings that the effects of social–structural position, as represented by such components of occupational self-direction as substantive complexity and closeness of supervision, have relatively contemporaneous effects on such aspects of psychological functioning as ideational flexibility and distress, whereas the reciprocal effects of these aspects of psychological functioning on job conditions tend to be lagged.

2. "Intellectual flexibility," the SEM measure of intellectual functioning used in the Kohn and Schooler (1983) studies, is defined as cognitive flexibility in coping with the intellectual demands of a complex situation. Its indices include (1) a summary score for performance on the Embedded Figures Test (Witkin, Dyk, Faterson, Goodenough, & Karp, 1962); (2) the interviewer's appraisal of the participant's intelligence; (3) the frequency of agreement with agree–disagree questions (because some of the questions included in the battery are stated positively and others negatively, an overall tendency to agree suggests that the participant is not thinking carefully about and is less differentiating about the questions); (4) the degree to which the answer to the question "What are all of the arguments you can think of for or against allowing cigarette commercials on TV?" provided reasons for both sides of the argument; and (5) the answer to a question about how to decide between two alternative locations for a hamburger stand (with answer adequacy being judged by a concern with potential costs, potential sales, and the understand-

ing that profits result from the difference between the two). The intellectual flexibility measure was highly correlated ($r = .86$, $p < .0001$) with a standard cognitive functioning factor based on standard cognitive tests introduced in the 1994 survey (i.e., immediate recall, category fluency, number series, verbal meaning, identical pictures, and different uses; Schooler, Mulatu, & Oates, 1999).

REFERENCES

Adler, N., & Ostrove, J. M. (1999). Socioeconomic status and health: What we know and what we don't. *Annals of the New York Academy of Sciences, 896*, 3–15.

Adler, N. E., Marmot, M., McEwan, B. S., & Stewart, J. (Eds.). (1999). *Annals of the New York Academy of Sciences: Vol. 896. Socioeconomic status and health in industrialized nations.* New York: New York Academy of Sciences.

Attwell, P. (1987). The deskilling controversy. *Work and Occupations, 14*, 323–346.

Biswas, U. N., & Pandey, J. (1996). Mobility and perception of socioeconomic status among tribal and caste group. *Journal of Cross-Cultural Psychology, 27*, 200–215.

Burkam, D. T., Ready, D. D., Lee, V. E., & LoGerfo, L. F. (2004). Social-class differences in summer learning between kindergarten and first grade: Model specification and estimation. *Sociology of Education, 77*, 1–31.

Caudill, W. A. (1973). The influence of social structure and culture on human behavior in modern Japan. *Journal of Nervous and Mental Disease, 157*, 240–257.

Cohen, D. (2001). Cultural variation: Considerations and implications. *Psychological Bulletin, 127*, 451–471.

Dickens, W. T., & Flynn, J. R. (2001). Heritability estimates versus large environmental effects: The IQ paradox resolved. *Psychological Review, 108*, 346–69.

Duckitt, J. (1992). Education and authoritarianism among English- and Afrikaans-speaking White South Africans. *Journal of Social Psychology, 132*, 701–708.

Entwisle, D. R., Alexander, K. L., & Olsen, L. S. (1997). *Children, schools, and inequality.* Boulder, CO: Westview Press.

Faiola, A. (2004, August 31). Japanese women live, and like it, on their own: Gender roles shift as many stay single. *The Washington Post*, p. A01.

Farnen, R. F., & Meleon, J. D. (2000). *Democracy, authoritarianism and education: A cross-national empirical survey.* New York: Palgrave Macmillan.

Flynn, J. R. (1987). Massive IQ gains in 14 nations: What IQ tests really measure. *Psychological Bulletin, 101*, 171–191.

Form, W. (1987). On the degradation of job skills. *Annual Review of Sociology, 13*, 29–47.

Freeman, M. A. (1997). Demographic correlates of individualism and collectivism: A study of social values in Sri Lanka. *Journal of Cross-Cultural Psychology, 28*, 321–341.

Gallo, L. C., & Matthews, K. A. (2003). Understanding the association between socioeconomic status and physical health: Do negative emotions play a role? *Psychological Bulletin, 129*, 10–51.

Goldstone, J. (1987). Cultural orthodoxy, risk and innovation: The divergence of East and West in the early modern world. *Sociological Theory, 5*, 119–135.

Greenough, W. T., Cohen, N. J., & Juraska, J. M. (1999). New neurons in old brains: Learning to survive? *Nature Neuroscience, 2*, 203–205.

Heyns, B. (1978). *Summer learning and the effects of schooling.* New York: Academic Press.

Inglehart, R., & Baker, W. E. (2000). Modernization, cultural change, and the persistence of traditional values. *American Sociological Review, 65*, 19–51.

Inkeles, A. (1960). Industrial man: The relation of status to experience, perception, and value. *American Journal of Sociology, 66*, 1–31.

Inkeles, A. (1969). Making men modern: On the causes and consequences of individual change in six developing countries. *American Journal of Sociology, 75*, 208–225.

Inkeles, A. (1983). *Exploring individual modernity.* New York: Columbia University Press.

Inkeles, A., & Smith, D. H. (1974). *Becoming modern: Individual changes in six developing countries.* Cambridge, MA: Harvard University Press.

Joreskog, K. G. (1973). A general method for estimating a linear structural equation system. In A. S. Goldberger & O. D. Duncan (Eds.), *Structural equation models in the social sciences* (pp. 85–112). New York: Seminar Press.

Kempermann, G., Kuhn, H. G., & Gage, F. H. (1997). More hippocampal neurons in adult mice living in an enriched environment. *Nature, 386*, 493–495.

Kohn, M. L. (1959). Social class and parental values. *American Journal of Sociology, 64*, 337–351.

Kohn, M. L., Kazimierz, M., Slomczynski, K. J., Khmelko, V., Mach, B. W., Paniotto, V., et al. (1997). Social structure and personality under conditions of radical social change: A comparative analysis of Poland and Ukraine. *American Sociological Review, 62*, 614–638.

Kohn, M. L., & Schooler, C. (1983). *Work and personality: An inquiry into the impact of social stratification.* Norwood, NJ: Ablex.

Kohn, M. L., & Slomczyski, K. M. (1990). *Social structure and self-direction: A comparative analysis of the United States and Poland.* Oxford, UK: Blackwell.

Kroeber, A. L. (1930). Caste. *Encyclopedia of the social sciences* (Vol. 3, pp. 254–257). New York: Macmillan.

Kunovich, R. M. (2004). Social structural position and prejudice: An exploration of cross-national differences in regression slopes. *Social Science Research, 33*, 20–44.

Lebra, T. S. (1984). *Japanese women: Constraint and fulfillment*. Honolulu: University of Hawaii Press.

Lowe, J. G., McHenry, R. D., & Pease, R. W., Jr. (1985). *Webster's ninth new collegiate dictionary*. Springfield, MA: Merriam-Webster.

Luke, T. W. (1991). The discourse of development: A genealogy of "developing nations" and the discipline of modernity. *Current Perspectives in Social Theory, 11*, 271–293.

Macfarlane, A. (1986). *Marriage and love in England: Modes of reproduction 1300–1840*. Oxford, UK: Blackwell.

Marmot, M. (1999). Epidemiology of socioeconomic status and health: Are determinants within countries the same as between countries? *Annals of the New York Academy of Sciences, 896*, 16–29.

Marmot, M., Ryff, C. D., Bumpass, L. L. Shipley, M., & Marks, N. F. (1997). Social inequalities in health: Next questions and converging evidence. *Social Science Medicine, 44*, 901–910.

McLeod, J. D., & Kessler, R. C. (1990). Socioeconomic status differences in vulnerability to undesirable life events. *Journal of Health and Social Behavior, 31*, 162–172.

Merton, R. K. (1957a). The role set: Problems in sociological theory. *British Journal of Sociology, 8*, 106–120.

Merton, R. K. (1957b). *Social theory and social structure*. New York: Free Press.

Miech, R., Essex, M. J., & Goldsmith, H. H. (2001). Socioeconomic status and the adjustment to school: The role of self-regulation during early childhood. *Sociology of Education, 74*, 102–120.

Miller, J., Schooler, C., Kohn, M. L., & Miller, K. A. (1979). Women and work: The psychological effects of occupational conditions. *American Journal of Sociology, 85*, 66–94.

Mulatu, M. S., & Schooler, C. (2002). Causal connections between SES and health: Reciprocal effects and mediating mechanisms. *Journal of Health and Social Development, 43*, 22–41.

Nakane, C. (1970). *Japanese society*. Berkeley: University of California Press.

Naoi, A., & Schooler, C. (1985). Occupational conditions and psychological functioning in Japan. *American Journal of Sociology, 90*, 729–752.

Naoi, M., & Schooler, C. (1990). Psychological consequences of occupational conditions among Japanese wives. *Social Psychology Quarterly, 58*, 100–116.

Neisser, U. (1998). Introduction: Rising test scores and what they mean. In *The rising curve: Long-term gains in IQ and related measures* (pp. 3–22). Washington, DC: American Psychological Association.

Nisbet, R. (2003). *The geography of thought: How Asians and Westerners think differently . . . and Why*. New York: Free Press.

Nisbett, R. E., & Cohen, D. (1996). *Culture of honor: The psychology of violence in the South*. Boulder, CO: Westview Press.

Ogburn, W. F. (1964). Social evolution reconsidered. In

O. D. Duncan (Ed.), *On culture and social change: Selected papers* (pp. 17–32). Chicago: University of Chicago Press.

Pearlin, L. I., & Kohn, M. L. (1966). Social class, occupation, and parental values: A cross-national study. *American Sociological Review, 31*, 466–479.

Penn, R., Michael, R., Rose, & Rubery, J. (1994). *Skill and occupational change*. Oxford, UK: Oxford University Press.

Ray, J. J. (1979). A short balanced F scale. *Journal of Social Psychology, 109*, 309–310.

Ridington, R. (1988). Knowledge, power, and the individual in subarctic hunting societies. *American Anthropologist, 90*, 98–110.

Schneirla, T. C. (1951). The "levels" concepts in the study of social organization in animals. In J. Rohrer & M. Sherif (Eds.), *Social psychology of the crossroads* (pp. 83–120). New York: Harper.

Schooler, C. (1972). Social antecedents of adult psychological functioning. *American Journal of Sociology, 78*, 299–322.

Schooler, C. (1976). Serfdom's legacy: An ethnic continuum. *American Journal of Sociology, 81*, 1265–1286.

Schooler, C. (1984). Psychological effects of complex environments during the life span: A review and theory. *Intelligence, 8*, 259–281.

Schooler, C. (1989). Social structural effects and experimental situations: Mutual lessons of cognitive and social science. In K. W. Schaie & C. Schooler (Eds.), *Social structure and aging: Psychological processes* (pp. 129–147). Hillsdale, NJ: Erlbaum.

Schooler, C. (1990a). Psychosocial factors and effective cognitive functioning through the life span. In J. E. Birren & K. W. Schaie (Eds.), *Handbook of the psychology of aging* (pp. 347–358). Orlando, FL: Academic Press.

Schooler, C. (1990b). Individualism and the historical and social–structural determinants of people's concern over self-directedness and efficacy. In J. Rodin, C. Schooler, & K. W. Schaie (Eds.), *Self directedness and efficacy: Causes and effects throughout the life course* (pp. 19–44). Hillsdale, NJ: Erlbaum.

Schooler, C. (1994). A working conceptualization of social structure: Mertonian roots and psychological and sociocultural relationships. *Social Psychology Quarterly, 57*, 262–273.

Schooler, C. (1996). William Caudill and the reproduction of culture: Infant, child and maternal behavior in Japan and the U.S. In D. Shwalb & B. Shwalb (Eds.), *Japanese childrearing: Two generations of scholarship* (pp. 139–163). New York: Guilford Press.

Schooler, C. (1998). Environmental complexity and the Flynn effect. In U. Neisser (Ed.), *The rising curve: Long-term gains in IQ and related measures* (pp. 67–79). Washington, DC: American Psychological Association.

Schooler, C. (2007). The effects of the cognitive complexity of occupational conditions and leisure time activities on the intellectual functioning of older adults. In W. Chodzko-Zajko & A. Kramer (Eds.), *Aging, exercise and cognition: Enhancing cognitive and brain plasticity of older adults.* Champaign, IL: Human Kinetics.

Schooler, C., & Mulatu, M. S. (2001). The reciprocal effects of leisure time activities and intellectual functioning in older people: A longitudinal analysis. *Psychology and Aging, 16*, 466–482.

Schooler, C., Mulatu, M. S., & Oates, G. (1999). The continuing effects of substantively complex work on the intellectual functioning of older workers. *Psychology and Aging, 14*, 483–506.

Schooler, C., Mulatu, M. S., & Oates, G. (2004). Effects of occupational self-direction on the intellectual functioning and self-directed orientations of older workers: Findings and implications for individuals and societies. *American Journal of Sociology, 110*, 161–197.

Schooler, C., & Naoi, M. (1988). The psychological effects of traditional and of economically peripheral job settings in Japan. *American Journal of Sociology, 94*, 335–355.

Schooler, C., & Smith, K. C. (1978). . . . and a Japanese wife: Social antecedents of women's role values in Japan. *Sex Roles, 4*, 23–41.

Sears, D. O. (1987). Implications of the life-span approach for research on attitudes of social cognition. In R. P. Abeles (Ed.), *Life span perspectives and social psychology* (pp. 17–60). Hillsdale, NJ: Erlbaum.

Sewell, W. H., Hauser, R. M., Springer, K. W., & Hauser, T. S. (2001). *As we age: A review of the Wisconsin Longitudinal Study, 1957–2001.* Madison: Center for Demography and Ecology, University of Wisconsin–Madison.

Simpson, M. (1972). Authoritarianism and education: A comparative approach. *Sociometry, 35*, 223–234.

Stansfeld, S. A., Head, J., & Marmot, M. (1998). Explaining social class differences in depression and well-being. *Social Psychiatry and Psychiatric Epidemiology, 33*, 1–9.

Tawney, R. H. (1963). *Religion and the rise of capitalism.* Gloucester, MA: Smith.

United States Department of Labor. (1965). *Dictionary of occupational titles.* Washington, DC: U.S. Government Printing Office.

Wallerstein, I. (1974). The rise and future demise of the world capitalist system: Concepts for comparative analysis. *Comparative Studies in Social History, 16*, 287–415.

Weber, M. (1958). *The Protestant ethic and the spirit of capitalism.* New York: Scribner.

Witkin, H. A., Dyk, R. B., Faterson, H. F., Goodenough, D. R., & Karp, S. A. (1962). *Psychological differentiation: Studies of development.* New York: Wiley.

Woodburn, J. (1982). Egalitarian societies. *Man, 17*, 431–451.

PART IV

ACQUISITION AND CHANGE OF CULTURE

CHAPTER 16

Food and Eating

PAUL ROZIN

As its name indicates, with "cultural" modifying "psychology," cultural psychology is a branch of psychology. Although extending the scope and depth of psychology, it has appropriately accepted the organization that psychology has imposed on its phenomena. That orientation, unlike the orientation in anthropology or zoology, focuses on basic underlying processes, such as perception, attention, cognition, and emotion. Indeed, the document proposing this volume notes that its middle section will be organized "in terms of domains of cultural-psychological empirical research. There will be sections on identities, cognition, emotion and motivation, interaction and social relationships, and socialization." The process orientation that has dominated psychology for more than a century, documented by P. Rozin (in press), has proved very productive. But, especially with the reemergence of mind as the central concern of psychology in the late 20th century, the process orientation has focused almost entirely on the features of minds, at the cost of ignoring the domains of life, the institutions, cultural environments and practices that constitute most of daily life (P. Rozin, in press). It is these latter aspects that have dominated the fine ethnographies provided by anthropologists over the century, and that formed the empirical basis for the serious consideration of culture within psychology.

The fields of cognitive science and evolutionary psychology, following on changes in orientation to animal learning, have become more involved with domain-specific adaptations. It seems appropriate to at least raise the possibility of a different organization of cultural psychology. This would organize the field around the major domains of life: eating, sex, protection (including housing and clothing), parenting, etc. Unfortunately, it is virtually impossible to accomplish both a process and life domain segmentation of a field at the same time. However, for this volume, at least two exceptions to the process approach have been incorporated: one is a chapter on religion, and the other, this chapter on the domain of food and eating. Although food is clearly central to both culture and human biology, it has been little studied by psychologists in general, or by cultural psychologists specifically. This state of affairs results primarily from the process orientation in the field, as well as long-term (but diminishing) assumptions about the adequacy of domain general principles to account for behavior. This chapter attempts to organize what we know about food and culture, and to argue for a central role for the study of food and eating in cultural psychology.

Because the study of food (except for obesity, eating disorders, and the regulation of intake) is almost absent from psychology, I provide here a set of references to orient a reader to what is known about this area, principally from disciplines other than psychology—from the anthropological/evolutionary perspective: Diamond (1996), Harris (1985), Harris and Ross (1987), Katz (1982), and P. Rozin (1982); from a more general cultural perspective: DeGarine (1972), Mead, (1943), and Messer (1984); from the ethnographic perspective (e.g., especially informative food-related ethnographies): Meigs (1984), Ohnuki-Tierney (1993), and Whitehead (2000); from a sociological perspective: Beardsworth and Keil (1995), Murcott (1983), and Maurer and Sobal (1995); and from a more psychological and biological perspective: Booth (1994), Logue (2004), Meiselman and MacFie (1996), P. Rozin (1976; P. Rozin & Schulkin, 1990), and Shepherd and Raats (2006). Important cultural–historical perspectives are provided by Kass (1994), Levenstein (1988, 1993), Simoons (1991), and Whorton (1982). A few authors provide a broad, general perspective, including Barker (1982), Fischler (1990), Katz (2004), Kiple and Ornelas (2000), and Meiselman (2000).

THE FOOD–EATING DOMAIN

Food has to do with one of the basic domains of survival. It is central in animal life: food search, identification, and ingestion probably accounts for most of the waking time of most animals. Food selection is perhaps *the* single most important force in animal evolution; if you want to know as much as you can about an unknown animal, the best thing to ask, other than about its phylogenetic classification, is "What does it eat?" This single fact is highly informative about the sense organs, physiology of the digestive system, motor abilities, and learning or cognitive capacities. Animals that eat a very narrow range of foods are highly tuned to detect and appropriate their prey: Examples are anteaters, the carnivorous mammals, and specialized herbivores, such as pandas and koalas. More generalist animals have a broader but less specialized set of skills and structures, and are generally more well developed in what we loosely call intelligence (see Milton's [1993] article on the relation between brain size and diet in monkeys). A generalist animal faces a great set of challenges: finding combinations of foods that are nutritive, bal-

anced, and minimally toxic. I can imagine no other task that is more intellectually demanding, though, surely, mastering complex social organizations (e.g., Humphrey, 1976) is also deeply complex and challenging (and sometimes related to feeding patterns or strategies). So a first reason to be interested in food in cultural psychology is that it is such an important part of our primate heritage and so closely linked to intelligence.

A second reason that suggests food as an important area of study follows from the recent increase of interest in affect in psychology. Food is one of the major sources of affect. Eating is at the same time satisfying and threatening. It is a necessary and frequent part of remaining alive, because it provides the only source of energy and life-sustaining nutrients. On the other hand, many of the possible edibles in the world are toxic or are vehicles for dangerous microorganisms. Presumably, for this reason, people (and other animals) feel very strongly about what goes in their mouths; they are rarely neutral on this point. The stakes are high. For humans, another dimension amplifies the affective response to foods. It is widely believed in traditional cultures that a person takes on the properties of the foods he or she eats ("You are what you eat"). In this context, eating can have moral import, and can affect a person's personality and fortunes. "You are what you eat" is an eminently sensible idea; when we mix two things (in this case, a person and the food she eats), it is natural to believe that the product reflects both of the constituents. Although modern biological science makes clear that there are no grounds for believing that properties such as moral status or personality could be transmitted by the molecules that result from the process of digestion, it has been shown that even educated Westerners believe, implicitly, that one takes on the properties of what one eats. Nemeroff and Rozin (1989) asked two groups of American students to read a few paragraphs about a culture, then answer questions about the people in that culture. Both groups read the same description, except that one culture was described as eating boar and hunting, but not eating, marine turtle, and the other as eating marine turtle and hunting, but not eating, boar. The boar-eaters were later rated as having more hair, and as being more aggressive, faster runners, and showing other boar properties (and fewer turtle properties) than the turtle-eaters.

Other arguments for a cultural psychology of food and eating derive directly from human issues, and human culture. Food selection and procurement figure prominently in almost all theories of the evolution of humans, with a shift from a more plant-dominated forest diet to a diet with more animal protein in the savannah environment. Animals are generally harder foods to procure, so that more demands are made on motor capacities and sensory abilities. But a diet relying on animals does relieve a creature of the risks of dietary imbalance. All animals are made of roughly the same molecules, so almost any animal is a good source of nutrition. Not so for plants, which are often incomplete or imbalanced sources of nutrients for animals, and must be eaten in appropriate combinations. For the human omnivore, seeking animal food but still consuming a wide range of plant foods, there are two challenges: procurement of food (most challenging for animal prey) and appropriate food selection (most challenging to the degree of reliance on plant foods).

If there is *a* prominent advance that set humans on the course to elaborated culture, it is surely the development of agriculture and domestication (Diamond, 1996). These powerful human advances, made primarily some 4,000 to 10,000 years ago, provided humans with a steady and efficient food supply. This allowed for larger aggregations of humans, and for the specialization of labor inside and outside the food domain that prompted all sorts of technological advances (e.g., guns and steel, as Diamond eloquently argues). So, in the evolution of human culture, food provides a critical opportunity for extended development of other domains of life, including all sorts of crafts, aesthetic practices, and high technologies.

In contemporary human life, work and food are usually the two major categories of waking activities. Activity logs from 14 cultures, painstakingly documented by Szalai (1972), reveal that (for three cultures that I have tabulated—Peru, the United States, and France in the early 1970s) at 13.2% of total time (including food-related activities: eating, shopping, preparation, cleanup), food is third behind sleep (36.7%) and work (16%). And, of course, much of work is devoted to earning money or trade that is ultimately spent on food. Indeed, among the traditional cultures of the world, including China and India, themselves about a third of humanity, food is the principal source of expenditures, amounting to about 50% of total expenditures (Samuelson, 1990). In more developed cultures, such as Western Europe and North America, food drops down to 20% or considerably less of total expenditures, but these cultures constitute a minority of the world.

So two more reasons for being interested in food, besides its importance in animal life and evolution and its high affective loading, is its importance in both human evolution (biologically and culturally) and its importance in contemporary daily life.

There are further, discipline-related reasons for the study of food to be of particular interest to psychologists in general, and to cultural psychologists in particular. First, food is a major subject of thought, because the need for it is so compelling, and obtaining it is so challenging. It is likely that many of the features of intelligence so important for humans arose first in solving problems in the domain of food. "What is edible and what is not" is one of the most critical problems facing the young human omnivore. Powerful plastic adaptations to discover the effects of ingested food (e.g., conditioned taste aversions) stand out among learning abilities, and use of food as reinforcement is the central technique of the psychology of learning. Siegal (1996) has argued that in child development, the first domain in which nascent intellectual abilities appear often concerns food and the detection of toxicity.

Second, food and eating are unique among our basic biological systems with respect to human culture. The other systems, including breathing, excretion and sex, maintain much of their nonhuman primate character even in elaborated human cultures. It is the remarkable stability of human mating systems under the impact of powerful cultural change that puts mate selection at the center of evolutionary psychology (Buss, 2004). Food, on the other hand, is the one biological system that has been massively transformed by culture into a range of meanings and practices, cuisines, social events, such that the nutritional function of food is often overshadowed by its social functions. There is nothing quite like dinner, let alone a dinner "party," for our other biological functions. This unique elaboration of food is the subject of Leon Kass's (1994) remarkable book, *The Hungry Soul*, in which he documents the transformation of food from a source of nutrition to a socially meaningful substance in biblical through European history. As Kass notes: "An activity that is inherently ugly is beautified by graceful deed and tactful speech. An activity that is violent and destructive is tamed by gentle manner that keeps its destructive character mostly out of sight. An activity that deforms and dissolves living forms is given form-ality of its own by the work of the human intellect" (p. 154). Or "We eat as if we don't have to, we exploit an animal necessity, as a ballerina exploits gravity" (p. 158).

Third, a remarkable thing has happened to the world of food in developed cultures toward the end of the 20th century. Technological advances have virtually inverted our food environment, so that our adaptations to our ancestral environment are now often maladaptive. This is discussed in a later section.

THE BIOLOGICAL FOOD SYSTEM: THE HUMAN GENERALIST AND SOME FOOD UNIVERSALS

The food generalist faces a daunting food choice problem. Obtaining adequate nutrition involves satisfying the body's persistent need for some 40 nutrients, including many specific amino acids, some fatty acids, vitamins, minerals and water. In the course of satisfying these nutritional constraints, the generalist must also attain adequate energy from a mixture of proteins, fats, and carbohydrates. This set of nutritional requirements can be met easily if there is a fair amount of animal food in the diet, but also by choosing a broad diet among plant foods. However, the generalist faces a dilemma, because in the course of sampling the potential food environment widely, he is likely to encounter potential foods with toxic components or harmful microorganisms. The former are more likely in plants, the latter in animal foods. The risks of eating broadly are high, as are the benefits resulting from the ability to survive in diverse environments. There are no simple ways to avoid toxins and infective agents reliably on sensory grounds, nor to avoid potential foods that have minimal nutritional value. For the most part, this must be learned.

The food generalist, particularly the mammalian generalist (as exemplified by the relatively well studied domestic rat, *Rattus norvegicus*, and human beings), faces serious challenges in both the selection of a balanced diet and the avoidance of harmful or useless potential foods. He is equipped with some bio-

logical adaptations to aid in what must ultimately be primarily a process of acquisition. One set of genetically produced adaptations establish at a modest level some of the adaptations characteristic of specialist animals for particular foods or nutrients (P. Rozin, 1976; P. Rozin & Schulkin, 1990). In full form, this type of adaptation includes an internal state detector, which indicates a need for a certain nutrient, and a sensory detection system, which identifies the presence of that substance in the environment. For a koala, a "univore" surviving almost entirely on eucalyptus leaves, one simple system of this sort is all that is necessary for a complete food selection system: an internal detector indicating a need for food (e.g., "hunger"), and a sensory ability to recognize appropriate food (in this case, a "eucalyptus detector"). Acquisition of energy guarantees acquisition of necessary nutrients.

There are some genetically prepared biological aids to food selection in the mammalian generalist, what have been termed "specialists" within the generalist (P. Rozin, 1976). Thus, for water, there is a specific system that signals a need for water ("thirst") and a specific recognition of the sensory characteristics of water. There is also a dedicated taste system for sodium ions, a critical mineral requirement, and there is some evidence for a central detector system to indicate a need for sodium (Richter, 1956; Denton, 1982; Schulkin, 1991). It is possible that there are a few other specific mineral identification and detection systems. There is a well-investigated energy-state detection system, signaled by an internal state usually described as "hunger." Although there are no very reliable sensory indications of the presence or absence of energy in a potential food, the sweet taste is a reasonable indicator of the presence of sugars, and the detection of fatty textures also indicates the presence of calories in the form of fat. Finally, a bitter detection system allows for rejection of classes of entities that include common toxins.

Overall, in the sensory domain, then, there is strong evidence for an innate preference associated with sweet (sugars), and an innate aversion to bitter, associated with toxins. These innate preferences and aversions have been clearly demonstrated in newborn infants (Steiner, 1979; Rosenstein & Oster, 1988). As well, there are indications of innate preferences for salt at some concentrations (Beauchamp, 1981). A definite preference for fatty textures is probably innate but has not been demonstrated in newborns. The combined sweet and fat preferences result in strong adult preferences for mixtures of the two (Drewnowski & Greenwood, 1983). Two well documented infant taste aversions are not as easy to tie to nutritional adaptations. An innate and present-at-birth aversion to sour (acid) tastes (Steiner, 1979; Rosenstein & Oster, 1988) does not correspond to any obvious threat to health; it could perhaps represent a bias to avoid unripe fruit in favor of more nutritive ripe fruit. Aversions to chemical irritants (such as chili pepper), prominent in young children, are probably present at birth. It is not clear what these are protective of, because most natural irritants are not harmful. In short, a suite of probably innate taste biases *help* the generalist to solve the food selection problem, but they do not solve the problem. None are effective with respect to microbially contaminated food, and there are safe and nutritive natural entities that trigger the innate avoidance systems.

So far as we know, unlike the hedonically marked and innately biased taste system, and some similar adaptations in the common chemical sense and perception of oral texture, there are no strongly marked innate olfactory biases (Bartoshuk, 1990). The most likely candidate would be an innate avoidance of decay odor, because of its association with potentially harmful microbes. There is no evidence that such a system exists; indeed, young children seem attracted to decayed material, including feces (P. Rozin, Hammer, Oster, Horowitz, & Marmara, 1986). Children of about 2 years of age or less will put virtually anything in their mouths, including what is described as and appears to be feces.

Sensory biases do not exhaust the innate behavioral repertoire of the generalist. It is in the nature of the generalist to be both interested in new potential foods and cautious about them, because they may be toxic or infected, or simply poor sources of nutrition. This combination of risks and benefits manifests (in rats and humans, where it has been studied most) in an interplay between fear of the new (neophobia) and attraction to the new (neophilia). Nowhere is this more apparent than in the behaviors of wild rats (Barnett, 1956). What is familiar is safe, but it restricts the nutritional horizon in ways that may be maladaptive as the environment changes. A common "solution" to what I have called the "generalist's dilemma" is the cautious sampling of potential new foods.

Finally, an impressive set of adaptations aid the generalist in discovering the nutritional consequences of things ingested. Unlike most forms of learning, in which the consequences of an action or experience are rapid, there is an inherent delay between the action/experience (eating) and its metabolic consequences in the food system. Digestion takes time. It is now well established that a robust learning system connects tastes with their delayed consequences. In its most prominent form, conditioned taste aversions, this system allows for the association between a taste and a negative consequence (e.g., nausea) that may occur even hours later (Garcia, Hankins, & Rusiniak, 1974; P. Rozin & Kalat, 1971). There is a corresponding, usually weaker ability to associate tastes with delayed positive (nutritional) consequences (Garcia, Ervin, Yorke, & Koelling, 1967; Sclafani, 1999).

The digestive system and other parts of the body (e.g., the fat stores) work along with behavioral adaptations to solve the problem of acquiring adequate nutrients and energy. Thus, the liver constitutes a short-term store of energy (in the form of glycogen), and fat deposits in the body form a long-term store. Together, they allow the animal to endure periods of food shortage, usually measured in hours (e.g., between meals), days, or weeks. Metabolic pathways, often predominantly in the liver, allow for detoxification of low levels of dietary toxins, the conversion of energy forms, such as the synthesis of fat from carbohydrate, and the synthesis of important molecules, such as proteins and some amino acids.

One cannot help but be impressed by the enormous variety of foods and eating patterns across humanity. Indeed, ethnic cuisines would have no appeal if we all ate the same things in the same ways. But the metabolic requirements and behavioral biases I have discussed do result in a substantial number of food/culinary universals or near universals in humans. One should also be open to considering *near* universals, because human ingenuity has allowed the invasion of very inhospitable environments, such as the Arctic, that severely constrain nutritional options.

The frequent need for energy, water, and nutrients guarantees that all humans eat (and drink) rather frequently, normally more than once a day. Given that humans are not adapted to consume very low calorie density foods, such as leaves, they almost always eat rather energy-rich foods in concentrated periods of time, called meals (Pliner & Rozin, 2000). Although meals are not necessary (as opposed to continuous grazing) nutritionally, our digestive system is adapted to consuming and processing much more food than is immediately needed, and time can be spent more efficiently (from the point of view of attending to other needs, conserving energy, and avoiding predation) if eating activities are clustered in time. The availability of animal foods, and elaborate preparations of foods, encourage organization of eating in terms of meals.

Virtually all human beings consume some combination of plant and animal foods. In most cases, males are more involved in the procurement of animal foods, and females in the procurement of plant foods, with females more involved in the preparation of foods for ingestion. Eating at meals is usually a social occasion. Sharing of food is a form of bonding—throughout the world, one shares food with those with whom one is close, and this sharing ("shared substance") reinforces the closeness. Thus, food is interpersonally important. Although to some degree foods are consumed raw in all cultures, there is some processing of many foods before ingestion. This includes physical changes (removing shells, grinding), mixing of foods, and cooking. Almost all groups of humans can be described as having a cuisine: a set of rules about eating, and a set of "recipes" for the preparation of foods. These are discussed later, but include, among other things, the addition of group-specific characteristic flavors ("flavor principles") to staples (E. Rozin, 1982). Similarly, almost all human groups exploit some staple grain as a cheap source of energy. Finally, food is universally used as a reward for children and adults, and cuisines and food habits constitute part of a group's identity.

THE TRANSFORMED BIOLOGICAL MOTIVE: PREADAPTATION AND THE FUNCTIONS AND MEANINGS OF FOOD IN CULTURAL CONTEXT

Leon Kass (1994) captures the major transformation in eating by humans with the contrast between the German verbs *fressen*, eating by animals, and *essen*, for eating by humans. Unlike almost all other animals, humans bring food to their mouth rather than bringing their mouth to the food. Humans eat using implements, have table "manners," engage in complex social/informational exchanges during eating (at meals), elaborate foods extensively before eating them, and eat foods in specific orders. In short, eating is an expression of human civilization. Food has become much more than nutrition. As noted in the introduction, food is unique among the biological domains in the degree to which it has been transformed culturally. Food is used by humans for much more than nutrition.

Preadaptation, the process that accounts for the expansion of the food domain in the history of human cultures, was appreciated by Darwin and has been expressed in fuller form by some more modern evolutionists, particularly Bock (1959) and Mayr (1960). It involves the use of an already existent (usually evolved) structure for a new purpose. According to Mayr, preadaptation is the main source of evolutionary novelties and the principal process in speciation. It essentially involves a recombination of existing structures and genes rather than creation of new genes by mutation. One of the finest examples of preadaptation has to do with the food system. The mouth, with its elaborations of teeth and tongue, is an aperture designed to take in nutrients (and air). Clearly, the tongue and teeth have evolved to facilitate the processing of food. But in human evolution, the teeth and tongue, and the entire oral cavity and its link to the respiratory system, are utilized by the language system for the expression of speech. It is noteworthy that the teeth and tongue did not evolve to facilitate language, but were rather opportunistically used by the speech system. To take another example relevant to food, a good argument can be made that the species of plants and animals that were domesticated thousands of years ago were selected by humans because they were preadapted, in terms of social organization, mode of reproduction, and so on, to be useful to, and manageable by, humans.

Preadaptation is even more fundamental in cultural evolution than it is in biological evolution (P. Rozin, 1999a). This is because variation in cultural evolution can be directed by purpose, whereas in biological evolution, the occurrence of variations is dependent on random processes. If a cultural tradition, practice, artifact, or institution might be adaptive in a new context, it can just be transplanted. One does not have to wait for the opportunity to arise by generation of random variants (a very unlikely event, if the use in a new context requires a series of adaptations). Thus, one can combine the virtues of the calculator and typewriter to create a computer, or apply a culinary technique discovered in one culture to another. The flowering of food from nutrition to a complex expression of civilization (Kass, 1994) has taken place along a number of lines, presumably to different degrees and in different temporal orders of evolution in different cultures (Figure 16.1). Early in human evolution, food became an entity of social significance. The meal became a center for social interaction. Food became central to important cultural events. Food sharing became explicit and implicit forms of expression of interpersonal intimacy. Food became a marker of the status of the individual (as in the Hindu caste system, or the public consumption of expensive foods), and a form of group identity. Note the description of British sailors as "limeys," Germans as "krauts," and French as "frogs." Food enters the aesthetic domain as cuisine, taking its place next to other human activities with lesser links to our fundamental biology, such as literature, music, and art. Cuisines elaborate the flavors and presentation of food in ways that can hardly be described, in most cases, as motivated by improved nutritional properties. Rather, it is appeal to the palate and the eye.

Food becomes an integral part of the moral/ religious domain, such as when it is used in religious ritual (e.g., taking the host in the Catholic church, the Jewish laws of Kashrut). In Hindu India, with more than 800 million people, food can be considered a form of "moral currency"; Appadurai (1981) describes it as a "biomoral" substance. The caste system, which ranks people according to moral purity, is largely defined and defended in terms of food

transactions designed to prevent the food of those less morally pure to become consumed by those higher in the system (Marriott, 1968). In the West, for example, the United States, the moral role of food is muted, though overeating, fast foods, fatty foods, and most clearly cigarettes, take on moral overtones (Stein & Nemeroff, 1995; P. Rozin, 1999b).

Finally, in addition to expanded roles for food as art form, moral, and social vehicle, the vocabulary associated with food is co-opted as a means of describing things that have nothing to do with food; that is, food has a metaphoric function. In fact, food is one of the major sources of metaphor (Lakoff & Johnson, 1980), such as when we say that "Janet is sweet," or "Let's get to the meat of the paper." Metaphor is, of course, a quintessential example of preadaptation: export of a word from its original context to other contexts.

DISGUST AS AN EXAMPLE OF PREADAPTATION AND THE CULTURAL EVOLUTION OF THE FOOD SYSTEM

The role of food as a foundation system to be elaborated in various cultural contexts through the principle of preadaptation is well illustrated in the cultural history of the emotion of disgust (see P. Rozin, Haidt, McCauley, & Imada, 1997; P. Rozin, Haidt, & McCauley, 2000, for reviews). Disgust is and has always been regarded as one of five to 10 basic emotions by psychologists. It is featured by Darwin (1872/ 1965) in *The Expression of Emotions in Man and Animals*, and figures centrally in Izard's (1977), Tomkins's (1963), and Ekman's (1992) general perspectives on emotion. Following on Ekman's conception of basic emotions, disgust is characterized as having a particular hardwired pattern of expression, psychophysio-

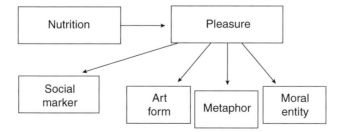

FIGURE 16.1. Food preadaptation.

logical response, and behavior. The expression focuses around the nose and mouth, and includes raising of the upper lip, wrinkling of the nose, and often a gaping that involves a drop of the lower jaw and tongue extension (Ekman & Friesen, 1975; P. Rozin, Lowery, & Ebert, 1994). These gestures contribute to the functional outcome of ejecting materials from the mouth and closing the nasal passages. They are quite common among the mammals in general. The psychophysiological event that accompanies the elicitation and experience of disgust is nausea. The behavior is withdrawal from the source of disgust.

In nonhuman animals, disgust is elicited by foods or potential foods that have been experienced to have an "unpleasant" taste; bitter tastes seem innately to elicit the disgust facial expression. The function of the expression seems to both expel or turn away from an offending food and to communicate this food quality to conspecifics. Baeyens, Kaes, Eelen, and Silverans (1996) have demonstrated that humans can acquire a dislike for a beverage (taste) when they consume it at the same time as another, visible person who is making a "disgust" face.

It is clear that in its origin, disgust is a food-related emotion: (1) That is how it functions, virtually exclusively, in nonhuman animals and human infants; (2) in terms of its Latin origins, the word in English (and some other languages) actually means "bad taste"; (3) the nausea that typically accompanies disgust and helps to define it is a response that specifically functions to discourage ingestion; and (4) the facial expression clearly functions to expel food and odors.

In light of these observations, it is quite remarkable that the elicitors of disgust in humans include a wide range of events, only a minority of which can be traced to food. Elicitors include contact with death or filth, many body products, disliked individuals, and the experience of certain activities deemed to be immoral (e.g., sexual perversions or child abuse). We (P. Rozin & Fallon, 1987; P. Rozin et al., 1997; P. Rozin, Haidt, & McCauley, 2000) have proposed an account based on preadaptation whereby, through culture history (or cultural evolution) and perhaps in normal socialization, a series of stages of expansion of the meaning and elicitors of disgust occurs. Whereas the meanings and elicitors of disgust expand, the basic program (expression, behavior, physiological response) remains roughly the same.

In our posited first stage (see Figure 16.2), elicitors of disgust remain potential foods, but the feature of the food that promotes disgust is not its sensory properties, but the nature or origin of the food (P. Rozin & Fallon, 1987). Thus, a quintessentially disgusting food, such as a cockroach or worm, has usually never been tasted. It is the idea of what it is; it is offensive. Perhaps, the idea is that that incorporation of offensive objects might make the self offensive, by the "You are what you eat" principle.

A particularly interesting feature of this ideational disgust, which we call "core disgust," is that ideationally disgusting entities are "contagious"; that is, they follow the sympathetic magical law of contagion: "Once in contact, always in contact" (Frazer, 1890/1922; Tylor, 1871/1974; Mauss, 1902/1972; P. Rozin, Millman, & Nemeroff, 1986; P. Rozin & Nemeroff, 1990). If a disgusting potential food (e.g., a worm or cockroach) touches an otherwise edible entity, it renders it inedible and in fact disgusting. This property, although characteristic of ideational disgust, does not hold for the original distasteful (e.g., bitter) dis-

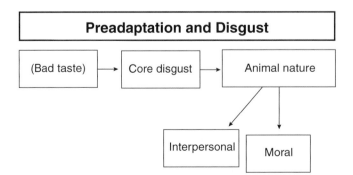

FIGURE 16.2. Preadaptation: Cultural evolution of disgust.

gust elicitors. Because contagion is characteristic of all ideational disgust elicitors and is not characteristic of the more primitive bad taste "disgusts," we use the terminology *distastes* for bad tastes, and reserve disgust for the culturally acquired rejections that show the contagion property. The contagion property appears to be universal among adult humans but absent in animals or in children younger than about 4 years of age. It seems to be a universal cultural acquisition, perhaps supported by its adaptive advantage in discouraging consumption of infected foods. It is notable, as Angyal (1941) pointed out, that almost all core disgust foods are of animal origin. It is these same foods that have the highest risk as vehicles for transmitting infectious agents.

Feces appears to be the universal core disgust substance. It does not qualify as an innate distaste, since it is not rejected by infants (or most animals; P. Rozin, Hammer, et al., 1986); rather, it is a universally acquired human disgust, with its own fundamental developmental concomitant, toilet training.

We believe that disgust is co-opted as a cultural tool to establish culturally supported aversions or prohibitions by endowing the relevant objects with disgust properties. If a forbidden entity becomes disgusting, it will be naturally avoided, and no rules or formal punishments need be invoked. Such is clearly the case with the outcome of toilet training. A previously attractive substance becomes powerfully disgusting.

By our account, the range of disgust expands from its initial food base to include three other categories of events or elicitors. First, following on the focus on animal foods, it is extended to a wide range of animal features—features that humans share with animals. It is a frequent theme in cultural narratives, rituals, and beliefs that humans are not animals and are superior to animals. Any reminder of the animal nature of humans then becomes undesirable. One animal feature is particularly aversive to humans: their mortality (Becker, 1973; Pyszczynski, Greenberg, & Solomon, 1997). Disgust seems to be used as a device to distract humans from reminders of their mortality. By helping to distance humans from their own animal nature, and from animals, it seems to assist in a major goal that develops cross-culturally as humans evolve. That mortality is at the base of what we will call "animal nature disgust" is supported by two observations: (1) the quintessential odor of disgust is the odor of decay of animal

matter, and that is the odor of death; and (2) psychometrically, disgust reactions to death and things associated with death are among the very best predictors of general disgust sensitivity (Haidt, McCauley, & Rozin, 1994). The rejection of animal nature "stage" of disgust fits with the nature of the civilizing process, as described by the distinguished culture historian, Norbert Elias (1939/1978): "People in the course of the civilizing process, seek to suppress in themselves every characteristic that they feel to be animal" (p. 120).

We have identified two other "domains" or "stages" of disgust; we are not at all sure whether there is a regular order in their developmental or cultural acquisition. One is interpersonal disgust (Figure 16.2), a disgust response to contact with most other individual humans, hence clearly not related to animal nature rejection. Contact, the more intimate the more disgusting, with strangers, disliked persons, or persons from outside one's own group seem to elicit this type of disgust, which accounts for why "used food" is highly unpopular, as is used clothing, by many people in many cultures. Presumably, this type of disgust has the adaptive value of strengthening ingroup connections and weakening those with outgroups.

Finally, disgust is used to one degree or another depending on the culture to support moral principles; hence, moral disgust. Disgust can be engaged to reinforce a morally cultural based prohibition. The degree to which this occurs seems to be related to the type of moral system a culture has.

Shweder, Much, Mahapatra, and Park (1997) have proposed that three types of moral systems exist across cultures (see Table 16.1). The autonomy system holds that an activity is immoral if it interferes with the rights of an-

TABLE 16.1. Correspondence between Moral Systems and Moral Emotions: The CAD Triad Hypothesis

Rhetoric	Focal concepts	Emotion
Community	Duty, hierarchy, interdependence	Contempt
Autonomy	Harm, rights, justice	Anger
Divinity	Sacred order, natural order, purity	Disgust

Note. Based on Shweder et al. (1997) and P. Rozin, Lowery, et al. (1999).

other person. It describes Western moral systems quite well. The community system identifies immorality as violation of hierarchical structures, such as addressing a respected elder informally. The divinity system considers as immoral any action that reduces one's own or another's purity (divinity). The community and divinity systems are robust parts of morality in many traditional cultures, as demonstrated by Shweder et al. for Hindu Indians. The emotions that involve moral condemnation of others are typically anger, contempt, and disgust. We (P. Rozin, Lowery, et al., 1999) have pointed out that there is a satisfying mapping of these three emotions onto Shweder et al.'s (1997) three systems, with anger associated with autonomy, contempt with community, and disgust with divinity (Table 16.1). We have demonstrated a correspondence between moral offenses of each type and both the emotion words and emotion expressions for each of the three emotions, in both the United States and Japan. Clearly, in a culture in which divinity is an important source of moral principles, disgust will be an important moral emotion. This is illustrated in studies by Haidt, Koller, and Dias (1993), in which they inquired of upper middle-class and lower class Americans and Brazilians whether it was immoral to eat roadkill dog. All respondents felt disgust, but only the middle-class Americans allowed that this was not an immoral act, because nobody was hurt (autonomy was not violated). Because they did not accept a divinity moral system, disgust was not considered a sufficient condition to designate something as immoral.

I have just given a sense of the incredible elaboration of the simple "Get this out of my mouth" emotion into a "Get this away from my soul" emotion. A transition from a "body" to a "soul" emotion—a rich description of this broad function of disgust is described and documented by William I. Miller (1997) in his excellent book, *The Anatomy of Disgust*. This same type of expansion of meanings for food (as opposed to disgust) in European history is described in Leon Kass's *The Hungry Soul* (1994).

Kass (1994) provides a particularly graphic illustration of food, disgust, and civilization. In a typical meal situation in many cultures, individuals face each other while eating. They place food into their mouths, the interior of which is generally regarded as disgusting by others. Furthermore, the mass of chewed food in the

mouth is itself disgusting (both interpersonally and because of its involvement with body secretions, etc.). Remarkably, due to the virtuosity of eating as informed by table manners, this exchange goes on face-to-face without either partner being exposed to any disgust stimuli. More remarkably, the individuals are often conversing while eating, using the same hole to speak that they use to ingest food; still, neither the inside of the mouth nor the ingested food is seen by the partner!

One final interesting feature of disgust in its culturally elaborated form is that it is often funny. Many jokes and cartoons engage disgust, and disgust is typically at the core of humor for young male children. How is it that a negative emotion becomes a source of amusement? Our proposal is that it is one of many manifestations that humans enjoy "constrained" negative events (what we have called "benign masochism"), that is, events that signal threat but are not really threatening (P. Rozin, 1990a). When a well-dressed person other than oneself or partners steps in "dog-doo," it is sort of amusing; not so for the self.

By the same process of preadaptation that expands disgust elicitors in culture history, the process of contagion is carried along with the new elicitors. Thus, contact with an immoral person shows contagion properties; people do not wish to wear Hitler's sweater (P. Rozin, Millman, et al., 1986; P. Rozin & Nemeroff, 1990; Nemeroff & Rozin, 2000).

A comparison of the status of disgust in the United States and India is instructive. Disgust is centered in the core and animal nature domain in the United States, with some extension into the interpersonal domain, and minimal moral disgust. In Hindu India, on the other hand, a good part of disgust engages the interpersonal and moral domain, as illustrated by the caste system, and there is relative insensitivity to animal nature disgust; at least, there is less of a response to contact with death.

CULTURE AND BIOLOGY: SOME FOOD CASE HISTORIES

In this section, I briefly consider the history of some human foods to illustrate how biological, cultural, and psychological factors interact in the cultural evolution of foods (see P. Rozin, 1982, for a more systematic discussion of this issue).

Sugar

The cultural history of sugar is a paradigmatic illustration of how a simple biological predisposition, the preference for a sweet taste, is amplified and elaborated by culture. The innate sweet preference encourages the search for this stimulus and learning about where and when it can be found. In conjunction with the development of agriculture, the desire motivates in humans the cultivation of crops, primarily ripe fruits, that provide this desirable taste experience. Much later in human history, the technology to extract the source of sweetness, sugars, from their natural plant sources allows for the experience of an even more desirable sweet experience. As well, this important advance opens a wide door for expansion of the domain of acceptable foods, because sugar can be added to foods that are otherwise much less palatable, such as coffee or chocolate, and to enhance the taste of traditional dishes.

The search for a source of easily extractable sugar (sugar cane) was a main motivation for the colonization of the tropical Americas by Europeans, and the availability of cheap sugar introduced it to the middle and lower classes, and transformed cuisine in many ways. The extensive culinary and social implications of the availability of inexpensive sugar are well documented by Sidney Mintz (1985) in his book, *Sweetness and Power*. Further technological advances allowed for extraction of sugars from sources other than sugar cane, including sugar beets and corn.

Finally, in the food-flooded modern, developed world, where the calories signaled by the sweet taste are often avoided as opposed to sought, there is the development of artificial sweeteners, uncoupling the taste from the calories that usually go with it, allowing for the experience of the pleasure of sweetness without the calories. All of these extensive advances, with major implications for cuisine and society, are motivated quite directly by the biological predisposition for sweet tastes.

Chocolate

One of the great culinary creations of culture, chocolate, represents a more elaborate version of the amplification illustrated by sugar. It illustrates the creation of a "superfood," motivated by twin biological predispositions for sweet tastes and fatty texture, both indicators of caloric value. The great appeal of chocolate, one of the favorite foods in the Western world, has to do with its sweetness, fatty texture, aroma, and melt-in-the-mouth quality. Importantly, none of these features are obvious in the wild chocolate bean. So, unlike the case for sugar, the cultural evolution of chocolate involved discovery and development of a potential in a natural product. This extremely complex technology involves both modifying the natural product to enhance some of its properties and adding other things (particularly sugar, sometimes milk and vanilla) to improve palatability and produce variety. The natural chocolate bean is extremely bitter and has neither the aroma nor the fatty texture of commercial chocolate. It was ground and consumed as a beverage in close to its natural form by the Indians of Mesoamerica, well before the arrival of Cortez (see Coe & Coe, 1996, for the history of chocolate). This was an innately unpalatable beverage, an acquired taste.

Brought to Europe by the early Spanish explorers, chocolate was transformed into a luscious food by Western Europeans, and later Americans, in a complex process that involves many stages and, critically, depends on the availability of cheap sugar. The result is a food, source of calories and nutrients that is among the most popular in the Western world, and is presently the most craved substance in North America (Weingarten & Elston, 1991; P. Rozin, Levine, & Stoess, 1991).

The story of chocolate, like that of sugar but more so, is the story of the amplification and elaboration of biological predispositions. The difference is that the aspects of chocolate that satisfy these predispositions are not apparent in the natural product. It is of particular cultural and psychological interest that although chocolate is raised in tropical areas, particularly Africa, South America, and parts of Asia, the great desire for it and consumption of it is in the very countries that cannot grow it: Europe, the United States, and Canada. This may be explained, in part, on economic grounds: Chocolate is expensive, and the tropical countries in which it grows are not wealthy.

Chili Pepper

Chili pepper is probably the most widely consumed spice in the world, other than garlic (if one chooses to consider garlic a spice). It is eaten on a daily basis, usually as part of a seasoning sauce used with almost all savory foods by more than 2 billion people every day. It is an essential part of the basic flavoring ("flavor principle"; see the section on cuisine) of most tropical and semitropical cuisines in the world. The contrast with chocolate and sugar is striking, because unlike these two popular foods, chili pepper is innately aversive on account of its oral irritant properties. So chili pepper illustrates the reversal of an innate aversion, a case where culture overwhelms and reverses a biological predisposition (see P. Rozin, 1990a, for a detailed consideration of psychological and cultural aspects of chili use).

All chili peppers come from the Americas and were introduced to Europe by the early explorers of the Americas. They spread later to Africa and Asia. The innately aversive irritation of the peppers, caused by a family of chemicals called capsaicins, were bred out of the imported peppers. This probably happened first in Hungary, and the result was what we now call sweet peppers, which became a mainstay of Mediterranean cuisines. But, in spite of the availability of such mild peppers, it was the "hot" peppers that spread to tropical and semitropical Africa and Asia. It is a remarkable feature of history, and particularly culinary history, that such a "bad tasting" product achieved so much success, particularly when other foods from the Americas, including tomatoes and potatoes, experienced substantial resistance before adoption in Europe and other countries.

The story of the chili pepper and the widespread adoption of other innately unpalatable substances, such as black pepper, ginger, tobacco, and coffee, raise two very important questions for cultural psychology. First, what are the cultural or biological adaptive values of this widespread practice, and second, how does culture manage to accomplish the hedonic reversal? As to adaptive value, there are possible accounts but no certain solutions (reviewed in Rozin, 1990a). Billing and Sherman (1998) have made a good case for the antimicrobial value of spices in general, including chili pepper. Other accounts, each with minimal evidence, suggest nutritional values, thermoregulatory (cooling) effects, and coverage of the taste of spoilage.

From the perspective of cultural psychology, the particular interest of chili pepper and other innately aversive substances and activities is how they are socialized. And most critically, it is extremely clear that people consume chili pepper because they like its taste; that is, cultural processes lead to a hedonic reversal in which an innately aversive sensation becomes a pleasant sensation! People do not consume chili pepper like a medicine, because they think it is good for them. They consume it because they like it.

We do not have an adequate account of how this happens (reviewed in Rozin, 1990a), but given the generality of cultural adoption of initially aversive substances and activities, I briefly discuss the causes of hedonic reversal for the chili pepper as a model system. A whole family of accounts link chili pepper ingestion to positive effects it produces, including sweating and lowered body temperature, and induced parasympathetic activity (including salivation, gastric secretion, and lowered heart rate) and endogenous opiate release in the brain. All of these effects do occur; the question is their role in the acquisition of liking. To learn from these effects (and somehow, via this learning, transform the hedonic response), repeated exposure is necessary. Normally, when an aversive event or substance is encountered, it is subsequently avoided. So one important effect of culture is to produce an environment, social and physical, in which there is repeated consumption of food with chili pepper in it. Is this a sufficient condition (e.g., Zajonc's [1968] well-documented "process" of "mere exposure")?

The answer is clearly "no"; fieldwork and preference tests in the field (P. Rozin & Schiller, 1980) indicate that whereas all Mexicans in a village over the age of 6 or so years like the burn of chili pepper, not a single animal in the same village does so. This in spite of the fact that the dogs, pigs, and chickens consume the daily garbage, which regularly includes stale staple foods and dishes, and excess salsa (the chili pepper–based sauce that is placed on most savory foods; P. Rozin & Kennel, 1983). The reversal of the innate aversion for chili pepper, and almost certainly other entities, seems to be an almost uniquely human accomplishment, and to involve culture as an essential ingredient.

Field measurements (Rozin & Schiller, 1980) indicate that very young Mexican children do not like chili pepper, and that a liking for the hot taste occurs somewhere around 4–6 years of age. There are two reasonable, not conflicting, accounts. One is social: In the meal setting, the entire family consumes food with chili pepper in it, or with an accompanying sauce to be added to the foods. There is no overt pressure at the table to consume hot pepper. But the young child observes that older siblings and all adults consume it with gusto, and this experience may in some way produce the hedonic reversal.

A second account, which we call "benign masochism" (P. Rozin & Schiller, 1980; P. Rozin, 1990a), puts chili-liking together with a whole set of uniquely human activities, in which pleasure is produced by the elicitation of negative experiences and/or emotions: riding roller coasters, recreational parachute jumping, going to sad movies, smoking cigarettes, drinking black coffee. The idea is that humans, and only humans, seem to get pleasure out of the fact their body is signaling danger/rejection to them, but they know they are really safe. This body–mind disparity seems to induce pleasure. The case is particularly clear for roller-coaster riding. We have some evidence that this might be the case for the chili pepper, because we have shown that any individual's most preferred level of "burn" for the chili pepper is the level just slightly below the level of aversive pain (just as the best roller coaster is the scariest, within constraints; Rozin & Schiller, 1980). It is worth noting that disgust humor, discussed earlier, is another possible example of benign masochism.

The important lesson from chili pepper as an example of a learned reversal of innate aversions is that, at a minimum, it invokes cultural mechanisms at three levels: (1) the availability of the substance or experience, (2) the continued exposure to it in spite of its initial negative effects, and (3) in some yet to be fully understood way, the accomplishment of the hedonic reversal.

Ironically, yet another account for hedonic reversal involves endogenous opiate secretion that invokes an opponent process model. According to this view (P. Rozin, 1990a), the adaptive opponent system, which is generally employed to adapt to certain types of events that disturb equilibrium, is over-activated and produces a reversal. Such an account has been used to account for addiction (Solomon, 1980).

Milk

Milk is necessarily the first food of mammals. Until the development of animal domestication and then dairying by humans, milk was a unique food available only to baby mammals. In the contemporary human world, milk and derivative dairy products form an important part of the diet in many cultures. It is notably absent from most East Asian cuisines but present in some form in most others as a food for children and adults. Milk illustrates a very important point about the relation of biology to culture. The culture history of dairy products shows both how biological constraints affect cultural evolution and institutions, and, importantly, how culture affects our biology. This dual-direction effect is the focus of this short section on milk.

Because milk is unavailable as a food past nursing in the predomestication environment, it would be problematic to have adult mammals seeking their first food. A number of mechanisms have evolved to accomplish not only the weaning from milk but also some decline in its preference (reviewed in P. Rozin and Pelchat, 1988). The most relevant mechanism is genetically programmed lactose intolerance (see Simoons, 1969, 1970). The only carbohydrate in mammalian milk (with a few minor exceptions) is lactose, a sugar that is the combination of two simpler sugars, glucose and galactose. Lactose is found only in milk. Lactose, which cannot be absorbed directly, is broken into its two utilizable subcomponents by the gut enzyme, lactase. This enzyme, present in the gut of virtually all mammals, is deprogrammed such that it gradually disappears at about the time of weaning of the species in question. Undigested lactose ferments in the hind gut, producing gas pains and diarrhea, and interfering with absorption of some of the nutrients in milk. These unpleasant symptoms very likely contribute to the weaning process. Preagricultural humans were therefore like all other mammals and unable to utilize milk effectively after weaning.

Domestication made milk available as an adult food. There is convincing evidence, largely from the work of Frederick Simoons (1969, 1970), that two very different types of adaptations occurred since the origin of domestication to encourage the availability of milk and its products in the postweaning human diet. First, cultural innovations adapted to a biological limitation (adult lactose intolerance) by digesting milk outside of the body, breaking down the lactose into its utilizable components before ingestion. This was done with microorganisms and results in products such as cheese and yogurt. These appropriately termed "cultured" products make the carbohydrate in milk utilizable and bypass the negative symptoms.

A second set of biological adaptations occurred subsequent to the rise of dairying. In a group of cultures primarily from Northern Europe, but also including some pastoral groups in Africa, the availability of dairy food set up a situation in which the ability to digest milk was adaptive. There is a single gene mutation that, when it occurs, blocks the deprogramming of lactase production at weaning. In these cultures, the occurrence of this mutation improved survivability, and gradually the gene frequency rose. The result is that most people of Northern European origin (and a few African groups) retain their lactase and can drink raw milk throughout their lives. They are lactose tolerant adults. Hence, a cultural advance changed the adaptive landscape for humans and induced a genetic change in some groups of humans.

The main point is the dual direction of culture–biology change so well illustrated by milk. Many issues related to dairy products may engage cultural psychology, but these are not be dealt with here. Of particular interest is why Chinese cuisine, one of the world's major cuisines, includes no dairy products. This may have a cultural–historical explanation: The Chinese were ruled by despised Mongols for a long period and the Mongols are heavy dairy consumers.

Meat

Meat should be a subject of special interest to psychologists, because it is a quintessential example of the interesting and important state of ambivalence. It is at the same time the most tabooed and the most favored food across the human race. Meat is a charged entity, imbued with multiple meanings. Because it is the food whose composition is most similar to that of humans, it is the most complete of foods. But this same similarity makes meat most likely to be the host to microorganisms that also find a happy home in humans. Meat is most nutritive and most infective. Obtaining meat involves hunting and killing animals, an act that requires great skill and is at the same time morally questionable. The anthropologist Stanley Tambiah (1969) elaborated some of these points in a well-known paper entitled "Animals Are Good to Think and Good to Pro-

hibit." He might as well have replaced the word *think* with *eat*.

Meat, represented in terms of the most favored parts of animals, is in traditional societies often restricted for the consumption of males, or the more important males. At the same time, in some cultures, some religions, and among some individuals within meat-eating cultures, prohibition of all meat is practiced. Vegetarianism has a long history and a wide geographical presence. Meat is the only general category of foods that is widely prohibited. Almost all objects of food disgust cross-culturally are animals or animal products (Angyal, 1941; P. Rozin & Fallon, 1987). This can, perhaps, be related to the role of disgust in denying our animal nature, as well as in the "You are what you eat" principle (eat an animal and become animal-like; Nemeroff & Rozin, 1989). Of course, cannibalism, often the most negatively regarded human food practice, is a special example of meat eating.

The place of meat in human life has been treated by a number of authors, including Marvin Harris (1985), from an evolutionary perspective; Frederick Simoons (1961/1994) from the cultural–geographic perspective, with a focus on meat taboos; Julia Twigg (1983) from the vegetarian perspective, and other authors in more general treatments (e.g., Beardsworth & Keil, 1997; Fiddes, 1991; P. Rozin, 2004).

CUISINE

Eating involves incorporating substance; humans typically do something to the things they find in the world before consuming them. Some of this amounts to physical preparation such as peeling or cutting, but much involves more elaborate transformations, including mixing, grinding, cooking, and flavoring. These behaviors conveniently often leave substantial records that can be examined by archeologists (unlike sex, for example); it is not as good as writing, but it is a meaningful record. Of course, when combined with writing, the food domain results in recipes and cookbooks.

We can use the word *cuisine* to represent the body of shared rules, beliefs, and practices relating to food within any culture. Regularities are sufficiently great within cultures that we can usually identify the culture by examining what is eaten.

At the level of the "dish," Elisabeth Rozin (1982) points out that there are three components: staple foods, processing techniques, and flavorings. She notes that most cuisines add a particular set of flavoring ingredients to most savory dishes, and calls these "flavor principles." Thus, Southern Italian cuisine is characterized by tomato, sweet pepper, olive oil, and oregano as flavorings. Chinese cuisine typically flavors with soy sauce, ginger root, and rice wine, and Mexican cuisine characteristically uses chili pepper with either lime or tomato. Flavor principles provide a distinctiveness/identity to the foods of a particular group, and offer a sense of comfort and familiarity. They may also serve as a means to introduce a new staple food into a cuisine by making it taste familiar with the traditional flavor principle (E. Rozin & Rozin, 1981).

The meal is another component of cuisine. Meals have an internal structure, varying from a single dish of combined ingredients to sequences of foods, as in the appetizer–entrée–dessert sequence common in many Western cuisines (see Douglas & Nicod, 1974, for an analysis of the British meal). In many traditional cultures, the various meals are similar in content and structure, with breakfast as warmed over dinner. In many Western cultures, a separate first meal, breakfast, has its own foods and flavors. Howard Schutz (1989) has pointed out that cultures' "appropriateness" rules have to do with what foods can be mixed or eaten together, proper sequences of foods, and foods for particular times or occasions.

The social eating situation is a third aspect of cuisine. There are issues of who eats with whom, order of eating (e.g., children first), and rules for leaving the table and for what is supposed to be discussed during the meal. These very elaborate traditions are treated in the next section.

CIVILIZED EATING

One of the most striking things about the food world that varies a great deal across cultures is the etiquette of eating, or table manners. As Kass (1994) and Elias (1939/1978) point out, the meal is one of the special areas in which humans display and celebrate the fact that they are civilized. Most modern humans do not eat like animals. They sit at tables, use utensils, respect and do not touch the food on the plates of others, refrain from calling attention to their bodily functions while eating, and observe complex rules of social interaction. Civilized eating is highly complex and requires great skill. Both Kass and Elias indicate that in civilized eating, the biological aspects of eating are suppressed (see the earlier discussion of suppression of disgust during eating). The learning of table manners by children is surely one of the more difficult aspects of growing up.

All of these civilizations of the daily meal are yet more elaborated in the special food occasions, such as attending restaurants, feasts, dinner parties, or weddings (Kass, 1994). And the etiquette and subtle meanings of eatings are particularly elaborated in Hindu–Indian culture (Khare, 1976).

FOOD SOCIALIZATION: WEANING AND TOILET TRAINING

With breast-feeding and careful monitoring of the human infant by its mother, little can go wrong with its food world in the first year. Evidence suggests that for the first year or two of life, children will put anything they find into their mouth (P. Rozin, Hammer, et al., 1986). This potentially dangerous tendency is neutralized by maternal vigilance. It seems that the most important thing a child has to learn in the early years is what *not* to eat. Of course, in addition to familial vigilance, the environment can be scoured so that the child does not encounter dangerous things.

Freud correctly noted two of the major events of early childhood: weaning and toilet training. One is about food, and the other is a consequence of eating. Weaning is a necessary event, and toilet training, though not literally necessary, is universal. Both involve denying a child a pleasure, and both can be problematic. Both are problems solved in very diverse ways in different cultures, at different ages, with different degrees of attention and harshness. Because Freud saw these two events as central in the formation of personality, they received great attention in a cross-cultural context for at least a generation of field anthropology. As with many other features of a highly overdetermined developmental trajectory, normal children can and do typically become trained following a wide range of weaning and toilet training procedures. These are things that have to be done, but how they are done is not highly constrained in terms of much higher benefits or costs for one technique as opposed to another. Indeed, a related issue, bottle- or breast-feeding, has occupied an enormous amount of research attention in psychological and medical research in the developed world.

The most important aspects of both toilet training and weaning is that they demand attention, are usually taken seriously by adults, and are accomplished in accordance with a rather complex set of belief structures and practices. They are about food and are major milestones in early life. Ironically, no doubt in part due to the attention they received by Freud, developmental psychology in the last part of the 20th century paid scant attention to these two fundamental processes (P. Rozin, in press).

The acquisition of table manners and food traditions is another important aspect of food socialization that has been little studied by psychologists. Birch, Billman, and Richards (1984) reported that the category of special foods eaten at breakfast in the United States becomes distinctive and separate for children in the later preschool years. P. Rozin, Fallon, and Augustoni-Ziskind (1986) reported that until the later preschool years, children in the United States do not understand or incorporate a variety of food-mixing prohibitions; thus, the young preschool child who likes food A (e.g., steak) and food B (e.g., ice cream) will like A + B. Cuisine is not that simple (Schutz, 1989).

PREFERENCES: FORMATION AND TRANSMISSION

Food is one of the domains in which preferences are salient. Most foods are either liked or disliked; relatively few produce a neutral response. It is quite remarkable that although preferences for food, music, and a wide range of activities are a very important part of life (and economics), they are studied little by psychologists, cultural or otherwise (P. Rozin, in press). The question for all preferences (leaving aside love and preferences for other people) is, how do they get formed? What makes us like some things and dislike others? The food domain is a natural place to study this, because there are so many food preferences, they are public, and they are usually open for discussion (e.g., unlike sexual preferences). Surely, one of the major distinctive features of a culture is its cuisine and associated food preferences. If we

know someone is particularly fond of rice and soy sauce, we can make a good guess that they are from East or Southeast Asia.

Whereas there are surely large cross-cultural differences in food preferences, there is also wide variation within cultures. There is no point in trying to quantify and compare these differences; it all depends on which foods are being studied. Variance in preference for tofu is going to be largely intercultural between Chinese and Americans. But, for the same two cultures, variance in preferences for broccoli might well be primarily explained intraculturally.

Given the generalist background of humans, it is unlikely that most preferences are accounted for in terms of genetic endowment. Two other natural reasons might be critical early experiences and the early environment, as controlled and instantiated largely by the parents. Of course, the human mammal would be poorly served by a tendency to develop strong and permanent preferences for early foods. This would have led to a focus on milk, a food unavailable in the ancestral environment after weaning. That adult food preferences are largely formed in the first 6 years of life is a common Western view, perhaps a derivative of Freud's focus on what he designated the critical first 6 years. So far as I know, there is no evidence that the first 6 years are any more important than the next, or the next 6 years after that.

Both genetic and early experience accounts predict substantial parent–child correlations in food preferences. Remarkably, they are in fact very low. Results from Americans suggest values averaging around .15 for preferences for specific foods, comparing the preferences of parents (or the midpoint of mother and father) and the preference of their adult child (Pliner, 1983; P. Rozin, 1991). Similar results appear for music preference, whereas correlations for values such as attitudes to abortion are notably higher (P. Rozin, 1991). Cavalli-Sforza, Feldman, Chen, and Dornbusch (1982) identified three routes for transmission of preferences: vertical (parent–child), horizontal (peer influence), and oblique (e.g., teacher–student, media–child). The low parent–child correlations suggest substantial roles for peers, teachers, heroes, and culturewide forces.

It is not surprising that parents, peers, and other cultural forces produce certain within-culture commonalities in preferences. Not at all clear is what produces within-culture differences. We do not have a set of well-documented mechanisms, although mere exposure (Zajonc, 1968; Pliner, 1982), some types of evaluative conditioning (Martin & Levey, 1978; deHouwer, Thomas, & Baeyens, 2001), and "social influence" (whatever that means; e.g., Birch (1980); Birch, Zimmerman, & Hind, 1980; Baeyens et al., 1996; Duncker, 1938) are surely involved (for reviews, see Birch, Fisher, & Grimm-Thomas, 1996; P. Rozin, 1988, 1990b).

Peer influences are obviously important in the development of food preferences in some cultures, perhaps especially in adolescence. There is some surprising evidence of its absence in food and music preferences in some American contexts (Rozin, Riklis, & Margolis, 2003).

Of course there is more to transmission than preference. Attitudes toward food and eating, including their importance in comparison to other activities, and the balance of worries and pleasures about eating vary considerably not only between cultures (e.g., between France and the United States; P. Rozin, Fischler, Imada, Sarubin, & Wrzesniewski, 1999) but also within cultures. Recent ethnographic data suggest that some of the major differences in food attitudes between Americans and Southern Europeans can be traced to differences in the types of interactions that occur around the dinner table (Ochs, Pontecorvo, & Fasulo, 1996). The Italian family eating environment is much more oriented toward the shared pleasure of eating, and less toward concerns about food, health, and coaxing children or making bargains to promote healthier eating. This work is a promising beginning for systematic studies of food socialization in a cultural context.

THE INVERSION OF THE ANCESTRAL FOOD WORLD AND THE OBESITY EPIDEMIC

A particular problem of general interest to cultural psychology and cultural studies has to do with the stresses and dislocations that occur in human life as a result of major and rapid culture advances, especially in technology. For example, the rapid increase in the power and accessibility of the Internet and e-mail have produced much more rapid and widespread links among people around the world, allowing a rumor to spread around the world in hours,

as opposed to years. Although most news that individuals received was vetted through a chain of other people or, more recently, newspapers and other media, an individual can now spread "news," accurate or not, directly to consumers around the world. Modern societies have yet to figure out how to compensate for the potential dangers of instant communication and rapid transmission of diseases because of extensive international travel, or how to control weapons of mass destruction.

We are, both biologically and culturally, adapted more to our ancestral food environment than to our very recent, developed world cultural environment. Enormous challenges to humans have emerged in the food domain as a result of technological advances. The inversions are laid out in Table 16.2. An ancestral environment in which food was in relatively short supply has been replaced by an environment in which cheap food is abundant and always available. An ancestral environment that offered a modest variety of potential foods, mixed with many acutely dangerous potential foods, has been replaced by an environment offering an extraordinary range of safe food choices; I venture that the contemporary urban food supermarket has more different types of foods available than were ever available to anyone on earth even 30 years ago! In the ancestral environment, the foods available evolved under complex adaptation pressures and were rarely (except for animal foods) very calorie dense; in the contemporary environment, foods of extraordinary caloric density and extraordinarily appealing sensory properties are available; chocolate is a prime example. There is nothing so palatable or calorie dense in the natural plant world. In the ancestral environment, we had to work to obtain food; in the contemporary environment, minimal calorie expenditure is necessary. In the ancestral environment, there was a rather close temporal link (measured usually in hours) between ingestion of a food and appreciation of its consequences (nutritional virtues or toxicity).

In the contemporary environment, acute risks of imbalance or toxicity are minimized by cultural means, such as sanitation systems and preservatives. The generally remote food risks in contemporary developed cultures are described as consequences for life expectancy that result from particular patterns of food choice; these are measured in decades, not in hours. The epidemiological revolution is largely re-

TABLE 16.2. Contrast between Human Ancestral Food Environment and Contemporary Developed World Food Environment

Feature	Ancestral environment	Contemporary developed world environment
Availability	Modestly short supply	Wildly abundant
Variety	Modest	Extraordinary: almost all edibles and cultural elaborations of them available to everyone
Super foods	Nonexistent, except for animal foods	Widely available via technological advance (e.g., grain flours, chocolate)
Energy expenditure necessary to obtain food	Substantial	Minimal
Cost	Substantial in terms of time and energy expenditure	Minimal
Consequences of foods: Epidemiological revolution	Apparent within hours of ingestion	Not apparent at all, culturally informed re: effects decades later
Suitability for evaluating foods	Adapted to short-term consequence evaluation	Inability to process and understand complex long term food risk information

sponsible for this change. Only in the contemporary environment do we get information in the form of risk or probabilities of the long-term effects of dietary patterns from epidemiological and other cultural resources. But we are not evolved to make this sort of evaluation; we did not originally live that long, and the short-term effects of foods were our predominant concern. Cultures have yet to adapt to this source of information. Individuals are not educated about even the basics of probability or the nature of science, and are unable to evaluate the importance of communicated information about risks. Hence, the cultural transformations that occurred largely in the 20th century have rendered our biological heritage, finely tuned to our ancestral environment, worse than useless. And the technological advances (e.g., in epidemiology) have not been compensated by lay education that would allow us to comprehend them and behave adaptively with respect to them; we do not teach nutrition, probability, and associated risk–benefit analysis, and we do not teach how science works, which would allow individuals to interpret intelligently the findings of specific studies broadcast in the media.

The result of these mismatches has been an "epidemic" of obesity and widespread dieting, and concern about eating a healthy diet. It is our biological heritage—and that of most if not all animals—to expend as little energy as possible to obtain adequate nutrition and protec-

tion, because energy expenditure requires more energy intake, which itself consumes energy and increases the probability of being prey for other species (Elner & Hughes, 1978; Krebs & Davies, 1997). Furthermore, in the natural world, there is generally a bias to consume food when it is available, since it is often scarce, and undernutrition is a greater threat than overnutrition. Our biological tendencies to eat when food is available and to expend as little energy as possible have become destructive in the modern developed world, where food is palatable, plentiful, and available with minimal energy expenditure.

One result of all of these forces, particularly in the United States, is a great ambivalence about eating, with concerns about obesity tempering the potential enjoyment of a highly palatable, omnipresent, and inexpensive food world (Rodin, Silberstein, & Striegel-Moore, 1985; P. Rozin, Bauer, & Catanese, 2003).

My French colleague Claude Fischler and I, along with a number of students, have taken on the task of examining how different cultures deal with the mismatch between the ancestral and contemporary, developed world food environment, focusing on France and the United States. We have argued that France has been more successful in creating or maintaining compensatory cultural institutions (P. Rozin, Fischler, et al., 1999; P. Rozin, Kabnick, Pete, Fischler, & Shields, 2003; summarized in P. Rozin, 2005), because traditional features of cultural food-related and other institutions in France offer a better buffer to the changes in the food environment. The evidence for greater success in France is not only the substantially lower level of obesity and overweight in France but also a much lower incidence of death due to cardiovascular disease. Our observations and measurements suggest that the French situation is more successful than the American one of the following reasons:

1. The French food environment discourages overeating by offering smaller portions and discouraging snacking (P. Rozin, Kabnick, et al., 2003).
2. The cultural geography of living styles in France, including especially the availability of food sources (stores) locally and within walking distance of most homes, and the greater inconveniences and expenses associated with the use of automobiles, probably leads to greater energy expenditure in daily life in France.
3. The traditional French attitudes toward food focus more on the experience of eating and less on the (health) consequences of eating, leading to less conflict and worry about eating, and more pleasure.
4. Certain deep differences in cultural values with respect to food tend to reduce the impact of easy availability of inexpensive, varied, and highly palatable foods (Stearns, 1997; P. Rozin, 2005). These cultural values include:
   a. An emphasis on moderation as the reigning principle for eating in France, as opposed to abundance in the United States. The striking contrast is illustrated by the quintessential American eating holiday, Thanksgiving, in which being overstuffed seems to be a sign of a successful dinner. As well, the "all you can eat" restaurant is common in the United States and rare in France (P. Rozin, Kabnick, et al., 2003).
   b. A related emphasis on food quality in France and food quantity in the United States. In a sense, love and caring are expressed more in terms of quantity of food offered in the United States versus quality of food in France.
   c. Collective food values are more prominent in France, whereas individualized food values are prominent in the United

States. This may result from the strong individualism/Protestant traditions in the United States. As a result, Americans prefer to be offered a much wider variety of minor variants of the same food (Rozin, Fischler, Shields, & Masson, 2006), and are much more inclined in a restaurant to do their own mixing and matching of main meat dish and vegetable accompaniments, and more individualized seasoning of foods (salt, pepper, ketchup, mustard, etc.).
   d. Americans are more motivated to spend money and arrange their lives to minimize effort and maximize convenience, which has the result of spending less energy. The French are more inclined to spend more money on maximizing joy, that is, having memorable and relatively unique experiences. This corresponds to the important distinction between comforts and pleasures made by Scitovsky (1976/1992).
   e. Americans are more inclined to conceive of health as heavily influenced by environmental influences (e.g., electric power lines, environmental toxins, foods), whereas the French see health more as a matter of internal balance (Payer, 1996).

In short, our analysis indicates that the greater success of the French in resisting both the promotion of overeating and inactivity in the modern world results from a combination of differences in cultural values and in the arrangement of the environment. Most of the differences described here operate to preserve the pleasures of eating, reduce exaggerated worries about eating, and promote weight control in the French as opposed to Americans. It is not that the French have developed better compensatory mechanisms for the modern food environment, but that food institutions already in place have increased resistance to these changes.

FOOD AND SEX

I have argued that food plays a special role in cultural psychology because of the ways cultures have transformed the food domain. In contrast, sex plays a prominent role in evolutionary psychology, because of the many basic similarities in the construal and contexts of sexual behavior in the ancestral and modern environments. Yet there are important and fundamental similarities between these two domains. From the point of view of behavior, food is the critical domain for individual survival, and sex, for species survival. Both are incorporative; except for breathing, these are the two domains in which we take into our bodies material substances from outside our bodies. In both domains, there is great sensitivity about what gets in; there is great pleasure when the "right" stuff gets in, and great aversion, fear, and disgust when the "wrong" stuff gets in.

Contamination and purity are important in the thinking within both domains. Both sex and food involve sharing substance with another person. This is obvious for sex (and may include shared saliva). For food, shared substance occurs in three senses: eating a food prepared by another person, and eating together with another person (perhaps from the same plate or taking bites from the same entity) and, in societies that practice cannibalism, eating another person—either as a demeaning act (analogous to rape) or as an intimate, incorporative act of preserving a loved one within oneself. Alan Fiske (personal communication, January 16, 1991) has pointed out that eating is commonly used as a metaphor for sexual relations in many cultures, and that rules concerning food and sex are often either parallel or mutually determinative. For example, South Asians of higher caste abhor sharing food or drink with people of lower caste and women having sexual relations with men of lower caste. For men in some West African cultures, it is taboo to eat, drink, or share tobacco or kola with the husband of any woman with whom they have sex. They believe that to do so would kill the husband. Conversely, a woman must never cook food for a man who eats with another man with whom she has sexual relations. In several West African pastoralist societies, warriors have sexual relations with some women and eat food cooked by others, but they cannot be seen eating by the women with whom they have sex. In Western cultures, dinner dates and patterns of food sharing may be considered part of sexual foreplay.

Meigs's (1984) analysis of the food taboos of the Hua of Papua New Guinea is an exemplary demonstration of mixed nutritive and sexual meanings of foods. Foods are believed to be vehicles for "vital essence," deriving from both their origins and the people who have handled them. There is great concern that pubescent males be protected from feminization by foods. Hence, they are not allowed to consume any food raised or prepared by a fertile woman. Furthermore, a whole set of foods that are believed to be feminine, and hence feminizing, are prohibited during this period. Meigs assembled a list of such foods, and noted that, as a group, they are reddish in color and soft in texture.

Sex and food each have their relevant aperture, though the mouth is, in many cultures, shared in both food and sex functions. Parallels between the vagina and the mouth are obvious, including common terminology (labia and lips). The high sensitivity of women to vaginal intrusion by foreign and potentially contaminating objects parallels the sense of oral intrusion for such objects by both males and females (P. Rozin, Nemeroff, Horowitz, Gordon, & Voet, 1995).

Finally, at least in American English, there are important metaphorical exchanges of food and sex words. *Eat* has sexual connotations; the word *meat* is sometimes used to refer to women in a sexual context and is also used to refer to male genitals.

SOME IMPORTANT GENERAL ISSUES THAT CAN BE WELL-ADDRESSED IN THE FOOD DOMAIN

Many basic issues in psychology are present in both food and other domains. In some cases, the food domain may provide a particularly convenient area for study of such issues; in other cases, insights from the study of food and eating may contribute to general understanding, or greater understanding of another domain of life. A few of these general issues are considered here.

Food and Environment

The amount of food consumed, and the choice of food are both influenced by many factors, some of which fall within the domains of physiology, psychology, and culture. Perhaps the single most important determinant, mundane as it may be, is the environment. One can only eat foods that are available in the environment. Generally, if food is accessible and at least mildly palatable, people will eat it. The availability of food is principally a result of economic factors and sociocultural traditions and institutions. The previous analysis of the "French paradox" suggests a major role for differences in the physical and social environments of the United States and France. The idea that people eat what is available does not excite the imagination, nor does it encourage psychological theory. That it has not been given much attention in the psychological study of food and eating is perhaps a manifestation of a "fundamental attribution error." In most psychological studies, what is at issue, given the presence of food or food choices, is how people think and behave. But recent work on food, much from within psychology, has focused on the environment, particularly portion size as a main determinant of food intake. A number of investigators have pointed this out in recent years (Hill & Peters, 1998; Rolls, 2003; P. Rozin, Kabnick, et al., 2003; Wansink, 2004), and have documented cultural differences in this area (Rozin, Kabnick, et al., 2003) and recent American historical trends toward larger portion size (Rolls, 2003; Young & Nestle, 1995). Portion size, and more general issues of food availability and context (Meiselman, 1996), fall heavily into the domain of cultural psychology.

Food, Social Class, and Social Structure

The foods consumed, and attitudes toward food, vary across social classes. This area represents an interface between psychology and sociology. Cultural psychology must address social structure and social class, because these are psychologically important manifestations of culture. The social structure of Hindu India has an enormous influence on food transactions, as mediated by the caste system (Appadurai, 1981; Marriott, 1968). Changes in food habits within any culture usually take place over decades or even centuries, and typically move from one class to another. Thus, for example, in Europe, chocolate moved from upper to lower classes. Economic factors (rarity and high cost) partly account for this, as well as a general tendency for lower classes to imitate the behavior of higher classes. On the other hand, some foods, including chili pepper and, more generally, highly spiced foods, have often moved from the lower to the upper classes. The popularity of ethnic cuisines among well-off Americans in recent decades represents a movement from lower to higher classes.

Finally, in modern American society, principally among more educated and wealthy groups (Leichter, 1997), the idea of healthy eating and exercise has taken hold. This often acquires a moral tinge, what has been called "secular" morality by Solomon Katz (1997).

Food as Symbol

Symbolism has always held a fascination in psychology, partly because both metaphors and symbols seem such a central part of human life (e.g., Lakoff & Johnson, 1980). Food, because of its centrality in life, and because it is incorporated into the body, is a major source for symbols and metaphors. For example, rice plays a central role in Japanese life and thought, over and above its nutritional importance (Ohnuki-Tierney, 1993). Food is at the center of many taboos, many of which seem to serve functions outside the domain of nutrition (e.g., Douglas, 1966).

Globalization and Starvation

An important general issue that is well illustrated in the food domain is globalization. Technological advances and globalization have made calories inexpensive (Drewnowski, 1999), have led to a market that caters precisely to individual tastes (Kahn & McAlister, 1997), and have generally transformed the world of food and nutrition (Sobal, 1999). What used to be local food risks have become well-publicized, international fears, with mad cow disease as a clear example (Fischler, 1999). Modern food technology and the modern car-based environment has fostered a situation in which convenience has become a prime commodity. It is likely that the inherent and biologically predisposed laziness of all animals, including humans, is being catered to more and more effectively. It may soon be possible to accomplish eating, entertainment, and other major activities with a minimal of energy expenditure. It was once good to be lazy, but it may not be any more, in terms of either quality of life or longevity. In the meantime, technological advances have greatly improved the safety and shelf-life of foods, introduced a massive variety of highly palatable foods, cut food prices, and made it easy to deliver any type of food almost anywhere in the world. Food is a major area for the study of globalization. The successful penetration of McDonald's into vastly different cultures argues for both important food universals, and a certain cultural sensitivity motivated by the profit motive (Watson, 1997).

At the same time that all of this is happening, along with the surplus of cheap and nutritive food in the developed world, there are still major problems with starvation in the less developed world. It is generally agreed that starvation is a complex product of politics, and economics, sometimes exacerbated by specific cultural practices or preferences. But the major problem today seems to be one of distribution of already produced food to the locations where it is most needed, and this has to do with economics, politics, and culture.

CONCLUSIONS

Food is basic, and it is about biology, psychology (individual experience), and culture. There are many universals and many major culture differences. Cultural evolution is particularly robust in the food domain, and preadaptation of foundational food system features is rampant. The food system presents particular challenges and particular opportunities for cultural psychology. The cross-cultural and historical records are good, especially because food is so central in archeology and ethnography. The biological constraints and predispositions are well understood. What we need is for more researchers to take up the challenge.

REFERENCES

Angyal, A. (1941). Disgust and related aversions. *Journal of Abnormal and Social Psychology, 36,* 393–412.

Appadurai, A. (1981). Gastro-politics in Hindu South Asia. *American Ethnologist, 8,* 494–511.

Baeyens, F., Kaes, B., Eelen, P., & Silverans, P. (1996). Observational evaluative conditioning of an embedded stimulus element. *European Journal of Social Psychology, 26,* 15–28.

Barker, L. M. (Ed.) (1982). *The psychobiology of human food selection.* Bridgeport, CT: AVI.

Barnett, S. A. (1956). Behaviour components in the feeding of wild and laboratory rats. *Behaviour, 9,* 24–43.

Bartoshuk, L. M. (1990). Distinctions between taste and smell relevant to the role of experience. In E. D. Capaldi & T. L. Powley (Eds.), *Taste, experience and feeding* (pp. 62–72). Washington, DC: American Psychological Association.

Beardsworth, A., & Keil, T. (1997). *Sociology on the menu.* London: Routledge.

Beauchamp, G. K. (1981). Ontogenesis of taste preference. In D. Walcher & N. Kretchmer (Eds.), *Food, nutrition and evolution* (pp. 49–57). New York: Masson.

Becker, E. (1973). *The denial of death.* New York: Free Press.

Billing, J., & Sherman, P. W. (1998). Antimicrobial functions of spices: Why some like it hot. *Quarterly Review of Biology, 73,* 3–49.

Birch, L. L. (1980). Effect of peer model's food choices and eating behaviors on pre-schoolers food preferences. *Child Development, 51,* 489–496.

Birch, L. L., Billman, J., & Richards, S. S. (1984). Time of day influences food acceptability. *Appetite, 5,* 109–116.

Birch, L. L., Fisher, J. O., & Grimm-Thomas, K. (1996). The development of children's eating habits. In H. L. Meiselman & H. J. H. MacFie (Eds.), *Food choice, acceptance and consumption* (pp. 161–206). London: Blackie.

Birch, L. L., Zimmerman, S. I., & Hind, H. (1980). The influence of social-affective context on the formation of children's food preferences. *Child Development, 51,* 856–861.

Bock, W. J. (1959). Preadaptation and multiple evolutionary pathways. *Evolution, 13,* 194–211.

Booth, D. A. (1994). *Psychology of nutrition.* London: Taylor & Francis.

Buss, D. (2004). *Evolutionary psychology. The new science of the mind* (2nd ed.). Boston: Allyn & Bacon.

Cavalli-Sforza, L. L., Feldman, M. W., Chen, K. H., & Dornbusch, S. M. (1982). Theory and observation in cultural transmission, *Science, 218,* 19–27.

Coe, S. D., & Coe, M. D. (1996). *The true history of chocolate.* London: Thames & Hudson.

Darwin, C. R. (1965). *The expression of emotions in man and animals.* Chicago: University of Chicago Press. (Original work published 1872)

DeGarine, I. (1972). The socio-cultural aspects of nutrition. *Ecology of Food and Nutrition, 1,* 143–163.

deHouwer, J., Thomas, S., & Baeyens, F. (2001). Associative learning of likes and dislikes: A review of 25 years of research on human evaluative conditioning. *Psychological Bulletin, 127,* 853–869.

Denton, D. A. (1982). *The hunger for salt.* Berlin: Springer-Verlag.

Diamond, J. (1996). *Guns, germs, and steel: The fates of human societies.* New York: Norton.

Douglas, M. (1966). *Purity and danger.* London: Routledge.

Douglas, M., & Nicod, M. (1974). Taking the biscuit: The structure of British meals. *New Society, 30,* 744–747.

Drewnowski, A. (1999). Fat and sugar in the global diet: Dietary diversity in the nutrition transition. In R. Grew (Ed.), *Food in global history* (pp. 194–206). Boulder, CO: Westview Press.

Drewnowski, A., & Greenwood, M. R. C. (1983).

Cream and sugar: Human preferences for high-fat foods. *Physiology and Behavior, 30,* 629–633.

Duncker, K. (1938). Experimental modifications of children's food preferences through social suggestion. *Journal of Abnormal and Social Psychology, 33,* 489–507.

Ekman, P. (1992). An argument for basic emotions. *Cognition and Emotion, 6,* 169–200.

Ekman, P., & Friesen, W. V. (1975). *Unmasking the face.* Englewood Cliffs, NJ: Prentice-Hall.

Elias, N. (1978). *The history of manners: Vol. 1. The civilizing process* (E. Jephcott, Trans.). New York: Pantheon Books. (Original work published 1939).

Elner, R. W., & Hughes, R. N. (1978). Energy maximization in the diet of the shore crab, *Carcinus maenus. Journal of Animal Ecology, 47,* 103–116.

Fiddes, N. (1991). *Meat. A natural symbol.* London: Routledge.

Fischler, C. (1990). *L'homnivore.* Paris: Editions Odile Jacob.

Fischler, C. (1999). The "mad cow" crisis: A global perspective. In R. Grew (Ed.), *Food in global history* (pp. 207–213). Boulder, CO: Westview Press.

Frazer, J. G. (1922). *The golden bough: A study in magic and religion* (abridged ed., T. H. Gaster, Ed.). New York: Macmillan. (Original work published 1890)

Garcia, J., Ervin, F. R., Yorke, C. H., & Koelling, R. A. (1967). Conditioning with delayed vitamin injection. *Science, 155,* 716–718.

Garcia, J., Hankins, W. G., & Rusiniak, K. W. (1974). Behavioral regulation of the milieu interne in man and rat. *Science, 185,* 824–831.

Haidt, J., Koller, S., & Dias, M. (1993). Affect, culture, and morality, or is it wrong to eat your dog? *Journal of Personality and Social Psychology, 65,* 613–628.

Haidt, J., McCauley, C. R., & Rozin, P. (1994). A scale to measure disgust sensitivity. *Personality and Individual Differences, 16,* 701–713.

Harris, M. (1985). *Good to eat: Riddles of food and culture.* New York: Simon & Schuster.

Harris, M., & Ross, E. (Eds.). (1987). *Food and evolution.* Philadelphia: Temple University Press.

Hill, J. O., & Peters, J. C. (1998). Environmental contributions to the obesity epidemic. *Science, 280,* 1371–1374.

Humphrey, N. K. (1976). The social function of intellect. In P. P. G. Bateson & R. A. Hinde (Eds.), *Growing points in ethology* (pp. 303–317). Cambridge, UK: Cambridge University Press.

Izard, C. E. (1977). *Human emotions.* New York: Plenum Press.

Kahn, B. E., & McAlister, L. (1997). *Grocery revolution: The new focus on the consumer.* Reading, MA: Addison-Wesley.

Kass, L. (1994). *The hungry soul.* New York: Free Press.

Katz, S. H. (1982). Food, behavior and biocultural evolution. In L. M. Barker (Ed.), *The psychobiology of human food selection* (pp. 171–188). Westport, CT: AVI.

Katz, S. H. (1997). Secular morality. In A. Brandt & P. Rozin (Eds.), *Morality and health* (pp. 297–330). New York: Routledge.

Katz, S. (Ed.). (2004). *Encyclopedia of food.* New York: Scribner.

Khare, R. S. (1976). *The Hindu hearth and home.* Durham, NC: Carolina Academic Press.

Kiple, K. F., & Ornelas, K. C. (Eds.). (2000). *Cambridge world history of food.* Cambridge, UK: Cambridge University Press.

Krebs, J. R., & Davies, N. B. (Eds.). (1997). *Behavioural ecology* (4th ed.). Oxford, UK: Blackwell Scientific.

Lakoff, G., & Johnson, M. (1980). *Metaphors we live by.* Chicago: University of Chicago Press.

Leichter, H. M. (1997). Lifestyle correctness and the new secular morality. In A. Brandt & P. Rozin (Eds.), *Morality and health* (pp. 359–378). New York: Routledge.

Levenstein, H. (1988). *Revolution at the table. The transformation of the American diet.* New York: Oxford University Press.

Levenstein, H. (1993). *Paradox of plenty. A social history of eating in modern America.* New York: Oxford University Press.

Logue, A. W. (2004). *The psychology of eating and drinking* (3rd ed.). New York: Brunner-Routledge.

Marriott, M. (1968). Caste ranking and food transactions: A matrix analysis. In M. Singer & B. S. Cohn (Eds.), *Structure and change in Indian society* (pp. 133–171). Chicago: Aldine.

Martin, I., & Levey, A. B. (1978). Evaluative conditioning. *Advances in Behaviour Research and Therapy, 1,* 57–102.

Mauss, M. (1972). *A general theory of magic* (R. Brain, Trans.). New York: Norton. (Original work published 1902)

Maurer, D., & Sobal, J. (Eds.). (1995). *Eating agendas: Food and nutrition as social problems.* New York: deGruyter.

Mayr, E. (1960). The emergence of evolutionary novelties. In S. Tax (Ed.), *Evolution after Darwin: Vol. 1. The evolution of life* (pp. 349–380). Chicago: University of Chicago Press.

Mead, M. (1943). The problem of changings food habits. *Bulletin of the National Research Council, 108,* 20–31.

Meigs, A. S. (1984). *Food, sex, and pollution: A New Guinea religion.* New Brunswick, NJ: Rutgers University Press.

Meiselman, H. L. (1996). The contextual basis for food acceptance, food choice, and food intake: The food, the situation, and the individual. In: H. L. Meiselman & H. L. H. MacFie (Eds.), *Food choice, acceptance and consumption* (pp. 239–263). London: Blackie.

Meiselman, H. L. (Ed.). (2000). *Dimensions of the meal. The science, culture, business, and art of eating.* Gaithersburg, MD: Aspen.

Meiselman, H. L., & MacFie, H. L. H. (Eds.). (1996).

Food choice, acceptance and consumption. London: Blackie.

Messer, E. (1984). Anthropological perspectives on diet. *Annual Review of Anthropology, 13,* 205–249.

Miller, W. I. (1997). *The anatomy of disgust.* Cambridge, MA: Harvard University Press.

Milton, K. (1993, August). Diet and primate evolution. *Scientific American,* pp. 86–93.

Mintz, S. W. (1985). *Sweetness and power.* New York: Viking.

Murcott, A. (Ed.). (1983). *The sociology of food and eating.* London: Gower.

Nemeroff, C., & Rozin, P. (1989). "You are what you eat": Applying the demand-free "impressions" technique to an unacknowledged belief. *Ethos: Journal of Psychological Anthropology, 17,* 50–69.

Nemeroff, C., & Rozin, P. (2000). The makings of the magical mind. In K. S. Rosengren, C. N. Johnson, & P. L. Harris (Eds.), *Imagining the impossible: Magical, scientific, and religious thinking in children* (pp. 1–34). New York: Cambridge University Press.

Ochs, E., Pontecorvo, C., & Fasulo, A. (1996). Socializing taste. *Ethnos: Journal of Psychological Anthropology, 61,* 7–46.

Ohnuki-Tierney, E. (1993). *Rice as self: Japanese identities through time.* Princeton, NJ: Princeton University Press.

Payer, L. (1996). *Medicine and culture.* New York: Holt.

Pliner, P. (1982). The effects of mere exposure on liking for edible substances. *Appetite, 3,* 283–290.

Pliner, P. (1983). Family resemblance in food preferences. *Journal of Nutrition Education, 15,* 137–140.

Pliner, P., & Rozin, P. (2000). The psychology of the meal. In H. Meiselman (Ed.), *Dimensions of the meal: The science, culture, business, and art of eating* (pp. 19–46). Gaithersburg, MD: Aspen.

Pyszczynski, T., Greenberg, J., & Solomon, S. (1997). Why do we need what we need?: A terror management perspective on the roots of human social motivation. *Psychological Inquiry, 8,* 1–20

Richter, C. P. (1956). Salt appetite of mammals: Its dependence on instinct and metabolism. In *L'instinct dans le comportement des animaux et de l'homme* (pp. 577–629). Paris: Masson.

Rodin, J. Silberstein, L. R., & Striegel-Moore, R. H. (1985). Women and weight: A normative discontent. In T. B. Sonderegger (Ed.), *Nebraska Symposium on Motivation: Vol. 32. Psychology and Gender* (pp. 267–307). Lincoln: University of Nebraska Press.

Rolls, B. J. (2003). The supersizing of America: Portion size and the obesity epidemic. *Nutrition Today, 38,* 42–53.

Rosenstein, D., & Oster, H. (1988). Differential facial responses to four basic tastes in newborns. *Child Development, 59,* 1555–1568.

Rozin, E. (1982). The structure of cuisine. In L. M. Barker (Ed.), *The psychobiology of human food selection* (pp. 189–203). Westport, CT: AVI.

Rozin, E., & Rozin, P. (1981). Culinary themes and variations. *Natural History, 90*(2), 6–14.

Rozin, P. (1976). The selection of food by rats, humans and other animals. In J. Rosenblatt, R. A. Hinde, C. Beer, & E. Shaw (Eds.), *Advances in the study of behavior* (Vol. 6, pp. 21–76). New York: Academic Press.

Rozin, P. (1982). Human food selection: The interaction of biology, culture and individual experience. In L. M. Barker (Eds.), *The psychobiology of human food selection* (pp. 225–254). Westport, CT: AVI.

Rozin, P. (1988). Social learning about foods by humans. In T. Zentall & B. G. Galef, Jr. (Eds.), *Social learning: A comparative approach* (pp. 165–187). Hillsdale, NJ: Erlbaum.

Rozin, P. (1990a). Getting to like the burn of chili pepper: Biological, psychological and cultural perspectives. In B. G. Green, J. R. Mason, & M. R. Kare (Eds.), *Chemical senses: Vol. 2. Irritation* (pp. 231–269). New York: Marcel Dekker.

Rozin, P. (1990b). Development in the food domain. *Developmental Psychology, 26,* 555–562.

Rozin, P. (1991). Family resemblance in food and other domains: The family paradox and the role of parental congruence. *Appetite, 16,* 93–102.

Rozin, P. (1999a). Preadaptation and the puzzles and properties of pleasure. In D. Kahneman, E. Diener, & N. Schwarz (Eds.), *Well-being: The foundations of hedonic psychology* (pp. 109–133). New York: Russell Sage Foundation.

Rozin, P. (1999b). The process of moralization. *Psychological Science, 10,* 218–221.

Rozin, P. (2004). Meat. In S. Katz (Ed.), *Encyclopedia of food* (pp. 666–671). New York: Scribner.

Rozin, P. (2005). The meaning of food in our lives: A cross-cultural perspective on eating and well-being. *Journal of Nutrition Education and Behavior, 37,* S107–S112.

Rozin, P. (in press). Domain denigration and process preference in academic psychology. *Perspectives on Psychological Science*

Rozin, P., Bauer, R., & Catanese, D. (2003). Attitudes to food and eating in American college students in six different regions of the United States. *Journal of Personality and Social Psychology, 85,* 132–141.

Rozin, P., & Fallon, A. E. (1987). A perspective on disgust. *Psychological Review, 94*(1), 23–41.

Rozin, P., Fallon, A. E., & Augustoni-Ziskind, M. (1986). The child's conception of food: Development of categories of accepted and rejected substances. *Journal of Nutrition Education, 18,* 75–81.

Rozin, P., Fischler, C., Imada, S., Sarubin, A., & Wrzesniewski, A. (1999). Attitudes to food and the role of food in life: Comparisons of Flemish Belgium, France, Japan and the United States. *Appetite, 33,* 163–180.

Rozin, P., Fischler, C., Shields, C., & Masson, E. (2006). Attitudes toward large numbers of choices in the food domain: A cross-cultural study of five countries in Europe and the USA. *Appetite, 46,* 304–308.

Rozin, P., Haidt, J., & McCauley, C. R. (2000). Disgust. In M. Lewis & J. Haviland (Eds.), *Handbook of emotions, second edition* (pp. 637–653). New York: Guilford Press.

Rozin, P., Haidt, J., McCauley, C. R., & Imada, S. (1997). The cultural evolution of disgust. In H. M. Macbeth (Ed.), *Food preferences and taste: Continuity and change* (pp. 65–82). Oxford, UK: Berghahn.

Rozin, P., Hammer, L., Oster, H., Horowitz, T., & Marmara, V. (1986). The child's conception of food: Differentiation of categories of rejected substances in the 1.4 to 5 year age range. *Appetite, 7,* 141–151.

Rozin P, Kabnick, K., Pete, E., Fischler, C., Shields, C. (2003). The ecology of eating: smaller portion sizes in France than in the United States help explain the French paradox. *Psychological Science, 14,* 450–454.

Rozin, P., & Kalat, J. W. (1971). Specific hungers and poison avoidance as adaptive specializations of learning. *Psychological Review, 78,* 459–486.

Rozin, P., & Kennel, K. (1983). Acquired preferences for piquant foods by chimpanzees. *Appetite, 4,* 69–77.

Rozin, P., Levine, E., & Stoess, C. (1991). Chocolate craving and liking. *Appetite, 17,* 199–212.

Rozin, P., Lowery, L., Imada, S., & Haidt, J. (1999). The CAD triad hypothesis: A mapping between three other-directed moral emotions (contempt, anger, disgust) and three moral ethics (community, autonomy, divinity). *Journal of Personality and Social Psychology, 76,* 574–586.

Rozin, P., Millman, L., & Nemeroff, C. (1986). Operation of the laws of sympathetic magic in disgust and other domains. *Journal of Personality and Social Psychology, 50,* 703–712.

Rozin, P., & Nemeroff, C. J. (1990). The laws of sympathetic magic: A psychological analysis of similarity and contagion. In J. Stigler, G. Herdt, & R. A. Shweder (Eds.), *Cultural psychology: Essays on comparative human development* (pp. 205–232). Cambridge, UK: Cambridge University Press.

Rozin, P., Nemeroff, C., Horowitz, M., Gordon, B., & Voet, W. (1995). The borders of the self: Contamination sensitivity and potency of the mouth, other apertures and body parts. *Journal of Research in Personality, 29,* 318–340.

Rozin, P., & Pelchat, M. L. (1988). Memories of mammaries: Adaptations to weaning from milk in mammals. In A. N. Epstein & A. Morrison (Eds.), *Advances in psychobiology* (Vol. 13, pp. 1–29). New York: Academic Press.

Rozin, P., Riklis, J., & Margolis, L. (2003). Mutual exposure or close peer relationships do not seem to foster increased similarity in food, music or television program preferences. *Appetite, 42,* 41–48.

Rozin, P., & Schiller, D. (1980). The nature and acquisition of a preference for chili pepper by humans. *Motivation and Emotion, 4,* 77–101.

Rozin, P., & Schulkin, J. (1990). Food selection. In E. M. Stricker (Ed.), *Handbook of behavioral neurobiology: Vol. 10. Food and water intake* (pp. 297–328). New York: Plenum Press.

Samuelson, R. J. (Ed.). (1990). *The economist book of vital world statistics.* New York: Random House.

Schulkin, J. (1991). *Sodium hunger. The search for a salty taste.* Cambridge, UK: Cambridge University Press.

Schutz, H. G. (1989). Beyond preference: Appropriateness as a measure of contextual acceptance of food. In D. M. H. Thomson (Ed.), *Food acceptability* (pp. 115–134). Essex, UK: Elsevier.

Scitovsky T. (1992). *The joyless economy: The psychology of human satisfaction* (rev ed.). Oxford, UK: Oxford University Press. (Original work published 1976)

Sclafani, A. (1999). Macronutrient-conditioned flavor preferences. In H.-R. Berthoud & R. J. Seeley (Eds.), *Neural control of macronutrient selection* (pp. 93–106). Boca Raton, FL: CRC Press.

Shepherd, R., & Raats, M. M. (Eds.). (2006). *Psychology of food choice.* Wallingford, UK: CABI.

Shweder, R. A., Much, N. C., Mahapatra, M., & Park, L. (1997). The "big three" of morality (autonomy, community, divinity), and the "big three" explanations of suffering. In A. Brandt & P. Rozin (Eds.), *Morality and health* (pp. 119–169). New York: Routledge.

Siegal, M. (1997). Becoming mindful of food. *Current Directions in Psychological Science, 4,* 177–181.

Simoons, F. J. (1969). Primary adult lactose intolerance and the milk drinking habit: A problem and biological and cultural interrelations: I. Review of the medical research. *American Journal of Digestive Diseases, 14,* 819–836.

Simoons, F. J. (1970). Primary adult lactose intolerance and the milk drinking habit: A problem and biological and cultural interrelations: II. A cultural–historical hypothesis. *American Journal of Digestive Diseases, 15,* 695–710.

Simoons, F. J. (1991). *Food in China: A cultural and historical inquiry.* Boca Raton, FL: CRC Press.

Simoons, F. J. (1994). *Eat not this flesh: Food avoidances from prehistory to the present.* Madison: University of Wisconsin Press (Original work published 1961)

Sobal, J. (1999). Food system globalization, eating transformations, and nutrition transitions. In R. Grew (Ed.), *Food in global history* (pp. 171–193). Boulder, CO: Westview Press.

Solomon, R. L. (1980). The opponent process theory of acquired motivation. *American Psychologist, 35,* 691–712.

Stearns, P. N. (1997). *Fat history. Bodies and beauty in the modern West.* New York: New York University Press.

Stein, R. L., & Nemeroff, C. J. (1995). Moral overtones of food: Judgments of others based on what they eat. *Personality and Social Psychology Bulletin, 21,* 480–490.

Steiner, J. E. (1979). Human facial expressions in response to taste and smell stimulation. In H. W. Reese & L. P. Lipsitt (Eds.), *Advances in child development and behavior* (Vol. 13, pp. 257–295.) New York: Academic Press.

Szalai, A. (Ed.) (1972). *The use of time: Daily activities of urban and suburban populations in twelve countries.* The Hague: Mouton.

Tambiah, S. J. (1969). Animals are good to think and good to prohibit. *Ethnology, 8,* 423–459.

Tomkins, S. S. (1963). *Affect, imagery, consciousness: Vol. 2. The negative affects.* New York: Springer.

Twigg, J. (1983). Vegetarianism and the meanings of meat. In A. Murcott (Ed.), *The sociology of food and eating: Essays on the sociological significance of food* (pp. 18–30). London: Gower.

Tylor, E. B. (1974). *Primitive culture: Researches into the development of mythology, philosophy, religion, art and custom.* New York: Gordon Press. (Original work published 1871)

Wansink, B. (2004). Environmental factors that increase food intake and consumption volume of unknowing consumers. *Annual Review of Nutrition, 24,* 455–479.

Watson, J. L. (Ed.). (1997). *Golden arches East: McDonald's in East Asia.* Stanford, CA: Stanford University Press.

Weingarten, H. P., & Elston, D. (1991). A survey of cravings in a student sample. *Appetite, 17,* 167–175.

Whitehead, H. (2000). *Food rules. Hunting, sharing, and tabooing game in Papua New Guinea.* Ann Arbor: University of Michigan Press.

Whorton, J. C. (1982). *Crusaders for fitness.* Princeton, NJ: Princeton University Press.

Young, L. R., & Nestle, M. (1995). Portion size in dietary assessment: Issues and policy implications. *Nutrition Reviews, 53*(6), 149–158

Zajonc, R. B. (1968). Attitudinal effects of mere exposure. *Journal of Personality and Social Psychology, 9*(2), 1–27.

CHAPTER 17

Religion's Social
and Cognitive Landscape
An Evolutionary Perspective

SCOTT ATRAN

Le XXIème siècle sera religieux ou ne sera pas
[The 21st century will be religious or will not *be*].
—André Malraux

This chapter explores religion's social and cognitive landscape from an evolutionary perspective. Explaining religion is a serious problem for any evolutionary account of human thought and society. Religious practice is costly in terms of material sacrifice (at least one's prayer time), emotional expenditure (inciting fears and hopes), and cognitive effort (maintaining both factual and counterintuitive networks of beliefs). Adaptationist arguments usually attempt to offset the apparent functional disadvantages of religion with even greater functional advantages, such as maintenance of personal well-being and group solidarity.

The main thesis in this chapter, however, is that religion is not an evolutionary adaptation per se, but a recurring *by-product* of the complex evolutionary landscape that sets cognitive, emotional, and material conditions for ordinary human interactions. The conceptual foundations of religion are intuitively given by task-specific, panhuman cognitive domains, including folk mechanics, folk biology, and folk psychology. Core religious beliefs minimally violate ordinary intuitions about the world, with its inescapable problems. Cultural manipulations of humans' innate hypersensitivity to agency in folk psychology are especially important for understanding the supernatural. Be-

417

cause supernatural beliefs minimally violate and readily activate intuitively given modular processes, they are more likely to survive transmission across minds under a wide range of different environments and learning conditions, and to become recurrent and enduring aspects of human cultures. Because religious beliefs cannot be deductively or inductively validated, validation occurs only by ritually addressing the very emotions motivating religion, although ritual modes may differ appreciably in literate and large-scale societies versus small-scale societies that rely more heavily on iconic representations and face-to-face contact.

Enabling people to imagine minimally impossible supernatural worlds helps to solve existential problems, including death and deception. In the competition for moral allegiance, secular ideologies are at a disadvantage. For if people learn that all apparent commitment is self-interested convenience or worse, manipulation for the self-interest of others, then their commitment is debased and withers. Noninstrumental or "sacred" values appear to rouse hearts and minds passionately to break out of this viciously rational cycle of self-interest, and to adopt group interests that may benefit individuals in the long run, though compulsory adherence to such values can also encourage cultural intolerance and protracted political conflict.

INTRODUCTION

Ever since Edward Gibbon's (1845/1776) *Decline and Fall of the Roman Empire*, scientists and secularly minded scholars have been predicting, or pushing for, the ultimate demise of religion (cf. Dawkins, 2006; Dennett, 2006; Harris, 2006). But, if anything, religious fervor is increasing across the globe. New religious movements (NRMs) continue to arise at a furious pace—perhaps at the rate of two or three per day (Lester, 2002). There are now nearly 2 billion self-proclaimed Christians (about one-third of humanity), 25% of whom are Pentecostals or charismatics (people who stay in mainstream Protestant and Catholic churches and have adopted Pentecostal practices, e.g., healings, speaking in tongues, casting out demons and laying hands upon the sick; Goodstein, 2000, p. 24). In Africa, for example, the Winner's Church, a Pentecostal church

that celebrates newfound market wealth and success, is only a dozen years old (N. Onishi, 2002) but already has more than 50,000 members in 32 branches on the continent. During the same period, the Falun Gong, a Buddhist offshoot, has grown to perhaps 100 million adherents in East Asia and the Al Qaeda-led *jihadi* movement has spread across the Muslim world.

The United States—the world's most economically powerful and scientifically advanced society—is also one of the world's most professedly religious societies. Evangelical Christians and fundamentalists include about 25% of Americans (Talbot, 2000, p. 36) who, together with charismatics, comprise about 40% of the American population. About the same number believe that God speaks to them directly (H. Bloom, 1999, pp. 120–123). Among Americans, 90% pray for God's intervention in life and 90% believe God cares for them (H. Bloom, 1999); 69% believe in angels, and at least 50% believe in ghosts, the devil, and the literal interpretation of Genesis (polls cited in Pinker, 1997; Dennett, 1995). Even in Western Europe, the most secular of societies, more than 60% of the population believe in the soul (Humphrey, 1995).

An underlying reason for religion's endurance is that science treats humans and intentions only as incidental elements in the universe, whereas for religion they are central. Science is not particularly well-suited to deal with people's existential anxieties—death, deception, sudden catastrophe, loneliness, or longing for love or justice. It cannot tell us what we *ought* to do, only what we can do. Religion thrives because it addresses people's yearnings and society's moral needs. Other factors in religion's persistence as humankind's provisional evolutionary destiny involve naturally selected elements of human cognition. These include the inherent susceptibility of religious beliefs to modularized (innate, universal, domain-specific) conceptual processing systems, such as folk psychology, that favor survival and recurrence of the supernatural within and across minds and societies.

Although science may never replace religion, science can help us understand how religions are structured in individual minds (brains) and across societies (cultures), and also, in a strictly material sense, why religious belief endures. In every society,[1] it appears, there are the following:

1. Widespread counterfactual and counterintuitive belief in supernatural agents (gods, ghosts, goblins, etc.).
2. Hard-to-fake public expressions of costly material commitments to supernatural agents, that is, offering and sacrifice (offerings of goods, property, time, life).
3. Mastery by supernatural agents of people's existential anxieties (death, deception, disease, catastrophe, pain, loneliness, injustice, want, loss).
4. Ritualized, rhythmic sensory coordination of items 1, 2, and 3, that is, communion (congregation, intimate fellowship, etc.).

In all societies an evolutionary canalization and convergence of items 1, 2, 3, and 4 tends toward what I refer to as "religion"; that is, passionate communal displays of costly commitments to counterintuitive worlds governed by supernatural agents (Atran, 2002). Although these facets of religion emerge in all known cultures and animate the majority of individual human beings in the world, there are considerable individual and cultural differences in the degree of religious commitment. (But an analysis of the origin and nature of these intriguing and important differences must be left for another time.)

These four conditions do not constitute necessary and sufficient features of "religion." Rather, they comprise a stipulative (working) framework that delimits a causally interconnected set of pancultural phenomena that comprises the object of our study (Atran & Norenzayan, 2004). One may choose to call phenomena that fall under this set of conditions "religion" or not; however, for my purposes their joint satisfaction is what I mean by the term. Nevertheless, this working framework is offered as an adequate conceptualization that roughly corresponds to what most scholars consider religion.

Cognitive theories of religion primarily concern item 1. These concentrate almost entirely on the micropsychological processes of cultural transmission, the processes that causally generate, transform, and connect chains of mental and public representations into "cultures," and parts of culture such as religion. Cognitive theories attempt to explain religious belief and practice as cultural manipulations of ordinary psychological processes of categorization, reasoning, and remembering (Sperber, 1975;

Atran, 1990; Lawson & McCauley, 1990; Boyer, 1994; Andresen, 2001; Pyysiäinen & Anttonen, 2002). Empirical studies in this area have almost wholly concerned memory and cognitive constraints on the structuration and transmission of religious beliefs (J. Barrett & Keil, 1996; Barrett & Nyhoff, 2001; Boyer & Ramble, 2001; Owsianiecki, Upal, Sloan, & Tweney, 2005). They do not account for the emotional involvement that leads people to sacrifice to others what is dear to themselves, including labor, limb, and life. Such theories are often short on motive and unable to distinguish Mickey Mouse from Moses, cartoon fantasy from religious belief (Atran, 1998, p. 602; cf. Boyer, 2000). They fail to tell us why, in general, the greater the sacrifice of personal self-interest for apparently absurd group beliefs—as in Abraham offering up his beloved son to an invisible being—the more others trust in one's religious commitment (Kierkegaard, 1843/1955).

Commitment theories of religion primarily concern item 2. These focus almost exclusively on the macroinstitutional dynamics of socially distributed traits, rules, norms, and other cultural prototypes. Commitment theories attempt to explain the apparent altruism and emotional sacrifice of immediate self-interest accompanying religion in terms of long-term benefits to the individual (Alexander, 1987; Irons, 1996; Nesse, 2001) or group (Boehm, 1999; Sober & Wilson, 1998; D. S. Wilson, 2002; Boyd & Richerson, 2005)—benefits that supposedly contribute to genetic fitness or cultural survival. Empirical studies have almost wholly concentrated on material measures of individual and group costs and benefits. They do not account for the cognitive peculiarity of the culturally universal belief in beings who are imperceptible in principle, and who change the world via causes that are materially and logically inscrutable in principle. They do not distinguish Marxism from monotheism, secular ideologies from religious belief.

Experiential theories primarily concern item 3. These mainly target states of altered consciousness and personal sensations. Empirical studies focus on tracking participants' neurophysiological responses during episodes of religious experience and recording individual reports of trance, meditation, vision, revelation, and the like (Persinger, 1987; Beit-Hallahmi & Argyle, 1997; d'Aquili & Newberg, 1999; Joseph, 2002). Cognitive structures of the human mind/brain in general, and cognitions of agency in particular, are described either cognitively in simpleminded terms (binary oppositions, holistic vs. analytical tensions, hierarchical organization, etc.) or in psychoanalytic terms that have little input from, or pertinence to, recent findings of cognitive and developmental psychology.

Performance theories primarily concern item 4. These attend to the psychosocial dynamics of liturgy and ritual practice, that is, to the affective character and sociological implications of what Durkheim (1912/1995) called "collective effervescence." Empirical studies have almost wholly focused on normative and ceremonial expressions of religion. They underplay more mundane cognitive processes of categorization, reasoning, and decision making that underlie all religious beliefs and commitments, and that make such beliefs and commitments comprehensible (Barth, 1975; V. Turner, 1969; Tambiah, 1981; Rappaport, 1999; Watanabee & Smuts, 1999).

Now, if (1) supernatural agents are cognitively salient, and possess omniscient and omnipotent powers, and (2) there is sufficient costly signaling from people within a community to convince others that commitment to the supernatural is genuine, then (3) the supernatural can be invoked to ease existential anxieties, such as death and deception, that forever threaten human life everywhere and from which no enduring rational escape is possible. However, conceptions of the supernatural invariably involve the interruption or violation of universal cognitive principles that govern ordinary human perception and understanding of the everyday world. Consequently, religious beliefs and experiences cannot be reliably validated (or disconfirmed as false) through consistent logical deduction or consistent empirical induction.

Validation occurs only by (4) collectively satisfying the emotions that motivate religion in the first place. Through a "collective effervescence" (Durkheim, 1912/1995), communal rituals rhythmically coordinate emotional validation of, and commitment to, moral truths in worlds governed by supernatural agents. Through the sensory pageantry of movement, sound, smell, touch, and sight, religious rituals affectively coordinate actors' minds and bodies into convergent expressions of public sentiment (cf. Tinbergen, 1951)—a sort of N–person

bonding that communicates moral consensus as sacred, transcending all reason and doubt (Rappaport, 1999). But for those left outside the religious consensus, it may seem that "cruelty and intolerance to those who do not belong to it are natural to every religion" (Freud, 1921/1955).

The rituals that accompany all religions almost always include music and other sorts of voluntary rhythmic stimulations. Even the Taliban, which banned nearly every sort of collective sensory stimulation, systematically used *a capella* chants to cement adherence to their religious fraternity.[2] Prayers in all religions employ the same gests of submission: outstretched arms with chest exposed and throat bared, genuflection, prostration, and so on. These are pretty much the same bodily expressions that other social animals display to signal submission, including our simian cousins and canine friends. But for humans such gests are not merely symbolic: In embodying them people actually provoke in themselves feelings of submission and humbleness before a greater power. Other common ritual acts that socially coordinate bodily movements among members of a congregation include sway and dance. The emotional unity created during these performances underscores the commitment to sacrifice a bit of oneself for others—not necessarily in the here and now, but as an open-ended promise to help others in any number of ways when they may need it most.

To evoke a strong and intimate sense of community, members of a religious community often create families of fictive kin. For example, from Paris suburbs to Indonesian jungles, the Mujahedin I have interviewed who profess religious commitment to martyrdom actions (suicide attacks) come from almost every walk of life and socioeconomic background (which is why global profiling across cells of suicide bombers is a waste of time); however, within each cell of typically 8–12 people, all tend to eat the same sort of food, sport the same clothing, chant the same slogans, and share the same daily rites and routines. Through incorporation of recruits into relatively small and closeted cells—emotionally tight-knit brotherhoods—religiously inspired terror organizations create a family of cellmates who are just as willing to sacrifice for one another as is a parent for a child. These culturally contrived cell loyalties mimic and (at least temporarily) override genetically based fidelities to kin, while securing belief in sacrifice to a larger group cause. And this can even mutate over the Internet into a virtual family whose members may be physically remote from one another, but who are as emotionally linked and primed for mutual sacrifice as any real family or group of friends (Atran & Stern, 2005).[3]

In the final tally, eruptive emotions are often stronger and more convincing than careful reason—perhaps because evolution selected our emotions to wax when we believe ourselves to be faced with inescapable problems of survival. Failure to figure in the emotional costs and payoffs associated with those aspects of life that are not rationally controllable—including death and deception, heartbreak and loneliness, catastrophe and want, injustice and lack of fairness—reduces any purely cognitive theory of religion to barely more than an account of how people are able to assimilate all manner of fictional reverie.

WHY IS RELIGION AN EVOLUTIONARY DILEMMA?

Religion is a serious riddle for any evolutionary account of human thought and society. From an evolutionary standpoint, the reasons for why religion should not exist are patent: Religion is materially expensive, and it is unrelentingly counterfactual and even counterintuitive. Religious practice is costly in terms of material sacrifice (at least one's prayer time), emotional expenditure (inciting fears and hopes), and cognitive effort (maintaining both factual and counterintuitive networks of beliefs). Summing up the anthropological literature on religious offerings, Raymond Firth (1963, pp. 13–16) concludes that "sacrifice is giving something up at a cost. . . . 'afford it or not,' the attitude seems to be."[4]

In all religions, argued the empirical philosopher and religious believer Thomas Hobbes, there are bodiless but sentient souls and spirits that act intentionally, though not in ways that can be verified empirically or understood logically. As for "one infinite, omnipotent, and eternal God," even the enlightened "choose rather to confess He is incomprehensible and above their understanding than to define His nature by 'spirit incorporeal,' and then confess their definition to be unintelligible" (1651/1901, Vol. 1, part XII, p. 69). (This "incompre-

hensibility" is strongly related to the technical notion of "counterintuitiveness" that I discuss a bit later on.)

If people literally applied counterfactual and counterintuitive religious principles and prescriptions to factual navigation of everyday environments they would likely be either dead or in the afterlife in very short order—probably in too short order for individuals to reproduce and the species to survive. Imagine creatures who always truly believed that the dead lived on and the meek were advantaged over the strong, or that one could arbitrarily suspend the known physical and biological laws of the universe with a prayer (or for those less institutionalized, by crossing one's fingers). Their fitness value would be close to nil. The trick is in knowing how and when to suspend factual belief without countermanding the facts and compromising survival. But why take the risk of neglecting the facts at all, even in exceptional circumstances?

As for costly material commitment to the supernatural, there cannot be individual fitness advantages of the sort that part-for-whole sacrifice among animals may convey (Burkert, 1996) given that the probability of certifiably obtaining the desired outcome, such as a rewarding afterlife or freedom from catastrophe, ranges between zero and chance. For a bear to sacrifice its paw in a trap by gnawing it off, a lizard to leave behind its tail for a predator, or a bee to die by stinging an intruder to save the hive, seem reasonable trade-offs for survival. Yet what could be the calculated gain from the following:

- Years of toil to build gigantic structures that house only dead bones (Egyptian, Mesoamerican, and Cambodian pyramids)?
- Giving up one's sheep (Hebrews) or camels (Bedouin) or cows (Nuer of Sudan) or chickens (Highland Maya) or pigs (Melanesian tribes, Ancient Greeks), or buffaloes (South Indian tribes)?
- Dispatching wives when husbands die (Hindus, Incas, Solomon Islanders)?
- Slaying one's own healthy and desired offspring (the first born of Phoenicia and Carthage, Pawnee and Iroquois maidens, Inca and Postclassic Mayan boys and girls, children of South India's tribal Lambadi)?
- Chopping off a finger for dead warriors or relatives (Dani of New Guinea, Crow and other American Plains Indians)?

- Burning one's house and all other possessions for a family member drowned, crushed by a tree, or killed by a tiger (Nāga tribes of Assam)?
- Knocking out one's own teeth (Australian aboriginals)?
- Making elaborate but evanescent sand designs (Navajo, tribes of Central Australia)?
- Giving up one's life to keep Fridays (Muslims) or Saturdays (Jews) or Sundays (Christians) holy?

Try to come up with an adaptive logic that generates a unitary explanation for all of these phenomena, or for just stopping whatever one is doing to murmur often incomprehensible words while gesticulating several times a day. As Bill Gates aptly surmised, "Just in terms of allocation of time resources, religion is not very efficient. There's a lot more I could be doing on a Sunday morning" (cited in Keillor, 1999).

Evolution cannot account for religion simply as an adaptation for some ancestral task that is "hardwired" into us. There is no gene for the complex of beliefs and behaviors that make up religion, any more than there is a gene for science; nor is their likely any genetic complex with law-like or systematic qualities that is responsible for most religious belief or behavior. It is rash and very likely wrong to infer that because nearly every historically successful human society was religiously based (especially popular in sociobiology) nature selected a propensity for religion because ancestral tribes that believed themselves favored in battle by the gods were victorious over other tribes. For if one seriously considers the beliefs of people who think they are favored by the gods and how they behave as a result, then one has got a good chunk of human belief and behavior to cover.

ADAPTATIONIST THEORIES OF RELIGION

Adaptationist arguments usually attempt to offset the apparent functional disadvantages of religion with even greater functional advantages. Adaptationists study traits within specific ecological contexts and evaluate whether a current trait produces the highest reproductive success given the alternative strategies available. This has yet to be determined for any religious trait. Nor have researchers examined religions' ability to respond to the selective

pressures of diverse ecological contexts. In other words, to date, most of the adaptationist literature on religion is largely theoretical and offers only a few empirical tests (for exceptions see Sosis, 2000; Sosis & Bressler, 2003; Bering & Borklund, 2004).

Social Control

Behavioral ecologists have argued that evolution is a competitive process in which selection occurs at the individual, rather than the group, level (Dawkins & Krebs, 1978; cf. Barrett, Dunbar, & Lycett, 2001). From this vantage, selective pressures should favor deceptive strategies when individuals can exploit other group members for individual advantage. Thus, interactions between signalers and receivers should escalate in an evolutionary arms race in which signalers attempt to influence the behaviors of receivers to their own advantage, and receivers attempt to recognize deception and resist manipulation that is not in their best interests. The result of such escalation would be increasingly complex ritual behaviors as senders attempt to deceive receivers, and receivers seek to determine the truthfulness of senders' signals.

Cronk (1994) applied this reasoning to explore human moral systems cross-culturally. In contrast to previous work that emphasized how moral systems enhance cooperation within groups (Alexander, 1987), Cronk observed that despite the benefits of mutualism (a relationship between two species that benefits both), there are still conflicts of interests within groups. As a result of these conflicts, moral statements can be used to manipulate others to benefit the signalers at a cost to the receivers. Cronk argues that religion can be used by elites to maintain social control, noting that this claim is supported by the classic cross-cultural study by Swanson (1960), who found inegalitarian societies to be more likely than egalitarian societies to believe in moralizing and punishing gods. Cronk follows Krebs and Dawkins (1984), who claimed that cooperative signals should be simple, whereas manipulative signals should be more elaborate, with greater repetition. Thus, religious communities concerned with conquest, control, and conversion should have more elaborate and repetitive displays than communities with little interest in "convincing any nongroup members of their correctness." But this hypothesis yet has to be reliably tested.

Costly Signaling Theory

Some researchers have observed that the hypothesized "arms race" between deceivers and receivers does not always occur. For example, when a direct link between signal and underlying condition exists, as between physical size and vocal signal frequency, deception is precluded (Johnstone, 1998). Zahavi (1975) argued that even in the absence of such direct physical linkage, it is possible to ensure signal reliability *if signals are differentially costly to produce*. In other words, signals expressing phenotypic condition can be honest if the costs to lower quality organisms of imitating the signals of higher quality organisms outweigh the benefits that can be achieved (Grafen, 1990).

Various researchers have proposed the application of costly signaling theory to religious ritual to explain how social cohesion is promoted by religion or, more generally, how nonkin groups manage to cooperate in order to compete with rival groups (Irons, 1996; Sosis & Alcorta, 2003; Bulbulia, 2004). These researchers view religion's ability to promote solidarity as its primary function but recognize that social bonding is not an end in itself; by increasing solidarity religion facilitates intragroup cooperation. Indeed, Irons (2001) argued that the primary adaptive benefit of religion is its ability to promote cooperation and overcome problems of collective action that humans have faced throughout their evolutionary history, including cooperative hunting, food sharing, defense, and warfare. When faced with the conditions of collective action, the incentive to claim falsely that one will cooperate is especially high, because individuals can achieve their greatest gains by refraining from cooperation when others cooperate. Although everyone may gain if all group members invest in the cooperative goal, attainment of such large-scale cooperation is often difficult to achieve without social mechanisms limiting the potential to free ride on the efforts of others. Therefore, whenever an individual can achieve net benefits from defection, the only credible signals of cooperative intentions are those that are "costly to fake"; otherwise, they can easily be imitated by free riders, who do not intend to invest in the cooperative pursuit.

The costly signaling theory of ritual posits that religious behaviors or rituals are costly-to-fake signals that advertise an individual's level of commitment to a religious group. Preferred signalers are those who are highly committed to the goals and ideals of the group, which typically include ingroup altruism. Cooperation is facilitated because those who are uncommitted can be avoided as partners in collective action, because they will find it too expensive to pay the costs of religious behavior. In ethnohistorical studies on 19th-century U.S. communes and economic field experiments on Israeli kibbutzim, Sosis and colleagues have demonstrated a positive association between participation in religious ritual and enhanced cooperation (Sosis & Bressler, 2003; Sosis & Ruffle, 2004); however, they have yet to examine how the high levels of cooperation observed within religious communities translate into individual fitness gains.

Ritual Healing Theory

McClenon (2002) offers an intriguing theory of the evolution of religion. He notes that ancestral primates undoubtedly used rudimentary rituals to alleviate social stress. Social grooming in nonhuman primates, as well as the ritualized hand gestures of hominoids and the chimpanzee "rain dance" described by Goodall (1986) all constitute such rituals. McClenon argues that hominins developed more complex rituals that produced therapeutic altered states of consciousness. He claims, citing Winkelman (1992), that shamanic healing "was present in all regions of the world at some time in their hunting and gathering past." According to McClenon (2002), those who were most suggestible in our evolutionary past would have benefited most from shamanic healing ceremonies, resulting in lower morbidity and mortality rates. Accepting the efficacy of shamanistic healing would have been particularly valuable to birthing mothers, thus directly contributing to reproductive success. He concluded that suggestibility and hypnotizability confer adaptive advantages on those who possess these traits.

McClenon's theory (2002) integrates several critical features of religion and suggests a linkage between proximate neurophysiological mechanisms of religious ritual and evolutionary causation. First, it addresses what most believe to be the earliest form of religion, shamanism. Although Irons and Chagnon (2002) have shown how Yanomamo shamanistic religion and beliefs can be understood as costly signals of commitment, the costly signaling theory of religion does not account for why shamanistic religion should focus on healing. In-deed, the second important contribution of the ritual healing theory is that it accounts for why religion is universally associated with health and healing practices. There is an extensive lit-erature showing a negative relationship be-tween religious practice and belief, and mor-bidity and mortality rates (Hummer, Rogers, Narn, & Ellison, 1999; Levin, 1994; Matthews et al., 1998). The ritual healing theory of reli-gion offers possible insights into this relation-ship.

The Symbolic Species

Deacon (1997) has proposed an alternative evolutionary theory of religion that situates the origins of human religious ritual in our unique social structure. Observing that humans are the only pair-bonded primate with significant pa-ternal investment to live in large, multimale groups, he notes that the inherent difficulty of maintaining pair-bonds when females are in close proximity to other potential mates proba-bly accounts for its rarity across species. Dea-con further argues that the risk of cuckoldry is compounded by the human foraging ecology: Males cannot continually mate during periods of high female fertility, because male and fe-male resource acquisition often occurs sepa-rately. Deacon proposes that symbolic culture arose in response to this dilemma so as to rep-resent a social contract for which prior index-ical communication (e.g., calls, display behav-iors) was insufficient. Rituals allowed a shift from indexical signs that connect abstractions with objects to signs that connect two abstrac-tions. Religious ritual achieves this by inducing new "gestalts" and binding abstractions through emotions. For example, marriage ritu-als link the abstraction of future behaviors re-garding sexual fidelity to the community and are sanctified through emotional associations. Deacon—in line with Durkheim (1912/1995), Rappaport (1999), and Burkert (1996)—main-tains that ritual is the foundation of the social contract and enables the extensive reciprocal relationships that make human life, as we know it, possible. Deacon's hypothesis of hominid pair-bonding as the evolutionary driv-ing force for religious ritual remains highly speculative, although broader research into how ritual can cement commitment in intersexual relationships is likely to have a promising in evolutionary psychology.

Ritual and Emotion

The work of Alcorta and Sosis (2005) focuses on religion as an adaptive complex intimately linked to the neural plasticity of hominids. These authors identify four traits of religion re-current across cultures including (1) belief sys-tems incorporating supernatural agents and counterintuitive concepts; (2) communal ritual, (3) separation of the sacred and the profane; and (4) adolescence as a preferred developmen-tal period for religious transmission. They pro-pose both ontogenetic and neurophysiological proximate mechanisms underlying religious be-liefs and behaviors, arguing that the critical ele-ment differentiating religious from nonhuman ritual is the conditioned association of emotion and abstract symbols. Incorporation of music as a central component of human ritual is criti-cal to this process, and to the evolution of both protosymbolic thought and human religious systems. These authors propose neurophysio-logical mechanisms involved in the emotional valencing of symbolic systems and argue that the brain plasticity of human adolescence con-stitutes an "experience-expectant" develop-mental period for ritual conditioning of sacred symbols. The emotional charging of beliefs re-garding social relationships subsequently drives behavioral choices. Food and sleep de-privation, fear, physical ordeals, and drugs in-crease neurophysiological impacts in terms of memory, reward learning, and emotional charging of stimuli. Alcorta and Sosis maintain that religious ritual, and the emotion-ally valenced symbolic systems it engenders, evolved to extend communication and coordi-nation of social relations across time and space.

Alcorta and Sosis (2005) argue that far from being an evolutionary by-product, religion rep-resents a critical adaptive complex—the emo-tional charging of beliefs in ritual being one key component—that evolved in response to eco-logical challenges faced by early human popu-lations. The still largely untested assumption is that individual fitness benefits resulted from both participation in ritual itself and the coop-erative activities it enabled. The empathy and shared emotional charging experienced in rites of passage supposedly give valence the cogni-tive schemas associated with sacred things, such as counterintuitive supernatural beliefs.

In summary, adaptationist theories of reli-gion, such as costly signaling of social commit-ment, ritual healing to alleviate social stress, and symbolic and emotional bonding theories, help us to understand potentially important mechanisms for generating social cohesion in the evolutionary competition for survival. But despite claims that various functional accounts singly or collectively produce an evolutionary explanation of religion, at best they represent (still largely speculative and untested) compatibility arguments about the social benefits of accommodating the various bits and pieces of beliefs and behaviors that characteristically figure in religion, as well as in many other aspects of social life (hunting and gathering, agricultural and trade associations, political ideology and government, musical ensembles and sports teams, etc.). There is no account of how the characteristically supernatural worlds that manage people's existential dilemmas are actually produced and/or predictably structured.

Some Other Evolutionary Accounts: Sociobiology, Group Selection, and Memetics

Other evolutionary approaches to religion and culture include sociobiology (Harris, 1974; E. O. Wilson, 1978), group selection theory (Sober & Wilson, 1998; Boehm, 1999), and memetics (Dawkins, 1976; Dennett, 1997). Proposals from these alternative approaches are often "mind-blind" to the cognitive constraints on religious beliefs and practices, viewing religion and culture as bundles of functionally integrated, fitness-bearing traits: for example, packages of environment-induced rituals (the material infrastructure underlying ideational superstructure), machine-like patternings of collective norms (worldviews), or partnerships of invasive and authorless ideas (memeplexes).

Proponents of these alternatives do not deny that minds have causally "proximate" roles in generating religious behaviors—as they may in generating economic behaviors—or that cognition may form part of some "ultimate" explanation of religion. Nevertheless, a common claim is that a meaningful causal account of such behaviors requires initial focus on measurable relationships between putative fitness-motivating factors in religious behaviors and ostensible fitness consequences (Dennett, 1995, pp. 358–359; Sober & Wilson, 1998, pp. 182, 193; cf. Lumsden & Wilson, 1981): for example, between individuals needing protein in animal-poor environments and ritual human sacrifice (E. O. Wilson, 1978; Harris, 1974),

between ideas endeavoring to propagate themselves and proselytizing for altruism (Lynch, 1996; Blackmore, 1999), or between groups competing for survival and Judaism's alleged cultural and genetic separatism to create eugenically a master race of economic calculators (MacDonald, 1998; D. S. Wilson, 2002). These arguments are presented through selective use of anecdotal evidence rather than being reliably tested and demonstrated.

Thus, despite sociobiological claims to the canons of "scientific materialism," the causal account that is supposed to produce religious practices (e.g., Aztec cannibalistic sacrifice) from their ostensible material functions (e.g., compensating for lack of large game as sources of protein in Mesoamerica) are wholly mysterious (e.g., How does eating someone generate the idea or formation of a pyramid or priest?). Moreover, similar practices often arise or endure independently, or regardless of material need: For example, the African Azande said they just preferred the taste of human meat (Evans-Pritchard, 1960), and game was abundant for Mesoamerica's Lowland Maya, who also practiced human sacrifice (deLanda, 1566/ 1985; Atran, Lois, & Ucan Ek', 2004).

It is also notoriously difficult to establish measurable criteria by which whole cultures/ societies or worldviews/memeplexes can have fitness consequences.[5] Functional accounts are often synthetic abstractions, for example, a lone anthropologist's normative digest of some culture that in reality has no clear boundaries and no systematically identifiable structural functions. Indeed, most reported "norms" are too semantically open-ended to have specific contents, such as the Ten Commandments: Even members of the same church congregation fail to provide interpretations of the Ten Commandments that other congregation members consistently recognize as being interpretations of the Ten Commandments (Atran, 2001). There are no "replicating" or even definite or definable cultural units for natural selection and vertical (transgenerational) or horizontal (contemporaneous) transmission (e.g., memes can be anything, from a gender marker to a partial tune, cell phone, cooking recipe, political philosophy, etc.). These facts render implausible attempts to explain religions (or cultures with a religious element) as discrete or integrated functional systems (for reviews of specific arguments, see Atran, 2001, 2002, 2005; Atran & Norenzayan, 2004).[6]

In brief, religious sacrifice generally runs counter to calculations of immediate utility, such that future promises are not discounted in favor of present rewards. In some cases, sacrifice is extreme. Although such cases tend to be rare, they are often held by society as religiously ideal: for example, sacrificing one's own life or nearest kin. Researchers sometimes take such cases as prima facie evidence of "true" (nonkin) social altruism (Rappaport, 1999; Kuper, 1996), or group selection, wherein individual fitness decreases so that overall group fitness can increase (relative to the overall fitness of other, competing groups; Sober & Wilson, 1998; D. S. Wilson, 2002). But this may be an illusion.

A telling example is contemporary suicide terrorism (Atran 2003). Consider the "oath to *jihad*" taken by people who join *Harkat al-Ansar*, a Pakistani-based ally of Al-Qaeda, which affirms that by their sacrifice, enlistees help secure the future of their "family" of fictive kin: "Each [martyr] has a special place— among them are brothers, just as there are sons and those even more dear" (cited in Rhode & Chivers, 2002, p. A1). In the case of religiously inspired suicide terrorism, these sentiments are purposely manipulated by organizational leaders, guides, and trainers to the advantage of the manipulating elites rather than to the individual (much as the fast food or soft drink industries manipulate innate desires for naturally scarce commodities such as fatty foods and sugar to ends that reduce personal fitness but benefit the manipulating institution). No "group selection" is involved for the sake of the cultural "superorganism" (D. S. Wilson, 2002; cf. Kroeber, 1923/1963), like a bee for its hive, only cognitive and emotional manipulation of some individuals by others. In evolutionary terms, quest for status and dignity may represent proximate means to the ultimate end of gaining resources, but as with other proximate means (e.g., passionate love), they may become emotionally manipulated ends in themselves (Tooby & Cosmides, 1992).

RELIGION AS EVOLUTIONARY BY-PRODUCT

There are many different and even contrary explanations for why religion exists in terms of beneficial functions served. These include functions of social (bolstering group solidarity, group competition), economic (sustaining public goods, surplus production), political (mass opiate, rebellion's stimulant), intellectual (e.g., explain mysteries, encourage credulity), health and well-being (increase life expectancy, accept death), and emotional (terrorizing, allaying anxiety) utility. Many of these functions have prevailed in one cultural context or another, yet all have also been true of cultural phenomena besides religion.

Such descriptions of religion often help to explain insightfully how and why given religious beliefs and practices help to provide competitive advantages over other sorts of ideologies and behaviors for cultural survival. Still, these accounts provide little explanatory insight into cognitive selection factors responsible for the ease of acquisition of religious concepts by children, or for the facility with which religious practices and beliefs are transmitted across individuals. They have little to say about which beliefs and practices—all things being equal—are most likely to recur in different cultures and most disposed to cultural variation and elaboration. None predicts the following cognitive peculiarities of religion:

- Why do *agent* concepts predominate in religion?
- Why are *supernatural-agent* concepts culturally universal?
- Why are *some* supernatural agent concepts *inherently better* candidates for cultural selection than others?
- Why is it necessary, and how it is possible, to *validate* belief in supernatural agent concepts that are logically and factually inscrutable?
- How is it possible to prevent people from deciding that the existing moral order is simply wrong or *arbitrary*, and from stealthily *defecting* from the social consensus through *deception*, thus fatally compromising social cohesion?

This argument does not imply that religious beliefs and practices cannot perform social functions, or that the successful performance of such functions does not contribute to the survival and spread of religious traditions. Indeed, there is substantial evidence that religious beliefs and practices often alleviate potentially dysfunctional stress and anxiety (Ben-Amos, 1994; Worthington, Kurusu, McCullough, & Sandage, 1996), and maintain social cohesion in the face of real or perceived conflict (Allport, 1956; Pyszczynski, Greenberg, & Solomon,

1999). It does imply that social functions are not phylogenetically responsible for the cognitive structure and cultural recurrence of religion.

The general idea is that religion is not an evolutionary adaptation per se but a recurring cultural by-product of the complex evolutionary landscape that sets cognitive, emotional and material conditions for ordinary human interactions (Kirkpatrick, 1999; Boyer, 2001; Atran, 2002; Pinker, 2004). Religion exploits ordinary cognitive processes to passionately display costly devotion to counterintuitive worlds governed by supernatural agents. The conceptual foundations of religion are intuitively given by task-specific, panhuman cognitive domains, including folkmechanics, folkbiology, and folkpsychology. Core religious beliefs minimally violate ordinary notions about how the world is, with all of its inescapable problems, thus enabling people to imagine minimally impossible supernatural worlds that solve existential problems, including death and deception.

Supernatural agents, such as ghosts, the Abrahamic Deity, and the Devil, are much like human agents psychologically (belief, desire, promise, inference, decision, emotion) and biologically (sight, hearing, feel, taste, smell, coordination) but lack material substance and some associated physical constraints. These imaginary worlds are close enough to factual, everyday worlds to be not only perceptually compelling and conceptually tractable but also surprising enough to capture attention, prime memory, and "contagiously" spread from mind to mind. This gives beliefs in the supernatural and associated behaviors an advantage in the competition for cultural survival.

Supernatural beliefs and behaviors gain coherence and further advantage when they focus on the management of people's existential anxieties. Religion has endured in nearly all cultures and most individuals because humans are faced with problems they cannot solve. As people routinely interact, they naturally tend to exploit various mundane cognitive faculties in special ways to solve an array of inescapable, existential problems that have no apparent worldly solution. Consider death. Because we have cognitive abilities to travel in time and track memory, we are automatically aware of death everywhere. Physical death is something that organisms have evolved to avoid. People seek some kind of a long-term solution to this

looming prospect, but there is none. That's the "tragedy of cognition." Lucretius and Epicurus thought they could solve this through reason. They said, "Look, what does it matter? We weren't alive for infinite generations before we were born. It doesn't bother us. Why should we be worried about the infinite generations that will come after us?" Nobody bought that line of reasoning, because anyone who is alive has got something to lose (cf. Kahneman & Tversky, 1979).

Another existential problem is deception. Recent experiments in developmental psychology show that children are aware of deception at least by age 3 (and perhaps as early as 15 months; K. Onishi & Baillargeon, 2005). If you have rocks and plants and bodies of water before you and say, "Oh, there's no piece of iron there," "That's not wet," or "That's not really a tree," someone can come along and say, "Look, you're nuts; I can touch it; I can show you it's a piece of iron." For commonsense physical events, we have ways of verifying what is real or not. For moral judgments, we have nothing comparable. If someone says, "Oh, he should be a beggar and he should be a king," or "Murder is bad and capital punishment is good," what is there in the world to prove this so? If nothing is sure, how will people ever get on with one another, especially nonkin? How can they build societies and come to trust one another, so they will not defect? One solution involves inventing a minimally counterintuitive world governed by deities, who watch over people to make sure that there will be no defectors or shirkers.

All of this is not to say that *the* function of religion is to promise resolution of all outstanding existential anxieties, any more than *the* function of religion is to neutralize moral relativity and establish social order to give meaning to an otherwise arbitrary existence, to explain the unobservable origins of things, and so on. Religion has no evolutionary functions per se. Rather, existential anxieties and moral sentiments constitute—by virtue of evolution—ineluctable elements of the human condition, and the cognitive invention, cultural selection, and historical survival of religious beliefs are due in part to success in simultaneously accommodating these evolutionarily disparate elements. To be sure, there are evolutionarily adapted behaviors (e.g., costly signaling, ritual engagement) that contribute to the production and endurance of religious beliefs and behaviors, including those that carry likely fitness benefits for individuals (e.g., mental health and psychological well-being, cooperation and friendship) as they bond to form cohesive and competitive social groups. But religion is both psychologically much more and behaviorally much less than the product of naturally selected mechanisms that generate intragroup cooperation for intergroup competition.

THE SUPERNATURAL AGENT: HAIR-TRIGGER FOLKPSYCHOLOGY

Religions invariably center on supernatural *agent* concepts, such as gods, goblins, angels, ancestor spirits, and jinns. Granted, nondeistic "theologies" such as Buddhism and Taoism doctrinally eschew personifying the supernatural or animating nature with supernatural causes. Nevertheless, common folk who espouse these faiths routinely entertain belief in an array of gods and spirits that behave counterintuitively in ways that are inscrutable to factual or logical reasoning.[7] Even Buddhist monks ritually ward off malevolent deities by invoking benevolent ones, and conceive altered states of nature as awesome.[8]

Mundane agent concepts are central players in what cognitive and developmental psychologists refer to as "folkpsychology" and the "theory of mind." A reasonable speculation is that hair-trigger agency evolved so that humans respond "automatically" under conditions of uncertainty to potential threats (and opportunities) by intelligent predators (and protectors). From this evolutionary perspective, agency is a sort of "innate releasing mechanism" (Tinbergen, 1951) whose proper evolutionary domain encompasses animate objects, but which inadvertently extends to moving dots on computer screens, voices in the wind, faces in the clouds, and virtually any complex design or uncertain circumstance of unknown origin (Guthrie, 1993; cf. Hume, 1757/1956).

A number of experiments show that children and adults spontaneously interpret the contingent movements of dots and geometrical forms on a screen as interacting agents with distinct goals and internal motivations for reaching those goals (Heider & Simmel, 1944; Premack & Premack, 1995; P. Bloom & Veres, 1999; Csibra, Gergely, Biró, Koós, & Brockbank, 1999). Such a biologically prepared, or "modu-lar," processing program would provide a rapid and economical reaction to a wide—but not unlimited—range of stimuli that would have been statistically associated with the presence of agents in ancestral environments. Mistakes, or "false positives," would usually carry little cost, whereas a true response could provide the margin of survival (Seligman, 1971; Geary & Huffman, 2002).

Our brains may be trip-wired to spot lurkers (and to seek protectors) when conditions of uncertainty prevail (when startled, at night, in unfamiliar places, during a sudden catastrophe, and in the face of solitude, illness, prospects of death, etc.). Plausibly, the most dangerous and deceptive predator for the genus *Homo* since the Late Pleistocene has been *Homo* itself, which may have engaged in a spiraling behavioral and cognitive arms race of individual and group conflicts (Alexander, 1989). Given the constant menace of enemies within and without, concealment, deception, and the ability to generate and recognize false beliefs in others would favor survival. In potentially dangerous or uncertain circumstances, it would be best to anticipate and fear the worst of all likely possibilities: presence of a deviously intelligent predator.

From an evolutionary perspective, argues Stewart Guthrie (1993), it is better to be safe than sorry regarding the detection of agency under conditions of uncertainty. This cognitive proclivity would favor emergence of malevolent deities in all cultures, just as a countervailing Darwinian propensity to attach to protective caregivers would favor apparition of benevolent deities. Thus, for the Carajá Indians of Central Brazil, intimidating or unsure regions of the local ecology are religiously avoided: "The earth and underworld are inhabited by supernaturals. . . . There are two kinds. Many are amiable and beautiful beings who have friendly relations with humans. . . . Others are ugly and dangerous monsters who cannot be placated. Their woods are avoided and nobody fishes in their pools" (Lipkind, 1940, p. 249). Similar descriptions of supernaturals appear in ethnographic reports throughout the Americas, Africa, Eurasia, and Oceania (Atran, 2002).

In addition, humans *conceptually create* information to mimic and manipulate conditions in ancestral environments that originally produced and triggered evolved cognitive and emotional dispositions (Sperber, 1996). Humans habitually "fool" their own innate releasing programs, such as when people become sexually aroused by makeup (which artificially highlights sexually appealing characteristics), fabricated perfumes, or undulating lines drawn on paper or dots arranged on a computer screen, that is, pornographic pictures.[9] Indeed, much of human culture—for better or worse—can be arguably attributed to focused stimulations and manipulations of our species' innate proclivities. Such manipulations can serve cultural ends far removed from the ancestral adaptive tasks that originally gave rise to those cognitive and emotional faculties triggered, although manipulations for religion often centrally involve the collective engagement of existential desires (e.g., wanting security) and anxieties (e.g., fearing death).

Recently, a number of devout American Catholics eyed the image of Mother Teresa in a cinnamon bun sold at a shop in Tennessee. Latinos in Houston prayed before a vision of the Virgin of Guadalupe, whereas Anglos saw only the dried remnants of melted ice cream on a pavement. Cuban exiles in Miami spotted the Virgin in windows, curtains, and television afterimages as long as there was hope of keeping young Elian Gonzalez from returning to godless Cuba. And on the day of the World Trade Center bombing, newspapers showed photos of smoke billowing from one of the towers that "seems to bring into focus the face of the Evil One, complete with beard and horns and malignant expression, symbolizing to many the hideous nature of the deed that wreaked horror and terror upon an unsuspecting city" ("Bedeviling: Did Satan Rear His Ugly Face?," *Philadelphia Daily News*, September 14, 2001). In all these cases, there is culturally conditioned emotional priming in anticipation of agency. This priming, in turn, amplifies the information value of otherwise doubtful, poor, and fragmentary agency-relevant stimuli. This enables the stimuli (e.g., cloud formations, pastry, ice-cream conformations) to achieve the mimimal threshold for triggering hyperactive facial recognition and body-movement recognition schemas that humans possess.

In summary, supernatural agents are readily conjured up, perhaps because natural selection has trip-wired cognitive schemas for agency detection in the face of uncertainty. Uncertainty is omnipresent; so, too, is a hair-trigger agency–

detection mechanism that readily promotes supernatural interpretation and is susceptible to various forms of cultural manipulation. Cultural manipulation of this modular mechanism and priming facilitate and direct the process. Because the phenomena created readily activate intuitively given modular processes, they are more likely to survive transmission from mind to mind under a wide range of different environments and learning conditions than entities and information that are harder to process (Atran & Sperber, 1991; Boyer, 2000). As a result, they are more likely to become enduring aspects of human cultures, such as belief in the supernatural.

COUNTERINTUITIVE WORLDS

The supernatural occupies counterintuitive worlds that are not merely counterfactual in the sense of physically implausible or nonexistent. Rather, the supernatural literally lacks truth conditions. A counterintuitive notion can take the surface form of a proposition (e.g., "Omnipotence [i.e., God] is insubstantial"), but the structure of human semantics is such that no specific meaning can be given to the expression, and no specific inferences generated from it (or, equivalently, any and all meanings and inferences can be attached to it). The meanings and inferences associated with the subject (omnipotence = physical power) of a counterintuitive expression contradict those associated with the predicate (insubstantial = lack of physical substance), as in the expressions "The bachelor is married" or "The deceased is alive."

Aristotle (1963) was the first to point out in his *Categories* that such counterintuitive expressions cannot even be judged false, because no set of truth conditions could ever be definitely associated with them. He gave the example of "two-footed knowledge." According to Aristotle, "two-footed" could be sensibly (truly or falsely) applied to all animals, but not to any sort of knowledge, because knowledge falls under the ontological category of nonsubstantial things, whereas being two-footed falls under the altogether distinct ontological category of substantial things. Trying to put together things from different ontological categories produces a "category mistake."[10] Cognitive and developmental psychologists experimentally have shown that children across cultures do not violate such categorical constraints on language learning when attempting to learn the meaning of words (Keil, 1979; Walker, 1992).

All the world's cultures have attention-arresting religious myths because they are counterintuitive in this technical sense. Still, people in all cultures also recognize that such beliefs are counterintuitive, whether or not they are religious believers (Atran, 1996). In our society, for example, Catholics and non-Catholics alike are unquestionably aware of the difference between Christ's body and ordinary wafers, or between Christ's blood and ordinary wine. Likewise, the Native American Cowlitz are well aware of the difference between the deity Coyote and everyday coyotes, or between Old Man Wild Cherry Bark and ordinary wild cherry bark (Jacobs, 1934, pp. 126–133).

Religious beliefs are counterintuitive because they violate what studies in cognitive anthropology and developmental psychology indicate are universal expectations about the world's everyday structure, including such basic categories of "intuitive ontology" (i.e., the ordinary ontology of the everyday world that is built into the language learner's semantic system) as person, animal, plant, and substance (Atran, 1989). They are generally inconsistent with fact-based knowledge, though not randomly so. Beliefs about invisible creatures who transform themselves at will or perceive events that are distant in time or space flatly contradict factual assumptions about physical, biological, and psychological phenomena (Atran & Sperber, 1991). But apart from these few extraordinary and surprising features, such beings remain unsurprising and ordinary in terms of their beliefs, desires, reasonings, and behaviors. Consequently, these remarkable but tractable beliefs more likely will be retained and transmitted in a population than random departures from common sense, thus becoming part of the group's culture. Insofar as category violations shake basic notions of ontology they are attention-arresting, hence memorable; but only if the resultant impossible worlds remain bridged to the everyday world can information about them be readily be stored, evoked, and transmitted.

As a result, religious concepts need little in the way of overt cultural representation or instruction to be learned and transmitted. A few fragmentary narrative descriptions or episodes suffice to mobilize an enormously rich network of implicit background beliefs (Boyer, 1994, 2001). For instance, if God is explicitly described as being jealous and able to move mountains, He is therefore implicitly known to have other emotions, such as anger and joy, and other powers, such as the ability to see and touch mountains, or to lift and see most anything smaller than a mountain, such as a person, pot, pig, or pea.

Invocation of supernatural agents implicates two cognitive aspects of religious belief: (1) activation of naturally selected conceptual modules, and (2) failed assignment to universal categories of ordinary ontology. Conceptual modules are activated by stimuli that fall into a few intuitive knowledge domains, including folkmechanics (inert object boundaries and movements), folkbiology (species configurations and relationships), and folkpsychology (interactive and goal-directed behavior). Ordinary ontological categories are generated by further, more specific activation of conceptual modules. Among the universal categories of ordinary ontology are *person, animal, plant, substance*.[11]

To give an example, sudden movement of an object stirred by the wind may trigger the agent-detection system that operates over the domain of folkpsychology, and a ghost invoked to interpret this possibly purposeful event. In normal circumstances, a sudden movement of wind might activate cognitive processing for agents, but would soon deactivate upon further analysis ("it's only the wind"). But in the case of (bodiless) supernatural agents, the object-boundary detectors (edge, contour, etc.) that operate over the domain of folkmechanics, and which are required to identify the agent, cannot be activated. The same cognitive conditions operate when supernatural beings and events, like ghosts or gods, are evoked in religious ceremonies, whether or not there is any actual triggering event (e.g., a sudden movement of unknown origin or other uncertain happening). In such cases, assignment to the person or animal category cannot be completed, because ghosts and gods have counterintuitive properties (e.g., movements and emotions without physical bodies). This results in a potentially endless, open-textured evocation of possible meanings and inferences to interpret the event; however, the process can be provisionally stopped, and the semantic content somewhat specified, in a given context (e.g., a Sunday sermon that fixes interpretation of a Biblical passage on some particular community event in the preceding week).

Ordinary ontological categories always involve more specific processing over the folkmechanics domain (nonliving objects and events).

- Only substance involves further processing that is exclusive to folkmechanics.
- Plant involves additional processing over the folkbiological domain (every organism is assigned to one and only one folk species).
- Animal involves supplemental processing over the domains of folkbiology (every animal is assigned uniquely to a folk species) and folkpsychology (animal behavior is scrutinized as indicating predator or prey, and possibly friend or foe).
- Person involves more specific processing over the folkpsychological domain (human behavior is scrutinized as indicating friend or foe, and possibly predator or prey), and the folkbiological domain (essentialized group assignments, e.g., race and ethnicity).

The relationship between conceptual modules and ontological categories is represented as a matrix in Table 17.1. Changing the intuitive relationship expressed in any cell generates what Pascal Boyer (2000) calls a "minimal counterintuition." For example, switching the cell (− folkpsychology, substance) to (+ folkpsychology, substance) yields a thinking talisman, whereas switching (+ folkpsychology, person) to (− folkpsychology, person) yields an unthinking zombie (cf. J. Barrett, 2000).

These are general, but not exclusive, conditions on supernatural beings and events. Inter-

vening perceptual, contextual or psycho-thematic factors, however, can change the odds. Thus, certain natural substances— mountains, seas, clouds, sun, moon, planets— are associated with perceptions of great size or distance, and with conceptions of grandeur and continuous or recurring duration. They are, as Freud surmised, psychologically privileged objects for focusing the thoughts and emotions evoked by existential anxieties such as death and eternity. Violation of fundamental social norms also readily lends itself to religious interpretation (e.g., ritual incest, fratricide, status reversal).

Finally, supernatural agent concepts tend to be emotionally powerful because they trigger evolutionary survival templates. This also makes them attention arresting and memorable. For example, an all-knowing bloodthirsty deity is a better candidate for cultural survival than a do-nothing deity, however omniscient. In the next section, I address some of the cognitive processes that contribute to the cultural survival of supernatural beliefs.

CULTURAL SURVIVAL: MEMORY EXPERIMENTS WITH COUNTERINTUITIVE BELIEFS

Many factors are important in determining the extent to which ideas achieve a cultural level of distribution. Some are ecological, including the rate of prior exposure to an idea in a population, physical and social facilitators and barriers to communication and imitation, and institutional structures that reinforce or suppress an idea. One complex of psychological factors concerns the apparent sensitivity to religious ideas in young children. Research with American and European children indicates that

TABLE 17.1. Mundane Relations between Naturally Selected Conceptual Domains and Universal Categories of Ordinary Ontology.

Ontological categories	Conceptual domains and associated properties				
	Folkmechanics	Folkbiology		Folkpsychology	
				Psychophysical (e.g., hunger, thirst, etc.)	Epistemic (e.g., believe, know, etc.)
	Inert	Vegetative	Animate		
Person	+	+	+	+	+
Animal	+	+	+	+	−
Plant	+	+	−	−	−
Substance	+	−	−	−	−

Note. Changing the relation in any one cell (+ to −, or − to +) yields a minimal, supernatural counterintuition.

through grade 1 (age 6–7), most children think that God is present everywhere, can hear prayers and see everything, and is near when they feel troubled or happy. This lends credence to the Jesuit mantra: "Give me a child till the age of 7 and I'll give you a Believer for life." Sentiments about God's pervasiveness in life seem to degrade with age unless institutionally supported, and God's presence and guidance become associated more with danger and difficulties (Thun, 1963; Goldman, 1964; Tamminen, 1994).

Of all cognitive factors, however, mnemonic power may be the single most important one at any age (Sperber, 1996). In oral traditions that have characterized most human cultures throughout history, an idea that is not memorable cannot be transmitted and cannot achieve cultural success (Rubin, 1995). Moreover, even if two ideas pass a minimal test of memorability, a *more* memorable idea has a transmission advantage over a less memorable one (all else being equal). This advantage, even if small at the start, accumulates from generation to generation of transmission, leading to massive differences in cultural success at the end.

One of the earliest accounts of memorability and the transmission of counterintuitive cultural narratives was Bartlett's (1932) classic study of "The War of the Ghosts." Bartlett examined the ways British university students remembered, then transmitted a Native American folktale. Over successive retellings of the story, some culturally unfamiliar items or events were dropped. Perhaps Bartlett's most striking finding was that the very notion of the ghosts—so central to the story—was gradually eliminated from the retellings, suggesting that counterintuitive elements are at a cognitive disadvantage. Other unfamiliar items were distorted, being replaced by more familiar items (e.g., a canoe replaced by a rowboat).

In recent years, though, growing theoretical and empirical work suggest that minimally counterintuitive concepts are cognitively optimal; that is, they enjoy a cognitive advantage in memory and transmission in communication. In one series of experiments, J. Barrett and Nyhoff (2001) asked participants to remember and to retell Native American folktales containing both natural and nonnatural events or objects. Content analysis showed that participants remembered 92% of minimally counterintuitive items but only 71% of intuitive items.[12] These results, contrary to the findings in Bartlett's classic experiments, seem to indicate that minimally counterintuitive beliefs are better recalled and transmitted than intuitive ones.

Importantly, the effect of counterintuitiveness on recall is not linear. Too many ontological violations render a concept too counterintuitive to be comprehensible and memorable. Boyer and Ramble (2001) demonstrated that concepts with too many violations were recalled less well than those that were minimally counterintuitive. These results could be observed immediately after exposure, as well as after a 3-month delay, in cultural samples as diverse as the Midwestern United States, France, Gabon, and Nepal. Consistent with the idea that this memory advantage is related to cultural success, a review of anthropological literature indicates that religious concepts with too many ontological violations are rather rare (Boyer, 1994).

Although suggestive, these studies leave several issues unresolved. For one: why do minimally counterintuitive concepts not occupy most of the narrative structure of religions, folktales, and myths? Even casual perusal of culturally successful materials, such as the Bible, Hindu *Veda*, or Maya *Popul Vuh*, suggests that counterintuitive concepts and occurrences are a minority. The Bible is a succession of mundane events—walking, eating, sleeping, dreaming, copulating, dying, marrying, fighting, and suffering storms and drought—interspersed with a few counterintuitive occurrences, such as miracles and appearances of supernatural agents (e.g., God, angels, and ghosts). One possible explanation for this is that counterintuitive ideas are transmitted in narrative structures. To the extent that narratives with too many counterintuitive elements are at a cognitive disadvantage, cognitive selection at the narrative level would favor minimally counterintuitive narrative structures.

In one study that tested this hypothesis, Norenzayan, Atran, Faulkner, and Schaller (2006) analyzed folktales possessing many of the counterintuitive aspects of religious stories. They examined (1) the cognitive structure of Grimm Brothers' folktales, and (2) the relative cultural success of each tale. The hypothesized nonlinear relation between the frequency of counterintuitive elements and cultural success was confirmed (Figure 17.1). Minimally counterintuitive folktales (containing two to three supernatural events or objects) consti-

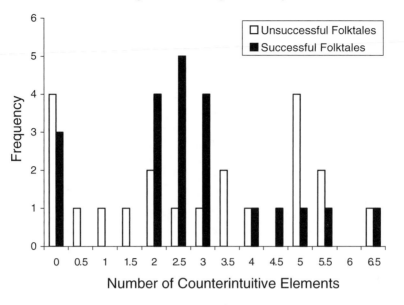

FIGURE 17.1. Frequency distribution of counterintuitive elements contained in samples of culturally successful and unsuccessful folktales.

tuted 76.5% of culturally successful sample, whereas stories with fewer counterintuitive elements (scores < 2), and with excessive numbers of counterintuitive elements (scores > 3) constituted only 30% and 33% of the culturally successful sample, respectively. Overall, minimal counterintuitiveness predicted cultural success of folktales accurately 75% of the time. Perceived memorability and ease of transmission, but not other features of the folktale (e.g., whether the tale contains a moral lesson, interest value to children), partly mediated the relationship between minimal counterintuitiveness and cultural success. Whereas results indicate that cultural success is a nonlinear (inverted U-shape) function of the number of counterintuitive elements, success was not predicted by unusual narrative elements that are otherwise intuitive.

If memorability is the critical variable that mediates the effect of minimal counterintuitiveness on cultural success, than minimally counterintuitive knowledge structures should enjoy superior memory in the long run. To test this hypothesis more directly in a related study, Norenzayan, Atran, and Hansen (2005; reported in Atran & Norenzayan, 2004) examined the short- and long-term memorability of knowledge structures that systematically varied in the proportion of coun-

terintuitive elements. Their methodology differed from prior studies by employing "basic level" concepts (e.g., thirsty door) that are cognitively privileged (Rosch, Mervis, Grey, Johnson, & Boyes-Braem, 1976), and most commonly found in supernatural narratives. Participants were not cued to expect unusual events or to transmit interesting stories to others. Instead, Rosche et al. used a standard memory paradigm to measure recall.

The study examined the memorability of intuitive (INT) and minimally counterintuitive (MCI) beliefs and belief sets over a period of a week. Two-word statements that represented INT and MCI items were generated. Each statement consisted of a concept and one property that modified it. INT statements were created with use of a property appropriate to the ontological category (e.g., closing door). MCI statements were created with the concept modified by a property transferred from *another* ontological category (e.g., thirsty door). This procedure explicitly operationalizes minimal counterintuitiveness as the transfer of a property associated with the core conceptual domains of folkphysics, folkbiology, folkpsychology, from an appropriate ontological category of person, animal, plant, substance, to an inappropriate one (Atran & Norenzayan, 2004). For example, a "thirsty door" transfers a folkbiological property (thirst) from its proper category (animal) to an improper category (inert object/substance).

U.S. students rated these beliefs on degree of supernaturalness using a 6-point Likert scale, with MCI beliefs significantly more likely than INT beliefs to be associated with supernaturalness. Although no differences were found in immediate recall, after 1-week delay minimally counterintuitive knowledge structures led to superior recall relative to all intuitive or maximally counterintuitive structures,[13] replicating the curvilinear function found in the folktale analysis. With Yukatek Maya speakers, minimally counterintuitive beliefs were again more resilient than intuitive ones. A follow-up study revealed no reliable differences between the Yukatek recall pattern after 1 week and after 3 months (Atran & Norenzayan, 2004), indicating a cultural stabilization of the recall pattern.

In brief, minimally counterintuitive beliefs, as long as they come in small proportions, help people remember and presumably transmit the intuitive statements. A small proportion of minimally counterintuitive beliefs give the story a mnemonic advantage over stories with no counterintuitive beliefs, or with far too many counterintuitive beliefs. This dual aspect of supernatural beliefs and belief sets— commonsensical and counterintuitive—renders them intuitively compelling yet fantastic, eminently recognizable but surprising. Such beliefs grab attention, activate intuition, and mobilize inference in ways that greatly facilitate their mnemonic retention, social transmission, cultural selection, and historical survival. When emotional valence is added, these relevant mysteries (Sperber, 1996) become irresistibly catchy (Heath & Sternberg, 2001).

MODES OF RELIGIOSITY: AN ANTHROPOLOGICAL APPROACH TO RELIGIOUS TRANSMISSION

Religious traditions also involve the transmission of more complex and cross-culturally diverse concepts and practices, including ritual form (McCauley & Lawson, 2002), that present a further challenge to adherents' cognitive systems that go beyond mnemonic processing of intuitive and counterintuitive ideas. Why do religious beliefs become complex and challenging? And why is it so important to adherents that their own particular versions of "the truth" should transcend all others?

According to Harvey Whitehouse (2000, 2004), two factors greatly increase the chances that knowledge will be recalled. One is repetition. Repeating information increases the likelihood that it will be remembered. The other is arousal. Shocking or upsetting events are more likely to be recalled later than dull and unremarkable ones. But these two routes to remembering give rise to rather different kinds of recall. According to Whitehouse, religious traditions exploit these two kinds of memories in ways that have considerable consequences for the way religious concepts are formed and transmitted, and for the way religious traditions, as social institutions, are organized and spread.

In the doctrinal mode (Figure 17.2), religious practices tend to be frequently repeated and routine, such as daily prayer, weekly services, or annual celebrations. Frequent repetition supposedly builds an accurate memory routine for the ritual's abstract, schematic organization, or "script," such as the formulaic order of events in a Moslem prayer, Catholic mass or Jewish Passover. Participants customarily perform these scripted actions almost automatically but retain little long-term memory of the changing details and contents of the rites in question, such as who was actually present or what exactly was preached on a given occasion. Particular details and contents of scripted actions can vary substantially from one ritual performance to another. Yet the schematic sequence of events repeats with fairly high fidelity over time.

By tuning out the scripted routine, and forgetting changing details, participants are able to turn their attention to the "semantic" structure and "logical" implications of religious doctrine presented in exegesis, argumentation, and sermonizing. The repetitive routine is usually directed by a rigid social hierarchy. Routinization minimizes the risks of unintended innovations; hierarchization enhances monitoring, policing, and sanctioning of nonconformity. This normalizing design encourages indoctrination and preservation of orthodoxy. It also favors identification with masses of anonymous worshippers, which often promotes univeralist and humanist notions of common fellowship.

In contrast to the "logocentric iconophobia" of the doctrinal mode (Whitehouse, 2000, p. 156), the imagistic mode (Figure 17.3) relies mainly on unverbalized, emotionally arousing

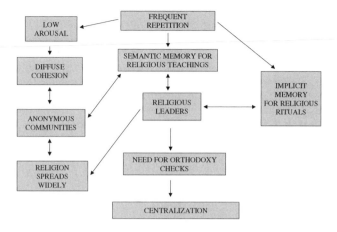

1. Frequent repetition activates semantic memory for religious teachings.
2. Semantic memory for religious teachings and the presence of religious leaders are mutually reinforcing features.
3. The presence of religious leaders implies a need for orthodoxy checks.
4. Frequent repetition leads to implicit memory for religious rituals.
5. Implicit memory for religious rituals enhances the survival potential of authoritative teachings stored in semantic memory.
6. The need for orthodoxy checks encourages religious centralization.
7. Semantic memory for religious teachings leads to anonymous religious communities.
8. The presence of religious leaders is conducive to the religion spreading widely.

FIGURE 17.2. Schematic presentation of the doctrinal mode of religious transmission.

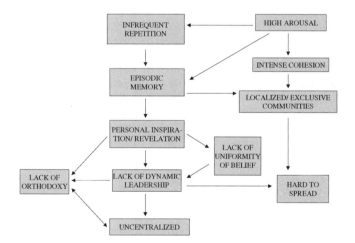

1. Infrequent repetition and high arousal activate episodic memory.
2. Activation of episodic memory triggers spontaneous exegetical reflection.
3. SER leads to a diversity of religious representations.
4. SER and representational diversity inhibit dynamic leadership.
5. Lack of dynamic leadership, lack of centralization, and lack of orthodoxy are mutually reinforcing.
6. High arousal fosters intense cohesion.
7. Intense cohesion and episodic memory foster localized, exclusive communites.
8. Localized/exclusive communities and lack of dynamic leadership inhibit spread/ dissemination.

FIGURE 17.3. Schematic presentation of the imagistic mode of religious transmission.

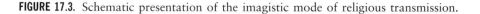

experiences and "episodic memory" of a spatiotemporally localized and autobiographical sort. The most sacred and revelatory rites in the imagistic mode are highly arousing, once-in-a-lifetime episodes.[14] These are often physically excruciating and sensorially invasive: hideous masks and grotesquely painted dancers, horrifying cries and hoots, piercing whistles and pounding drums, overexposure to direct sunlight and heat or darkness and cold, extended sleep and food deprivation, anonymous pummeling and deep body laceration, and so forth. Possible examples of what Whitehouse (2000) calls "rites of terror" include initiations among Native American Cheyenne and Arapaho (Lowie, 1924), Navajo (Kluckholn & Leighton, 1946/1974), Walbiri (Meggitt, 1965) and other aboriginals of the Central Australian Desert (Spencer & Gillen, 1904), Mountain Ok Baktaman (Barth, 1975) and Ilahita Arapesh of Highland Papua New Guinea (Tuzin, 1982), and Ituri Forest Pygmies in the African Congo (Turnbull, 1962). Although Whitehouse avoids equating the doctrinal, or "digital," mode with large-scale Western religions or literacy, and the imagistic, or "analogic," mode with small-scale tribal religions and cults, he argues that imagistic rituals are historically primary, dating at least to Upper Paleolithic cave art (see M. Turner, 1996).[15]

METAREPRESENTING COUNTERINTUITIVE WORLDS: A THEORY-OF-MIND EXPERIMENT

If counterintuitive beliefs arise by violating innately given expectations about how the world is built, how can we possibly bypass our own hardwiring to form counterintuitive religious beliefs? The answer is that we do not entirely bypass commonsense understanding, but we conceptually parasitize it to transcend it. This occurs through the cognitive process of metarepresentation.

Humans have a metarepresentational ability to form representations of representations. This allows people to understand a drawing or picture of someone or something as a drawing or picture, and not as the real thing. It lets us imagine fiction and gives us an ability to think about being in different situations and to decide which options are best for the purposes at hand, *without our having to actually live through (or die in) the situations we imagine*. It affords us the capacity to *model the world in different ways and to conscientiously change the world by entertaining new models* that we invent, evaluate, and implement. It enables us to become aware of our experienced past and imagined future as past or future events distinct from the present we represent to ourselves, and so permits us to reflect on our own existence. It allows people to comprehend and interact with one another's minds.

Metarepresentation also lets people retain half-understood ideas; children come to terms with the world in similar ways when they hear a new word. By embedding half-baked (quasi-propositional) ideas in other factual and commonsense beliefs, these ideas can simmer through personal and cultural belief systems and change them (Sperber, 1985; Atran & Sperber, 1991). A half-understood word or idea is initially retained metarepresentationally, as standing in for other ideas we already have in mind. Supernatural ideas always remain metarepresentational.

After Dennett (1978), most researchers in folkpsychology, or "theory of mind," maintain that attribution of mental states, such as belief and desire, to other persons requires metarepresentational reasoning about false beliefs. Not before the child can understand that other people's beliefs are *only* representations—and not just recordings of the way things are—can he or she entertain and assess other people's representations as veridical or fictional, truly informative or deceptive, exact or exaggerated, or worth changing one's own mind for or ignoring. Only then can the child appreciate that God thinks differently from most people, in that only God's beliefs are always true.

In one of the few studies to replicate findings on "theory of mind" in a small-scale society (cf. Avis & Harris, 1991), Knight, Sousa, Barrett, and Atran (2004) showed 48 Yukatek-speaking children (26 boys, 22 girls) a tortilla container and told them, "Usually tortillas are inside this box, but I ate them and put these shorts inside." They asked each child in random order what a person, God, the sun (*k'in*), principal forest spirits (*yumil k'ax'ob'*, "Masters of the Forest"), and other minor spirits (*chiichi'*) would think was in the box. As with American children (L. Barrett et al., 2001), the youngest Yukatek (age 4 years) overwhelmingly attribute true beliefs to both God and people in equal measure. After age 5, the children attribute mostly false beliefs to people but continue to attribute mostly true beliefs to

God. Thus, 33% of the 4-year-olds said that people would think tortillas were in the container, versus 77% of 7-year-olds. In contrast, no significant correlation was detected between answers for God and age.

Collapsing over ages, Yukatek children attribute true beliefs according to a hierarchy of human and divine minds, one in which humans and minor spirits are seen as easier to deceive. Mental states of humans were perceived as different from those of God, and those of Masters of the Forest and the Sun god. God is seen as all-knowing, and local religious entities fall somewhere in the middle (Figure 17.4). Lowland Maya believe God and forest spirits to be powerful, knowledgeable agents that punish people who overexploit forest species. For adults, such beliefs have measurable behavioral consequences for biodiversity, forest sustainability, and so forth (Atran et al., 2002). From an early age, people may reliably attribute to supernaturals cognitive properties that are *different* from those of their parents and other people.

In summary, metarepresentational abilities, which are intimately bound to fully developed cognitions of agency and intention, also allow people to entertain, recognize, and evaluate the differences between true and false beliefs. Given the ever-present menace of enemies within and without, concealment, deception, and the ability to generate false beliefs and recognize them in others would favor survival. But because representations of agency and intention include representations of false belief and deception, human society is forever under threat of moral defection.

If some better ideology is likely to be available somewhere down the line, then, reasoning by backward induction, there is no more justified reason to accept the current ideology than convenience. As it happens, the very same metacognitive aptitude that initiates this problem also provides a resolution through metarepresentation of minimally counterintuitive worlds. Invoking supernatural agents who may have true beliefs that people ordinarily lack creates the arational conditions for people to steadfastly commit to one another in a moral order that goes beyond apparent reason and self-conscious interest. In the limiting case, an omniscient and omnipotent agent (e.g., the supreme deity of the Abrahamic religions) can ultimately detect and punish cheaters, defectors,

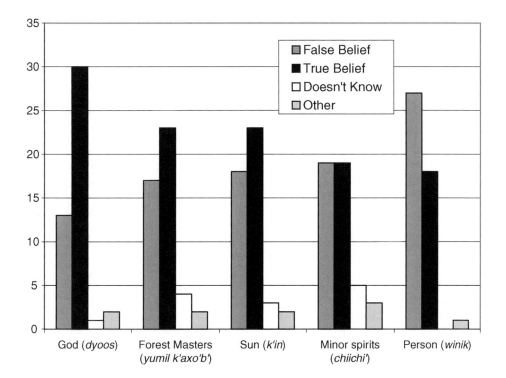

FIGURE 17.4. What's in the container?: Yukatek Maya children's responses to false belief task.

and free riders, no matter how devious (Frank, 1988; Dennett, 1997).

In the competition for moral allegiance, secular ideologies are at a disadvantage. For if people learn that all apparent commitment is self-interested convenience or worse, manipulation for the self-interest of others, then their commitment is debased and withers. Especially in times of vulnerability and stress, social deception and defection in the pursuit of self-preservation are therefore more likely to occur, as Ibn Khaldûn noted long ago (1318/1958, Vol. 2, part III, p. 41). Religion passionately rouses hearts and minds to break out of this viciously rational cycle of self-interest, and to adopt group interests that may benefit individuals in the long run. Commitment to the supernatural underpins the "organic solidarity" (Durkheim, 1912/1995) that makes social life more than simply a contract among calculating individuals. Commitment to the supernatural is further sustained by the relieving of pervasive existential anxieties, to which I now turn.

EXISTENTIAL ANXIETY: AN EXPERIMENT ON WHAT MOTIVATES RELIGIOUS BELIEF

If supernatural agents are cognitively salient and possess hidden knowledge and powers, then they can be invoked to ease existential anxieties, such as death and deception, that forever threaten human life everywhere. To test this, Norenzayan, Hansen, and Atran (reported in Atran & Norenzayan, 2004; Norenzayan & Hansen, 2006) built on a study by Cahill, Prins, Weber, and McGaugh (1994) dealing with the effects of adrenaline (adrenergic activation) on memory.

The hypothesis was that existential anxieties (particularly death) deeply affect not only how people remember events but also their propensity to interpret events in terms of supernatural agency. Each of three groups of college students was primed with one of three different stories (Table 17.2): Cahill et al.'s (1994) uneventful story (neutral prime), their stressful story (death prime), and another uneventful story whose event-structure matched the other two stories but included a prayer scene (religious prime). Afterwards, each group of subjects read a *New York Times* article (October 2, 2001) whose lead-in ran: "Researchers at Columbia University, expressing surprise at their own findings, are reporting that women at an

in vitro fertilization clinic in Korea had a higher pregnancy rate when, unknown to the patients, total strangers were asked to pray for their success." The article was provided under the guise of being a story about "media portrayals of scientific studies." Finally, students rated strength of their belief in God and the power of supernatural intervention (prayer) on a 9-point scale.

Results show that strength of belief in God's existence and in the efficacy of supernatural intervention (Figure 17.5) are reliably stronger after exposure to the death prime than to either to the neutral or religious prime (no significant differences between either uneventful story). This effect held even after controlling for religious background and prior degree of religious identification. In a cross-cultural follow-up, 75 Yukatek-speaking Maya villagers were tested with stories matched for event structure but modified to fit Maya cultural circumstances. They were also asked to recall the priming events. We (Atran & Norenzayan, 2004) found no differences among primes for belief in the existence of God and spirits (near the ceiling in this very religious society). However, subjects' belief in efficacy of prayer for invoking the deities was significantly greater with the death prime than with religious or neutral primes. Awareness of death more strongly motivates religiosity than mere exposure to emotionally nonstressful religious scenes, such as praying. This supports the claim that emotionally eruptive existential anxieties motivate supernatural beliefs.[16]

According to terror management theory (TMT), cultural worldview is a principal buffer against the terror of death. TMT experiments show that thoughts of death function to get people to reinforce their cultural (including religious) worldview and derogate alien worldviews (Greenberg et al., 1990; Pyszczynski et al., 1999). In this view, then, awareness of death should enhance belief in a worldview-consistent deity but diminish belief in a worldview-threatening deity. An alternative view is that the need for belief in supernatural agency overrides worldview defense needs for death-aware subjects.

To test these competing views, Norenzayan, Hansen, and Atran (reported in Atran & Norenzayan, 2004) told 73 American undergraduates that the prayer groups described in the first experiment described earlier were Buddhists in Taiwan, Korea, and Japan. Supernatu-

TABLE 17.2. Three Stories with Matching Events Used to Prime Feelings of Religiosity: Neutral (Uneventful), Death (Stressful), Religious (Prayer Scene)

Neutral	Death	Religious
1 A mother and her son are leaving home in the morning.	A mother and her son are leaving home in the morning.	A mother and her son are leaving home in the morning.
2 She is taking him to visit his father's workplace.	She is taking him to visit his father's workplace.	She is taking him to visit his father's workplace.
3 The father is a laboratory technician at Victory Memorial Hospital.	The father is a laboratory technician at Victory Memorial Hospital.	The father is a laboratory technician at Victory Memorial Hospital.
4 They check before crossing a busy road.	They check before crossing a busy road.	They check before crossing a busy road.
5 While walking along, the boy sees some wrecked cars in a junkyard, which he finds interesting.	While crossing the road, the boy is caught in a terrible accident, which critically injures him.	While walking along, the boy sees a well-dressed man stop by a homeless woman, falling on his knees before her, weeping.
6 At the hospital, the staff are preparing for a practice disaster drill, which the boy will watch.	At the hospital, the staff prepare the emergency room, to which the boy is rushed.	At the hospital, the boy's father shows him around his lab. The boy listens politely, but his thoughts are elsewhere.
7 An image from a brain scan machine used in the drill attracts the boy's interest.	An image from a brain scan machine used in a trauma situation shows severe bleeding in the boy's brain.	An image from a brain scan that he sees reminds him of something in the homeless woman's face.
8 All morning long, a surgical team practices the disaster drill procedures.	All morning long, a surgical team struggles to save the boy's life.	On his way around the hospital, the boy glances into the hospital's chapel, where he sees the well-dressed man sitting alone.
9 Makeup artists are able to create realistic-looking injuries on actors for the drill.	Specialized surgeons are able to reattach the boy's severed feet, but can not stop his internal hemorrhaging.	With elbows on his knees, and his head in his hands, the man moves his lips silently. The boy wants to sit beside him, but his father leads him away.
10 After the drill, while the father watches the boy, the mother leaves to phone her other child's preschool.	After the surgery, while the father stays by the dead boy, the mother leaves to phone her other child's preschool.	After a brief tour of the hospital, while the father watches the boy, the mother leaves to phone her other child's preschool.
11 Running a little late, she phones the preschool to tell them she will soon pick up her child.	Barely able to talk, she phones the preschool to tell them she will soon pick up her child.	Running a little late, she phones the preschool to tell them she will soon pick up her child.
12 Heading to pick up her child, she hails a taxi at the number nine bus stop.	Heading to pick up her child, she hails a taxi at the number nine bus stop.	Heading to pick up her child, she hails a taxi at the number nine bus stop.

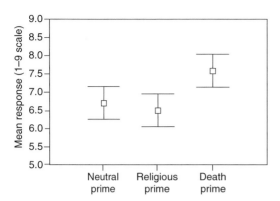

FIGURE 17.5. Strength of belief in supernatural power after priming (neutral, religious, or death), then reading a newspaper article about effects of prayer on pregnancy. Vertical bars represent margin of error at $p = .05$.

ral belief was measured either shortly after the primes or after a significant delay between the primes and the belief measures. When the primes were recently activated, as expected, there was a stronger belief in the power of Buddhist prayer in the death prime than in the control prime. Remarkably, death-primed subjects who previously self-identified as strong believers in Christianity were *more* likely to believe in the power of Buddhist prayer. In the neutral (control) condition, there was no correlation between Christian identification and belief in Buddhist prayer. Given a choice between supernatural belief versus rejecting an alien worldview (Buddhism), Christians chose the former. This finding is difficult to explain simply in terms of bolstering a cultural (in this case, Christian-centered) worldview.[17]

There was no evidence for differences in recall of priming events after subjects rated their strength of belief in God and the efficacy of supernatural intervention. With this in mind, note that uncontrollable arousal mediated by adrenergic activation (e.g., subjects chronically exposed to death scenes) can lead to posttraumatic stress disorder if there is no lessening of terror and arousal within hours; however, adrenergic blockers (e.g., propranolol, guanfacine, and possibly antidepressants) can interrupt neuronal imprinting for long-term symptoms, as can cognitive-behavioral therapy (work by Charles Marmar, discussed in McReady, 2002, p. 9). A plausible hypothesis is that heightened expression of religiosity fol-

lowing exposure to death scenes that provoke existential anxieties may also serve this blocking function. The further claim—that not only do existential anxieties spur supernatural belief but also these beliefs are in turn affectively validated by assuaging the very emotions that motivate belief in the supernatural—has yet to be tested.

SACRED VALUES IN DECISION MAKING AND THE LIMITS OF RATIONAL CHOICE

Religious behavior often seems to be motivated by *sacred values* (SVs). A sacred value incorporates moral and ethical beliefs and "independently of its prospect of success." Max Weber (1978, Vol. 1, p. 24) distinguishes the non-instrumental "value rationality" of religions and transcendent political ideologies from the "instrumental rationality" of *realpolitik* and the marketplace. Instrumental rationality involves strict cost–benefit calculations regarding goals, and entails abandoning or adjusting goals if costs for realizing them are too high. For Immanuel Kant (1788/1997), virtuous religious behavior is its own reward, and attempts to base it on utility nullifies its moral worth.

High-cost personal sacrifices to (nonkin) others in society seem to be typically motivated by, and framed in terms of, noninstrumental values. This includes Jihadist conceptions of martyrdom, which also involve a moral commitment to kill infidels for the sake of God. One review indicated that "only a minority of human violence can be understood as rational, instrumental behavior aimed at securing or protecting material rewards" (Baumeister, Smart, & Boden, 1996, p. 5). Historically, religiously motivated violence tends to underpin the most intractable and enduring conflicts within and between cultures (Allport, 1956) and civilizations (Huntington, 1997).

Political scientists and economists acknowledge the role of religious values in coordinating groups for economic, social, and political activities, and in providing people with immunity that goes with action in large numbers (Schelling, 1963). From a rational-choice perspective, such values operate instrumentally to form convergent trust among masses of people with disparate interests and preferences (Hardin, 1995), thus reducing "transaction costs" that would otherwise be needed to mobilize them (Fukuyama, 1995). Others (Horowitz, 1984; Varshney, 2003) grant the instrumental value of "ethnicity"—and values rooted in other ascriptive (birth-based) identities such as religion and language—but ask: "Why would ethnicity be the basis for mobilization at all?" And why does the mobilization of these values energize the most enduring and intractable conflicts between groups (Cohen, 2002)? This suggests that noninstrumental values possess inherent qualities that instrumental values may lack (passion, obligation), and that these two sorts of values can interact in intricate ways. (Of course, one can always recast noninstrumental values in instrumental terms, just as one can always frame any perceptual or conceptual relationship in terms of "similarity"; but the issue is whether doing so helps or hinders explanatory power to predict further judgments and decisions.)

Psychologists have recently developed controlled ways of testing ideas about allied notions of "protected values" and "taboo trade-offs" (Fiske & Tetlock, 1997). Tetlock (2000) described a protected value as "any value that a moral community implicitly or explicitly treats as possessing infinite or transcendental significance that precludes comparisons, trade-offs . . . with bounded or secular values." Despite more than a decade of research on protected values and decision making, knowledge of their influence is quite limited. What is clear is that protected values have a privileged link to moral outrage and other emotions (Baron & Spranca, 1997), especially when a person holding a sacred value is offered a secular value or trade-off, such as selling one's child or selling futures betting on acts of terrorism (Medin, Schwartz, Blok, & Birnbaum, 1999, Tetlock, 2003).

One claim is that SVs are associated with deontological, or moral obligation, requirements rather than consequentialist rules that strictly weigh benefits against costs or link means to ends. People with SVs often say that one has a moral obligation to act, independent of likelihood of success, "because I couldn't live with myself if I didn't." But there is little analysis of the mental accounting involved in quantity insensitivity (cf. Baron & Greene, 1996) or of the stability of values across decision frames (Fischhoff et al., 1980): For example, a medical decision framed as one of survival may be insensitive to cost, but not when couched in terms of a marginal increase in prospects for survival (Tversky, Slovic, & Sattath, 1988). Tanner and Medin (2004) find protected values to be associated with elimination of otherwise robust framing effects, such as favoring choices framed as gains over those framed as losses. Beyond this, there is little consensus. Moreover, analyses that have been done are primarily with "standard" laboratory populations of university students, using fictional scenarios—a practice that sometimes produces results that do not readily generalize to other populations and methods (Medin & Atran, 2004; cf. Henrich et al., 2001).

Some tentative studies couple world events and people with SVs who engage in heroism or suicide terrorism to underline the importance of morally motivated decision making (Atran, 2004; Skitka & Mullen, 2002). But significant empirical and theoretical challenges remain. For example, researchers note (Baron & Spranca, 1997; Tetlock, 2003) that although people who ostensibly hold SVs sometimes seem to treat them as having infinite utility (e.g., in refusing to consider trade-offs), this implies that people with such values should spend literally all their time and effort protecting and promoting that value. Moreover, infinite utility is incompatible with any sort of "preference schedule": Expected utilities are weighted averages, which makes little sense when one of the terms is infinite.

Thus some have suggested these values are only pseudosacred (Baron & Leshner, 2000; Thompson & Gonzalez, 1997); others have noted that people with SVs may nonetheless engage in indirect trade-offs (McGraw & Tetlock, 2005; Tetlock, 2000). One may be tempted to think of sacred values as self-serving "posturing," but the reality of acts such as suicide bombings and a monk's self-immolation undermines this stance (Gambetta, 2005). Moreover, SVs necessary to an individual's identity may take on truly absolute value only when value-related identity seems gravely threatened (e.g., via humiliation), just as food may take on absolute value only when sustenance for life is threatened.

For example, our research team (Atran, 2006a; Ginges, Atran, Medin, & Shikaki, in press) recently conducted studies indicating that instrumental approaches to resolving political disputes are suboptimal when protagonists transform the issues or resources under dispute into essential moral values, that is, values that a moral community treats as possessing transcendental significance that precludes comparisons or tradeoffs with instrumental values of realpolitik or the marketplace. Instrumental decision making involves strict cost–benefit calculations regarding goals and entails abandoning or adjusting goals if costs of realizing them are too high. We found that emotional outrage and support for violent opposition to compromise over sacred values is (1) not mitigated by offering instrumental incentives to compromise but (2) is decreased when the adversary makes instrumentally irrelevant compromises of their own sacred values.

In a survey of Jewish Israelis living in the West Bank and Gaza (settlers, $N = 601$) conducted in August 2005, days before Israel's withdrawal from Gaza, we randomly presented participants with one of several hypothetical peace deals. All involved Israeli withdrawal from 99% of the West Bank and Gaza in exchange for peace. We identified a subset of participants (46%) who had transformed land into an essential value; they believed that it was never permissible for the Jewish people to "give up" part of the "Land of Israel," no matter how extreme the circumstance. For these participants, all deals thus involved a "taboo" trade-off. Some deals involved an added instrumental incentive, such as money or the promise of a life free of violence (taboo+), while in other deals Palestinians also made a "taboo" trade-off over one of their own sacred values in a manner that neither added instrumental value to Israel nor detracted from the taboo nature of the deal being considered ("tragic"). From a rational perspective, the taboo+ deal is improved relative to the taboo deal and thus violent opposition to the tragic deal should be weaker. However, we observed the following order of support for violence: taboo+ > taboo > tragic (see Figure 17.6A), where those evaluating the tragic deal showed less support for violent opposition than the other two conditions. An analysis of intensity of emotional outrage again found that taboo+ > taboo > tragic (see Figure 17.6C); those evaluating the tragic deal were least likely to report anger or disgust at the prospect of the deal being signed.

These results were replicated in a survey of Palestinian refugees ($N = 535$) in Gaza and the West Bank conducted in late December 2005, 1 month before Hamas was elected to power. In this experiment, hypothetical peace deals (see supporting online materials) all violated the Palestinian "right of return," a key issue in the conflict (Shamir & Shikaki, 2005). For the 80% of participants who believed this was an essential value, we once more observed that for violent opposition the order between conditions was taboo+ > taboo > tragic, where those evaluating a "tragic" deal showed lowest support for violent opposition (see Figure 17.6B). Further, the same order was found for two measures ostensibly unrelated to the experiment: (1) the belief that Islam condones suicide attacks, and (2) reports of joy at hearing of a suicide attack (see de Quervain et al., 2004, for evidence of for joy as a neurophysiological correlate of revenge). Compared to refugees who had earlier evaluated a taboo or taboo+ deal, those who had evaluated a tragic deal believed less that Islam condoned suicide attacks and were less likely to report feeling joy at hearing of a suicide attack (see Figure 17.6D). In neither the settler nor the refugee studies did participants responding to the "tragic" deals regard these deals as more implementable than participants evaluating taboo or taboo+ deals.

These experiments reveal that in political disputes where sources of conflict are cultural, such as the Israeli–Palestinian conflict or emerging clashes between the Muslim and Judeo-Christian world, violent opposition to compromise solutions may be exacerbated rather than decreased by insisting on instrumentally driven tradeoffs, while noninstrumental symbolic compromises may reduce support for violence.[18]

Or consider religiously motivated terrorism. Most terrorists who have been studied—including would-be or captured suicide bombers—fail to show any psychopathology or sociopathy, and are generally at least as educated and economically well-off as their surrounding populations (Krueger & Maleckova, 2003; Atran, 2003; Stern, 2003; Sageman, 2004; Merari, 2005). Such findings are often taken to support the idea that terrorist action—including self-destruction—derives from rational decisions to optimize strategies for attaining sociopolitical goals (Pape, 2005; Madsen, 2004; M. Bloom, 2005): the religious "bargain" of mostly young men dying for a promising afterlife (Stark, 2000); ultimate sacrifice as maximizing the goal of improving lives of fam-

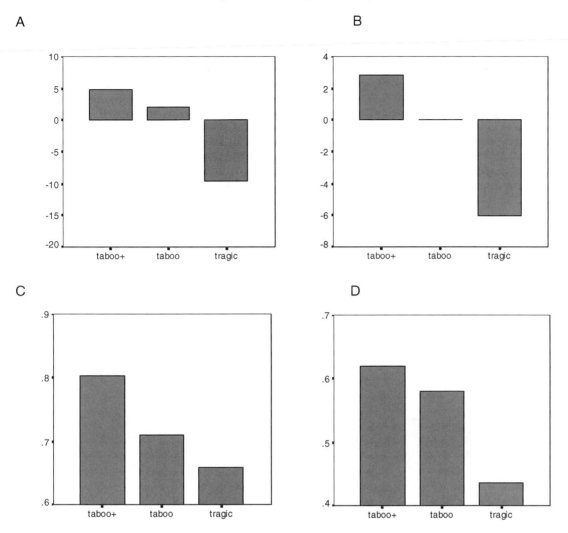

FIGURE 17.6. Predictions of the percentage of the population who would use violence to oppose: a peace deal perceived to violate a sacred value (taboo condition); the taboo deal plus an added instrumental incentive (taboo+); or the taboo deal plus a sacred value concession without instrumental value, from the adversary (tragic) for (A) Israeli settlers (linear trend $F[1,195] = 5.698$, $P = .018$) and (B) Palestinian refugees ($F[1, 384] = 7.201$, $P = .008$). Parallel results obtained for emotional reactions by: (C) settlers reporting anger or disgust at an Israeli leader who would agree to the tradeoff being evaluated ($F[1, 260] = 4.436$, $P = .036$); and (D) refugees reporting "joy" at hearing of a suicide bombing according to the type of tradeoff being evaluated ($F[1, 418] = 7.48$, $P = .007$). The trend of emotional intensity and support for violence in each case, taboo+ > taboo > tragic, could not be predicted by an instrumental account of human behavior.

ily or compatriots, which offsets the "opportunity cost" of an educated life lost prematurely (Azzam, 2005; cf. Becker, 1968); and "trading life" for a social identity that is affirmed in death but devalued by continued living (Harrison, 2006; cf. Akerlof & Kranton, 2000).

These speculations are theoretically plausible; however, no empirical study involving structured interviews or experiments with religious suicide terrorists has ever put these speculations to empirical test. Rather than obey a utilitarian "logic of rational consequence," these actors perhaps more closely follow a "logic of moral appropriateness" (Hoffman & McCormick, 2004). For example, I recently interviewed 12 self-identified recruits for martyr attack from the Hamas Block at al-Najah University in Nablus (which provides more suicide bombers than any other demographic group of Palestinians) and six members each of Hamas and Al Aqsa' Martyrs Brigades in Gaza's Jabaliyah refugee camp. All were asked questions of the sort, "So what if your family were to be killed in retaliation for your action?" or "What if your father were dying and your mother found out your plans for a martyrdom attack and asked you to delay until the family could get back on its feet?" To a person they answer along lines that there is duty to family but duty to God cannot be postponed. But most of those interviewed also say that if a roadside bomb can produce the same damage (i.e., without causing the deaths of any members of the group), then it is preferable. More recent interviews with leaders and foot soldiers of Indonesia's Jemaah Islamiyah, Al-Qaeda's mainly ally in Southeast Asia, show similar results (cf. Atran & Stern, 2005; Atran, 2006b).[19] In short, when the focus is on the act itself, they may be even anti consequentialist, but when the focus is on the enemy, consequentialism emerges.

In summary, whereas study of judgment and decision making has greatly advanced (for reviews, see Kahneman, 2003; Markman & Medin, 2002; Schneider & Shanteau, 2003), much more is known about decision-making facets of economic behavior than about morally motivated behavior, especially religiously motivated social and political behavior. I hope this will change given the critical importance of religious values in human judgment and decision making, and their crucial involvement in personal well-being, cultural survival, and political conflict.

CONCLUSION: EVOLUTION'S CANALIZING LANDSCAPE

Think metaphorically of humankind's evolutionary history as a landscape formed by different mountain ridges. This landscape functions everywhere to canalize, but not determine, individual and cultural development. It greatly reduces the possible sources of religious expression into structures that constantly reappear across history and societies.

This landscape is shaped by natural selection. It is ancestrally defined by specific sets of affective, social, and cognitive features—different mountain ridges. Each ridge has a distinct contour, with various peaks whose heights reflect evolutionary time. One such evolutionary ridge encompasses panhuman emotional faculties, or "affect programs." Some of these affect programs, such as surprise and fear, date at least to the emergence of reptiles. Others, such as grief and guilt, may be unique to humans. Another ridge includes social interaction schemas. Some schemas may go far back in evolutionary time, such as those involved in detecting predators and seeking protectors, or which govern direct "tit-for-tat" reciprocity ("You scratch my back, I'll scratch yours"). Other social interaction schemas seem unique to humans, such as committing to nonkin. Still another ridge encompasses panhuman mental faculties, or cognitive "modules," such as folkmechanics, folkbiology, and folkpsychology. Folkmechanics is this ridge's oldest part, with links to amphibian brains. Folkpsychology is the newest, foreshadowed among apes. Only humans appear to metarepresent multiple models of other minds and worlds (Tomasello, Kruger, & Ratner, 1993), including the supernatural.

Human experience lies along this evolutionary landscape, usually converging on more or less the same life paths—much as rain that falls anywhere in a mountain valley landscape drains into a limited set of lakes or rivers (Kauffman, 1993; Sperber, 1996). As humans randomly interact and "walk" through this landscape, they naturally tend toward certain forms of cultural life, including religious paths. Cultures and religions do not exist apart from the individual minds that constitute them and the environments that constrain them, any more than a physical path exists apart from the organisms that tread and groove it, and the surrounding ecology that restricts its location and course. Individual minds mutually interact within this converging landscape in an open-ended time horizon, exploiting its features in distinctive ways to produce the religious and cultural diversity we see in the world and throughout human history.[20]

Nevertheless, all religions follow the same structural contours. They invoke supernatural agents to deal with emotionally eruptive existential anxieties, such as loneliness, calamity, and death. They have malevolent and predatory deities, as well as more benevolent and protective ones. These systematically, but minimally, violate modularized expectations about folkmechanics, folkbiology, and folkpsychology. And religions communally validate counterintuitive beliefs through musical rituals and other rhythmic coordinations of affective body states. Finally, these landscape features are mutually constraining. They include evolved constraints on emotional feelings and displays, modularized conceptual and mnemonic processing, and social commitments that attend to information about cooperators, protectors, predators, and prey. Religious and cultural life is pervaded and largely constituted by the manipulation of these landscape features—for good or bad.

ACKNOWLEDGMENTS

Thanks to Richard Sosis for the material in the section "adaptationist Theories of Religion" (apart from "Other Functionalist Accounts"); Ara Norenzayan for contributions to the sections "Cultural Survival" and "Existential Anxiety" and for Figures 17.1 and 17.5; Harvey Whitehouse for information in the section "Modes of Religiosity" and for Figures 17.2 and 17.3; Nicola Knight and Paulo Sousa for analyses in the section "Metarepresenting Counterintuitive Worlds" and for Figure 17.4; and Jeremy Ginges and Douglas Medin for ideas and insights in the section "Sacred Values in Decision Making." My appreciation also to the National Science Foundation for research support on some of the issues discussed in this chapter (Grant Nos. SBR 9707761, SBR 0132469, SBR 0424629, BCS-0446738, and SBE-0527396).

NOTES

1. No conceptual distinction is made here between "culture" and "society" or "mind" and "brain."

2. In a survey of persons who reported a religious experience (Greeley, 1975), music emerges as the single most important elicitor of the experience. Listeners as young as 3 years old reliably associate basic or primary emotions to musical structures, such as happiness, sadness, fear and anger (Trainor & Trehub, 1992; Panksepp, 1993).

3. According to the European Interactive Advertising Association, the Internet increasingly represents the essential media for the 15–24 age group, which is "the holy grail" for most advertisers: "European Youth Ditching TV and Radio for Web," *European Tech Wire* (retrieved June 24, 2005, from *www.europeantechwire.com/etw/2005/06/24/*). Personal bonds formed online without physical contact appear to generate solid reputations for trustworthiness and the same deep commitment generated by physical intimacy, but often faster and over a wider set of personal relations (Resnick & Zeckhauser, 2002). A recent study of online dating by researchers at the University of Bath indicates that the Internet allows men to manifest emotions that cement durable relationships in ways that are easier than face-to-face contact: "Internet Dating Much More Successful Than Thought," online press release, University of Bath, February 2005 (*www.eurekalert.org/pub_releases/2005-02/uob-idm021305.php*). The Web also lets women enter into chat rooms with men who would otherwise shun female contact, and it empowers a minority of two in dialogue with the sentiment that they can span the world.

4. Although calculations of economic or political utility often influence religious practices (Stark, 2000), religious sacrifice usually costs something for the persons on whose behalf the offering is made. That is why "sacrifice of wild animals which can be regarded as the free gift of nature is rarely allowable or efficient" (Robertson Smith, 1894, p. 466). Thus, for the Nuer of Sudan, substituting a highly valued item (cow) by one less-valued (fowl or vegetable) is allowable only to a point, after which "a religious accounting might reveal that the spirits and ghosts were expecting a long overdue proper sacrifice, because accounts were out of balance so to speak" (Evans-Pritchard, 1940, p. 26). In many cases, the first or best products of one's livelihood goes to the gods, as with the first fruits of the Hebrews or the most perfect maize kernels of the Maya. Most, if not all, societies specify obligatory circumstances under which religious sacrifice must be performed, regardless of economics.

5. As Dan Sperber (1996) asked in an open communication to the Evolution and Human Behavior Society: "Is fitness a matter of having descendants with a recognizable ideology? Of population size? Of variations in size (expansion)? Of duration? Of some weighted combination of size and duration? What of social systems that expand rapidly at the expense of heritability (empires)?" Without answers to such questions (and none seem forthcoming) the idea of societal-level fitness is hopelessly vague.

6. In a student project in Michigan, Sara Konrath compared interpretations of cultural sayings (e.g., "Let a thousand flowers bloom") among 26 control subjects

and 32 subjects with autism. Subjects with autism were significantly more likely to paraphrase closely and repeat content from the original statement (e.g., "Don't cut flowers before they bloom"). Controls were more likely to infer a wider range of cultural meanings, with little replicated content (e.g., "Go with the flow," "Everyone should have equal opportunity")—a finding consistent with previous results from East Asians (who were familiar with "Let a thousand flowers bloom" as Mao's credo; Atran 2001). Only subjects with autism, who lack inferential capacity normally associated with theory of mind (ToM), came close to being "meme machines." They may be excellent replicators of literal meaning, but they are poor transmitters of cultural meaning. (To deal with deficits in counterfactual thinking, St. Paul's Church in Alabama [Trenton Diocese] has a special program for people with autism: "The church requires that children who receive Holy Communion be able to recognize the difference between ordinary bread and the Eucharist. . . . The St. Paul's program was designed to teach the difference" (Rev. Sam Sirianni, cited in A. Raboteau, "Celebrating a Milestone," *Austism Society of Alabama, National and World New Forum*, retrieved June 25, 2000, from *www.autism-alabama.org/ubb/forum2/html/000145.html*). With some exceptions, ideas do not reproduce or replicate in minds in the same way that genes replicate in DNA. They do not generally spread from mind to mind by imitation. It is biologically prepared, culturally enhanced, richly structured minds that generate and transform recurrent convergent ideas from often fragmentary and highly variable input (Sperber & Hirschfeld, 2004; Atran, Medin, & Ross, 2005).

7. Although the Buddha and the buddhas are not regarded as gods, Buddhists clearly conceive of them as "counterintuitive agents" (Pyysiännen, 2003). In Sri Lanka, Sinhalese relics of the Buddha have miraculous powers. In India, China, Japan, Thailand, and Vietnam, magic mountains and forests are associated with the Buddha; literature and folklore in every Buddhist tradition recount amazing events surrounding the Buddha and the buddhas.

8. Experiments with adults in the United States (J. Barrett & Keil, 1996) and India (J. Barrett, 1998) further illustrate the gap between theological doctrine and actual psychological processing of religious concepts. When asked to describe their deities, subjects in both cultures produced abstract and consensual theological descriptions of gods as being able to do anything, to anticipate and react to everything at once, always to know the right thing to do, and to be able to dispense entirely with perceptual information and calculation. When asked to respond to narratives about these same gods, the same subjects described the deities as being in only one place at a time, puzzling over alternative courses of action, and looking for evidence in order to decide what to do (e.g., to save Johnny first, who's praying for help because his foot is stuck in a river in the United States and the water is rapidly rising, or to save little Mary

first, whom He has seen fall on railroad tracks in Australia where a train is fast approaching).

9. An example from ethology offers a parallel. Many bird species have nests parasitized by other species. Thus, the cuckoo deposits eggs in passerine nests, tricking the foster parents into incubating and feeding the cuckoo's young. Nestling European cuckoos often dwarf their host parents (Hamilton & Orians, 1965): "The young cuckoo, with its huge gape and loud begging call, has evidently evolved in exaggerated form the stimuli which elicit the feeding response of parent passerine birds. . . . This, like lipstick in the courtship of mankind, demonstrates successful exploitation by means of a 'super-stimulus' " (Lack, 1968). Late nestling cuckoos have evolved perceptible signals to *manipulate* the passerine nervous system by initiating and then arresting or interrupting normal processing. In this way, cuckoos are able to subvert and to co-opt the passerine's modularized survival mechanisms.

10. For Aristotle, the world that could be properly described in ordinary Greek was the world that is (nomologically). This led him to conflate the world's ontological structure (what philosophy and science consider to be the ultimate "stuff" composing the world) with the semantic structure of language (the constraints governing the ordinary relations between words and thoughts). More recent philosophers interpret the notion of a category mistake to be a logical or semantic "type confusion" (Sommers, 1963; Pap, 1963).

11. According to Boyer (1994, 2000), bodiless supernaturals are counterintuitive because they think and act but lack physical substance. The matter is not so simple. First, experiments with infants and adults indicate that ordinary intuitions about causal agents do not require knowledge or perception of material substance, only the expectation (perhaps never actually realized) that there *ultimately is* a physical source of intentional action (Csibra et al., 1999). Ontological violations block such expectations being realized *even in principle* (e.g., invisible agents versus heard but unseen beings). They countermand rules for eventual processing, not actual perception. Second, not all mental states are equally bound to ordinary intuitions about bodies. Recent studies with American school children indicate that children from five years on more readily attribute epistemic mental states (see, think, know) to beings in the afterlife than psychobiological mental states (hunger, thirst, sleepiness; Bering & Bjorklund, 2002). Ordinary distinctions between mind and body (e.g., dreaming) thus seem to provide at least *some* intuitive support for extraordinary beings with disembodied minds (Hobbes, 1651/1901).

12. J. Barrett and Nyhoff (2001, p. 79) list as common items "a being that can see or hear things that are not too far away"; "a species that will die if it doesn't get enough nourishment or if it is severely damaged"; "an object that is easy to see under normal lighting conditions." Such items fall so far below ordinary expectations that communication should carry some new or sa-

lient information that J. Barrett and Nyhoff (2001, pp. 82–83) report: "common items were remembered so poorly relative to other items. . . . In some instances of retelling these items, participants tried to make the common property sound exciting or unusual." In other words, some subjects tried to meet minimum conditions of relevance (Sperber & Wilson, 1995). For the most part, common items failed these minimum standards for successful communication.

13. Maximally counterintuitive statements (MXCI) were created by modifying a concept with two properties taken from another ontological category (e.g., squinting wilting brick). To control for memory differences on two versus three-word items, for each MXCI statement, a matching statement was generated, with only one of the properties being counterintuitive (e.g., chattering climbing pig).

14. Psychologists familiar with Tulving's (1972) original semantic–episodic distinction may find this confusing, because both types of memory were supposed to be verbal and propositional. According to Whitehouse, highly infrequent episodes seem to be engraved in detail in participants' minds, confidently and forever, as especially vivid "flashbulb memories" (Brown & Kullick, 1982) akin to the memories of Americans who experienced such personally momentous social events as, the Kennedy assassinations, the explosion of the Challenger Space Shuttle, or 9/11 (though it is not clear that the psychologist's notion of flashbulb memory is entirely appropriate inasmuch as many so-called flashbulb memories seem to endure and stabilize more through narrative consolidation, including via "TV priority," rather than relived emotion; Neisser & Harsch, 1992).

15. Figure 17.3 indicates that emotionally arousing and unusual experiences, or "rites of terror," will lead to idiosyncratic beliefs or a "lack of uniformity." Shinobu Kitayama (personal communication) suggests an alternate hypothesis: For these highly arousing, ambiguous experiences, people will rely on culturally supplied explanations and narratives to make sense of their "once in a lifetime" experiences. If that were so, highly imagistic, arousing, unusual, or ambiguous experiences may lead to uniformity within a culture, because people would rely on common culturally supplied narratives to make sense of the event. This may be true of revival meetings. In any event more work is needed.

16. In control conditions, equally anxiety-provoking scenarios (e.g., a visit to the dentist, where dental pain is experienced) did not lead to stronger supernatural belief. Moreover, whenever stronger anxiety was found in the mortality salience condition, controlling for self-reported anxiety (measured on the PANAS scale) failed to eliminate the effect (Norenzayan & Hansen, 2006).

17. One interpretation is that if supernatural intervention works for Buddhism, this would confirm the feasibility of a similar intervention by a Christian god. But further experiments by Hansen and Norenzayan provide compelling evidence that (1) Christians are un-

willing to believe in Buddha or shamanic spirits in control conditions, and they believe in God far more than they believe in Buddha or spirits and (2) Christian subjects shift toward more belief in Buddha and spirits under mortality salience. Moreover, identification with Christian faith is uncorrelated with belief in Buddha and spirits in control conditions, but *positively* correlated under mortality salience. One possibility that is not ruled out by these experiments is that Christians may believe that if Buddha or shamanic spirits exist, so does God or Jesus. This interpretation is not that different from what we suggest, namely, that people are generally open to the supernatural, no matter who the deity is, under mortality salience. It is clear that people are *not* derogating culturally other deities. This contrasts markedly with TMT claims that, under mortality salience, people derogate other cultures.

18. One alternative interpretation of the data is to argue that the Palestinians' "sacred value" trade-offs in the tragic condition signaled greater willingness to compromise on their part. If that were the case, the "tragic" condition might be superior *instrumentally* to the other two conditions, because participants could find it easier to believe that the deal would be peacefully and successfully implemented. To test this interpretation, participants were asked whether they believed that the deal they had been presented with would be "peacefully and successfully implemented." Responses were scored 1 for *yes*, .5 for *not sure*, and 0 for *no*. The data showed that this alternative interpretation did not hold.

19. For a sample set of questions and responses, see S. Atran, "The Emir: An interview with the Abu Bakr Ba'asyir, alleged leader of *Jemaah Islamiyah*," *Spotlight on Terrorism* (Jamestown Foundation), September 15, 2005; available at *jamestown.org/terrorism/news/article.php?articleid=2369782.*

20. The working notion of "religion" used here—a group's costly commitment to a counterintuitive world of supernatural beings who manage people's existential anxieties—is not meant to *define* religion or to delimit its natural scope and limits. It is used only to circumscribe roughly what people would ordinarily include the term. As with Darwin's use of the commonsense notion of species, which first focused his attention, subsequent discoveries revealed only rough correspondence between the commonsense construct (species) and historically contingent patterns of evolution (more or less geographically isolated and interbreeding populations). Darwin continued with a traditional circumscription of "species," while denying it any special ontological status or reality, using it only as a heuristic notion that could ground attention as diverse and often inconclusive scientific analyses advanced (Atran, 1998). Likewise, this working characterization and account of "religion" may help to orient research, but it should not be mistaken for a final point of reference and explanation. The chosen conduit metaphor is of an evolutionary landscape that constrains (initially randomly) interacting humans, as they "walk" through life, onto converging life

paths that involve cognitions of supernatural agents who deal with emotionally eruptive existential anxieties and regulate long-term social commitments. Within this framework, an explanatory account, or "theory," of religion, would build from the "bottom-up" in terms of the cognitive, emotional, and social microprocesses that assemble interacting individuals into religious traditions. In the end, "religion," like "culture," may turn out to be more of a analytic hodgepodge of "family resemblances" than a natural kind with systematic properties (on "culture," see Atran et al., 2005).

REFERENCES

Akerlof, G., & Kranton, R. (2000). Economics and identity. *Quarterly Journal of Economics*, 115, 715–753.

Alcorta, C., & Sosis, R. (2005). Ritual, emotion, and sacred symbols: The evolution of religion as an adaptive complex. *Human Nature*, 16, 323–359.

Alexander, R. (1987). *The biology of moral systems*. New York: Aldine de Gruyter.

Alexander, R. (1989). Evolution of the human psyche. In C. Stringer (Ed.), *The human revolution*. Edinburgh: University of Edinburgh Press.

Allport, G. (1956). *The nature of prejudice*. Cambridge, MA: Harvard University Press.

Andresen, J. (Ed.). (2001). *Religion in mind*. New York: Cambridge University Press.

Aristotle. (1963). *Aristotle: Categories and de Interpretatione* (J. L. Ackrill, Trans.). Oxford, UK: Clarendon.

Atran, S. (1989). Basic conceptual domains. *Mind and Language*, 4, 7–16.

Atran, S. (1990). *Cognitive foundations of natural history*. Cambridge, UK: Cambridge University Press.

Atran, S. (1996). Modes of thinking about living kinds: Science, symbolism and common sense. In D. Olson & N. Torrance (Eds.), *Modes of thought: Explorations in culture and cognition*. New York: Cambridge University Press.

Atran, S. (1998). Folkbiology and the anthropology of science. *Behavioral and Brain Sciences*, 21, 547–609.

Atran, S. (2001). The trouble with memes. *Human Nature*, 12, 351–381.

Atran, S. (2002). *In gods we trust*. New York: Oxford University Press.

Atran, S. (2003). Genesis of suicide terrorism. *Science*, 299, 1534–1539.

Atran, S. (2004, October). *Tuning out Hell's harpists: Interviews with Hamas*. Paper presented to the Permanent Monitoring Panel on Terrorism, World Federation of Scientists, Geneva. Retrieved on November 19, 2006, from *www.sitemaker.umich.edu/satran/files/satran0105.pdf*

Atran, S. (2005). Adaptationism in human cognition: Strong, spurious, or weak? *Mind and Language*, 20, 39–67.

Atran, S. (2006a, April). *Global Network Terrorism*.

Part 1: Sacred values and radicalization. Briefing to the National Security Council, White House, Washington, DC. Available at *www.au.af.mil/au/awc/awcgate/whitehouse/atrannsc-042806.pdf*

Atran, S. (2006b). The moral logic and growth of suicide terrorism. *The Washington Quarterly*, 29, 127–147.

Atran, S., Lois, X., & Ucan Ek', E. (2004). *Plants of the Petén Itza' Maya* (University of Michigan Memoirs, No. 38). Ann Arbor: University of Michigan Museum of Anthropology Publications.

Atran, S., Medin, D., & Ross, N. (2005). The cultural mind: Ecological decision making and cultural modeling within and across populations. *Psychological Review*, 112(4), 744–776.

Atran, S., Medin, D., Ross, N., Lynch, E., Vapnarsky, V., Ucan Ek', E., et al. (2002). Folkecology, cultural epidemiology, and the spirit of the commons. *Current Anthropology*, 43, 421–450.

Atran, S., & Norenzayan, A. (2004). Religion's evolutionary landscape: Counterintuition, commitment, compassion, communion. *Behavioral and Brain Sciences*, 27, 713–770.

Atran, S., & Sperber, D. (1991). Learning without teaching: Its place in culture. In L. Tolchinsky-Landsmann (Ed.), *Culture, schooling and psychological development*. Norwood, NJ: Ablex.

Atran, S., & Stern, J. (2005). Small groups find fatal purpose through the web. *Nature*, 436, 620.

Avis, J., & Harris, P. (1991). Belief–desire reasoning among Baka children. *Child Development*, 62, 460–467.

Azzam, J.-P. (2005). Suicide-bombing as intergenerational investment. *Public Choice*, 122, 177–198.

Baron, J., & Greene, J. (1996). Determinants of insensitivity to quantity in valuation of public goods. *Journal of Experimental Psychology: Applied*, 2, 107–125.

Baron, J., & Leshner, S. (2000). How serious are expressions of protected values? *Journal of Experimental Psychology: Applied*, 6, 183–194.

Baron, J., & Spranca, M. (1997). Protected values. *Organizational Behavior and Human Decision Processes*, 70, 1–16.

Barrett, J. (1998). Cognitive constraints on Hindu concepts of the divine. *Journal for the Scientific Study of Religion*, 37, 608–619.

Barrett, J. (2000). Exploring the natural foundations of religion. *Trends in Cognitive Sciences*, 4, 29–34.

Barrett, J., & Keil, F. (1996). Conceptualizing a nonnatural entity. *Cognitive Psychology*, 31, 219–247.

Barrett, J., & Nyhoff, M. (2001). Spreading nonnatural concepts. *Journal of Cognition and Culture*, 1, 69–100.

Barrett, L., Dunbar, R., & Lycett, J. (2001). *Human evolutionary psychology*. Basingstoke, UK: Macmillan.

Bartlett, F. (1932). *Remembering*. Cambridge, UK: Cambridge University Press.

Barth, F. (1975). *Ritual and knowledge among the*

Baktaman of New Guinea. New Haven, CT: Yale University Press.

Baumeister, R., Smart, L., & Boden, J. (1996). Relation of threatened egotism to violence and aggression. *Psychological Review, 103*, 5–23.

Becker, G. (1968). Crime and punishment: An economic approach. *Journal of Political Economy, 76*, 169–217.

Beit-Hallahmi, B., & Argyle, M. (1997). *The psychology of religious behavior, belief, and experience*. London: Routledge.

Ben-Amos, P. G. (1994). The promise of greatness: Women and power in an Edo spirit possession cult. In T. Blakely, W. van Beek, & D. Thomson (Eds.), *Religion in Africa*. Portsmouth, NH: Heinemann.

Bering, J., & Bjorklund, D. (2002, March). *Simulation constraints on the development of death representation*. Paper presented at the conference, "Minds and Gods," Ann Arbor, University of Michigan and John Templeton Foundation.

Bering, J., & Bjorklund, D. (2004). The natural emergence of reasoning about the afterlife as a developmental regularity. *Developmental Psychology, 40*, 217–233.

Blackmore, S. (1999). *The meme machine*. Oxford, UK: Oxford University Press.

Bloom, H. (1999, June 14). Billy Graham. *Time Magazine*, pp. 120–123.

Bloom, M. (2005). *Dying to kill: The allure of suicide terrorism*. New York: Columbia University Press.

Bloom, P., & Veres, C. (1999). The perceived intentionality of groups. *Cognition, 71*, B1–B9.

Boehm, C. (1999). *Hierarchy in the forest*. Cambridge, MA: Harvard University Press.

Boyd, R., & Richerson, P. (2005). *The origin and evolution of cultures*. New York: Oxford University Press.

Boyer, P. (1994). *The naturalness of religious ideas*. Berkeley: University of California Press.

Boyer, P. (2000). Functional origins of religious concepts. *Journal of the Royal Anthropological Institute, 6*, 195–214.

Boyer, P. (2001). *Religion explained*. New York: Basic Books.

Boyer, P., & Ramble, C. (2001). Cognitive templates for religious concepts. *Cognitive Science, 25*, 535–564.

Brown, R., & Kulick, J. (1982). Flashbulb memory. In U. Neiser (Ed.), *Memory observed: Remembering in natural contexts*. San Francisco: Freeman.

Bulbulia, J. (2004). Religious costs as adaptations that signal altruistic intention. *Evolution and Cognition, 10*, 19–38.

Burkert, W. (1996). *Creation of the sacred*. Cambridge, MA: Harvard University Press.

Cahill, L., Prins, B., Weber, M., & McGaugh, J. (1994). Beta-adrenergic activation and memory for emotional events. *Nature, 371*, 702–704.

Cohen, S. (2002). India, Pakistan, and Kashmir. *Journal of Strategic Studies, 25*, 32–60.

Cronk, L. (1994). Evolutionary theories of morality and the manipulative use of signals. *Zygon, 29*, 81–101.

Csibra, G., Gergely, G., Bíró, S., Koós, O., & Brockbank, M. (1999). Goal attribution without agency cues. *Cognition, 72*, 237–267.

d'Aquili, E., & Newberg, A. (1999). *The mystical mind*. Minneapolis: Fortress Press.

Dawkins, R. (1976). *The selfish gene*. New York: Oxford University Press.

Dawkins, R. (1998). *Unweaving the rainbow*. Boston: Houghton Mifflin.

Dawkins, R. (2006). *The God delusion*. Boston: Houghton Mifflin.

Dawkins R., & Krebs J. R. (1978). Animal signals: Information or manipulation? In J. R. Krebs & N. Davies (Eds.), *Behavioural ecology: An evolutionary approach* (1st ed.). Oxford, UK: Blackwell.

Deacon T. (1997). *The symbolic species*. New York: Norton.

de Landa, D. (1985). *Relación de la cosas de Yucatán*. In M. Rivera Dorado (Ed.), *Crónicas de America* (Vol. 7). Madrid: Historia 16 (Original work composed in 1566)

Dennett, D. (1978). Response to Premack and Woodruff: Does the chimpanzee have a theory of mind? *Behavioral and Brain Sciences, 4*, 568–570.

Dennett, D. (1995). *Darwin's dangerous idea*. New York: Simon & Schuster.

Dennett, D. (1997). Appraising grace: What evolutionary good is God? *The Sciences, 37*, 39–44.

Dennett, D. (2006). *Breaking the spell: Religion as a natural phenomenon*. New York: Viking.

de Quervain, D., Fischbacher, U., Treyer, V., Schellhammer, M., Schnyder, U., Buck, A., et al. (2004). The neural basis of altruistic punishment. *Science, 305*, 1254–1258.

Durkheim, É. (1995). *The elementary forms of religious life*. New York: Free Press. (Original work published 1912)

Evans-Pritchard, E. (1940). *The Nuer*. Oxford, UK: Oxford University Press.

Evans-Pritchard, E. (1960). Zande cannibalism. *Journal of the Royal Anthropological Institute, 90*, 238–258.

Firth, R. (1963). Offering and sacrifice. *Journal of the Royal Anthropological Institute, 93*, 12–24.

Fischoff, B., Slovic, P., & Lichtenstein, S. (1980). Knowing what you want: Measuring labile variables. In T. Wallstein (Ed.), *Cognitive processes in choice and decision behavior*. Hillsdale, NJ: Erlbaum.

Fiske, A., & Tetlock, P. (1997). Taboo tradeoffs: Reactions to transactions that transgress the spheres of jutice. *Political Psychology, 18*, 255–297.

Frank, R. (1988). *Passions within reason*. New York: Norton.

Freud, S. (1955). *Group psychology and the analysis of the Ego*. In J. Strachey (Ed.), *The standard edition of the complete psychological works of Sigmund Freud* (Vol. 18). London: Hogarth Press. (Original work published 1921)

Fukuyama, F. (1995). *Trust*. New York: Free Press.

Gambetta, D. (2005). *Making sense of suicide missions*. New York: Oxford University Press.

Geary, D., & Huffman, K. (2002). Brain and cognitive evolution. *Psychological Bulletin, 128,* 667–698.

Gibbon, E. (1845). *Decline and fall of the Roman empire* (6 vols.). London: International Book Company. (Original work published 1776–1788)

Ginges, J., Atran, S., Medin, D., & Shikaki, K. (in press). Sacred bounds on rational resolution of conflict. *Proceedings of the National Academy of Sciences of the USA.*

Grafen, A. (1990). Biological signals as handicaps. *Journal of Theoretical Biology, 144,* 517–546.

Goldman, R. (1964). *Religious thinking from childhood to adolescence.* London: Routledge & Kegan Paul.

Goodall, J. (1986). *The chimpanzees of Gombe: Patterns of behavior.* Cambridge, MA: Harvard University Press.

Goodstein, L. (2000, January 1). A direct line to God in an impersonal era. *New York Times,* p. 24.

Greeley, A. (1975). *The sociology of the paranormal.* London: Sage.

Greenberg, J., Pyszczynski, T., Solomon, S., Rosenblatt, A., Veeder, M., Kirkland, S., et al. (1990). Evidence for terror management theory II. *Journal of Personality and Social Psychology, 58,* 308–318.

Guthrie, S. (1993). *Faces in the clouds: A new theory of religion.* New York: Oxford University Press.

Hamilton, W., & Orians, G. (1965). Evolution of brood parasitism in altricial birds. *Condor, 67,* 361–382.

Hardin, R. (1995). *One for all: The logic of group conflict.* Princeton, NJ: Princeton University Press.

Harris, M. (1974). *Cows, pigs, wars, and witches.* New York: Random House.

Harris, S. (2006). *Letter to a Christian nation.* New York: Knopf.

Harrison, M. (2006). An economist looks at suicide terrorism. *World Economics, 7*(3), 1–15.

Heath, C., & Sternberg, E. (2001). Emotional selection in memes: The case of urban legends. *Journal of Personality and Social Psychology, 81,* 1028–1041.

Heider, F., & Simmel, S. (1944). An experimental study of apparent behavior. *American Journal of Psychology, 57,* 243–259.

Henrich, J., Boyd, R., Bowles, S., Camerer, C., Fehr, E., & Gintis, H. (2001). In search of *Homo economicus:* Behavioral experiments in 15 small-scale societies. *American Economic Review, 91,* 73–78.

Hobbes, T. (1901). *Leviathan.* New York: Dutton. (Original work published 1651)

Hoffman, B., & McCormick, G. (2004). Terrorism, signaling, and suicide attack. *Studies in Conflict and Terrorism, 27,* 243–281.

Horowitz, D. (1984). *Ethnic groups in conflict.* Berkeley: University of California Press.

Hume, D. (1956). *The natural history of religion.* Stanford, CA: Stanford University Press. (Original work published 1757)

Hummer, R., Rogers, R., Narn, C., & Ellison C. (1999). Religious involvement and U.S. adult mortality. *Demography, 36,* 273–285.

Humphrey, N. (1995). *Soul searching: Human nature and supernatural belief.,* London: Chatto & Windus.

Huntington, S. (1997). *The clash of civilizations.* New York: Simon & Schuster.

Ibn Khaldûn. (1958). *The Muqaddimah* (3 vols.). London: Routledge & Kegan Paul. (Original work composed in 1318)

Irons, W. (1996). Morality, religion, and human nature. In W. Richardson & W. Wildman (Eds.), *Religion and science.* New York: Routledge.

Irons, W. (2001). Religion as a hard-to-fake sign of commitment. In R. Nesse (Ed.), *Evolution and the capacity for commitment.* New York: Russell Sage Foundation.

Irons, W., & Chagnon, N. (2002, June 19–23). *The unseen order: How religion works as a hard-to-fake sign of commitment.* Paper presented at Human Behavior and Evolution Society meeting, Rutgers University, New Brunswick, NJ.

Jacobs, M. (1934). *Northwest Sahaptin texts.* New York: Columbia University Press.

Johnstone, R. (1998). Game theory and communication. In L. Dugatkin & H. Reeve (Eds.), *Game theory and animal behavior.* New York: Oxford University Press.

Joseph, R. (Ed.). (2002). *NeuroTheology.* San Jose, CA: University of California Press.

Kahneman, D. (2003). Maps of bounded rationality: Psychology for behavioral economics. *American Economic Review, 93,* 1449–1475.

Kahneman, D., & Tversky, A. (1979). Prospect theory: An analysis of decision under risk. *Econometrica, 47,* 263–291.

Kant, I. (1997). *Critique of practical reason.* Cambridge, UK: Cambridge University Press. (Original work published in 1788)

Kauffman, S. (1993). *The origins of order.* New York: Oxford University Press.

Keil, F. (1979). *Semantic and conceptual development.* Cambridge, MA: Harvard University Press.

Keillor, G. (1999, Jun 14). Faith at the speed of light. *Time Magazine.*

Kierkegaard, S. (1955). *Fear and trembling and the sickness unto death.* New York: Doubleday. (Original work published 1843)

Kirkpatrick, L. (1999). Toward an evolutionary psychology of religion and personality. *Journal of Personality, 67,* 921–952.

Kluckholn, C., & Leighton, D. (1974). *The Navaho.* Cambridge, MA: Harvard University Press. (Original work published 1946)

Knight, N., Sousa, P., Barrett, J., & Atran, S. (2004). Children's attributions of beliefs to humans and God: Cross-cultural evidence. *Cognitive Science, 28,* 117–126.

Krebs J. R., & Dawkins, R. (1984). Animal signals: Mind-reading and manipulation. In J. R. Krebs & N. Davies (Eds.), *Behavioural ecology: An evolutionary approach* (2nd ed.). Oxford, UK: Blackwell.

Kroeber, A. L. (1963). *Anthropology: Culture patterns and processes.* New York: Harcourt, Brace & World. (Original work published 1923)

Krueger, A., & Malecková, J. (2003). Seeking the roots of terror. *Chronicle of Higher Education.* Retrieved June 6, 2003 from *chronicle.com/free/v49/i39/39b01001.htm*

Kuper, A. (1996). *The chosen primate.* Cambridge, MA: Harvard University Press.

Lack, D. (1968). *Ecological adaptations for breeding in birds.* London: Methuen.

Lawson, E. T., & McCauley, R. (1990). *Rethinking religion.* New York: Cambridge University Press.

Lester, T. (2002, February 8). Supernatural selection. *The Atlantic Monthly.*

Levin, J. (1994). Religion and health. *Social Science Medicine, 38,* 1475–1482.

Lipkind, W. (1940). Carajá cosmography. *Journal of American Folk-Lore, 53,* 248–251.

Lowie, R. (1924). *Primitive religion.* New York: Boni & Liveright.

Lumsden, C., & Wilson, E. (1981). *Genes, mind and culture.* Cambridge, MA: Harvard University Press.

Lynch, A. (1996). *Thought contagion.* New York: Basic Books.

MacDonald, K. (1998). *Separation and its discontents: Toward an evolutionary theory of Anti-Semitism.* Westport, CT: Praeger.

Madsen, J. (2004). The rationale of suicide attack. *Risq* (online). Retrieved September, 2004 from *www.risq.org/modules.php?name=News&file=print&sid=367*

Markman, A., & Medin, D. (2002). Decision making. In H. Pashler (Series Ed.), & D. Medin (Vol. Ed.), *Steven's handbook of experimental psychology.* New York: Wiley.

Matthews, D., McCullough, M., Larson, D., Koenig, H., Swyers, J., & Milano, M. (1998). Religious commitment and health status. *Archives of Family Medicine, 7,* 188–124.

McCauley, R., & Lawson, E. T. (2003). *Bringing ritual to mind.* New York: Cambridge University Press.

McClenon, J. (2002). *Wondrous healing: Shamanism, human evolution and the origin of religion.* DeKalb: Northern Illinois University Press.

McGraw, A., & Tetlock, P. (2005). Relational framing: The power to render acceptable transactions unacceptable and unacceptable transactions acceptable. *Journal of Consumer Psychology, 15,* 2–16.

McReady, N. (2002, February). Adrenergic blockers shortly after trauma can block PTSD. *Clinical Psychiatry News,* pp.

Medin, D., & Atran, S. (2004). The native mind: Biological categorization and reasoning in development and across cultures. *Psychological Review, 111,* 960–983.

Medin, D., Schwartz, H., Blok, S., & Birnbaum, L. (1999). The semantic side of decision making. *Psychonomic Bulletin and Review, 6,* 562–569.

Meggitt, M. (1965). *The desert people: A study of the Walbiri of central Australia.* Chicago: University of Chicago Press.

Merari, A. (2005). Social, organization, and psychological factors in suicide terrorism. In T. Bjorgo (Ed.), *Root causes of suicide terrorism.* New York: Routledge.

Neisser, U., & Harsch, N. (1992). Phantom flashbulbs. In E. Winograd & U. Neisser (Eds.), *Affect and accuracy in recall.* Cambridge, UK: Cambridge University Press.

Nesse, R. (Ed.). (2001). *Evolution and the capacity for commitment.* New York: Russell Sage Foundation.

Norenzayan, A., Atran, S., Faulkner, J., & Schaller, M. (2006). Memory and mystery: Cultural selection of minimallu counterintuitive narratives. *Cognitive Science, 30,* 1–23.

Norenzayan, A., & Hansen, I. (2006). Belief in supernatural agents in the face of death. *Personality and Social Psychology Bulletin, 32,* 174–187.

Onishi, K., & Baillargeon, R. (2005). Do 15-month-old infants understand false beliefs? *Science, 308,* 255–25.

Onishi, N. (2002). Africans fill churches that celebrate wealth. *New York Times,* March 13.

Owsianiecki, L., Upal, M. A., Sloan, D. J., & Tweney, R. (2005). Role of context in the recall of counterintuitive concepts. *Journal of Cognition and Culture, 5,* 215–240.

Panksepp, J. (1993). Emotional source of "chills" induced by music. *Music Perception, 13,* 171–207.

Pap, A. (1963). Types and meaninglessness. *Mind, 69,* 41–54.

Pape, R. (2003). *Dying to win: The strategic logic of suicide terrorism.* New York: Random House.

Persinger, M. (1987). *Neurophysiological bases of God beliefs.* New York: Praeger.

Pinker, S. (1997). *How the mind works.* New York: Norton.

Pinker, S. (2004, October 29). *The evolutionary psychology of religion.* Paper presented at the annual meeting of the Freedom from Religion Foundation, Madison, WI. Available online at *pinker.wjh.harvard.edu/articles/media/2004_10_29_religion.htm*

Premack, D., & Premack, A. (1995). Origins of social competence. In M. Gazzaniga (Ed.), *The cognitive neurosciences.* Cambridge, MA: MIT Press.

Pyszczynski, T., Greenberg, J., & Solomon, S. (1999). A dual process model of defense against conscious and unconscious death-related thoughts: An extension of terror management theory. *Psychological Review, 106,* 835–845.

Pyysiäinen, I. (2003). Buddhism, religion, and the concept of "God." *Numen, 50,* 147–171.

Pyysiäinen, I., & Anttonen, V. (Eds.). (2002). *Current approaches in the cognitive science of religion.* London: Continuum.

Rappaport, R. (1999). *Ritual and religion in the mak-*

ing of humanity. New York: Cambridge University Press.

Resnick, P., & Zeckhauser, R. (2002). Trust among strangers in internet interactions. In M. Baye (Ed.), *Advances in Applied Microeconomics, 11.* Amsterdam: Elsevier Science.

Rhode, D., & Chivers, C. (2002, March 17). Qaeda's grocery lists and manuals of killing. *New York Times,* p. A1.

Robertson Smith, W. (1894). *Lectures on the religion of the Semites* London: Adam & Charles Black.

Rosch, E., Mervis, C., Grey, W., Johnson, D., & Boyes-Braem, P. (1976). Basic objects in natural categories. *Cognitive Psychology, 8,* 382–439.

Rubin, D. (1995). *Memory in oral traditions.* New York: Oxford University Press.

Sageman, M. (2004). *Understanding terror networks.* Philadelphia: University of Pennsylvania Press.

Schelling, T. (1963). *The strategy of conflict.* New York: Oxford University Press.

Schneider, S., & Shanteau, J. (Eds.). (2003). *Emerging perspectives on judgment and decision research.* Cambridge, UK: Cambridge University Press.

Seligman, S. (1971). Phobias and preparedness. *Behavioral Therapy, 2,* 307–320.

Shamir, J., & Shikaki, K. (2005). Public opinion in the Israeli-Palestinian two-level game. *Journal of Peace Research, 42,* 311–328.

Skitka, L., & Mullen, E. (2002). The dark side of moral conviction. *Analyses of Social Issues and Public Policy, 2,* 35–41.

Sober, E., & Wilson, D. S. (1998). *Unto others.* Cambridge, MA: Harvard University Press.

Sommers, F. (1963). Types and ontology. *Philosophical Review, 72,* 327–363.

Sosis, R. (2000). Religion and intragroup cooperation: Preliminary results of a comparative analysis of utopian communities. *Cross-Cultural Research, 34,* 70–87.

Sosis, R., & Alcorta, C. (2003). Signaling, solidarity, and the sacred: The evolution of religious behavior. *Evolutionary Anthropology, 12,* 264–274.

Sosis, R., & Bressler, E. (2003). Cooperation and commune longevity: A test of the costly signaling theory of religion. *Cross-Cultural Research, 37,* 211–239.

Sosis, R., & Ruffle, B. (2004). Ideology, religion, and the evolution of cooperation: Field experiments on Israeli kibbutzim. *Research in Economic Anthropology, 23,* 87–115.

Spencer, B., & Gillen, F. (1904). *The Northern tribes of Central Australia.* London: Macmillan.

Sperber, D. (1975). *Rethinking symbolism.* Cambridge, UK: Cambridge University Press.

Sperber, D. (1985). Anthropology and psychology: Towards an epidemiology of representations. *Man, 20,* 73–89.

Sperber, D. (1996). *Explaining culture.* Oxford, UK: Blackwell.

Sperber, D., & Hirschfeld, L. (2004). The cognitive foundations of cultural stability and diversity. *Trends in Cognitive Sciences, 8,* 40–46.

Sperber, D., & Wilson, D. (1995). *Relevance: Communication and cognition* (2nd ed.). Oxford, UK: Blackwell.

Stark, R. (2000). *The rise of Christianity.* Princeton, NJ: Princeton University Press.

Stern, J. (2003). *Terror in the name of God: Why religious militants kill.* New York: HarperCollins.

Swanson, G. (1960). *The birth of the gods.* Ann Arbor: University of Michigan Press.

Talbot, M. (2000, February 27). A mighty fortress. *New York Times Magazine,* p. 34.

Tambiah, S. (1981). *A performative approach to ritual.* London: British Academy.

Tamminen, K. (1994). Religious experiences in childhood and adolescence. *International Journal for the Psychology of Religion, 4,* 61–85.

Tanner, C., & Medin, D. (2004). Protected values: No omission bias and no framing effects. *Psychonomic Bulletin and Review, 11,* 185–191.

Tetlock, P. (2000). Coping with trade-offs: Psychological constraints and political implications. In S. Lupia, M. McCubbins, & S. Popkin (Eds.), *Political reasoning and choice.* Berkeley: University of California Press.

Tetlock, P. (2003). Thinking the unthinkable: Sacred values and taboo cognitions. *Trends in Cognitive Sciences, 7,* 320–324.

Thompson, L., & Gonzalez, R. (1997). Environmental disputes: Competition for scarce resources and clashing of values. In M. Bazerman & D. Messick (Eds.), *Environment, ethics, and behavior: The psychology of environmental valuation and degradation.* San Francisco: New Lexington Press.

Thun, T. (1963). *Die religiose Entscheidung der Jugend.* The Hague: Mouton.

Tinbergen, N. (1951). *The study of instinct.* London: Oxford University Press.

Tomasello, M., Kruger, A., & Ratner, H. (1993). Cultural learning. *Behavioral and Brain Sciences, 16,* 495–511.

Tooby, J., & Cosmides, L. (1992). The psychological foundations of culture. In J. Barkow, L. Cosmides, & J. Tooby (Eds.), *The adapted mind: Evolutionary psychology and the generation of culture.* New York: Oxford University Press.

Trainor, L., & Trehub, S. (1992). The development of referential meaning in music. *Music Perception, 9,* 455–470.

Tulving, E. (1972). Episodic and semantic memory. In E. Tulving & W. Donaldson (Eds.), *Organization of memory.* New York: Academic Press.

Turnbull, C. (1962). *The forest people: A study of the pygmies of the Congo.* New York: Simon & Schuster.

Turner, M. (1996). *The literary mind: Origins of thought and language.* Oxford, UK: Oxford University Press.

Turner, V. (1969). *The ritual process.* New York: Aldine.

Tuzin, D. (1982). Ritual violence among the Ilahita Arapesh. In G. Herdt (Ed.), *Rituals of manhood:*

Male initiation in Papua New Guinea. Berkeley: University of California Press.

Tversky, A., Slovic, P., & Sattath, S. (1988). Contingent weighting in judgment and choice. *Psychological Review, 95,* 371–384.

Varshney, A. (2003). Nationalism, ethnic conflict and rationality. *Perspectives on Politics, 1,* 85–99.

Walker, S. (1992). Supernatural beliefs, natural kinds and conceptual structure. *Memory and Cognition, 20,* 655–662.

Watanabee, J., & Smuts, B. (1999). Explaining ritual without explaining it away. *American Anthropologist, 101,* 98–112.

Weber, M. (1978). *Economy and society* (G. Roth & C. Wittich, Eds.). Berkeley: University of California Press.

Whitehouse, H. (2000). *Arguments and icons.* Oxford, UK: Oxford University Press.

Whitehouse, H. (2004). *Modes of religiosity: A cognitive theory of religious transmission.* Walnut Creek, CA: AltaMira Press.

Wilson, D. S. (2002). *Darwin's cathedral.* Chicago: University of Chicago Press.

Wilson, E. O. (1978). *On human nature.* Cambridge, MA: Harvard University Press.

Winkelman, M. (1992). *Shamans, priests, and witches: A cross-cultural study of magico-religious practitioners.* (Anthropological Research Papers, No. 44). Tempe: Arizona State University.

Worthington, E., Kurusu, T., McCullough, M., & Sandage, S. (1996). Empirical research on religion and psychotherapeutic processes of outcomes. *Psychological Bulletin, 19,* 448–487.

Zahavi, A. (1975). Mate selection: A selection for a handicap. *Journal of Theoretical Biology, 53,* 205–214.

CHAPTER 18

Cultural Evolution and the Shaping of Cultural Diversity

LESLEY NEWSON
PETER J. RICHERSON
ROBERT BOYD

This chapter focuses on the way that cultures change and how cultural diversity is created, maintained, and lost. Human culture is the inevitable result of the way our species acquires its behavior. We are extremely social animals, and an overwhelming proportion of our behavior is socially learned. The behavior of other animals is largely a product of innate, evolved determinants of behavior combined with individual learning. They make quite modest use of social learning, whereas we acquire a massive cultural repertoire from the people with whom we associate (Richerson & Boyd, 2005, Chap. 2). Expertise in exploiting our environment, values about what matters in life, and even feelings about whom to trust and whom to hate are mostly "absorbed" from those around us.

What is more, we are very adept at transmitting cultural information to others, not only through frank teaching but also through the constant social interaction characteristic of human life: mutual observation and casual conversation during which behaviors and beliefs are seen, described, evaluated, and generally gossiped about. As Rogoff, Paradise, Mejia Arauz, Correa-Chavez, and Angelillo (2003) note, teaching in traditional cultures is not like formal schoolwork or the school-like teaching seen in modern societies and families. Children learn by close observation, followed by concrete participation in the activities of everyday life, gaining greater participation as they master more complex skills. Adults teach in the sense that they tolerate children's participation and lightly guide and structure children's learning experiences.

Cultural diversity inevitably develops in the course of cultural transmission. Individuals are constantly misremembering and thus varying some piece of culture, as well as making more deliberate variations. Learners often put their own personal twist on what they have been taught. Once such a new "cultural variant" exists, there is a tendency for it to be preserved. A woman's children may pick up a variant she created and spread it among their friends at school, who might then pass it on to their families. If such cultural processes were all that were operating, cultural diversity would increase without bound. In fact, although cultural diversity is great, it is not boundless. Other social processes operate to select and winnow away less useful cultural variants. This results in members of the same culture and subculture sharing a large proportion of their cultural information.

The sharing of cultural information allows groups of humans to interact and to cooperate effectively, so it is essential that some processes act to limit diversity. If such processes did not exist, human societies could not function as they do. Languages and dialects are the canonical examples of shared cultural information. For members of a social network to be able to communicate, their vocabulary and grammar has to overlap to a large extent. Thus, conformity to common usage acts powerfully to limit linguistic diversity. Variation in language usage does exist at the individual level, but the bulk of the variation is concentrated between communities that historically had little reason or opportunity to communicate with one another. When groups do not interact, their languages evolve separately and in time become mutually unintelligible. Linguistic conformity and diversity are especially important in explaining patterns of cultural change. Much cultural transmission involves language, and much cultural variation thus follows patterns of linguistic variation (Pagel & Mace, 2004). Of course, the spread of cultural variants can defy linguistic barriers, especially in the current "global village"; a great majority of the world's people know that Coca-Cola is a soft drink and that a Big Mac is a certain American-style meat sandwich. However, as a general rule, cultural diversity between communities must exist because some tools, techniques, and economic practices are suited to the situation of a given community and some are not. As cultures change, they adapt, with less successful cultural variants being forgotten or modified.

Our objective in this chapter is to dissect the process of cultural change, and the divergence and merging of cultures by describing the complex concatenation of forces that shape cultural diversity—forces that, for example, act to wipe out whole languages and technologies, while constantly spawning new dialects and new technologies. We draw a number of qualitative inferences from theory and available data, but the quantitative study of the dynamics of cultural diversity is still in its infancy.

The current pattern of cultural diversity among our species is the result of the changes in the knowledge, practices, and beliefs that have occurred over the last 70,000 years or so. Genetic evidence revealing how closely related all modern humans are suggests that we are descended from a relatively small population with limited individual and subcultural variation (Harpending et al., 1998). Between 50 and 100,000 years ago this population began to grow and spread, first in Africa, then across the world. With this expansion came a diversification of languages, subsistence systems, patterns of social organization, and other cultural features. As more complex societies began to evolve about 5,000 years ago, subcultures—classes, castes, occupational groups, and religious faiths—began to diversify *within* cultures to a degree not seen in earlier tribal scale societies. Meanwhile the growth of complex societies began to sweep away the former diversity *between* small-scale societies. Each of the many elements making up the vast body of information comprising a population's culture can change in a variety of ways, so the potential for creating new combinations of ways to perceive and interact with the physical world is staggering. On top of that, there are many possible variations on how to define social interaction, interaction with the biological environment, and so on.

We are not aware of any comprehensive attempt to quantify cultural diversity and its change through time, although many partial catalogues exist (e.g., Fearon, 2003). Jorgensen's (1980) classic study of the ethnographic diversity of Western North American Indians analyzes the patterns of covariation to be found among the different dimension of culture in his dataset. Cultural anthropology textbooks use various simplifying schemes to sketch the spatiotemporal patterns of diversity (Johnson & Earle, 2000). Many studies have been drawn from the Human Relations Area Files, a large database of ethnographic and historical data (Murdock, 1967, *www.yale.edu/hraf/*).

A number of researchers have attempted to infer the history of related groups of peoples by employing the methods used by biologists to determine the evolutionary descent of species (Cavalli-Sforza, 2000; Moylan, Graham, Borgerhoff Mulder, Nunn, & Håkansson, 2005; Pagel & Mace, 2004). These studies are often based on linguistic data; we probably know more about language change and diversity than about any other segment of culture (Nettle, 1999), except perhaps technology (Basalla, 1988; Needham, 1987). The Centre for the Evolutionary Analysis of Cultural Behavior, based at University College London, has begun the project of constructing quantitative databases of archaeological data (*www.ceacb.ucl.ac.uk/home/*), but, as with biodiversity, the many dimensions of cultural diversity defy easy analysis (Dunn, Terill, Reesink, Foley, & Levinson, 2005).

Our approach to describing cultural change is to view it as an evolutionary process. However it is important first to point out that we do not use the word *evolution* in the sense first used by the 19th century founders of anthropology to mean *progress* from less complex to more complex societies (Burrow, 1966). We use it in the sense used by Darwin. Just as people acquire their genes from their parents, they acquire their culture from the people they encounter. They model their behavior on that of significant others in their lives. These cultural "models" may actively communicate values, skills, and information; they may be passive objects of imitation or emulation, or they may play some intermediate "teaching" role (Rogoff et al., 2003). Whichever way transmission occurs, the models from whom an individual acquires his or her culture are limited in number, a small sample drawn from the larger population. In principle, any individual might learn some element of culture from any other individual in the world, but in practice we usually model our behavior on the behavior of a limited number of people from our own culture and subculture. In principle, an individual can invent a completely novel and personal body of knowledge, beliefs, and values, but in practice people make only marginal changes in the culture they inherit from others.

The transmission of culture between individuals is the engine of cultural replication and change but, for the most part, what any single individual member says or does has little impact on the process of change. Culture and cultural change are best viewed as population-level phenomena. Single individuals are largely prisoners of the culture they inherit but the decisions they make, and the outcomes of those decisions, are what drive cultural evolution. Summed over a *population* of individuals and over some span of time, some culturally characteristic behaviors, beliefs, and values become more common in the population, whereas others become less common, and still others disappear altogether. New cultural characteristics arise and either "survive" and spread through the population or fade away.

Thus, the all-important population-level phenomena of cultural evolution that we describe here emerge from the aggregation of myriad events and decisions at the individual level. A long tradition of social, cognitive, and developmental-psychological research provides us with a basic understanding of cultural transmission, of how information is learned and processed, and how cultural norms are adopted and developed by individuals and groups (e.g., Asch, 1951; Bandura, 1986; Bloom, 2000; Festinger, Schachter, & Back, 1950; Newcomb, 1943; Newcomb, Koenig, Flacks, & Warwick, 1967; Rogers, 1995; Sherif & Murphy, 1936; Tomasello, 1999). Cultural psychologists, by investigating the degree of diversity between and within populations, observe the effects of cultural variation on behavior.

A massive gulf exists between the individual-level social interactions during which cultural variants are acquired and modified and the long-term population-level changes that cause two groups of people to become "culturally different." However this gulf can be bridged by methods developed by population geneticists to study genetic evolution. Viewed at the population level, "Culture" (i.e., the pool of cultural information associated with a population) has a certain formal similarity to the pool of genes associated with a species. Theorists have therefore capitalized on this similarity to create mathematical models of the cultural evolutionary process (e.g., Boyd & Richerson, 1985; Cavalli-Sforza & Feldman, 1981). Evolutionary biology also furnishes inspiration for empirical investigations of cultural evolution (Baum, Richerson, Efferson, & Paciotti, 2004; Insko et al., 1983; Jacobs & Campbell, 1961; McElreath et al., 2005).

In other words, applying these methods provides the opportunity to investigate cultural change in much the same way that changes in the composition of a population's gene pool can be investigated. Studying culture in this way is not "biological reductionist" in the sense that it relies on an assumption that individuals are biologically determined to acquire specific behaviors (Richerson & Boyd, 2005).

What it does rely on is the assumption that humans are genetically adapted to acquire some of the cultural characteristics of the people with whom they associate. Few would disagree with this. Undoubtedly genes play some role in the directions in which cultures evolve, but this role is limited. For example, the human senses of taste and smell undoubtedly place constraints on the evolution of diets, but this is far from deterministic. Many cultures have evolved cuisines rich in spices and aromas that generate alarm and disgust in the "untutored" palate. In the very long run, cultures actually create the environments to which its members must adapt genetically. This leads to the co-evolution of genes with culture.

The main purpose of theoretical models of cultural evolution is to investigate the large-scale and long-term consequences of the aggregate of individual-level events. However, cultural evolutionary analysis can also be performed in reverse; given a characteristic, such as the human propensity to cooperate in large groups of distantly related people, models can help to investigate what sorts of individual-level properties might give rise to such an outcome. Only in the simplest cases is this exercise trivial. By using mathematical models to create predictions about cultural evolution that can then be tested, cultural psychology will more fully develop its potential as an experimental science.

Evolutionary analysis of culture provides an answer to the commonest criticism leveled at cultural explanations of human behavior—that they are not actually explanatory. The suggestion that people behave according to the dictates of their cultures is little more than description, and many social scientists are more impressed by the power of explanatory systems, such as economics and behavioral ecology, which allow deep causal analyses of human behavior. The fact that cultural variation exists is important in its own right, but these social scientists also want to explain how the variations arise. Cultural evolution undertakes to provide this explanation. The basic format of evolutionary analyses is a virtuous circle. Individuals in one sense are prisoners of their cultures. What we believe, how we behave, and so on, are largely based on what we acquire from our culture. But, at the same time, our decisions about which elements of the culture we encounter to adopt and the effects of those decisions upon our lives are the most important motors of cultural diversification. In the long run, culture is shaped by the actions its individual members and the consequences of those actions.

Evolutionary theory and empirical studies allow us to describe the behaviors and processes that maintain and destroy cultural variation. We review this work with an emphasis on contemporary cultural change. Losses of cultural diversity due to the apparent assimilation of smaller cultures and the "globalization" of some aspects of culture are often noted. On the other hand, new variations arise and many old variants stubbornly resist conversion to modernity. Commentators commonly express the fear that cultural change in the modern world will inevitably lead to homogeneity as the members of smaller cultures are assimilated into larger ones. We argue that the processes of cultural evolution will ensure that cultural diversity is maintained. The pattern of cultural diversity has changed and is likely to change further, however, so it is likely that culturally different groups will become less distinct.

THE CAPACITY FOR CUMULATIVE CULTURE

For the last 30 years or so, most of the scholars who have applied Darwinian thinking to human behavior have investigated the evolution of psychological mechanisms acquired via the genetic rather than the cultural inheritance system. Insights developed in the 1960s and 1970s into how natural selection acts on behavioral genes (Hamilton, 1964; Trivers, 1971, 1972; Williams, 1966) have led to a revolution in our understanding of the reproductive and social behavior of nonhuman animals and have formed the theoretical basis of many investigations of human behavior. The idea that evolved psychological mechanisms interact with environmental circumstances to produce specific behaviors inspired many testable hypotheses, and much fruitful science has been accomplished (e.g., Buss, 1999; Cronk, Chagnon, & Irons, 2000), but inevitably the extent to which such studies can explain human behavior is limited.

We humans undoubtedly possess many genetically evolved psychological mechanisms that allow us to make sense of the environment, and that structure the ways we perceive information from our senses. We share many of these cognitive capacities with other animals. But among the evolved mechanisms unique to humans, the most important the ones govern the way we acquire, use, modify, abandon and pass on cultural information. Behavioral characteristics acquired through our genetic inheritance cannot begin to explain the complexity and diversity of human behavior. Humans thrive in a wide variety of natural habitats, consuming a wide variety of diets and constructing a complicated variety of social systems. Yet among the 6 or so billion humans worldwide there is far less *genetic* diversity than among the fewer than 200,000 chimpanzees occupying African forests (H. Kaessmann & Pääbo, 2002; H. Kaessmann, Wiebe, & Pääbo, 1999; Tamura & Nei, 1993).

The classical explanation for greater diversity of human behavior is that individual humans *learn* behavior from one another rather than rely on instinct. This is also too simplistic. Animal species as diverse as rats, pigeons, and fish, as well as chimpanzees, have been found to acquire behaviors through social learning (Moore, 1996). Once a behavior exists in a population, the likelihood increases that the behavior will be exhibited by members of subsequent generations. This can result in persistent differences between the behaviors observed in separate groups of animals. Such behavioral diversity, which cannot be explained by genetic or environmental differences, is by many definitions evidence of culture (Byrne et al., 2004). Comparisons of the behaviors observed in the six most widely studied chimpanzee populations revealed that each community possesses a distinctive repertoire of behaviors that, if observed in human populations, would be reported as cultural differences (Whiten et al., 1999). However, the chimpanzee cultural repertoire is very limited compared to the powerful technologies and complex institutions that characterize human cultures.

Human cultures are more complex because they are the product of many generations of *accumulated* cultural change. The cultures of other animals—even of chimpanzees—show at most very modest signs of cumulative improvement (Boyd & Richerson, 1996). Useful behaviors may be acquired through social learning, but these are all behaviors that the individuals could, and often do, learn on their own. In human cultures, by contrast, each newborn member has access to a vast body of knowledge and

know-how that is far greater than a single individual could learn by experience, even in several lifetimes of experience. Learning and invention enables individuals to contribute to the body of cultural knowledge, but no one starts from scratch. Just as *genetic* evolution is the accumulation of small changes in *genes* that gave an advantage to the organisms that carried them, *cultural* evolution is a process that allows useful *cultural* variants to be acquired, improved upon, then passed on. Small success builds on small success.

Experimental studies comparing human and chimpanzee abilities to acquire behaviors by social transmission show that we are the more adept imitators by a large margin (Tomasello, 1996; Whiten & Custance, 1996). The behavior of apes who have observed a demonstration suggests that they rarely copy a precise procedure but are inclined to use it as a guide to developing their own solution to a problem (Whiten & Custance, 1996). Children, on the other hand, are such faithful imitators that they have been found to persist in using a demonstrated technique for obtaining a reward that apes soon abandon for a more efficient method of their own devising. Many years of observing chimpanzees in the wild has yielded little evidence of what might be construed as one chimpanzee trying to tell another something useful (Byrne, 1995); however, for a more generous interpretation of chimpanzee social learning, see Boesch (2003). High-fidelity imitation and evaluative communication or teaching (Castro & Toro, 2004) seem to be a derived package of cognitive and motivational traits that provide the psychological foundation for our complex cultural repertoires.

Cultural diversity in humans grows directly out of the cumulative evolution of complex cultural repertoires. Part of this diversity is due to historical happenstance. Cultures evolve in partial isolation and tend to diverge from one another as small differences accumulate generation by generation. The purest examples are from the symbolic part of cultural repertoires, such as language (Bettinger, Boyd, & Richerson, 1996; Labov, 2001; Logan & Schmittou, 1998; Nettle, 1999; Thomason, 2001), whereas variants such as technical skills are influenced by environmental factors. When populations live in different habitats, adaptive processes of cultural change lead to diversification, because variants appropriate to the respective habitats are most likely to be adopted.

Adaptive cultural change can, of course, also lead to convergence when populations live in similar environments (Johnson & Earle, 2000). Groups that make their living in a desert will likely develop some similar practices whether the desert is in Australia or Tunisia. However, adaptive processes also leave ample room for historical factors that maintains variation between populations, even if their survival problems are similar. Complex cultural adaptations can vary along many dimensions. The "design topography" is probably quite rough and likely to lead to many local optima. For example, the problem of carrying and storing water can be solved in a number of ways, and a culture that has already developed the skill of weaving waterproof baskets may never acquire the technology for producing pottery and vice versa. Partially isolated cultures evolve along different trajectories even if the only processes operating are adaptive and deterministic (Boyd & Richerson, 1992a).

An ability and desire to influence and to be influenced are important elements of the psychological processes that govern the transmission of cultural information, but again, there are more complexities. If the transmission of cultural information were simply a matter of demonstration by those who are knowledgeable and faithful copying by those who are naive, cultural evolution would be slow and very similar to biological evolution. Copying errors would be the only source of variation and variants would be selected by natural selection alone. Cultural evolution is rapid and allows rapid adaptation, because the human capacity for culture includes psychological mechanisms that enable individuals to introduce variation and make better than random choices between the cultural variants to which they are exposed (Durham, 1991; Richerson & Boyd, 2005). Classic social-psychological investigations of social influence and persuasion have show that there is a fair amount of consistency in the social conditions that result in individuals and groups remembering some things and forgetting others, or adopting some norms and attitudes and eschewing others (Asch, 1951; Hovland, Janis, & Kelley, 1953; Sherif & Murphy, 1936). As we argue later, it is likely that the "decisions" this involves also rely on evolved psychological mechanisms that increase the likelihood of individuals ending up with the optimum arrangement of beliefs and behaviors that their culture has to offer.

BIOLOGICAL AND CULTURAL EVOLUTION

The molecular mechanics of the biological inheritance system are now well understood and the idea that a physical substance (DNA) carries inherited information has become part of mass culture. Richard Dawkins (1976) proposed a Darwinian analysis of cultural change in which "memes" are analogous to genes. Dawkins envisaged memes to be discrete replicators that spread through a population and which can be worked on by natural selection. One problem with this way of thinking about cultural evolution is the variableness of cultural variants. Some are discrete units of information (e.g., the fact that chili peppers are safe to eat despite their sensory effects), but others (e.g., beliefs about what constitutes appropriate work for a lady) are more complex and perhaps cannot be faithfully transferred from mind to mind (Sperber, 1996, Chap. 5).

We cannot, at least not yet, define the nature of a "meme" or even know whether it is useful to think of culture as a collection of units, but this lack of understanding does not prevent a Darwinian analysis of cultural change. Many schemes for transmitting heritable variation are susceptible to a broadly Darwinian analysis (Richerson & Boyd, 2005, pp. 80–94). Remember that Darwin laid the foundations of evolutionary analysis with no knowledge of genes, what they do, or how they mutate. For the evolution of an information system to be analyzed, only two criteria need be met: (1) The system must contain characteristics that can be passed on (i.e., inherited), and (2) these characteristics must vary between individuals in a population. Darwin recognized that variants continue in a population as long as they continue to be inherited, and that the probability of their recurrence in the next generation can be affected by a number of forces. Exactly the same can be said about the information, technology, beliefs, ideas, preferences, habits, expertise, and all the other potentially variable elements that make up culture. The key to evolutionary analysis is identifying and investigating the forces that affect the continuity of cultural characteristics and the emergence of new ones.

The variability of cultural elements is undoubtedly shaped to some extent by preferences laid down by human genetic inheritance (Barkow, Cosmides, & Tooby, 1992; Daly & Wilson, 1983; Durham, 1991), but when it comes to deciding how to behave, culture routinely overwhelms biology. For example, military training (Richerson & Boyd, 1999) and religious indoctrination (Wilson, 2002) often lead people to perform feats of altruism on behalf of their community, fellow believers, or a whole nation, without in anyway benefiting their "selfish genes." More prosaically, individuals are routinely persuaded to endure pain to behave according culture's norms. For example, many Western women feel compelled to dance while wearing 3-inch stiletto heels. Given the permanent problems with the feet and back that this has been observed to cause (Rudicel, 1994), the wearing of currently fashionable female footwear bears a disturbing similarity to the foot-binding practices in 19th-century China (Brown, 2004). The need to avoid causing more immediate or severe damage does seem to set limits on cultural evolution, however. Actual amputation of healthy feet and a preference for hand walking are unlikely to become cultural norms.

The constraints that the human genetic endowment places on cultural evolution have to be seen in the context of the effect that culture has had on the composition of that endowment. The practices and preferences that a population acquires through cultural evolution also affect the selection of genes, such as when a cultural preference for certain physical characteristics makes it more likely that an individual with these traits is chosen as a sexual partner, or less likely that she is chosen as a victim of infanticide.

Gene selection can also occur as a result of two less direct mechanisms. First, the adoption of a cultural practice can result in some individuals thriving at the expense of others. For example, populations that learned how to extract a nutritious food source (milk) from domesticated grazing animals were better equipped to exploit the grassland habitat, but not all members of the population would have benefited equally. Those lucky enough to have a genetic makeup that enabled them to continue drinking milk beyond the age of weaning were better able to tolerate the new food. After a number of generations, the migration or poor survival of individuals who could not produce the enzyme that breaks down the milk sugar (lactose) would have made the genotype that confers lactose tolerance virtually universal in populations for which milk is an important component of the diet (Simoons, 1969, 1970). Sec-

ond, the practices of a population may alter the environment in such a way that the selective pressures on the population are changed. An example of this is the increase in the incidence of the sickle-cell genes in West African populations that began to cultivate yams (Durham, 1991). The growing of yams required the cutting of clearings in the rain forest. This increased the amount of standing water, which in turn increased the prevalence of malaria-carrying mosquitoes. And this, in turn, increased the relative chances of survival of individuals who were protected from malaria because they carried a sickle-cell gene.

The preferences and practices inherited culturally can also shield transmitted characteristics from the action of natural selection (Laland, Richerson, & Boyd, 1996). For example, if the range of a species of animal widens to include regions with colder climates, those individuals whose physiology and anatomy make them better able to withstand the cold have a selective advantage. In the case of humans, individuals with a round, high surface-to-volume ratio body shape require less energy to remain warm than do individuals who are tall and thin. However, clothing, fire, and other culturally evolved methods of protecting against the cold reduce the selective pressure exerted by nature and allow a population to maintain a wider variety of body shapes or to evolve toward body shape that meets a *culturally* evolved preference rather than one that is environmentally expedient. Culture enables groups of humans to create (and constantly recreate) the ecological niche they inhabit (Odling-Smee, Laland, & Feldman, 2003). Inevitably, as in all ecological niches, the composition of the gene pool changes as some individuals achieve greater reproductive success. These genetic changes can then influence the course of cultural evolution.

The coevolution of genes and culture creates opportunities for behaviors to evolve that could not have evolved through the action of natural selection on genes alone. Modern human behavior is the product of many hundreds of generations of interplay between the genetic and cultural inheritance systems. In chimpanzee groups, powerful, successful alpha males usually mate with all the females in their group, as they become fertile, and are aggressive to rival males. Stronger males therefore have more offspring than weaker ones, and their male offspring are likely to inherit not only the father's strength but also genes that promote taking advantage of strength. The evolution of a group of primates with the capacity for culture (e.g., our early hominid ancestors) can go in a quite different direction. The females of such a group might *culturally* evolve a preference for males who are not promiscuous, who help provision their offspring, and who are reluctant to fight. In this *cultural* environment, females may still prefer large strong capable males, but they especially favor those with genes that endow them with a tendency to suppress sexual and competitive aggression to devote effort to productive activities.

Biological evolution can explain altruism between kin and individuals who develop a long history of reciprocal mutual aid, but the extensive cooperation seen in humans between nonrelatives is a puzzle from the point of view of standard evolutionary theory. Gene–culture coevolution provides an explanation for the evolution of behaviors that allow humans to create cooperative social groupings of nonrelatives (Richerson, Boyd, & Henrich, 2003), but it is not the only explanation entertained by evolutionists (Henrich et al., 2003). Groups that interact infrequently can evolve very different cultural traditions and institutions. The ones with cultures that enable or encourage their members to behave more effectively will thrive at the expense of groups that are less culturally well endowed. Therefore, cultural evolution is more susceptible to group selection than is genetic variation. Groups that developed traditions of punishing selfish behavior that was detrimental to the group as a whole may well have been more successful than groups that tolerated more individualistic behavior. Genes that facilitate cooperation could have arisen in such groups, because the cultural environment would have favored individuals who were more docile and willing to behave in accordance with cultural norms. Repeated coevolutionary cycles eventually could drastically modify the psychological mechanisms that influence human social interaction (Boyd & Richerson, 1992b; Boyd, Gintis, Bowles, & Richerson, 2003).

Note that sharing knowledge with others is potentially a form of altruism and also a potential means of exploiting others by propagating self-serving ideas (Cohen & Vandello, 2001). Language vastly expanded our capacity to transmit both useful and deceptive information to others (Knight, Studdert-Kennedy, & Hurford, 2000). Complex culture can arise only if members of a group socialize their youngsters to be informed and "properly behaved" fellow members of their cultural group, and it can only be maintained if a large enough group of individuals continues to hold, share, and pass on the information possessed by the group. The number of people needed to support cultures of hunter-gatherers is surprisingly large, as Henrich (2004) shows in his comparison of the technological complexity of a number of hunter-gatherer cultures. When Europeans first encountered the aborigines inhabiting Tasmania, their population of 4,000 had a very limited tool kit compared to that of mainland aborigines. Archeological investigation has revealed that during the 10,000 to 12,000 years since rising sea levels caused Tasmania to be cut off from the mainland, the isolated islanders gradually lost many skills their ancestors had possessed, including fishing and the making of clothes.

The diversity of languages and other symbolic elements of culture is interesting in this light because divergence of language essentially socially isolates groups. Why did a characteristic evolve that places constraints the complexity of culture? In small-scale societies, the people who are subject to the same norms of cooperation also speak the same language or dialect. Did rapid change in language become established because the resulting dialect variation serves to protect the members of a cultural group from members of groups with which they no longer regularly communicate? When groups can no longer effectively communicate, members are less likely to inadvertently betray their own group's cultural secrets to competing groups, and they are also unlikely to be manipulated by malign advice or comments from competitors. In modern contexts, linguistic variation grows rapidly along social fault lines, generating new linguistic diversity, and perhaps protecting and generating other forms of cultural diversity (Labov, 2001). Contrariwise, the establishment of standard forms of speech via education and mass media is arguably responsible for the emergence of national sentiments and the destruction of much small-scale cultural variation in the large societies of the modern period (Anderson, 1991). Most likely, the social psychology that we deploy in deciding whom to trust for purposes of imitation and teaching has innate elements that were built by gene–culture coevolution.

That humans are highly cooperative animals is supported both by common experience and experimental evidence. People may complain about the selfishness and dishonesty they encounter, but the fact that such behavior is considered worthy of complaint is telling. Our societies only function because there is a general level of trust, an expectation that we will be trusted, and a willingness to identify and punish individuals who behave in an untrustworthy way. To investigate the nature of human cooperativeness, economists have developed games for people to play in the laboratory that give subjects the opportunity to behave selfishly or cooperatively in an environment where social cues that encourage cooperation can be controlled.

One of these games, Ultimatum, is played between two players who are never known to each other. One player is randomly selected to be the "proposer," with the task of proposing how a sum of money will be divided. The other, the "responder," can accept this division or reject it. If the proposal is rejected, neither player gets any money. This game played between selfish rationalists would result in the proposer getting the maximum share possible and the responder accepting whatever remains; even a 99 to 1 split would be accepted by a selfish rationalist, because anything is better than nothing. The overwhelming conclusion of these studies when carried out in Western populations is that humans do not behave like selfish rationalists. Most proposers share the money 50–50, and many responders reject offers smaller than 25–30% of the proposer's windfall.

In a series of studies that exemplify current quantitative cross-cultural research, Henrich et al. (2004) took the Ultimatum game to 15 cultures with varying degrees of integration into the global economic system. They found that the more contact and integration the groups had with modern market economies, the more likely their members were to choose a 50–50 distribution. The more isolated the culture, the more likely their members were to propose and accept offers that those in market economies would find unfair or bizarre. The family-based Machiguengan culture of southeastern Peru both propose and accept very low offers, and members of the Gnau and Au culture of Papua New Guinea make offers of a larger then 50% share. (The larger offers were likely to be refused because, in this culture, accepting such offers would make the responder uncomfortably indebted to the proposer.) The 50–50 split commonly agreed upon by members of market economies perhaps reflects a greater exposure to the cultural tradition of fair dealing with strangers that allows modern markets to operate. Even if a concept of how to deal with strangers is partly a cultural construct, however, in none of the cultures did players behave like selfish rationalists—hence, the conclusion that humans possess a genetically evolved tendency to behave cooperatively. The innate tendencies are reinforced, however, by culturally evolved practices that promote cooperation and trust.

Human social instincts also include what may be thought of as cultural tools, such as the capacity to acquire rapidly a sophisticated symbolic system of exchanging information (language), a tendency to categorize human groups on the basis of appearance or dialect, or symbolic markers such as dress (Gil-White, 2001; Richerson & Boyd, 2001), and a set of preferences or biases that influence which cultural variants an individual chooses to acquire (Richerson & Boyd, 2005). These preferences serve as a quick means of choosing which cultural variants to acquire. Such shortcuts are necessary because, as cultures accumulate values, skills, knowledge, and so forth, their members have an increasingly wide choice of variants to adopt. This makes it increasingly difficult, and eventually impossible, for members to even be aware of every cultural variant available. If humans had spent a large proportion of their time investigating the value of each variant, culture would have ceased to be effective as a way of enabling individuals to gain expertise rapidly. Individuals who made reasonably good decisions quickly would have been more successful than those who made bad decisions and *also more successful* those who made good decisions but only after much deliberation (Gigerenzer & Goldstein, 1996). The ability to make sensible judgments quickly would have been reflected in the number of children an individual produced, so natural selection would have favored individuals with innate preferences that made such behavior most likely.

One obvious rule of thumb to follow when deciding whether to replace a cultural variant would be to avoid replacing a familiar belief or behavior with a new one, unless there is a good reason to do so. There are also often practical reasons for maintaining the status quo. Standardizing driving practices worldwide, so that everyone drives on the left-hand side of the road, may bring long-term benefits, but the short-term expense and chaos it would bring has caused few countries to even contemplate it. In many domains, however, humans readily investigate novel cultural variants. Judging by the alacrity with which people embrace unfamiliar foods, be it "ethnic cuisine" or Western "fast food," we are relatively unconservative in our taste in food. Historical inertia is profoundly important in characterizing a culture, but individuals who fear novelty and doggedly follow old ways would have been at a disadvantage compared to those willing to consider promising innovations.

One reason for suspecting that a new cultural variant is worthwhile is that other people have adopted it. The social provenance of a variant is usually easier to establish than its actual worth, and it is reasonable to assume that at least some of the individuals who adopted the variant would have taken the trouble to evaluate its worth. A good rule of thumb to follow when contemplating what cultural variants to adopt is to imitate behaviors that are popular with people similar to oneself, who seem confident in what they are doing or are considered worthy of admiration (Boyd & Richerson, 1985; Henrich & Gil-White, 2001). Research generally supports the existence of such preferences in people's conformity to social norms (Asch, 1956; Sherif & Murphy, 1936) and adoption of attitudes (Chaiken, 1979; Simons, Berkowitz, & Moyer, 1970; Wright, 1966).

The transmission of cultural information depends on which cultural variants individuals acquire, so, at the population level, these preferences can be seen as "forces" that influence the direction of cultural evolution. The magnitude and interaction of a number of forces affect the ways that cultures change.

THE PROCESSES OF CULTURAL EVOLUTION

Any particular bit of cultural variation is likely to be subject to a complex of processes, with some tending to increase its future representation in the culture, and others, decrease it. It is impossible to predict precisely how a culture is likely to change because of the complex concatenation of forces that influences this change. This does not mean, however, that cultural change is unfathomable; it is complex but not random. The evolutionary analysis of cultural evolution follows the same pattern as genetic

evolution, although the details are considerably different.

First of all, consider the inheritance system. In the *genetic* inheritance system, the information, coded in genes, is transmitted from parents to offspring with considerable fidelity. The transmission process itself merely recreates the population from generation to generation, with no change in the frequencies of genes. The cultural inheritance system is not nearly so rigid. Transmission of cultural information can be from parents to offspring, from other adults to children, or among people of similar age and experience. Cavalli-Sforza and Feldman (1981), following the terminology used by epidemiologists, termed the three prototypical types of transmission as follows: *vertical*, *oblique*, and *horizontal*, respectively. To the extent that such patterns of transmission operate by faithful teaching or imitation, the looser structure of cultural transmission still acts to replicate the status quo. As in the genetic inheritance system, the transmission process itself does not affect the frequency of cultural variants. Whether a transmitted vertically, horizontally, or obliquely, cultural variant is still passed on.

Evolution occurs in both the genetic and cultural inheritance system because of forces that cause the frequency of variants in the population to change. Some of the forces are the same in both systems, so it is worthwhile to look for a moment at the simpler genetic evolutionary process.

The extent to which a *gene* is present in the next generation depends on four forces:

1. *Natural selection*—The genes of individuals who are more efficient converters of environmental resources to offspring are more highly represented in the offspring generation.
2. *Mutation*—Copying errors and damage to genes cause random changes to individual genes, slightly reducing the level of parental genes and generally increasing genetic diversity.
3. *Drift*—All populations are finite, so there is never a perfectly probabilistic distribution of parental genes for reasons that have nothing to do with their effects on the organisms that possess them.
4. *Migration*—Flows of genes between subpopulations who might be adapted to slightly different environmental conditions

reduce the effect of natural selection and drift.

The basic task for cultural evolutionists is the same as that of evolutionary biologists: to identify and investigate the forces that affect the transmission of characteristics in a population (in this case, the *cultural* characteristics) using mathematical models and empirical investigation. The purpose of the models is not to produce precise descriptions or predictions of cultural change, but to investigate the operation of forces at the population level. They are useful in the same way that meteorological models are useful for forecasting (but not precisely predicting) future weather. The systems that affect weather are so complex that even vastly complex models cannot predict the detail of weather and climate change. However, relatively simple models provide useful broad-brush explanations and forecasts that improve as our understanding of meteorological processes increases.

First of all, changes in the frequency of cultural variants that occur over time are influenced by the same four forces identified as influencing the remolding of the combination of genetic variants that exist in a population:

1. *Natural selection*—The prevalence of variants decline if they are possessed by people who have fewer offspring.
2. *Mutation*—Random changes in cultural variants occur when learners do not reproduce them accurately.
3. *Drift*—The flow and transmission of cultural information cannot be completely uniform throughout a population, so inevitably there are random differences in the cultural variants to which groups are exposed. Groups within a culture whose members have little contact with one another increasingly diverge.
4. *Migration*—New variants to a population via migration result in decreased prevalence of the old ones.

The evolution of culture differs from the evolution of genes most strikingly in being subject to what we call "decision-making forces." Because cultural transmission is spread out over a significant fraction of our lives, the cultural variants we adopt are influenced by the behavioral choices of the individuals taking part in our social interactions. Our choices (consciously or unconsciously) about what we say or display to the people with whom we interact affect which of our behaviors and beliefs they are exposed to. Once a cultural variant has been displayed, its transmission then depends on the choice made (consciously or unconsciously) by each observer. Will he adopt it, ignore it, dismiss it, reject it, not notice it, or forget it? Evolved cultural acquisition tools create innate preferences or "biases" that incline a person to adopt some variants rather than others. These biases, operating in each individual member of a culture, sort among existing cultural variants, causing some to increase in frequency and others to decrease. Donald Campbell (1965) called biases "vicarious selectors," because he imagined that the biases themselves ultimately arise from the action of natural selection on the genetic and cultural features of the biases. Vicarious selectors evolve because being naturally selected is a costly business, and behavioral mechanisms to anticipate and forestall it are favored. However, the higher order effects vary depending on the type of bias.

Innate cultural acquisition tools are undoubtedly shaped and sharpened by learning, both individual and social learning. For example, once a child reaches adolescence, she may begin to imitate her parents less and abandon some vertically acquired cultural variants in favor of those of her peers or teachers. This change may occur because her culture expects adolescents to begin to ignore parental influence, but the adolescent may also have had personal experiences that lead her to realize that her parents' judgments are often not reliable in some areas. And there might also be an innate component to teenage rebellion. In ancestral populations, children who began to question parental authority once they approached sexual maturity may have had greater reproductive success than those who maintained childish compliance. Any genes that encouraged "teenage rebellious" behavior would then have been genetically selected.

Establishing the factors that influence the adoption and development of social norms by individuals and by groups has been the aim of much very fruitful research in social psychology. Although most social psychologists have not approached the study from an evolutionary perspective, their findings are consistent with the operation of psychological mechanisms that evolved, because they encouraged quick and reasonably effective decisions on which cultural variants to acquire (Gigerenzer & Goldstein, 1996). For example, the "elaboration likelihood model" of Petty and Cacioppo (1986) describes two routes by which exposure to a message leads (or fails to lead) to a change in attitude. In taking what they call the "central route to attitude change," an individual decides to take up a new cultural variant by considering the content of a persuasive message. However, the "peripheral route to attitude change" provides an alternative decision-making mechanism for those who are unable or lack the motivation to elaborate on the content of the message. Instead, a quick assessment of peripheral cues (e.g., pleasant images or emotions, or indicators of expertise) associated with the source of the message and its delivery provides the basis of evaluation. Attitudes formed by the peripheral route are, however, less stable and less likely to predict behavior than those formed by the central route.

Boyd and Richerson (1985) considered three "learning biases" that arise from the way individuals decide which cultural variants to adopt.

1. *Content-based bias*—Individuals choose to adopt a cultural variant based on consideration of the variant itself. Essentially they take the "central route" (Petty & Cacioppo, 1986) to choosing a cultural variant. Some variants are clearly useful or superior to the alternatives. When the best choice is not so obvious, learners can weigh costs and benefits or determine how consistently a new variant compares with those that have already been adopted.

2. *Model-based bias*—Individuals can choose to adopt cultural variants based on consideration of the social provenance of the variant. In many cases, it may be more expedient for a learner to avoid the trouble of weighing whether a cultural variant is worth adopting and simply look at others who have adopted it and determine whether they are worthy of imitation. Are they happy, confident, and successful in terms with which the learner identifies? The literature on persuasion provides ample evidence that such considerations are very influential in individuals' decisions (e.g., Perloff, 2003). Prestige systems are usually based on symbols with which members of a culture identify. People in a given culture or subculture share a common definition of "prestige" and the behavior that defines it. For example, some English speakers (consciously or unconsciously) attach more significant to informa-

tion delivered with a "posh" accent, whereas others may favor other accents.

3. *Frequency-based bias*—Individuals can choose to adopt a cultural variant based on considering how popular it is. Very common variants are likely to have been adopted and kept for good reason (Henrich & Boyd, 1998). Individuals with a tendency to copy the most popular behavior are therefore likely to benefit from the experience of their fellow group members. In many cases, conforming also prevents a naive individual from inadvertently breaking some implicit rule of cooperation and risking punishment by fellow group members. Even if the practical benefits of a variant may be limited, there are social benefits associated with sharing the attitudes of other members of one's social network. If all of your friends have taken the trouble to learn the goal-scoring record of every member of the Premier League, it is a good idea to do the same, or risk having nothing to talk about in the pub on Friday nights. The classic social-psychological experiments of Asch, Sherif, and others established the tendency of humans to adjust their behavior to that of the people around them, and demonstrated the persistence of behaviors and beliefs thus acquired (Asch, 1956; Festinger et al., 1950; Newcomb, 1943; Newcomb et al., 1967; Sherif & Murphy, 1936). More recent research has attempted to characterize the group processes that contribute to the formation and change of social norms (Moreland, Levine, & McMinn, 2001; Postmes, Haslam, & Swaab, 2005).

A learner can only adopt cultural variants that are actually on display, so cultural transmission is also subject to "communicator biases." Individuals can choose when and to whom they display or communicate the variants in their cultural repertoire.

1. *Situation-based bias*—A tendency to conform to group norms limits the behaviors a person displays based on whether he or she is observed and the social situation. This reinforces the conformist bias on the part of the observers. Research in stereotyping has shown that cultural traditions influence how members of a culture behave in front of members of not only other cultures but also specific groups within their own culture based on sex, age, and occupation (Allport, 1954).

2. *Observer-based bias*—There is evidence

that evolved mechanisms influence contributions to a conversation. When asked what reproductive advice would be appropriate in a range of situations, mothers were more inclined to encourage behavior consistent with reproductive success if they were primed to think in terms of giving advice to a daughter rather than to a friend (Newson, 2003; Newson, Postmes, Lea, & Webley, 2005). Innate tendencies may also influence how an individual behaves in front of a group versus an individual, or with close friends versus strangers.

Human beings, acting as individuals or in groups, actively attempt to direct or influence cultural change. This introduces two more forces.

1. *Innovation*—Individuals occasionally invent a new cultural variant or (more often) modify an existing one rather than faithfully copying one of the existing cultural variants. The deliberate engineering of more appropriate genes has only begun to be a factor in biological evolution, but adjusting and improving cultural variants is an important force in cultural evolution. Individuals can mix social and individual learning in a way that is reminiscent of Lamarck's (and Darwin's) ideas about organic inheritance (Boyd & Richerson, 1989). Innovation usually takes more effort and is more risky than adopting cultural variants used by others, so it is more likely to occur when existing variants are inefficient. Perhaps existing variants are difficult to understand or to imitate correctly. Changes in the physical or cultural environment may have made them less appropriate. It is in the interest of societies to encourage innovation, because new variants that are more effective can then be copied by others, and the whole society potentially benefits. Populations are likely to be more successful if they evolve institutions that reward successful scholars and inventors and nurture those that show promise. A society that rewards its merely technically competent physicians more richly and more consistently than creative, talented biomedical and social researchers is likely to evolve an increasingly costly, cumbersome, and inefficient health system.

2. *Group decision making*—Conformity and group processes create the tendency for individuals within a network to agree on the cultural variants to adopt, but when the interests

of group members diverge, culturally evolved institutions for collective decision making may be employed (Boehm, 1996). Procedures involved in these more formal decision-making methods also influence cultural change. For example, decisions made through a referendum process are likely to differ from those made by committees of appointed experts. The extent to which a population employs formal decision-making processes is therefore also likely to affect the way a culture changes.

In summary then, cultural evolution is influenced by the same five factors that influence biological evolution:

1. Vertical transmission of variants (from parent to child)
2. Natural selection
3. Mutation
4. Drift
5. Migration

Added to this is the effect of the pattern of cultural variant transmission, which is more complex than the transmission of genetic information. As well as being transmitted from parent to child, cultural variants can be transmitted:

1. Between peers (horizontal transmission).
2. From older/more experienced nonparents to younger/less experienced individuals (oblique transmission).

Because of the greater complexity of cultural transmission, additional forces influence changes in frequency of cultural variants in a population:

1. Bias on the part of the person acquiring the cultural information (learning biases):
   - Content-based bias (based on an evaluation of the variant itself).
   - Model-based bias (based on an evaluation of the prestige or success of the source of the variant).
   - Frequency-based bias (based on an evaluation of the popularity of the variant).
2. Bias on the part of the person displaying or communicating the cultural information (communicator biases):
   - Situation-based bias (based on the communication's evaluation of the social situation).
   - Observer-based bias (based on the com-

municator's evaluation of the observers present).

3. Explicit attempts by members of a culture to influence cultural change:
   - Innovation—the invention of a new cultural variant that may potentially replace older ones.
   - Group decision-making processes—their nature and extent.

This concatenation of forces averaged over a population drives the cultural change the population experiences. By analyzing cultural change in terms of these forces, it is possible to explain patterns of historical cultural change broadly and to make testable predictions about changes in characteristics of cultures, such as patterns of diversity.

THE DYNAMICS OF CULTURAL DIVERSITY

Just as some genes are not passed on and disappear during the course of biological evolution, some cultural variants are ignored and eventually forgotten as culture evolves. However, new cultural variants are also constantly being created. Among the cultural evolutionary forces mentioned earlier, some act to generate cultural variants, whereas others cause variants to become extinct by the selection of some at the expense of others. There are also forces that have no effect on the total number of variants but do influence the way they are distributed. If "cultural diversity" is defined as the number of cultural variants available to members of a population, we can analyze changes in diversity by looking at the balance between the forces that generate new cultural variants and those that select between them. If "cultural diversity" is defined as the extent of cultural difference between groups or regions, we analyze it by looking at the balance between forces that disperse variants and those that create barriers to their dispersal.

Looking at the processes of cultural evolution one by one:

1. *Natural selection*—Any force that selects between variants reduces diversity. Selection normally acts to constrain variation within a culture. Many variants are passed from parents to offspring, so those that are associated with individuals who fail to thrive and produce offspring have a tendency to become less common

in a population. An extreme example is the values and beliefs of cults that requires their members to practice mass suicide or strict celibacy. Cultural variants associated with such groups are less likely to be passed on to future generations. An exception occurs when frequency-dependent selection favors rare types. As labor becomes increasingly divided in a society, for example, natural selection disfavors skills that are too common with respect to economic demand and favors scarcer skills. Complex societies have evolved an ever-increasing division of labor, and a good deal of within-culture diversity is the result of division of labor. Intersociety trade is important in most human societies, leading to some division of labor between societies. If all else is equal, intersociety division of labor reduces diversity within societies and increases it between societies.

Trade aside, selection has complex effects on intersocietal cultural diversity. Much between-societies cultural diversity is due to cultures adapting to local conditions. By the Late Pleistocene, anatomically modern hunter-gatherers had spread to virtually all the world's habitable landmasses, developing a considerable diversity of subsistence strategies (Klein, 1999). Adaptive divergence is limited to the extent that societies in similar environments acquire similar adaptations (Johnson & Earle, 2000). But adaptive convergence is never complete, in part because environments are never exactly alike (Diamond, 1997) and probably in part because, like other complex design problems, the same functions can be realized more or less equally well by rather different arrangements (Boyd & Richerson, 1992a). Modern developed nations are a case in point. Despite much convergence, the G-8 nations (the world's richest economies) retain many distinctive differences in every aspect of their societies.

2. *Mutation*—Random copying errors are the ultimate source of variation in genetic systems, and random errors in cultural transmission play a similar role. Random errors tend to increase diversity both within and between cultures. However, as Henrich (2004) has shown, the errors that occur in cultural transmission also limit the diversity of culture by limiting the complexity of cultural traits. Complex, multi-component cultural traits are more likely to be transmitted with fatal errors. Small populations are more likely to lack the rare, highly skilled individuals who can recognize and re-

pair mistakes that develop as complex techniques are passed on, so, as mentioned earlier, the internal complexity of the culture that a population can sustain is limited by its size. Henrich reviews evidence that sophisticated watercraft was lost not only on Tasmania but also on other small islands in Oceania despite their importance to subsistence on the islands that retained them. Under these assumptions, errors will cause similar losses in different small-scale societies, reducing the scope for both between-group and within-group diversity. Techniques for storing cultural information outside the human mind, such as in texts or pictures, can counteract this effect, allowing small communities, such as a scientific subdiscipline, to maintain a large store of complex knowledge (Barth, 1990; Donald, 1991).

3. *Drift*—When cultural variants are rare or seldom used in a population, there is a random chance that they will be forgotten, creating the cultural analogue of genetic drift. Drift, therefore, is a force that decreases the total number of cultural variants. Since the effects of drift are random and affect different cultures independently, diversity between cultures is increased by drift. Again, techniques for creating external stores for cultural information counter the effect.

4. *Migration*—Spatial and social mobility cause people who have adopted different cultural variants to interact. This increases cultural diversity on the local level, because a mix of culturally different people increases the number of variants to which individuals in each group can be exposed, but it has no effect on the overall number of cultural variants that exist. The cultural diversity between groups is reduced by migration.

Conquest is a special case of migration; the military or commercial conquest of culturally different populations often leads to considerable reductions in diversity. This is well documented in the case of languages (Nettle, 1999). For example, the European conquest of the Americas led to the loss of most Amerindian languages to Spanish and English. Foster's (1960) study of the spread of other elements of Spanish culture to Latin America is a classic. A rather limited subset of Spanish culture penetrated the New World, giving Latin America anomalously low cultural diversity along many dimensions besides language. The ethnographic record suggests that such conquests are an ancient factor in patterns of diversity (R. C.

Kelly, 1985; Knauft, 1985). In the contemporary world, global mass communication makes European, and especially American, culture known to practically everyone.

5. *Bias on the part of the person acquiring the cultural information (learning biases)*—These selective forces in which individuals choose to adopt only some cultural variants, while ignoring or abandoning others, generally bring an overall decrease in the diversity of cultural variants.

• *Content-based bias*—This is highly analogous to natural selection. A new cultural variant that is widely perceived to bring practical benefits will be widely adopted, thus decreasing cultural diversity. An example of this is the widespread adoption in Europe of the potato as a staple crop during the 17th and 18th centuries. In many farming areas, choosing to plant potatoes over other crops increased the amount of food a peasant family could produce and the number of children it could successfully raise. In the case of the potato, the benefits were found to be exaggerated, and the farmers' dependence on the crop resulted in widespread famine when potato blight destroyed crops in the 19th century. Nevertheless, cultivation of the new crop had contributed to a rapid population expansion that prompted the migration of Europeans to other continents.

The diversity-reducing effect of content-based bias is mitigated by individual or group differences, both learned and genetic. If some groups of Europeans had been genetically ill-equipped to digest potatoes, then they would have not adopted the crop. Most human populations outside of the traditional dairying populations of western Eurasia and Africa cannot digest milk sugar (Durham, 1991). Thus, in eastern Eurasia an alternate technology based on soybean products evolved to fill roughly the same nutritional niche as milk. Much cultural diversity exists because literal and figurative tastes differ. Adaptive diversification and convergence proceed in roughly the same way they do with natural selection.

• *Model-based biases*—The imitation of individuals deemed by a group or subculture to be good models has the effect of decreasing diversity within that group, while increasing diversity between groups that have different criteria for choosing good models. The effect is, therefore, like that of conformity bias. Symbolic systems are a very rich source of between-group diversity because of the arbitrary nature of symbols. High status can be symbolized by elaborate tattoos, as in Polynesia, or by "designer clothes," as in today's global commercial culture. Linguistic diversity is the most striking example.

• *Frequency-based bias*—Conforming to cultural norms by adopting the most common cultural variants in the cultural or subcultural group decreases diversity within groups and helps to maintain diversity between groups when migration occurs, because migrants begin to adopt the most common variants in the population they have joined.

6. *Communicator biases*—Individuals choosing the circumstances in which to display a cultural variant limits the number of cultural variants available for adoption. The effect varies, however, depending on the type of bias.

• *Situation-based bias*—Potential cultural models that regulate behavior depending on the social situation tends to reinforce ritual behavior, decreasing diversity within each social situation, but emphasizing differences between them. For example, "office worker behavior" may be similar in many different business organizations and quite different from the "factory worker behavior" in another part of the same organization. In both cases, the behavior displayed is likely to change substantially when individuals leave work to be with their families or take part in leisure activities. The long-term population-level effects of this have not been the subject of systematic investigation.

• *Observer-based bias*—Potential cultural models regulating their own behavior depending on who is watching is a barrier to the transmission of cultural variants and tends to decrease diversity within groups. For example, children mostly see adults displaying cultural variants that adults deem appropriate for them to see. However, this also tends to increase diversity between groups. Children then behave differently from adults, at least while adults are present. Again, the long-term population-level effects of the tendency of individuals to regulate their behavior in response to the observers present have not yet been subject to systematic investigation, however, so it is only possible to speculate on how this force may influence cultural evolution.

7. *Innovation*—The invention of new cultural variants is a force that increases diversity. New variants that are clearly superior to older variants may replace them, but often inventions increase choice and cultural complexity. For example, the invention of the automobile replaced bicycles and horses for many purposes, but the riding of bicycles and horses is still part of modern culture.

8. *Formal group decision-making processes*—When a group decision-making process is well supported by the group, it has the power to limit cultural diversity within the group and increase it between groups. Members cease to have the choice of whether to adopt a cultural variant. For example, if a decision to ban pornography is made and effectively enforced, the use of pornography cannot be adopted by group members. However, a group decision-making process is unlikely to maintain the support of the group if its decisions are unpopular with members, or if the decisions put the group at a disadvantage compared to other groups. Subcultures can often persist and even thrive in the face of considerable repression. For example, Handelman (1995) describes how the Russian Thieves' World organized crime community persisted in the face of Imperial and Soviet repression. One might have thought that authoritarian societies that invest much in police "services" and have heavy punishment for deviance might at least be free of organized crime. However, the Thieves' World rather successfully resisted suppression, much as the ethnically based prison and youth gangs thrive in the United States despite (or perhaps because of) long prison terms.

It may be the case that groups using similar group decision-making processes tend to make similar decisions. It is commonly alleged by some politicians, for example, that democracies are less likely to declare war. If this were the case, then finding effective means of group decision-making would have the effect of reducing cultural diversity between groups. Certain group decisions may support diversity. The most obvious would be decisions that specifically protect minority cultures. The U.S. Bill of Rights protects religion and speech, ensuring protections for many kinds of cultural variation. Swiss federalism provides for canton-level autonomy in many matters. Many group decisions have complex effects upon cultural diversity. Economic growth policies tend to bring modernity's effects on diversity, reducing local diversity in many aspects of culture, while increasing the diversity of occupations and spawning many medium-size subgroups, such as businesses and government bureaucracies.

REPRISE: EFFECTS OF MODERNIZATION

Modern communication and transportation technologies, and the development of global markets, have profoundly changed the social environments in which culture is propagated (Inkeles, 1983). By examining how these changes affect the balance of cultural evolutionary forces, we can estimate how these changes affect cultural diversity (Henrich et al., 2001; Shoumatoff, 2005).

In theory, modern communication could allow social influence to be centralized and the dissemination of cultural ideas to be dominated by a small number of powerful individuals or groups that could decide to suppress the dissemination of some cultural variants, while attractively presenting others. Even if such individuals had no malign intentions, their activities could, in theory, destroy diversity and create a homogenized global culture.

This is unlikely to be the case in practice, however, because whether a cultural variant is adopted or ignored depends on the decision-making processes in the minds of potential recipients of the information. Evidence suggests that increasing the means by which the information can be transmitted has little effect on these processes. For example, the wide-scale acquisition of mobile phone use behavior, which brought substantial changes to the lives of many people, did not occur immediately as a result of exposure to advertising and news of the new technology. The pattern of adoption traced the same S-shaped curve (Massini, 2004) as the adoption of hybrid corn among Midwestern farmers in the 1940s (Griliches, 1957), suggesting that the spread of mobile phone use largely took place by diffusion as nonusers modeled their behavior on those who had adopted the new technology. Their decisions were the result of some combination of model-based and frequency-based bias cultural transmission. Content-based bias undoubtedly also played a role. The rate of adoption was slightly influenced by variations in the cost of buying and using mobile phones, suggesting that at least some people partly based their decision on an analysis of costs and benefits.

Henrich (2001) has found that biased cultural transmission dominates in practically all cases of the diffusion of innovations.

Mass communication, therefore, may well hasten the spread of a useful new cultural variant at the *population* level, because it makes it possible to expose many people to the new cultural variant simultaneously, but *individuals* still go through the same process when deciding whether to adopt a new variant. This is substantially based upon observations of earlier adopters.

New technologies that threaten to reduce cultural variation may also provide means of preserving or increasing it. For example, random error in the transmission of cultural information (mutation) is a source of cultural variation that is potentially much reduced by computers, photocopiers, printers, and the equipment for audio and video recording and copying. Centrally planned educational syllabuses, textbooks, and standard exams attempt to ensure that all students in a population are exposed to more or less the same things in the same way. What consumers of information actually *learn*, however, cannot be controlled, and it may be that information reproduction technology actually *increases* the likelihood of errors in the transmission of cultural information. Cultural transmission occurs when a cultural variant is reproduced in a *human mind*, not on paper or disk. Simply presenting many people with many identical copies of accurately stored information does not ensure error-free transmission of the same cultural variant to every one of them. It fact, it vastly decreases the amount of information to which people can be exposed. Potential learners can choose where to direct their attention.

Although not decreasing the net amount of cultural variation, changes in social interaction can reduce diversity between groups and regions. This shift began with the development of agriculture. Pagel and Mace (2004) have suggested that human subpopulations continually secede and diverge from larger groups to better control some defensible resources. In a simple society of nomadic foragers, cultural divisions create geographical separation, because the physical environment is the source of the resources. The more resource-rich the physical environment, therefore, the larger the number of cultures it can support. The development of technologies that increase the resources extracted from the environment inevitably allow a greater diversity of cultures to occupy a given area. The development of agriculture increased the carrying capacity of some habitats enough to allow the growth of population centers of unprecedented size and density. This brought changes in the pattern of cultural diversity, with different cultures and subcultures inhabiting the same geographical space.

Some diversity of social roles does exist within mobile foraging cultures, primarily based on age and gender (R. L. Kelly, 1995), but all members of a cultural group exploit the same habitat or habitats, so they must all acquire more or less the same knowledge and skills. In sedentary societies, members have more opportunity to invest time and resources in modifying their home environment, creating artificial habitat diversity within a geographical region and increasingly making their living by exploitation of a range of *culturally* created niches. Those exploiting the "farming" niche needed to acquire different knowledge and skills than tradesmen, artisans, and soldiers. Cultural divisions therefore develop between occupational categories. Just as those who share a niche in the natural environment share a desire to defend the physical resources present within their territory, those who exploit the same cultural niche share a desire to control access to the resources that their skills and knowledge allow them to acquire.

Modernization amplifies and extends the changes that began with the advent of agriculture. Before modernization, most people migrated as part of their family or social group. Modernization brings *individual* spatial and social mobility (Bongaarts & Watkins, 1976; Zelinsky, 1971). Individuals migrate to urban centers to work in factories and often leave their region or country of birth. Children attend school and have less exposure to the cultural variants of their parents and more exposure to nonfamily culture. In the terms developed by cultural evolutionists, oblique and horizontal transmission increases and vertical transmission declines.

The increasing inclination of Western mothers to return work soon after giving birth causes nonparental exposure to begin earlier in a child's life. In many cases, this results in infants being exposed to cultural variants from nannies and day care assistants who are temporary or first-generation immigrants. Mass communication further increases the proportion of nonparental cultural trans-

mission. More and more of the cultural variants available to members of a modernizing society are transmitted between people who are not kin, friends, countrymen, or even acquaintances. Young people are therefore less likely to follow the ways of their parents and more likely to create novel recombinations of diverse cultural variants. As the modernization process continues, the choice of occupations, educational specializations, and ultimately leisure pursuits available to young people increases. Individuals whose genetic inheritance is very similar might end up with a very different cultural endowment.

One consequence of the decrease in interaction between kin that accompanies modernization may be the fundamental cultural change that is characteristic of modernizing societies; people begin to limit the number of children they produce and birthrates decline sharply (Newson et al., 2005). Social interactions between kin are more likely than interaction between friends or work colleagues to include encouragement or to reward behavior likely to lead to the expansion of the family (Newson et al., in press). In modern social networks, in which there is little contact between kin, the content of social influence is far less pronatal. Natural selection, therefore, favors people who have not embraced modernity, or who have adopted other cultural variants associated with modernity but not the belief that it is better to have a small family. Anabaptist populations, for example, have a high birthrate and are increasing rapidly because enjoy the prosperity associated with life in modern North America but resist cultural influences from outside their kinship-based communities (Richerson & Boyd, 2005, Chap. 5).

The size of modern populations and complexity of cultures and subcultures sharing the same space, resources, and problems have forced increased use of formal group decision making. Councils and representative bodies are by no means an innovation of modern cultures and have been observed in foraging societies (Boehm, 1996), but as societies become more complex, increasingly sophisticated institutions are necessary to reconcile the interests of individuals and groups that have access to, or desire access to, the same space and resources. Individuals and groups that are culturally very different increasingly share problems and must agree on solutions. Inevitably the increased use of decision-making bodies reduces cultural diversity, because these bodies are authorized to limit the cultural variants available to the populations they represent.

The need to find compromises and to make decisions that can be justified to all interested parties influences the decision-making process and inevitably the decisions themselves. Judgments must appear rational and consistent, and (where possible) be supported by evidence and appeal to a set of values appreciated by all the interested parties. The success of a formal decision-making body depends on the extent to which the population approves of the choices it provides. One form of group decision-making process that is an innovation of modern societies is the survey or opinion poll, through which putative "decision makers" can be guided on the decision to make. How the various, formal decision-making processes might affect cultural change has not yet been studied by evolutionists.

The technological and social changes associated with modernization increase rather than decrease the range of cultural variants available for individuals to acquire. Paradoxically, this can give the impression of reduced cultural diversity. Although the choice is wide, the same range of choices is increasingly available all over the world, particularly in urban areas. The cultural institutions, practices, and values necessary to allow culturally diverse groups to cohabit contribute to this impression. There is cultural-evolutionary convergence on variants, such as convertible currencies, a publicly acknowledged criminal code with formal trials of those accused of transgressions, evidence-based decision making, tolerance of diversity, and respect for individual choice that make effective and peaceful transactions possible.

SUMMARY AND CONCLUSION

It is useful to think of culture as a collection of "cultural variants" maintained in the minds or records of members of a population. This is analogous to the genes—the collection of "genetic variants" maintained in the gene pool of a species. Cultural change occurs by a process of evolution, as described by Darwin, which is analogous to but different in detail from biological evolution. Darwinian theory and mathematical modeling tools used by population geneticists to understand changes in the gene pool over time can be used to understand and model cultural change.

It is transmission of cultural information from individual mind to individual mind that maintains culture variants in a population, and it is the increased adoption of some variants (including new variants) compared to others that drives cultural change. The adoption of cultural variants is not random; remembering a fact, developing an opinion, or learning a skill is the result of a conscious or unconscious decision by an individual. The pattern of adoption of cultural variants has been the subject of investigation by social psychologists, and the findings are consistent with humans having evolved psychological mechanisms that bias decision making to increase the likelihood of an individual acquiring useful rather than maladaptive cultural variants. At the population level, these biases can be seen as forces that influence the direction of cultural evolution. Our ability to understand cultural differences and change can be improved by systematic observations of the forces driving cultural evolution and the creation of testable hypotheses that predict outcomes as a result of social and environmental change. This creates huge scope for research in quantitative ethnography and cultural psychology. The topic may be almost endlessly complex, but it is correspondingly endlessly fascinating, and our understanding can improve with study.

Modernization brings rapid cultural change, and we have presented here a demonstration of how cultural-evolutionary theory can be used to examine how modernization affects cultural diversity. Although it is often suggested that modernization reduces cultural diversity, an evolutionary analysis suggests a more mixed picture. If "diversity" is defined as the number and variety of cultural variants available for individuals to acquire, modernization undoubtedly increases diversity. If, however, "diversity" is seen as regional differences in available culture variants, then it has decreased. In small-scale societies, the complexity and diversity of culture within societies is small, but the diversity between small, local groups is large. Waves of modernization over the last few thousand years have created complex cultures with substantial diversity within them, but they destroy much small-scale variation in the course of their expansion. The formation of intermixing cultural groups, which began with the advent of agriculture and creation of population centers, increases rapidly with modernization.

REFERENCES

Allport, G. W. (1954). *The nature of prejudice.* Cambridge, MA: Addison-Wesley.

Anderson, B. (1991). *Imagined communities: Reflections on the origin and spread of nationalism* (Rev. and extended ed.). London: Verso.

Asch, S. E. (1951). Effects of group pressure upon the modification and distortion of judgments. In H. Guetzkow (Ed.), *Groups, leadership and men* (pp. 39–76). Pittsburgh: Carnegie Press.

Asch, S. E. (1956). Studies of independence and conformity: I. A minority of one against a unanimous majority. *Psychological Monographs, 70.*

Bandura, A. (1986). *Social foundations of thought and action: A social cognitive theory.* Englewood Cliffs, NJ: Prentice-Hall.

Barkow, J. H., Cosmides, L., & Tooby, J. (1992). *The adapted mind: Evolutionary psychology and the generation of culture.* New York: Oxford University Press.

Barth, F. (1990). Guru and the conjurer: Transactions in knowledge and the shaping of culture in Southeast Asia and Melanesia. *Man, 25*(4), 640–653.

Basalla, G. (1988). *The evolution of technology.* Cambridge, UK: Cambridge University Press.

Baum, W. M., Richerson, P. J., Efferson, C. M., & Paciotti, B. M. (2004). An experimental model of cultural evolution including traditions of rule giving and rule following. *Evolution and Human Behavior, 25,* 305–326.

Bettinger, R. L., Boyd, R., & Richerson, P. J. (1996). Style, function, and cultural evolutionary processes. In H. D. G. Maschner (Ed.), *Darwinian archaeologies* (pp. 133–164). New York: Plenum Press.

Bloom, P. (2000). *How children learn the meanings of words.* Cambridge, MA: MIT Press.

Boehm, C. (1996). Emergency decisions, cultural-selection mechanics, and group selection. *Current Anthropology, 37*(5), 763–793.

Boesch, C. (2003). Is culture a golden barrier between human and chimpanzee? *Evolutionary Anthropology, 12,* 82–91.

Bongaarts, J., & Watkins, S. C. (1996). Social interactions and contemporary fertility transitions. *Population and Development Review, 22*(4), 639–682.

Boyd, R., Gintis, H., Bowles, S., & Richerson, P. J. (2003). The evolution of altruistic punishment. *Proceeding of the National Academy of Sciences USA, 100,* 3531–3535.

Boyd, R., & Richerson, P. J. (1985). *Culture and the evolutionary process.* Chicago: University of Chicago Press.

Boyd, R., & Richerson, P. J. (1989). Social learning as an adaptation. *Lectures on Mathematics in the Life Sciences, 20,* 1–26.

Boyd, R., & Richerson, P. J. (1992a). How microevolutionary processes give rise to history. In M. H. Nitecki & D. V. Nitecki (Eds.), *History and evolution* (pp. 179–209). Albany: State University of New York Press.

Boyd, R., & Richerson, P. J. (1992b). Punishment allows the evolution of cooperation (or anything else) in sizable groups. *Ethology and Sociobiology, 13*(3), 171–195.

Boyd, R., & Richerson, P. J. (1996). Why culture is common but cultural evolution is rare. *Proceedings of the British Academy, 88,* 73–93.

Brown, M. J. (2004). *Is Taiwan Chinese?: The impact of culture, power, and migration on changing identities.* Berkeley: University of California Press.

Burrow, J. W. (1966). *Evolution and society: A study in Victorian social theory.* Cambridge, UK: Cambridge University Press.

Buss, D. M. (1999). *Evolutionary psychology: The new science of the mind.* Boston: Allyn & Bacon.

Byrne, R. (1995). *The thinking ape: Evolutionary origins of intelligence.* Oxford, UK: Oxford University Press.

Byrne, R., Barnard, P. J., Davidson, I., Janik, V. M., McGrew, W. C., Miklosi, A., et al. (2004). Understanding culture across species. *Trends in Cognitive Sciences, 8,* 341–346.

Campbell, D. T. (1965). Variation and selective retention in socio-cultural evolution. In H. R. Barringer, G. I. Blanksten, & R. W. Mack (Eds.), *Social change in developing areas: A reinterpretation of evolutionary theory* (pp. 19–49). Cambridge, MA: Schenkman.

Castro, L., & Toro, M. (2004). The evolution of culture: From primate social learning to human culture. *Proceedings of the National Academy of Science USA, 101*(27), 10235–10240.

Cavalli-Sforza, L. L. (2000). *Genes, peoples, and languages.* Farrar, Straus & Giroux.

Cavalli-Sforza, L. L., & Feldman, M. W. (1981). *Cultural transmission and evolution: A quantitative approach.* Princeton, NJ: Princeton University Press.

Chaiken, S. (1979). Communicator's physical attractiveness and persuasion. *Journal of Personality and Social Psychology, 37,* 1387–1397.

Cohen, D., & Vandello, J. (2001). Honor and "faking" honorability. In R. M. Nesse (Ed.), *Evolution and the capacity for commitment* (pp. 163–185). New York: Russell Sage Foundation.

Cronk, L., Chagnon, N. A., & Irons, W. (2000). *Adaptation and human behavior: An anthropological perspective.* New York: de Gruyter.

Daly, M., & Wilson, M. (1983). *Sex, evolution and behavior.* Boston: Willard Grant.

Dawkins, R. (1976). *The selfish gene.* Oxford, UK: Oxford University Press.

Diamond, J. (1997). *Guns, germs, and steel: The fates of human societies.* New York: Norton.

Donald, M. (1991). *Origins of the modern mind: Three stages in the evolution of culture and cognition.* Cambridge, MA: Harvard University Press.

Dunn, M., Terrill, A., Reesink, G., Foley, R. A., & Levinson, S. C. (2005). Structural phylogenetics and the reconstruction of ancient language history. *Science*, *309*, 2072–2075.

Durham, W. H. (1991). *Coevolution: Genes, culture, and human diversity*. Stanford, CA: Stanford University Press.

Fearon, J. D. (2003). Ethnic and cultural diversity by country. *Journal of Economic Growth*, *8*(2), 195–222.

Festinger, L., Schachter, S., & Back, K. (1950). *Social pressures in informal groups: A study of a housing community*. New York: Harper.

Foster, G. M. (1960). *Culture and conquest: America's Spanish heritage*. New York: Wenner-Gren Foundation for Anthropological Research.

Gigerenzer, G., & Goldstein, D. G. (1996). Reasoning the fast and frugal way: Models of bounded rationality. *Psychological Review*, *103*(4), 650–669.

Gil-White, F. J. (2001). Are ethnic groups biological "species" to the human brain?: Essentialism in our cognition of some social categories. *Current Anthropology*, *42*(4), 515–554.

Griliches, Z. (1957). Hybrid corn: An exploration of the economics of technological change. *Econometrica*, *48*, 501–522.

Hamilton, W. D. (1964). Genetic evolution of social behavior I, II. *Journal of Theoretical Biology*, *7*(1), 1–52.

Handelman, S. (1995). *Comrade criminal: Russia's new Mafiya*. New Haven, CT: Yale University Press.

Harpending, H. C., Batzer, M. A., Gurven, M., Jorde, L. B., Rogers, A. R., & Sherry, S. T. (1998). Genetic traces of ancient demography. *Proceedings of the National Academy of Sciences USA*, *95*(4), 1961–1967.

Henrich, J. (2001). Cultural transmission and the diffusion of innovations: Adoption dynamics indicate that biased cultural transmission is the predominate force in behavioral change. *American Anthropologist*, *103*(4), 992–1013.

Henrich, J. (2004). Demography and cultural evolution: Why adaptive cultural processes produced maladaptive losses in Tasmania. *American Antiquity*, *69*(2), 197–221.

Henrich, J., & Boyd, R. (1998). The evolution of conformist transmission and the emergence of between-group differences. *Evolution and Human Behavior*, *19*(4), 215–241.

Henrich, J., Boyd, R., Bowles, S., Camerer, C., Fehr, E., Gintis, H., et al. (2001). In search of *Homo economicus*: Behavioral experiments in 15 small-scale societies. *American Economic Review*, *91*(2), 73–78.

Henrich, J., Boyd, R., Bowles, S., Camerer, C., Fehr, E., & Gintis, H. (2004). *Foundations of human sociality: Economic experiments and ethnographic evidence from fifteen small-scale societies*. Oxford, UK: Oxford university Press.

Henrich, J., & Gil-White, F. J. (2001). The evolution of prestige—Freely conferred deference as a mechanism for enhancing the benefits of cultural transmission. *Evolution and Human Behavior*, *22*(3), 165–196.

Henrich, J., Bowles, S., Boyd, R. T., Hopfensitz, A., Richerson, P. J., Sigmund, K., et al. (2003). Group report: The cultural and genetic evolution of human cooperation. In P. Hammerstein (Ed.), *Genetic and cultural evolution of cooperation* (pp. 445–468). Cambridge, MA: MIT Press.

Hovland, C. I., Janis, I. L., & Kelley, H. H. (1953). *Communication and persuasion: Psychological studies of opinion change*. New Haven, CT: Yale University Press.

Inkeles, A. (1983). *Exploring individual modernity*. New York: Columbia University Press.

Insko, C. A., Gilmore, R., Drenan, S., Lipsitz, A., Moehle, D., & Thibaut, J. (1983). Trade versus expropriation in open groups: A comparison of two type of social power. *Journal of Personality and Social Psychology*, *44*, 977–999.

Jacobs, R. C., & Campbell, D. T. (1961). The perpetuation of an arbitrary tradition through several generations of laboratory microculture. *Journal of Abnormal and Social Psychology*, *62*, 649–568.

Johnson, A. W., & Earle, T. K. (2000). *The evolution of human societies: From foraging group to agrarian state* (2nd ed.). Stanford, CA: Stanford University Press.

Jorgensen, J. G. (1980). *Western Indians: Comparative environments, languages, and cultures of 172 Western American Indian Tribes*. San Francisco: Freeman.

Kaessmann, H., & Pääbo, S. (2002). The genetical history of humans and the great apes. *Journal of Internal Medicine*, *251*, 1–18.

Kaessmann, H., Wiebe, V., & Pääbo, S. (1999). Extensive nuclear DNA sequence diversity among chimpanzees. *Science*, *286*, 1159–1162.

Kelly, R. C. (1985). *The Nuer conquest: The structure and development of an expansionist system*. Ann Arbor: University of Michigan Press.

Kelly, R. L. (1995). *The foraging spectrum: Diversity in hunter-gatherer lifeways*. Washington, DC: Smithsonian Institution Press.

Klein, R. G. (1999). *The human career: Human biological and cultural origins* (2nd ed.). Chicago: University of Chicago.

Knauft, B. M. (1985). *Good company and violence: Sorcery and social action in a Lowland New Guinea society*. Berkeley: University of California Press.

Knight, C., Studdert-Kennedy, M., & Hurford, J. R. (2000). *The evolutionary emergence of language: Social function and the origins of linguistic form*. Cambridge, UK: Cambridge University Press.

Labov, W. (2001). *Principles of linguistic change: Social factors* (Vol. 29). Malden, MA: Blackwell.

Laland, K. N., Richerson, P. J., & Boyd, R. (1996). Developing a theory of animal social learning. In C. M. Heyes & B. G. Galef, Jr. (Eds.), *Social learning in animals: The roots of culture* (pp. 129–154). San Diego: Academic Press.

Logan, M. H., & Schmittou, D. A. (1998, Summer). The uniqueness of Crow art: A glimpse into the history of an embattled people. *Montana: The Magazine of Western History*, pp. 58–71.

Massini, S. (2004). The diffusion of mobile telephony in Italy and the UK: An empirical investigation. *Economics of Innovation and New Technology*, 13, 251–277.

McElreath, R., Lubell, M., Richerson, P. J. M., Baum, W., Edsten, E., Waring, T., et al. (2005). Applying formal models to the laboratory study of social learning: The impact of task difficulty and environmental fluctuation. *Evolution and Human Behavior*, 26, 483–508.

Moore, B. R. (1996). The evolution of imitative learning. In C. M. Heyes & B. G. Galef, Jr. (Eds.), *Social learning in animals: The roots of culture* (pp. 245–265). San Diego: Academic Press.

Moreland, R. L., Levine, J. M., & McMinn, J. G. (2001). Self-categorization and work group socialization. In M. A. Hogg & D. Terry (Eds.), *Social identity processes in organizational contexts* (pp. 87–100). Philadelphia: Psychology Press.

Moylan, J. W., Graham, C. M., Borgerhoff Mulder, M., Nunn, C. L., & Håkansson, N. T. (2005). Cultural traits and linguistic trees: Phylogenetic signal in East Africa. In C. P. Lipo, M. J. O'Brien, M. Collard, & S. J. Shennan (Eds.), *Mapping our ancestors: Phylogenetic approaches in anthropology and prehistory* (pp. 33–52). New York: Aldine.

Murdock, G. P. (1967). *Ethnographic atlas*. Pittsburgh: University of Pittsburgh Press.

Needham, J. (1987). *Science and civilization in China: Vol. 5. Part 7. The gunpowder epic*. Cambridge, UK: Cambridge University Press.

Nettle, D. (1999). *Linguistic diversity*. Oxford, UK: Oxford University Press.

Newcomb, T. M. (1943). *Personality and social change*. New York: Holt, Rinehart & Winston.

Newcomb, T. M., Koenig, L. E., Flacks, R., & Warwick, D. P. (1967). *Persistence and change: Bennington College and its Students after twenty-five years*. New York: Wiley.

Newson, L. (2003). *Kin, culture, and reproductive decisions*. Unpublished doctoral dissertation, University of Exeter, Exeter, UK.

Newson, L., Postmes, T., Lea, S. E. G., & Webley, P. (2005). Why are modern families small?: Toward an evolutionary and cultural explanation for the demographic transition. *Personality and Social Psychology Review*, 9, 360–375.

Newson, L., Postmes, T., Lea, S. E. G., Webley, P., Richerson, P. J., & McElrath, R. (in press). Influences on communication about reproduction: The cultural evolution of low fertility. *Evolution and Human Behavior*.

Odling-Smee, F. J., Laland, K. N., & Feldman, M. W. (2003). *Niche construction: The neglected process in evolution* (Vol. 37). Princeton, NJ: Princeton University Press.

Pagel, M., & Mace, R. (2004). The cultural wealth of nations. *Nature*, 428, 276–278.

Perloff, R. M. (2003). *The dynamics of persuasion: Communication and attitudes in the 21st century*. London: Erlbaum.

Petty, R. E., & Cacioppo, J. T. (1986). The elaboration likelihood model of persuasion. In L. Berkowitz (Ed.), *Advances in experimental social psychology* (Vol. 19, pp. 123–205). New York: Academic Press.

Postmes, T., Haslam, S. A., & Swaab, R. (2005). Social influence in small groups: An interactive model of social identity formation. *European Review of Social Psychology*, 16, 1–42.

Richerson, P. J., & Boyd, R. (1999). Complex societies—The evolutionary origins of a crude superorganism. *Human Nature*, 10(3), 253–289.

Richerson, P. J., & Boyd, R. (2001). The evolution of subjective commitment to groups: A tribal instincts hypothesis. In R. M. Nesse (Ed.), *Evolution and the capacity for commitment* (pp. 186–220). New York: Russell Sage Foundation.

Richerson, P. J., & Boyd, R. (2005). *Not by genes alone: How culture transformed human evolution*. Chicago: University of Chicago Press.

Richerson, P. J., Boyd, R., & Henrich, J. (2003). Cultural evolution of human cooperation. In P. Hammerstein (Ed.), *Genetic and cultural evolution of cooperation* (pp. 357–388). Berlin: MIT Press.

Rogers, E. M. (1995). *Diffusion of innovations* (4th ed.). New York: Free Press.

Rogoff, B., Paradise, R., K., Mejia Arauz, R., Correa-Chavez, M., & Angelillo, C. (2003). Firsthand learning through intent participation. *Annual Review of Psychology*, 54, 175–203.

Rudicel, S. A. (1994). The shod foot and its implications for American women. *Journal of the Southern Orthopaedic Association*, 3, 268–272.

Sherif, M., & Murphy, G. (1936). *The psychology of social norms*. New York/London: Harper & Brothers.

Shoumatoff, A. (2005). *Dispatches from the vanishing world*. Retrieved July 17, 2005, from *www.dispatchesfromthevanishingworld.com/*

Simons, H. W., Berkowitz, N. N., & Moyer, R. J. S., (1970). Similarity, credibility and attitude change: A review and a theory. *Psychological Bulletin*, 73, 1–16.

Simoons, F. J. (1969). Primary adult lactose intolerance and the milking habit: A problem in biologic and cultural interrelations: I. Review of the medical research. *American Journal of Digestive Diseases*, 14(12), 819–836.

Simoons, F. J. (1970). Primary adult lactose intolerance and the milking habit: A problem in biologic and cultural interrelations: II. A culture historical hypothesis. *American Journal of Digestive Diseases*, 15(8), 695–710.

Sperber, D. (1996). *Explaining culture: A naturalistic approach*. Oxford, UK: Blackwell.

Tamura, K., & Nei, M. (1993). Estimation of the number of nucleotide substitutions in the control region of mitochondrial DNC in humans and chimpanzees. *Molecular Biology and Evolution, 10*(3), 512–526.

Thomason, S. G. (2001). *Language contact*. Washington, DC: Georgetown University Press.

Tomasello, M. (1996). Do apes ape? In C. M. Heyes & B. G. Galef, Jr. (Eds.), *Social learning in animals: The roots of culture* (pp. 319–346). New York: Academic Press.

Tomasello, M. (1999). *The cultural origins of human cognition*. Cambridge, MA: Harvard University Press.

Trivers, R. (1972). Parental investment and sexual selection. In B. Campbell (Ed.), *Sexual selection and the descent of man* (pp. 136–139). Chicago: Aldine.

Trivers, R. L. (1971). The evolution of reciprocal altruism. *Quarterly Review of Biology, 46*(1), 35–57.

Whiten, A., & Custance, D. (1996). Studies of imitation in chimpanzees and children. In C. M. Heyes & B. G.

Galef, Jr. (Eds.), *Social learning in animals: The roots of culture* (pp. 291–318). New York: Academic Press.

Whiten, A., Goodall, J., McGrew, W. C., Nishida, T., Reynolds, V., Sugiyama, Y., et al. (1999). Cultures in chimpanzees. *Nature, 399,* 682–685.

Williams, G. C. (1966). *Adaptation and natural selection: A critique of some current evolutionary thought*. Princeton, NJ: Princeton University Press.

Wilson, D. S. (2002). *Darwin's cathedral: Evolution, religion, and the nature of society*. Chicago: University of Chicago Press.

Wright, P. (1966). Attitude change under direct and indirect interpersonal influence. *Human Relations, 19,* 199–211.

Zelinsky, W. (1971). The hypothesis of the mobility transition. *Geographical Review, 61,* 219–249.

CHAPTER 19

Cultural Psychology
of Moral Development

JOAN G. MILLER

Morality is central to culture. As noted by Shweder, "culture" involves "community-specific ideas about what is true, good, beautiful and efficient that are . . . constitutive of different ways of life, and play a part in the self-understanding of members of the community" (1999, p. 212). Whereas it is widely agreed that culture involves shared moral commitments (e.g., D'Andrade, 1984; Strauss & Quinn, 1997), the issue of whether morality is culturally variable remains controversial. The concern is raised by many psychological theorists that acknowledging cultural variability in morality leads to the stance of an extreme moral relativism, and that cultural approaches to morality embody passive views of the individual (e.g., Turiel, 2002). Work from the perspective of cultural psychology challenges this conclusion. Documenting qualitative cultural variation in moral outlooks, this work draws implications for expanding basic psychological theory in the area of morality, addressing challenges about how to understand moral development in ways that both avoid extreme moral relativism and embody a dynamic view of the individual and culture.

The goal of this chapter is to provide a critical analysis of research on culture and morality, identifying contributions of work in this domain. The first section presents an overview of mainstream psychological theories of moral development, with a focus on understanding why, despite their attention to cultural issues, theorists in this tradition reject the idea of any significant cultural variation as existing in moral outlooks. This is followed by an overview of key theoretical assumptions of cultural psychology, as well as a review of empirical work documenting cultural variation in moral outlooks. In turn, the final section of the chapter identifies new directions for research on moral development.

APPROACHES TO MORAL DEVELOPMENT IN MAINSTREAM TRADITION

Psychological approaches to moral development tend to treat morality as based on criteria that individuals perceive to be above social consensus, rather than merely on rules, norms, or other societal standards. It is assumed that the issues individuals consider to be moral are concerns that they regard as involving right or wrong, and as going beyond what is merely normative or socially accepted. Thus, from this

477

perspective, it is recognized that morality transcends societal standards and differs from mere social conventions. However, although these assumptions about the formal criteria defining morality are widely shared, controversy exists concerning the content issues that individuals invest with moral force. Whereas it is assumed within work in cultural psychology that the content of morality shows significant cultural variation, the content of morality is assumed to be universal within mainstream psychological viewpoints.

Discussion below focuses on the theoretical models of moral development forwarded in the most clearly developed and influential mainstream psychological theories of morality: the cognitive-developmental framework of Kohlberg, the distinct domain perspective of Turiel, and the morality of caring framework of Gilligan. Although the theories differ in their views of the content of morality and of the ontogenetic processes through which morality arises, they share a stance of defining morality as emerging through developmental processes that do not depend on cultural input and of downplaying the role of culturally variable content assumptions as impacting on moral codes.

Cognitive-Developmental Model of Kohlberg

Kohlberg's cognitive-developmental model of moral development has been the most conceptually influential framework in the field, inspiring most of the later work that followed (Kohlberg, 1969, 1971, 1981). The model grounds morality in philosophical arguments that Kohlberg saw as providing an objective basis for morality and is distinguished by its formulation of a compelling stage model. Groundbreaking in its time and dominating research on moral development in developmental psychology for many decades, the Kohlbergian model offers a universalistic approach. Strikingly, however, this universalism is based, not on ignoring culture, but on rejecting, both on theoretical and empirical grounds, the validity of cultural approaches to morality.

Part of the Cognitive Revolution in psychology and drawing heavily on Piagetian theory, Kohlberg forwarded a model that offered a sharp break with the then-dominant behaviorist and psychoanalytic models of morality (e.g., Berkowitz, 1964; Eysenck, 1961; Freud, 1930). Piaget had rejected behaviorist and maturational approaches because, in his view, they treat knowledge as merely a copy of information supplied by the environment. He furthermore assumed that cultural approaches resemble behaviorist perspectives in embodying a passive view of the child (Piaget, 1932, 1973). Kohlberg adopted these same assumptions, agreeing with the Piagetian premise that the active construction of knowledge is antithetical to cultural learning (Kohlberg, 1971).

However, beyond this concern shared by Kohlberg and Piaget that cultural approaches assume a passive view of development, Kohlberg raised additional concerns about the problematic stance of a relativistic morality that he felt inhered in giving weight to culture. Thus, he criticized the "relativist point of view" held by anthropologists as assuming "the validity of every set of norms for the people whose lives are guided by them" (Kohlberg, 1971, p. 159). Citing an argument by Brandt, he maintained that such a stance leads to the condoning of abusive practices merely because of their normative acceptability:

> It does not follow directly from the fact that the Romans approved of infanticide and we do not, that infanticide was really right for them and really wrong for us or that it is neither right nor wrong for everybody. (Brandt, 1959, p. 84; cited in Kohlberg, 1971, p. 159)

Kohlberg also pointed to the logical contradiction of relativistic appeals for tolerance of other people's beliefs as a stance that treats the principle of toleration itself in nonrelative terms.

To construct a universalistic morality, Kohlberg grounded his theoretical model in logical arguments based on Western philosophical premises (Rawls, 1971). Drawing from the Kantian concept of the categorical imperative, Kohlberg argued for the necessity of excluding relationship-based and affective considerations from morality. In this view, to be moral, an outlook must meet the formal criteria of being universally applicable, prescriptive, and capable of being applied in an impartial and impersonal manner. Such a morality is seen as excluding any considerations that relate to one's social position or to any type of affective considerations.

The six-stage developmental sequence of moral development forwarded by Kohlberg

(1969) treats role-related and affective types of considerations as lower forms of reasoning that individuals emphasize at earlier, premoral levels of development. In this model, the most developmentally primitive stance forms the preconventional level, focused on affective and other self-interested concerns, including a stance of avoiding punishment (Stage 1) and of instrumental exchange (Stage 2). In turn, the developmentally more advanced conventional level encompasses relationship and role-related considerations, including a focus on social role expectations (Stage 3) and on the rule of law and other societal-level concerns (Stage 4). Finally, the developmentally highest level, the only level at which reasoning is considered fully moral in nature, includes both a stage focused on individual rights that have been agreed upon by the whole society (Stage 5) and a stage focused on self-chosen principles of justice, human rights, and respect for the dignity of individual persons (Stage 6). The methodology utilized in research on the Kohlbergian model involves presenting individuals with hypothetical moral dilemmas that embody justice issues and assessing individuals' open-ended reasoning in resolving these dilemmas. Although successful in evoking highly reflective moral reasoning, the emphasis in this methodology on the verbal articulation of responses introduces a complexity for children and other populations with limited education.

The Kohlbergian model has been subject to extensive cross-cultural testing that Kohlberg and his colleagues have interpreted as supporting the universality of the Kohlbergian claims, despite the consistent findings of extensive cross-cultural variation in the observed distribution of moral reasoning (Snarey, 1985). Thus, for example, in an early report of cross-cultural findings, Kohlberg (1971) noted that whereas most U.S. respondents by age 16 had reached the postconventional level of moral development, in both Taiwan and Mexico, the dominant form of reasoning reached by this age was only at the conventional level. This type of result showing that higher levels of moral development were only reached in sociocultural communities marked by characteristics such as Westernization, higher education, and urbanization was interpreted as evidence that particular environments are more stimulating than other sociocultural settings and thus push cognitive development faster and further.

This developmental perspective on cultural differences adopted by Kohlberg provided a framework for interpreting the marked cross-cultural differences in moral reasoning as reflecting variation in the individual's rate of development but not in the fundamental concepts that comprise morality. Although critics charged that the Kohlbergian scheme was biased in its grounding in Western liberal, secular cultural assumptions (e.g., Simpson, 1974; Sullivan, 1977) and may have been insufficiently sensitive to the adaptive demands of different sociocultural settings (e.g., Edwards, 1975; Harkness, Edwards, & Super, 1981) or to response biases linked to socioeconomic status (e.g., Buck-Morss, 1975), theorists in the Kohlbergian tradition remained unmoved by these critiques, finding the evidence of cross-cultural variation to be fully compatible with their claims of a universal developmental progression of justice morality (Kohlberg, Levine, & Hewer, 1983). As will be seen in the later discussion of research in cultural psychology, only when the fundamental conceptual assumptions of the Kohlbergian model were subject to a culturally based conceptual broadening were more fundamental cultural challenges to the Kohlbergian model articulated.

Distinct Domain Framework

The distinct domain framework developed originally by Turiel (1983, 1998a), but associated with a growing number of theorists (e.g., Turiel, Smetana, & Killen, 1991; Nucci, 2002; Smetana, 1995), challenges the developmental claims of the Kohlbergian model, while retaining its universalism. The Kohlbergian model portrays the development of moral understandings as involving a process of cognitive differentiation in which individuals hold one dominant form of understanding at any given time, with developmentally more adequate later understandings arising through transformation of developmentally less adequate earlier understandings. Thus, conventional understandings emerge as a replacement for preconventional understandings, and moral understandings emerge as a replacement for conventional understandings. Challenging this view, distinct domain theorists argue, in contrast, that social experience is always multifaceted, with different types of understandings applied to different types of social behaviors. Thus, rather than viewing one type of outlook as replacing another over development, the distinct domain theory maintains that at any given point in development, individuals apply different forms of understanding to different types of social issues.

As in both Kohlbergian and Piagetian theory, theorists in the distinct domain tradition assume that morality centers on content issues involving harm, justice, and individual rights, and that moral development occurs through self-constructive processes that do not depend on cultural input. As in Kohlbergian theory, it is also assumed that cultural approaches to morality inevitably lead to an extreme moral relativism and are antithetical to the active construction of knowledge. In contrast to the Kohlbergian view, however, the self-constructive processes underlying moral judgment are seen as entailing relatively simple inductive judgments rather than the complex deductive judgments assumed within the Kohlbergian framework. It is assumed that issues involving harm and injustice are categorized as moral, issues involving social coordination, as social conventions, and issues that involve neither type of concern are categorized as matters of personal choice.

Methodologically, work within the distinct domain perspective utilizes simplified methodologies for assessing moral reasoning that uncover greater developmental competencies than are apparent with the Kohlbergian protocol (Turiel, 1983). Utilizing child-friendly testing procedures, the methodology focuses on the child's ability to distinguish between different types of social rules, rather than, as in Kohlbergian testing, on their open-ended response justifications. Thus, for example, to assess whether a child categorizes an issue such as hitting in moral terms, short-answer response questions may be asked to assess whether the child treats the rule against hitting as nonchangeable (e.g., "Would it be okay to change this rule?"), non-culturally-relative (e.g., "Would it be okay to have a different rule about this in another school?"), and nonlegitimately subject to regulation (e.g., "Is this the person's own business?").

Research by theorists in the distinct domain tradition has tended to focus on clear-cut "prototypical" issues and to uncover findings that individuals in all cultures have the ability to distinguish between issues of morality, convention, and personal choice, and that this ability is evident in children as young as preschool age (Turiel, 1983, 1998a). Such findings are interpreted as supporting the model's claim that judgments of harm and injustice take a universal form that is unaffected by cultural influences. As I discuss later, however, work within cultural psychology has challenged this conclusion in examining a broader range of types of issues. This latter work, as will be seen, not only provides evidence that conceptions of morality extend beyond issues of harm and justice but also that judgments of harm and justice vary depending on culturally variable content assumptions.

Morality of Caring Framework of Gilligan

The morality of caring framework developed by Gilligan (1977, 1982) offers a compelling cultural critique of Kohlbergian theory, as well as of related assumptions in the distinct domain perspective, both in its argument for the need to treat morality as extending to issues of caring, rather than as limited to the avoidance of harm and injustice, and in its assertion that perspectives on morality are gender-related. However, although conceptually broadening the scope of the moral domain in these ways, the framework retains a universalistic emphasis. The morality of caring is formulated in culturally invariant terms and issues of gender variation treated as fundamentally the same across all cultures.

From the perspective of the morality of caring framework, the argument is made for the need to treat issues of caring in fully moral terms rather than to limit the scope of morality to the prohibition-oriented issues of justice. Drawing on psychodynamic formulations and attachment theory, the perspective maintains that the distinctive socialization experiences of males and females lead to the development of contrasting senses of self and morality (Gilligan & Wiggins, 1988). In identifying with their mothers and in having experiences in family interaction that emphasize interpersonal responsiveness, girls are seen as developing a connected sense of self and an associated morality of caring. This sense of self and morality, however, becomes problematic at adolescence, when the girl finds that it conflicts with the autonomous sense of self valued in the larger culture. In contrast, although males are seen as attached to their mothers, they are assumed to identify with their fathers. Desiring to overcome the inequality that they experience in relation to their fathers, males are seen as developing an autonomous sense of self and associated morality of justice.

The model assumes that although there exist two rather than only one type of moral perspective (i.e., moralities of both justice and of caring), the form of these perspectives is culturally invariant. As Gilligan argues, "All people are born into a situation of inequality and no child survives in the absence of adult connection. Since everyone is vulnerable both to oppression and to abandonment, two stories about morality recur in human experience" (Gilligan & Wiggins, 1988, p. 281). The universality of morality is assumed to reflect the universality of gender-related developmental processes, as well as the cross-culturally common experience of gender bias. Any observed cross-cultural variation in the moralities of caring and of justice is assumed to represent only a minor difference in relative emphasis and not in the basic form of either type of morality.

In testing the claims of the morality of caring framework, Gilligan and her colleagues typically tap moral reasoning in the context of real life rather than hypothetical situations and employ interpretive data analysis techniques that involve the qualitative assessment of open-ended interview data. Support for the claim of gender differences was uncovered in early research undertaken by Gilligan and her colleagues (Gilligan, 1982; Gilligan, Ward, & Taylor, 1988). However, subsequent studies by a broader range of investigators have tended to find little or no evidence of gender variation (Thomas, 1986; Walker, 1984; Walker, Pitts, Hennig, & Matsuba, 1995).

The universality of the morality of caring framework has been assumed rather than subjected to explicit cross-cultural empirical testing. Although some studies have been conducted by Gilligan and her colleagues with ethnic minority populations within the United States (e.g., Bardige, Ward, Gilligan, Taylor, & Cohen, 1988; Ward, 1988), no known work undertaken in this tradition has tested the assumed cross-cultural universality of this form of morality. The studies conducted with ethnic/minority populations have in some cases called into question claims about the morality of caring being gender-related (Stack, 1986), as well as, most recently, highlighted the links drawn between caring and social justice among African American respondents (Walker & Snarey, 2004). However, there has been no direct chal-

lenge to the morality of caring itself. This result reflects the tendency for research to focus only on any references to caring rather than to consider qualitative cultural variation in the nature of caring responses. As will be seen, in tapping caring in ways that are more sensitive to the contrasting cultural meanings underlying caring responses and to contextual variation in care-based reasoning, work in cultural psychology reveals the existence of qualitatively variable forms of the morality of caring.

Summary

Drawing initial inspiration from the seminal theoretical model of Kohlberg, mainstream psychological theories in recent years have increasingly embraced the distinct domain perspective, a viewpoint that retains the focus on the morality of justice but treats justice understandings as coexisting with understandings of social conventions and personal issues. Arguments forward by Gilligan for the existence of a morality of caring are also highly influential in contemporary work, although such a morality generally is no longer considered to be gender related but rather is seen as embraced by both males and females. Differing in their focus, these various mainstream perspectives share a universalistic emphasis that treats culture as incompatible with the requirements of morality.

KEY ASSUMPTIONS OF WORK ON MORAL DEVELOPMENT WITHIN CULTURAL PSYCHOLOGY

This section presents a brief overview of some of the key theoretical premises of cultural psychology and of the underlying assumptions of work on moral development from a cultural psychology perspective. Consideration of these assumptions makes clear respects in which a cultural focus embodies the constructivism and contextual sensitivity of mainstream psychological models of morality, while giving greater weight to cultural influences on the content of moral codes.

Mutual Constitution of Culture and Psychological Processes

Cultural psychology has at times been characterized as a subfield or area of specialization in psychology, and this type of view may be inad-

vertently implied by the present contrast between the "mainstream" tradition of work on
moral development and perspectives within
cultural psychology. This terminology, however, is used only to distinguish approaches
characterized by different theoretical assumptions about the role of culture in basic psychological theory, and not to distinguish different
areas of specialization or fields of study. Work
within cultural psychology is defined fundamentally by its conceptual commitments to a
view of culture as central in human experience
and cuts across all areas of psychology rather
than representing a subfield of the discipline.

The core of cultural psychology is the
premise that cultural and psychological processes are mutually constitutive (Cole, 1990,
1996; Markus, Kitayama, & Heiman, 1996;
J. G. Miller, 1997, 1999; Shweder, 1990;
Shweder & Sullivan, 1990, 1993). It is not
only assumed that culture depends on communities of intentional agents but also that
psychological processes require cultural experience for their developmental emergence.
With the exception of certain innate propensities that are evident early in infancy, the
emergence and maintenance of most psychological processes are seen as dependent on
cultural input. Cultural meanings which involve processes of mediation and internalization, are viewed as impacting on individuals'
psychological understandings and affecting
their cognition and behavior:

> Cultural, institutional, and historical forces are
> "imported" into individuals' actions by virtue of
> using cultural tools, on the one hand, and
> sociocultural settings are created and recreated
> through individuals' use of mediational means, on
> the other. The resulting picture is one in which,
> because of the role cultural tools play in mediated
> action, it is virtually impossible for us to act in a
> way that is not socio-culturally situated. (Wertsch,
> 1995, p. 90)

From this perspective, it is recognized that, although children assume an active role in making sense of their experience, this experience is,
in part, culturally patterned. As Bruner (1973)
notes, whereas it was recognized during the
Cognitive Revolution that individuals go beyond the information given in contributing
meanings to experience, the essential role of
culture in this meaning-making process was
not fully apparent:

> What was obvious from the start was perhaps too
> obvious to be fully appreciated. . . . The symbolic
> systems that individuals used in constructing
> meaning were systems that were already in place,
> already "there," deeply entrenched in culture and
> language. . . . When we enter human life, it is as if
> we walk on stage into a play whose enactment is
> already in progress—a play whose somewhat
> open plot determines what parts we may play and
> toward what denouements we may be heading.
> (Bruner, 1990, pp. 11, 34)

Within cultural psychology, it is assumed that
whereas individuals' understandings of the
world and participation in it are mediated by
cultural symbols, there is no one-to-one relationship between cultural meanings and individual understandings (J. G. Miller, 1997). In
contrast to the claims made by various theorists in the cognitive-developmental and distinct domain traditions (Turiel, 2002), cultural-
psychological approaches do not treat the individual in passive terms or assume that there exists a one-to-one mapping between cultural
meanings and individual understandings.
Rather, cultural psychology embodies an active
view of the agent, while also treating this agent
as fundamentally socioculturally embedded
rather than as a pristine processor of information (Schwartz, 1981).

Dynamic Views of Culture and Psychology

From an ecological perspective, culture is
conceptualized in functional terms as adapted
to the objective affordances and constraints
of different environments (Berry, Poortinga,
Segall, & Dasen, 1992; Bronfenbrenner,
1979). In an early, highly influential example
of this type of model, in the Six Culture Project, cultural practices are treated as functionally related to the objective requirements set
by different ecological conditions, with psychological processes seen as mediating between the culture and the physical environment (Whiting & Whiting, 1975). Thus,
linkages in this investigation were demonstrated among rich natural ecologies, societies
with complex social structures, and child-
rearing practices that emphasize competitiveness. Ecological approaches to culture are essential in calling attention to the contrasting
adaptive demands of different settings, thus
challenging a view that treats the contexts for
human development as universal.

Although not downplaying the importance of ecological views of culture, work in cultural psychology emphasizes the need to understand culture also in symbolic terms (Geertz, 1973; Shweder & LeVine, 1984). From such a perspective, culture is seen as a system of symbolic meanings that are embodied in artifacts and practices, and that bear an open rather than fully determinate relationship to objective constraints (Shweder, 1984). Culture is also understood as reflecting, in part, nonfunctional considerations rather than being exclusively functionally based (LeVine, 1984). Such a perspective implies that cultural values and activities cannot be explained exclusively by reference to objective ecological conditions. To give an example, research indicates that Japanese educators tend to consider the preschool practice of having many children assigned to a given teacher as functional in providing children with experience in and promoting their knowledge about being good members of a group (Tobin, Wu, & Davidson, 1989). This symbolic value, however, is less central in U.S. contexts in which preschool educators tend to consider it beneficial to have fewer children assigned to a given teacher, so that the children may be accorded more individual attention and more opportunities to exercise individual decision making. Thus, whereas both types of preschool classroom practices may be considered adaptive, the basis of their functionality cannot be understood merely by reference to objective constraints, such as school resources, but requires also taking into account nonfunctional values, such as pedagogical viewpoints, related to goals for the children's development.

Within cultural psychology, not only is culture seen as affecting the meanings of contexts, and the practices through which contexts are structured, but psychological processes themselves are also recognized as being contextually dependent (J. G. Miller, 1997, 2002). It is assumed that cultural influences on psychological phenomena depend on contextual considerations and should not necessarily be assumed to be highly generalized. Thus, it must be understood, that because a psychological process is in part culturally constituted does not imply that the psychological process, or that any observed cross-cultural variation, is contextually invariant. Rather, the argument is for the need to give weight *both* to culture, as shared meanings and practices, and to context, as objective affordances and constraints, in psychological explanation rather than to reduce one type of consideration to the other.

Conceptions of the Moral

In terms of assumptions related specifically to understanding moral development, theorists in cultural psychology acknowledge commonality and variability in conceptions of both moral and nonrational influences on moral outlooks. These assumptions give rise to a culturally broadened view of diversity rather than to an extreme moral relativism (Miller, 2001).

Formal versus Content-Based Definitions of the Moral

Work in cultural psychology distinguishes between formal and content-based definitions of the moral. Issues of morality are seen as distinguishable from issues of mere social convention by formal criteria such as their perceived generalizability, impersonality, unalterability, and ahistorical qualities (Pool, Shweder, & Much, 1983; Turiel, 1983). Thus, a rule seen in moral as opposed to conventional terms is assumed to apply in all similar social contexts rather than, as in the case of convention, to depend on local customs and norms. Equally, what is moral is considered to be impersonal in the sense that it does not depend on an individual or society recognizing it as such. Whereas issues of morality are seen as nonalterable by social consensus and as historically invariant, issues of social convention are seen as alterable by social consensus and as historically contingent. Areas of behavior that are perceived to be beyond the scope of legitimate social regulation and, thus, considered issues of neither morality nor social convention, are understood as matters of personal choice.

Note that in distinguishing between different types of social understandings on the basis of these formal criteria, researchers in cultural psychology and in the mainstream traditions of work on moral development are rejecting a purely emotivist stance on morality, as might be found in certain behaviorist approaches (Berkowitz, 1964), or a purely conventional stance on morality, as might be found in certain social-psychological work that makes no distinction between morality and mere normative conformity (e.g., Darley & Pittman, 2003; Taylor, 2003). Although the influence of affective factors on moral reasoning is not denied (Haidt, 2001; Kagan, 1984), what is moral is considered by the individual to be based on criteria that go beyond mere self-interest or instrumental gain.

However, whereas mainstream and cultural-psychological approaches agree on similar formal definitions of the moral, cultural-psychological approaches treat the relationship between the form and content of morality as potentially culturally variable, whereas it is assumed to be cross-culturally invariant within mainstream approaches (J. G. Miller, 2006; Shweder, 1982). This, then, constitutes the most central point of contrast between the two traditions. Mainstream theories assume that issues of harm, justice, and welfare have the same fundamental meaning and are categorized in the same terms universally. In contrast, work from a cultural psychology suggests that the content invested with moral force extends beyond the issues of harm, rights, and welfare concerns, and that the same types of content issues may be categorized in different terms depending on culturally variable meanings and practices.

Importance of Nonrational Considerations

Reflecting their cognitive-developmental roots, mainstream psychological theories of moral development emphasize the rational nature of moral judgment. Moral reasoning is portrayed as fundamentally similar to other types of cognitive inference, in being based on deductive or inductive processing of information. Thus, if individuals draw different moral inferences based on the same information (e.g., if it is morally acceptable in one cultural population to have an abortion and in another it is not), this difference is likely to arise ultimately from variation in individuals' knowledge about the nature of the harm involved and to be resolvable, at least potentially, by individuals obtaining more scientific facts about the situation (Turiel, Killen, & Helwig, 1987). From this perspective, moral outlooks are considered to be ultimately reconcilable (i.e., it is assumed that if all individuals had the same information and were able to process this information cognitively in an equally accurate and nonbiased manner, their understandings of the "facts" of situations would be the same, as would their moral judgments (Turiel et al., 1987).

Whereas work within cultural psychology acknowledges both the rational and affectively based inference processes that inform moral judgment, attention is also given to the nonrational judgments that enter into weighting of information and that invariably reflect considerations of value rather than purely reflections of the "facts" of given situations. To give an example, whether abortion is considered a moral violation or a matter of the woman's personal discretion depends in part on culturally and subculturally variable conceptions of which entities in the world are to be considered persons and entitled to protection from harm (Shweder, Mahapatra, & Miller, 1987). This delineation of personhood (i.e., the question of when to consider human life as beginning) represents a matter of value that can never be decided based on biological considerations alone. Likewise, in another example, the criteria that underlie the moral appraisal that it is appropriate for parents to read their 10-year-old child's report card without prior permission but not to read their child's diary reflect culturally variable conceptions of what constitute "territories" of the self (e.g., Do they extend to one's mail?) and of what constitutes harm (e.g., Does reading this particular information constitute a violation of the child's privacy or an appropriate expression of concern?). The types of cultural meanings that inform these judgments embody nonrational assumptions that cannot be merely controlled or held constant when evaluating differences in moral outlook. Thus, to attempt to hold them constant when appraising cultural differences in moral outlook, a stance recently advocated by theorists in the distinct domain tradition, would mean adopting a stance that bleaches culture of its meaning (J. G. Miller, 2006).

Although much of the resistance to culture in mainstream approaches to moral development stems from a concern that cultural approaches invariably lead to extreme forms of relativism, this is not the stance adopted within cultural psychology. As noted, the type of position adopted in work on moral development within cultural psychology does not eschew comparative evaluation of cultural practices or equate moral acceptability with the social acceptance of particular practices. Rather, it recognizes that the cultural meanings given to particular practices affect their implications and must therefore be given greater, though still not absolute, weight in evaluating their moral status.

RESEARCH ON CULTURE AND MORAL DEVELOPMENT

Research on culture and moral development centers not merely on assessing the universality of psychological theories of moral development but on expanding the psychological constructs and process explanation invoked in understanding moral outlooks. As will be seen, this work highlights the need to expand present psychological models of morality to recognize qualitative variability in basic moral constructs and outlooks.

Justice Reasoning

Issues of justice have a central role in all psychological theories of morality, with the moral status of justice unchallenged even in theories such as that of Gilligan, which sees the scope of morality as expanded to encompass other types of concerns, such as caring. The central role of justice in any morality is equally not called into question in work in cultural psychology. Rather, on an abstract or formal level, the ideas of both justice and harm are assumed to exist in all moral codes, with the idea of justice seen as the abstract rule of treating like cases alike and the idea of harm as that of avoiding harm (Shweder et al., 1987). However, as cultural theorists have noted, at this abstract level, justice and harm are compatible with a wide range of cultural diversity in moral outlooks, because cultural communities fill in notions of harm and justice in markedly culturally variable ways.

Commonalities

The universality of at least of some moral concern with justice is seen in the mention of justice concerns in moral reasoning early in development, and in at least some commonality in justice reasoning in concrete cases. Thus, cross-cultural commonality tends to be observed in justice judgments in cross-cultural research that utilizes content issues involving "prototypical" cases in which there is considerable cross-cultural agreement about the meaning of the situations portrayed (Turiel, 1983). This can be seen, for example, in control issues included in cross-cultural research that involve issues such as theft or arbitrary assault, which are portrayed as undertaken in a voluntary and intentional way under decontextualized circum-

stances that include no mention of any alternative motivation or meaning to the behavior. Thus, for example, both Indian and U.S. adult populations have been shown to agree that taking another person's property without their permission represents a moral violation that involves justice violations and includes a violation of property rights (J. G. Miller, Bersoff, & Harwood, 1990; Shweder et al., 1987). Notably, awareness of justice violations is documented in research that utilizes similar prototypical vignettes with young children. Thus, in research involving children as young as 3 years old both in the United States (Smetana, 1981; Smetana, Schlagman, & Adams, 1993) and in different Asian cultures (Song, Smetana, & Kim, 1987; Yau & Smetana, 2003), children identify acts involving arbitrary assault and violation of property rights as justice violations that have moral rather than merely conventional status.

Research of this type supports the idea that justice concerns form part of morality universally. However, it does not indicate that, universally, justice concerns will invariably be accorded the same priority as other types of competing moral issues, that individuals will be held accountable to the same degree cross-culturally for justice breaches, or that the same issues will be conceptualized as involving justice concerns. It is in these areas of instantiating justice judgments in the concrete contexts of everyday moral reasoning that cultural variation in justice morality is shown to exist.

Variation in Priority Given to Justice Relative to Competing Moral Issues

In terms of priority given to justice judgments compared to other types of competing issues, cross-cultural research indicates that even in cases in which there is substantial cross-cultural agreement about the moral status of the justice issue involved, cross-cultural variation may result from differential priority being given to justice issues compared to other salient, competing moral concerns. Such a tendency may be seen, for example, in the following qualitative response given by a respondent to a Kohlbergian hypothetical dilemma that involved the issue of whether a son should let his father spend money for his own personal uses that the son had earned, and that the father had promised to let the son use to pay for attending camp. A Kenyan respondent is responsive to the justice issue embodied in the vignette (i.e., the breach of a promise by the father) but gives priority to the son's duty to be responsive to his father's wishes and authority:

> [If a father breaks his word], it will cause hatred because the son will be angry, saying, "I wanted to follow my own intentions, but my father cheated: he permitted me and then refused me." . . . So it is bad. . . . [However,] the one for the son is worse. Imagine a child disobeying my own words, is he really normal? (Edwards, 1986, p. 425)

The Kohlbergian scoring protocol, it may be noted, was not sensitive to this type of differential weighting of justice and competing moral concerns, and would have scored this as a nonmoral conventional stance. This type of stance, failing to appreciate the moral character of conflicting concerns, may have contributed to the skewed distribution of moral reasoning observed cross-culturally (Snarey, 1985).

Other evidence that there may be relatively greater priority given to interpersonal considerations compared to competing justice concerns in collectivist cultures is supported by experimentally controlled research that presented samples of U.S. and Indian adult and child populations with hypothetical conflict situations in which fulfillment of a justice issue conflicts with fulfillment of a competing interpersonal responsibility (J. G. Miller & Bersoff, 1992). An idiographic procedure was utilized in constructing the conflict situations to ensure that individuals viewed the individual justice and interpersonal breaches as equivalent in their seriousness and as tapping a range of issues, from major life-threatening concerns to minor issues. There was a common trend to give priority to the justice issues in the case of the life-threatening breaches (i.e., that pitted taking a life against saving a life). However, in a pattern congruent with the cross-cultural Kohlbergian trends reported earlier, marked cross-cultural differences were observed in the case of the non-life-threatening breaches. Thus, the Indian respondents tended more frequently to give priority to the competing interpersonal obligations than did the U.S. respondents. For example, whereas all of the U.S. respondents judged that it was morally wrong to steal a train ticket, even if this was the only way to fulfill the interpersonal responsibility of attending a best friend's wedding, a majority of the Indian re-

spondents judged that it was morally required to participate as planned in the wedding, even if this meant having to engage in the justice breach of stealing the ticket.

While supporting the universality of a moral concern with issues of justice, this research challenges claims that justice issues invariably take priority over competing moral concerns, an assumption that has been made in past theorizing based on the Kantian notion of perfect versus imperfect duties (Gert, 1988; Kant, 1797/1964; Urmson, 1958). From this latter perspective, justice is considered a "perfect" duty that may be fully realizable, in that it involves prohibition-oriented concerns (i.e., not to violate another's rights or to harm another). In contrast, helping and issues of family and friendship obligations are considered "imperfect" or "superogatory" concerns. The latter are considered desirable to undertake, but because of their positive orientation (i.e., calling for positive responsiveness to someone else's needs), they are too unbounded in scope to be fully realizable and must therefore always be somewhat delimited in scope. The present evidence highlights the need to recognize that whereas this type of formal distinction may be drawn between negative versus positive duties, the cultural meaning given to these two types of issues is crucial in how they are weighted in moral judgment, and not merely their status as positive versus negative obligations (J. G. Miller, 1991).

Variation in Weighting of Contextual Factors

Cross-cultural research on social attribution has documented marked cross-cultural differences in social inference. Thus, it has been demonstrated that there tends to be a greater emphasis on explaining social behavior in terms of dispositional traits of the person in individualistic cultures, whereas in collectivist cultures more weight is given in social attribution to social role relations and other contextual factors (Cousins, 1989; J. G. Miller, 1984; Shweder & Bourne, 1984). In terms of moral reasoning, these cross-cultural differences related to folk theories of the agent's relationship to the surround translate into variation in judgments of moral accountability or responsibility.

Judgments of accountability are presupposed in moral reasoning, in that they bear on the intentional nature of behavior. The domain of rule-governed behavior involves voluntary action in which the agent is judged to have sufficient control over his or her behavior to be held accountable for performing it. From this perspective, an agent cannot be held accountable for a behavior that is a mere occurrence or involuntary event; only if it is judged that an agent could have acted otherwise or prevented a particular behavior can he or she be held accountable for having engaged in this behavior. Thus, as research has shown, persons tend to be judged less responsible for a given behavior to the extent that the behavior is understood to be unintended, the agent is seen as lacking the capacities to understand the consequences of his or her behavior or to control its execution, or the behavior is seen as under the control of situational influences (Darley & Zanna, 1982; Fincham & Jaspars, 1980; Heider, 1958).

Research evidence suggests that in tending to view behavior as more situationaly influenced than U.S. populations, Indians tend more frequently to treat contextual factors as extenuating circumstances that reduce agents' accountability for justice violations (Bersoff & Miller, 1993). Thus, it has been shown that Indian adult and child populations more frequently absolve agents of accountability for what they perceive to be harmful or unjust behavior to the extent that this behavior is undertaken either under emotional duress or in the context of agent immaturity. For example, whereas both Indian and U.S. respondents agree that breaking into a locked house constitutes a moral violation, Indians more frequently than Americans maintain that agents should not be held morally accountable for such a breach if the agent had been frightened by an unexpected noise.

Variation in Definitions of Harm and Injustice

Perhaps most fundamentally, cultural variation in justice reasoning reflects the contrasting cultural theories of the person, of social relations, and of their interrelationship that affect how harm and justice are defined in concrete cases. Notably this variation is not just a matter of individuals having different available information but of contrasting definitions of personhood and harm that cannot be merely adjudicated by reference to the "facts" of situations.

Within Hindu Indian culture the persons seen as entitled to protection from harm extends to all forms of life (Vasudev & Hummel,

1987). Rather than a matter of mere personal choice, refraining from eating or otherwise harming animals is considered a moral and not merely a personal issue. Likewise, in other cases, the domains of the self that are seen as entitled to protection from harm may be drawn more broadly in collectivist than in individualistic cultures, resulting in acts that have a moral status in individualistic cultures not seen as entailing issue of harms or rights violations in collectivist cultures. Thus, for example, with respect to issues of family inheritance, in assuming that females should be accorded equal status as males, U.S. adults consider an inheritance practice that disadvantages the female to be a violation of her rights (Shweder et al., 1987). In contrast, in treating male–female relations in more differentiated terms, Indian adults consider it appropriate and thus not a moral violation for females to have lesser inheritance than males. It may be further noted that within cultures of honor, such as found in certain communities within the U.S. South, conceptions of personhood are so intertwined with social reputation that harm to reputation tends to be perceived as inseparable from harm to the self (Cohen & Nisbett, 1997; Vandello & Cohen, 2003).

Interpersonal Morality

Interpersonal morality pertains to responsibilities that exist to meet the needs of others and is therefore a type of "positive" morality that contrasts with the "negative" or prohibition-oriented morality of justice. Whereas justice morality involves refraining from acts of harm or injustice, interpersonal morality involves showing positive responsiveness to the needs of others. Interpersonal responsiveness has always been considered an aspect of morality, because it concerns issues of welfare; however, at least within the Kantian tradition that informs the work of theorists such as Kohlberg and Turiel, it has been assumed to have a superordinate or discretionary status rather than the fully obligatory character of justice morality (Kahn, 1992).

As noted earlier, in forwarding her model of a morality of caring, Gilligan (1982) challenged these Kantian assumptions and argued for the need to recognize caring as a qualitative, distinct form of morality that differs from that of justice but is fully moral in character. Thus, she maintained that the morality of caring is not subordinate to that of justice. She also argued that the morality of caring is based on a type of affective commitment or "co-feeling" that is oriented toward welfare concerns and is not vulnerable to self-serving and non-welfare-oriented emotions.

I mention the contributions of cultural research to demonstrate that moralities of caring take distinctive forms, and that the form of the morality of caring identified by Gilligan and her colleagues represents a culturally distinctive perspective grounded in the individualism of U.S. culture. Strikingly, this work also provides direct insight into the nature of caring responses among U.S. populations, suggesting that morality of caring responses are more contingent than assumed.

To assess the perceived moral status of caring, research conducted among U.S. and Indian adult and child populations tapped perceived responsibilities to meet the needs of others in cases involving low sacrifice or cost to the helper, and varying role relationships and levels of need (Miller et al., 1990; see also J. G. Miller & Luthar, 1989; J. G. Miller & Bersoff, 1994, 1995). In both cultures, helping tended to be seen as highly desirable and as a perceived responsibility. Among the U.S. respondents, the dominant tendency was to treat helping as a matter for personal decision making, whereas among Indian respondents, helping tended to be seen as an issue that is legitimately subject to social regulation. The trends observed among the U.S. respondents call attention to respects in which the approach to caring adopted in Gilligan's model embodies a voluntaristic approach to interpersonal responsibilities that is consonant, at least in this respect, with the aretaic model of helping assumed in the Kantian tradition, and that is in accord with the emphasis on personal freedom of choice in U.S. culture. In contrast, they point to the existence in India of a tendency to accord interpersonal responsibilities a more obligatory moral status, one that accords it the same status as issues of justice, a pattern predicted by neither the aretaic model of the Kantian framework nor Gilligan's portrayal of the morality of caring.

Gilligan herself emphasized the freely given nature of interpersonal responsiveness in the morality of caring, viewing caring responses as based not on role obligations but on affectively grounded personal commitments, providing a reliable basis for moral commitments that is not affected by nonmoral emotions. A cross-cultural study conducted among U.S. and Indian adults, utilized a between-participant manipulation to assess the impact of personal affinity and liking on perceived interpersonal responsibilities (J. G. Miller & Bersoff, 1998). Both U.S. and Indian respondents judged that moral responsibilities of parents to their young children were unaffected by such nonmoral affective considerations (i.e., the responsibility to meet a need of one's child is unaffected by how much personal affinity and liking one has for the child). However, in the case of adult siblings, friends, and even adult troop leaders to their child Scouts, U.S. adults judged that the responsibility to help was less when the relationship involved low personal affinity and liking compared with high personal affinity and liking. Thus, for example, U.S. respondents judged that a man had less moral responsibility to help his brother move into a new apartment if the man and his brother shared few common tastes and interests, and were not affectively close, compared with a situation in which they shared many tastes and interests, and had a warm and affectionate relationship. In contrast, the moral responsibility to help was not found to be contingent on such nonmoral considerations among the Indian respondents. These results suggest that the morality of caring as it exists among middle-class European American respondents is more contingent on nonmoral affective considerations than previously assumed, and, in this respect, somewhat vulnerable to the unreliability assumed by Kantian theorists to inhere in any affectively based morality. In contrast, the results suggest that the type of role-based perspective emphasized among middle-class Hindu Indian respondents is less contingent on nonmoral affective preferences.

Research conducted among U.S. populations of different religious backgrounds extends this work by suggesting that the pattern observed among U.S. respondents may reflect, at least in part, the value placed within Christianity on acting in accord with one's mental states (Cohen & Rozin, 2001). It was documented that, compared to Jewish respondents, Christian respondents make a more negative appraisal of the moral character of a hypothetical agent who behaves in ways that are responsive to the needs of his elderly parents whom he dislikes. These findings, which were demonstrated in other types of moral appraisal as well, not only point to possible within-culture sources of variation in interpersonal morality but also identify some of the specific ways that Christian doctrine may have impact on the results observed in the cross-cultural investigation by J. G. Miller and Bersoff (1998), a study undertaken among a predominately Christian U.S. population.

More generally, the consistent pattern of cross-cultural differences observed in these various studies highlights the need to broaden the theoretical framework of Gilligan to take into account the observed cross-cultural variation. The responses observed among the U.S. and the Indian respondents both represent moralities of caring and encompass what theorists have characterized as types of *Gemeinschaft* concerns (Snarey & Keljo, 1991). However, whereas the approach captured in Gilligan's theoretical model privileges a voluntaristic approach to caring of an agent acting outside of role obligations, the approach captured in the work described earlier in India privileges an agent attuned to what are perceived to be natural duties associated with his or her social roles. This insight led to the proposal for expanding the theoretical constructs invoked to understand interpersonal morality, with the type of approach captured in Gilligan's model termed an "individually oriented" perspective and that observed in India termed a more "duty-based" perspective (J. G. Miller, 1994). Notably, the point of these conceptual labels is to call for an expansion of theory in this area and not to make assertions about uniform differences in moral orientation (J. G. Miller, 2006). In arguing that the morality of caring can take a "duty-based" form, no claim is being made that Indians always emphasis duty in moral reasoning, just as when Gilligan argued for the existence of a "morality of caring," she was not claiming that women in all cases emphasize caring in moral reasoning.

Although the available research to date is limited, evidence suggests that modes of caring found in other collectivist cultures differ in distinctive ways from both the morality of caring framework identified among U.S. respondents and that observed in the Indian research discussed earlier. To give some examples, work has uncovered among Japanese populations an emphasis on an approach to interpersonal morality that centers on issues on *omoiyari*, or empathy within one's ingroup (Shimizu, 2001). For example, such a stance is reflected in the

following response of an adolescent boy who does not report a case of vandalism by another student to the teachers; the boy takes such action in empathizing with the student's desire to retain a supportive relationship with his mother, the school nurse—a relationship that would be disrupted by such a report:

> You see if I became their enemy (by accusing them), they would feel uncomfortable to see my mother. . . . So although they destroy school property, I would feel bad for them if they lost someone with whom they could talk about their problems. (Shimizu, 2001, p. 463)

In turn, work with Chinese populations illustrates an approach to interpersonal morality that privileges what is perceived to be the innate, affectively grounded moral tendency of *jen*, "the deep affection for kin rooted in filial piety and extended through the family circle to all men" (Dien, 1982, p. 334). This can be seen, for example, in the invocation of the concept of *jen* by a Chinese respondent in reasoning about the Heinz dilemma:

> Even though the law did not set limit to the price of the drug, the druggist should not set the price so high because the druggist should have the feeling of distress at the suffering of others. He knows pretty well that the drug is used to cure people in danger, and if the price is so high, the poor people couldn't afford to buy it and would therefore lose their lives. So, the price should not be set so high based on *jen*. In addition, in making the drug, the druggist should hold a "doctor-with-a-parental-heart" attitude. Otherwise, the social consequences are likely to be disastrous. (Ma, 1997, p. 107)

Although this type of response would be scored at the conventional level in the Kohlbergian approach, as critics have pointed out and as argued here, it represents a type of alternative, communitarian postconventional morality.

Moralities of Divinity

Treating morality as secular in nature, the dominant psychological theories of morality assume that religious concerns have no role in morality. Within the mainstream frameworks, religion is excluded from morality, because it is seen as based on faith rather than on rationality. Although it is empirically observed that spiritual concerns are mentioned in open-ended reasoning, such concerns are considered to be merely conventional rather than moral in nature. Cultural research demonstrates, in contrast, that spiritual concerns are integrally related to concerns with justice and caring, and are therefore the core to lay conceptions of morality.

Evidence for this claim may be seen, for example, in research on moral exemplars. Thus, in an indepth qualitative study of the perspectives of individuals who identified as having shown extraordinary moral commitment, Colby and Damon (1992) observed that many of these individuals attributed their value commitments to their religious faith. Such a stance is illustrated in the following explanation given by a respondent who ascribes the years she devoted to caring for the poor to her conversion to fundamentalist Christianity: "I didn't know how I was doing it or why, but I know the Holy Spirit was leading me, saying, 'You have to help them, you have to help them' " (p. 354). As reflected in this response, many individuals attributed their stamina in being able to make the type of personal sacrifice entailed in living morally exemplary lives to their faith and saw serving God as part of the justification for their actions. Similar results have been observed in the case of populations who maintain a predominately secular outlook. Thus, for example, Walker et al. (1995) found that concerns with religion, faith, and spirituality commonly informed the lay conceptions of morality held by adolescents and adults from the Vancouver area of Canada, a region that is highly secular. In this investigation, religion was observed to provide justifications for a morality built on ideas of justice and welfare, including concerns that focused on issues of reward and punishment, such as fear of eternal damnation; concerns that appeared to include some conventional elements, such as the importance of church and fellow believers; and concerns that involved moral principles such as *agape* love.

Spiritual outlooks have been shown to motivate not only commitments to moralities based on justice or caring but also to entail distinctive epistemological assumptions that impact on how issues of justice and caring are understood at different ages. Such trends were documented, for example, in a study examining the responses of Nepalese Buddhist monks to the Kohlbergian Heinz moral dilemma (Huebner & Garrod, 1991, 1993). Reflecting outlooks framed by Buddhist conceptions of karma, at younger ages, respondents centered on the negative karma that would ensue from Heinz stealing the drug. As a young adolescent argued, "If you create negative actions (bad karma), then you will become sick or die and when you die, then you will go to the animal realism or to the hell realms . . . or you will be born into very bad future lives with much sickness and no money" (1993, p. 180). In contrast, at older ages, karma entered into moral judgments in affecting the reasons why life is to be valued. Thus, in assuming that all beings continue to exist in some form endlessly, an older adolescent justified saving Heinz's wife's life out of concern for her contributions to society:

> If the person dies, then that person will no longer be around. He will go on to another existence, but maybe he will be an animal or in another part of the world. Anyway, he will never be exactly the same again. This is the way it is, and so we must protect people from dying. If it is for two more years, or even as short as three months, this person can still do some good things. He can help another person. (Huebner & Garrod, 1991, p. 181)

In these responses, the central concept is not one of a perceived right to life, as observed typically among respondents from a Judeo-Christian background, but rather the unique qualities distinguishing different lives.

Importantly, cultural evidence also demonstrates that spiritual outlooks not only support moralities of justice and of caring but also constitute their own distinctive form of morality. Thus, Shweder, Much, Mahapatra, and Park (1997) established that there exist three and not merely two, broad forms of moral orientation: (1) an ethics of "autonomy" that involves issues of harm, rights, and justice, and that has been the center of both Kohlbergian research and that in the distinct domain tradition; (2) an ethics of "community" that involves responsiveness to the needs of others, and that has been the focus both in Gilligan's morality of caring model and in more cultural approaches to caring; and (3) an ethics of "divinity" that has tended to be considered exclusively a conventional type of orientation. The morality of divinity involves concerns with issues such as the sacred order, sin, purity, pollution, and sanctity that bear on protection of the human soul from spiritual degradation and on promotion of spiritual refinement. Evidence for the existence of this ethic may be seen in themes that were spontaneously mentioned in reasoning about everyday behavioral events among an orthodox Hindu Indian sample and a secular U.S. sample (Shweder et al., 1997). In certain cases, concerns with divinity were common across the two cultural populations, with both U.S. and Indian respondents raising concerns primarily involving divinity in the case of the issue of incest. In other cases, the concerns tended to be culturally variable, with, for example, the secular U.S. population tending to consider eating beef as involving the absence of harm and the orthodox Hindu Indian population centering on the spiritual degradation that would ensue from such behavior. The morality of divinity has also been shown to be distinguishable from the moralities of autonomy and of community in terms of its emotional meanings. Thus, research conducted among U.S. and Japanese college students demonstrates that disgust is associated with violations of purity–sanctity, a central concern in the morality of divinity, whereas anger is linked to the individual rights' violations associated with the morality of autonomy, and contempt is linked to the violation of communal codes in the morality of community (Rozin, Lowery, Imada, & Haidt, 1999).

Work on themes of divinity also highlights the need to understand morality as extending beyond issues involving harm or welfare and demonstrates that perceptions of harm or welfare are culturally variable. In this regard, research conducted among a U.S. and a Brazilian population of lower socioeconomic status demonstrates that issues perceived to involve extremely disgusting or disrespectful actions, such as using the national flag for a bathroom rag or eating the family dog, are perceived as moral violations, even though such actions are regarded as principally involving concerns related to divinity and not harm (Haidt, Koller, & Dias, 1993). Thus, within the Brazilian population, moral judgment was more closely predicted by asking whether the respondent was "bothered" personally by the action than by asking whether anyone was harmed. Work by Jensen (1997, 1998) has further documented that whether or not harm is even seen as existing in a given situation depends on spiritual outlooks. This trend is illustrated in work comparing moral judgments of the orthodox Hindu Indian practice of *sati*. Whereas orthodox U.S.

respondents treated such behavior as an issue of moral harm, many of the orthodox Indians viewed it as virtuous behavior. As one orthodox Hindu informant commented:

> *Sati* is morally right. . . . The wife dies with her husband in order to (preserve) her chasitity and (show) her devotion to her husband. (Jensen, 1998, p. 101)

Work of this type notably highlights the need to recognize that whether or not harm is even perceived to exist depends in part on culturally and religiously based value commitments.

Summary

Cultural work demonstrates that marked cross-cultural variation exists in justice reasoning that reflects contrasting weighting of competing moral and nonmoral concerns, and culturally variable assumptions concerning the nature of persons, harm, and territories of the self entitled to protection from harm. This work also documents that forms of interpersonal morality are culturally variable; indeed, the framework proposed by Gilligan is itself a culturally bound model. Culturally variable forms of interpersonal morality differ in important respects, among others, such as their emphasis on personal choice, contingency on nonmoral considerations, and weight accorded to affective considerations. Importantly, cultural work is also highlighting the need to expand the scope of the moral domain to encompass concerns involving divinity. Such concerns constitute a distinctive form of morality that embraces conceptions of spiritual concerns that transcend issues of harm.

NEW DIRECTIONS

In terms of promising new directions, cultural work on moral development is further examining the nature of moral reasoning in everyday contexts, exploring issues of power dynamics and culture conflict, and contributing to an understanding of the developmental processes through which moral outlooks emerge. Select examples of this work are briefly discussed below as I highlight some of the new theoretical insights and methodological approaches that distinguish work in this area.

Morality in Everyday Contexts

In examining moral development in relation to a wider range of everyday situations, cultural work is contributing to further conceptual broadening of the scope of the moral domain. One example of this type of approach is found in a recent series of studies that examined reasoning about real-life ecological issues, such as the 1990 Exxon *Valdez* oil spill, among children of different sociocultural backgrounds and different everyday relationships to the natural environment (Howe & Kahn, 1996; Kahn, 1997, 1998, 1999). Age-related changes were observed among U.S. children, with second graders tending to emphasize a "homocentric" form of reasoning that focuses on implications of harm to the ecology relative to human welfare (e.g., that polluting nature would get people sick), and fifth-grade and eighth-grade students placing greater emphasis on "biocentric" reasoning that treats nature itself as having moral standing or an intrinsic right to be protected from harm. In contrast, homocentric forms of reasoning tend to be emphasized among children from the Brazilian Amazon. Providing evidence to suggest that universally moral and not merely conventional reasoning is applied to protecting the natural world from harm, this work also highlights the varied sociocultural processes that impact on children's outlooks. Thus, whereas the perspective of the U.S. sample appears to reflect in part the emphasis placed on ecological concerns in the curriculum of U.S. schools and popular culture, the outlooks of children from the Brazilian Amazon appear to stem, at least in part, from individuals' sense of being more dependent on nature for their immediate physical survival.

In another example of approaches to understanding morality in everyday contexts, an ethnographic study examined the processes by which youth organizations create moral experiences that are instrumental in participant's adaptation in the larger community (Heath, 1996). Norms that develop in such organizations promote moral values, such as a sense of fair processes, as well as family-like relationships of caring. Such outlooks are reflected, for example, in the everyday conversations among members of an all-male, African American inner-city basketball team in reflecting on how they saw their coach as getting them to do what was considered right. Work of this type points to the value of understanding moral values as they emerge in everyday behavioral interaction and conversational interchange, rather than conducting studies focused explicitly on moral reasoning tasks.

Power Dynamics and Culture Conflict

In terms of new directions, cultural work also focuses on integrating a concern with cultural meanings and practices, and a concern with power dynamics. It is recognized that cultural meanings and practices may in some cases constitute instruments of domination, in which groups in subordinate positions suffer discrimination and have unequal access to resources (e.g., Abu-Lughod, 1993; Appadurai, 1988; Turiel, 1998b, 2002). However, cultural also emphasizes work that relationships of unequal power need to be understood in the context of culturally variable meanings and practices.

In the area of dissent, research demonstrates that cultural practices are framed in ways that take into account distinctive cultural emphases; thus, they do not in all cases privilege what is assumed in mainstream psychological theories of morality to be the universal moral value of individual equality. This type of trend was observed, for example, in a comparative study examining conceptions of everyday family roles and of feminism among samples of middle-aged women from Japan and the U.S. (Schaberg, 2002). Although the Japanese women expressed dissent with the gender role practices of their society, their concerns did not map directly onto the concerns with seeking greater freedom of choice and equality expressed by U.S. respondents. Valuing reciprocal interdependence in family relationships, the Japanese women criticized the family role expectations of their society as insufficiently flexible and called for greater accommodation in gender role expectations. However, they rejected the egalitarian model of marital relations emphasized by U.S. respondents. The Japanese respondents also forwarded a moral critique of what they viewed as the individual-centered and, in their eyes, somewhat selfish stance of U.S. feminism, and called for a form of feminism that, differing from that emphasized within the United States, entailed a greater commitment to social activism and contributing to the community.

In another example, an ethnographically based sociolinguistic study of Hindu Indian family life likewise documented respects in which dissent tends to be framed in culturally distinctive ways that may give priority to social hierarchy rather than treat all persons as morally equal (Much, 1997). Such a trend may be illustrated in the example of an adolescent son in a Brahmin family who temporarily stopped wearing the holy symbol of the Sacred Thread. The son's reported motives were to challenge the moral meanings given to that symbol and to express his own personal view that wearing such a symbol represented merely an unimportant matter of social convention rather than a moral duty. However, in framing dissent in this way, the son notably did not call into question more fundamental commitments of his cultural community to the principle of hierarchy and to the importance of caste identity.

These same types of concerns with attending both to power dynamics and culturally variable meanings is also evident in work examining culture conflict in the context of immigration (Shweder, Minow, & Markus, 2002). This work, like that preceding it, focuses on the challenge of identifying standards for moral appraisal that, while being sensitive to issues of harm and abuse, recognize that their identification must proceed in culturally sensitive ways. In this regard, as Shweder, Markus, Minow, and Kessel (1997) have pointed out, problems arise when the legal system and other public institutions enforcing particular U.S. outlooks on values such as equality, child rights, and so on, end up overriding the contrasting outlooks and everyday practices of immigrant populations. In examining this type of issue, Shweder (2002) critically examined the meanings associated with a practice, such as female genital alteration, that, while treated as a universal issue of harm by various feminist scholars and governmental institutions, is invested with cultural meanings and embodied in everyday cultural practices that give it value as a sign of female identity and maturity. In other examples, Kim and Markus (2002) critically examine the cultural emphasis on verbal expression in particular U.S. mainstream cultural contexts, which gives rise to cultural practices that may infringe on what may be seen as a "freedom of silence" in immigrant groups that place a greater value on nonverbal modes of communication.

Notably, work in this general area of power dynamics and culture conflict is of value in addressing not only this central theoretical challenge of how to integrate a concern with cultural meanings and power dynamics in moral appraisal of cultural practices but also the question of moral relativism that has been central in psychological work on moral development. It argues for the need to recognize the complex, yet necessary, questions that arise in moral appraisal of cultural practices. Embodying what might be characterized as a pragmatic rather than extreme form of moral relativism, this type of cultural psychology stance does not eschew comparative cultural appraisal but maintains that such appraisal must proceed with as complete as possible an understanding of local cultural viewpoints, including that of the observer. As Shweder comments:

> Cultural psychology fully acknowledges that there is no way to avoid making critical judgments about good and bad, right and wrong, true and false, efficient and inefficient. . . . Any culture deserving of respect, must be defensible in the face of criticism from "outside." . . . One of the distinctive features of cultural psychology is that it is willing to try to make that defense, representing the "inside" point of view in such a way that it can be understood, perhaps appreciated, or at the very least tolerated from an "outside" point of view. (2000a, p. 216)

The resultant stance calls for a more pluralistic view of cultural diversity than that embodied in the mainstream perspectives on moral development in psychology, or in many contemporary public institutions. It acknowledges the existence at an abstract moral level of moral universals, including concerns with "justice, beneficence, autonomy, sacrifice, liberty, loyalty, sanctity, duty" (Shweder, 2000b, p. 164), while also recognizing that these goods are instantiated in culturally distinctive ways and cannot be maximized simultaneously.

Enculturation and Moral Development

Finally, another important new direction for work on moral development is to contribute to an understanding of the processes through which moral meanings are embodied and communicated in everyday practices. This work increasingly not only focuses on discourse practices as contexts for child socialization but also attends to language use and normative shifts that impact on the changing moral outlooks of adults.

Work with child populations is calling attention to the role of discourse practices as contexts in which children come to understand, as well as to participate in creating, shared moral outlooks that are salient within their cultural communities. In early groundbreaking work in this area, Much and Shweder (1978) documented that children tacitly display, as well as come to develop, their ability to distinguish between different types of rules as a function of how they and others in their social environments respond to their behavior. Thus, kindergartners and their teachers offered distinctive types of justifications to breaches of different types of social rules. Both children and teachers tended to respond to breaches of social conventions with statements concerning the applicability of the relevant rule. For example, a child defended his violation of the rule that children were to play outside by citing his cold as a plausible exception to the rule—"My mother said! I just got a sore throat!"—only to be rebuffed by a teacher who offered an alternative interpretation of the prevailing rule—"Well, if you can't go out, then you stay home because you're sick" (Much & Shweder, 1978, p. 21). In contrast, children responded to breaches of moral rules, a type of rule that is considered absolute, in ways that either denied that the act occurred or that redefined the act to make the agent nonblameworthy. Thus, for example, a child accused of stealing a peer's chair responded that because the chair was empty, she did not steal it, she merely "sat in it" (p. 37). Notably, this type of conversational interchange, with its opportunities for feedback and negotiation, functioned in a tacit way that conveyed powerful culturally variable moral messages, even though it was not viewed by any of the participants as involving issues of morality.

Cultural work is also focusing on how everyday socialization practices in the family and larger community embody particular moral values. Thus, for example, recent sociolinguistic work among families from Taiwan has documented an emphasis on disciplinary practices that communicate a moral sense of shame (Fung, 1999; Fung & Chen, 2001). This may be seen in the following example of a mother and older sister's verbal shaming responses to a 3-year-old child who has committed the breach of approaching the researcher's camcorder. The mother threatens to ostracize and withdraw love from her child, commenting, "We don't want you; you stand here. Mama is mad. Look how ugly your crying will be on tape"—a stance underscored by the 5-

year-old sister joining in with the chant, "Ugly monster, ugly monster" (Fung, 1999, p. 193). This type of moral emphasis notably is also evident in other everyday socialization practices, with Taiwanese mothers using personal storytelling as an opportunity to communicate moral lessons through spontaneously narrating examples of children's past transgressions, a trend not observed among European American mothers, who tend more frequently to use such interaction as an opportunity for entertainment and affirmation of the child's sense of self and promotion of their self-esteem (P. J. Miller, Wiley, Fung, & Liang, 1997). More generally, cultural work is pointing to the role of culture in assigning children to different everyday socialization contexts that affect their moral outlooks. Thus, for example, Edwards (1985) has pointed to the role of everyday experiences in sibling caregiving in various African rural communities as opportunities for the socialization of responsibility, whereas cross-national comparisons have pointed to the role of voluntary work commitments for adolescents in promoting a sense of civic responsibility (Flanagan, Bowes, Jonsson, Csapo, & Shblanova, 1998).

Notably, work by Rozin (1999) on "moralization" examines processes by which affective preferences are converted into moral commitments among adult and not merely child members of a culture. Thus, Rozin traces how common cultural practices, such as cigarette smoking or even overeating, that may be associated with negative affective reactions such as disgust, can take on moral overtones for individuals through not only rational reflection but also a range of societal practices that call negative attention to such behavior, such as a cigarette tax, initiating scientific inquiry to uncover new information about processes that affect the behavior and the implementation of new legal regulations. Such processes of cultural change in the perceived moral status of particular behaviors can occur relatively rapidly, with the moralization of attitudes toward smoking occurring across three generations of Americans within a 20- to 40-year period, and morally coloring people's perceptions (Rozin & Singh, 1999). Thus, in a striking illustration of such an effect, U.S. college students tend to judge people who eat primarily high-fat diets to be less considerate than people who eat primarily fruits and vegetables (Stein & Nemeroff, 1995).

Summary

In terms of new directions, research on moral development is increasingly examining moral outlooks reflected in a wide range of real-life issues and everyday cultural settings. Integrating a concern with power dynamics with an attention to cultural meanings and practices, this work provides insight into processes of resistance and dissent, as well as issues of cultural conflict. New process accounts that are also being developed not only highlight the everyday practices and modes of social interaction that impact on children's developing moral outlooks but also provide insights into the affectively and culturally grounded processes by which moral outlooks change at a societal level that affects the outlooks of adults.

CONCLUSION

Research on moral development in cultural psychology highlights the need to expand contemporary mainstream psychological theories of morality, to make them more culturally inclusive, and to pay increased attention to the role of cultural meanings and everyday practices in the developmental emergence of moral outlooks. Rather than leading to an extreme form of moral relativism, work in this tradition underscores the importance of becoming more aware of the discretionary aspects of one's own cultural outlooks and of appraising alternative cultural commitments in ways that are appreciative of their coherence and sense. Generative in nature and increasingly addressing real-world applications, work on moral development in cultural psychology underscores the inseparable interrelationships between culture, morality, and lived experience.

REFERENCES

Abu-Lughod, L. (1993). *Writing women's worlds: Bedouin stories.* Berkeley: University of California Press.

Appadurai, A. (1988). Putting hierarchy in its place. *Cultural Anthropology, 3,* 36–49.

Bardige, B., Ward, J. V., Gilligan, C., Taylor, J., & Cohen, G. (1988). Moral concerns and considerations of urban youth. In C. Gilligan, J. V. Ward, & J. Taylor (Eds.), *Mapping the moral domain* (pp. 159–173). Cambridge, MA: Harvard University Press.

Berkowitz, L. (1964). *Development of motives and values in a child.* New York: Basic Books.

Berry, J. W., Poortinga, Y. H., Segall, M. H., & Dasen, P. R. (1992). *Cross-cultural psychology: Research and applications.* Cambridge, UK: Cambridge University Press.

Bersoff, D. M., & Miller, J. G. (1993). Culture, context, and the development of moral accountability judgments. *Developmental Psychology, 29*(4), 664–676.

Brandt, R. B. (1959). *Ethical theory.* Upper Saddle River, NJ: Prentice Hall.

Bronfenbrenner, U. (1979). *The ecology of human development: Experiments by nature and design.* Cambridge, MA: Harvard University Press.

Bruner, J. S. (1973). Going beyond the information given. In J. M. Anglin (Ed.), *Beyond the information given: Studies in the psychology of knowing* (pp. 218–238). New York: Norton.

Bruner, J. (1990). *Acts of meaning.* Cambridge, MA: Harvard University Press.

Buck-Morss, S. (1975). Socio-economic bias in Piaget's theory: Implications for cross-cultural studies. *Human Development, 18,* 35–49.

Cohen, D., & Nisbett, R. E. (1997). Field experiments examining the culture of honor: The role of institutions in perpetuating norms about violence. *Personality and Social Psychology Bulletin, 23*(11), 1188–1199.

Colby, A., & Damon, W. (1992). *Some do care: Contemporary lives of moral commitment.* New York: Free Press.

Cole, M. (1990). Cultural psychology: A once and future discipline? In J. J. Berman (Ed.), *Nebraska Symposium on Motivation: Vol. 38. Cross-cultural perspectives* (pp. 279–335). Lincoln: University of Nebraska Press.

Cole, M. (1996). *Cultural psychology: A once and future discipline.* Cambridge, MA: Harvard University Press.

Cousins, S. D. (1989). Culture and self-perception in Japan and the United States. *Journal of Personality and Social Psychology, 56,* 124–131.

D'Andrade, R. G. (1984). Cultural meaning systems. In R. A. Shweder & R. A. LeVine (Eds.), *Culture theory: Essays on mind, self, and emotion* (pp. 88–119). New York: Cambridge University Press.

Darley, J. M., & Pittman, T. S. (2003). The psychology of compensatory and retributive justice. *Personality and Social Psychology Review, 7*(4), 324–336.

Darley, J., & Zanna, M. (1982). Making moral judgments. *American Scientist, 70,* 515–521.

Dien, D. S.-F. (1982). A Chinese perspective on Kohlberg's theory of moral development. *Developmental Review, 2,* 331–341.

Edwards, C. P. (1975). Societal complexity and moral development: A Kenyan study. *Ethos, 3*(4), 505–527.

Edwards, C. P. (1985). Another style of competence: The caregiving child. In A. D. Vogel & G. F. Melson (Eds.), *The origins of nurturance* (pp. 95–121). New York: Erlbaum.

Edwards, C. (1986). Cross-cultural research on

Kohlberg's stages: The basis for consensus. In S. Modgil & C. Modgil (Eds.), *Kohlberg: Consensus and controversy* (pp. 419–430). Philadelphia: Falmer Press.

Eysenck, H. J. (1961). *Handbook of abnormal psychology: An experimental approach*. New York: Basic Books.

Fincham, F., & Jaspars, J. (1980). Attribution of responsibility: From man the scientist to man as lawyer. In L. Berkowitz (Ed.), *Advances in experimental social psychology* (Vol. 13, pp. 82–138). San Diego, CA: Academic Press.

Flanagan, C., Bowes, J. M., Jonsson, B., Csapo, B., & Shblanova, E. (1998). Ties that bind: Correlates of adolescents' civic commitment in seven countries. *Journal of Social Issues, 54*(3), 457–475.

Freud, S. (1930). *Civilization and its discontents*. London: Hogarth Press.

Fung, H. (1999). Becoming a moral child: The socialization of shame among young Chinese children. *Ethos, 27*(2), 180–209.

Fung, H., & Chen, E. C. (2001). Across time and beyond skin: Self and transgression in the everyday socialization of shame among Taiwanese preschool children. *Social Development, 10*(3), 420–437.

Geertz, C. (1973). *The interpretation of cultures*. New York: Basic Books.

Gert, B. (1988). *Morality: A new justification of the moral rules*. New York: Oxford University Press.

Gilligan, C. (1977). In a different voice: Women's conceptions of self and of morality. *Harvard Educational Review, 47*(4), 481–517.

Gilligan, C. (1982). *In a different voice: Psychological theory and women's development*. Cambridge, MA: Harvard University Press.

Gilligan, C., Ward, J. V., & Taylor, J. (Eds.). (1988). *Mapping the moral domain*. Cambridge, MA: Harvard University Press.

Gilligan, C., & Wiggins, G. (1988). The origins of morality in early childhood relationships. In C. Gilligan, J. Ward, & J. Taylor (Eds.), *Mapping the moral domain: A contribution of women's thinking to psychological theory and education* (pp. 111–138). Cambridge, MA: Harvard University Press.

Haidt, J. (2001). The emotional dog and its rational tail: A social intuitionist approach to moral judgment. *Psychological Review, 108*(4), 814–834.

Haidt, J., Koller, S. H., & Dias, M. G. (1993). Affect, culture, and morality, or is it wrong to eat your dog? *Journal of Personality and Social Psychology, 65*(4), 613–628.

Harkness, S., Edwards, C. P., & Super, C. M. (1981). Social roles and moral reasoning: A case study in a rural African community. *Developmental Psychology, 17*(5), 595–603.

Heath, S. B. (1996). Ruling places: Adaptation in development by inner-city youth. In R. Jessor, A. Colby, & R. A. Shweder (Eds.), *Ethnography and human development: Context and meaning in social inquiry* (pp. 225–251). Chicago: University of Chicago Press.

Heider, F. (1958). *The psychology of interpersonal relations*. New York: Wiley.

Howe, C. C., & Kahn, P. H. (1996). Along the Rio Negro: Brazilian children's environmental views and values. *Developmental Psychology, 32*(6), 978–987.

Huebner, A., & Garrod, A. (1991). Moral reasoning in a Karmic world. *Human Development, 34*, 341–352.

Huebner, A. M., & Garrod, A. C. (1993). Moral reasoning among Tibetan Monks: A study of Buddhist adolescents and young adults in Nepal. *Journal of Cross-Cultural Psychology, 24*(2), 167–185.

Jensen, L. A. (1997). Different worldviews, different morals: America's culture war divide. *Human Development, 40*(6), 325–344.

Jensen, L. A. (1998). Moral divisions within countries between orthodoxy and progressivism: India and the United States. *Journal for the Scientific Study of Religion, 37*(1), 90–107.

Kagan, J. (1984). *The nature of the child*. New York: Basic Books.

Kahn, P. H. (1992). Children's obligatory and discretionary moral judgments. *Child Development, 63*, 416–430.

Kahn, P. H. (1997). Bayous and jungle rivers: Cross-cultural perspectives on children's environmental moral reasoning. In H. D. Saltzstein (Ed.), *Culture as a context for moral development: New perspectives on the particular and the universal* (pp. 23–36). San Francisco: Jossey-Bass.

Kahn, P. (1998). Children's moral and ecological reasoning about the Prince William Sound oil spill. *Developmental Psychology, 33*(6), 1091–1096.

Kahn, P. (1999). *The human relationship with nature: Development and culture*. Cambridge, MA: MIT Press.

Kant, I. (1964). *The doctrine of virtue*. Chicago: University of Chicago Press. (Original work published 1797)

Kim, H. S., & Markus, H. R. (2002). Freedom of speech and freedom of silence: An analysis of talking as a cultural practice. In R. Shweder, M. Minow, & H. R. Markus (Eds.), *Engaging cultural differences: The multicultural challenge in liberal democracies* (pp. 432–452). New York: Russell Sage Foundation.

Kohlberg, L. (1969). Stage and sequence: The cognitive-developmental approach to socialization. In D. A. Goslin (Ed.), *Handbook of socialization theory* (pp. 347–380). Chicago: Rand McNally.

Kohlberg, L. (1971). From *is* to *ought*: How to commit the naturalistic fallacy and get away with it in the study of moral development. In T. Mischel (Ed.), *Cognitive development and epistemology* (pp. 151–236). New York: Academic Press.

Kohlberg, L. (1981). *The philosophy of moral development: Moral stages and the idea of justice* (Vol. 1). New York: Harper & Row.

Kohlberg, L., Levine, C., & Hewer, A. (1983). Moral stages: A current formulation and a response to critics. In J. A. Meacham (Ed.), *Contributions to human development* (Vol. 10, pp. 1–177). Basel, Switzerland: Karger.

LeVine, R. A. (1984). Properties of culture: An ethnographic view. In R. A. Shweder & R. A. LeVine (Eds.), *Culture theory: Essays on mind, self, and emotion* (pp. 67–87). New York: Cambridge University Press.

Ma, H. K. (1997). The affective and cognitive aspects of moral development: A Chinese perspective. In H. Kao & D. Sinha (Eds.), *Asian perspectives on psychology* (pp. 93–109). Thousand Oaks, CA: Sage.

Markus, H. R., Kitayama, S., & Heiman, R. J. (1996). Culture and "basic" psychological principles. In E. Higgins & A. Kruglanski (Eds.), *Social psychology: Handbook of basic principles* (pp. 857–913). New York: Guilford Press.

Miller, J. G. (1984). Culture and the development of everyday social explanation. *Journal of Personality and Social Psychology, 46*(5), 961–978.

Miller, J. G. (1991). A cultural perspective on the morality of beneficence and interpersonal responsibility. In S. Ting-Toomey & F. Korzenny (Eds.), *International and intercultural communication annual* (Vol. 15, pp. 11–27). Newbury Park, CA: Sage.

Miller, J. G. (1994). Cultural diversity in the morality of caring: Individually oriented versus duty-based interpersonal moral codes. *Cross-Cultural Research, 28*(1), 3–39.

Miller, J. G. (1997). Theoretical issues in cultural psychology. In J. W. Berry, Y. H. Poortinga, & J. Pandey (Eds.), *Handbook of cross-cultural psychology: Vol. 1. Theory and method* (2nd ed., pp. 85–128). Boston, MA: Allyn & Bacon.

Miller, J. G. (1999). Cultural psychology: Implications for basic psychological theory. *Psychological Science, 10*(2), 85–91.

Miller, J. G. (2001). Culture and moral development. In D. Matsumoto (Ed.), *The handbook of culture and psychology* (pp. 151–169). New York: Oxford University Press.

Miller, J. G. (2002). Bringing culture to basic psychological theory: Beyond individualism and collectivism: Comment on Oyserman et al. (2002). *Psychological Bulletin, 128*(1), 97–109.

Miller, J. G. (2006). Insights into moral development from cultural psychology. In M. Killen & J. Smetana (Eds.), *Handbook of moral development* (pp. 375–398). Mahwah, NJ: Erlbaum.

Miller, J. G., & Bersoff, D. M. (1992). Culture and moral judgment: How are conflicts between justice and interpersonal responsibilities resolved? *Journal of Personality and Social Psychology, 62*(4), 541–554.

Miller, J. G., & Bersoff, D. M. (1994). Cultural influences on the moral status of reciprocity and the discounting of endogenous motivation [Special issue: The self and the collective]. *Personality and Social Psychology Bulletin, 20*(5), 592–602.

Miller, J. G., & Bersoff, D. M. (1995). Development in the context of everyday family relationships: Culture, interpersonal morality, and adaptation. In M. Killen & D. Hart (Eds.), *Morality in everyday life: Developmental perspectives* (pp. 259–282). New York: Cambridge University Press.

Miller, J. G., & Bersoff, D. M. (1999). The role of liking in perceptions of the moral responsibility to help: A cultural perspective. *Journal of Experimental Social Psychology, 34*(5), 443–469.

Miller, J. G., Bersoff, D. M., & Harwood, R. L. (1990). Perceptions of social responsibilities in India and in the United States: Moral imperatives or personal decisions? *Journal of Personality and Social Psychology, 58*(1), 33–47.

Miller, J. G., & Luthar, S. (1989). Issues of interpersonal responsibility and accountability: A comparison of Indians' and Americans' moral judgments. *Social Cognition, 7*(3), 237–261.

Miller, P. J., Wiley, A. R., Fung, H., & Liang, C.-H. (1997). Personal storytelling as a medium of socialization in Chinese and American families. *Child Development, 68*(3), 557–568.

Much, N. C. (1997). A semiotic view of socialisation, lifespan development and cultural psychology: With vignettes from the moral culture of traditional Hindu households [Special issue: Cultural constructions and social cognition: Emerging themes]. *Psychology and Developing Societies, 9*(1), 65–106.

Much, N. C., & Shweder, R. A. (1978). Speaking of rules: The analysis of culture in breach. In W. Damon (Ed.), *New directions for child development: Moral development* (Vol. 2, pp. 19–39). San Francisco: Jossey-Bass.

Nucci, L. P. (2002). The development of moral reasoning. In U. Goswami (Ed.), *Blackwell handbook of childhood cognitive development* (pp. 303–325). Malden, MA: Blackwell.

Piaget, J. (1932). *The moral judgment of the child*. London: Routledge & Kegan Paul.

Piaget, J. (1973). Need and significance of cross-cultural studies in genetic psychology. In J. W. Berry & P. R. Dasen (Eds.), *Culture and cognition: Readings in cross-cultural psychology* (pp. 299–309). London: Methuen.

Pool, D. L., Shweder, R. A., & Much, N. C. (1983). Culture as a cognitive system: Differentiated rule understandings in children and other savages. In E. T. Higgins, D. N. Ruble, & W. W. Hartup (Eds.), *Social cognition and social development: A sociocultural perspective* (pp. 193–213). New York: Cambridge University Press.

Rawls, J. (1971). *Justice as fairness*. Cambridge, MA: Harvard University Press.

Rozin, P. (1999). The process of moralization. *Psychological Science, 10*(3), 218–221.

Rozin, P., Lowery, L., Imada, S., & Haidt, J. (1999). The CAD triad hypothesis: A mapping between three moral emotions (contempt, anger, disgust) and three moral codes (community, autonomy, divinity). *Journal of Personality and Social Psychology, 76*(4), 574–586.

Rozin, P., & Singh, L. (1999). The moralization of cigarette smoking in the United States. *Journal of Consumer Psychology, 8*(3), 321–337.

Schaberg, L. (2002). *Toward a cultural broadening of feminist theory: A comparison of everyday outlooks on social roles, dissent, and feminism among United States and Japanese adults.* Unpublished doctoral dissertation, University of Michigan, Ann Arbor.

Schwartz, T. (1981). The acquisition of culture. *Ethos, 9,* 4–17.

Shimizu, H. (2001). Japanese adolescent boys' senses of empathy (*omoiyari*) and Carol Gilligan's perspectives on the morality of care: A phenomenological approach. *Culture and Psychology, 7*(4), 453–475.

Shweder, R. A. (1982). Beyond self-constructed knowledge: The study of culture and morality. *Merrill–Palmer Quarterly, 28*(1), 41–69.

Shweder, R. A. (1984). Anthropology's romantic rebellion against the enlightenment, or there's more to thinking than reason and evidence. In R. A. Shweder & R. A. LeVine (Eds.), *Culture theory: Essays on mind, self, and emotion* (pp. 27–66). Cambridge, UK: Cambridge University Press.

Shweder, R. A. (1990). Cultural psychology—What is it? In J. W. Stigler, R. A. Shweder, & G. Herdt (Eds.), *Cultural psychology: Essays on comparative human development* (pp. 27–66). New York: Cambridge University Press.

Shweder, R. A. (1999). Cultural psychology. In R. A. Wilson & F. C. Keil (Eds.), *The MIT encyclopedia of the cognitive sciences* (pp. 211–213). Cambridge, MA: MIT Press.

Shweder, R. A. (2000a). The psychology of practice and the practice of the three psychologies. *Asian Journal of Social Psychology, 3,* 207–222.

Shweder, R. A. (2000b). Moral maps, "First World" conceits and the new evangelists. In L. Harrison & S. P. Huntington (Eds.), *Culture matters: How values shape human progress* (pp. 158–177). New York: Basic Books.

Shweder, R. A. (2002). What about "female genital mutilation"?: And why understanding culture matters in the first place. In R. A. Shweder, M. Minow, & H. R. Markus (Eds.), *Engaging cultural differences: The multicultural challenge in liberal democracies* (pp. 216–251). New York: Russell Sage Foundation.

Shweder, R. A., & Bourne, E. J. (1984). Does the concept of the person vary cross-culturally? In R. A. Shweder & R. A. Levine (Eds.), *Culture theory: Essays on mind, self, and emotion* (pp. 158–199). New York: Cambridge University Press.

Shweder, R. A., & LeVine, R. A. (1984). Culture theory: Essays on mind, self, and emotion. Cambridge, UK: Cambridge University Press.

Shweder, R. A., Mahapatra, M., & Miller, J. G. (1987). Culture and moral development. In J, Kagan & S. Lamb (Eds.), *The emergence of morality in young children* (pp. 1–83). Chicago: University of Chicago Press.

Shweder, R. A., Markus, H. R., Minow, M. L., & Kessel, F. (1997). The free exercise of culture: Ethnic customs, assimilation and American law. *Newsletter of the Social Science Research Council, 51*(4), 61–67.

Shweder, R. A., Minow, M., & Markus, H. (Eds.). (2002). *Engaging cultural differences: The multicultural challenge in liberal democracies.* New York: Russell Sage Foundation.

Shweder, R. A., Much, N. C., Mahapatra, M., & Park, L. (1997). The "big three" of morality (autonomy, community, divinity) and the "big three" explanations of suffering. In A. M. Brandt (Ed.), *Morality and health* (pp. 119–169). New York: Routledge.

Shweder, R. A., & Sullivan, M. A. (1990). The semiotic subject of cultural psychology. In L. A. Pervin (Ed.), *Handbook of personality: Theory and research* (pp. 399–416). New York: Guilford Press.

Shweder, R. A., & Sullivan, M. A. (1993). Cultural psychology: Who needs it? *Annual Review of Psychology, 44,* 497–527.

Simpson, E. L. (1974). Moral development research: A case study of scientific cultural bias. *Human Development, 17*(2), 81–106.

Smetana, J. G. (1981). Preschool children's conceptions of moral and social rules. *Child Development, 52*(4), 1333–1336.

Smetana, J. (1995). Morality in context: Abstractions, ambiguities and applications. In R. Vasta (Ed.), *Annals of child development: A research annual* (pp. 83–130). Philadelphia: Jessica Kingsley.

Smetana, J. G., Schlagman, N., & Adams, P. W. (1993). Preschool children's judgments about hypothetical and actual transgressions. *Child Development, 64,* 202–214.

Snarey, J. R. (1985). Cross-cultural universality of social-moral development: A critical review of Kohlbergian research. *Psychological Bulletin, 97*(2), 202–232.

Snarey, J., & Keljo, K. (1991). In a *Gemeinschaft* voice: The cross-cultural expansion of moral development theory. In W. M. Kurtines & J. L. Gewirtz (Eds.), *Handbook of moral behavior and development: Vol. 1. Theory* (pp. 395–424). Hillsdale, NJ: Erlbaum.

Song, M.-J., Smetana, J., & Kim, S. Y. (1987). Korean children's conceptions of moral and conventional transgressions. *Developmental Psychology, 23*(4), 377–382.

Stack, C. B. (1986). The culture of gender: Women and men of color. *Signs, 11*(2), 321–324.

Stein, R., & Nemeroff, C. J. (1995). Moral overtones of food: Judgments of others based on what they eat. *Personality and Social Psychology Bulletin, 21*(5), 480–490.

Strauss, C., & Quinn, N. (1997). *A cognitive theory of cultural meaning.* New York: Cambridge University Press.

Sullivan, E. V. (1977). A study of Kohlberg's structural theory of moral development: A critique of liberal social science ideology. *Human Development, 20*(6), 352–376.

Taylor, A. J. W. (2003). Justice as a basic human need. *New Ideas in Psychology, 21*(3), 209–219.

Thomas, S. J. (1986). Estimating gender differences in the comprehension and preference of moral issues. *Developmental Review, 6,* 165–180.

Tobin, J. J., Wu, D. Y. H., & Davidson, D. H. (1989). *Preschool in three cultures: Japan, China, and the United States.* New Haven, CT: Yale University Press.

Turiel, E. (1983). *The development of social knowledge: Morality and convention.* Cambridge, UK: Cambridge University Press.

Turiel, E. (1998a). The development of morality. In N. Eisenberg (Ed.), *Handbook of child psychology: Social, emotional, and personality development* (Vol. 3, pp. 863–892). New York: Wiley.

Turiel, E. (1998b). Notes from the underground: Culture, conflict, and subversion. In J. Langer & M. Killen (Eds.), *Piaget, evolution, and development* (pp. 271–296). Mahwah, NJ: Erlbaum.

Turiel, E. (2002). *The culture of morality: Social development, context, and conflict.* New York: Cambridge University Press.

Turiel, E., Killen, M., & Helwig, C. C. (1987). Morality: Its structure, functions, and vagaries. In J. Kagan & S. Lamb (Eds.), *The emergence of morality in young children* (pp. 155–243). Chicago: University of Chicago Press.

Turiel, E., Smetana, J. G., & Killen, M. (1991). Social contexts in social cognitive development. In W. M. Kurtines & J. L. Gewirtz (Eds.), *Handbook of moral behavior and development: Vol. 2. Research* (pp. 307–332). Hillsdale, NJ: Erlbaum.

Urmson, J. C. (1958). Saints and heroes. In A. I. Melden (Ed.), *Essays in moral philosophy* (pp. 198–216). Seattle: University of Washington Press.

Vandello, J. A., & Cohen, D. (2003). Male honor and female fidelity: Implicit cultural scripts that perpetuate domestic violence. *Journal of Personality and Social Psychology, 84*(5), 997–1010.

Vasudev, J., & Hummel, R. C. (1987). Moral stage sequence and principled reasoning in an Indian sample. *Human Development, 30*(2), 105–118.

Walker, L. J. (1984). Sex differences in the development of moral reasoning: A critical review. *Child Development, 55*(3), 677–691.

Walker, L. J., Pitts, R. C., Hennig, K. H., & Matsuba, M. K. (1995). Reasoning about morality and real-life moral problems. In M. Killen & D. Hart (Eds.), *Morality in everyday life: Developmental perspectives* (pp. 371–407). New York: Cambridge University Press.

Walker, V. S., & Snarey, J. R. (Eds.). (2004). *Race-ing moral formation: African American perspectives on care and justice.* New York: Teachers College Press.

Ward, J. V. (1988). Urban adolescents' conceptions of violence. In C. Gillian, J. V. Ward, & J. Taylor (Eds.), *Mapping the moral domain* (pp. 175–200). Cambridge, MA: Harvard University Press.

Wertsch, J. V. (1995). Sociocultural research in the copyright age. *Culture and Psychology, 1,* 81–102.

Whiting, B. B., & Whiting, J. W. (1975). *Children of six cultures: A psycho-cultural analysis.* Cambridge, MA: Harvard University Press.

Yau, J., & Smetana, J. G. (2003). Conceptions of moral, social-conventional, and personal events among Chinese preschoolers in Hong Kong. *Child Development, 74*(3), 647–658.

CHAPTER 20

Situating the Child in Context
Attachment Relationships and Self-Regulation in Different Cultures

GILDA A. MORELLI
FRED ROTHBAUM

01.23.97 *I am on a forest trail somewhere in the Ituri Rain Forest.[1] I am about a half a kilometer from Oboobi's camp and still I can hear shrieks of delight and hilarity as Efe men, women, and children prepare for what promises to be a night's worth of dancing at a local village. Everyone is celebrating a good rice harvest after a long hunger season. I know what to expect—women braiding hair and body painting anyone who asks, children practicing their dance steps, little ones wearing newly woven waist belts. What I didn't expect however was Kamisiku wearing a coveted shirt I gave to my friend Oboobi for this event. A bit surprised and maybe even a little bit angry, I asked Oboobi why Kamisiku had my shirt on. "Well," she replied, "she asked for it, and I couldn't deny her." But I said, "Now you'll go to the dance mbuchi" (in this instance meaning without a top to wear).*

A few months later I sit with my husband under the stars enjoying the quiet that comes with darkness. So the rustling of leaves on the forest path comes as a surprise because it heralds a late night visitor. "Hodi," we hear, "usiangopa, mihaiko balozi" (Hello, don't be afraid, I am not a spirit). Standing in the forest opening is Oboobi carrying a 20 liter container of palm oil and 10 kilograms of plantains (a goodly amount of desirable food). As she sits, Oboobi tells us of her good luck getting the food and asks if we would store it for her so she doesn't have to share it away with the other families in her camp.

Sharing is an assumed part of Efe life; it is part of what it means to be an Efe. Infants' experiences with sharing begin as soon as they are born, with camp members participating in their care. But, what is sharing? Is Oboobi acting out of obligation when she gives her shirt away and out of choice when she hides her food? Is the latter but not the former an autonomous action?

We start our chapter with Oboobi and the decisions she makes because they crystallize for us some of the thorny issues we consider in this chapter on attachment and self-regulation—issues of autonomy, internalization, and integration. These issues are closely tied to cultural differences in "healthy" development and "mature" ways of being in the world—fundamental concerns of this chapter.

Much of the research on attachment relationships and self-regulation builds on longstanding philosophical and theoretical traditions that prioritize the individual and the psychological processes of autonomy and internal cohesion (of which internalization and integration are the basis).[2] This theoretical legacy may be one reason why the antecedents of attachment relationships and of self-regulation—sensitive and responsive parenting—are similar, and why attachment and self-regulation lead to similar forms of later social competence (Miller, 2004). We do not doubt that these relations exist—at least for children growing up in communities that emphasize autonomous and internally cohesive ways of being in the world. However, in communities that emphasize other ways of being, antecedents and consequences may be different.

In this chapter we examine traditional accounts of attachment relationships and self-regulation in infancy and early childhood, as well as the experiences that foster their healthy development. Of primary interest is whether personal qualities such as autonomy and internal cohesion are important to the development of these psychological processes in people everywhere. We begin with a brief review of self-determination theory, because the psychological needs described by this theory (e.g., autonomy), as well as the process of developing autonomous forms of motivation (internalization and integration), are also cornerstones of the development of healthy attachment relationships and self-regulation. These Western-oriented traditions consider the self as agentic—an organizer of action and an integrative center of experience (Ryan, Kuhl, & Deci, 1997; Sroufe, 1996), internally controlled, and relatively unchanging across contexts. We next present a view on self-systems prevalent in non-Western communities that takes into account ways of being a person in the world that emphasizes qualities such as harmony and interdependence rather than autonomy and independence. What is important to this self is the self-in-context, and we consider the implications of this self-system for the psychological processes associated with attachment relationships and self-regulation, as well as the care experiences underlying their development. We end with a consideration of self-coherence and its relation to different notions of the self.

TRADITIONAL (WESTERN) THEORIES

Self-Determination Theory

What motivates people to carry out activities that—unlike exploration and novelty seeking—are not inherently or intrinsically satisfying? Why, for example, does a child give up her chair to a visitor, only to be left sitting on the floor? Why does a father use the little money he has to send his youngest son but not his oldest daughter to school? And why does a mother participate in genital cutting ceremonies to mark her daughter's transition to adulthood? Self-determination theory addresses these questions.

Scholars working in this tradition believe that behavior is governed by external forces (the child might be punished if she did not let the visitor sit in her chair) or by personal volition (a child explores the environment because she wants to and chooses to do it). What distinguishes motivations along this continuum is the extent to which regulations are perceived as autonomous (Ryan & Deci, 2000a, 2000b). Self-determined regulations are freely chosen (internalized), fully integrated with other aspects of self, and experienced as authentic. On the other hand, regulations that are neither internalized nor integrated are a "controlled regulation . . . executed without being processed, coordinated, or endorsed by self" (Ryan et al., 1997, p. 707).

The need for autonomy, one of three universal needs posited by self-determination theorists, is best met in infancy and early childhood by caregivers who are appropriately contingent and receptive to their child's signals; who structure and support their child's endeavors in nonintrusive, unobtrusive, and fittingly challenging ways—following the child's lead and fostering her sense of control and competence; who respects the child as a separate person with a will of her own; and who are warm and positive in their involvements. Grolnick and Ryan (1989) consider as exemplars of good parenting adults who value autonomy as a goal first and foremost, even at the expense of obedience and conformity; who rely on encouragement, praise, and reasoning to motivate children; and who are nondirective, preferring not to impose their will—including when children are in problem-solving and decision-making situations. When the need for autonomy is met, the person is more integrated intrapsychically (actions, thoughts, and feelings originate from self and internally cohere) and socially (Deci & Ryan, 2000).

There is a great similarity between self-determination theory and traditional accounts of attachment relationships and self-regulation in the prioritizing of personal agency, control, and internal cohesion, and in the qualities of care important to the development of these processes. The need for autonomy lies at the heart of all three theories.

Attachment Theory

05.16.96 I am within meters of Afukbe's camp, and as is customary I announce my arrival with a chorus of hodis and greet people by shaking their hands asking while doing so if they have "beaten the morning"—unashinda. As I approach the chief's family, I see that his daughter is there with her toddler son. The toddler is clearly alarmed by my approach, but still his mother stretches out his arm and hand to allow me to shake it. However, as she does so, he digs in his heels, arches his back, and lets out a howl that rivals any I've heard before. The camp is utterly amused by this and begins to tease the child as he takes refuge behind his mother's back, dragging her breast with him. I am nonplussed. The Efe often get children to do things by telling them that the "white woman" is going to take them away if they don't, and I have sent many an unfamiliar child galloping into the arms of someone they know, tears streaming down their faces. I sit next to the chief, and watch amusedly as the toddler first peeks at me with breast in mouth, and slowly comes out from hiding to sit on his mom's lap. His mom takes the opportunity to tell him how I gave his grandfather medicine when he was sick, shows him the shirt I brought to welcome him, and asks him to greet me. His mom again stretches out his hand, and this time he allows me to shake it.[3]

Attachment theory is concerned with a child's developing sense of self, other people, and relationships (Sroufe, 1996; Weinfield, Sroufe, Egeland, & Carlson, 1999), and it is psychology's most influential theory of relatedness. Confidence in self, what to look forward to from others, and the capacity for close relationships develop during the first year of life, based on a child's history of experiences with the people who care for him. These experiences, and the beliefs and expectations that develop from them, are represented by the child as "internal working models" (Bretherton, 1992). Early care experiences also play a role in the regulatory abilities the child develops, and together the child's internal working model and regulatory abilities form the basis for how well

he or she functions now and later on in life, both personally and interpersonally (Sroufe, 1996).

The core tenets of attachment theory originate in the work of Bowlby. He focused initially on the protective functions of the attachment system that promote infant survival (in order to reproduce). Accordingly, attachment system behaviors consisted of "any form of behavior that results in a person attaining or maintaining proximity to some other clearly identified individual who is conceived of as better able to cope with the world. It is most obvious whenever the person is frightened, fatigued, or sick, and is assuaged by comforting and caregiving" (Bowlby, 1988, pp. 26–27). However, Bowlby, along with Ainsworth and others, increasingly recognized the importance of broadening the function and set goal of the attachment system beyond infant survival and proximity to include the support of the infant's innate drive for exploration and mastery of the inanimate and social world made possible by "felt security" (Ainsworth & Bowlby, 1991).

Ainsworth's contributions to attachment theory included the concept of secure base, maternal sensitivity to infant signals, and patterns of infant attachment relationship; she also developed a procedure to test empirically assumptions related to attachment theory (Bretherton, 1992). This procedure, known as the Strange Situation, assesses individual differences in infants' relationships with their caregivers when stressed (Ainsworth, Blehar, Waters, & Wahl, 1978). Particular attention is paid to how well infants organize their attachment and exploratory behaviors when reunited with their caregiver after a short period of time alone or with an unfamiliar person (secure base phenomenon, see below). Infants who respond to their caregiver positively upon her return and who are able to use their caregiver as a base from which to explore the environment are characterized as being secure in their relationship. Insecure infants, in contrast, do not seek contact with their caregiver on her return (avoidant) or they are not able to become calm in her presence (ambivalent), and they do not use their caregiver as a secure base.

Attachment Relationships and the Secure Base from Which to Explore

Attachment theory places great importance on the child's ability to explore the environment and aspects of the child's relationship with caregivers that makes this possible. Exploration with the support of caring others is one way the child is able to gather information about her inanimate and social environment and develop mastery over it. This mastery is important to the child's developing sense of self as competent and autonomous.

Exploration in and of itself does not promote autonomy in the child; the quality of the child's attachment relationship must be considered as well; in fact, it is the balance between exploration and attachment that matters. Healthy autonomy develops when the child is able to use his caregiver as a "secure base" from which to explore the environment, because he feels sufficiently protected and comforted by her presence. Children who do not experience this felt security—who neither view their caregiver as someone they can trust nor themselves as worthy of support—are not able to achieve the same confidence in their mastery of the environment, in themselves, and in others (Weinfield et al., 1999).

The attachment and exploration systems work in tandem, balancing one another, with activation of one reducing activation of the other (Ainsworth et al., 1978; Bowlby, 1982). Together they function to keep the infant out of harm's way and to enable him to explore the environment when all is safe. Although at any moment attachment and exploration are in opposition, over time they are complementary, and "infants who are effectively dependent will become effectively independent" (Weinfield et al., 1999, p. 76). As Bretherton writes, "Confidence in the mother's physical and psychological availability appears to lay the groundwork for autonomous exploration and problem solving, coupled with the expectation that help will be forthcoming when needed" (Bretherton, 1985, p. 21).

Sensitive Care and Security of Attachment Relationships

The ability of children to organize their attachment behaviors to balance their need for protection and felt security with their need for exploration, mastery, and autonomy relate to their history of care. The aspect of caregiving receiving the most attention is a mother's sensitivity and responsiveness to her infant and young child (Ainsworth et al., 1978; de Wolff & van IJzendoorn, 1997).

Bretherton (1987) described *sensitivity* as "maternal respect for the child's autonomy" (p. 1075) and three of the four scales developed by Ainsworth (1976) to evaluate caregiving emphasize autonomy supporting practices. For example, Ainsworth included in her description of the acceptance scale a mother who "values the fact that the baby has a will of its own, even when it opposes hers, . . . finds his anger worthy of respect, . . . [and] respect[s] the baby as a separate, autonomous person (p. 4). She noted in her cooperation scale that the "mother views her baby as a separate, active autonomous person, whose wishes and activities have a validity of their own. . . . She avoids situations in which she might have to impose her will on him" (p. 4). Finally, for her sensitivity scale, Ainsworth stated that "it is a good thing for a baby to gain some feeling of efficacy. She nearly always gives the baby what he indicates he wants" (pp. 3–4). This conceptualization of sensitive and responsive caregiving is still the "gold standard" in the field.

Competence and Attachment Relationships

Attachment theorists maintain that sensitive and responsive caregivers foster children's confidence to act effectively and autonomously both in early childhood and later in development. Children with different care histories fall short of developing the qualities that foster personal and interpersonal competence.

Research linking attachment security and competence support this claim, although the strength of the association between the two is modest. Thompson (1998) suggests that lack of theoretical clarity is partly responsible for this modest relation; attachment relationships should not foreshadow all aspects of later competence. He argues that there is little theoretical reason to expect a child's attachment relationship to predict later cognitive ability, but there is every reason to expect it to predict later aspects of social and emotional competence that relate to a child's representation of self, others, and relationships.

Children with secure attachment histories, compared to their insecure age mates, display more confidence and self-esteem, persistence in problem-solving tasks, and mature forms of exploration (Cassidy, 1988; Cassidy & Kobak, 1988; Grossmann, Grossmann, & Zimmermann, 1999; Matas, Arend, & Sroufe, 1978; Nezworski, 1983, cited in Wienfield et al.,

1999; Sroufe, Fox, & Pancake, 1983). Children with insecure attachment histories not only score lower on all of these measures but also higher on measures of other behavior problems. They are more likely to seek the attention and the physical closeness of adults at the expense of peer relations and to rely extensively on these adults for help.

Children with secure histories also enjoy more positive relationships with their parents and peers than do young children with insecure histories. These children experience more mutually rewarding experiences with their mothers (Thompson, 1998); they are more competent in their interactions with familiar peers and more popular with them (Ladd, 1999; Sroufe, 1983), and they are more social with unfamiliar adults than agemates with less secure attachment histories, perhaps because of their expertise in exploring the interpersonal environment (Thompson, 1998).

Self-Regulation Theory

10.15.96 I watch as EmaKpendule quietly enters camp with her three children following close behind. The sun is setting and they've been gone since early morning gathering food from the forest floor. This hunger season has been quite severe—taking its toll on the young and old alike. Kependule, the oldest at age 4, looks around and sees other children helping their mothers, and joins her mother, who is emptying the basket of fruits and nuts. But as she does so she starts to cry—she is hungry and there is little to show for their day's labor. Tears stream down her face, and every so often I hear a muffled sob, yet she continues to help, but now she is placing food on a plate for herself and her sisters. The three of them sit in a circle with the plate of food in the middle. Kependule picks out just a few morsels and the second oldest does the same; neither says anything as the youngest takes much of what is there. Only a few minutes go by before they finish eating, and when they are done, they stumble into their hut to help their mother prepare their sleeping mats. As they settle down for the night, I hear Kependule tell her sisters, "We shouldn't cry, tomorrow we won't be hungry. We will go to the water Uala and catch lots of fish."

How children like Kpendule develop culturally appropriate ways of acting and feeling is of interest to researchers studying self-regulation. Examples of self-regulation are evident in the scene just described: Kpendule joining her mother as she empties the basket of food, taking a small amount of food from the communal bowl, and modulating her distress. Many researchers maintain that the development of self-regulatory processes involves a gradual shift from external to internal mechanisms of control, and they are interested in how this occurs and the consequences of it.

The first signs of children's ability to self-regulate—to act appropriately on their own, by their own choosing, in a flexible and adaptive way—are evident in early childhood (Eisenberg, 2002; Grolnick, McMenamy, & Kurowski, 1999; Kopp, 2001). Early regulatory capacities lay the groundwork for later ones. Infants regulate their states of arousal in the first months of life, and how well they do this relates to their exploration and mastery of the environment at this age. As toddlers, children begin to develop social standards of control and compliance, and as young children they appropriate moral codes of conduct. These emergent regulatory abilities collectively support the young child's developing sense of autonomy—a person with an "independent identity and self-sufficient behavior" (Calkins, Smith, Gill, & Johnson, 1998, p. 351). Contributing to these early accomplishments is the care children receive: "The movement towards autonomy and self-regulation is viewed as rooted in the quality of the earlier infant–caregiver relationship" (Sroufe, 1996, p. 204).

There is no unified literature on self-regulation. Rather, researchers typically examine emotional regulation or behavioral regulation, although some study both, and most acknowledge their interrelatedness (e.g., Calkins, 2004; Eisenberg, 2002; Kochanska, Coy, & Murray, 2001; Stifter, Spinrad, & Braungart-Rieker, 1999). Investigators interested in emotional regulation rely on notions of temperament and, in particular, the constructs of effortful control (temperament that is managed voluntarily) and reactivity (fearfulness, impulsivity) (e.g., Rothbart, 1989; Rothbart & Derryberry, 1981). Investigators interested in behavioral self-regulation draw on self-determination theory. Yet these researchers concur that autonomy is a developmental goal and agree on the type of care that supports its development.

Regulation of Emotional Expressiveness

Theorists concerned with emotional development agree that emotion regulation is goal-directed and functional in nature (Eisenberg & Morris, 2002).[4] Emotional regulation is evident early in the life of the child, and it is a central organizing construct, embedded in many other developments (Sroufe, 1979). At first, infants rely mostly on caregivers to manage their affective states (Thompson, 1994), but with time, infants assume more responsibility, and by early childhood, emotion regulation is largely self-initiated. Self-regulation theorists place great emphasis on this shift toward increased autonomy.

The quality of infants' experiences with their caregivers is important to the development of emotional self-regulation. What matters is whether caregivers are sensitive and responsive, rejecting, or act unpredictably in response to infants' emotional signals—especially during times of heightened arousal when infants are feeling threatened. Attachment theorists believe that infants develop a style of emotional expressiveness that best maintains their relationship with close others—a style that develops into strategies for regulating emotions (Cassidy, 1994). When infants are cared for in a sensitive and responsive manner, they learn that it is acceptable for them to express positive and negative emotions, and that seeking help from close others to regulate emotions is an effective strategy. Infants with this attachment history are likely to remain organized in the face of stress, to trust themselves to regulate their emotions, and to be open and flexible in their expression of emotions as they grow up. By comparison, infants with insecure attachment histories are less confident in expressing emotions or they express emotions inappropriately because of the unavailability or unpredictability of their care providers. As children, they are likely to mistrust themselves to regulate their emotion and they respond to stress in rigid or inefficient ways.

There is empirical support for this view. Children with insecure compared to secure attachment histories are more prone to express negative emotions as infants (distress and fearfulness) and are more aggressive as young children (Diener, Mangelsdorf, McHale, & Frosch, 2002; Grossmann et al., 1999; Kochanska, 2001; Weinfield et al., 1999). Moreover, children with insecure attachment histories are more likely to remember negative events, whereas their agemates with secure histories are more likely to remember positive events (Belsky, Spritz, & Crnic, 1996). The expression of negative emotions, as well as the attention to negative events that is observed in children with insecure attachment histories, point to heightened negative emotionality.

Regulation of Behavior

Behavioral self-regulation rests on the development of accomplishments that occur around the second year of life, such as voluntary control and awareness of standards, along with an ability to evaluate and to adapt one's actions accordingly (Kopp, 2001). One of the more well-studied examples of behavioral self-regulation is compliance to a caregiver's request (Kochanska et al., 2001). Compliance is a heterogeneous construct entailing types that are motivationally distinct: committed and situational compliance (Kochanska et al., 2001). In committed compliance, the child wholeheartedly embraces the caregiver's agenda and endorses it as his own; in situational compliance, the child does not embrace the caregiver's agenda and his compliance is sustained by the caregiver's control.

Eagerly embracing another's agenda, the hallmark of committed compliance, indicates that the child experiences the action as personally endorsed and self-generated (Kochanska et al., 2001). This nascent sense of autonomy is important for the development of internalization and integration (Ryan & Deci, 2000b). By comparison, when a child does not experience a sense of control over the action, as is the case with situational compliance, the action is experienced as an externally controlled regulation, without being processed, coordinated, or endorsed by self (Ryan et al., 1997).

Regulation Strategies

How well children regulate their emotions and behaviors partly depends on their effortful control—the ability to "willfully or voluntarily inhibit, activate, or change (modulate) attention and behavior" (Eisenberg, Smith, Sadovsky, & Spinrad, 2004, p. 260). One measure of effortful control includes indices of attention shifting (or distraction). Infants and young children who use this strategy express less negative emotion (distress, anger; Bridges, Grolnick, & Connell, 1997; Calkins & Johnson, 1998; Grolnick, Bridges, & Connell, 1996; Tronick, 1989) and are able to delay gratification longer (Eisenberg et al., 2004) than peers using other self-regulatory strategies.

Using a composite measure of effortful control that included an assessment of attentional control, Kochanska, Murray, and Harlan (2000) found that higher effortful control at 22 months predicted better regulation of anger (during frustrating situations) at 22 and 33 months, and joy (during pleasurable situations) at 33 months. Effortful control is also positively related to young children's committed compliance and to aspects of moral development associated with it, and negatively related to externalizing behaviors in early school-age children (Kochanska, 2001; Kochanska et al., 2001; Kochanska, Murray, & Coy, 1997).[5]

Whereas shifting attention is considered one of the more adaptive self-regulation strategies, moving closer to or making contact with an adult, or waiting for a person to intervene, are examples of less adaptive self-regulation strategies, especially for older children. As children get older, there should be a "greater reliance on solitary or intraindividual strategies of regulation/control" (Eisenberg & Morris, 2002, p. 199). These two classes of strategies represent the ends of an autonomy continuum from self-reliant and active to stimulus-bound and passive (Grolnick et al., 1999). A particularly important aspect of autonomous regulation is the ability to use strategies flexibly depending on the context. A child who is able to do this is able to "experience emotions over a range of intensities without the feeling of being out of control" (Bridges & Grolnick, 1995, p. 205).

The type of care that fosters adaptive self-regulatory abilities also fosters healthy attachment relationships.[6] This care is supportive, warm, sensitive, responsive, nonintrusive (asking if the child needs help, making suggestions, offering explanations), and emotionally positive. In contrast is care that is intrusive, directive (telling the child what to do or physically making the child do something), and emotionally negative (angry, hostile, demeaning). Young children whose mothers are involved with them in positive ways are more likely to rely on adaptive regulation strategies, are less distressed in situations meant to elicit negative emotions, show more committed compliance, and score higher on measures of conscience than are children with mothers who are less positive and supportive of them (e.g., Calkins & Johnson, 1998; Feldman, Greenbaum, & Yirmiya, 1999; Kochanska & Murray, 2000; Silverman & Ippolito, 1995).

Scholars provide many reasons why positive care fosters adaptive regulatory abilities and the competencies associated with them, but what is basic to all is the view that this type of parenting is a minimal threat to the child's autonomy and in fact supports its development. Often cited is the explanation that sensitive care provides children with varied opportunities to observe and practice valued ways of regulating emotions and behavior on their own, with a sense of self-discovery and self-confidence. By contrast, care that thwarts children's autonomous functioning deprives them of the feeling that they have a say in things—a sense of choice and control that comes when children are able to mobilize resources they want (when others respond to their bids and follow their lead). What contributes to these feelings of choice and control is parents who are willing to negotiate or share power with their child (Crockenberg & Litman, 1990).

Our discussion of healthy attachment relationships and adaptive self-regulation says a lot about valued ways of being a person in middle-class U.S. and Western European communities. Attachment relationships and self-regulation are conceptualized in ways that make sense given the values of the people most often studied and of the researchers who most often study them. However, other ways of being a person in the world reflect ethics besides autonomy, such as ethics of community (duty, hierarchy) and divinity (sacred order, natural order) (Shweder, Much, Mahapatra, & Park, 1997), and this raises questions about the appropriateness of Western-based notions of healthy development for people who live by these ethics. We now consider the self more broadly than how it is portrayed by the theories and research we reviewed earlier, examining "the way culture, community, and psyche become coordinated and make each other possible" (Shweder et al., 2000, p. 868). We then consider attachment relationships and self-regulation from this perspective.

MULTIPLE SELFWAYS— MULTIPLE DEVELOPMENTAL PATHWAYS

The *self* determines what a person notices, thinks about, feels, and remembers; how and why a person relates to others; what it means to be an acceptable, good, and moral person; and how a person organizes, interprets, and makes sense of experiences. This means that the experience and expression of self is integral to psychological processes such as attachment and self-regulation. The self develops as infants and children take part in the day-to-day life of their community—in culturally organized practices, routines, and traditions that provide opportunities to develop valued ways of being a person in the world (Rogoff, 1990). Cultural practices and contexts are one side of a "two-sided thing" (Shweder et al., 2000, p. 874), the other side is the mentalities associated with them. Mentalities are what we know, want, feel, value, and believe. They give form and meaning to practices and are reflected in them.

An Efe example illustrates how practices and mentalities relate, and how community members foster the development of similarly minded infants and children. As soon as infants are able to toddle, around 8 or 9 months of age, they are asked to carry bits of food and other delectable items to different camp members. When the infant places the item in the person's hand, the person immediately places it back in the infant's hand and asks the infant to return it to the person who sent it, or to give it to someone else. It is not unusual for this to go on for awhile and everyone seems to enjoy it. Infants are engaged in this "game" until they are about a year old. When asked about this routine, camp members say that it is important for children to learn when they are young the value and practice of sharing, particularly when this means giving away desirable items to the people with whom they live. Sharing is critical to the survival of the Efe: People must depend on each other for many things, especially food, because the success of a hunt or a gathering expedition is never guaranteed. But sharing is more than this: It connects people to one another, making public, confirming, and authenticating social relationships; it is a way to express affection, friendship, and good will.

Ways of being a person in the world are culturally and historically grounded and at the same time personal: *personal* because of the peculiarities of an individual's experiences; *cultural* because people of a community participate in a system of practices and beliefs that foster a shared understanding of valued ways of acting, feeling, and thinking; and *historical* because cultural practices and beliefs are "passed down" from one generation to the next. Generational transmission is not a passive process. Individuals reproduce, as well as produce, aspects of culture, which is as dynamic as the people who constitute and are

constituted by them. Markus, Mullally, and Kitayama (1997) refer to "self" and "selfway" to distinguish between the personal and cultural–historical aspects of self (although this distinction does not imply that these aspects of self are divisible). Selfway is a characteristic way of being a person in the world that develops because of the culturally mediated experiences people of a community have in common. Self is the personalization of this characteristic way.

The relation between self and selfway is nicely illustrated in a conversation one of us had with a U.S. middle-class mother of European descent who was asked to tell us where her young infant slept and why (Morelli, Rogoff, Oppenheimer, & Goldsmith, 1992). She hesitated at first, then told me that her 1-year-old son sleeps with herself and her husband. She laughed awkwardly and quickly added that no one knew this, especially her mother, who would have been very upset had she known. This mother decided not to participate in a practice common to people like herself and promoted by experts in the field. Still, she was aware of what was expected of her, and her resistance to the practice of sleeping in a bed (and even a room) separate from her infant was a source of concern.

Cultural Patterning of Selfways and Self

Two well-researched selfways, independence and interdependence, were once considered to be opposites. The former emphasizes autonomy (internal control, individual choice, personal agency) and the latter, heteronomy (conformity, obligation, reciprocity, and loyalty).[7] However, for all of us, agency, choice, loyalty, and obligation are important in certain situations at certain times in our lives. As researchers acknowledged this, it began to make less sense to think of selfways in dichotomous ways. The revision in thinking, and the research that led to it, suggests that individuals develop heterogeneous orientations—with different emphases on independent and interdependent orientations in different contexts (e.g., Shweder et al., 2000). But how these qualities are experienced and expressed by people relate to the culture's predominant value system: "Although independence and interdependence are viewed as dimensions of functioning in any culture, they are expected to take on different meanings when they are part of different cultural value systems" (Raeff, 1997, pp. 212–

213; see also Markus et al., 1997; Shweder et al., 2000).

Autonomy is the ethic that underlies the independent selfway and North Americans' and Western Europeans' views of the self. What these people notice, how they make sense of it, and what they do as a result are likely to rest more on their perceived personal qualities, such as traits, attributes, and talents, than on situational or relational qualities. These personal qualities are the defining feature of self for this selfway and are the source of self-knowledge (Suh, 2000). Reference to and affirmation of these qualities, which promote a tendency toward self-expression and self-enhancement are likely to support the self-determining attitude required for being a valued person (Shweder et al., 2000).

People living elsewhere rely on different ethics to justify their way of being. The ethics of community prevalent in many East Asian societies places great value on virtues such as respect, duty, and obligation, privileges situational and interpersonal qualities, and underlies the interdependent selfway. What is important to this self is the self-in-context, especially the interpersonal context. For example, Miller (1984) observed that older Indian children relied more on contextual factors to explain social situations, whereas older children in the United States relied more on individual, stable, personality traits. Ip and Bond (1995) found that Chinese participants referred more often to social roles when describing themselves than did North American participants. And Japanese students were twice as likely as European American students to include other people in their self-descriptions (50% compared to 24%) (Markus et al., 1997). People in communities with this ethic prioritize harmonious connections, which require knowing and meeting the expectations of others (Weisz, Rothbaum, & Blackburn, 1984a). Expressions of self-criticism and the need for self-improvement make possible this moral good, as do acts to fit in socially (Weisz, Rothbaum, & Blackburn, 1984b). Self-expansive actions, of which expressions of happiness are an example (Kitayama, Karasawa, & Mesquita, 2004), and acts that call attention to self or emphasize the distinct and uniqueness of self, threaten harmony.

The ethics by which people live relate not only to how competencies are defined but also to how they develop. Keller and colleagues postulated that competencies such as healthy attachment and adaptive self-regulation develop along one of two developmental pathways (Greenfield, Keller, Fuligni, & Maynard, 2003; Keller, 2003). They proposed a component model of parenting made up of different parenting systems, including body contact, body stimulation, object stimulation, and face-to-face exchange. The way practices relate within and across systems suggest two parenting styles. The proximal style emphasizes bodily closeness, and the distal style emphasizes physical separateness and distance. These styles are related respectively to the development of an interdependent and independent selfway (Keller, Lohaus, Volker, Cappenberg, & Chasiotis, 2004; Rothbaum & Trommsdorff, 2006). Another formulation of developmental pathways is provided by Rothbaum, Pott, Azuma, Miyake, and Weisz (2000), who suggest that close relationships in Japan are characterized by efforts to achieve "symbiotic harmony," and that relationships in the United States are characterized by efforts to achieve "generative tension." Rather than depicting these cultures as differing in their investment in relationships, they review evidence suggesting that they differ in the meaning and dynamics of relationships.

We now consider young children's attachment relationships and self-regulation growing up in societies where ethics like community are important. In doing so, we revisit the thesis that healthy development inevitably involves internalization and integration (internal cohesion) that are critical to autonomous functioning. We proceed cautiously, however, because the cultures we refer to as living by ethics of community differ in how this ethic is experienced and expressed in everyday life, as do cultures living by ethics of autonomy.

BROADENING OUR THINKING ABOUT ATTACHMENT RELATIONSHIPS

We begin by asking whether our understanding of attachment relationships changes when we include in our theories people whose way of being a person are rooted in ethics of community or divinity—where what they notice, feel, think about, and remember are motivated by situational and interpersonal considerations more often than not. We accept the challenge implied by LeVine and Norman (2001) when they said,

"The study of attachment . . . gave rise to an approach as blind to culture as any other in psychology" (p. 86). Below, we reexamine central tenets of attachment theory, this time considering research in communities where autonomy is not as central a concern.

Our thesis goes beyond suggesting that culturally informed research just consider the possibility that the circumstances of a child's life, including cultural circumstances, relate only to the quality of the attachment relationship. Rather, it must also consider the very premises underlying traditional attachment theory. We posit that the very essence—the very meaning—of attachment relationships is related to ethics by which people live. Among people living by ethics of community, attachment relationships are based more on goals involving interdependence—harmony, duty, and obligation. Accordingly, the attachment system is more undermined by inability to depend on and fit in with others than on inability to gain autonomy. The care experiences that foster this type of attachment relationship and related competence are also fundamentally different (Rothbaum, Weisz, Pott, Miyake, & Morelli, 2000).

The Secure Base from Which to Explore and Security of Attachment Relationships

At the heart of the notion of attachment security is the concept of a secure base. "For both Bowlby and Ainsworth, to be attached is to use someone preferentially as a secure base from which to explore" (Waters & Cummings, 2000, p. 165). We maintain that attachment theorists' conceptualization of the secure base reflects the Western emphasis on exploration and the belief that exploration leads to an independent selfway. As noted by Seifer and Schiller (1995), "Secure base behavior provides a context in which differentiation of self and other can take place" (p. 149). Japanese attachment experts are less likely to emphasize a dynamic that is so centered on individuation. According to Takahashi (1990, p. 29), "Mothers' effectiveness in serving a secure base function well represents the quality of attachment only in the American culture, in which social independence or self-reliance is emphasized."

Few studies have adopted emic or derived etic methods (culturally sensitive measures) when examining the nature of security in non-Western ("majority world") cultures.[8] To our knowledge, only Harwood, Miller, and Irizarry (1995) have used open-ended methods to explore indigenous concepts pertaining to the nature of the secure base. These investigators focused on the key attachment theory concept of optimal balance (alternating between exploration/autonomy and attachment/relatedness). They found that "Puerto Rican mothers conceptualized optimal balance in terms of . . . a contextually appropriate balancing of calm, respectful attentiveness with positive engagement in interpersonal relationships [rather than] . . . in terms of autonomy and relatedness" (p. 112). As expected, the balance of autonomy and relatedness was the primary theme emerging from the interviews with the Anglo mothers.

In summarizing their findings, Harwood and colleagues (1995) comment: "The construct of security versus insecurity has become equated in U.S. psychology with a host of culturally valued qualities that are specific to the socialization goals of our highly individualistic society, thus limiting their cross cultural meaningfulness" (p. 114). This captures well our concerns about current conceptualizations of security—that they are grounded in independent ways of being and the emphasis on autonomy. In Puerto Rico, people live by ethics of community and are relatively more concerned with respect, duty, and obligation. For them, attachment has more to do with awareness of persons and situations in which these values must be exhibited.

Observations of infants in different cultures suggest that there may be a biological basis to the link between attachment and exploration (Van IJzendoorn & Sagi, 1999). However, the extent to which exploration occurs, and the primacy of the link between attachment and exploration, varies across cultures. Japanese babies have repeatedly been observed to engage in less exploratory activity than U.S. babies, including in the Strange Situation (reviewed in Rothbaum, Weiss, Pott, Miyake, & Morelli, 2000). Moreover, whereas Japanese babies are more oriented to their mothers in circumstances involving both distress and positive emotions, U.S. infants are more oriented to the environment in such circumstances (Bornstein, Azuma, Tamis-LeMonda, & Ogino, 1990; Friedlmeier & Trommsdorff, 1999).

Whereas the link between attachment and exploration behavioral systems is seen as primary in many middle-class U.S. and Western

European communities, the link between the attachment and dependence behavioral systems appears primary in majority world communities, including Japan and Puerto Rico. Just as exploration during infancy fosters ethics of autonomy, dependence fosters ethics of community. In Japan there is a greater emphasis on accommodation or "social fittedness" (Emde, 1992) and related qualities including empathy with others, compliance with their wishes, and responsiveness to social cues and norms. Support for our view of attachment in the life of Japanese children comes from the study of *amae*, an indigenous Japanese concept that refers to relationships involving both attachment and dependence (Doi, 1989; Emde, 1992; Okonogi, 1992). According to Doi (1992) *amae* means "to depend and presume upon another's love or bask in another's indulgence" (p. 8); *amae* is "what an infant feels when seeking his or her mother." The parallels between *amae* and attachment in their developmental course, antecedents, consequences, and role in adaptation (Emde, 1992; Okonogi, 1992; Rothbaum, Kakinuma, Nagaoka, & Azuma, 2005), led Doi to conclude: "The concept of attachment which was introduced by John Bowlby . . . obviously covers the same area as *amae*" (1989, p. 350).

The view that *amae* is an attachment-related construct for relationships in Japan is supported by research that uses a modified separation–reunion paradigm with preschool children (Mizuta, Zahn-Waxler, Cole, & Hiruma, 1996). Mothers and their children were observed during preseparation and reunion episodes for attachment (e.g., proximity, anxiety, and avoidance) and *amae*-related behaviors (e.g., dependence). The emotion language mothers and children used when talking about past separations and reunions was noted as well. The researchers observed that compared to U.S. children, Japanese children exhibited more dependent behavior characteristic of *amae* when reunited with their mothers; following the reunion, Japanese mothers and their children expressed more feelings of sadness due to separation (presumably related to interpersonal loss) and less feelings of fear (presumably related to perceived danger) than their U.S. counterparts. Mizuta and colleagues speculated that, for the Japanese children, attachment has more to do with meeting *amae* needs (for indulgence and interdependence) than meeting needs for autonomy and exploration.

Whereas separation activates the attachment system in both cultures, activation is associated with threats to very different needs. Japanese children's *amae* behaviors on reunion signaled their perception that their needs for indulgence and interdependence were threatened, and Japanese mothers responded to them by engaging their *amae*-related behaviors (providing proximal reassurances), presumably to reaffirm the relationship. *Amae*, the authors conclude, "may be an appropriate means of deactivating an attachment system aroused by interpersonal loss more than exploratory risk" (p. 156). Findings with adults also indicate a closer link between attachment and *amae* in Japan than in the United States (Kondo-Ikemura & Matsuoka, 1999).

These cultural differences in views regarding children's relationships may relate to the higher levels of "insecure–ambivalent" babies and lower levels of "insecure–avoidant" babies in Japan than in the United States (Van IJzendoorn & Sagi, 1999). There are many similarities between descriptions of insecure–ambivalent behaviors and behaviors widely regarded as adaptive in Japan, including exaggerated cute and babyish behaviors (Main & Cassidy, 1988), extreme expressions of need for care and attention, extensive clinging and proximity seeking, helpless dependency (Cassidy & Berlin, 1994), extreme passivity, blurring of boundaries between self and other (Weinfield et al., 1999), and failure to engage in exploration (Ainsworth et al., 1978). Many of these features of ambivalent behavior characterize the normal *amae* relationship in Japan (Doi, 1973; Kondo-Ikemura & Matsuoka, 1999; Lebra, 1994; Mizuta et al., 1996).

Sensitive Care and Security of Attachment Relationships?

Carlson and Harwood (2003) found that, as predicted, mothers' physical control related to insecure attachment in Anglo American families, but not in Puerto Rican families: "The highest ratings of physical control were associated with secure 12-month attachment status for these middle-class Puerto Rican dyads. This apparently paradoxical finding highlights the need for culturally specific definitions of sensitive caregiving" (p. 17). These findings stand in stark contrast to Western findings, reviewed earlier, that responsive, nonintrusive, autonomy-fostering maternal practices hold the key to secure attachment. According to Carlson and Harwood, physical control is part of a larger system of practices and beliefs among Puerto Rican mothers. "Teaching infants to be attentive, calm, and well behaved requires considerably more physical prompting and control than teaching infants to be assertive and self-confident. Thus it appears that maternal use of physical control may be regulated by maternal socialization goals" (p. 18).

Interestingly, parental control, directiveness, and strictness are more valued and emphasized in many cultural and ethnic communities— African American, Korean, Chinese, and Iranian—than they are among European Americans (Carlson & Harwood, 2003). Members of all of these groups subscribe to a selfway that emphasizes the importance of accommodating oneself to the needs of others and to situational demands, and seeking harmony with others. Children who have experienced controlling caregiving are more likely to find security in relationships characterized by clearly prescribed role expectations, where their own and their partner's accommodation will cement close ties. Future research may show an association between parental control and security in all of these cultural groups. By contrast, Western attachment theorists maintain that efforts to physically control, shape, or interfere with infants' activity are associated with insensitivity and insecurity. The link between autonomy fostering and security—which is assumed to be universal by attachment theorists (Allen & Land, 1999; Belsky, Rosenberger, & Crnic, 1995)—may be a predominantly Western phenomenon (cf. Dennis, Cole, Zahn-Waxler, & Mizuta, 2002).

Cultural studies suggest as well that the timing of caregivers' response to babies' signals may not be the same across cultures. Western investigators evaluate caregiver's behavior in terms of its responsiveness—how contingent the response is (immediately after) to the child's overt signal. By contrast, studies in other cultures emphasize the ways caregivers anticipate shifts in a baby's emotional state and respond proactively (or respond to very subtle and covert signals). Anticipatory responsiveness is reported among the Japanese (Rothbaum, Nagoaka, & Ponte, 2005; Trommsdorff & Friedlmeier, 2003), the Nso of Cameroon (Voelker, Yovsi, & Keller, 1998), and Puerto Ricans and Central American immigrants in the United States (Harwood, 1992). Under-

lying U.S. caregivers' reliance on responsiveness is their emphasis on children's autonomy, children's responsibility for clarifying their needs, and the value of children's explicit signals. Underlying Japanese caregivers' reliance on anticipation is their emphasis on children's dependence on others, caregivers' responsibility for clarifying children's needs, and the value of caregivers' assumptions about children's needs (Rothbaum et al., 2005).

Cultural differences in proactive compared to reactive responses to babies' signals may reflect prioritization of selfways emphasizing harmony and context-embeddedness versus autonomy and individuation (Keller et al., 2003). Proactive caregiving may pave the way for attachment relationships that emphasize interdependence, extreme empathy, merger of self and other, and heightened attentiveness and sensitivity to situational demands.

Competence and Attachment Relationships?

Just as there are differences in the nature of security and practices fostering it, there are differences in competencies that follow from security. Attachment theorists emphasize Western values and behaviors associated with autonomy, including exploration, self-assertion, self-esteem, and independence. By contrast, "from [an East Asian] perspective, an assertive, autonomous . . . person is immature and uncultivated" (Fiske, Kitayama, Markus, & Nisbett, 1998, p. 923).

Other investigators also highlight cultural differences in conceptions of competence. Keller (2003) notes that Western-based ideas of competence—which emphasize individual ability, cultivation of the individual mind, exploration, discovery, and personal achievement—are fundamentally different from conceptions seen in many other societies, such as the Baolue of the Ivory Coast, A-Chew of Zambia, Nso of Cameroon, Cree of Alaska, Hindu of India, and Chinese of mainland China and Taiwan. In these majority world societies, competence is considered "as moral self-cultivation, a social contribution, discouraging individual celebration of achievement . . . [and] as communal achievements, including the ability to maintain social harmony implying social respect and acceptance of social roles" (p. 289).

Other cultural studies support Keller's view. In their conversations with mothers, Harwood et al. (1995) found that Anglo mothers' views of social competence centered on self-maximization and independence, as seen in their emphasis on autonomy, happiness, confidence, and exploration. For Puerto Rican mothers, social competence involved "proper demeanor" and interdependence, as seen in their emphasis on respect, obedience, calmness, politeness, gentleness, and kindness. "Proper demeanor" refers to more than appropriate ways of relating to others; it also refers to what is described in English as "teachable." It involves a receptivity to one's elders "in order to become skilled in the interpersonal and rhetorical competencies that will someday be expected of the well-socialized adult" (p. 98). If attachment research had its origins in non-Western cultures, we suspect that qualities such as proper demeanor (and *sunao*—a similar Japanese construct) would be considered universal consequences of security.

BROADENING OUR THINKING ABOUT SELF-REGULATION

Eisenberg and Zhou (2000) raise the possibility that "people in individualistic and collective cultures differ in their standards for emotion regulation, beliefs and values regarding an optimal state, or attention to and perception of their own emotional state" (p. 169). We elaborate on this observation, examining self-regulation mostly in African and East and Southeast Asian communities. For these people, the *self* in *self*-regulation is less concerned with internal attributes and qualities and more concerned with situational circumstances. Adaptive self-regulation in these communities, like healthy, close relationships, more often includes efforts to achieve relational harmony than personal autonomy. Regulatory processes reflect a heightened concern with interpersonal contexts (self-presentation to gain acceptance) compared to personal contexts (delay of gratification when alone). Because of this, they are likely to differ in form, function, meaning, and circumstances of occurrence.

Self-Regulation of Emotions and Behavior

When people live by ethics of autonomy, emotional expressiveness[9] often draws attention to their inner qualities and attributes. These emotions cover the gamut from positive to negative, including frustration and anger. Positive emotions are perhaps the most desirable be-

cause they foster and protect personal esteem, which sustains the autonomous self (Mesquita, 2003). This is not like the emotional expression of people for whom community is paramount. For them, socially engaging emotions that bind people together (e.g., empathy and shame) are valued. Positive emotions are valued by people who live by ethics of community when they foster and strengthen social ties, as seen in many Asian societies, for example (Kitayama, Markus, & Kurokawa, 2000). Ego-based, socially disengaging emotions that disrupt harmony, such as anger, frustration, and pride, are seen negatively (Kitayama et al., 2004; Markus & Kitayama, 1991). These people have a heightened awareness of their audience's expectations, and regulatory processes are attuned to situational cues and reflect more consideration of social norms than of personal attitudes and beliefs (Kitayama & Markus, 1999). Adaptive self-regulation leads to responsive coordination with others and, ultimately, relational harmony.

There is evidence to support this view. Japanese students and community members were asked what they would do if offended by another person. Common answers included doing nothing, taking responsibility for the offense, and seeking closeness to the offender, all of which reflect concerns about relational harmony and efforts to repair the relationship. By comparison, American students were more likely to blame the offender (69%)—a disengaging response (Mesquita, Karasawa, Haire, & Izumi, 2002, cited in Kitayama et al., 2004). Japanese students also said that they experience more interpersonally engaged emotions in everyday social situations and generally felt more positive when they did; the valence of the emotion (whether shame or empathy) mattered less to them. By comparison, North American students preferred positive emotions—emotional valence was key—and were generally more positive when experiencing interpersonally disengaged emotions (those reflecting independence).

Even at young ages, children's experience and expression of emotions are consistent with the ethics of the society in which they live. Among Indonesians, the expression of negative emotions is infrequent, but when they are expressed, young children's healthy functioning is compromised. Third-grade Indonesian children are likely to respond to family members' relatively nonhostile, low-key negative emotions with poorer performance on measures of self-regulation (attentional control and inhibitory control), sympathy, and externalizing behaviors, according to their parents. Family members' expression of positive emotions, however, was not related to children's enhanced functioning, unlike what is often observed in the United States (Eisenberg, Liew, & Pidada, 2001). Compared to North American preschoolers, Japanese preschoolers responded to hypothetical emotionally challenging situations (involving interpersonal conflict and distress) with fewer references to anger and aggression, highlighting Japanese children's desire not to harm others (Zahn-Waxler, Friedman, Cole, Mizuta, & Hiruma, 1996). When asked what they would do in the situation, North American, but not Japanese, preschoolers said they would avoid the person involved—a disengaging strategy.

Emotional regulation sometimes takes place at the level of appraisal (what a person notices and attends to), minimizing expressions of disruptive emotions. We see this among the Utku Inuits (Briggs, 1970), Tahitians (Levy, 1973), and Nepali Tamang (Cole & Tamang, 1998). Six- to 9-year-old Tamang children participating in a study similar to the one by Zahn-Waxler and colleagues (1996) just described reported feeling "okay" when asked about these emotionally challenging situations. Their responses suggested that the situations were not appraised as emotionally significant to them, which is consistent with the peaceful and calm demeanor valued by the Tamang. By contrast, for the Chhetri-Brahmin children participating in this study, regulation took place at the level of expression. Although these children consistently reported feelings of anger in these situations, they said that they would mask their emotion so others would not know about them (show no facial signs of the felt emotion).

Children living in other East Asian and Southeast Asian communities such as Korea, China, and Thailand, are often described as overregulated in their emotional expressions compared to their North American agemates. Chen and her colleagues (1998) found that Chinese 2-year-olds scored higher on measures of behavioral inhibition in their reaction to a scary object in a laboratory situation than did Canadian toddlers. Almost half of the Chinese children did not even touch the object (47%), whereas most Canadian toddlers did (88%). The shyer (behaviorally inhibited) the Chinese child, the more likely was his mother to express warm and accepting attitudes toward him,

which was untrue of Canadian mothers of shy children.

Historically, shyness among the Chinese was considered mature and sensitive, unlike expressiveness, which was regarded as nonadaptive and immature regulation (Ho, 1986). Shy children fared well in terms of peer acceptance, leadership, and academic achievement (Chen, Cen, Li, & He, 2005; Chen et al., 2003). By contrast, shy North American children do not fare well; they are more prone to internalizing problems such as social withdrawal and depression (Eisenberg, 2002), are regarded as socially inept or immature, and have poor peer relations (Eisenberg & Zhou, 2000). However, today in China, the shy child is doing less well. Chen et al. (2005) examined measures of elementary school–age children's social and academic functioning, including shyness, at three different points in time—1990, 1998, and 2002. Whereas shyness in the 1990 cohort was associated with positive outcomes like those just noted, in the 2002 cohort it was not. Rather, shyness was correlated with peer rejection, school problems, and depression. Shyness, once traditionally valued and encouraged, is now seen as an impediment to developing qualities, such as social assertion and initiative, that many consider necessary for success in China's increasingly capitalistic system.

The emotion of feeling-with-others, or empathy, is important for connecting people with one another (Saarni, 1997); in fact, it may be considered the quintessential interpersonally engaging emotion. Empathetic-related responses take into account, and accommodate to, the needs of the other in appropriate, prosocial ways (Roberts & Strayer, 1996). In Japan, empathy helps a person "avoid inconveniencing, annoying, or imposing on others" (Clancy, 1986, pp. 233–234). Japanese mothers consider empathy, as well as obedience and good manners, a self-regulatory function that increases with the age of the child (Rothbaum, Kakinuma, et al., 2005; Kashiwagi, 1988, cited in Ujiie, 1997).

Placing the burden of understanding people's needs and intentions on the listener may support the development of empathy and, more broadly, the sensitivity and responsiveness to others that are important to the regulatory processes maintaining relational harmony. A good listener must notice and attend to the speaker and other relevant situational cues to intuit what another has on his or her mind. Japanese mothers help children learn this competency by telling them directly what others are thinking and feeling in various situations (Clancy, 1986). Similarly, among the Kaluli of New Guinea, mothers speak for their babies, teaching them what to say in social situations (Ochs & Schieffelin, 1984).

In many U.S. middle-class families, by comparison, the speaker rather than the listener is responsible for effective communication. The speaker must make himself heard and understood—regulating the volume, animation, and persistence of the messages to make it clear what he is trying to say. An example of U.S. children's responsibilities as speakers is observed in a study where European American middle-class mothers and Efe mothers were asked to show their child how to work a difficult toy, then asked to shift their attention from their child to the researcher to answer some questions (Morelli, Verhoef, & Anderson, 1996). Representative of the U.S. children was Sara, who marched back and forth, breaking the line of vision between her mother and the researcher, chanting "Look at me, look at me." Finally Sara grabbed her mother's face in her hands, turned it toward her face and yelled, "Look at me!" This child was responsible for regulating her expressiveness to communicate her needs and did so using overt actions and distal verbal strategies. The Efe children depend more on relatively subtle behaviors, such as increased proximity, gentle touch, and postural shifts that relied on their mothers to make sense of their needs, and that did not disrupt the flow of adult activity (see also Rogoff, Mistry, Goncu, & Mosier, 1993).

Empathetic expressiveness is an important element of social relations for people everywhere. Two-year-old German and Japanese girls expressed comparable levels of empathy (when one's own emotional reaction is congruent with the emotional reaction of the other) in a situation designed to elicit this emotion—when a playmate (stranger) expressed sadness over a broken toy (Trommsdorff, 1995). However, compared to the German girls, the Japanese girls were more distressed (upset, anxious, uneasy) by their playmate's sadness and were less likely to recover from it (stayed tense) even though their mothers were as likely to respond contingently to their distress (Friedlmeier & Trommsdorff, 1999). By Western standards the distress reaction of the Japanese girls would represent difficulty in adaptively regulating empathy, leading to overarousal, which is considered aversive and is thought to promote a concern about one's self at the expense of a concern for others (Eisenberg, Smith, et al., 2004). This was true for the German girls; for the Japanese girls, feelings of empathy-related distress did not interfere with their ability to act in a prosocial manner toward the playmate (Trommsdorff & Kornadt, 2003). In other contexts, distress may cause Japanese children to focus on themselves, but distress in empathetic contexts seems to be associated with increased concern for others.

In this study, the Japanese girls were more likely to regulate their distress by seeking physical closeness with their mothers than were the German girls, who were more likely to use eye contact. Unlike the German girls, the Japanese girls did not approach the playmate; they remained close to their mothers, leaving it up to the playmate to approach them. Similarly, young Chinese children stayed closer to their mothers in novel situations meant to elicit stress than did Canadian children (Chen et al., 1998). Physical proximity as a regulation strategy is considered immature by Westerners; however, it is more compatible with people concerned with relational harmony, and it is consistent with many other aspects of care—such as co-sleeping, co-bathing, and prolonged periods of holding—that maximize proximity. Heightened proximity is likely accompanied by lower levels of autonomy (Rothbaum & Trommsdorff, 2006). Distal forms of closeness such as eye-to-eye contact by comparison are more compatible with autonomous self-regulation, which in the West is a hallmark of maturity.

Fitting in, rather than standing out, is important as well to relational harmony (Rothbaum, Weisz, & Snyder, 1982). The practice of self-criticism is one way to achieve fit. Self-criticism shows that a person is aware of her shortcomings and is willing to improve on them (Mesquita, 2003; Shweder et al., 2000). This involves sensitivity to the expectations of others and to the demands of the situation (e.g., see Chao, 1992). We see signs of self-criticism in East Asian children starting at an early age. Stigler, Smith, and Mao (1985) found that Chinese elementary school students rated their competence in the cognitive, physical, and general domains lower than did their North American agemates. In school, Japanese children are given time to reflect on what was not done to meet idealized standards and to consider ways to improve in the future (Heine, Markus, Lehman, & Kitayama, 1999). Among the Chinese, mothers speak of themselves as more rejecting and less accepting of their children than do Canadian mothers (Chen et al., 1998), and they use storytelling to talk about their children's transgressions in ways that are highly critical of the child (P. J. Miller, Fung, & Mintz, 1996). Similarly, Korean parents make clear that their children do not fulfill their hopes (Markus et al., 1997).

Self-discipline in the form of perseverance and endurance makes it possible for East Asian children to strive to meet the expectations of others. The Koreans have a term—*sugohaseyo*—that captures this ethos: "No matter hard you work, you can always work harder" (Grant & Dweck, 2001, p. 207). Tobin, Wu, and Davidson (1989) describe a scene in which Chinese preschoolers, working silently for 20 minutes, build, tear down piece by piece, and rebuild structures exactly as they appear in a picture. This attention to order and regimentation is seen as an important part of children's learning self-regulation, discipline, and social harmony. But one U.S. preschool teacher remarked, upon viewing a videotape of these children, "I guess what bothers me most is that there is such an overemphasis on order and on behaving properly at the cost of stamping out the children's creativity . . . instead of [allowing them] to play in a natural, imaginative way" (p. 92). In the West, this type of persistence would probably not be characterized as adaptive self-regulation, because it does not appear to be autonomous and flexible.

Because of their emphasis on self-improvement, many East Asians attribute their achievements to effort rather than ability. For example, fifth-grade Korean children were more likely to say that they would work harder if they experienced an academic setback than were their North American agemates (Grant & Dweck, 2001). This is consistent with the Japanese notion of "becoming better" (Heine et al., 1999, p. 771). When a person's efforts are not enough to meet the expectations of others, he is likely to experience great distress—high self-blame and negative affect—in part because he is acutely aware of and sensitive to other's opinion of him, and his failures reflect poorly on close others. Unlike Western standards, this distress would not be seen as a failure to self-regulate adaptively, because it motivates children to persevere in their attempts toward self-improvement (Chang, 2001).

East Asian and African adults' encouragement of compliance further indicates that they link self-regulation with relational harmony. Japanese mothers cajole their children into complying by relying on appeals to empathy (how they are hurt by the situation), social disapproval, and withdrawal of attention by ignoring the child. Clancy (1986) describes a Japanese mother coaxing a child to do what she was told by offering to help the child, doing it along with the child, or watching as the child performed the assigned task. U.S. parents, in comparison, use ego-enhancing strategies such as praise, encouragement, and reference to the child's accomplishments to motivate children to do what they are told (see review by Abe & Izard, 1999; see also Dennis et al., 2002).

Japanese adults tend not to view children's resistance to requests as establishing personal boundaries or seeking autonomy, but rather as selfishness and egocentrism (Yamada, 2004) or as a sign of the child's immaturity: "He is only a child, he'll have time to brush his teeth when he is older" (Osterweil & Nagano, 1991, p. 369). This does not mean that Japanese parents are less tolerant of children's resistance; rather, they attribute it less to needs for autonomy and more to needs for maturity (Lebra, 1994). In several African communities, noncompliance is considered a moral transgression (Nsamenang, 1992). In middle-class U.S. communities, however, noncompliance is sometimes considered a sign that the child is acting autonomously. Older children are seen as showing more mature forms of noncompliance such as bargaining and negotiation, and mothers' responses to their children's noncompliance changes accordingly (Kuczynski, Kochanska, Radke-Yarrow, & Girnius-Brown, 1987). Mothers of children using these more mature noncompliance strategies are more likely to countermand by reasoning and counternegotiation. Ujiie (1997) notes that U.S. parents' encouragement of the child not to comply with seemingly unfair requests—which he calls assertive autonomy—is difficult for many Japanese to understand or accept, because this goes against the virtue of adjusting one's needs to the needs of the group. Ujiie notes that Japanese comments such as "He is assertive" or "He has a self" are typically pejorative.

Developmental Pathway to Interdependent Self-Regulation

Keller, Yovsi, et al. (2004) explored the premise that East Asian and African children's early care experiences underlie the development of self-regulatory processes that reflect heightened concerns with relational harmony. They examined the maternal correlates of infants' and toddlers' self-regulation in communities differing in their emphasis on autonomy and community—the Nso of Cameroon (representative of an interdependent cultural pathway) and Greek infants of Greece (representative of an independent cultural pathway). They identified two styles of parenting associated with these different ethics (Keller, Lohaus, et al., 1999) and argued that the distal style, with its emphasis on face-to-face contact and object play, was more likely to foster in children a concern with issues of personal autonomy and separateness; the proximal style, with its emphasis on bodily closeness, in contrast, was more likely to foster in children a concern with issues of heteronomy and relatedness.

Keller, Yovsi, et al. (2004) reasoned as well that the timing of accomplishments such as self-regulation (e.g., committed compliance) and self-recognition would depend in part on the importance of the ethics by which people lived. Compliance is extremely important among many East Asians and Africans; the press for early compliance is noted in the Gusii of Kenya (LeVine, 2004), the Efe of the Democratic Republic of Congo (Morelli, 1997), among children living in Nyansongo in Kenya, and among the Chinese (Chao & Tseng, 2002; Chen et al., 2003). Similarly, Japanese babies are pressed to develop indirect speech forms, assumedly to help fit in and not offend (Clancy, 1986). For example, the Japanese language allows a speaker to negate entire sentences once spoken to make an assertion less direct, perhaps in response to the listener's expression. Japanese people rarely disagree or say "no" in public to avoid offending another or others. Self-recognition, by contrast, is consistent with a child's sense of self as separate and autonomous, and the early press for self-recognition is more often seen among Western parents.

Keller, Yovsi, et al. (2004) found that, within culture, the proximal parenting style relates to the development of self-regulation and the distal parenting style, to the development of self-recognition. Between-culture differences were also found: The Nso infants, who experience greater proximal contact, develop self-regulation earlier than do Greek babies, and Greek babies, who experience greater distal contact, develop self-recognition earlier than do Nso infants; that is, the caregiving practices that predict later self-recognition and self-regulation are similar across cultures, but the

emphasis on these caregiving practices and the emergence of the developmental outcomes with which they are linked differ. Keller, Yovsi, et al. relate the cultural differences in caregiving and in their developmental outcomes to differences between the communities in their prevailing ethics, namely, the Nso emphasis on interdependence (i.e., concerns with community) and the Greek emphasis on independence (i.e., concerns with autonomy).

Broadening Our Conceptions of Good Care

The proximal versus distal style of parenting is one of several useful ways of distinguishing between the care practices of communities that live by different ethics. Another valuable distinction is between types of sensitivity. In the West, sensitivity is equated with a host of caregiving characteristics, including contingent responsiveness to children's signals, as well as promptness, cooperation, availability, and following the child's lead. This interactive style is believed to promote autonomy, because the child perceives herself as in control and competent, certain that caring others are available if the need arises. However, the nature of sensitivity varies across cultures, and this may have implications for self-regulation and the processes associated with its development.

Cameroonian and German mothers, for example, differ in their sensitivity to positive and negative infant signals. Cameroonian mothers are more sensitive to infants' signs of distress, and German mothers, to infants' positive signals (Voelker et al., 1998). Similar differences between non-Western and Western mothers are reported by Friedlmeier and Trommsdorff (1999) and LeVine (2004). LeVine's findings indicate that Gusii mothers of Kenya are more sensitive to their baby's distressed vocalizations than are middle-class U.S. mothers, and that Gusii babies cry less than the U.S. babies. The Gusii practice of maintaining nearly constant contact with babies in the first year of life allows mothers to respond quickly to their infant's distress. Gusii mothers are shocked by videos of American mothers allowing infants to cry, even momentarily. For Gusii mothers, prevention of crying through continuous contact is morally mandated. Yet Gusii mothers show little responsiveness to positive signals. Unlike middle-class U.S. mothers, they do not amplify positive expressions of emotions but turn away from infants who are getting positively excited, so as to calm and soothe them (LeVine, 2004).

Sensitivity in non-Western cultures may be more proactive, with adults and even children anticipating others' distress, or recognizing nascent signs of it, and taking measures to avoid it. There is evidence of this among the Efe, where adults sometimes comfort infants even before they are noticeably upset (Morelli, Henry, & Baldwin, 2002); so too among the Nso (Keller, Yovsi, & Voelker, 2002) and the Guisii (LeVine, 2004). In Japan, preschool teachers emphasize the importance of anticipating children's needs and see the child's role as waiting for the teacher to meet their needs (Rothbaum, Nagoaka, & Ponte, 2005). Anticipatory responsiveness breaks down the child leads/adult follows interactive style, prioritizing less the child's control, and making more ambiguous the distinction between self and other. The U.S. preschool teachers in the previous study reported that anticipation undermined the development of self-expression, self-assertion, and autonomy in young children.

Like parental sensitivity, parental control has different meaning and implications for self-regulation in other cultures. Control includes expressions of warmth in many societies living by ethics of community. For example, Chinese parents and teachers govern—*guan*—children by taking control, directing their behaviors, and placing demands on them (Tobin et al., 1989). *Guan* also means to love and to care for, and it is viewed in a positive light by adults and children alike. Japanese and Korean adolescents associate parental control (*guan*) with warmth and acceptance (Chao & Tseng, 2002). Control for many Asians is rooted in notions of family hierarchy, respect, obligation, and self-sacrifice. In contrast, control for many North Americans is negatively associated with feelings of closeness (measured in terms of cohe-

siveness; Nomura, Noguchi, Saito, & Tezuka, 1995). For them, control is antithetical to self-determination and positive caregiving, because it is rooted in heteronomy, inequality, and restrictiveness.

Because human qualities such as attachment and self-regulation take on very different forms and have different meanings, it should not be surprising that they develop in systematically different ways. In some communities, social development is fostered by distal parenting, sensitive responsiveness, and autonomy fostering practices. In other communities, social development is fostered by proximal parenting, sensitive anticipation, and authoritarian control.

REFLECTIONS ON COHERENCE: CONSISTENCY OR FLEXIBILITY

According to Western theorists, secure attachments and successful self-regulation are predicated on a coherent self. Although all cultures may value self-coherence, we believe there are important differences in the meaning of *coherence* and conceptions of self. Here we review evidence that Western laypersons and researchers emphasize intraindividual consistency across persons, situations, and time, whereas non-Western laypersons and researchers emphasize extraindividual flexibility across roles and contexts (Heine, 2001). Moreover, we attempt to show that theories of attachment and self-regulation are grounded in Western notions of self-coherence that highlight the all important role of autonomy. We also consider how attachment and self-regulation might be understood differently when non-Western notions of self-coherence, which rely much less on notions of autonomy, are adopted (see Table 20.1).

TABLE 20.1. Cultural Differences in Conceptions of Coherence

	Locus	Stability	Process	Central principle/value	One self/ many selves
Western coherence	Intraindividual	Consistency (across time, place, and person)	Internalization, integration	Autonomy	Notion of core authentic self
Non-Western (majority world) coherence	Extraindividual	Flexibility (across time, place, and person)	Balance between demands of different relationships	Community/ harmony	Importance of different roles in different contexts

Research on Coherence

In the West, the self is viewed as relatively un-changing across situations and stable across time, and consistency is seen as essential to healthy functioning (Heine, 2001; Suh, 2002). Many Western theories of social functioning are predicated on this notion of self-consistency (see Kitayama & Markus, 1999, for a review). Consistency is much less valued in East Asia, where "an individual's relation-ships and roles take precedence over abstracted and internalized attributes, such as attitudes, traits and abilities. . . . It is important for the East Asian self to be able to determine what the role requirements are for a given situation and to adjust self accordingly" (Heine, 2001, p. 886).

Evidence of greater emphasis on internal self-consistency in Western than non-Western communities comes from various quarters. In the West, individual attitudes are typically more powerful predictors of behavior than are social norms (Triandis, 1995). Belief in attitude–behavior consistency is more pro-nounced among Australians than Japanese— indeed, Japanese are more likely to align their actions with others' beliefs than with their own (Kashima, Siegel, Tanaka, & Kashima, 1992), and Japanese manifest less susceptibility to dis-sonance (less consistency between one's own attitudes and behavior) than do Canadians (Heine & Lehman, 1997).

Whereas, for North Americans, self-coherence is evident in the consistency of un-derlying attitudes and dispositions, coherence for East Asians is evident in "attunement of the self with the social surrounding. . . . It is this self in a specific social context that predomi-nates in subjective experience" (Kitayama & Markus, 1999, p. 264). There is greater consis-tency among American than among Korean students' self-views across social roles, such as son, daughter, and friend (Suh, 2000), and across hypothetical situations (Suh, 2002). Similarly there is more consistency for Ameri-cans than for Japanese when making self-descriptions when different people are in the room with them (Kanagawa, Cross, & Markus, 2001), and when they are describing their personal versus public selves (see Kitayama & Markus, 1999).

Underlying different representations of cohe-sion are differences in attention, perception, and reasoning. Fiske et al. (1998) cite several studies indicating a tendency toward linear, analytic, decontextualized information pro-cessing in the West, and holistic, context-dependent information processing in the East. Eastern thought is often dialectical—in this context one thing is true, whereas in another context the opposite is true, or the middle way is endorsed (Nisbett, Peng, Choi, Norenzayan, & Ara, 2001).

Coherence in Attachment and Self-Regulation Theory

Coherence is a central construct in Western the-ories of attachment and self-regulation. In ad-dition to entailing consistency between internal psychological characteristics (beliefs, emotions, dispositions, goals, etc.), the coherent self de-picted in these theories is autonomous, unified, integrated, and authentic, as opposed to exter-nally driven, inconsistent, fragmented, and false.

In attachment theory, children's coherence is most evident in their "internal working model"—the stable, integrated set of expecta-tions and experiences pertaining to relation-ships and the self. A coherent model is one link-ing attachment and autonomy (i.e., it depicts a caregiver who fosters the child's autonomy by sensitively responding to needs for security). Adult attachment is assessed by the Adult At-tachment Interview, which relies on the notion of coherent discourse—the consistency, clarity, succinctness, and most importantly, the meaningfulness of the attachment narrative. In-dividuals must fully own and integrate positive and negative aspects of experience for their narratives to be coherent. Autonomy allows for a sense of ownership of inner experience and integration of the narrative. This is evident in the term used for the most secure and coherent adult attachment category—*autonomous* (Fonagy, 1999; Main & Goldwyn, 1998).

In Western self-regulation theory, coherence is typically conceptualized as integration. It is sometimes operationalized as correlations be-tween different self-regulatory constructs (in-volving emotional control, compliance, delay, etc.), or by one construct (compliance) over dif-ferent situations or over time (Kochanska & Murray, 2000). Little attention is devoted to contextual factors. Self-coherence and success-ful self-regulation emerge when the individual freely and autonomously chooses goals, be-cause such goals can be fully integrated with other self-endorsed goals (Baumeister & Vohs, 2003; Eisenberg, Smith, et al., 2004; Ryan & Deci, 2000b).

More recent theories of self-regulation, particularly theories of social cognition in adults (see Cervone & Shoda, 1999, for reviews), place greater emphasis on situational differences than do the self-regulation theories focused on in this chapter. However, these theories depict situations and perceptions of situations as modifiable by self (Cervone & Shoda, 1999; Heine, 2001), they do not depict situations as part of self, and they link self-regulation with autonomy. These are quintessential features of Western self-coherence.

A very different notion of coherence in non-Western cultures is not predicated on ethics of autonomy, but on ethics of community, and, more specifically, on an emphasis not only on harmony, but also on respect, duty, obligation, and proper demeanor. Unlike values associated with autonomy (choice, freedom, agency), values associated with community are closely tied to specific persons (role relationships), places, and situations (public/formal vs. private/informal). They are meaningless when stripped of role and context. What makes the self coherent is not internalization, but coordination with others in the community. Coherence is less predicated on an independent, unitary, authentic sense of self, and more on an interdependent sense of self that is always mindful of particular others and particular contexts in which the self is situated: "Normative demands . . . [are] perceived to be part and parcel of the self" (Kitayama & Markus, 1999, pp. 265–266).

The implications for attachment and self-regulation are profound. When coherence is defined in terms of community and harmony, relationships do not primarily serve to foster the self's goals, but rather to determine the self's roles. Without roles there is no self-coherence. As a result, coherence is less likely to be experienced or expressed as consistency. Consistency in self-regulation in different situations (public and private), or with different persons (ingroup and outgroup members), would not be seen as a marker of authenticity of self, but rather as a sign of incoherence and immaturity. Such behavior ignores the press for modifying one's behavior to accommodate to interpersonal and contextual demands (Fiske et al., 1998; Heine, 2001; Kitayama & Markus, 1999).

The Role of Balance in Coherence

Despite their emphasis on consistency, Western theorists are very focused on internal conflicts. Conflict is central to psychodynamic theory and was a major concern of behaviorists, including cognitive behaviorists. Healthy development is seen as the ability to link or integrate competing desires. This is seen in attachment theorists' emphasis on the trade-off between the desire for attachment and the desire for autonomy (which, early in life, is manifested as exploration). The more secure the attachment, the more the child ventures outward, and the more the child ventures outward, the more she experiences fear and seeks security/attachment figures. Optimal functioning occurs when these competing needs are balanced and integrated. Self-regulation theorists' central thesis is very similar: that there is a trade-off between socially desirable behaviors (attention, compliance, delay of gratification) and autonomy, and optimal functioning represents the balance and integration of the two. Autonomy is seen as leading to compliance ("committed" compliance), and compliance is seen as setting the stage for autonomy. In both theories, the key phenomena of interest (attachment and aspects of self-regulation) are inextricably linked with autonomy; the quality of the linkage determines the coherence of the organism. Both theories' depiction of autonomy as the phenomenon with which all other processes must be balanced stems from the assumption of an independent selfway, and the equating of coherence with internal, autonomous integration of different aspects of self.

Conceptions of balance in non-Western communities have little to do with autonomy. The attachment balance in these communities is between attachment and role responsibilities. Harwood and colleagues (1995) emphasize the balance between closeness and "respectful attentiveness," and investigators focused on Japan emphasize the balance between closeness and formal, role-prescribed behavior (Kitayama & Markus, 1999; Rothbaum & Kakinuma, 2004). The central conflict involves different roles and contexts more so than different internal desires. The individual who has secure intimate relationships is more capable of fulfilling formal duties and role responsibilities, and of balancing different relationships (Heine, 2001; Rothbaum & Kakinuma, 2004). Similarly, self-regulation is a balance between soft-hearted, self-sympathetic behavior and hard-hearted, disciplined behavior; the ability to know with whom and when to engage in each type of behavior constitutes self-coherence and effective regulation (Kitayama & Markus, 1999).

Western conceptions of attachment and self-regulation, which are predicated on an independent selfway, treat autonomy as central, and community and context as relatively peripheral. Non-Western conceptions, which are predicated on an interdependent selfway, treat the ability to act appropriately with different persons in different situations as central. Coherence in this case is located at the interface of self and context rather than internally. It is based less on free will, individual choice, and autonomous ownership of different ways of being, and more on fitting the self (different aspects of self) with contextual realities. Whereas autonomy is the connective tissue that allows for coherence in the West, context appropriateness is the connective tissue that allows for coherence in many non-Western communities. In the latter communities, coherence of attachment is evident when children know with whom and in what situations they can be intimate and dependent, and with whom and in what situations they must be reserved and accommodating. The situated self is always mindful of the particular persons and settings in which she is embedded.

CONCLUSION: JUST TWO PATHWAYS?

In this chapter we have taken to task Western theories of attachment and self-regulation for their assumption of a single pathway to valued forms of security and regulation. However, we may be vulnerable to a similar charge: The assumption of two distinct pathways may not do justice to the diversity of models of attachment and self-regulation, as well as to underlying conceptions of coherence that characterize human functioning worldwide.

There are competing views about the number of pathways that should be entertained in cultural studies: Some theorists feel more strongly than we do about the pervasiveness of two relatively distinct pathways (e.g., Greenfield et al., 2003). These investigators tend to lump together diverse cultures into two relatively separate pathways—typically, those from North America, and Northern and Western Eu-

rope, and those from the rest of the world. Other theorists accept the two-pathway paradigm but argue for subdivisions within them, sometimes as hybrid forms that combine elements of both categories (e.g., Kağitçibaşi, 1996). Still others leave open the possibility of new, as yet unidentified pathways, while acknowledging the substantial evidence currently supporting the two-pathway view (e.g., Saraswathi, 2003). Finally, there is another set of views antithetical to the ones noted that question any press to identify larger pathways; for these theorists, each community is unique and cannot meaningfully be grouped with any other along comprehensive dimensions (e.g., Gergen, Gulerce, Lock, & Misra, 1996).

In this chapter, our assumptions frequently conform to the first of these views—two relatively distinct cultural pathways. Yet we believe that science is best served when researchers leave open the possibility of many pathways, not just two. We described the majority world as living by ethics of community without strong justification for combining such diverse communities in a single category, and we sometimes defined these communities in terms of what they do *not* value (e.g., autonomy). When we defined these communities in terms of what they do value—harmony, community, accommodation—we did not acknowledge that these communities may differ in how they make sense of these constructs. We need to accept the possibility of new pathways as well as "subdivisions" within the two prevailing pathways.

Our understanding of attachment and self-regulation will be hindered, not advanced, by searching for *the* alternative to Western theories of these constructs. It will also be hindered if we resist attempts to identify "ways of being" common to people of different communities, and if we are unwilling to cluster these communities based on these qualities. Clustering has served to highlight some of the most important and valuable distinctions that we have developed in cultural studies (e.g., individualism–collectivism; independence–interdependence), and it is an indispensable tool for making sense of the remarkable variation that characterizes humanity. The problem with these distinctions is that they tend to be used in ways that oversimplify; the solution is to resist that tendency and to be continuously mindful of exceptions that elucidate the complexities.

We began this chapter by considering one community—the Efe hunters and gatherers of the Democratic Republic of Congo—that challenges Western assumptions about attachment and self-regulation. We might have talked about them in a way that implied they best fit the interdependent pathway, living by ethics of community. But we are not completely convinced of this characterization. The Efe are self-reliant and independent in ways consistent with qualities typically associated with people who live by ethics of autonomy. This may be in part because of the way they make a living—hunting and gathering (Barry, Bacon, & Child, 1959). They are also an emotionally expressive people—expressing emotions publicly for all to witness. Gilda A. Morelli remembers with great amusement the sheepish look on Kebe's face as the sounds of his angry wife grew louder as she approached our village. It appears that the moment she heard that Kebe was visiting with us instead of hunting, she expressed her great annoyance with him by yelling loudly and gesticulating widely, and continued to do so on her march from her camp to our village, about a kilometer. The seemingly unrestrained expressions of emotions such as anger are quite common among the Efe, and it took some time for us to get use to this.

Although this portrayal may be construed as an example of the need for a subdivision of the interdependent pathway, we would like to consider the possibility that it represents a third pathway, in which self–other tensions are navigated in a way not characteristic of the two identified pathways. Among the Efe, interdependence seems so profound that it is taken for granted—a given—and little appears to threaten it in any obvious way—certainly not acts that call attention to self or emphasize the distinct and uniqueness of self. Perhaps a closer study of acts that threaten survival, literally, may help us better understand the Efe selfway. We do not have a readily available script to describe this selfway, but we think it is worth considering ways to do so. We hope that this chapter contributes to this endeavor and, by doing so, points to other possible pathways to attachment and self-regulation.

NOTES

1. Gilda A. Morelli has lived and worked with the Efe of the Ituri Rain Forest of the Democratic Republic

of Congo since 1981. The vignettes about them were taken from her field notes spanning over two decades. The names used are typical Efe names, but there is no correspondence between the name and the persons described in the scene. The Efe make a living by hunting and gathering forest foods, and working in local villages in exchange for agricultural goods such as rice and peanuts. To some they are known as "Pygmies" but this is a term they find pejorative.

2. In this part of the chapter, the theories, perspectives, and research referenced (unless noted) were developed primarily in English-speaking (United States, Canada, Australia, and New Zealand) and Western and Northern European communities, and are referred to by most as "Western" theories. We typically do not use this qualifier for the sake of simplicity in the sections on self-determination theory, attachment relationships, and self-regulation.

3. We juxtapose vignettes describing Efe children's experiences with accounts of children's experiences described by Western theorists concerned with attachment and self-regulation. These theorists assume that the experiences they describe are common to all children. We hope the vignettes call attention to differences, as well as to similarities, between what occurs in one community and what is assumed to be universal.

4. Eisenberg and Spinrad (2004) define *emotion regulation* as "the process of initiating, avoiding, inhibiting, maintaining, or modulating the occurrence, form, intensity, or duration of internal feeling states, emotion-related physiological, attentional processes, motivational states, and/or behavioral concomitants of emotion in the service of accomplishing affect-related biological or social adaptation or achieving individual goals" (p. 338). This definition is like that used by Grolick, McMenamy, and Kurowski (1999), but other conceptualizations exist (e.g., Cole, Martin, & Dennis, 2004).

5. Recent research examines how psychological processes such as temperament or effortful control moderate or mediate the relation between security of attachment or maternal interactive style and behavioral regulation (e.g., Feldman, Greenbaum, & Yirmiya, 1999; Kochanska & Knaack, 2003). We do not review this research, because the findings do not alter the gist of what we have to say.

6. Much of the research we consider examines maternal interactive style in structured situations, most often in a laboratory setting, which asks the mother to play with her child, teach her child how to work a toy or play a game, or to get her child to do a task such as "cleanup." Children's emotional expression is usually observed in situations that are frustrating (waiting to get a toy or food) or upsetting (child is restrained). Children's compliance is typically assessed in cleanup tasks or delay tasks with mother present, conscience, in terms of compliance in the absence of an adult, and responses to items that assess the "moral self" or to hypothetical moral situations.

7. A similar distinction is made between individual-

istic and collectivistic societies, with people in individualistic societies characterized as independent, and those in collectivistic societies, as interdependent.

8. The expression "majority world" is used in the remainder of the chapter to refer to the overwhelming majority of the world's cultures and the vast majority of the world's population, including, but not limited to, Asian, African, southern and eastern European, and Hispanic/Latino communities. We do not believe that there is homogeneity between or within these countries, but they have in common being neglected by prevailing theories and evidence, which are based overwhelmingly on studies of Western cultures.

9. What people notice and attend to includes appraising the situation, which contributes significantly to their emotional experience and expression (Mesquita, 2003).

REFERENCES

Abe, J., & Izard, C. (1999). Compliance, noncompliance strategies, and the correlates of compliance in 5-year-old Japanese and American children. *Social Development*, 8(1), 1–20.

Ainsworth, M. D. (1976). *Systems for rating maternal care behavior*. Princeton, NJ: Educational Testing Service Test Collection.

Ainsworth, M. D., Blehar, M. C., Waters, E., & Wahl, S. (1978). *Patterns of attachment: A psychological study of the Strange Situation*. Hillsdale, NJ: Erlbaum.

Ainsworth, M. D., & Bowlby, J. (1991). An ethological approach to personality development. *American Psychologist*, 46(4), 333–341.

Allen, J. P., & Land, D. (1999). Attachment in adolescence. In J. Cassidy & P. R. Shaver (Eds.), *Handbook of attachment* (pp. 319–335). New York: Guilford Press.

Barry, B. I., Bacon, I. L., & Child, M. K. (1959). Relation of child training to subsistence economy. *American Anthropologist*, 61(1), 51–63.

Baumeister, R. F., & Vohs, K. D. (2003). Willpower, choice, and self-control. In G. Loewenstein, D. Read, & R. F. Baumeister (Eds.), *Time and decision: Economic and psychological perspectives on intertemporal choice* (pp. 201–216). New York: Russell Sage Foundation.

Belsky, J., Rosenberger, K., & Crnic, K. (1995). The origins of attachment security: "Classical" and contextual determinants. In S. Goldberg, R. Muir, & J. Kerr (Eds.), *Attachment theory: Social, developmental, and clinical perspectives* (pp. 153–183). Hillsdale, NJ: Analytic Press.

Belsky, J., Spritz, B., & Crnic, K. (1996). Infant attachment security and affective–cognitive information processing at age 3. *Psychological Science*, 7, 111–114.

Bornstein, M. H., Azuma, H., Tamis-LeMonda, C., & Ogino, M. (1990). Mother and infant activity and interaction in Japan and in the United States: I. A comparative macroanalysis of naturalistic exchanges. *International Journal of Behavioral Development*, 13(3), 267–287.

Bowlby, J. (1982). *Attachment and loss* (Vol. 1, 2nd ed.). New York: Basic Books.

Bowlby, J. (1988). *A secure base: Parent–child attachment and healthy human development*. New York: Basic Books.

Bretherton, I. (1985). Attachment theory: Retrospect and prospect. *Monographs of the Society for Research in Child Development*, 50(1), 3–39.

Bretherton, I. (1987). New perspectives on attachment relations: Security, communication and internal working models. In J. Osofsky (Ed.), *Handbook of infant development* (pp. 1061–1100). New York: Wiley.

Bretherton, I. (1992). The origins of attachment theory: John Bowlby and Mary Ainsworth. *Developmental Psychology*, 28, 759–775.

Bridges, L. J., & Grolnick, W. S. (1995). The development of emotional self-regulation in infancy and early childhood. In N. Eisenberg (Ed.), *Social development: Review of personality and social psychology* (pp. 185–211). Thousand Oaks, CA: Sage.

Bridges, L. J., Grolnick, W. S., & Connell, J. P. (1997). Infant emotion regulation with mothers and fathers. *Infant Behavior and Development*, 20(1), 47–57.

Briggs, J. L. (1970). *Never in anger: Portrait of an Eskimo family*. Cambridge, MA: Harvard University Press.

Calkins, S. D. (2004). Early attachment processes and the development of emotional self-regulation. In R. F. Baumeister & K. D. Vohs (Eds.), *Handbook of self-regulation: Research, theory, and applications* (pp. 324–339). New York: Guilford Press.

Calkins, S. D., & Johnson, M. C. (1998). Toddler regulation of distress to frustrating events: Temperamental and maternal correlates. *Infant Behavior and Development*, 21(3), 379–395.

Calkins, S. D., Smith, C. L., Gill, K. L., & Johnson, M. C. (1998). Maternal interactive style across contexts: Relations to emotional, behavioral and physiological regulation during toddlerhood. *Social Development*, 7, 250–369.

Carlson, V. J., & Harwood, R. L. (2003). Attachment, culture, and the caregiving system: The cultural patterning of everyday experiences among Anglo and Puerto Rican mother–infant pairs. *Infant Mental Health Journal*, 24(1), 53–73.

Cassidy, J. (1988). Child–mother attachment and the self in six-year-olds. *Child Development*, 59, 121–134.

Cassidy, J. (1994). Emotion regulation: Influences of attachment relationships. *Monographs of Society for Research in Child Development*, 59, 228–249.

Cassidy, J., & Berlin, L. (1994). The insecure/ambivalent pattern of attachment: Theory and research. *Child Development*, 65, 971–991.

Cassidy, J., & Kobak, R. R. (1988). Avoidance and its

relation to other defensive processes. In J. Belsky & T. Nezworski (Eds.), *Clinical implications of attachment* (pp. 300–323). Hillsdale, NJ: Erlbaum.

Cervone, D., & Shoda, Y. (1999). *The coherence of personality: Social-cognitive bases of consistency, variability, and organization.* New York: Guilford Press.

Chang, E. C. (2001). Cultural influences on optimism and pessimism: Differences in Western and Eastern construals of the self. In *Optimism and pessimism: Implications for theory, research, and practice* (pp. 257–280). Washington, DC: American Psychological Association.

Chao, R. K. (1992). Immigrant Chinese mothers and European American mothers: Their aims of control and other child rearing aspects related to school achievement. *Dissertation Abstracts International, 53*(6-A), 1787–1788.

Chao, R. K., & Tseng, V. (2002). Parenting of Asians. In M. H. Bornstein (Ed.), *Handbook of parenting: Vol. 4. Social conditions and applied parenting* (2nd ed., pp. 59–93). Mahwah, NJ: Erlbaum.

Chen, X., Cen, G., Li, D., & He, Y. (2005). Social functioning and adjustment in Chinese children: The imprint of historical time. *Child Development, 76*(1), 182–195.

Chen, X., Rubin, K., Cen, G., Hastings, P. D., Chen, H., & Stewart, S. L. (1998). Child-rearing attitudes and behavioral inhibition in Chinese and Canadian toddlers: A cross-cultural study. *Developmental Psychology, 34*(4), 677–686.

Chen, X., Rubin, K. H., Liu, M., Chen, H., Wang, L., Li, D., et al. (2003). Compliance in Chinese and Canadian toddlers: A cross-cultural study. *International Journal of Behavioral Development, 27*(5), 428–436.

Clancy, P. M. (1986). The acquisition of communicative style in Japanese. In G. Schieffelin & E. Ochs (Eds.), *Language socialization across cultures* (pp. 213–250). New York: Cambridge University Press.

Cole, P. M., Martin, S. E., & Dennis, T. A. (2004). Emotion regulation as a scientific construct: Methodological challenges and directions for child development research. *Child Development, 75*(2), 317–333.

Cole, P. M., & Tamang, B. L. (1998). Nepali children's ideas about emotional displays in hypothetical challenges. *Developmental Psychology, 34*, 640–646.

Crockenberg, S., & Litman, C. (1990). Autonomy as competence in 2-year-olds: Maternal correlates of child defiance, compliance, and self-assertion. *Developmental Psychology, 26*(6), 961–971.

de Wolff, M. S., & van IJzendoorn, M. H. (1997). Sensitivity and attachment: A meta-analysis on parental antecedents of infant attachment. *Child Development, 68*, 571–591.

Deci, E. L., & Ryan, R. M. (2000). The "what" and "why" of goal pursuits: Human needs and self-determination of behavior. *Psychoanalytic Inquiry, 11*(3), 227–268.

Dennis, T. A., Cole, P. M., Zahn-Waxler, C., & Mizuta, I. (2002). Self in context: Autonomy and relatedness in Japanese and U.S. mother–preschooler dyads. *Child Development, 73*(6), 1803–1817.

Diener, M. L., Mangelsdorf, S. C., McHale, J. L., & Frosch, C. A. (2002). Infants' behavioral strategies for emotion regulation with fathers and mothers: Associations with emotional expressions and attachment quality. *Infancy, 3*(2), 153–174.

Doi, T. (1973). *Anatomy of dependence.* Tokyo: Kodansha International Press.

Doi, T. (1989). The concept of *amae* and its psychoanalytic implications. *International Review of Psychoanalysis, 16*, 349–354.

Doi, T. (1992). On the concept of *amae. Infant Mental Health Journal, 13*(1), 7–11.

Eisenberg, N. (2002). Emotion-related regulation and its relation to quality of social functioning. In W. W. Hartup & R. A. Weinberg (Eds.), *Child psychology in retrospect and prospect: In celebration of the 75th anniversary of the Institute of Child Development* (Vol. 32, pp. 133–171). Mahwah, NJ: Erlbaum.

Eisenberg, N., Liew, J., & Pidada, S. U. (2001). The relations of parental emotional expressivity with the quality of Indonesian children's social functioning. *Emotion, 1*(2), 116–136.

Eisenberg, N., & Morris, S. A. (2002). Children's emotion-related regulation. In R. V. Kail (Ed.), *Advances in child development and behavior* (Vol. 30, pp. 189–229). San Diego: Academic Press.

Eisenberg, N., Smith, C. L., Sadovsky, A., & Spinrad, T. L. (2004). Effortful control: Relations with emotion regulation, adjustment, and socialization in childhood. In R. F. Baumeister (Ed.), *Handbook of self-regulation: Research, theory, and applications* (pp. 259–282). New York: Guilford Press.

Eisenberg, N., & Spinrad, T. L. (2004). Emotion-related regulation: Sharpening the definition. *Child Development, 75*(2), 334–339.

Eisenberg, N., & Zhou, Q. (2000). Regulation from a developmental perspective. *Psychological Inquiry, 11*(3), 166–177.

Emde, R. N. (1992). *Amae,* intimacy, and the early moral self. *Infant Mental Health Journal, 13*(1), 34–42.

Feldman, R., Greenbaum, C. W., & Yirmiya, N. (1999). Mother–infant affect synchrony as an antecedent of the emergence of self-control. *Developmental Psychology, 35*(5), 223–231.

Fiske, A., Kitayama, S., Markus, H., & Nisbett, R. (1998). The cultural matrix of social psychology. In D. Gilbert, S. Fiske, & G. Lindzey (Eds.), *The handbook of social psychology* (4th ed., Vol. 2, pp. 915–981). Boston: McGraw-Hill.

Fonagy, P. (1999, May). *Transgenerational consistencies of attachment: A new theory.* Paper presented at the American Psychoanalytic Association Meeting, Washington, DC.

Friedlmeier, W., & Trommsdorff, G. (1999). Emotion regulation in early childhood: A cross-cultural comparison between German and Japanese toddlers.

Journal of Cross-Cultural Psychology, 30(6), 684–711.

Gergen, K. L., Gulerce, A., Lock, A., & Misra, G. (1996). Psychological science in cultural context. *American Psychologist, 51*, 496–503.

Grant, H., & Dweck, C. (2001). Cross-cultural response to failure: Considering outcome attributions with different goals. In F. Salili & C. Chiu (Eds.), *Student motivation: The culture and context of learning* (pp. 203–219). Dordrecht, The Netherlands: Kluwer Academic.

Greenfield, P. M., Keller, H., Fuligni, A., & Maynard, A. (2003). Cultural pathways through universal development. *Annual Review of Psychology, 54* (1), 461–490.

Grolnick, W. S., Bridges, L. J., & Connell, J. P. (1996). Emotion regulation in two-year-olds: Strategies and emotional expressions in four contexts. *Child Development, 67* (3), 928–941.

Grolnick, W. S., McMenamy, J. M., & Kurowski, C. O. (1999). Emotional self-regulation in infancy and toddlerhood. In L. Balter & C. Tamis-LeMonda (Eds.), *Child psychology: A handbook of contemporary issues* (pp. 3–22). Philadelphia: Psychology Press.

Grolnick, W. S., & Ryan, R. M. (1989). Parental styles associated with children's self-regulation and competence in school. *Journal of Educational Psychology, 81*(2), 143–154.

Grossmann, K. E., Grossmann, K., Zimmermann, P. (1999). A wider view of attachment and exploration: Stability and change during the years of immaturity. In J. Cassidy & P. R. Shaver (Eds.), *Handbook of attachment: Theory, research, and clinical applications* (pp. 760–786). New York: Guilford Press.

Harwood, R. L. (1992). The influence of culturally derived values on Anglo and Puerto Rican mothers' perceptions of attachment behavior. *Child Development, 63*, 822–839.

Harwood, R. L., Miller, J. G., & Irizarry, N. L. (1995). *Culture and attachment: Perceptions of the child in context.* New York: Guilford Press.

Heine, S. J. (2001). Self as cultural product: An examination of East Asian and North American selves. *Journal of Personality, 69*, 881–906.

Heine, S. J., & Lehman, D. R. (1997). Culture, dissonance, and self-affirmation. *Personality and Social Psychology Bulletin, 23*, 389–400.

Heine, S. J., Markus, H. R., Lehman, D. R., & Kitayama, S. (1999). Is there a universal need for positive self-regard? *Psychological Review, 106*(4), 766–794.

Ho, D. F. (1986). Chinese pattern of socialization: A critical review. In M. H. Bond (Ed.), *The psychology of Chinese people* (pp. 1–37). New York: Oxford University Press.

Ip, G. W. M., & Bond, M. H. (1995). Culture, values, and the spontaneous self-concept. *Asian Journal of Psychology, 1*(1), 29–35.

Kağitçibaşi, C. (1996). *Family and human development across cultures.* Mahwah, NJ: Erlbaum.

Kanagawa, C., Cross, S. E., & Markus, H. R. (2001). "Who am I?": The cultural psychology of the conceptual self. *Personality and Social Psychology Bulletin, 27*, 90–103.

Kashima, Y., Siegel, M., Tanaka, K., & Kashima, E. S. (1992). Do people believe behaviors are consistent with attitudes?: Toward a cultural psychology of attribution processes. *British Journal of Social Psychology, 31*, 111–124.

Keller, H. (2003). Socialization for competence: Cultural models of infancy. *Human Development, 46*, 288–311.

Keller, H., Lohaus, A., Kuensemueller, P., Abels, M., Yovsi, R., Voelker, S., et al. (2004). The bioculture of parenting: Evidence from five cultural communities. *Parenting: Science and Practice, 4*(1), 25–50.

Keller, H., Lohaus, A., Volker, S., Cappenberg, M., & Chasiotis, A. (1999). Temporal contingency as an independent component of parenting behavior. *Child Development, 70*(2), 474–485.

Keller, H., Papaligoura, Z., Kuensemueller, P., Voelker, S., Papaeliou, C., Lohaus, A., et al. (2003). Concepts of mother–infant interaction in Greece and Germany. *Journal of Cross-Cultural Psychology, 34*(6), 677–689.

Keller, H., Yovsi, R., Borke, J., Kartner, J., Jensen, H., & Papligoura, Z. (2004). Developmental consequences of early parenting experiences: Self-recognition and self-regulation in three cultural communities. *Child Development, 75*(6), 1745–1760.

Keller, H., Yovsi, R. D., & Voelker, S. (2002). The role of motor stimulation in parental ethnotheories. *Journal of Cross-Cultural Psychology, 33*, 398–445.

Kitayama, S., Karasawa, M., & Mesquita, B. (2004). Collective and personal processes in regulating emotions: Emotion and self in Japan and the U.S. In P. Philippot & R. S. Feldman (Eds.), *The regulation of emotion* (pp. 251–273). Mahwah, NJ: Erlbaum.

Kitayama, S., & Markus, H. R. (1999). Yin and yang of the Japanese self: The cultural psychology of personality coherence. In D. Cervone & Y. Shoda (Eds.), *The coherence of personality: Social-cognitive bases of consistency, variability, and organization* (pp. 242–302). New York: Guilford Press.

Kitayama, S., Markus, H. R., & Kurokawa, M. (2000). Culture, emotion, and well-being: Good feelings in Japan and the United States. *Cognition and Emotion, 14*(1), 93–124.

Kochanska, G. (2001). Emotional development in children with different attachment histories: The first three years. *Child Development, 72*(2), 474–490.

Kochanska, G., Coy, K. C., & Murray, K. T. (2001). The development of self-regulation in the first four years of life. *Child Development, 72*(4), 1091–1111.

Kochanska, G., & Knaack, A. (2003). Effortful control as a personality characteristic of young children: Antecedents, correlates, and consequences. *Journal of Personality, 71*, 1087–1112.

Kochanska, G., & Murray, K. T. (2000). Mother–child mutually responsive orientation and conscience development: From toddler to early school age. *Child Development, 71*(2), 417–431.

Kochanska, G., Murray, K. T., & Coy, K. C. (1997). Inhibitory control as a contributor to conscience in childhood: From toddler to early school age. *Child Development, 68*(2), 263–277.

Kochanska, G., Murray, K. L., & Harlan, E. T. (2000). Effortful control in early childhood: Continuity and change, antecedents, and implications for social development. *Developmental Psychology, 36*, 220–232.

Kondo-Ikemura, K., & Matsuoka, Y. (1999, April). *The characteristics of attachment styles in Japanese students.* Paper presented at the Society for Research in Child Development, Albuquerque, NM.

Kopp, C. B. (2001). Self-regulation in childhood. In N. Eisenberg, N. J. Smelser, & P. B. Baltes (Eds.), *International encyclopedia of the behavioral and social sciences* (pp. 13862–13866). New York: Elsevier.

Kuczynski, L., Kochanska, G., Radke-Yarrow, M., & Girnius-Brown, O. (1987). A developmental interpretation of young children's noncompliance. *Developmental Psychology, 23*, 799–806.

Ladd, G. W. (1999). Peer relationships and social competence during early and middle childhood. *Annual Review of Psychology, 50*, 333–359.

Lebra, T. S. (1994). Mother and child in Japanese socialization: A Japan–U.S. comparison. In P. M. Greenfield & R. R. Cocking (Eds.), *Cross-cultural roots of minority child development* (pp. 259–274). Hillsdale, NJ: Erlbaum.

LeVine, R. A. (2004). Challenging the expert: Findings from an African study of infant care and development. In U. P. Gielen & J. L. Roopnarine (Eds.), *Childhood and adolescence in cross-cultural perspectives*. Westport, CT: Praeger.

LeVine, R. A., & Norman, K. (2001). The infant's acquisition of culture: Early attachment reexamined in anthropological perspective. In C. C. Moore & H. F. Matthews (Eds.), *The psychology of cultural experience* (pp. 83–103). New York: Cambridge University Press.

Levy, R. I. (1973). *Tahitians: Mind and experience in the Society Islands.* Chicago: University of Chicago Press.

Main, M., & Cassidy, J. (1988). Categories of response to reunion with the parent at age 6: Predictable from infant attachment classifications and stable over a 1-month period. *Developmental Psychology, 24*, 1–12.

Main, M., & Goldwyn, R. (1998). *Adult attachment classification system.* Unpublished manuscript, University of California, Berkeley.

Markus, H. R., & Kitayama, S. (1991). Culture and the self: Implications for cognition, emotion, and motivation. *Psychological Review, 98*, 224–253.

Markus, H. R., Mullally, P. R., & Kitayama, S. (1997). Self-ways: Diversity in modes of cultural participation. In U. Neisser & D. Jopling (Eds.), *The conceptual self in context* (pp. 13–61). Cambridge, UK: Cambridge University Press.

Matas, L., Arend, R., & Sroufe, L. A. (1978). Continuity of adaptation in the second year: The relationship between quality of attachment and later competence. *Child Development, 49*, 547–556.

Mesquita, B. (2003). Emotions as dynamic cultural phenomena. In R. J. Davidson, K. R. Scherer, & H. H. Goldsmith (Eds.), *Handbook of affective sciences* (pp. 871–890). Oxford, UK: Oxford University Press.

Mesquita, B., Karasawa, M., Haire, A., & Izumi, S. (2002). *The emotion process as a function of cultural models: A comparison between American, Mexican, and Japanese cultures.* Unpublished manuscript, Wakeforest University, Winston-Salem, NC.

Miller, J. G. (1984). Culture and the development of everyday social explanation. *Journal of Personality and Social Psychology, 45*(6), 961–978.

Miller, J. G. (2004). The cultural deep structure of psychological theories of social development. In R. Sternberg & E. Grigorenko (Eds.), *Culture and competence* (pp. 111–138). Washington, DC: American Psychological Association.

Miller, P. J., Fung, H., & Mintz, J. (1996). Self-construction through narrative practices: A Chinese and American comparison of early socialization. *Ethos, 24*(2), 237–280.

Mizuta, I., Zahn-Waxler, C., Cole, P. M., & Hiruma, N. (1996). A cross-cultural study of preschoolers' attachment: Security and sensitivity in Japanese and U.S. dyads. *International Journal of Behavioral Development, 19*, 141–159.

Morelli, G. (1997). Growing up female in a forager community. In M. E. Morbeck, A. Galloway, & A. Zihlman (Eds.), *Life history, females and evolution.* Princeton, NJ: Princeton University Press.

Morelli, G., Henry, P. I., & Baldwin, H. (2002, November). *Different caregivers but similar care among the Efe foragers: Are there different ways to conceptualize consistency of care?* Paper presented at the American Anthropological Association, New Orleans, LA.

Morelli, G., Rogoff, B., Oppenheimer, G., & Goldsmith, D. (1992). Cultural variations in infants' sleeping arrangements: Questions of independence. *Developmental Psychology, 28*, 604–613.

Morelli, G., Verhoef, H., & Anderson, C. (1996, August). *Please don't interrupt me, I'm talking: Community variation in the way children share the attention of their caregivers with others.* Paper presented at the International Society for the Study of Behavioral Development, Québec, Canada.

Nezworski, M. T. (1983). *Continuity in adaptation into the fourth year: Individual differences in curiosity and exploratory behavior of preschool children.* Unpublished doctoral dissertation, University of Minnesota, Minneapolis.

Nisbett, R. E., Peng, K., Choi, I., & Norenzayan, A. (2001). Culture and systems of thought: Holistic versus analytic cognition. *Psychological Review, 108*(2), 291–310.

Nomura, N., Noguchi, Y., Saito, S., & Tezuka, I. (1995). Family characteristics and dynamics in Japan and the United States: A preliminary report from the family environment scale. *International Journal of Intercultural Relations, 19*, 59–86.

Nsamenang, A. B. (1992). *Human development in cultural context: A Third World perspective.* Newbury Park, CA: Sage.

Ochs, E., & Schieffelin, B. (1984). Language acquisition and socialization: Three developmental stories and their implications. In R. Shweder & R. A. LeVine (Eds.), *Culture theory: Essays on mind, self and emotion* (pp. 276–320). Chicago: University of Chicago Press.

Okonogi, K. (1992). *Amae* as seen in diverse interpersonal interactions. *Infant Mental Health Journal, 13*, 18–25.

Osterweil, Z., & Nagano, K. N. (1991). Maternal views on autonomy: Japan and Israel. *Journal of Cross-Cultural Psychology, 22*, 362–375.

Raeff, C. (1997). Individuals in relationships: Cultural values, children's social interactions, and the development of an American individualistic self. *Developmental Review, 17*, 205–238.

Roberts, W., & Strayer, J. (1996). Empathy, emotional expressiveness, and prosocial behavior. *Child Development, 67*(2), 449–470.

Rogoff, B. (1990). *Apprenticeship in thinking.* New York: Oxford University Press.

Rogoff, B., Mistry, J., Goncu, A., & Mosier, C. (1993). Guided participation in cultural activity by toddlers and caregivers. *Monographs of the Society for Research in Child Development, 58*(8, Serial No. 236).

Rothbart, M. K. (1989). Temperament and development. In G. A. Kohnstamm, J. E. Bates, & M. K. Rothbart (Eds.), *Temperament in childhood* (pp. 187–247). New York: Wiley.

Rothbart, M. K., & Derryberry, D. (1981). Development of individual differences in temperament. In M. E. Lamb & A. L. Brown (Eds.), *Advances in developmental psychology* (pp. 37–86). Hillsdale, NJ: Erlbaum.

Rothbaum, F., & Kakinuma, M. (2004). *Amae* and attachment: Security in cultural context. *Human Development, 47*, 34–39.

Rothbaum, F., Kakinuma, M., Nagaoka, M., & Azuma, H. (2005). *Attachment and* amae: *Parent–child closeness in the US and Japan.* Unpublished manuscript, Tufts University, Medford, MA.

Rothbaum, F., Nagaoka, R., & Ponte, I. (2005). *Caregiver sensitivity in cultural context: Japanese and US teachers' beliefs about anticipating and responding to children's needs.* Unpublished manuscript, Tufts University, Medford, MA.

Rothbaum, F., Pott, M., Azuma, H., Miyake, K., & Weisz, J. (2000). The development of close relationships in Japan and the US: Pathways of symbiotic harmony and generative tension. *Child Development, 71*, 1121–1142.

Rothbaum, F., & Trommsdorff, G. (2006). Do roots and wings complement or oppose one another?: The socialization of relatedness and autonomy in cultural context. In J. E. Grusec & P. D. Hastings (Eds.), *The handbook of socialization* (pp. 461–489). New York: Guilford Press.

Rothbaum, F., Weiss, J., Pott, M., Miyake, K., & Morelli, G. (2000). Attachment and culture: Security in the United States and Japan. *American Psychologist, 55*, 1093–1104.

Rothbaum, F., Weisz, J., & Snyder, S. (1982). Changing the world and changing the self: A two-process model of perceived control. *Journal of Personality and Social Psychology, 42*, 5–37.

Ryan, R. M., & Deci, E. L. (2000a). The darker and brighter sides of human existence: Basic psychological needs as a unifying concept. *Psychological Inquiry, 11*(4), 319–338.

Ryan, R. M., & Deci, E. L. (2000b). Self-determination theory and the facilitation of intrinsic motivation, social development, and well-being. *American Psychologist, 55*(1), 68–78.

Ryan, R. M., Kuhl, J., & Deci, E. L. (1997). Nature and autonomy: Organizational view of social and neurobiological aspects of self-regulation in behavior and development. *Development and Psychopathology, 9*, 701–728.

Saarni, C. (1997). Emotional competence and self-regulation in childhood. In P. Salovey & D. J. Sluyter (Eds.), *Emotional development and emotional intelligence: Educational implications* (pp. 35–66). New York: Basic Books.

Saraswathi, T. S. (2003). *Cross-cultural perspectives in human development: Theory, research and applications.* Thousand Oaks, CA: Sage.

Seifer, R., & Schiller, M. (1995). The role of parenting sensitivity, infant temperament, and dyadic interaction in attachment theory and assessment. In E. Waters, B. Vaughn, G. Posada, & K. Kondo-Ikemura (Eds.), *Caregiving, cultural, and cognitive perspectives on secure-base behavior and working models* (pp. 146–147). *Monographs of the Society for Research in Child Development, 60*(2–3, Serial No. 244).

Shweder, R. A., Goodnow, J. J., Hatano, G., LeVine, R. A., Markus, H. R., & Miller, P. J. (2000). The cultural psychology of development: One mind, many mentalities. In W. Damon & R. M. Lerner (Eds.), *Handbook of child psychology, Vol. 1. Theoretical models of human development* (5th ed., pp. 865–937). New York: Wiley.

Shweder, R. A., Much, N. C., Mahapatra, M., & Park, L. (1997). The "Big Three" of morality (autonomy, community, divinity) and the "Big Three" explanations of suffering. In A. M. Brandt & P. Rozin (Eds.), *Morality and health* (pp. 119–169). New York: Routledge.

Silverman, I. W., & Ippolito, M. F. (1995). Maternal antecedents of delay ability in young children. *Journal of Applied Developmental Psychology, 16,* 569–591.

Sroufe, L. A. (1979). Socioemotional development. In J. Osofsky (Ed.), *Handbook of infant development* (pp. 462–516). New York: Wiley.

Sroufe, L. A. (1983). Infant–caregiver attachment and patterns of adaptation in preschool: The roots of maladaptation and competence. In M. Perlmutter (Ed.), *The Minnesota Symposia on Child Psychology: Development and policy concerning children with specific needs* (pp. 41–83). Hillsdale, NJ: Erlbaum.

Sroufe, L. A. (1996). *Emotional development: The organization of emotional life in the early years.* New York: Cambridge University Press.

Sroufe, L. A., Fox, N. A., & Pancake, V. (1983). Attachment and dependency in developmental perspective. *Child Development, 54,* 1615–1627.

Stifter, C. A., Spinrad, T. L., & Braungart-Rieker, J. M. (1999). Toward a developmental model of child compliance: The role of emotion regulation in infancy. *Child Development, 70*(1), 21–32.

Stigler, J. W., Smith, S., & Mao, L. (1985). The self-perception of competence by Chinese children. *Child Development, 56,* 1259–1270.

Suh, E. M. (2000). Self, the hyphen between culture and subjective well-being. In E. Diener & E. M. Suh (Eds.), *Culture and subjective well-being* (pp. 63–86). Cambridge, MA: MIT Press.

Suh, E. M. (2002). Culture, identity consistency, and subjective well-being. *Journal of Personality and Social Psychology, 83,* 1378–1391.

Takahashi, K. (1990). Are the key assumptions of the "Strange Situation" procedure universal?: A view from Japanese research. *Human Development, 33,* 23–30.

Thompson, R. A. (1994). Emotion regulation: A theme in search of definition. In N. A. Fox (Ed.), *Monographs of the Society for Research in Child Development, 59,* 25–52.

Thompson, R. A. (1998). Early sociopersonality development. In W. Damon & E. Eisenberg (Eds.), *Handbook of child development: Vol. 3. Social, emotional, and personality development* (pp. 177–235). New York: Wiley.

Tobin, J. J., Wu, D. Y. H., & Davidson, D. H. (1989). *Preschool in three cultures.* New Haven, CT: Yale University Press.

Triandis, H. C. (1995). *Individualism and collectivism.* Boulder, CO: Westview Press.

Trommsdorff, G. (1995). Person–context relations as developmental conditions for empathy and prosocial action: A cross-cultural analysis. In T. A. Kindermann & J. Valsiner (Eds.), *Development of person–context relations* (pp. 113–146). Hillsdale, NJ: Erlbaum.

Trommsdorff, G., & Friedlmeier, W. (2003). *Maternal sensitivity and preschool children's emotion regulation in Japan and Germany.* Unpublished manuscript, University of Konstanz, Konstanz, Germany.

Trommsdorff, G., & Kornadt, H. J. (2003). Parent–child relations in cross-cultural perspective. In L. Kuczynski (Ed.), *Handbook of dynamics in parent–child relations* (pp. 271–306). London: Sage.

Tronick, E. Z. (1989). Emotions and emotional communication in infancy. *American Psychologist, 44*(2), 112–119.

Ujiie, T. (1997). How do Japanese mothers treat children's negativism? *Journal of Applied Developmental Psychology, 18*(4), 467–483.

Van IJzendoorn, M. H., & Sagi, A. (1999). Cross-cultural patterns of attachment: The universal and contextual dimensions. In J. Cassidy & P. R. Shaver (Eds.), *Handbook of attachment: Theory, research, and clinical applications* (pp. 713–734). New York: Guilford Press.

Voelker, S., Yovsi, R., & Keller, H. (1998). *Maternal interaction quality as assessed by non trained raters from different cultural backgrounds.* Paper presented at the 15th Biennial ISSBD meetings, Bern, Switzerland.

Waters, E., & Cummings, E. M. (2000). A secure base from which to explore close relationships. *Child Development, 71*(1), 164–172.

Weinfield, N. S., Sroufe, A. L., Egeland, B., & Carlson, E. A. (1999). The nature of individual differences in infant–caregiver attachment. In J. Cassidy & P. R. Shaver (Eds.), *Handbook of attachment: Theory, research, and clinical applications* (pp. 68–88). New York: Guilford Press.

Weisz, J. R., Rothbaum, F. M., & Blackburn, T. C. (1984a). Standing out and standing in: The psychology of control in America and Japan. *American Psychologist, 39,* 955–969.

Weisz, J. R., Rothbaum, F. M., & Blackburn, T. C. (1984b). Swapping recipes for control. *American Psychologist, 39,* 974–975.

Yamada, H. (2004). Japanese mothers' views of young children's areas of personal discretion. *Child Development, 75*(1), 164–179.

Zahn-Waxler, C., Friedman, R. J., Cole, P., Mizuta, I., & Hiruma, N. (1996). Japanese and United States preschool children's responses to conflict and distress. *Child Development, 67,* 2462–2477.

CHAPTER 21

Biocultural Co-Construction of Developmental Plasticity across the Lifespan

SHU-CHEN LI

Historically, the nature–nurture controversy has been debated for centuries, dividing the fields of behavioral and neurobiological development (for reviews, see Meaney, 2001; Rensberger, 1983). On the nature side, nativists argue that human development is determined by innate factors, such as genetic endowment and brain maturation. On the nurture side, the empiricists see development as the result of experience and learning, and that individuals at the beginning of life are more or less capable of acquiring what the environment provides. Although interactionism has also been proposed as an alternative to steer research and public views away from the simple but false dichotomy, the nature–nurture debate continues and has even intensified since the publication of two working drafts of human genome sequence at the turn of the 21st century (International Human Genome Sequencing Consortium, 2001; Venter et al., 2001).

Instead of polarizing toward either end, the aim of this chapter is to approach the age-old nature–nurture debate through the lens of biocultural co-constructivism (Baltes, Rösler, & Reuter-Lorenz, 2006; Li, 2003; Li & Lindenberger, 2002). Although there are certainly biologically based limits on behavior and cognition, it is also important to consider brains as open, dynamic information processors that are receptive to sociocultural influences. The fundamental proposition of biocultural co-constructivism is that contextualized experiences shape the functional dynamics of brain–behavior reciprocity. Building on general, species-typical neurobiological predispositions that are evolved through brain evolution, during ontogeny brains obtain information about the world and are shaped by it through embodied and embedded experiential tuning. The term "embodiment" as used here refers to the notion that brains sense and perceive stimulations from the external world through bodily sensory and motor processes, whereas the term "embedding" refers to the fact that most of the information that brains process is socioculturally contextualized (cf. A. Clark, 1999, for a review of embodiment; see

Hatano & Wertsch, 2001, for review of socio-cultural contextualization). Therefore, lifespan development of behavior and cognition should not automatically be considered solely as the maturation or aging of basic information-processing mechanisms and their neurobiological substrates.

Conceptions of environmental, cultural, and behavioral factors interacting with the biological inheritance of human development have long philosophical traditions. For instance, Tetens (1777) assigned extraordinary plasticity to human nature, thus stipulating opportunities for environmental, cultural, and individual regulation during life ontogeny. At the evolutionary phylogenetic level, St. George Jackson Mivart (1871) suggested that behavioral changes and adaptation precede and affect natural selection. Among modern behavioral development researchers there is the consensus that individual ontogeny is hierarchically organized within an open developmental system that has multiple levels of contexts (e.g., the endogenous neurobiological context and the exogenous family, school, and sociocultural contexts). Consequently, developmental phenomena need to be investigated by jointly considering interactions between endogenous and exogenous processes at various levels (e.g., Alexander, 1969; Anastasi, 1958; Baltes, 1979; Baltes & Singer, 2001; Bronfenbrenner, 1979; Bronfenbrenner & Ceci, 1994; Gottlieb, 1976, 1998; Magnusson, 1988, 1996; Schaie, 1965).

A general awareness of co-constructive notions in and of itself is, however, not enough to resolve the nature–nurture and brain–behavior controversies. The integration of experiential and cultural influences into the day-to-day research practices of neurosciences requires that reciprocal interactive processes implementing biocultural co-construction of brain, mind, and behavior at different levels be further specified. Lacking specifications of such cross-level reciprocal interactions, in part, has been one of the reasons why the nature–nurture debate has continued, because mechanisms of mutual influences between biology and culture during the processes of brain evolution and ontogeny are not made explicit (cf. Ingold, 1998; King, 2000). Cross-level frameworks that explicate reciprocal interactions of developmental plasticity across different levels and time scales are thus needed to foster integration of research from related subfields of developmental and life sciences.

BEYOND RESOURCES: CULTURE'S ACTIVE ROLE IN DEVELOPMENT

Culture has most commonly been conceived as a socially inherited body of man-made material artifacts, knowledge, values, and beliefs accumulated from the past of a given social group that functions as resources to coordinate current human life among individuals and between individuals and the physical environment (e.g., D'Andrade, 1996; Herskovitz, 1948; Tylor, 1874). If only the "resource" aspect is emphasized—as is the case in most generic definitions—then culture is merely the static and passive product of past civilization that is utilized to support the current ways of human life. Some scholars criticized the inadequacy of such notions of culture that view it as merely the supplement of biologically based capacities. The main concern of these criticisms is that a static resource view of culture could not address the intertwined relations of culture and biology in the course of human phylogeny and individual ontogeny (e.g., Geertz, 1973).

Culture as Collective Social Processes

The accumulation of cultural resources can be considered as a dynamic process that involves the so-called "ratchet effect" or "cumulative cultural evolution" (Tomasello, 1999). During such a process, individuals of a given cultural group progressively made modifications to the inherited body of cultural resources. Consequently, the inherited cultural resources become more complex, encompassing a wider range of adaptive functions. Furthermore, at the ontogenetic level, ongoing collective social dynamics (i.e., face-to-face interpersonal interactions, other social interactions derived from them, and shared intentionality) constructs the shared social reality in present societies (Berger & Luckmann, 1967; Searle, 1995). The process aspect of culture is particularly emphasized in recent research on cognitive engineering of the workplace and interactive minds (e.g., Baltes & Staudinger, 1996; Hutchins, 1995). For instance, the routines, habits, and performance criteria of a given workplace are not always static across even relatively short periods (i.e., weeks or months); rather, they are constructed online with the intentions, thoughts, and behaviors of members in the group affecting each other to shape the collective "working culture." Bringing the collective social processing aspect of culture to the foreground makes obvious the social interactions taking place in the individual's proximal developmental context as part of the processes mediating cultural influences on brain, cognitive, and behavioral development.

Culture as Developmentally Relevant

One other somewhat implicit but consistent feature in modern conceptions of culture is its relevancy for individual development. For instance, Williams (1973) pointed out that many of these notions arise from terms referring to processes that help organisms *grow*. For instance, culture has been considered as an integral part of the "garden for development" (Cole, 1999) or "developmental niche" (Gauvain, 1995, 1998; Super & Harkness, 1986), that edify individual development to minimize the distance between the individual's attained and potential levels of performance (Vygotsky, 1978). Highlighting developmental relevancy as distinct from the resource and process aspects of culture emphasizes the active role and function of cultural resources, together with the social processes generating them in individual development. Different cultures (or subcultures within a culture) can differ in the level of resources (or opportunities), as well as constraints, they put forward for individual development in profiles of behavioral expressions, in the constellations and processes of interactive minds, and in their receptivity to modifications by individual behaviors and new technological advances (Baltes & Singer, 2001).

To explicitly consider the dynamics of biocultural co-constructive influences on lifespan development, the three distinct but related aspects of culture (resource, process, and developmental relevancy) need to be simultaneously highlighted. Culture, thus, can be reconsidered as ongoing collective social processes that generate social, psychological, linguistic, symbolic, material, and technological resources that influence human development via reciprocal mechanisms feeding back into individuals' moment-to-moment microgenesis, lifespan ontogeny involving mind–brain interaction, and human phylogeny involving culture–gene coevolution (Li, 2003). Defined as such, culture is not just the passive product of socially inherited resources of human civilizations, such as

tools, technology, language, knowledge, art, customs, values, and beliefs that are accumulated over the past. Rather, it is the "cogenerator" of culture–gene coevolution during human phylogeny in the long run, and together with behavioral, cognitive, and neurobiological plasticity, it is the active "coproducer" of brain, cognitive, and behavioral development during individual lifespan ontogeny.

RELATIVE CONTRIBUTIONS OF BIOLOGY AND CULTURE ACROSS THE LIFESPAN

Human development reflect the interactions between three classes of processes: (1) species-typical neurobiological and cultural evolutionary processes; (2) normative, age-graded, socialization-typical ontogenetic processes with which the individual acquires shared pragmatic knowledge (e.g., basic language and arithmetic skills) of a given sociocultural group; and (3) idiosyncratic (non-normative) influence of person-specific professional expertise and skills that result, at least in part, from the individual's self-selected and constructed personal life experiences and history (Li & Freund, 2005; Baltes & Smith, 2004). Developmentalists and lifespan researchers generally appreciate the fact that both biological and socialization processes contribute to individual ontogeny, and that multiple classes of processes at different levels affect development. However, the dynamical shift in the relative contributions of biology and culture across different periods of life is a topic that is rarely considered. Baltes (1997) made an effort to propose a framework for considering the interplay of biology and culture in lifespan development by specifying three principles (see Figure 21.1).

The first principle suggests that biology-based plasticity decreases after maturity. This is presumably due to the lack of evolutionary selection pressure on survival in the postreproductive phase of life; therefore, beneficial evolutionary selection affording optimal functioning (in the sense of basic biological potential) was less operative for later periods of life as genetic evolution proceeded. Second, more and more culture is required to extend human development to higher levels of functioning and older ages. By increases in cultural resources, for instance, via the process of cumulative cultural evolution (Tomasello, 1999), the

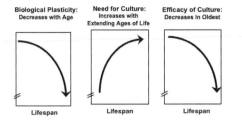

FIGURE 21.1. Schematic representation of principles about the dynamic interplay between biology and culture across the lifespan. Adapted from Baltes (1997). Copyright 1997 by the American Psychological Association. Adapted by permission.

window of ontogenetic time and opportunities can be extended and expanded for more individuals into older ages. However, at the same time, it should also be kept in mind that the cultural conditions and resources required for reaching increasingly higher levels of functioning and older ages increase as well. The third principle states that cultural impact or efficiency varies by age. Specifically, as decline in neurobiological functions limits the effectiveness of cultural influences, the efficacy of cultural resources decreases with increasing age during adult development. Thus, it takes more and more resources and support to produce the same level of cognitive performance in old age. Examples drawn from lifespan cognitive devel-

opment are reviewed in the following section to illustrate these principles.

Differential Trajectories and Dynamic Organization of Intellectual Abilities

The differential trajectories and dynamic organization of different aspects of intellectual abilities across the lifespan are two illustrations of the dynamic interplay between biology and culture in the domain of cognitive development. Dual-component theories of intelligence distinguish between fluid cognitive mechanics, which reflect the operations of the relatively more neurobiology-based information-processing mechanisms (e.g., processing speed, working memory, and attention), and crystallized cognitive pragmatics (e.g., language and practical skills), which are the outgrowth of experience- and culture-based knowledge (e.g., Baltes, Lindenberger, & Standinger, 1998; Cattell, 1971; Horn, 1968). Cross-sectional age gradients and longitudinal age trajectories (e.g., McArdle, Ferrer-Caja, Hamagami, & Woodcock, 2002) of these two domains of intellectual abilities generally show a lead–lag pattern across the lifespan. As an example, empirical cross-sectional age gradients, covering the age range from 6 to 89 years plotted in Figure 21.2 show that the more biology-based fluid cognitive mechanics develop and decline earlier than the more culture-based crystallized cognitive

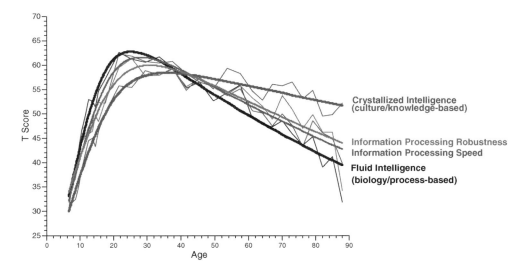

FIGURE 21.2. Fitted empirical age gradients of two broad domains of intellectual abilities along with gradients of basic processing speed and processing robustness. Adapted from Li et al. (2004). Copyright 2004 by Blackwell. Adapted by permission.

pragmatics. The maximum performances of cognitive mechanics and the associated basic information-processing mechanisms (e.g., processing speed and robustness) are achieved by individuals in their mid-20s, whereas the maximum performances of cognitive pragmatics (e.g., culture-based verbal knowledge) are achieved by individuals in their mid-40s and remain stable until 70 years of age, at which point they also decline (Li et al., 2004).

Applying Baltes's (1997) framework to intellectual development, a further proposition can be made. During childhood and old age, neurobiological influences on behavior and cognition are strong; thus, individual differences are affected relatively more by species-typical neurobiological constraints. In adulthood, when the optimal efficacy of neurobiological mechanisms is reached and maintained, individual differences are affected relatively more by socioculturally contextualized experiences that individuals accumulate through their personal life histories (see Figure 21.3). During life periods when there are strong biological constraints on basic information-processing mechanisms underlying the acquisition and expression of culture-based knowledge, the different facets of intelligence and their constituent basic information-processing mechanisms are expected to correlate more highly with each other than in periods when neurobiological efficacy functions at (or above) threshold level.

This proposition suggests that variations in the relative contributions of biology and culture are contributing factors to the differentiation (diversifying) and dedifferentiation (dediversifying) of intellectual abilities, which is an empirical phenomenon that has been discussed in cognitive-developmental psychology since the 1940s (e.g., Balinsky, 1941; Baltes, Cornelius, Spiro, Nesselroade, & Willis, 1980; Garrett, 1946; Reinert, 1970). This proposition is further supported by recent cross-sectional and longitudinal findings. For instance, in a cross-sectional lifespan sample, the amount of covariance shared among the more biologically based aspects of basic cognitive processes (e.g., indicated by information-processing speed of visual and memory search, response competition, and choice reactions), the more biologically based intellectual abilities (memory, reasoning, perceptual speed), and the more culture-based abilities (e.g., verbal knowledge and verbal fluency) were observed to be higher at both ends of the lifespan than in adulthood (see Figure 21.4, which plots the lifespan functions of correlations between basic information-processing speed and two broad domains of intellectual abilities separately). Applying a dynamic structural modeling technique (i.e., statistical methods that analyze the relations between age-related processes of change) to the longitudinal data from the Berlin Aging Study, Ghisletta and Lindenberger (2003) demonstrated that aging-related declines in the pragmatic knowledge of intelligence (indexed by culture-based verbal knowl-

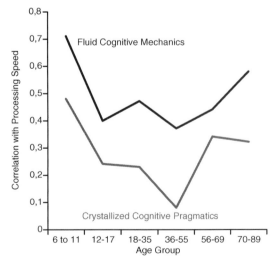

FIGURE 21.4. Stronger correlation between basic information-processing speed and two facts of intellectual abilities in childhood and old age than in adulthood. Adapted from Li et al. (2004). Copyright 2004 by Blackwell. Adapted by permission.

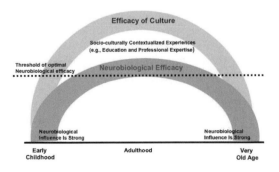

FIGURE 21.3. Schematic representation of the relative contributions of neurobiological constraints and sociocultural contextualized experiences on individual differences across the lifespan.

edge) are correlated with changes in the cognitive mechanics (indexed basic cognitive processing speed), with the cognitive mechanics being the leading factor. This suggests that, in old age, neurobiological correlates of declining basic information-processing speed constrain the expression of socioculturally acquired knowledge.

CROSS-LEVEL RECIPROCAL INTERACTIONS OF DEVELOPMENTAL PLASTICITY

Parallel to the concept of lifespan variations in the relative contributions of biology and culture to development, a related more recent framework focuses on the reciprocal interactions of developmental plasticity across levels (Li, 2003). As schematically shown in Figure 21.5, an integral whole of biocultural influences on lifespan brain and behavioral development can be implemented through reciprocal interactive processes and developmental plasticity that are simultaneously embedded within three timescales (i.e., phylogenetic, ontogenetic, and microgenetic times) encompassing multiple levels (i.e., sociocultural, behavioral, cognitive, neurobiological, and genetic). Individual ontogeny throughout life in this framework is considered as a dynamic process that is cumulatively traced out by moment-to-moment experiences and activities taking place through reciprocal interactions across the behavioral, cognitive, and neurobiological levels on the microgenetic timescale. These moment-to-moment microgenetic events are couched within (1) the proximal developmental context involving culturally embedded social interactions and situations on the lifespan ontogenetic timescale and (2) the distal context of culture–gene coevolution occurring on the long-term phylogenetic timescale.

More specifically, the framework of cross-level dynamic biocultural co-constructivism particularly highlights the reciprocal influences between interactive processes and developmental plasticity at different levels occurring on different timescales. This is depicted in Figure 21.5 by the dynamic joining of the feed-downward and feed-upward processes across the different levels and timescales, thus generating an integral whole of biocultural co-

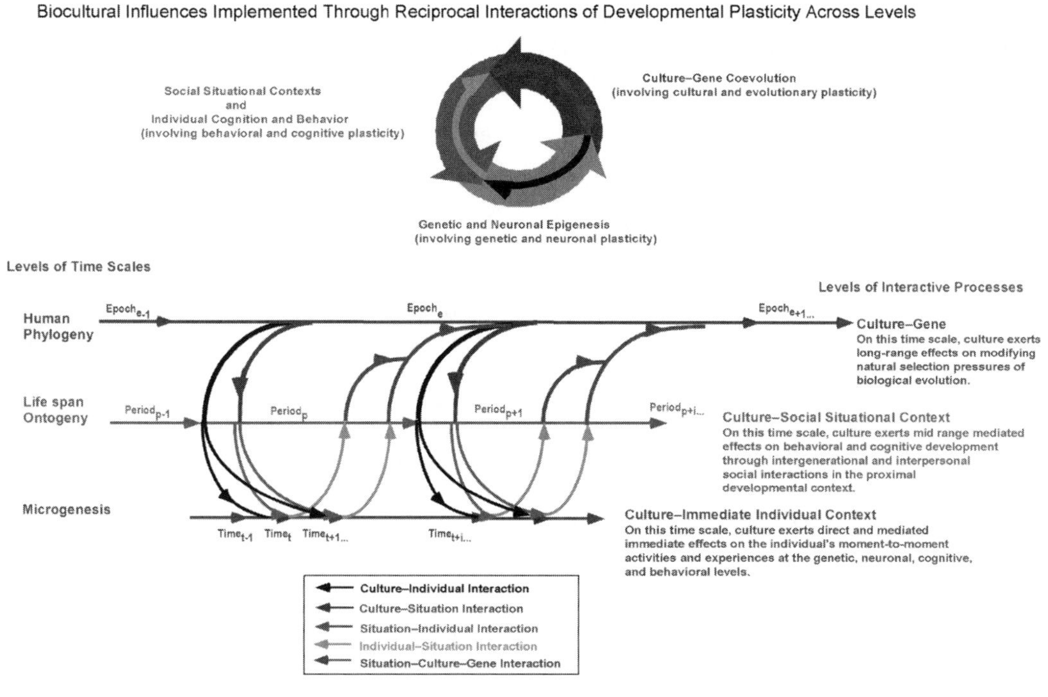

FIGURE 21.5. Schematic representation of biocultural co-construction of developmental plasticity across levels. Adapted from Li (2003). Copyright 2003 by the American Psychological Association. Adapted by permission.

constructive influences on human development. Feed-downward influences denote cultural factors arising from human phylogeny affecting individual moment-to-moment experiences at the behavioral, cognitive, and neurobiological levels. Feed-upward influences represent neurobiologically implemented individual cognition and behavior that contribute to collective social dynamics and cultural change.

Regarding feed-downward influences, *culture–individual interaction* highlights the direct influences of culture on behavior and cognition through the individual's firsthand personal experiences with the physical or formal properties of culture-specific artifacts and symbolic tools evolved over the human phylogenetic time. The phonological and orthographical properties of languages are examples of formal characteristics of culture-specific linguistic environments affecting the perceptual and neuronal aspects of language processing on the timescale of moment-to-moment activities. Other than directly influencing the individual, culture may first shape the social contexts and daily situations within which individual development takes place through *culture–situation interaction*. Culture-specific social customs, values, and concepts about the individual's identity are some examples. Through *situation–individual interaction*, the influences of culturally embedded social interactions (e.g., parent–child interaction, schooling, and peer interactions) mediate cultural impacts on the individual's moment-to-moment experiences. As for feed-upward influences, processes of cultural changes involve *individual–situation interaction* that cumulatively integrates moment-to-moment experiences at the genetic, neuronal, cognitive, and behavioral levels into an individual's ontogenetic history. Subsequently, processes of collective social dynamics played out in the individual ontogenetic histories of a society's members generate further culture–gene coevolution (Durham, 1991).

Contrary to the nativist view of innate and encapsulated genetic and neurobiological processes, across various subfields of life and developmental sciences there is a clear, reemerging zeitgeist of co-constructive conceptions that are accompanied by much recent empirical support for developmental plasticity at different levels. The remaining sections of this chapter review empirical evidence of developmental plasticity at different levels and examples of biocultural co-construction to illustrate these mechanisms.

Evolutionary Plasticity

It has recently been argued both on empirical and theoretical grounds that genetic programs and brain organizations reflect the sociocultural basis of evolution. The conventional coevolutionary theory has been extended by postulating a set of mediating mechanisms called "niche construction" to relate biological evolution and cultural changes to each other (Laland, Odling-Smee, & Feldman, 2000). Central to the concept of niche construction is the capacity of organisms and individuals to modify and construct the sources of natural selection in their environment via (1) learning and experience-dependent processes during individual ontogeny, and (2) processes of cultural change on another scale. For instance, the dairy farming culture selects for adult lactose tolerance and leads to populations in dairy farming societies with a higher percentage (i.e., more than 90%) of lactose absorbers in comparison to the percentage of lactose absorbers (i.e., less than 20%) in societies without dairy faming (Aoki, 1986; Feldman & Cavalli-Sforza, 1989).

A more recent study found evidence in support of a gene–culture coevolution between cattle milk protein genes and human lactase genes. The geographic patterns of variation in genes encoding the most important milk proteins in 70 native European cattle breeds showed substantial geographic coincidence with present-day lactose tolerance in Europeans. The diversity in cattle milk genes is higher in north-central Europe than in southern Europe and the Near East, and, correspondingly, lactose tolerance is higher in northern Europeans (Beja-Pereira et al., 2003).

Behavioral and Cognitive Plasticity

As for developmental plasticity at the behavioral and cognitive levels, various theories in the field of developmental psychology have emphasized the malleability of behavior and cognition by contextualized experiential factors (see Collins, Maccoby, Steinberg, Hetherington, & Bornstein, 2000). For instance, Vygotsky (1978) had already emphasized the role of social interactions in proximal developmental contexts, such as parent–child relations, peer relations, and schooling in promoting an individual's attained level of development toward a higher level of potential. More recently, sociocultural contextual approaches (e.g., Cole, 1999; Gauvain, 1995) have focused more specifically on cultural influences affecting these social interactions and their subsequent mediated effects on individual development. In a related but different vein, rather than focusing on cultural influences at a higher level, the relationship contextual approach (e.g., Reis, Collins, & Berscheid, 2000) examines fine-grained details (e.g., emotional and cognitive aspects) of different types of interpersonal relationships and their impact on child development. Still others focus on the linguistic environment as a main facet of culture-specific social interactions in an individual's proximal developmental context (e.g., K. Nelson, 1996). Cross-cultural studies on parenting style (Bornstein, Tal, & Tamis-LeMonda, 1991) found that differential emphases on interpersonal versus object orientation that were mediated through parent–child interactions in the Japanese and American cultures, respectively, affected the types of games and languages at which toddlers performed well in these two societies.

At the cognitive level, a series of recent cross-culture studies have demonstrated that different cultures foster different cognitive styles that, in turn, may affect the basic perceptual, cognitive (e.g., Kitayama, Duffy, Kawamura, & Larsen, 2003; Nisbett, Peng, Choi, & Norenzayan, 2001), and social attributional (Miyamoto & Kitayama, 2002) processes. As for cognitive plasticity across the lifespan, memory-training studies showed that older adults (ages 60–80) still displayed a fair amount of cognitive plasticity in improving their memory performance after training (Baltes & Kliegl, 1992) and that in very old age (i.e., age 80 years and older), marginal cognitive plasticity was still preserved (Singer, Lindenberger, & Baltes, 2003). However, the relative extent of cognitive plasticity was much more limited in old adults, in comparison both to young adults and to children. In a lifespan study of memory plasticity, Brehmer, Li, Müller, van Oertzen, and Lindenberger (in press) observed that the amount of memory performance gain after extensive memory training was highest in young adults (20–25 years), followed by school-age children (9–12 years), then older adults (65–78 years).

Neural and Genetic Plasticity

At the neuronal level of analysis in the field of neurobiology, behavior- and experience-dependent neuronal plasticity have attracted much research attention since Hebb's (1949) proposal of associative synaptic strengthening (i.e., the concept and later discovered phenomenon—neurons that fire frequently together wire together). For instance, it has been demonstrated that the brains of rats reared in environments affording broader ranges of experiences also show more complex synaptic structure with more synapses per neuron, than rats reared in less stimulating environment (e.g., Greenough & Black, 1992; for review, see Grossman, Churchill, Bates, Kleim, & Greenough, 2002; Rosenzweig, 1996). In humans, it was demonstrated that the overall cortical gyral patterns (patterns of brain gyral/sulcal relationship), though in part affected by genes (e.g., Pennington et al., 2000), may also be influenced by experiential factors (Bartley, Jones, & Weinberger, 1997). Another example involves the amygdala, a brain region very much implicated in social-cognitive developmental disorders (e.g., autism) and sometimes referred to as the "innate module" of social cognition (Baron-Cohen, 1995). Contrary to the innate notion, although the amygdala develops relatively early in human gestation (i.e., embryonic days 30–50), its separate nuclei do not start to differentiate until after birth, suggesting plasticity in the amygdala's responses to experiential influences (Kordower, Piecinski, & Rakic, 1992). Building on such evidence, some researchers have proposed concepts such as "neural constructivism" (Quartz & Sejnowski, 1997) or experience-induced neural plasticity (C. A. Nelson, 1999) to consider representational features of the synaptic connections as built from dynamic interactions between neural growth mechanisms, on the one hand, and experience-derived neural activity on the other.

Regarding developmental plasticity at the genetic level, there is a recent shift from the traditional view of unidirectional gene → protein information flow (Crick, 1958) to a probabilistic-epigenetic framework (Gottlieb, 1998). The key concept of this framework is bidirectional interactions among genes, neuronal activity, behavior, and environment. Environmental and experiential influences on genetic activities and expressions have been found in various studies (see review in Gottlieb,

1998). Of particularly interest here is the finding of maternal style modulating genetic effects on the offspring's reactions to stressors. Genetically highly reactive rhesus monkey infants raised by especially nurturant females exhibited much less deficit in early exploration and less accentuated responses to mild stressors than were otherwise typical for genetically highly reactive infants raised by normal or highly reactive females (Suomi, 1999).

Cortical Plasticity across the Lifespan

One important but less emphasized aspect of the evidence on plasticity is that neural plasticity occurs even after maturation, beyond infancy and early childhood (see C. A. Nelson, 2000, for review). Regarding plasticity during early development, accumulating data suggest that the functional specialization of the neocortex is established through subsequent epigenetic interactions with the immediate experiential context (Changeux, 1985; Edelman, 1987; Johnson, 2001; Kolb & Whishaw, 1998). Thus, experiential influences leave traces in developing brains capturing developmental effects that accumulate through the individual's moment-to-moment activities and experiences. For instance, it has been demonstrated that face processing is less localized or specialized (i.e., not as differentiated) in infants than in adults. In infants, face processing involves both left and right ventral visual pathways, whereas in adults, face processing primarily involves the right ventral visual pathway. Whereas adult brain activity shows specific sensitivity to upright human faces, no such sensitivity for face orientation is observed in young infants (de Haan, Pascalis, & Johnson, 2002).

Regarding plasticity after maturation, there is also increasing evidence for cortical and cognitive plasticity extending beyond the developing brain to other periods of the lifespan. Many recent data show that the adult brain can also adaptively change its structural and functional organization in response to accumulated developmental history reflecting daily experiences and aging. For instance, Maguire et al. (2000) found that the brain region involved in storing spatial representation of the environment (i.e., posterior hippocampi) of adults who had extensive spatial navigation experience (i.e., taxi drivers who navigate in big cities) was significantly larger in comparison to age controls. As

for functional plasticity during aging, a series of recent neuroimaging data found evidence for reorganization of cortical functions in old age. In comparison to the more clearly lateralized cortical information processing in young adults, people in their 60s and beyond showed bilateralized (bihemispheric) activity during memory retrieval (e.g., Cabeza, 2002; Cabeza et al., 1997) and during both verbal and spatial working memory processing (e.g., Reuter-Lorenz et al., 2000). It has been suggested that these data might indicate that the aging brain could "recruit" cortical areas in both hemispheres to compensate for neurocognitive declines during aging. Regarding structural plasticity in old age, recently neuroscience's century-old dogma that there is no addition of new neurons in the adult mammalian brain has also been revised. There is now evidence that increased environmental complexity stimulates the growth of new hippocampal neurons (i.e., neurogenesis) in the adult brains of various species, such as birds, rats, and humans (see Gross, 2000, for a review). Data also indicate that physical exercise training that increases aerobic fitness reduces aging-related loss in gray and white matter density (Colcombe et al., 2003).

In summary, sociocultural influences could have effects on the brain's structural and functional organization through early experiential "tuning" of synaptic connections and functional circuitry. In addition, though less flexible than in the early part of development, there is still marked cortical plasticity throughout most of the adult lifespan, both in terms of structural and functional plasticity. This opens up possibilities for cultural and experiential influences to be intimately integrated into the individual's cumulative developmental history, reflecting lifelong adaptations both to ongoing life experiences couched in the respective sociocultural context and to lifespan developmental change in the efficacy and integrity of the brain itself.

EXAMPLES OF BIOCULTURAL CO-CONSTRUCTION

Because the interdisciplinary research on biocultural co-construction of lifespan neurocognitive development is still in a very early developing stage, available studies are limited. Nevertheless, three sets of selective findings reviewed in this section demonstrate, particularly, the reciprocal influences of social contexts, culture-specific language environment, and expertise training.

Coevolution of Social Group Size, Language, and Brain

Focusing predominantly on the human phylogenetic scale, Dunbar (1993, 2003) showed that group size covaries with relative neocortical volume in nonhuman primates. This led to the proposal that the brain's encephalization is not driven by the cognitive demands of toolmaking, but by an intricate coevolving process between the growth in brain size and the need to manage increasing social bonding complexity associated with larger social group size. More recent data comparing the complexity of social structure in New World and Old World monkeys, in part, also supported this proposal. D. A. Clark, Mitra, and Wang (2001) found that the neocortical volume of Old World monkeys, as well as some orders of New World monkeys with more complex social structure resembling that of Old World monkeys, is larger than that of New World monkeys with less complex social structure. Furthermore, based on a similar percentage of daily time (20%) spent for social grooming in primate and social interactions in modern human populations, Dunbar (1993) also argued that language evolved to be a more efficient way for humans to deal with the increased social complexity associated with the larger human group size in comparison to that of the primates. The use of language as a communication medium further requires humans to evolve and develop competency in understanding and inferring the intentions of others (i.e., theory of mind; Baron-Cohen, 1995). The subsequent effect on the level of individual ontogeny, in turn, was for language to become part of the socially inherited, species-specific cultural resources for different societies to support individuals' interactions with each other and with the environment. Indeed, the linguistic relativity theory (Saunders & van Brakel, 1997; Whorf, 1956) contends that human understanding of the world is, in part, constructed through language.

Brain encephalization is also correlated with the extended juvenile periods in primates and humans (Joffe, 1997). It has been suggested that this relation may also arise from selection pressures associated with complex social dynamics, because young individuals of species

with more complex social structure need more efficient communication skills to manage more intricate social interactions. The acquisition of sophisticated communication skills, in turn, may benefit from an extended juvenile period during which the individual not only learns elaborate means of communication but also develops more fully proficiency in interpreting the behavior and intention of other species members (Bjorklund & Pellegrini, 2000). The extended juvenile period in humans, in turn, allows an extended amount of time and opportunities for intergenerational social interactions, operating in conjunction with language and other cultural resources, to influence brain and cognitive development.

Co-Construction of Cultural Knowledge and Cognitive and Neural Plasticity

Language is perhaps the most ubiquitous, pragmatic daily skill that individuals of a given sociocultural group acquire through socialization. Literally, the daily contexts of *Homo sapiens*, are overlaid by the linguistic environments in which we are either at home (i.e., mother language context) or in which we find ourselves (e.g., foreign language contexts). The specific features of different languages contribute to fine differentiations between different linguistic environments. A language-specific linguistic environment affects the development of language processes through formal (e.g., phonology, orthography, and verb morphology) or social-interactive (e.g., parental speech) aspects of language. For instance, infants show better generalizations to phonetic variants around the prototypes contained in their native languages, a phenomenon known as the "perceptual magnet effect" (Kuhl, Williams, Lacerda, Stevens, & Lindblom, 1992). Culture-specific language differences may also influence parental speech and subsequently affect patterns of semantic and cognitive development. For instance, the English and Korean languages differ in their verb morphology, among other things. English has a highly analytic structure, with relative little reliance on morphological variations. Nouns are generally obligatory in English sentences, and it is rare to construct sentences consisting of only an inflected verb, without nouns or pronouns. English-speaking parents thus focus heavily on object naming in conversations with their children. In contrast, the Korean language has rich verb morphology, with different verb endings marking important semantic distinctions. Thus Korean parental speech often consists of highly inflected verbs with few nouns. It has been suggested that differences in verb morphology between Korean and English may contribute to the developmental pattern of Korean children acquiring verbs that are relevant to the concepts of planning first, and nouns relevant for object categorization second, whereas the order of the developmental pattern is reversed in American children (Gopnik, Choi, & Baumberger, 1996).

Language acquisition at the behavioral level may have major implications for the functional architecture of the brain. Recent cognitive neuroscience findings indicate a dynamic shift in cortical organization over the course of language acquisition during childhood (see Neville et al., 1998, for a review). Similarly, the progressive developmental history of learning and using languages of different orthographical complexity throughout adult life leaves its trace at the cortical level. For instance, in comparison to the Italian language, English orthography is rather inconsistent, with complicated mappings of letters to sounds. Paulesu et al. (2000) recently found that Italian readers showed greater activation in the left superior temporal regions associated with phoneme processing, whereas English readers showed greater activations, particularly for nonwords, in the left posterior inferior temporal gyrus and anterior frontal gyrus, areas associated with word retrieval during both reading and naming tasks. These data suggest that acquiring the rather complex orthographical mapping of the English language impels English readers to invoke additional neurocognitive mechanisms involving word retrieval from semantic memory while reading.

Co-Construction of Person-Specific Expertise and Cognitive and Neural Plasticity

Throughout, it is emphasized that cognitive development across the lifespan has an ever increasingly strong component of individualization that likely cannot be entirely captured by individual differences in basic information-processing mechanisms and their neurobiological substrates. The case of individual differences in experiences and life histories reflecting socioculturally structured contextual influence can perhaps be best illustrated with respect to

occupational contexts. Different types of occupations engender, for instance, job-related stimulus and demand characteristics of varying complexity in individuals' daily job contexts and related experience-based outcomes. At the behavioral level, longitudinal studies have demonstrated reciprocal effects between the complexity of the occupational contexts and intellectual functioning in older adults (e.g., Schooler, Mulatu, & Oates, 1999; Schooler & Mulatu, 2004).

Another naturalistic setting for considering person-specific sociocultural influences on lifespan cognition is bilingualism (or multilingualism in general). As mentioned earlier, language is a representative aspect of general pragmatic knowledge that individuals of a given sociocultural group acquire. However, individuals may differ in their language expertise in terms of whether they need to master more than one language for their daily functioning. Child developmental and aging research have shown that the daily experience of processing two or more languages is associated with bilingual individuals' advantage in executive control functions that were measured by working memory or inhibition tasks (Bialystok, 2001; Bialystok, Craik, Klein, & Viswanathan, 2004).

Other than understanding the influences of sociocultural context on cognitive plasticity in natural settings, cognitive intervention studies reveal cognitive plasticity in individuals, even individuals in old age (see Kramer & Willis, 2002, for a review; Baltes & Lindenberger, 1988). Such research has primarily two goals. The first is to understand processes that underlie cognitive performance and its ontogeny. The second is to explore the range of what is possible in principle. In terms of memory plasticity in old age, memory training studies employing the testing-the-limit paradigm (an experimental paradigm that accesses individuals' current performance and maximum performance after extensive training) showed that older adults (from about 60 to 80 years) still displayed a fair level of cognitive plasticity and improved their associative memory by learning a culture-based mnemonic technique (i.e., the method of loci; Baltes & Kliegl, 1992). This technique is among the oldest mnemonic devices that was originated with the ancient Greeks around 500 B.C. When applying this mnemonic, the individuals learn to associate parts of the to-be-remembered material with different locations in a familiar place, in the order that the materials need to be recalled later. This method helps to improve memory for associations between memory events by linking them with the order of locations in the already familiar environment (see Bower, 1970, for classical review).

Aside from the demonstration of performance enhancement by acquiring special skills, these studies exemplify how training research using the testing-the-limit paradigm explores constraints on the zone (range) of potential development (Baltes, 1997). Thus, not unlike contemporary work in childhood, the focus is on maximum limits. Despite the continued plasticity in older ages, it could be shown that the cognitive plasticity of older individuals in the fourth age (i.e., 80 years and older) is markedly reduced in comparison to young adults (Singer et al., 2003). Extending the testing-the-limit memory training across the lifespan, the evidence shows that young children around 10 years of age have greater developmental reserve plasticity than older adults around 70 years of age (Brehmer et al., 2004).

In a way, expertise acquisition can be considered as long-term "testing-the-limit" type of training implemented in the natural settings of individuals' daily experiences. Expert performance is the result of intense practice extended for at least a minimum of 10 years for most domains of skills (Ericsson, Krampe, & Tesch-Römer, 1993). In the domain of music expertise, empirical evidence suggest that the long-term extended daily practice of older expert pianists helps to maintain their elite performance, in spite of age-related decline in basic cognitive processes (Krampe & Ericsson, 1996). There is also evidence that long-term acquisition of expertise leads to experience-induced cortical functional reorganization, in addition to behavioral changes. For instance, Elbert, Pantev, Wienbruch, Rockstroh, and Taub (1995) found that cortical representations of the fingers of the left hands of string players were larger than those of the right hand holding the bow, and this was particularly true for individuals who started playing the instrument early in life. Outside the domain of music, Maguire et al. (2000) found that given their extensive navigation experience, London taxi drivers' posterior hippocampi, a region of the brain involved in storing spatial representation of the environment, were significantly larger in comparison to same-age individuals who did not have as much navigation experience. Furthermore, when comparing drivers, the number of years spent as a taxi driver correlated positively with hippocampal volume. These data indicate that the adult brain still possesses functional plasticity, allowing the posterior hippocampus to expand to accommodate elaboration of environmental spatial representation in individuals who rely heavily on their navigation skills and have achieved a high level of navigation expertise in a particular environment.

CONCLUDING REMARKS

Admittedly, findings regarding sociocultural influences on lifespan neurocognitive development are still very limited and leave many gaps between the different levels of analyses at the current stage. Nevertheless, the fact that there are emerging co-constructive views and empirical evidence of developmental plasticity at various levels, as reviewed in this chapter, indicates that at least the possibilities for bridging these gaps are gradually on the rise.

Given neural plasticity that responds to lifespan developmental changes in the integrity of the brain itself, as well as lifelong adaptations to ongoing life experiences couched in the individual's own respective sociocultural context, future research needs to focus less on the commonly used localization approach to study neurocognitive processes, mainly by analyzing regional activation differences as a function of task conditions. Instead, lifespan changes and individual differences in brain–behavior mapping need to be considered more explicitly (Li & Lindenberger, 2002). For instance, instead of assuming that cortical regions and circuitry associated with particular functionalities in normal adult are very similar, if not identical, to those in developing children or old adults, lifespan changes in brain–behavior mapping need to be investigated and taken into account (e.g., Cabeza, 2002; Grady, McIntosh, & Craik, 2003; Karmiloff-Smith, 1998; Reuter-Lorenz, 2002; Schlaggar et al., 2002).

The biocultural co-constructive and adaptive nature of cognitive development cautions against an immediate interpretation of age differences in cognitive operations as solely driven by the growth and decline of basic information-processing mechanisms and their associated neurobiological mechanisms. The biocultural co-construction framework highlights lifespan variations in the relative contributions of biology and culture to cognitive functioning. In early cognitive development, idiosyncratic person-specific experiences tend to play a lesser role relative to contributions of species-typical neurobiological and age-normative sociocultural factors. In subsequent phases of lifespan development, however, life-history-specific influences may be more significant for understanding adult cognitive development and aging. In old age, because of the pervasiveness of biological decline, processes of greater generality are likely to reenter the system as powerful regulating forces of the developmental trajectories. Evidence reviewed in this chapter provides initial support for these propositions. Further empirical verifications will require combined age- and culture-comparative, cross-level designs that examine basic cognitive and neuronal processes in well-controlled laboratory settings, as well as studies of cognition in everyday functioning using ecologically valid tasks that reflect sociocultural specificities (e.g., Gopnik et al., 1996; Kelly, Miller, Fang, & Fang, 1999; Kitayama et al., 2003; Nisbett et al., 2001; Park, Nisbett, & Hedden, 1999; Paulesu et al., 2000; Snibbe, Kitayama, Markus, & Suzuki, 2003).

In conclusion, the existing empirical evidence of developmental plasticity at different levels presents a warning against the "pure reductionist approach" to the genetic and neuronal bases of mind and behavior that ignores the influences from cultural, experiential, and cumulative developmental contexts. The reason is clear: Genetic activities and neural mechanisms themselves possess remarkable plasticity awaiting sociocultural contexts to exert reciprocal influences on them and to be the "coauthors" of mind and behavior. People are more than mere biological organisms; human mind and behavior need to be understood in the proper context within a brain, in a body that lives in an eventful world abounding with objects and people. Indeed, the brain offers the necessary biophysical reality for individual cognition and action; it alone, however, is not sufficient to engender the mind or behavior. On the mind–brain continuum, the individual mind is the expression emerging from the personalized brain (Greenfield, 2000; Llinas & Churchland, 1996). The very processes for personalizing the biological faculty of the mind take place throughout lifespan development in environmental and sociocultural contexts, which entail intimate dynamical exchanges between nature and nurture, biology and culture.

REFERENCES

Alexander, T. (1969). *Children and adolescents: A biocultural approach to psychological development.* New York: Atherton Press.

Anastasi, A. (1958). Heredity, environment, and the question "How?" *Psychological Review, 65,* 197–208.

Aoki, K. (1986). A stochastic model of gene–culture co-evolution suggested by the "culture historical hypothesis" for the evolution of adult lactose absorption in humans. *Proceedings of the National Academy of Sciences USA, 83,* 2929–2933.

Balinsky, B. (1941). An analysis of the mental factors of various groups from mine to sixty. *Genetic Psychology Monographs, 23,* 191–234.

Baltes, P. B. (1979). Life-span developmental psychology: Some converging observations in history and theory. In P. B. Baltes & O. G. Brim (Eds.), *Life-span development and behavior* (pp. 255–279). New York: Academic Press.

Baltes, P. B. (1997). On the incomplete nature of human ontogeny: Selection, optimization, and compensation as foundation of developmental theory. *American Psychologist, 52,* 366–380.

Baltes, P. B., Cornelius, S. W., Spiro, A., Nesselroade, J. R., & Willis, S. L. (1980). Integration versus differentiation of fluid/crystallized intelligence in old age. *Developmental Psychology, 6,* 625–635.

Baltes, P. B., & Kliegl, R. (1992). Further testing of the limits of cognitive plasticity: Negative age differences in a mnemonic skill are robust. *Developmental Psychology, 28,* 121–125.

Baltes, P. B., & Lindenberger, U. (1988). On the range of cognitive plasticity in old age as a function of experience: 15 years of intervention research. *Behavior Therapy, 19,* 283–300.

Baltes, P. B., Lindenberger, U., & Staudinger, U. M. (1998). Life-span theory in developmental psychology. In W. Damon (Editor-in-Chief) & R. M. Lerner (Ed.), *Handbook of child psychology: Vol. 1. Theoretical models of human development* (pp. 1029–1041). New York: Wiley.

Baltes, P. B., Rösler, F., & Reuter-Lorenz, P. (2006). *Brain, mind, and culture: From interactionism to biocultural co-constructivism.* Cambridge University Press.

Baltes, P. B., & Singer, T. (2001). Plasticity and the aging mind: An exemplar of the biocultural orchestration of brain and behavior. *European Review, 9,* 59–76.

Baltes, P. B., & Smith, J. (2004). Lifespan psychology: From developmental contextualism to developmental biocultural co-constructivism. *Research on Human Development, 1,* 123–144.

Baltes, P. B., & Staudinger, U. M. (1996). *Interactive minds: Lifespan perspectives on the social foundation of cognition.* Cambridge, UK: Cambridge University Press.

Baron-Cohen, S. (1995). *Mindblindness: An essay on autism and theory of mind.* Cambridge, MA: MIT Press.

Bartley, A. J., Jones, D. W., & Weinberger, D. R. (1997). Genetic variability of human brain size and cortical gyral patterns. *Brain, 120,* 257–269.

Beja-Pereira, A., Luikart, G., England, P. R., Bradley, D. G., Jann, O. C., Bertorelle, G., et al. (2003). Gene-culture coevolution between cattle milk protein genes and human lactase genes. *Nature Genetics, 35,* 311–313.

Berger, P. L., & Luckmann, T. (1967). *The social construction of reality.* New York: Anchor-Doubleday.

Bialystok, E. (2001). *Bilingualism in development: Language, literacy, and cognition.* New York: Cambridge University Press.

Bialystok, E., Craik, F. I. M., Klein, R., & Viswanathan, M. (2004). Bilingualism, aging, and cognitive control: Evidence from the Simon task. *Psychology and Aging, 19,* 290–303.

Bjorklund, D. F., & Pellegrini, A. D. (2000). Child development and evolutionary psychology. *Child Development, 71,* 1687–1708.

Bornstein, M. H., Tal, J., & Tamis-LeMonda, C. S. (1991). Parenting in crosscultural perspective: The United States, France, and Japan. In M. H. Bornstein (Ed.), *Cultural approaches to parenting* (pp. 69–90). Hillsdale, NJ: Erlbaum.

Bower, G. H. (1970). Analysis of a mnemonic device. *American Scientist, 58,* 496–510.

Brehmer, Y., Li, S.-C., Müller, V., van Oertzen, T., & Lindenberger, U. (in press). Memory plasticity across the life span: Uncovering children's latent potential. *Developmental Psychology.*

Bronfenbrenner, U. (1979). *The ecology of human development.* Cambridge, MA: Harvard University Press.

Bronfenbrenner, U., & Ceci, S. J. (1994). Nature–nurture reconceptualized in developmental perspective: A bioecological model. *Psychological Review, 101,* 568–586.

Cabeza, R. (2002). Hemispheric asymmetry reduction in older adults: The Harold model. *Psychology and Aging, 17,* 85–100.

Cabeza, R., Grady, C. L., Nyberg, L., McIntosh, A. R., Tulving, E., Kapur, S., et al. (1997). Age-related differences in effective neural connectivity. *NeuroReport, 8,* 3479–3483.

Cattell, R. B. (1971). *Abilities: Their structure, growth and action.* Boston: Houghton Mifflin.

Changeux, J.-P. (1985). *Neuronal man.* New York: Oxford University Press.

Clark, A. (1999). An embodied cognitive science? *Trends in Cognitive Sciences, 3,* 345–351.

Clark, D. A., Mitra, P. P., & Wang, S. S. H. (2001). Scalable architecture in mammalian brains. *Nature, 411,* 189–193.

Colcombe, S. J., Erickson, K.-I., Raz, N., Webb, A. G., Cohen, N. J., McAuley, E., et al. (2003). Aerobic fitness reduces brain tissue loss in aging humans. *Journals of Gerontology, 58A,* M176–M180.

Cole, M. (1999). Culture in development. In M. H. Bornstein & M. E. Lamb (Eds.), *Developmental psychology: An advanced textbook* (pp. 73–123). Mahwah, NJ: Erlbaum.

Collins, W. A., Maccoby, E. E., Steinberg, L., Hetherington, E. M., & Bornstein, M. H. (2000). Contemporary research on parenting: The case for nature and nurture. *American Psychologist, 55,* 218–232.

Crick, F. H. C. (1958). On protein synthesis. In *Symposia of the Society for Experimental Biology: Vol. 12. The biological replication of macromolecules* (pp. 138–163). Cambridge, UK: Cambridge University Press.

D'Andrade, R. (1996). Culture. In A. Kuper & J. Kuper (Eds.), *Social science encyclopedia* (2nd ed., pp. 161–163). London: Routledge.

de Haan, M., Pascalis, O., & Johnson, M. H. (2002). Specialization of neural mechanisms underlying face recognition in human infants. *Journal of Cognitive Neuroscience, 14,* 199–209.

Dunbar, R. I. M. (1993). Co-evolution of neocortical size, group size, and language in humans. *Behavioral and Brain Sciences, 16,* 681–735.

Dunbar, R. I. M. (2003). The social brain: Mind, language, and society in evolutionary perspective. *Annual Review of Anthropology, 32,* 163–181.

Durham, W. H. (1991). *Coevolution: Gene, culture, and human diversity.* Stanford, CA: Stanford University Press.

Edelman, G. M. (1987). *Neural Darwinism: The theory of neuronal group selection.* New York: Basic Books.

Elbert, T., Pantev, C., Wienbruch, C., Rockstroh, B., & Taub, E. (1995). Increased cortical representation of the fingers of the left hand in string players. *Science, 270,* 305–307.

Ericsson, K. A., Krampe, R. T., & Tesch-Römer, K. (1993). The role of deliberate practice in the acquisition of expert performance. *Psychology Review, 100,* 363–406.

Feldman, M. W., & Cavalli-Sforza, L. L. (1989). On the theory of evolution under genetic and cultural transmission with application to the lactose absorption problem. In M. W. Feldmann (Ed.), *Mathematical evolutionary theory* (pp. 145–173). Princeton, NJ: Princeton University Press.

Garrett, H. E. (1946). A developmental theory of intelligence. *American Psychologist, 1,* 372–378.

Gauvain, M. (1995). Thinking in niches: Sociocultural influences on cognitive development. *Human Development, 38,* 24–45.

Gauvain, M. (1998). Cognitive development in social and cultural contexts. *Current Directions in Psychological Science, 7,* 188–192.

Geertz, C. (1973). *The interpretation of cultures.* New York: Basic Books.

Ghisletta, P., & Lindenberger, U. (2003). Age-based structural dynamics between perceptual speed and knowledge in the Berlin Aging Study: Direct evidence for abilities dedifferentiation in old age. *Psychology and Aging, 18,* 696–713.

Gopnik, A., Choi, S., & Baumberger, T. (1996). Cross-linguistic differences in early semantic and cognitive development. *Cognitive Development, 11,* 197–227.

Gottlieb, G. (1976). The roles of experience in the development of behavior and the nervous system. In G. Gottlieb (Ed.), *Neural and behavioral specificity* (pp. 25–54). New York: Academic Press.

Gottlieb, G. (1998). Normally occurring environmental and behavioral influences of gene activity: From central dogma to probabilistic epigenesis. *Psychological Review, 105,* 792–802.

Gottlieb, G. (2002). Developmental–behavioral initiation of evolutionary change. *Psychological Review, 109,* 211–218.

Grady, C. L., McIntosh, A. R., & Craik, F. I. M. (2003). Age-related differences in the functional connectivity of the hippocampus during memory encoding. *Hippocampus, 13,* 572–586.

Greenfield, S. (2000). *The private life of the brain.* New York: Penguin Press.

Greenough, W. T., & Black, J. E. (1992). Induction of brain structure by experience: Substrates for cognitive development. In M. R. Gunnar & C. A. Nelson (Eds.), *Minnesota Symposia on Child Psychology* (Vol. 24, pp. 155–200). Hillsdale, NJ: Erlbaum.

Gross, C. G. (2000). Neurogenesis in the adult brain: Death of a dogma. *Nature Reviews: Neuroscience, 1,* 67–73.

Grossman, A. W., Churchill, J. D., Bates, K. E., Kleim, J. A., & Greenough, W. T. (2002). A brain adaptation view of plasticity: is synaptic plasticity an overly limited concept? *Progress in Brain Research, 138,* 91–108.

Hatano, G., & Wertsch, J. V. (Eds.). (2001). Sociocultural approaches to cognitive development: The constitutions of culture in mind [Special issue]. *Human Development, 44.*

Hebb, D. O. (1949). *The organization of behavior.* New York: Wiley.

Herskovitz, M. J. (1948). *Man and his works: The science of cultural anthropology.* New York: Knopf.

Horn, J. L. (1968). Organization of abilities and the development of intelligence. *Psychological Review, 75,* 242–259.

Hutchins, E. (1995). *Cognition in the wild.* Cambridge, MA: MIT Press.

Ingold, T. (1998). From complementarity to obviation: On dissolving the boundaries between social and biological anthropology, archaeology and psychology. *Zeitschrift für Ethnologie, 123,* 21–52.

International Human Genome Sequencing Consortium. (2001). Initial sequencing and analyses of the human genome. *Nature, 409,* 860–921.

Joffe, T. H. (1997). Social pressures have selected for an extended juvenile period in primates. *Journal of Human Evolution, 32,* 593–605.

Johnson, M. H. (2001). Functional brain development in humans. *Nature Reviews: Neuroscience, 2,* 475–483.

Karmiloff-Smith, A. (1998). Development itself is the key to understanding developmental disorders. *Trends in Cognitive Sciences, 2,* 389–398.

Kelly, M. K., Miller, K, F., Fang, G., & Fang, G. (1999). When days are numbered: Calendar structure and the development of calendar processing in English and Chinese. *Journal of Experimental Child Psychology, 73,* 289–314.

King, B. J. (2000). Another frame shift: From cultural transmission to cultural co-construction. *Behavioral and Brain Sciences, 23,* 154–155.

Kitayama, S., Duffy, S., Kawamura, T., & Larsen, J. T. (2003). Perceiving an object and its context in different cultures: A cultural look at new look. *Psychological Science, 14,* 201–206.

Kolb, B., & Whishaw, I. Q. (1998). Brain plasticity and behavior. *Annual Review of Psychology, 49,* 43–64.

Kordower, J. H., Piecinski, P., & Rakic, P. (1992). Neurogenesis of the amygdala nuclear complex in the rhesus monkey. *Developmental Brain Research, 68,* 9–15.

Kramer, A. F. K., & Willis, S. L. (2002). Enhancing the cognitive vitality of older adults. *Current Directions of Psychological Sciences, 11,* 173–177.

Krampe, R. T., & Ericsson, K. A. (1996). Maintaining excellence: Deliberate practice and elite performance in young and older pianists. *Journal of Experimental Psychology: General, 125,* 331–359.

Kuhl, P. K., Williams, K. A., Lacerda, F., Stevens, K. N., & Lindblom, B. (1992). Linguistic experience alters phonetic perception in infants by 6 months of age. *Science, 255,* 606–608.

Laland, K. N., Odling-Smee, F. J., & Feldman, M. W. (2000). Niche construction, biological evolution, and cultural change. *Behavioral and Brain Sciences, 23,* 131–175.

Li, S.-C. (2003). Biocultural orchestration of developmental plasticity across levels: The interplay of biology and culture in shaping the mind and behavior across the life span. *Psychological Bulletin, 129,* 171–194.

Li, S.-C., & Freund, A. M. (2005). Advances in lifespan psychology: A focus on biocultural and personal influences. *Research in Human Development, 2,* 1–23.

Li, S.-C., & Lindenberger, U. (2002). Co-constructed functionality instead of functional normality: Dynamic biocultural co-construction of brain-behaviour mappings. *Behavioral and Brain Sciences, 25,* 761–762.

Li, S.-C., Lindenberger, U., Hommel, B., Aschersleben, G., Prinz, W., & Baltes, P. B. (2004). Transformations in the couplings among intellectual abilities and constituent cognitive processes across the life span. *Psychological Science, 15,* 155–163.

Llinas, R. R., & Churchland, P. S. (Eds.). (1996). *The mind–brain continuum: Sensory processes.* Cambridge, MA: MIT Press.

Magnusson, D. (1988). *Individual development from an interactional perspective: A longitudinal study.* Hillsdale, NJ: Erlbaum.

Magnusson, D. (Ed.). (1996). The lifespan development of individuals: Behavioral, neurobiological, and psychosocial perspectives: A Synthesis. Cambridge, UK: Cambridge University Press.

Maguire, E. A., Gadian, D. G., Johnsrude, I. S., Good, C. D., Ashburner, J., Frackowiak, R. S. J., et al. (2000). Navigation-related structural change in the hippocampi of taxi drivers. *Proceedings of the National Academy of Sciences of the USA, 97,* 4398–4403.

McArdle, J. J., Ferrer-Caja, E., Hamagami, F., & Woodcock, R. W. (2002). Comparative longitudinal structural analyses of the growth and decline of multiple intellectual abilities over the life span. *Developmental Psychology, 38,* 115–142.

Meaney, M. J. (2001). Nature, nurture, and the disunity of knowledge. *Annals of the New York Academy of Sciences, 935,* 50–61.

Mivart, G. J. (1871). *Genesis of species.* London: Macmillan.

Miyamoto, Y., & Kitayama, S. (2002). Cultural variation in correspondence bias: The critical role of attitude diagnosticity of socially constrained behavior. *Journal of Personality and Social Psychology, 83,* 1239–1248.

Nelson, C. A. (1999). Neural plasticity and human development. *Current Directions in Psychological Science, 8,* 42–45.

Nelson, C. A. (2000). Neural plasticity and human development: The role of early experience in sculpting memory systems. *Developmental Science, 3,* 115–136.

Nelson, K. (1996). *Language in cognitive development.* Cambridge, UK: Cambridge University Press.

Neville, H. J., Bavelier, D., Corina, D., Rauschecker, J., Karni, A., Lalwani, A., et al. (1998). Cerebral organization for language in deaf and hearing subjects: Biological constraints and effects of experience. *Proceedings of the National Academy of Sciences of the USA, 95,* 922–929.

Nisbett, R. E., Peng, K., Choi, I., & Norenzayan, A. (2001). Culture and systems of thought: Holistic versus analytic cognition. *Psychological Review, 108,* 291–310.

Park, D. C., Nisbett, R., & Hedden, T. (1999). Aging, culture, and cognition. *Journals of Gerontology: Series B, Psychological and Social Sciences, 54,* P75–P84.

Paulesu, E., McCrory, E., Fazio, F., Menoncello, L., Brunswick, N., Cappa, S. F., et al. (2000). A cultural effect on brain function. *Nature Neuroscience, 3,* 91–96.

Pennington, B. F., Filipek, P. A., Lefly, D., Chhabildas, N., Kennedy, D. N., Simon, J. H., et al. (2000). A twin MRI study of size variations in the human brain. *Journal of Cognitive Neuroscience, 12,* 223–232.

Quartz, S. R., & Sejnowski, T. J. (1997). The neural basis of cognitive development: A constructivist manifesto. *Behavioral and Brain Sciences, 20,* 537–596.

Reinert, G. (1970). Comparative factor analytic studies of intelligence throughout the life span. In L. R. Goulet & P. B. Baltes (Eds.), *Life-span developmental psychology: Research and theory* (pp. 476–484). New York: Academic Press.

Reis, H. T., Collins, W. A., & Berscheid, E. (2000). The relationship context of human behavior and development. *Psychological Bulletin, 126,* 844–872.

Rensberger, B. (1983). The nature–nurture debate, 1 & 2. *Science, 83,* 28–46.

Reuter-Lorenz, P. A. (2002). New visions of the aging mind and brain. *Trends in Cognitive Sciences, 6,* 394–400.

Reuter-Lorenz, P. A., Jonides, J., Smith, E., Marshuetz, C., Miller, A., Hartley, A., et al. (2000). Age differences in the frontal lateralization of verbal and spatial working memory revealed by PET. *Journal of Cognitive Neuroscience, 12,* 174–187.

Rosenzweig, M. R. (1996). Aspects of the search for neural mechanisms of memory. *Annual Review of Psychology, 47,* 1–32.

Saunders, B. A., & van Brakel, C. (1997). Are there nontrivial constraints on colour categorization? *Behavioral and Brain Sciences, 20,* 167–228.

Schaie, K. W. (1965). A general model for the study of developmental problems. *Psychological Bulletin, 64,* 92–107.

Schlaggar, B. L., Brown, T. T., Lugar, H. M., Visscher, K. M., Miezin, F. M., & Petersen, S. E. (2002). Functional neuroanatomical differences between adults and school-age children in the processing of single words. *Science, 296,* 1476–1479.

Schooler, C., & Mulatu, M. S. (2004). Occupational self-direction, intellectual functioning, and self-directed orientation in older workers: Findings and implications for individuals and societies. *American Journal of Sociology, 110,* 161–197.

Schooler, C., Mulatu, M. S., & Oates, G. (1999). The continuing effects of substantively complex work on the intellectual functioning of older workers. *Psychology and Aging, 14,* 483–506.

Searle, J. R. (1995). *The construction of social reality.* New York: Free Press.

Singer, T., Lindenberger, U., & Baltes, P. B. (2003). Plasticity of memory for new learning in very old age: A story of major loss? *Psychology & Aging, 18,* 306–318.

Snibbe, A. C., Kitayama, S., Markus, H. R., & Suzuki, T. (2003). They saw a game—a Japanese and American (football) field study. *Journal of Cross-Cultural Psychology, 34,* 581–595.

Suomi, S. (1999). Attachment in Rhesus monkeys. In J. Cassidy & P. R. Shaver (Ed.), *Handbook of attachment: Theory, research, and clinical applications* (pp. 181–197). New York: Guilford Press.

Super, C. M., & Harkness, S. (1986). The developmental niche: A conceptualization at the interface of child and culture. *International Journal of Behavioral Development, 9,* 545–569.

Tetens, J. N. (1777). *Philosophische Versuche über die menschliche Natur und ihre Entwicklung* [Philosophical experiments about human nature and its development]. Leipzig, Germany: Weidmanns Erben und Reich.

Tomasello, M. (1999). *The cultural origins of human cognition.* Cambridge, MA: Harvard University Press.

Tylor, E. B. (1874). Primitive culture: Researches into the development of mythology, philosophy, religion, language, art, and custom. London: Murray.

Venter, J. C. et al. (2001). The sequence of human genome. *Science, 291,* 1304–1351.

Vygotsky, L. S. (1978). *Mind in society.* Cambridge, MA: Harvard University Press.

Whorf, B. (1956). *Language, thought and reality.* Cambridge, MA: MIT Press.

Williams, R. (1973). *Keywords.* Oxford, UK: Oxford University Press.

PART V

COGNITION

CHAPTER 22

Intelligence and Culture

ROBERT J. STERNBERG

The study of culture and intelligence is based in part on the notion that behavior that in one cultural context is smart may be stupid in another cultural context (Cole, Gay, Glick, & Sharp, 1971; Sternberg, 2004a). Stating one's political views honestly and openly, for example, may win one the top political job, such as the presidency, in one culture, and the gallows in another.

One reason to study culture and intelligence is because they are so inextricably interlinked. Indeed, Tomasello (2001) has argued that culture is what, in large part, separates human from animal intelligence. Humans have evolved as they have, he believes, in part because of their cultural adaptations, which in turn develop even in infancy from about 9 months onward, from their ability to understand others as intentional agents.

The conceptualization, assessment, and development of intelligence cannot be fully or even meaningfully understood outside their cultural context. Work that seeks to study intelligence acontextually may impose an, often Western, investigator's view of the world on the rest of the world, frequently attempting to show that individuals who are more similar to the investigator are smarter than individuals who are less similar. Here, the term "Western" refers primarily to middle- to upper-middle-class North Americans and Western Europeans, so the term is used in a specific way, and not to refer to anyone who happens to live in the "West." For example, a test of intelligence developed and validated in one culture may or may not be equally valid, or even be valid at all, in another culture.

This chapter is divided into five parts. First, I define the main concepts of the chapter, *culture* and *intelligence*. Second, models of the relationship between culture and intelligence are specified. Third, the text introduces the chapter's ideas, including a description of some studies investigating various issues relating culture to intelligence. Fourth, I discuss cultural studies relevant to these ideas. Fifth, I consider whether "culture-fair" testing is possible, and finally, draw some conclusions.

WHAT IS CULTURE AND WHAT IS INTELLIGENCE?

Defining Culture

Because the topic of this chapter is culture and intelligence, it is necessary to define these constructs.

There have been many definitions of *culture* (e.g., Brislin, Lonner, & Thorndike, 1973; Kroeber & Kluckhohn, 1952), which is defined here as "the set of attitudes, values, beliefs and behaviors shared by a group of people, communicated form one generation to the next via language or some other means of communication (Barnouw, 1985)" (Matsumoto, 1994, p. 4). The term *culture* can be used in many ways and has a long history (Benedict, 1946; Boas, 1911; Mead, 1928; see Matsumoto, 1996). Berry, Poortinga, Segall, and Dasen (1992) described six uses of the term: descriptively to characterize a culture, historically to describe the traditions of a group, normatively to express rules and norms of a group, psychologically to emphasize how a group learns and solves problems, structurally to emphasize the organizational elements of a culture, and genetically to describe cultural origins.

Defining Intelligence

How is intelligence defined? Some psychologists, such as Edwin Boring (1923), have been content to define intelligence as whatever it is that tests of intelligence measure. This definition, unfortunately, is circular, because, according to it, the nature of intelligence determines what is tested, but what is tested must necessarily be determined by the nature of intelligence. Moreover, what different tests of intelligence test is not always the same thing. Different tests measure somewhat different constructs (Daniel, 1997, 2000; Embretson & McCollam, 2000; Kaufman, 2000; Kaufman & Lichtenberger, 1998), so it is not feasible to define intelligence by what tests test, as though they all measure the same thing.

Moreover, if intelligence were to turn out to be not quite the same thing from one culture to another, the definition would become totally vacuous, meaning as many different things as there are cultures. Tests, of course, can be translated. But what is to be translated? Obviously, a test of English vocabulary would not work well in Dholuo-speaking rural Kenya, such as in the town of Busia. So the words would, at least, need to be translated. But are the translated words that would be optimal on a test in English the same ones that would be optimal on a test in Dholuo? Are there even exact translations, given that the roots of the two languages are so different? Perhaps not. But then, is vocabulary for low-frequency words itself of equal importance to village residents in rural Busia, Kenya, and to residents of, say, Cambridge, Massachusetts? The residents of the town will probably never use any of those

complex words in their lives, and they may not even exist in their language. But to survive, those residents need to know how to farm under very difficult conditions, and a test of farming knowledge would be quite appropriate to them as a measure of their adaptive skills. Most of the readers of this chapter would have difficulty answering the farming vocabulary questions that would be relevant to their lives, even in translation. Boring's definition simply does not hold up well under close cultural scrutiny.

Historically, there are many different definitions of intelligence ("Intelligence and Its Measurement," 1921; Sternberg, 2000; Sternberg & Detterman, 1986). Over time, a consensus definition has tended to emphasize two important skills: adaptation to the environment and the ability to think and learn. In more recent times, a third component has been added to the definition, namely, understanding oneself and one's own skills, often referred to as *metacognition*. Broadly speaking, metacognition also includes theory of mind in general, or one's understanding of how other people's minds work as well. So a consensus of traditional definitions of *intelligence* is "the ability to adapt to the environment, to think and learn, and to understand oneself and others."

THEORIES OF INTELLIGENCE

Theories of intelligence are of two kinds: Explicit theories are proposed by investigators, and tested through and often suggested by empirical studies; implicit theories are folktheories—theories that people have in their heads.

Explicit theories and implicit theories are related in various ways. First, implicit theories of professionals serve as the bases for their explicit theories. Unfortunately, professionals, often unaware of this fact, so may not realize the extent to which their explicit theories are shaped and also limited by their implicit ones. Second, both kinds of theories are used in assessing intelligence. By far, more judgments are based on implicit theories—for example, judging candidates in job interviews, assessing acquaintances in casual encounters, evaluating partners in dating, evaluating potential business partners, and so forth. Third, laypeople and professionals alike tend to believe that implicit theories are somehow less "scientific" than explicit theories, although intelligence is in part a social construction, so it is not clear that implicit theories are less scientific. The science is in uncovering what they are. Finally, explicit theories are typically presented as being cross-culturally relevant, whereas such a claim is typically not made for implicit theories. But often tests of explicit theories across cultures assume rather than actually validate theories in the different cultures.

It may be that if Western norms and schooling spread across the world, then the explicit theories developed in the West will become more relevant around the world. But the trend toward Westernization is by no means the only trend in the world today. In much of the world, individuals are rebelling against what they see as an unwarranted and unwelcome encroachment of Westerners and Western values. So it is not clear just where things ultimately will go.

Explicit Theories of Intelligence

Conventional Psychometric Theories

Today, the most widely accepted traditional theories of intelligence are hierarchical ones. They build on the work of Charles Spearman (1904/1927), who proposed a factor of general intelligence (g), and of Louis Thurstone (1938), who proposed multiple factors of intelligence (verbal comprehension, number, verbal fluency, memory, perceptual speed, reasoning, spatial visualization). One such model, developed by Raymond Cattell (1971), proposed that general intelligence comprises two major subfactors: fluid ability (speed and accuracy of abstract reasoning, especially for novel problems) and crystallized ability (accumulated knowledge and vocabulary). Subsumed within these two major subfactors are other, more specific factors. A similar view was proposed by Philip E. Vernon (1969, 1971), who made a general division between practical–mechanical and verbal–educational abilities.

More recently, John B. Carroll (1993) proposed a hierarchical model of intelligence, based on his analysis of more than 460 data sets obtained between 1927 and 1987. His analysis encompasses more than 130,000 people from diverse walks of life and even countries of origin (although non-English-speaking countries are poorly represented among his data sets). The model Carroll proposed, based on his monumental undertaking, is a hierarchy

comprising three strata: Stratum I includes many narrow, specific abilities (e.g., spelling ability, speed of reasoning); Stratum II includes various broad abilities (e.g., fluid intelligence, crystallized intelligence); and Stratum III is just a single general intelligence, much like Spearman's g. Of these strata, the most interesting is Stratum II, which is neither too narrow nor too all-encompassing.

In addition to fluid intelligence and crystallized intelligence, Carroll includes in Stratum II learning and memory processes, visual perception, auditory perception, facile production of ideas (similar to verbal fluency), and speed (which includes both sheer speed of response and speed of accurate responding). Although Carroll does not break new ground, in that many of the abilities in his model have been mentioned in other theories, he does masterfully integrate a large and diverse factor-analytic literature, thereby giving great authority to his model. Whereas the factor-analytic approach has tended to emphasize the structures of intelligence, the information-processing approach has tended to emphasize the operations of intelligence.

Of course, there are many alternative theories of intelligence as well (Ceci, 1996; Spearman, 1904/1927; Thurstone, 1938), many of which are reviewed in Sternberg (1990, 2000). Consider just two of these.

Systems Theories

In recent times, some scholars have sought broader definitions of intelligence than was customary in the past. For example, Gardner (1983) does not believe in a single intelligence, but rather, in multiple intelligences. He has defined "multiple intelligences" as emanating from one's ability to work in multiple symbol systems, in particular, linguistic, logical–mathematical, spatial, musical, bodily-kinesthetic, naturalist, interpersonal, and intrapersonal. He has also speculated on the existence of an existential intelligence, which deals with broader questions of existence.

Each intelligence is a separate system of functioning. Nevertheless, these systems can interact to produce intelligent performance. For example, novelists rely heavily on linguistic intelligence but might use logical–mathematical intelligence in plotting story lines or checking for logical inconsistencies. Measuring intelligences separately may produce a profile of skills that is broader than would be obtained from, say, measuring verbal and mathematical abilities alone.

To identify particular intelligences, Gardner (1983) used converging operations, gathering evidence from multiple sources and types of data. The evidence includes (but is not limited to) the distinctive effects of localized brain damage on specific kinds of intelligences, distinctive patterns of development in each kind of intelligence across the lifespan, exceptional individuals (from both ends of the spectrum), and evolutionary history.

Gardner's theory (1983) is particularly relevant to those with cultural interests, because it puts into the realm of intelligence skills that traditional theories and cross-cultural investigations might neglect. For example, Romani (Gypsy) culture puts a large emphasis on the development of both musical and interpersonal skills. It also puts a heavy emphasis on oral storytelling skills (Fraser, 1995; Hancock, 1999). A traditional theory of intelligence would hold these skills as being outside the realm of intelligence. Thus, an illiterate Romani person might have trouble being classified as intelligent by traditional standards, because of the heavy emphasis in most tests of intelligence on understanding written verbal materials. But according to Gardner's theory, musical, interpersonal, and oral storytelling skills would all be relevant to the assessment of Romani intelligence, and potentially, anyone else's as well. Profiles comparing different peoples might therefore be quite different in Gardner's theory than in a traditional one. In a traditional theory, the development of such skills would be seen as outside the domain of intelligence. In essence, they simply would not "count."

Another theory arguing for a broader definition of intelligence is the theory of successful intelligence (see Sternberg, 1985, 1997, 1999b, for more details), which proposes its own definition of intelligence. The term "successful" intelligence is used to underscore the importance of understanding intelligence as a predictor of not only academic performance, in the tradition of Binet and Simon (1916), but also of success in life. This theory defines "successful" intelligence as the skills and knowledge needed for success in life, according to one's own definition of success, within one's sociocultural context. One acquires and utilizes these skills and this knowledge by capitalizing on strengths, by correcting or compensating for weaknesses, and by adapting to, shaping, or selecting environments through a balance of analytical, creative, and practical abilities.

In solving problems and making decisions, metacomponents, or higher order processes, determine what one is to do. Performance components actually do the work. And knowledge-acquisition components enable one to learn how to do it in the first place. Analytical intelligence results when components are applied to fairly abstract but familiar kinds of problems. Creative intelligence results when the components are applied to relatively novel tasks and situations. Practical intelligence results when the components are applied to experience for purposes of adaptation, shaping, and selection (e.g., Baltes, Dittmann-Kohli, & Dixon, 1984; Scribner, 1984, 1986; Sternberg et al., 2000).

Implicit Theories of Intelligence

Intelligence may be conceived in different ways in different cultures (see reviews in Serpell, 2000; and Sternberg & Kaufman, 1998). Such differences are important, because cultures evaluate their members, as well as members of others cultures, in terms of their own conceptions of intelligence.

The differences between Western and Eastern implicit theories of intelligence in many ways reflect the differences noted between Western and Eastern ways of thinking. In these terms, however, African conceptions would fit more into Eastern rather than Western views. For example, Markus and Kitayama (1991) have noted the greater tendency of Westerners to think in individualistic terms and of Easterners to think in collectivistic terms, and these differences are reflected in some ways in the implicit theories to be described. Moreover, Nisbett's (2003) characterization of differences between Western and Eastern cultures also apply, with Western views tending to be linear, context-independent, and less situated, and Eastern views tending to be more situated, nonlinear and dialectical, and context-dependent. If one accepts that implicit theories may drive people to socialize intelligence in different ways in different cultures, one may be inclined to test intelligence in differnt ways in different cultures, because parents may socialize the intelligence of children in different ways in different cultures (Sternberg & Suben, 1986).

In some cases, Western notions about intelligence are not shared by other cultures. For example, at the mental level, Western emphasis on speed of mental processing (Sternberg, Conway, Ketron, & Bernstein, 1981) is not shared in many cultures. Other cultures may even be suspicious of the quality of work that is done very quickly. Indeed, other cultures emphasize depth rather than speed of processing. They are not alone: Some prominent Western theorists have pointed out the importance of depth of processing for full command of material (e.g., Craik & Lockhart, 1972). Western tests often are narrowly constructed to reflect Western notions of the importance of time rather than any universal notion of its importance.

Often, Western investigators act as though their theories of intelligence—explicit or implicit—are not just proposals, but facts. For example, comparisons of intelligence across groups, as illustrated by Herrnstein and Murray (1994), assume that Western tests measure the same skills for all groups being compared and, moreover, are equally valid for all groups being compared. The result is that, typically, those groups that invent tests tend to do the best on them, then to feel intellectually superior to other groups. In this instance, Western groups might not do so well on tests created to measure adaptation in other environments. For example, their knowledge of natural herbal medications used to combat parasitic infections might be nil, but they would not sense any problem, because items measuring this knowledge would not appear on *their* tests.

In a study of implicit theories, Chen and Chen (1988) varied only the language. They explicitly compared the concepts of intelligence of Chinese graduates from Chinese-language versus English-language schools in Hong Kong. They found that both groups considered nonverbal reasoning skills as the most relevant skill for measuring intelligence. Verbal reasoning and social skills came next, and then numerical skill. Memory was seen as least important. The Chinese-language-schooled group, however, tended to rate verbal skills as less important than did the English-language-schooled group. Moreover, in an earlier study, Chen, Braithwaite, and Huang (1982) found that

Chinese students viewed memory for facts as important for intelligence, whereas Australian students viewed these skills as of only trivial importance.

Das (1994), also reviewing Eastern notions of intelligence, has suggested that in Buddhist and Hindu philosophies, intelligence not only involves waking up, noticing, recognizing, understanding, and comprehending, but also includes things such as determination, mental effort, and even feelings and opinions, in addition to more intellectual elements.

Differences between cultures in conceptions of intelligence have been recognized for some time. Gill and Keats (1980) noted that Australian university students value academic skills and the ability to adapt to new events as critical to intelligence, whereas Malay students value practical skills, as well as speed and creativity. Dasen (1984) found that Malay students emphasize both social and cognitive attributes in their conceptions of intelligence.

The differences between East and West may be due to differences in the kinds of skills valued by the two kinds of cultures (Srivastava & Misra, 1996). Western cultures and their schools emphasize what might be called "technological intelligence" (Mundy-Castle, 1974), so things such as artificial intelligence and so-called smart bombs are viewed, in some sense, as intelligent, or smart. African cultures place more emphasis on "social intelligence" (Mundy-Castle, 1974).

Western schooling also emphasizes other things (Srivastava & Misra, 1996), such as generalization, or going beyond the information given (Connolly & Bruner, 1974; Goodnow, 1976), speed (Sternberg, 1985), minimal moves to a solution (Newell & Simon, 1972), and creative thinking (Goodnow, 1976). Moreover, silence is interpreted as a lack of knowledge (Irvine, 1978). In contrast, the Wolof tribe in Africa views people of higher social class and distinction as speaking less (Irvine, 1978). This difference between the Wolof and Western notions suggests the usefulness of looking at African notions of intelligence as a possible contrast to U.S. notions.

Similar emphasis on social aspects of intelligence has been found as well among two other African groups—the Songhay of Mali and the Samia of Kenya (Putnam & Kilbride, 1980). The Yoruba, another African tribe, emphasize the importance of depth—of listening rather than just talking—to intelligence, and of being able to see all aspects of an issue and to place the issue in its proper overall context (Durojaiye, 1993).

Emphasis on the social aspects of intelligence is not limited to African cultures. Notions of intelligence in many Asian cultures also emphasize the social aspect of intelligence more than does the conventional Western or IQ-based notion (Azuma & Kashiwagi, 1987; Lutz, 1985; Poole, 1985; White, 1985).

In China, the Confucian perspective emphasizes the characteristic of benevolence and of doing what is right (Shi, 2004; Yang, 2001; Yang & Sternberg, 1997a). As in the Western notion, the intelligent person spends a great deal of effort in learning, enjoys learning, and persists in lifelong learning with a great deal of enthusiasm. The Taoist tradition, in contrast, emphasizes the importance of humility, freedom from conventional standards of judgment, and full knowledge of oneself, as well as of external conditions.

China is believed to be the first nation to employ widely tests of intelligence (Shi, 2004). Tests were used in ancient China for employment purposes. The tangram, which requires an individual to construct shapes, was first developed in the Song dynasty (Lin, 1980). Even young children were tested for their developmental skills, for example, by placing objects where they belong (Yan, 2001).

The difference between Eastern and Western conceptions of intelligence may persist even in the present day. Yang and Sternberg (1997b) studied contemporary Taiwanese Chinese conceptions of intelligence and found five factors underlying these conceptions: (1) a general cognitive factor, much like the *g* factor in conventional Western tests; (2) interpersonal intelligence (i.e., social competence); (3) intrapersonal intelligence; (4) intellectual self-assertion; and (5) intellectual self-effacement. In a related study, but with different results, Chen (1994) found three factors underlying Chinese conceptualizations of intelligence: (1) nonverbal reasoning ability, (2) verbal reasoning ability, and (3) rote memory. The difference may be due to different subpopulations of Chinese, to differences in methodology, or to differences in when the studies were done.

The factors uncovered in Taiwan differ substantially from those identified in U.S. people's conceptions of intelligence by Sternberg et al. (1981): (1) practical problem solving, (2) verbal ability, and (3) social competence. In both cases, however, people's implicit theories of intelligence seem to go quite far beyond what conventional psychometric intelligence tests measure. Of course, comparing the Chen (1994) study to the Sternberg et al. (1981) study simultaneously varies both language and culture.

Studies in Africa in fact provide yet another window on the substantial differences in conceptions of intelligence across cultures. Ruzgis and Grigorenko (1994) argued that, in Africa, conceptions of intelligence revolve largely around skills that help to facilitate and maintain harmonious and stable intergroup relations; intragroup relations are probably equally important and at times more important. For example, Serpell (1974, 1996) found that Chewa adults in Zambia emphasize social responsibilities, cooperativeness, and obedience as being important to intelligence; intelligent children are expected to be respectful of adults. Kenyan parents also emphasize responsible participation in family and social life as being important aspects of intelligence (Super & Harkness, 1982, 1986, 1993). In Zimbabwe, one word for intelligence, *ngware*, actually means to be prudent and cautious, particularly in social relationships. Among the Baoule, service to the family and community, and politeness toward and respect for elders are seen as key to intelligence (Dasen, 1984). In Zimbabwe, conceptions of intelligence are also represented by *njere* (in the Shona language) and *ukaliphile* (in the Ndebele language; Mpofu, 2004). The terms refer to behavior that is deliberate, socially responsible, positive, public-spirited, and altruistic (Chimhundu, 2001; Hadebe, 2001; Irvine, 1988; Mpofu, 1993, 2004). They also mean "wise," indicating that, as in Taiwanese Chinese culture (Yang & Sternberg, 1997a, 1997b), wisdom and intelligence are seen as closely related. Behavior is considered intelligent to the extent it benefits the community as a whole (Mpofu, 2004).

In India, words related to intelligence include *buddhi* (Sanskrit), which refers to awareness or consciousness (Baral & Das, 2004). Intelligence has been treated as a state, a process, or an entity in Indian philosophical literature (Srivastava & Misra, 2000). Das (1994) has referred to intelligence in Indian philosophy as pertaining to waking up, noticing, understanding, and comprehending.

In Latin America, implicit theories of teachers tend to emphasize academic skills as the main basis of intelligence (Kaplan, 1997). For example, in Argentina, Kaplan found that teachers emphasized the following as important to intelligence: good discipline, interest in learning, learning and thinking ability, and also coming from a stable home. Many teachers in this study also believed in the concept of a "bad head," that is, a head not suited to studying.

It is difficult to separate linguistic and conceptual differences in cross-cultural notions of intelligence. Converging operations can be used to achieve some separation; that is, different and diverse empirical operations can be employed to ascertain notions of intelligence. So one may ask in one study that people identify aspects of competence; in another, that they identify competent people; and in yet another study, that they characterize the meaning of "intelligence," and so forth.

The emphasis on the social aspects of intelligence is not limited to African cultures. Notions of intelligence in many Asian cultures also emphasize the social aspect of intelligence more than does the conventional Western or IQ-based notion (Azuma & Kashiwagi, 1987; Lutz, 1985; Poole, 1985; White, 1985).

It should be noted that neither African nor Asian notions emphasize exclusively social notions of intelligence. These conceptions of intelligence emphasize social skills much more than do conventional U.S. conceptions of intelligence, at the same time that they recognize the importance of cognitive aspects of intelligence. In a study of Kenyan conceptions of intelligence, Grigorenko et al. (2001) found that there are four distinct terms constituting conceptions of intelligence among rural Kenyans— *rieko* (knowledge and skills), *luoro* (respect), *winjo* (comprehension of how to handle real-life problems), *paro* (initiative)—with only the first directly referring to knowledge-based skills (including but not limited to academic endeavors).

Intelligence is viewed as being of great importance in many Western and some other cultures. This emphasis is not shared throughout the world. In Japan, for example, people rarely refer to an individual's level of intelligence at all (Sato, Namiki, Ando, & Hatano, 2004). Rather, there is much more emphasis on a person's motivation and diligence. Success is viewed as much more dependent on motivation than on intelligence (Sato et al., 2004). When

participants are given a task followed by success or failure feedback, Japanese students are more likely to attribute success to effort, good luck, or various situational factors, whereas American students are more likely to attribute success to their ability. In contrast, where as Japanese students are likely to attribute failure to lack of effort, the Americans attribute it to lack of ability (Miyamoto, 1985). Nevertheless, Japanese people do have a conception of intelligence. Factors emerging from a study of implicit theories were active social competence, processing efficiency, and receptive social competence (Azuma & Kashiwagi, 1987). None of the factors were considered to be innate.

It is important to realize, again, that there is no single overall U.S. conception of intelligence. Indeed, Okagaki and Sternberg (1993) found that different ethnic groups in San Jose, California, had rather different conceptions of what it means to be intelligent. For example, Latino parents of schoolchildren tended to emphasize the importance of social competence skills in their conceptions of intelligence, whereas Asian parents tended to emphasize rather heavily the importance of cognitive skills. Anglo parents also placed more emphasis on cognitive skills. Teachers, representing the dominant culture, emphasized more cognitive than social competence skills. The rank order of children of various groups' performance (including subgroups within the Latino and Asian groups) could be perfectly predicted by the extent to which their parents shared teachers' conceptions of intelligence. In other words, teachers tended to reward those children who were socialized into a view of intelligence that happened to correspond to their own.

Although researchers mostly emphasize lay implicit theories of intelligence in cultural studies, it is important to realize that expert implicit theories also differ. For example, Continental European thinking about intelligence, especially in French-speaking countries, was very heavily influenced by Piaget in the latter half of the 20th century, and this influence continues to be felt today (Lautrey & de Ribaupierre, 2004). Russian thinking was very heavily influenced by Vygotsky and Luria (Grigorenko, 2004). English thinking was very heavily influenced by Spearman (Deary & Smith, 2004), and North American thinking, by both Thurstone and Spearman (Sternberg, 2004c). Indian thinking was very heavily influenced by Eastern philosophy (Baral & Das, 2004).

MODELS OF THE RELATIONSHIP OF CULTURE TO INTELLIGENCE

Consider the four basic models of the relationship of culture to intelligence (Sternberg, 2004a; see also Sternberg, 1988, 1990) shown in Figure 22.1.

The models presented here differ in two key respects: whether there are cross-cultural differences in the nature of the mental processes and representations involved in adaptation that constitute intelligence, and whether there are differences in the instruments needed to measure intelligence (beyond simple translation or adaptation) as a result of cultural differences in the content required for adaptation.

In Model I, the nature of intelligence is the same across cultures, as are the tests used to measure intelligence. The theoretical positions of Jensen (1982, 1998) and Eysenck (1986) represent Model I types of positions. The argument is that the nature of intelligence is precisely the same cross-culturally, and that this nature can be assessed identically (using appropriate translations of text, where necessary) without regard to culture. For example, Jensen (1998) believes that general intelligence, or *g* (Spearman, 1927), is the same across time and place. What varies across time and place are its levels.

Model I is what is sometimes referred to as an "etic" approach to intelligence. One devises a measure or set of measures of a construct, then uses the measures in various cultures, sometimes doing minor adaptations to fit the measures to the culture (Carlstedt, Gustafsson, & Hautamäki, 2004; Deary & Smith, 2004; Demetriou & Papadopolous, 2004; Fernández-Ballesteros & Colom, 2004; Gulgoz & Kağitçibaşi, 2004; Rosas, 2004; Stankov, 2004; see, in general, essays in Sternberg, 2004b).

Model II represents a difference in the nature of intelligence but no difference in the instruments used to measure it. The measures used to assess intelligence are the same across cultures, but the outcomes obtained from using those measures are structurally different as a function of the culture being investigated. This approach is close to that taken by Nisbett (2003), who found that the same tests given in different cultures suggested that, across cultures, people think about problems in different ways.

In Model III, the dimensions of intelligence are the same, but the instruments of measurement are not. According to this view, measurement processes for a given attribute must be emic, that is, derived from within the context of the culture being studied rather than from outside it. This is not to say that the same instruments cannot be used across cultures, but when they are, the psychological meanings to be assigned to the scores will differ from one culture to another. This is the position taken in this chapter and in some earlier work (e.g., Sternberg, 1990).

According to this position, the components of intelligence and the mental representations on which they act are universal; that is, they are required for mental functioning in all cultures. For example, people in all cultures need to execute executive processes: (1) Recognize the existence of problems, (2) define what the problems are, (3) mentally represent the problems, (4) formulate one or more strategies for solving the problems, (5) allocate resources to solving the problems, (6) monitor solution of the problems, and (7) evaluate problem solving after it is done. What varies across cultures are the mental contents (i.e., types and items of knowledge) to which processes such as these are applied, and the judgments as to what are considered "intelligent" applications of the processes to these contents (Sternberg, 1997).

	Dimensions of Intelligence	
Relation	Same	Different
Tests of Intelligence — Same	Model I	Model II
Tests of Intelligence — Different	Model III	Model IV

FIGURE 22.1. Models of the relationship of culture to intelligence.

Thus, a wholly relativistic view of intelligence and culture would be inadequate. Some things are constant across cultures (mental representations and processes), whereas others are not (the contents to which they are applied and how their application is judged). Tests must be modified if they are to measure the same basic processes as they apply from one culture to another.

As a result, one can translate a particular test of intelligence, but there is no guarantee it will measure the same thing in one culture as in another. For example, a test that is highly novel in one culture or subculture may be quite familiar in the next. Even if the components of information processing are the same, the experiential novelty to which they are applied may be different. Moreover, the extent to which the given task is practically relevant to adaptation, shaping, and selection may differ. Hence, the components may be universal, but not necessarily the relative novelty or adaptive practicality of the components as applied to particular contents.

In Model IV, both the instruments and the ensuing dimensions of intelligence are different as a function of the culture under investigation. This position embraces the radical cultural relativist position (Berry, 1974) that intelligence can be understood and measured only as an indigenous construct within a given cultural context. It also embraces the position of Sarason and Doris (1979), who view intelligence largely as a cultural invention. In other words, nothing about intelligence is necessarily common across cultures.

Berry and Irvine (1986) have proposed four nested levels of the cultural context (in which intelligence and other hypothetical constructs reside). The broadest, ecological level, comprises the permanent or almost permanent characteristics that provide the backdrop for human action. The experiential context refers to the pattern of recurrent experiences within the ecological context that provides a basis for learning and development. The performance context comprises the limited set of environmental circumstances that account for particular behaviors at specific points in space and time. The narrowest, experimental context, comprises the environmental characteristics manipulated by psychologists and others to elicit particular responses or test scores.

STUDIES OF INTELLIGENCE IN ITS CULTURAL CONTEXTS

The previous discussion suggests that intelligence, understood wholly outside its cultural context, is a mythological construct. Some aspects of intelligence transcend cultures, namely, the mental processes underlying intelligence and the mental representations upon which they act. But these operations play themselves out in performance differently from one culture to another. As soon as one assesses performance, then, one is assessing mental processes and representations in a cultural context (Model III).

Most psychological research is done within a single culture. But single-cultural studies whose results are implicitly or even explicitly generalized across cultures potentially deprive the field in several ways. In particular, they may (1) introduce limited definitions of psychological phenomena and problems, (2) engender risks of unwarranted assumptions about the phenomena under investigation, (3) raise questions about cultural generalizability of findings, (4) engender risks of cultural imperialism, and (5) represent lost opportunities to collaborate and develop psychology around the world.

Many research programs demonstrate the potential hazards of single-culture research. For example, Greenfield (1997) found that it means a different thing to take a test among Mayan children than it does among most children in the United States. The Mayan expectation is that collaboration is permissible, and that it is rather unnatural *not* to collaborate. Clearly, only Model III or Model IV would apply if one accepted this difference as one that should be reflected in testing. Such a finding is consistent with the work of Markus and Kitayama (1991), suggesting different cultural constructions of the self in individualistic versus collectivistic cultures. Indeed, Nisbett (2003) has found that some cultures, especially Asian ones, tend to be more dialectical in their thinking, whereas European and North American cultures tend to be more linear. And individuals in different cultures may construct concepts in quite different ways, rendering results of concept formation or identification studies in a single culture suspect (Atran, 1999; Coley, Medin, Proffitt, Lynch, & Atran, 1999; Medin & Atran, 1999). Thus, groups may think about what appears superficially to be the same phenomenon—whether a concept or the taking of a test—differently. What appear to be differences in *g* may in fact be differences in cultural properties (Helms-Lorenz, Van de Vijver, & Poortinga, 2003). Helms-Lorenz et al. have argued that measured differences in intellectual performance may result from differences in cultural complexity, but complexity of a culture is extremely hard to define, and what appears to be simple or complex from the point of view of one culture may appear different from the point of view of another.

Many investigators have realized the importance of cultural context for the psychology of intelligence and cognition. These realizations have taken diverse forms. Indeed, Berry (1974) reviewed concepts of intelligence across a wide variety of cultural contexts, showing major differences across cultures.

Cole (1998) and Shweder (1991, 2002) have helped define cultural psychology as a field, distinguishing it from cross-cultural psychology (e.g., Irvine, 1979; Irvine & Berry, 1983; Marsella, Tharp, & Cibrorowski, 1979), which they believe tends to be somewhat less sensitive to differences among cultures. The studies described in this chapter represent both approaches, although our own studies are generally more in the "cultural" rather than "cross-cultural" tradition. Cole's overview of the field builds on his earlier work (Cole et al., 1971; Cole & Means, 1981; Cole & Scribner, 1974; Laboratory of Comparative Human Cognition, 1982), which showed how cognitive performance among populations, such as the Kpelle in Africa, can be both qualitatively and quantitatively different from that of the North Americans, who typically are tested in lab experiments on thinking and reasoning. What North Americans might think of as sophisticated thinking—for example, sorting taxonomically (as in a robin being a kind of bird)—might be viewed as unsophisticated by the Kpelle, whose functional performance on sorting tasks corresponded to the demands of their everyday life (as in a robin flying). Here, Model I would fail to find an important difference in the Kpelle versus traditional Western and specifically European and North American ways of thinking. In a related fashion, Bruner, Olver, and Greenfield (1966) found that among members of the Wolof tribe of Senegal, increasingly greater Western-style schooling was associated with greater use of taxonomic classification.

Cole's work built in turn upon earlier work, such as that of Luria (1931/1976), which showed that Asian peasants in the Soviet Union might not perform well on cognitive tasks because of their refusal to accept the tasks as they were presented. Models I and II would likely fail with such people, because people would be unwilling to accept the tests that are proposed to be universally applicable. Indeed, people in diverse cultures are presented with very diverse tasks in their lives. Gladwin (1970), studying the Puluwat who inhabit the Caroline Islands in the South Pacific, found that these individuals were able to master knowledge domains including wind and weather, ocean currents, and movements of the stars. They integrate this knowledge with mental maps of the islands to become highly respected navigators in their world.

In related work, Serpell (1979) designed a study to distinguish between a generalized perceptual deficit hypothesis and a more context-specific hypothesis for why children in certain cultures may show inferior perceptual abilities. He found that English children did better on a drawing task, but Zambian children did better on a wire-shaping task. Thus, children performed better on materials from their own environments that were more familiar to them.

Wagner (1978) had Moroccan and North American individuals remember patterns of Oriental rugs, and other individuals remembered pictures of everyday objects, such as a rooster and a fish. There was no evidence of a difference in memory structure, but evidence of a lack of difference depended precisely upon using tests that were appropriate to the cultural content of the individuals being studied. Moroccans, who have long experience in the rug trade, seemed to remember things in a different way than participants who did not have the Moroccans' skill in remembering rug patterns. In a related study, Kearins (1981) found that when asked to remember visuospatial displays, Anglo Australians used verbal (school-appropriate) strategies, whereas Aboriginals used visual (desert nomad–appropriate) strategies.

Goodnow (1962) found that for tasks using combinations and permutations, Chinese children with English schooling performed as well as or better than Europeans children; European children with Chinese schooling or those from very low-income families did somewhat worse than other children in their group. These results suggested that form of schooling primes children to excel in certain ways and not others (see also Goodnow, 1969).

Children from non-European or non–North American cultures do not always do worse on tests. Super (1976) found evidence that African infants sit and walk earlier than do their counterparts in the United States and Europe. But Super also found that mothers in the African cultures he studied made a self-conscious effort to teach their babies to sit and walk as early as possible. At more advanced levels of development, Stigler, Lee, Lucker, and Stevenson (1982; see also Stevenson & Stigler, 1994) found that Japanese and Chinese children had better developed mathematical skills than did North American children.

Carraher, Carraher, and Schliemann (1985) studied a group of children that is especially relevant for assessing intelligence as adaptation to the environment. This group of Brazilian street children is under great contextual pressure to form a successful street business. If they do not, they risk death at the hands of so-called "death squads," which may murder children who, unable to earn money, resort to robbing stores (or are suspected of resorting to robbing stores). Hence, if they are not intelligent in the sense of adapting to their environment, they risk death. The investigators found that the same children who are able to do the mathematics needed to run their street businesses are often barely able or unable to do school mathematics. In fact, the more abstracted and removed from real-world contexts the presentation of problems, the worse the children typically do on them. For children in school, the street context would be more removed from their lives. These results suggest that differences in context can have a powerful effect on performance. (See also Ceci & Roazzi, 1994; Nuñes, 1994; Saxe, 1990, for related work.) In this work, Models I and II would fail to reveal that tests adequately measuring skills in the Brazilian street children are not the tests typically used to measure such skills in more developed countries.

Such differences are not limited to Brazilian street children. Lave (1988) showed that Berkeley housewives who successfully could do the mathematics needed for comparison shopping in the supermarket were unable to do the same mathematics when placed in a classroom and given isomorphic problems presented in an abstract form. In other words, their problem was not at the level of mental processes but at the level of applying the processes in specific environmental contexts.

In summary, a variety of researchers have suggested that how one tests abilities, competences, and expertise can have a major effect on how "intelligent" students appear to be. Street children in Brazil, for example, need the same mathematical skills to solve problems involving discounts as do children in the United States about to take a high-stakes paper-and-pencil test of mathematical achievement. But the contexts in which they express these skills—hence, the contexts in which they can best display their knowledge on tests—are different (as in Model III described earlier). My colleagues and I have also done research suggesting that cultural context needs to be taken into account in testing for intelligence and its outcomes.

The measurement of intelligence may be viewed as occurring on a continuum from abilities to competencies to expertise (Sternberg, 1999a, 2003a, 2003b). All tests of intelligence, even the ones once believed to be culture-free, such as tests of abstract reasoning, measure skills that are at least in part acquired through the covariance and interaction of genes with environment. For example, a test of vocabulary found on intelligence tests is clearly a test of achievement. But so is a test of abstract reasoning, as shown by the Flynn effect, in which abstract reasoning skills showed substantial secular increases over the 20th century in diverse cultures around the world (Flynn, 1984, 1987). Hence, one can test knowledge as part of intelligence, but all tests of intelligence require knowledge, even if it is only knowing how to take the tests and to maximize one's score on them.

Children May Develop Contextually Important Skills at the Expense of Academic Ones

Many times, investigations of intelligence conducted in settings outside the developed world can yield a picture of intelligence that is quite at variance with the picture one would obtain from studies conducted only in the developed world. In a study in Usenge, Kenya, near the town of Kisumu, investigators studied school-age children's ability to adapt to their indigenous environment. They devised a test of practical intelligence for adaptation to the environment (see Sternberg & Grigorenko, 1997; Sternberg et al., 2001). The test of practical intelligence measured children's informal tacit knowledge for natural herbal medicines that the villagers believe can be used to fight various types of infections. Tacit knowledge is, roughly speaking, knowledge one needs to succeed in an environment, but it is usually not explicitly taught and often is not even verbalized (Sternberg et al., 2000). Children in the villages use their tacit knowledge of these medicines on average once a week in medicating themselves and others. More than 95% of the children suffer from parasitic illnesses. Thus, tests of how to use these medicines constitute effective measures of one aspect of practical intelligence as defined by the villagers, as well as their life circumstances in their environmental contexts. Note that the processes of intelligence are not different in Kenya. Children must still recognize the existence of an illness, define what it is, devise a strategy to combat it, and so forth. But the content to which the processes are applied—hence, the appropriate ways of testing these processes—may be quite different (as per Model III, described earlier).

Middle-class Westerners might find it quite a challenge to thrive or even survive in these contexts, or for that matter in the contexts of urban ghettos often not distant from their comfortable homes. For example, they would know how to use none of the natural herbal medicines to combat the diverse and abundant parasitic illnesses they might acquire in rural Kenya.

The investigators measured the Kenyan children's ability to identify the medicines, where they come from, what they are used for, and how they are dosed. They also administered to the children of the study the Raven Coloured Progressive Matrices Test (Raven, Court, & Raven, 1992), which is a measure of fluid or abstract reasoning–based abilities, as well as the Mill Hill Vocabulary Scale (Raven et al., 1992), which is a measure of crystallized or formal knowledge–based abilities. In addition, they gave the children a comparable test of vocabulary in their own Dholuo language. The children speak Dholuo in the home, English in the schools.

All correlations between the test of indigenous tacit knowledge and scores on fluid ability and crystallized ability tests were *negative*. The correlations with the tests of crystallized abilities were significantly so. In other words, the higher the children scored on the test of tacit knowledge, the lower they scored, on average, on the tests of crystallized abilities (vocabulary).

This surprising result can be interpreted various ways, but based on the ethnographic observations of the anthropologists on the team, Prince and Geissler (2001) concluded that a plausible scenario takes into account the expectations of families for their children. Many children drop out of school before graduation for financial or other reasons, and many families in the village do not particularly see the advantages of formal Western schooling. There is no reason they should, because the children in many families for the most part spend their lives farming or engaged in other occupations that make little or no use of Western schooling. These families emphasize teaching their children the indigenous informal knowledge that lead to successful adaptation in the environments in which they will really live. Children who spend their time learning the indigenous practical knowledge of the community may not always invest themselves heavily in doing well in school, whereas children who do well in school generally may invest themselves less heavily in learning the indigenous knowledge—hence, the negative correlations.

The Kenyan study suggests that the identification of a general factor of human intelligence may tell us more about how abilities interact with cultural patterns of schooling and society, and especially Western patterns of schooling and society, than about the structure of human abilities. In Western schooling, children typically study a variety of subject matter from an early age, thus developing skills in a variety of areas. This kind of schooling prepares the children to take a test of intelligence, which typically measures skills in a variety of areas. Often intelligence tests measure skills that children were expected to acquire a few years before taking the intelligence test. But as Rogoff (1990, 2003) and others have noted, this pattern of schooling is not universal and has not even been common for much of the history of humankind. Throughout history, and in many places still, schooling, especially for boys, takes the form of apprenticeships in which children learn a craft from an early age. They learn what they will need to know to succeed in a trade, but not a lot more. They are not simultaneously engaged in tasks that require the development of the particular blend of skills measured by conventional intelligence tests. Hence, it is less likely that one would observe a general factor in their scores, much as was discovered in Kenya.

What does a general factor mean anyway? Some years back, Vernon (1971) pointed out that the axes of a factor analysis do not necessarily reveal a latent structure of the mind, but rather represent a convenient way of characterizing the organization of mental abilities. Vernon believed that there was no single "right" orientation of axes; indeed, mathematically, an infinite number of orientations of axes can be fit to any solution in an exploratory factor analysis. Vernon's point seems perhaps to have been forgotten, or at least ignored, by later theorists.

Just as I argue here that the so-called *g* factor may partly reflect human interactions with cultural patterns, so has Tomasello (2001) argued that so-called *modularity of mind* may in part reflect human interactions with cultural patterns. This is not to dismiss the importance of biology. Rather, it is to emphasize its importance as it interacts with culture, rather than simply to view it as some kind of immutable effect that operates independently and outside of a cultural context.

The partial context specificity of intellectual performance does not apply only to countries far removed from North America or Europe. One can find the same on these continents, as was done in the studies of Yup'ik Eskimo children in southwestern Alaska.

Children May Have Substantial Practical Skills That Go Unrecognized in Academic Tests

Related, although certainly not identical, results appear in a study done among Yup'ik Eskimo children in southwestern Alaska (Grigorenko et al., 2004). The investigators assessed the importance of academic and practical intelligence in rural and semiurban Alaskan communities. They measured academic intelligence with conventional measures of fluid (the Cattell Culture Fair Test of *g*; Cattell & Cattell, 1973) and crystallized intelligence (the Mill Hill Vocabulary Scale; Raven et al., 1992). (These tests, to some extent, reflect a Western bias in terms of what counts as "intelligence.") They measured practical intelligence with a test of tacit knowledge of skills (hunting, fishing, dealing with weather conditions, picking and preserving plants, etc.) as acquired in rural Alaskan Yup'ik communities (the Yup'ik Scale of Practical Intelligence, YSPI). The semiurban children statistically significantly outperformed the rural children on the measure of crystal-

lized intelligence, but the rural children statistically significantly outperformed the semiurban children on the measure of the YSPI. The test of tacit knowledge skills was superior to the tests of academic intelligence in predicting practical skills as evaluated by adults and peers of the rural children (for whom the test was created), but not that of the semiurban children. This study, like the Kenya study, suggests the importance of practical intellectual skills for predicting adaptation to everyday environments. Can one find similar results in cultures that are urban and somewhat less remote from the kinds of cultures familiar to many readers?

Practical Intellectual Skills May Be Better Predictors of Health Than Academic Ones

In a study in Russia (Grigorenko & Sternberg, 2001), entirely distinct measures of analytical, creative, and practical intelligence (for details, see Grigorenko & Sternberg, 2001) were created, with at least two summative indicators for each construct. Principal components analysis, with both varimax and oblimin rotations, yielded clear-cut analytical, creative, and practical factors for the tests.

The main objective of this study was to predict, using the analytical, creative, and practical tests, mental and physical health among the Russian adults. Mental health was measured by widely used paper-and-pencil tests of depression and anxiety and physical health was measured by self-report. The best predictor of mental and physical health was the practical intelligence measure for mental and physical health, respectively. (Or, because the data are correlational, it may be that health predicts practical intelligence, although the connection here is less clear.) Analytical intelligence came second, and creative intelligence, third. All three contributed to prediction, however. Moreover, although the three abilities were the same (analytical, creative, practical); measuring them—especially the practical ones— required cultural adaptation that was appropriate for the Russian adults being tested (Model III).

The results in Russia emphasized the importance of studying health-related outcomes as one measure of successful adaptation to the environment. Health-related variables can affect people's ability to achieve their goals in life, or even to perform well on tests, as was found in Jamaica.

Physical Health May Moderate Performance on Assessments

When interpreting results, whether from developed or developing cultures, it is always important to take into account the physical health of the participants one is testing. In a study in Jamaica (Sternberg, Powell, McGrane, & McGregor, 1997), the investigators found that Jamaican schoolchildren who suffered from parasitic illnesses (for the most part, whipworm or *Ascaris*) did more poorly on higher level cognitive tests (e.g., working memory and reasoning) than did children who did not have these illnesses, even after controlling for socioeconomic status. The children with parasitic illnesses did better on fine-motor tasks, for reasons unknown to us.

Thus, many children were poor achievers not because they innately lacked abilities, but because they lacked the good health necessary to develop and display such abilities. A person who is moderately to seriously ill probably finds it more difficult to concentrate on reading or listening than if he or she is well. Children in developing countries are ill much, and even most, of the time. They simply cannot devote the same attentional and learning resources to schoolwork that well children have to devote. Here, as in Kenya, their health knowledge would be crucial for their adaptation to the environment. Testing that does not take into account health status is likely to give false impressions.

Do conventional tests, such as tests of working memory or of reasoning, measure all the skills that children in developing countries can bring to the table? Work done in Tanzania suggests that they do not.

Dynamic Testing May Reveal Cognitive Skills Not Revealed by Static Testing

A study in Tanzania (see Sternberg & Grigorenko, 1997, 2002; Sternberg et al., 2002) points out the risks of giving tests, scoring them, and interpreting the results as measures of some latent intellectual ability or abilities. Schoolchildren between the ages of 11 and 13 years near Bagamoyo, Tanzania, received tests, including a form-board classification test (a sorting task), a linear syllogisms test, and a Twenty Questions Test ("Find a Figure"), which measure the kinds of skills required on conventional tests of intelligence. Of course,

the investigators obtained scores that they could analyze and evaluate, ranking the children in terms of their supposed general or other abilities. However, they administered the tests dynamically rather than statically (Brown & Ferrara, 1985; Feuerstein, 1979; Grigorenko & Sternberg, 1998; Guthke, 1993; Haywood & Tzuriel, 1992; Lidz, 1991; Sternberg & Grigorenko, 2002; Tzuriel, 1995; Vygotsky, 1978).

Dynamic testing is like conventional static testing in that individuals are tested and inferences about their abilities are made. But dynamic tests differ in that children are given some kind of feedback to help them improve their performance. Vygotsky (1978) suggested that the children's ability to profit from the guided instruction they received during the testing session could serve as a measure of their zone of proximal development (ZPD), or the difference between their developed abilities and their latent capacities. In other words, testing and instruction are treated as being of one piece rather than as distinct processes. This integration makes sense in terms of traditional definitions of intelligence as the ability to learn ("Intelligence and Its Measurement," 1921; Sternberg & Detterman, 1986). A dynamic test directly measures processes of learning in the context of testing rather than measuring these processes indirectly as the product of past learning. Such measurement is especially important when not all children have had equal opportunities to learn in the past.

In the assessments, children were first given the ability tests. Experimental group children were then given an intervention. Control group children were not. The intervention consisted of a brief period of instruction in which children were able to learn skills that would potentially enable them to improve their scores. For example, in the 20 questions tasks, children were taught how a single true–false question could cut the space of possible correct solutions by half. Then all children—experimental and control groups—were tested again. Because the total time for instruction was less than an hour, one would not expect dramatic gains. Yet on average the gains from pre- to posttest in the experimental group were statistically significant, and significantly greater than those in the control group.

In the control group, the correlations between pre- and posttest scores were generally high. One would expect a high correlation, because there was no intervention; hence, the re-testing was largely a measure of alternate forms reliability. More importantly, scores on the pretest in the experimental group showed only weak, although significant, correlations with scores on the posttest. These correlations, which were significantly and substantially less than those in the control group, suggested that when tests are administered statically to children in developing countries, they may be rather unstable and easily subject to influences of training. The reason may be that the children are not accustomed to taking Western-style tests, so they profit quickly even from small amounts of instruction as to what is expected from them.

Of course, the more important question is not whether the scores changed or even correlated with each other; rather, how did they correlate with other cognitive measures? In other words, which test was a better predictor of transfer to other cognitive performances on tests of working memory, the pretest score or the posttest score? The investigators found the posttest score to be the better predictor of working memory in the experimental group. Children in the dynamic testing group improved significantly more than those in the control group (who did not receive intervening dynamic instruction between pre- and posttests).

In the Jamaica study described earlier, the investigators had failed to find effects of an antiparasitic medication, albendazole, on cognitive functioning. Might this have been because the testing was static rather than dynamic? Static testing tends to emphasize skills developed in the past. Children who suffer from parasitic illnesses often do not have the same opportunities as well children to profit from instruction and acquire skills. Dynamic testing emphasizes skills developed at the time of test. Indeed, the skills or knowledge are specifically taught at the time of test. Would dynamic testing show effects of medication (in this case, albendazole for hookworm and praziquantel for schistosomiasis) not shown by static testing?

The answer was "yes." Over time, treated children showed an advantage over children who did not receive treatment, and were closer after time had passed to the control (uninfected) group than were the untreated children. In other words, conventional static tests of intelligence may fail to reveal fully children's intellectual potentials. Thus, when tests are mod-

ified in different environments, as per Model III, one may wish to modify not only their content but also the form in which they are administered, as was done in the dynamic testing.

CULTURE-FAIR AND CULTURE-RELEVANT TESTING

A culture-fair test is equally appropriate for members of all cultures and comprises items that are equally fair to everyone. Believers in culture-fair tests generally follow Model I, described earlier, for the relation between culture and intelligence. This approach is illustrated by Zeidner, Matthews, and Roberts (2004), who state:

> As in other multicultural nations [besides Israel], research has been directed toward sociocultural differences in test scores. Because the tests are translated from English, any comparison of groups rests on the assumption that test adaptation is "culture-fair." . . . The basic principal [sic] guiding the development of all major Hebrew standardized test versions was to stay as close to the English original as possible, unless items lacked compatibility with Israeli culture or the psychometric attributes of the items in the Israeli samples needed upgrading. (p. 220)

In this approach, minor adaptations are made. For example, Israel uses a different calendar (the Jewish one) than does the United States; hence, an adaptation was made for the proper year and time references. But these differences are quite minor.

Researchers compared the performance of Jewish examinees of Western and Eastern (Asian/African) backgrounds and found that on the Wechsler Preschool and Primary Scale of Intelligence and Wechsler Intelligence Scale for Children—Revised (WISC-R) the children of Western origins outperformed the children of Eastern origins. The difference tended to increase with age (Lieblich, 1983; Minkowitch, Davis, & Bashi, 1982; Zeidner, 1985). Ethnic group had a larger effect than socioeconomic group, although both mattered.

Comparisons of Israeli Jewish children with Israeli Arab children showed an advantage for the Jewish children of approximately one standard deviation (Kugelmass & Lieblich, 1975; Kugelmass, Lieblich, & Bossik, 1974; Lieblich, 1983; Lieblich & Kugelmass, 1981). Christian Arab children tend to outscore Muslim and Druze students on Raven's Matrices (Bashi,

1976). Differences tend to be larger on nonverbal than on verbal tests.

Similar results have been found elsewhere. Savasir and Sahin (1995) found that Turkish children score about 12 points lower on the WISC-R than do American children. On the Gesell Developmental Schedules, Cantez and Girgin (1992) found that Turkish children generally lagged behind in the norms created for American children. In general, children from the educational systems in rural Turkey, which are less Westernized, have lower scores on translated Western intelligence and educational tests than those from educational systems in urbanized Turkey, which are more like Western systems (Kağitçibaşi, 1996; Kağitçibaşi, Sunar, & Bekman, 2001).

The etic approach is at least somewhat open to question. Because members of different cultures define intelligence differently, the very behaviors that may be considered intelligent in one culture may be viewed as unintelligent in another. Consider the concept of mental quickness. In mainstream U.S. culture, to say someone is "quick" is to say that the person is intelligent. Indeed, most group tests of intelligence are strictly timed. I found this out the hard way myself, when I failed to answer all or some of the items.

There can be no doubt that sometimes it is important to be fast. When you have not yet started writing a paper that is due the next day, it is definitely adaptive to be quick. An air traffic controller had better be fast if he or she values the lives of the passengers on the airplanes he or she is monitoring. In many cultures, however, quickness is not so valued. People elsewhere may believe that more intelligent people do not rush into things. In fact, early in the 20th century, a leading psychometric theoretician of intelligence, Louis Thurstone (1924), defined "intelligence" as the ability to withhold an instinctive response. In other words, the smart person does not rush into action but thinks first. Even in our own culture, no one is viewed as brilliant who decides on a marital partner, a job, or a place to live in the 20 to 30 seconds it might normally take to solve an intelligence test problem. So is it culturally fair to include a speed or timing component in an intelligence test?

Performance on tests that have been labeled "culture-fair" seems to be influenced by cultural factors. Examples are years of schooling and academic achievements (e.g., Ceci, 1996).

In summary, one must be careful when drawing conclusions about group differences in intelligence (Greenfield, 1997; Loehlin, 2000). The conclusions that appear to be justified on the surface may represent only a superficial analysis of group differences.

In the proposed model of culture and intelligence, Model III, tests are adapted in form and content to take into account the differences in adaptive tasks that individuals confront in diverse cultures, within and across countries. Individuals in other cultures often do not do well on our tests, nor would we do well on theirs. The processes of intelligence are universal, but their manifestations are not. Investigators who want best to understand, assess, and develop intelligence need to take into account the cultural contexts in which it operates. We cannot now create culture-free or culture-fair tests given our present state of knowledge. But we can create *culture-relevant tests*, and that should be our goal. Developing culture-fair tests based on each culture's own definition of intelligence may be an unrealistic goal. But it is possible to provide culture-relevant tests that require skills and knowledge that are relevant to the cultural experiences of the test takers. The content and procedures are appropriate to the cultural norms of the test takers. For example, 14-year-old boys performed poorly on a task when it was presented in terms of baking cupcakes. But they performed well when the task was framed in terms of charging batteries (Ceci & Bronfenbrenner, 1985). Brazilian maids had no difficulty with proportional reasoning when hypothetically purchasing food. But they had great difficulty with it when hypothetically purchasing medicinal herbs (Schliemann & Magalhües, 1990).

CONCLUSION

When cultural context is taken into account, (1) individuals are better recognized for and are better able to make use of their talents, (2) schools teach and assess children better, and (3) society utilizes rather than wastes the talents of its members. We can pretend to measure intelligence across cultures simply by translating Western tests and giving them to individuals in a variety of cultures. But such measurement is only pretense. We need to be careful even when we try to measure the intelligence of various cultural groups *within* a society.

ACKNOWLEDGMENTS

Preparation of this chapter was supported by the Partnership for Child Development, centered at Imperial College, University of London; the James S. McDonnell Foundation; the Institute of Educational Sciences (formerly the Office of Educational Research and Improvement), U.S. Department of Education; the United States Agency for International Development; the National Council for Eurasian and East European Studies; and the Spencer Foundation.

REFERENCES

Atran, S. (1999). Itzaj Maya folkbiological taxonomy: Cognitive universals and cultural particulars. In D. L. Medin & S. Atran (Eds.), *Folkbiology* (pp. 119–213). Cambridge, MA: MIT Press.

Azuma, H., & Kashiwagi, K. (1987). Descriptions for an intelligent person: A Japanese study. *Japanese Psychological Research, 29,* 17–26.

Baltes, P. B., Dittmann-Kohli, F., & Dixon, R. A. (1984). New perspectives on the development of intelligence in adulthood: Toward a dual-process conception and a model of selective optimization with compensation. In P. B. Baltes & O. G. Brim (Eds.), *Life-span development and behavior* (Vol. 6., pp. 33–76). New York: Academic Press.

Baral, B. D., & Das, J. P. (2004). Intelligence: What is indigenous to India and what is shared? In R. J. Sternberg (Ed.), *International handbook of intelligence* (pp. 270–301). New York: Cambridge University Press.

Barnouw, V. (1985). *Culture and personality.* Chicago: Dorsey Press.

Bashi, Y. (1976). *Verbal and nonverbal abilities of students in grades four, six, and eight in the Arab sector.* Jerusalem: School of Education, Hebrew University.

Benedict, R. (1946). *The crysanthemum and the sword.* Boston: Houghton Mifflin.

Berry, J. W. (1974). Radical cultural relativism and the concept of intelligence. In J. W. Berry & P. R. Dasen (Eds.), *Culture and cognition: Readings in cross-cultural psychology* (pp. 225–229). London: Methuen.

Berry, J. W., & Irvine, S. H. (1986). Bricolage: Savages do it daily. In R. J. Sternberg & R. K. Wagner (Eds.), *Practical intelligence: Nature and origins of competence in the everyday world* (pp. 271–306). New York: Cambridge University Press.

Berry, J. W., Poortinga, Y. H., Segall, M. H., & Dasen, P. R. (1992). *Cross-cultural psychology: Research and applications.* New York: Cambridge University Press.

Binet, A., & Simon, T. (1916). *The development of intelligence in children* (E. S. Kite, trans.). Baltimore: Williams & Wilkins.

Boas, F. (1911). *The mind of primitive man.* New York: Macmillan.

Boring, E. G. (1923, June 6). Intelligence as the tests test it. *New Republic,* 35–37.

Brislin, R. W., Lonner, W. J., & Thorndike, R. M. (Eds.). (1973). *Cross-cultural research methods.* New York: Wiley.

Brown, A. L., & Ferrara, R. A. (1985). Diagnosing zones of proximal development. In J. V. Wertsch (Ed.), *Culture, communication, and cognition: Vygotskian perspectives* (pp. 273–305). New York: Cambridge University Press.

Bruner, J. S., Olver, R. R., & Greenfield, P. M. (1966). *Studies in cognitive growth.* New York: Wiley.

Cantez, E., & Girgin, Y. (1992). Istanbul'da yasayan 3-11 yas grubundaki kiz va erkek cocuklara Gesell Testi'nin uygulanmiasindan elde edilen sonuclarin Gesell Gelisim Testi Normlari ile karsilastirilmasi ve normlara uygunlugunun arastirilmasi ile ilgili bir calisma. [A study about the comparison of the results obtained from the application of Gesell Development Schedules to 3- 11-year-old male and female children living in Istanbul with the norms of the Gesell Developmental Schedules]. Paper presented at the 8th Ulusal Psikoloji Kongresi Bilimsel Calismalari. Turkish Psychological Association, Ankara, Turkey.

Carlstedt, B., Gustafsson, J.-E., & Hautamäki, J. (2004). Intelligence—Theory, research, and testing in the Nordic countries. In R. J. Sternberg (Ed.), *International handbook of intelligence* (pp. 49–78). New York: Cambridge University Press.

Carraher, T. N., Carraher, D., & Schliemann, A. D. (1985). Mathematics in the streets and in schools. *British Journal of Developmental Psychology, 3,* 21–29.

Carroll, J. B. (1993). *Human cognitive abilities: A survey of factor-analytic studies.* New York: Cambridge University Press.

Cattell, R. B. (1971). *Abilities: Their structure, growth, and action.* Boston: Houghton Mifflin.

Cattell, R. B., & Cattell, A. K. S. (1973). *Measuring intelligence with the Culture Fair Tests.* Champaign, IL: Institute for Personality and Ability Testing.

Ceci, S. J. (1996). *On intelligence* (expanded ed.). Cambridge, MA: Harvard University Press.

Ceci, S. J., & Brofenbrenner, U. (1985). Don't forget to take the cupcakes out of the oven: Strategic time-monitoring, prospective memory and context. *Child Development, 56,* 175–190.

Ceci, S. J., & Roazzi, A. (1994). The effects of context on cognition: postcards from Brazil. In R. J. Sternberg & R. K. Wagner (Eds.), *Mind in context: Interactionist perspectives on human intelligence* (pp. 74–101). New York: Cambridge University Press.

Chen, M. J. (1994). Chinese and Australian concepts of intelligence. *Psychology and Developing Societies, 6,* 101–117.

Chen, M. J., Braithwaite, V., & Huang, J. T. (1982). Attributes of intelligent behaviour: Perceived relevance and difficulty by Australian and Chinese students. *Journal of Cross-Cultural Psychology, 13,* 139–156.

Chen, M. J., & Chen, H. C. (1988). Concepts of intelligence: A comparison of Chinese graduates from Chinese and English schools in Hong Kong. *International Journal of Psychology, 223*, 471–487.

Chimhundu, H. (Ed.). (2001). *Dura manzwi guru rechiShona.* Harare, Zimbabwe: College Press.

Cole, M. (1998). *Cultural psychology: A once and future discipline.* Cambridge, MA: Belknap.

Cole, M., Gay, J., Glick, J., & Sharp, D. W. (1971). *The cultural context of learning and thinking.* New York: Basic Books.

Cole, M., & Means, B. (1981). *Comparative studies of how people think.* Cambridge, MA: Harvard University Press.

Cole, M., & Scribner, S. (1974). *Culture and thought.* New York: Wiley.

Coley, J. D., Medin, D. L., Proffitt, J. B., Lynch, E., & Atran, S. (1999). Inductive reasoning in folkbiological thought. In D. L. Medin & S. Atran (Eds.), *Folkbiology* (pp. 205–232). Cambridge, MA: MIT Press.

Connolly, H., & Bruner, J. (1974). Competence: Its nature and nurture. In K. Connolly & J. Bruner (Eds.), *The growth of competence* (pp. 3–10). New York: Academic Press.

Craik, F. I. M., & Lockhart R. S. (1972). Levels of processing: A framework for memory research. *Journal of Verbal Learning and Verbal Behavior, 11*, 671–684.

Daniel, M. H. (1997). Intelligence testing: Status and trends. *American Psychologist, 52*, 1038–1045.

Daniel, M. H. (2000). Interpretation of intelligence test scores. In R. J. Sternberg (Ed.), *Handbook of intelligence* (pp. 477–491). New York: Cambridge University Press.

Das, J. P. (1994). Eastern views of intelligence. In R. J. Sternberg (Ed.), *Encyclopedia of intelligence* (pp. 91–97). New York: Macmillan.

Dasen, P. (1984). The cross-cultural study of intelligence: Piaget and the Baoule. *International Journal of Psychology, 19*, 407–434.

Deary, I. J., & Smith, P. (2004). Intelligence research and assessment in the United Kingdom. In R. J. Sternberg (Ed.), *International handbook of intelligence* (pp. 1–48). New York: Cambridge University Press.

Demetriou, A., & Papadopoulos, T. C. (2004). Human intelligence: From local models to universal theory. In R. J. Sternberg (Ed.), *International handbook of intelligence* (pp. 445–474). New York: Cambridge University Press.

Durojaiye, M. O. A. (1993). Indigenous psychology in Africa. In U. Kim & J. W. Berry (Eds.), *Indigenous psychologies: Research and experience in cultural context* (pp. 211–220). Newbury Park, CA: Sage.

Embretson, S. E., & McCollam, K. (2000). Psychometric approaches to the understanding and measurement of intelligence. In R. J. Sternberg (Ed.), *Handbook of intelligence* (pp. 423–444). New York: Cambridge University Press.

Eysenck, H. J. (1986). A theory of intelligence and the psychophysiology of cognition. In R. J. Sternberg (Ed.), *Advances in the psychology of human intelligence* (Vol. 3, pp. 1–34). Hillsdale, NJ: Erlbaum.

Feuerstein, R. (1979). *The dynamic assessment of retarded performers: The Learning Potential Assessment Device theory, instruments, and techniques.* Baltimore: University Park Press.

Fernández-Ballesteros, R., & Colom, R. (2004). The psychology of human intelligence in Spain. In R. J. Sternberg (Ed.), *International handbook of intelligence* (pp. 79–103). New York: Cambridge University Press.

Flynn, J. R. (1984). The mean IQ of Americans: Massive gains 1932 to 1978. *Psychological Bulletin, 95*, 29–51.

Flynn, J. R. (1987). Massive IQ gains in 14 nations. *Psychological Bulletin, 101*, 171–191.

Fraser, S. (Ed.). (1995). *The bell curve wars: Race, intelligence and the future of America.* New York: Basic Books.

Gardner, H. (1983). *Frames of mind: The theory of multiple intelligences.* New York: Basic Books.

Gill, R., & Keats, D. M. (1980). Elements of intellectual competence: Judgments by Australian and Malay university students. *Journal of Cross-Cultural Psychology, 11*, 233–243.

Gladwin, T. (1970). *East is a big bird.* Cambridge, MA: Harvard University Press.

Goodnow, J. J. (1962). A test of milieu effects with some of Piaget's tasks. *Psychological Monographs, 76*(serial No. 555).

Goodnow, J. J. (1969). Cultural variations in cognition skills. In D. R. Price-Williams (Ed.), *Cross-cultural studies* (pp. 246–264). Hardmondsworth, UK: Penguin.

Goodnow, J. J. (1976). The nature of intelligent behavior: Questions raised by cross-cultural studies. In L. Resnick (Ed.), *The nature of intelligence* (pp. 169–188). Hillsdale, NJ: Erlbaum.

Greenfield, P. M. (1997). You can't take it with you: Why abilities assessments don't cross cultures. *American Psychologist, 52*, 1115–1124.

Grigorenko, E. L. (2004). Is it possible to study intelligence without using the concept of intelligence?: An example from Soviet/Russian psychology. In R. J. Sternberg (Ed.), *International handbook of intelligence* (pp. 170–211). New York: Cambridge University Press.

Grigorenko, E. L., Geissler, P. W., Prince, R., Okatcha, F., Nokes, C., Kenny, D. A., et al. (2001). The organization of Luo conceptions of intelligence: A study of implicit theories in a Kenyan village. *International Journal of Behavior Development, 25*, 367–378.

Grigorenko, E. L, Meier, E., Lipka, J., Mohatt, G., Yanez, E., & Sternberg, R. J. (2004). The relationship between academic and practical intelligence: A case study of the tacit knowledge of Native American Yup'ik people in Alaska. *Learning and Individual Differences, 14*, 183–207.

Grigorenko, E. L., & Sternberg, R. J. (1998). Dynamic testing. *Psychological Bulletin, 124,* 75–111.

Grigorenko, E. L., & Sternberg, R. J. (2001). Analytical, creative, and practical intelligence as predictors of self-reported adaptive functioning: A case study in Russia. *Intelligence, 29,* 57–73.

Gulgoz, S., & Kağitçibaşi, C. (2004). Intelligence and intelligence testing in Turkey. In R. J. Sternberg (Ed.), *International handbook of intelligence* (pp. 248–269). New York: Cambridge University Press.

Guthke, J. (1993). Current trends in theories and assessment of intelligence. In J. H. M. Hamers, K. Sijtsma, & A. J. J. M. Ruijssenaars (Eds.), *Learning potential assessment* (pp. 13–20). Amsterdam: Swets & Zeitlinger.

Hadebe, S. (Ed.). (2001). *Isichamazwi.* Harare, Zimbabwe: College Press.

Hancock, T. (1999). The gender difference: Validity of standardized American tests in predicting MBA performance. *Journal of Education for Business, 75,* 91–94.

Haywood, H. C. & Tzuriel, D. (Eds.). (1992). *Interactive assessment.* New York: Springer-Verlag.

Helms-Lorenz, M., Van de Vijver, F. J. R., & Poortinga, Y. H. (2003). Cross-cultural differences in cognitive performance and Spearman's hypothesis: g or c? *Intelligence, 31,* 9–29.

Herrnstein, R., & Murray, C. (1994). *The bell curve.* New York: Free Press.

"Intelligence and its measurement": A symposium. (1921). *Journal of Educational Psychology, 12,* 123–147, 195–216, 271–275.

Irvine, J. T. (1978). "Wolof magical thinking": Culture and conservation revisited. *Journal of Cross-Cultural Psychology, 9,* 300–310.

Irvine, S. H. (1979). The place of factor analysis in cross-cultural methodology and its contribution to cognitive theory. In L. Eckensberger, W. Lonner, & Y. Poortinga (Eds.), *Cross-cultural contributions to psychology.* Amsterdam: Swets & Zeitlinger.

Irvine, S. H. (1988). Constructing the intellect of the Shona: A taxonomic approach. In J. W. Berry, S. H. Irvine, & E. B. Hunt (Eds.), *Indigenous cognitive functioning in a cultural context* (pp. 3–59). New York: Cambridge University Press.

Irvine, S. H., & Berry, J. W. (Eds.). (1983). *Human abilities in cultural context.* New York: Cambridge University Press.

Jensen, A. R. (1982). The chronometry of intelligence. In R. J. Sternberg (Ed.), *Advances in the psychology of human intelligence* (Vol. 1, pp. 255–310). Hillsdale, NJ: Erlbaum.

Jensen, A. R. (1998). *The g factor.* Westport, CT: Praeger-Greenwood.

Kağitçibaşi, Ç. (1996). *Family and human development across cultures: A view from the other side.* Mahwah, NJ: Erlbaum.

Kağitçibaşi, Ç., Sunar, D., & Bekman, S. (2001). Long-term effects of early intervention: Turkish low-income mothers and children. *Journal of Applied Developmental Psychology, 22,* 333–361.

Kaplan, K. (1997). Inteligencia, escuela y sociedad: Las categorias del juicio magisterial sbore la inteligencia [Intelligence, school, and society: The categories of the teachers' judgment about intelligence]. *Propuesta Educativa, 16,* 24–32.

Kaufman, A. S. (2000). Tests of intelligence. In R. J. Sternberg (Ed.), *Handbook of intelligence* (pp. 445–476). New York: Cambridge University Press.

Kaufman, A. S., & Lichtenberger, E. O. (1998). Intellectual assessment. In C. R. Reynolds (Ed.), *Comprehensive clinical psychology: Volume 4: Assessment* (pp. 203–238). Tarrytown, NY: Elsevier Science.

Kearins, J. M. (1981). Visual spatial memory in Australian Aboriginal children of desert regions. *Cognitive Psychology, 13,* 434–460.

Kroeber, A. L., & Kluckhohn, C. (1952). *Culture: A critical review of concepts and definitions.* Cambridge, MA: Peabody Museum.

Kugelmass, S., & Lieblich, A. (1975). *A developmental study of the Arab child in Israel: Scientific report* [Ford Foundation Grant 015.1261].

Kugelmass, S., Lieblich, A., & Bossik, D. (1974). Patterns of intellectual ability in Jewish and Arab children in Israel. *Journal of Cross-Cultural Psychology, 5,* 184–198.

Laboratory of Comparative Human Cognition. (1982). Culture and intelligence. In R. J. Sternberg (Ed.), *Handbook of human intelligence* (pp. 642–719). New York: Cambridge University Press.

Lautrey, J., & de Ribaupierre, A. (2004). Psychology of human intelligence in France and French-speaking Switzerland. In R. J. Sternberg (Ed.), *International handbook of intelligence* (pp. 104–134). New York: Cambridge University Press.

Lave, J. (1988). *Cognition in practice.* New York: Cambridge University Press.

Lidz, C. S. (1991). *Practitioner's guide to dynamic assessment.* New York: Guilford Press.

Lieblich, A. (1983). Intelligence patterns among ethnic and minority groups in Israel. In M. Nisan & U. Last (Eds.), *Between education and psychology* (pp. 335–357). Jerusalem: Magnes Press. (in Hebrew)

Lieblich, A., & Kugelmass, S. (1981). Patterns of intellectual ability of Arab school children in Israel. *Intelligence, 5,* 311–320.

Lin, C. T. (1980). A sketch on the methods of mental testing in ancient China. *Acta Psychological Sinica, 1,* 75–80. (in Chinese)

Loehlin, J. C. (2000). Group differences in intelligence. In R. J. Sternberg (Ed.), *Handbook of intelligence* (pp. 176–193). New York: Cambridge University Press.

Luria, A. R. (1976). Psychological expedition to central Asia. *Science, 74,* 383–384. (Original work published 1931)

Lutz, C. (1985). Ethnopsychology compared to what?: Explaining behaviour and consciousness among the Ifaluk. In G. M. White & J. Kirkpatrick (Eds.), *Per-*

son, self, and experience: Exploring Pacific ethnopsychologies (pp. 35–79). Berkeley: University of California Press.

Markus, H. R., & Kitayama, S. (1991). Culture and the self: Implications for cognition, emotion, and motivation. *Psychological Review, 98,* 224–253.

Marsella, A. J., Tharp, R., & Ciborowski, T. (Eds.). (1979). *Perspectives on cross-cultural psychology.* New York: Academic Press.

Matsumoto, D. (1994). *People: Psychology from a cultural perspective.* Pacific Grove, CA: Brooks/Cole.

Matsumoto, D. (1996). *Culture and psychology.* Pacific Grove, CA: Brooks/Cole.

Mead, M. (1928). *Coming of age in Samoa.* New York: Morrow.

Medin, D. L., & Atran, S. (Eds.). (1999). *Folkbiology.* Cambridge, MA: MIT Press.

Minkowitch, A., Davis, D., & Bashi, Y. (1982). *Success and failure in Israeli elementary education.* New Brunswick, NJ: Transaction.

Miyamoto, M. (1985). Parents' and children's beliefs and children's achievement and development. In R. Diaz-Guerrero (Ed.), *Cross-cultural and national studies in social psychology* (pp. 209–223). Amsterdam: Elsevier Science.

Mpofu, E. (1993). The context of mental testing and implications for psychoeducational practice in modern Zimbabwe. In W. Su (Ed.), *Proceedings of the second Afro-Asian psychological conference* (pp. 17–25). Beijing: University of Peking Press.

Mpofu, E. (2004). Intelligence in Zimbabwe. In R. J. Sternberg (Ed.), *International handbook of intelligence* (pp. 364–390). New York: Cambridge University Press.

Mundy-Castle, A. C. (1974). Social and technological intelligence in Western or Nonwestern cultures. *Universitas, 4,* 46–52.

Newell, A., & Simon, H. A. (1972). *Human problem solving.* Englewood Cliffs, NJ: Prentice Hall.

Nisbett, R. E. (2003). *The geography of thought: Why we think the way we do.* New York: Free Press.

Nuñes, T. (1994). Street intelligence. In R. J. Sternberg (Ed.), *Encyclopedia of human intelligence* (Vol. 2, pp. 1045–1049). New York: Macmillan.

Okagaki, L., & Sternberg, R. J. (1993). Parental beliefs and children's school performance. *Child Development, 64,* 36–56.

Poole, F. J. P. (1985). Coming into social being: Cultural images of infants in Bimin-Kuskusmin folk psychology. In G. M. White & J. Kirkpatrick (Eds.), *Person, self, and experience: Exploring Pacific ethnopsychologies* (pp. 183–244). Berkeley: University of California Press.

Prince, R. J., & Geissler P. W. (2001). Becoming "one who treats": A case study of a Luo healer and her grandson in western Kenya. *Educational Anthropology Quarterly, 32,* 447–471.

Putnam, D. B., & Kilbride, P. L. (1980). *A relativistic understanding of social intelligence among the Songhay of Mali and Smaia of Kenya.* Paper presented at the meeting of the Society for Cross-Cultural Research, Philadelphia, PA.

Raven, J. C., Court, J. H., & Raven, J. (1992). *Manual for Raven's Progressive Matrices and Mill Hill Vocabulary Scales.* Oxford, UK: Oxford Psychologists Press.

Rogoff, B. (1990). *Apprenticeship in thinking: Cognitive development in social context.* New York: Oxford University Press.

Rogoff, B. (2003). *The cultural nature of human development.* London: Oxford University Press.

Rosas, R. (2004). Intelligence research in Latin America. In R. J. Sternberg (Ed.), *International handbook of intelligence* (pp. 391–410). New York: Cambridge University Press.

Ruzgis, P. M., & Grigorenko, E. L. (1994). Cultural meaning systems, intelligence and personality. In R. J. Sternberg & P. Ruzgis (Eds.), *Personality and intelligence* (pp. 248–270). New York: Cambridge University Press.

Sarason, S. B., & Doris, J. (1979). *Educational handicap, public policy, and social history.* New York: Free Press.

Sato, T., Namiki, H., Ando, J., & Hatano, G. (2004). Japanese conception of and research on intelligence. In R. J. Sternberg (Ed.), *International handbook of intelligence* (pp. 302–324). New York: Cambridge University Press.

Savasir, L., & Sahin, N. (1995). *Wechsler Cocuklar icin Zeka Olcegi [Wechsler Intelligence Scale for Children].* Ankara: Turkish Psychological Association.

Saxe, G. B. (1990). *Culture and cognitive development: Studies in mathematical understanding.* Mahwah, NJ: Erlbaum.

Schliemann, A. D., & Magalhües, V. P. (1990). Proportional reasoning: From shops, to kitchens, laboratories, and, hopefully, schools. *Proceedings of the Fourteenth International Conference for the Psychology of Mathematics Education,* Oaxtepec, Mexico.

Scribner, S. (1984). Studying working intelligence. In B. Rogoff & J. Lave (Eds.), *Everyday cognition: Its development in social context* (pp. 9–40). Cambridge, MA: Harvard University Press.

Scribner, S. (1986). Thinking in action: Some characteristics of practical thought. In R. J. Sternberg & R. K. Wagner (Eds.), *Practical intelligence: Nature and origins of competence in the everyday world* (pp. 13–30). New York: Cambridge University Press.

Serpell, R. (1974). Aspects of intelligence in a developing country. *African Social Research, 17,* 576–596.

Serpell, R. (1979). How specific are perceptual skills? A cross-cultural study of pattern reproduction. *British Journal of Psychology, 70,* 365–380.

Serpell, R. (1996). Cultural models of childhood in indigenous socialization and formal schooling in Zambia. In C. P. Hwang & M. E. Lamb (Eds.), *Images of childhood* (pp. 129–142). Mahwah, NJ: Erlbaum.

Serpell, R. (2000). Intelligence and culture. In R. J. Sternberg (Ed.), *Handbook of intelligence* (pp. 549–580). New York: Cambridge University Press.

Shi, J. (2004). Diligence makes people smart: Chinese perspectives on intelligence. In R. J. Sternberg (Ed.), *International handbook of intelligence* (pp. 325–343). New York: Cambridge University Press.

Shweder, R. A. (1991). *Thinking through cultures: Multicultural expeditions in cultural psychology.* Cambridge, MA: Harvard University Press.

Shweder, R. A. (2002). *Engaging cultural differences: The multicultural challenge in liberal democracies.* New York: Russell Sage Foundation.

Spearman, C. (1927). *The abilities of man.* London: Macmillan.

Srivastava, S., & Misra, G. (1996). Changing perspectives on understanding intelligence: An appraisal. *Indian Psychological Abstracts and Reviews, 3.*

Srivastava, S., & Misra, G. (2000). *Culture and conceptualization of intelligence.* New Delhi: National Council of Educational Research and Training.

Stankov, L. (2004). Similar thoughts under different stars: Conceptions of intelligence in Australia. In R. J. Sternberg (Ed.), *International handbook of intelligence* (pp. 344–363). New York: Cambridge University Press.

Sternberg, R. J. (1985). *Beyond IQ: A triarchic theory of human intelligence.* New York: Cambridge University Press.

Sternberg, R. J. (1988). A triarchic view of intelligence in cross-cultural perspective. In S. H. Irvine & J. W. Berry (Eds.), *Human abilities in cultural context* (pp. 60–85). New York: Cambridge University Press.

Sternberg, R. J. (1990). *Metaphors of mind.* New York: Cambridge University Press.

Sternberg, R. J. (1997). *Successful intelligence.* New York: Plume.

Sternberg, R. J. (1999a). Intelligence as developing expertise. *Contemporary Educational Psychology, 24,* 359–375.

Sternberg, R. J. (1999b). The theory of successful intelligence. *Review of General Psychology, 3,* 292–316.

Sternberg, R. J. (2000). The holey grail of general intelligence. *Science, 289,* 399–401.

Sternberg, R. J. (2003a). What is an expert student? *Educational Researcher, 32*(8), 5–9.

Sternberg, R. J. (2003b). *Wisdom, intelligence, and creativity, synthesized.* New York: Cambridge University Press.

Sternberg, R. J. (2004a). Culture and intelligence. *American Psychologist, 59,* 325–338.

Sternberg, R. J. (Ed.). (2004b). *International handbook of intelligence.* New York: Cambridge University Press.

Sternberg, R. J. (2004c). North American approaches to intelligence. In R. J. Sternberg (Ed.), *International handbook of intelligence* (pp. 411–444). New York: Cambridge University Press.

Sternberg, R. J., Conway, B. E., Ketron, J. L., & Bernstein, M. (1981). People's conceptions of intelligence. *Journal of Personality and Social Psychology, 41,* 37–55.

Sternberg, R. J., & Detterman, D. K. (1986). *What is intelligence?* Norwood, NJ: Ablex.

Sternberg, R. J., Forsythe, G. B., Hedlund, J., Horvath, J., Snook, S., Williams, W. M., et al. (2000). *Practical intelligence in everyday life.* New York: Cambridge University Press.

Sternberg, R. J., & Grigorenko, E. L. (Eds.). (1997). *Intelligence, heredity, and environment.* New York: Cambridge University Press.

Sternberg, R. J., & Grigorenko, E. L. (2002). Just because we "know" it's true doesn't mean it's really true: A case study in Kenya. *Psychological Science Agenda, 15*(2), 8–10.

Sternberg, R. J., Grigorenko, E. L., Ngrosho, D., Tantufuye, E., Mbise, A., Nokes, C., et al. (2002). Assessing intellectual potential in rural Tanzanian school children. *Intelligence, 30,* 141–162.

Sternberg, R. J., & Kaufman J. C. (1998). Human abilities. *Annual Review of Psychology, 49,* 479–502.

Sternberg, R. J., Nokes, K., Geissler, P. W., Prince, R., Okatcha, F., Bundy, D. A., et al. (2001). The relationship between academic and practical intelligence: A case study in Kenya. *Intelligence, 29,* 401–418.

Sternberg, R. J., Powell, C., McGrane, P. A., & McGregor, S. (1997). Effects of a parasitic infection on cognitive functioning. *Journal of Experimental Psychology: Applied, 3,* 67–76.

Sternberg, R. J., & Suben, J. (1986). The socialization of intelligence. In M. Perlmutter (Ed.), *Perspectives on intellectual development: Vol. 19. Minnesota Symposia on Child Psychology* (pp. 201–235). Hillsdale, NJ: Erlbaum.

Stevenson, H. W., & Stigler, J. W. (1994). *The learning gap: Why our schools are failing and what we can learn from Japanese and Chinese education.* New York: Simon & Schuster.

Stigler, J. W., Lee, S., Lucker, G. W., & Stevenson, H. W. (1982). Curriculum and achievement in mathematics: A study of elementary school children in Japan, Taiwan, and the United States. *Journal of Educational Psychology, 74,* 315–322.

Super, C. M. (1976). Environmental effects on motor development: The case of African infant precocity. *Developmental Medicine and Child Neurology, 18,* 561–567.

Super, C. M., & Harkness, S. (1982). The development of affect in infancy and early childhood. In D. Wagner & H. Stevenson (Eds.), *Cultural perspectives on child development* (pp. 1–19). San Francisco: Freeman.

Super, C. M., & Harkness, S. (1986). The developmental niche: A conceptualization at the interface of child and culture. *International Journal of Behavioral Development, 9,* 545–569.

Super, C. M., & Harkness, S. (1993). The developmental niche: A conceptualization at the interface of child and culture. In R. A. Pierce & M. A. Black (Eds.), *Life-span development: A diversity reader* (pp. 61–77). Dubuque, IA: Kendall/Hunt.

Thurstone, L. L. (1924). *The nature of intelligence.* New York: Harcourt Brace.

Thurstone, L. L. (1938). *Primary mental abilities.* Chicago: University of Chicago Press.

Tomasello, M. (1999). *The cultural origins of human cognition.* Cambridge, MA: Harvard University Press.

Tzuriel, D. (1995). *Dynamic-interactive assessment: The legacy of L. S. Vygotsky and current developments.* Unpublished manuscript, Bar-Ilan University, Jerusalem, Israel.

Vernon, P. E. (1969). *Intelligence and cultural environment.* London: Methuen.

Vernon, P. E. (1971). *The structure of human abilities.* London: Methuen.

Vygotsky, L. S. (1978). *Mind in society: The development of higher psychological processes.* Cambridge, MA: Harvard University Press.

Wagner, D. A. (1978). Memories of Morocco: The influence of age, schooling, and environment on memory. *Cognitive Psychology, 10,* 1–28.

White, G. M. (1985). Premises and purposes in a Solomon Islands ethnopsychology. In G. M. White & J. Kirkpatrick (Eds.), *Person, self, and experience: Exploring Pacific ethnopsychologies* (pp. 328–366). Berkeley: University of California Press.

Yan, Z. (2001). *Yan's family rules—Piece of conduct.* In Chinese classic books series (multimedia version). Beijing: Beijing Yinguan Electronic Publishing. (in Chinese)

Yang, S.-Y. (2001). Conceptions of wisdom among Taiwanese Chinese. *Journal of Cross-Cultural Psychology, 32,* 662–680.

Yang, S.-Y., & Sternberg, R. J. (1997a). Conceptions of intelligence in ancient Chinese philosophy. *Journal of Theoretical and Philosophical Psychology, 17,* 101–119.

Yang, S.-Y., & Sternberg, R. J. (1997b). Taiwanese Chinese people's conceptions of intelligence. *Intelligence, 25,* 21–36.

Zeidner, M. (1985). A cross-cultural test of the situational bias hypothesis—the Israeli scene. *Evaluation and Program Planning, 8,* 367–376.

Zeidner, M., Matthews, G., & Roberts, R. D. (2004). Intelligence theory, assessment, and research: The Israeli experience. In R. J. Sternberg (Ed.), *International handbook of intelligence* (pp. 212–247). New York: Cambridge University Press.

CHAPTER 23

Perception and Cognition

ARA NORENZAYAN
INCHEOL CHOI
KAIPING PENG

For more than a century, most psychologists have based their discussions of human thinking on the cardinal assumption that basic cognitive processes are the same for all normal adult human beings, whether in the plains of Central Asia, the villages of East Africa, or the urban centers of Europe and North America. Cultural differences influence the content of minds, or the domains of thinking to which cognitive strategies are applied. For example, children in the Amazon might categorize snake varieties with the same interest that children in suburban America categorize video game varieties. Although *what* people think about varies considerably across cultures, the very *habits of thought*—the information processing strategies that people use recurrently to know the world around them—have been assumed to be the same everywhere.

Several historical developments in psychology have conspired to uphold cognitive universality as a foundational assumption in much of theorizing and research. First, the origins of psychology have been profoundly influenced by biology (Benjamin, 1988), leading to an assumption of universality in at least two respects: Much research on the biological basis of human psychology is conducted analogically in

other species. But if we begin with the view that humans in one culture share psychological mechanisms with other species, it follows that these same psychological mechanisms are assumed to be shared universally within humans themselves. Furthermore, to the extent psychology is grounded in biology, it inherits the theoretical foundation of evolutionary theory as well (Barkow, Cosmides, & Tooby, 1992; Pinker, 1997). Because evolutionary reasoning depends on the assumption of a shared, species-wide genome, this theoretical foundation encourages psychologists to accept psychic unity as a given rather than as a testable hypothesis. Learning theorists who influenced much of early experimental psychology in the mid-20th century also believed they were looking at mechanisms that applied not only to all humans but also to most other animals. The cognitive revolution, from its earliest development until nearly the end of the 20th century, rejected the learning theorists' behaviorism yet embraced the same universalistic position that was undoubtedly encouraged by the analogy between the human mind and the computer: Brain equaled hardware, cognitive procedures equaled operating principles and native software (Block, 1995). Because the "inputs" could be radically different across cultures given variation in ecological and social conditions, "outputs" in the form of beliefs and behaviors would also be radically different, without affecting the underlying cognitive architecture of the mind.

As the anthropologist Richard Shweder has observed, the major theoretical stances in 20th-century psychology presumed a "central processing device. The processor, it is imagined, stands over and above, or transcends, all the stuff upon which it operates. It engages all the stuff of culture, context, task and stimulus materials as its content" (1991, p. 80). But the idea of an autonomous "central processing device" that transcends ecology and context did not always dominate the landscape of psychology. Three major theoretical positions with a long history in psychology and the social sciences proposed that human thinking is profoundly attuned to the sociocultural contexts in which it naturally occurs.

The first challenge originated in none other than Wilhelm Wundt (1916), regarded as the founder of experimental psychology, who held the view that higher cognitive functions were affected by cultural practices, and that when cultures and histories diverged, cognitive processes also diverged. Thus, he proposed a cultural psychology that he termed *völkerpsychologie* or "folk psychology" to complement experimental psychology:

> [Folk psychology's] . . . problem relates to those mental products which are created by a community of human life [e.g., language, religion] and are, therefore, inexplicable in terms merely of individual consciousness, since they presuppose the reciprocal actions of many. . . . Individual consciousness is wholly incapable of giving us a history of the development of human thought, for it is conditioned by an earlier history concerning which it cannot in itself give us any knowledge. (p. 3)

A second significant early idea that culture fundamentally shapes thought was that of the influential Russian School of Lev Vygotsky (1978) and Alexander Luria (1971), and their associates in the West, including especially Michael Cole and his colleagues (e.g., Cole, 1996; Cole & Scribner, 1974). The Russian School continues to influence a wide range of contemporary research on culture and cognition (Cole & Hatano, Chapter 5, this volume; Hutchins, 1995; Lave & Wenger, 1991; Resnick, 1994;

Rogoff, 1990). According to Vygotsky, human cognition develops in a cultural context, which is the accumulated pattern of symbolic and nonsymbolic tool use throughout the historical existence of a group. To the extent that societies diverge in their historical trajectories, different activities and tools that become available then give rise to different cognitive tendencies.

A third influential idea elaborating the notion that culture influences thought has captured far more sustained attention in psychology and the social sciences than those of Wundt and possibly Vygotsky. The linguistic relativity hypothesis (Whorf, 1956) contends that the particular language people speak affects their thought processes. Given that linguistic conventions vary greatly across cultures, cognitive processes would also vary as a result.

As Tomasello has argued (1999), the idea that human cognition is fundamentally cultural can be understood in the context of an apparent puzzle in human evolutionary history. Humans are genetically highly similar to their primate relatives and, not surprisingly, share with them most of their basic cognitive repertoire. But superimposed on these similarities, humans distinctively possess a vast network of complex cognitive skills involving symbolic communication and complex reasoning skills, as well as elaborate tool use technologies, that are unprecedented in higher primate cognition. The puzzle is that these distinctive features of cognition and behavior emerged very recently, possibly no earlier than about 250,000 years ago (Foley & Lahr, 1997). Simply put, it is unlikely that so many of these human-specific sets of cognitive abilities arose by the usual slow processes of genetic variation and natural selection in such a short timescale. Rather, such rapid changes in cognition could be explained by the emergence of the evolutionarily novel human ability for transmitted culture that operates much faster than genetic transmission (Richerson & Boyd, 2005; Sperber, 1996). Cultural transmission allows information to be passed on not only genetically but also socially, through social learning mechanisms such as mimicry, imitation, instruction (Tomasello, Kruger, & Ratner, 1993), as well as by-products of communicative processes, such as gossip, conversations, and storytelling (Schaller, 2001). Thus, unlike the case of other primates, human children make use of a richly structured cultural context as they develop; this context channels their innate cognitive capacities in new directions and subsequently alters their behavior and cognition in profound ways (Norenzayan, Schaller, & Heine, 2006).

Human cognition is therefore culturally dependent in ways that other primate cognition is not. This dependence gives rise to cultural variation in cognition for two reasons. Human groups occupy vastly different ecological niches (Edgerton, 1971) that may evoke different cognitive habits to solve the same problems of human existence, and as a result, their social and psychological practices also diverge in response to the local conditions (D. Cohen, 2001). Moreover, the cognitive capacities that enable cultural transmission, such as imitation, are biased toward ingroup members, also encouraging the emergence of stable cultural variation (Henrich & Boyd, 1998).

This chapter reviews evidence concerning the assumption of universality of cognitive and perceptual processes (see Choi, Choi, & Norenzayan, 2004, for a review of cultural variation in judgment and decision making, not discussed in this chapter). The cross-cultural evidence reveals marked cultural differences in the cognitive strategies, or habits of thought, recruited to solve a given cognitive problem. Although researchers are only beginning to understand the mediating processes by which cultural experiences shape thinking, these cultural differences are likely tied to different construals of the self, ecological differences in visual environments, assumptions about the nature of the world, beliefs about the origins of knowledge, linguistic conventions, expertise or familiarity with certain domains of life but not others, and social practices that promote some cognitive strategies at the expense of others.

We focus on cultural variation in domain-general reasoning and perceptual processes, such as visual perception, attention, rule-based reasoning, exemplar-based classification, numerical reasoning, spatial reasoning, and perceptions of change. We do not examine the growing literature on cross-cultural regularity and variation in domain-specific reasoning. There are substantial regularities in some of the ways that people organize their perceptual and conceptual worlds, and these characteristic patterns are often observable from a very early age. The most convincing evidence deals with infants' understanding of the physical world (Baillargeon, 1995; Spelke, 1990; Spelke, Phillips, & Woodward, 1995), reasoning about biological entities across cultures by adults and

children (Berlin, Breedlove, & Raven, 1973; Medin, Unsworth, & Hirschfield, Chapter 25, this volume; Medin & Atran, 2004), and children's understanding of mental life across cultures (Avis & Harris, 1991; Callaghan et al., 2005; but see Lillard, 1998). For discussions of the cross-cultural evidence for domain-specific reasoning, see Atran, 1998; Atran, Medin, and Ross, 2005; Callaghan et al., 2005; Medin et al., Chapter 25, this volume; Medin and Atran, 2004; Nisbett and Norenzayan, 2002; Wellman, Cross, and Watson, 2001.

THE LINGUISTIC RELATIVITY HYPOTHESIS

The notion that cultural experiences influence thought is famously illustrated in the linguistic relativity, or Whorfian, hypothesis (Whorf, 1956), or the idea that the particular language people speak affects thought. After a period of intellectual stagnation and inconsistent results, a recent surge of systematic and compelling studies have examined and found some degree of support for this hypothesis (e.g., Levinson, 1996; Roberson, Davies, & Davidoff, 2000), although the precise psychological implications of these studies continue to be debated in the literature (e.g., Boroditsky, 2003; Levinson, Kita, Haun, & Rasch, 2002; Li & Gleitman, 2002; Gelman & Gallistel, 2004).

In an early attempt, Berlin and Kay (1969) examined color classification across cultures. They found that color names are assigned in terms of an orderly hierarchy. In the few cultures where there are only two color names, these are black and white. If a third color is added, it is red. The next three color terms are likely to be yellow, blue, and green, and so forth. Berlin and Kay also concluded that though boundaries of color terms vary across cultures and languages, the focal point of each basic color (e.g., the most prototypical red in an array of reds) is essentially the same. The work of Berlin and Kay has been interpreted to indicate that there is a universal, physiological basis to color classification.

The pioneering work of Heider and Oliver (1972; and subsequently Rosch) supported Berlin and Kay's analysis. Working with Dani tribesmen in New Guinea, whose language has only two basic color terms, Heider and Olivier showed color chips to Dani and English speakers, and then tested for recognition of the chips a few seconds later. Using this procedure, memory for color was largely independent of color vocabulary and, consistent with the proposal of Berlin and Kay, focal colors resulted in better memory than nonfocal colors for both English speakers (Americans) and the Dani. This work generally has been taken as clear evidence against the linguistic relativity hypothesis. However, it has been criticized on methodological grounds for its narrow scope and for lack of subsequent studies confirming the findings of the original studies with other tasks or linguistic groups (Hunt & Agnoli, 1991; Lucy, 1997; Lucy & Shweder, 1979; Saunders & van Brakel, 1997).

More recently, new research has emerged that questions the findings of Heider and Olivier (1972), and offers new evidence for the influence of linguistic color terms on color perception and memory. Roberson et al. (2000) sought to replicate and extend the original studies of Heider and Olivier (1972) with the Berinmo of Papua New Guinea, a hunter–gatherer people whose language has only five color terms. In a series of experiments, they found convergent lines of evidence for linguistic relativity in color perception and memory. Berinmo patterns of naming and memory were statistically more similar to each other than Berinmo memory was to English memory patterns; the recognition advantage for focal colors relative to nonfocal ones disappeared for both English speakers and Berinmo speakers when response bias was controlled for; category learning for focal versus nonfocal colors did not differ. These findings indicate that the Berinmo do not have an underlying cognitive organization of color that favors the foci of the eight English basic chromatic color categories (with the possible exception of focal red). Furthermore, Berinmo speakers' performance in color categorization was considerably poorer than that of English speakers, replicating Heider and Olivier's finding with the Dani. This was despite the fact that Berinmo and English speakers did not differ in a similar visual–spatial memory task that did not involve the color domain. This suggests that the poorer memory performance of the Dani and the Berinmo could be explained by their poorer color vocabularies rather than unfamiliarity with a formal test situation or lack of formal education, as Heider and Olivier suggested.

A recent effort to examine the linguistic relativity hypothesis in number marking was carried out by Lucy and his colleagues (Lucy, 1997; Lucy & Gaskins, 1997). Following an early study by Carroll and Casagrande (1958), they examined the extent to which linguistic differences in number marking affect thought. Yucatec Maya and many other languages (e.g., Chinese, Japanese) differ from English in number-marking patterns. In English, discrete shape is implicitly emphasized in many nouns. Therefore, English numerals directly modify their associated noun without shape information. In Yucatec, however, substance is implicitly emphasized in nouns, and Yucatec numerals are always accompanied by a numeral classifier that describes essential shape information needed to count the object. Does this differential emphasis on shape versus substance lead to different patterns of categorizing objects? In nonverbal classification tasks, participants were presented with a triad of objects that differed on substance or on shape (e.g., plastic box, cardboard box, a piece of cardboard). Consistent with the lexical structures of these two languages, Yucatec speakers showed a preference for material-based classification (cardboard box, cardboard), whereas English speakers showed a preference for shape-based classification (plastic box, cardboard box).

The effects of mathematical symbols on numerical reasoning (Dehaene, 1997) have been examined by K. F. Miller, Smith, Zhu, and Zhang (1995; see also K. F. Miller & Stigler, 1987). An interesting difference between the Chinese and English languages is that for certain blocks of numbers (especially the 10–20 block), the base-10 structure is less obvious in English than it is in Chinese. Does this structural difference between the two languages affect the way children learn to count? The answer is yes. The authors examined the development of counting in 3- to 5-year-old Chinese and American children. Results revealed a complex pattern of similarities and differences in number acquisition that indeed reflected the structural differences of English and Chinese counting systems. No differences in learning to count were found from 1 to 10, for which both cultures rely on rote learning and not-base-10 principles. But a difference emerged, favoring Chinese children, for counting in the second decade (10–20), where base-10 principles are first learned, and where Chinese has simpler and more consistent names for 10–20 that are more consistent with base-10 principles. No cultural differences were found for counting from 20 to 99, where both Chinese and English converge on a common structure of number names. Finally, no cultural differences were found in tasks consisting of object counting and simple mathematical problem solving. Thus, the cultural differences selectively emerged only when the structural differences in number naming were implicated in the number acquisition task.

Whether linguistic differences in counting systems affect numerical reasoning has been investigated in a more dramatic fashion among small-scale cultures that do not have an elaborate number marking system. In a recent study, Gordon (2004) examined reasoning among the Piraha, an Amazonian group that has a one–two–many counting system (see also Pica, Lerner, Izard, & Dehaene, 2004, for a similar study and similar results with the Munduruku of the Amazon). Two main findings emerged. First, counting tasks with varying cognitive demands showed that performance with quantities greater than three were poor. For example, Piraha speakers were shown an array of familiar items (e.g., sticks), and asked to match these items with the equivalent number of other familiar items (e.g., nuts). Results showed that Piraha speakers had great difficulty matching an array of items if the array contained more than three items.

Second, despite their poor counting performance for numbers that are not available in the Piraha counting system, participants' estimation errors in assessing the quantity of objects reflected a constant coefficient of variation; that is, the amount of error increased as a function of the magnitude of the target size. The ratio of this average error to the target size is a constant, suggesting adequate estimation of quantity. Piraha speakers' coefficient of variation was identical to that of English speakers. This indicates that Piraha speakers were sensitive to quantity, were trying hard to get the answers correct, but were insensitive to exactitude of numbers larger than three.

There is growing consensus in the literature that numerical thinking relies on two independent cognitive strategies: One is a primitive "analog" number sense that is sensitive to quantity but is limited in accuracy. This cognitive ability is independent of counting practices, can be shown to operate in human infants, and is shared by other nonlinguistic higher primates (e.g., Dehaene, 1997). Second, human infants appear to have a cognitive ability that is sensitive to the exactitude of small numbers, possibly up to about three items. But it is only with the emergence of linguistically coded counting systems and cultural practices of counting that children in some cultures are able to count with exactitude numbers larger than three (for other interpretations, see Carey, 2004; Gelman & Gallistel, 2004).

Another line of research, by Levinson (1996) focuses on linguistic variation in the coding of spatial location. Speakers of English and other Indo-European languages favor the use of body coordinates to represent the location of objects in relative terms (e.g., "The man is on the right of the house"). In contrast, other languages such as Guugu Yiimithirr (an Australian language) and Tzeltal (a Mayan language) favor absolute reference in fixed cardinal direction terms ("The man is west of the house"). Is this difference in linguistic convention implicated in cognition? Levinson and colleagues have examined this question in their program of research. In one study, they created nonlinguistic tasks that measured performance in locating objects and manipulated the sensitivity of the two spatial referent systems to rotation. As expected, speakers of Guugu Yiimithirr were unaffected by the rotation manipulation in locating objects accurately. English speakers, in contrast, were thrown off by the same rotation manipulation, being less accurate in locating the objects. In another study, Dutch and Tzeltal speakers were seated at a table and shown an arrow pointing either to the right (north) or to the left (south). They were then rotated 180° to a second table where they saw two arrows: one pointing to the left (north) and the other one pointing to the right (south). Participants were asked which arrow on the second table was like the one they saw before. Consistent with the spatial marking system of their languages, Dutch speakers chose the relative solution, whereas the Tzeltal speakers chose the absolute solution. Subsequent research has shown that contextual manipulations can induce English speakers to reason according to absolute spatial reference (Li & Gleitman, 2002). However this is not surprising given that cardinal location terms, although not salient, do exist in the English language. What is important is that habitual ways of reasoning are systematically related to the dominant ways of talking about space in a given culture.

Linguistic differences may affect reasoning not only about space but also about time. In

English, for example, time is discussed in *horizontal* terms, for example, when one says, "We are behind schedule," or "Let's move the meeting forward." In Mandarin, on the other hand, time is talked about in *vertical* terms: Earlier events are said to be *shàng* or "up," and later events are said to be *xià* or "down." In a series of experiments, Boroditsky (2001) investigated whether thinking about time is affected by this linguistic difference. In one study, English and Mandarin bilinguals were shown fish swimming either vertically or horizontally on a computer screen. Then participants were asked questions about time, such as "Does March come earlier or later than April?" Mandarin speakers were faster to confirm that March comes earlier than April after seeing the vertical movement of fish (which is consistent with the Mandarin linguistic coding of time), whereas English speakers showed the reverse pattern. Interestingly, another study showed that English speakers could be explicitly taught to think of time vertically, which then resulted in patterns of thinking characteristic of Mandarin speakers.

A well-known experimental attempt to test a linguistic relativity hypothesis is Alfred Bloom's (1981) work on counterfactual or hypothetical reasoning. Bloom noticed that the English language has an explicit linguistic device to code counterfactuals (the subjunctive mode; e.g., "If I were rich, I would travel the world"). Not so in the Chinese language, which instead expresses counterfactual meaning by relying on context, combined with the use of if . . . then statements. In a series of studies, Bloom gave English and Chinese speakers, as well as Chinese–English bilinguals, controlled counterfactual stories, and found that Chinese speakers did more poorly than English speakers in counterfactual reasoning. However, Au (1983) and L. G. Liu (1985) have criticized Bloom's work, raising questions about the accuracy of the Chinese translations of the stories. Furthermore, there is little doubt that Chinese are capable of counterfactual reasoning in everyday life. The question, then, is whether the presence or absence of a simple linguistic device to mark counterfactuals facilitates or discourages counterfactual reasoning (Hunt & Agnoli, 1991). As we see later, a case may be made that hypothetical reasoning is less prevalent in Chinese culture than among Westerners, though for reasons that may have more to do with factors other than differences in grammatical categories.

To summarize, after an initial period of mixed findings, growing evidence appears to favor the contention that linguistic differences affect thought. Although the strong version of the Whorfian hypothesis—that thinking is entirely determined by the particular language spoken in a community—has long been abandoned, less strong versions of the hypothesis have received empirical support in a variety of cognitive domains. Linguistic differences may result in habitually different ways of thinking, because different languages force their speakers to attend to strikingly different aspects of the world (Slobin, 1996). Although there are ongoing debates and controversies in this burgeoning new area of research (Hunt & Agnoli, 1991; Li & Gleitman, 2002; Gelman & Gallistel, 2004; Levinson et al., 2002), solid evidence has been found for the cognitive effect of linguistic differences in the coding of spatial location (Levinson, 1996), color categories (Roberson et al., 2000), and numerical reasoning (Gordon, 2004; K. F. Miller & Paredes, 1996; Pica et al., 2004). The work supporting linguistic relativity has profound implications for cognitive psychology and, more specifically, for the cultural mediation of thought. To the extent that societies have diverged in their linguistic conventions, so would cognitive processes, to some degree. Clearly, however, more research is needed to examine the pervasiveness of the influence of language on thought. Furthermore, the tools of experimental psychology can be profitably used to examine in more systematic detail the cognitive processes that mediate the linguistic shaping of thought. Finally, it is important to distinguish linguistic effects from other cultural effects on thought, for example, effects due to social practices, beliefs, or expertise in a domain. This is particularly challenging given that nonlinguistic cultural patterns and linguistic conventions tend to be confounded within the same populations.

DEDUCTIVE REASONING IN TRADITIONAL NONLITERATE SOCIETIES

According to the Vygotsky (1978), human cognition develops in a species-specific medium, that of culture, or the accumulated pattern of symbolic and nonsymbolic tool use of a social group. The various social activities that a child engages in interact with primitive, biologically given cognitive structures. The child gradually internalizes these social activities and develops ever more complex cognitive structures. Cultural variation in cognition emerges to the extent that societies experience different historical developments, which then lead to different social activities and tools, which in turn afford different thought processes that are congruent with the particular historical trajectories of societies.

A pioneering attempt to study how cultural–historical factors transform thought processes was an expedition to Central Asia by Luria (1971) in the early 1930s. The purpose of this project was to examine the effects of massive social and economic reforms in remote regions of Central Asia on the logical reasoning of Uzbek peasants. Luria presented simple syllogisms in a quasi-experimental format to four groups of people at different degrees of modernization: nonliterate women in remote villages, who did not participate in formal economic practices; nonliterate men engaged in traditional farming; young activists involved in collective farming (some of whom were minimally literate); and women attending teacher training schools (Scribner, 1977). If logical reasoning is a universal property of the mind that is impervious to historical changes, then no differences in logical reasoning would be observed among these four groups. However, to the extent that cognitive structures are transformed by historical change in socioeconomic and educational conditions, greater exposure to modernization would lead to more reliance on formal logic.

Luria (1971) found marked variation in logical reasoning. The strongest results emerged for syllogisms with contents *unfamiliar* to the villagers. Villagers living traditional lives had the most difficulty with problems that did not conform to their everyday experience, suggesting that their responses were driven by a concrete, knowledge-based approach to reasoning. In some extreme cases, this pattern led to the refusal of some individuals to engage in the logical reasoning task at all, on the grounds that the contents of the problems were unfamiliar, making the problem in principle unanswerable. For example, to one of Luria's unfamiliar problems—"In the far north all bears are white. Novaya Zemyla is in the far north.

What colors are the bears there?"—one participant responded, "But I don't know what kind of bears are there. I have not been there and I don't know. Look, why don't you ask old man X, he was there and he knows, he will tell you." (p. 271). In contrast, the same unfamiliar problems posed no difficulty to those who had some exposure to schooling.

Several studies on logical reasoning in traditional versus industrialized societies followed the Central Asian investigation by Luria. Most notable are studies conducted with the Kpelle and Vai in West Africa (Cole, Gay, Glick, & Sharp, 1971; Scribner, 1975; Scribner, 1977), as well as with Maya- and Spanish-speaking villagers in Yucatán, Mexico (Sharp & Cole, 1975, cited in Scribner, 1977). Several interesting conclusions can be drawn from the findings of Luria and these more recent studies. First, logical reasoning seems to be facilitated by Western-style schooling. Increases in performance are detected in people with 2–3 years of schooling. Second, when people are matched by age and schooling, there is little systematic cultural variation in performance among different nonliterate cultures. However, performance in such cultures is somewhat lower than that in comparable industrialized populations, such as the United States. Finally, the most important generalization is that the characteristic reasoning pattern in traditional societies is a preference for concrete thinking based on direct personal knowledge. Experimental evidence, as well as ethnographic accounts of everyday life, show that the low solution rates do not betray an absence of logical reasoning ability. Rather they indicate an unwillingness to *play the game of logic with the experimenter*, which dictates a hypothetical stance that is often inconsistent with personal knowledge. This fact is evident when the villagers are asked to justify their responses. Justifications overwhelmingly appeal to direct personal knowledge external to the logical problem itself. In the rare cases when people do mention the structure of the argument in their justifications, performance is high. This is true across individuals, as well as for each individual. Thus, whenever an individual agrees to play by the rules of logic, the capacity for logical reasoning with simple syllogisms is impeccable (Scribner, 1977).

However, as will become clear later in this chapter, this preference for concrete reasoning is not limited to nonliterate societies. Highly educated, industrialized East Asian samples in China and Korea also are more likely than comparable Western samples to favor concrete, intuitive, knowledge-based reasoning. Thus, the preference for formal logical reasoning prevalent in Western cultures may be only partly the result of the introduction of modern institutions such as industrialization. Other cultural factors that historically have been tied to the Western intellectual tradition, such as adversarial debate, contractual relationships, theoretical science, and formalization of knowledge, may account for the development of formal logical reasoning as a rhetorical system central to these activities (Becker, 1986; Lloyd, 1990; Nisbett, Peng, Choi, & Norenzayan, 2001).

CULTURAL DIFFERENCES IN PERCEPTION

Whereas Vygotsky and Luria examined higher level reasoning processes, other cross-cultural researchers have looked at whether the cultural environment affects perceptual processes. Segall, Campbell, and Herskovits (1966) investigated cultural differences in visual perception, particularly visual illusions. Here we focus on their findings regarding the famous Müller–Lyer illusion. Visual perception is a richly structured cognitive capacity with which every normal-sighted human being is biologically endowed. However, these biologically given visual processes may interact with the ecological properties of the external world, and learned habits of visual inference may be formed as a result of such dependence on ecological regularities. But to the extent that the ecological conditions in which people live diverge, culturally different habits of inference may emerge, even if the biological potential for vision is the same everywhere. Because people in the same cultural group share more or less the same ecological milieu, this question can best be answered by examining natural variation in ecological conditions across human cultures.

Segall et al. (1966) investigated this question, focusing on one ecological variable—the degree to which the visual environment is carpentered. They proposed the "carpentered world hypothesis." According to this idea, in industrialized cultures with a pervasive carpentered environment where right angles abound, people internalize several related perceptual tendencies: to interpret nonrectangular figures as rectangular, to perceive figures in perspective, and to interpret them as two-dimensional representations of three-dimensional objects. These tendencies should enhance the susceptibility to some visual illusions, including the Müller–Lyer illusion (see Figure 23.1). Segall et al. predicted that people in carpentered environments should be more susceptible to this illusion than people in noncarpentered environments. Over a 6-year period, psychologists and anthropologists administered visual tests that included European and North American samples, as well as samples in several African societies and the Philippines. The results supported the hypothesis: Although the susceptibility to the illusion was found across cultures, the average susceptibility to the Müller–Lyer illusion increased as a linear function of the degree to which the environment is carpentered. Subsequent research (Stewart van Leeuwen, 1973) showed that African school-age children in Zambia, who lived in an urban, carpentered environment, showed more susceptibility to the illusion than did children in a rural, uncarpentered region of Zambia.

Perceptual differences between urban industrialized groups and traditional populations have also been found by Witkin and Berry (1975). In this case, however, some traditional populations are more similar to industrialized groups than to other traditional populations. Witkin and his colleagues demonstrated that there are substantial individual differences in the extent to which people "differentiate" or decontextualize an object from the field in which it appears (Witkin, Dyk, Faterson, Goodenough, & Karp, 1974; Witkin et al., 1954). People who do this readily are "field independent" and people who do so with more

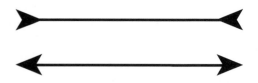

FIGURE 23.1. The Müller–Lyer illusion. Participants are asked to decide whether one of the two horizontal lines is longer than the other (in fact, they are exactly the same length). The angles-out version (top) is judged to be longer than the angles-in version (bottom).

difficulty are "field dependent." They had a number of tests to examine field dependence including the embedded figures test, which shows people's ability to separate a simple object from a more complex background, and the rod and frame test. In the latter test, participants look into a long box, at the end of which is a rod surrounded by a frame. The participant's task is to indicate when the rod is vertical. The rod and the frame can be tilted independently of one another. Field dependence is indicated by the extent to which the position of the frame influences judgments about the position of the rod.

Whereas Segall et al. (1966) examined the role of the physical environment, Witkin and his colleagues proposed that field dependence is in part the result of a social orientation toward people. An outward orientation toward the social environment encourages an orientation toward the field in general. Witkin and Berry (1975) found substantial cross-cultural differences in field dependence. Farmers who live in societies where they must coordinate their actions with others were found to be more field dependent than were people who hunt and gather, or herd animals for a living. The latter sorts of livelihoods require less coordination with the actions of others, and social, political, and economic role relations tend to be relatively simple. Industrialized peoples have levels of field dependence comparable to those of mobile hunter-gatherers and herders. Like mobile peoples, industrialized peoples have more freedom in their lives and relative simplicity in role relations. There is also experimental evidence that these different orientations cause different perceptual tendencies. Kühnen, Hannover, and Schubert (2001) temporarily induced independent versus interdependent self-construals among German participants. In the independent priming condition, participants thought about how they were different from their family and friends. In the interdependent priming condition, participants thought about their similarities to family and friends. Subsequently participants were given the embedded figures test that assesses perceptual processing devoid of any obvious social elements. As expected, an independent self-construal led to a more context-free or field-independent perceptual processing, whereas interdependent self-construal led to more context-bound or field-dependent processing.

HOLISTIC AND ANALYTIC REASONING

Nisbett and his colleagues have pursued the proposal that marked cultural differences in modes of reasoning may exist between not only modern industrialized and traditional populations but also the two industrialized cultural areas: the West (North America, Western Europe) and East Asia (China, Japan, and Korea). This research has been summarized by Nisbett and his colleagues (Nisbett, 2003; Nisbett & Masuda, 2003; Nisbett & Norenzayan, 2002; Nisbett et al., 2001; Peng & Nisbett, 1999) as holistic versus analytic reasoning.

Holistic thought involves an orientation to the context or field as a whole, including attention to relationships between a focal object and the field, and a preference for explaining and predicting events on the basis of such relationships. Holistic approaches rely on experience-based knowledge rather than abstract logic and are *dialectical*, meaning that there is an emphasis on change, a recognition of contradiction and the need for multiple perspectives, and a search for the "middle way" between opposing propositions. Analytic thought involves detachment of the object from its context, a tendency to focus on attributes of the object to assign it to categories, and a preference for using rules about the categories to explain and predict the object's behavior. Inferences rest in part on decontextualization of structure from content, use of formal logic, and avoidance of contradiction.

This distinction between habits of thought rests on a theoretical distinction made in psychology between two reasoning systems. One system is relatively associative, and its computations reflect similarity and contiguity (i.e., whether two stimuli share perceptual resemblance and co-occur in time); the other system relies on more abstract, symbolic representational systems, and its computations are a reflection of rule structure (e.g., Neisser, 1963; Sloman, 1996). The distinction that Witkin et al. (1975, 1974) made between "field dependence" and "field independence" in the perceptual realm, discussed earlier, resembles the cognitive distinction as well. The definition of Nisbett and his colleagues (2001) is meant to include both conceptual and perceptual aspects of the distinction, and also applies to the belief systems they regard as underlying those differences.

Although both systems of thought are in principle cognitively available to all normal adult humans, cultural experiences may encourage reliance on one system at the expense of another, giving rise to systematic cultural differences. These differences in cognitive orientation are believed to be rooted in the different social worlds of East Asians and Westerners today. East Asians are more interdependent in their socialization practices, values, and social behavior than people of European culture, who are in turn more independent. In studies in which participants are asked spontaneously to describe themselves, East Asian students generate self-descriptions that are more likely to reflect their social identities ("I am a Keio student") or refer to relationships ("I am a brother"). Americans more often generate self-descriptions that reflect abstract personality traits ("I am curious") than do Japanese participants (Cousins, 1989). Markus, Mullaly, and Kitayama (1997) found in one study that 50% of Japanese self-descriptions included references to ingroup members, in contrast to only 24% for Americans (see also Rhee, Uleman, Lee, & Roman, 1996). Social harmony is valued over debate and frank discussion in the East, to a far greater extent than in the West (Becker, 1986). (For reviews of the literature on social-psychological differences between Eastern and Western cultural contexts, see Bond, 1996; Fiske, Kitayama, Markus, & Nisbett, 1998; Kitayama, Duffy, & Uchida, Chapter 6, this volume; Markus & Kitayama, 1991; Triandis, 1989, 1995.)

If so, we might expect to find cognitive differences among contemporary peoples participating in Western and North American cultural contexts. Nisbett and his colleagues conducted a series of studies that investigated this idea. Most (but not all) experiments were conducted with college students, but similar results were obtained with nonstudent samples. East Asian participants were Chinese, Korean or Japanese, and were tested sometimes in their own countries in their native languages and sometimes in the United States. The great majority of "Westerners" studied were Americans. The results support several expectations in line with this hypothesis. Below we highlight some cross-cultural findings from this research.

Attention to Object versus Field

If Americans attend more to the object and less to the relations between the object and the field, we would expect them to be less field dependent than Asians. To test this possibility, Ji, Peng, and Nisbett (2000) gave the rod and frame test to Chinese and Americans matched for mathematical ability. Chinese were found to be more field dependent than Americans.

Masuda and Nisbett (2001) investigated attention to field versus focal object using a different paradigm. They showed underwater scenes to Japanese and American participants. Each scene consisted of rocks, plants, inert animals, small fish, and "focal" fish, which were larger, brighter, and faster moving than the others. Immediately after observing the scenes, participants were asked to describe what they had seen. Japanese typically began by referring to the context ("It looked like a river"), whereas Americans usually began by referring to the focal fish. Americans and Japanese made equal numbers of statements about the focal fish, but Japanese made about 70% more statements about the field and twice as many statements about relationships involving inert objects in the background. Participants were subsequently shown a number of objects, some of which had been in the original scenes and others which had not, and were asked to identify whether they had previously seen the object. Some of the objects were shown in their original environments, and others were shown in environments not seen before. This manipulation made no difference to the accuracy of Americans, but the performance of Japanese was less accurate when the background was different. Thus object and field appeared to have been bound for the Japanese (Chalfonte & Johnson, 1996; Hedden et al., 2000). When an object was removed from the context, their memory for the object was poorer.

In a related task, Masuda and Nisbett (2005) examined cultural differences in "change blindness," or a systematic failure to recognize marked changes in surroundings (Simons, 2000; Rensink, O'Regan, & Clark, 1997). For example, when people are asked to watch a videotape and count the number of ball passes between players, they consistently fail to notice the insertion of an unusual character into the scene, such as a person carrying an umbrella or even a person wearing a gorilla costume (Simons & Chabris, 1999). Furthermore, "change blindness" is evident even when participants are explicitly asked to search for changes in the visual field. Although participants often take a long time to detect major changes in a given scene, they are likely to detect changes in salient, focal objects faster than in objects of peripheral interest (Rensink et al., 1997). Masuda and Nisbett (2005) showed American and Japanese participants scenes in which changes occurred in focal object information (i.e., color and shape) and contextual information (i.e., background and objects' location), and participants were asked to identify changes in the scenes. Americans were more sensitive to focal object changes than to contextual changes, whereas East Asians were equally sensitive both to the focal object and to contextual information. This again reveals a greater tendency to attend to focal objects at the expense of the field among analytic thinkers.

More recently, Kitayama, Duffy, Kawamura, and Larsen (2003) developed a new paradigm to test cultural differences in perception. Participants were presented with a square frame, within which was shown a vertical line (see Figure 23.2). Participants were then shown another square frame of the same or different size and asked to draw a line identical to the first line in either absolute length (absolute task), or in proportion to the height of the surrounding frame (relative task). The absolute task is facilitated by the ability to decontextualize, whereas the relative task is facilitated by a contextualized mode of perceptual processing. The results indicated that Americans were more accurate in the absolute task, whereas Japanese

were more accurate in the relative task. In a subsequent study, Kitayama et al. showed that Japanese living in America and Americans living in Japan showed an intermediate pattern of accuracy, suggesting possible acculturation effects on perception (although other interpretations, such as self-selection, or different affordances of the perceptual environment are possible; see Kitayama et al., 2003).

Recently Chua, Boland, and Nisbett (2005) examined more precisely the mechanisms underlying cultural differences in attention. Chua et al. showed Chinese and American students (matched for age and field of study) photographs, each representing a focal object on a complex background (e.g., a tiger in a jungle), while students' eye movements were measured. The results showed that Americans fixated more on focal objects than did the Chinese, and looked at the focal objects more quickly. Furthermore, over time Chinese dispersed their attention to the background more than did the Americans. These findings support the idea that cultural experiences affect what people actually attend to in a scene.

Differing orientations of the self may explain the differential attentional and perceptual processing of East Asians and Westerners (Kühnen et al., 2001b). But could it also be that the perceptual environments of East Asia and the West contribute to these differences? If objects are more distinct from the field in the American

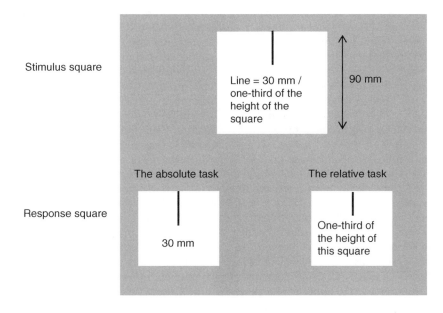

FIGURE 23.2. The framed-line test (Kitayama, Duffy, Kawamura, & Larsen, 2003).

perceptual environment, attention may be captured mainly by the object. On the other hand, if objects are embedded in the field and boundaries between objects are more ambiguous in the Japanese perceptual environment, attention may be dispersed to the whole field. Earlier we examined evidence for the notion that carpentered perceptual environments enhance vulnerability to certain kinds of visual illusions (Segall et al., 1966). Miyamoto, Nisbett, and Masuda (2006) similarly examined the perceptual environments of Japan and the United States. They took pictures of urban scenes in small, middle-size, and large cities in both countries, by randomly sampling places in each city. Using these pictures as stimuli, they analyzed the physical features of the scenes, and found that objects sampled in the United States stood out from the scenes, whereas objects sampled in Japan were embedded in the scenes.

Causal Explanation, Prediction, and Hindsight

Americans are more inclined to decontextualize the object from its context than are East Asians. We might therefore expect that Americans would be inclined to explain events by reference to properties of the object, and that East Asians would be inclined to explain the same events with reference to interactions between the object and the field. There is much evidence indicating that this is the case (for reviews see (Choi, Nisbett, & Norenzayan, 1999; Norenzayan & Nisbett, 2000). J. G. Miller (1984) showed that Americans were likely to explain both events that "had a good outcome" and events that "had a bad outcome" by invoking presumed properties of the actor. Hindu Indians explained the same events by reference to situational and contextual factors. Similarly, Morris and Peng (1994) and Lee, Hallahan, and Herzog (1996) have shown that Americans explain murders and sports events by invoking presumed dispositions of the individual, whereas Chinese and Hong Kong citizens explain the same events with reference to contextual factors.

Norenzayan, Choi, and Nisbett (2002) found that Korean participants were equally willing to make disposition-based predictions in the absence of contextual cues; however, Koreans were more responsive to contextual factors when making predictions about how people in general would be expected to behave in a given situation and, much more than American

participants, made use of their beliefs about situational power when making predictions about the behavior of a particular individual. Importantly, Norenzayan et al. found that Koreans and Americans endorsed beliefs about the causes of behavior that accorded with their explanations and predictions. Koreans placed more credence in situational theories than did Americans. Choi and Nisbett (1998) found similar results when they examined circumstances in which both Americans and Koreans showed a correspondence bias; that is, they mistakenly attributed behavior to dispositions of a target actor who was operating under social constraints. However, Koreans were much more willing than Americans to revise their mistaken inferences about dispositions. Several other studies have replicated this pattern of results, indicating that although correspondence bias can be shown to exist in East Asian groups, it is much weaker among not only Koreans but also Japanese (Masuda & Kitayama, 2004; Miyamoto & Kitayama, 2002), and Chinese (Knowles, Morris, & Chiu, 2001; for an exception, see Krull et al., 1999). Furthermore, these studies have found that East Asian groups are generally much more willing than Americans to revise their dispositional attributions when social constraints on the actor are salient (e.g., Miyamoto & Kitayama, 2002; see Choi et al., 1999, for a discussion of these issues).

Explanation patterns are different even for nonsocial events. Morris and Peng (1994) and Hong, Chiu, and Kung (1997) showed participants cartoon displays of fish moving in relation to one another in various ways. Chinese participants were more likely than Americans to see the behavior of the individual fish as being produced by external factors, whereas American participants were more inclined to see the behavior as being produced by internal factors. Peng and Knowles (2003) also found that Chinese students with no formal physics education were more likely to perceive causality to originate externally to the target object (e.g., gravity, medium, friction, field), whereas a similar group of Americans referred to causes internal to the object (e.g., shape, weight, inertia).

Sensitivity to the role of contextual factors and attention to the field may have additional consequences. In a series of experiments, Choi and Nisbett (1998) found that Koreans were more susceptible to *hindsight bias*, that is, the tendency to believe that one could have predicted some outcome that in fact one could not have predicted. Choi and Nisbett argued that the East Asians' greater susceptibility to this bias might be due to the holistic tendency to attend to an ever-increasing number of contextual factors, and to a tendency to model events causally less explicitly. When a large number of possible factors are attended to, and when these factors are not explicitly represented, any given outcome can be readily explained by drawing on any number of interrelated factors, leaving little room for surprise or the experience of inconsistency, thus maximizing hindsight.

The cultural difference in causal explanation was found not only in the locus of attribution but also in the amount of causal information people consider to explain a certain event. East Asians have holistic assumptions about the universe, dictating that all elements in the universe are somehow interconnected; consequently, an event or object cannot be understood in isolation from the whole. In contrast, Westerners hold that the universe consists of separate objects that can be understood in isolation from one another. Therefore, East Asians are expected to consider a greater amount of information than Westerners to explain a certain event. Choi, Dalal, Kim-Prieto, and Park (2003) conducted a series of studies to test this prediction. They provided European American, Asian American, and Korean participants with a short scenario of a murder incident, along with a list of 97 items of information that might or might not be relevant to the explanation of the incident. Then participants were asked to eliminate the irrelevant information from the list. Choi et al. hypothesized that East Asians would find it more difficult than would Westerners to judge a given piece of information irrelevant and "not connected," and to eliminate it from further consideration. They found the expected pattern, such that Koreans were less likely than European and Asian Americans to discard a given piece of information.

Similarity and Relationships versus Categories and Rules

East Asians are more likely to group objects on the basis of similarities and relationships among the objects, whereas Americans are more likely to group objects on the basis of categories and rules. Ji, Nisbett, and Zhang (2004) found that adults showed similar tendencies when asked about the association between words. Asked how strong the association was between words in a set, Chinese were more likely to find the association strong if there was a relationship between the words, either functional (e.g., pencil–notebook) or contextual (e.g., sky–sunshine), whereas Americans were more likely to find the association strong if the objects belonged to the same category (e.g., notebook–magazine).

Norenzayan, Smith, Kim, and Nisbett (2002) presented East Asians, Asian Americans, and European Americans with target objects and asked them to report whether the object was more similar to a group of objects to which it shared a strong family resemblance, or to a group of objects to which it could be assigned on the basis of an invariant unidimensional rule (see Figure 23.3). Thus, a schematic flower could be assigned to a group whose members it resembled most closely, or to a group whose members all shared a single feature that determined category membership (e.g., long stem). East Asians were more likely to regard the target as most similar to the group with which it shared a strong family resemblance, whereas Americans were more likely to regard the object as more similar to the group to which it could be assigned on the basis of the deterministic rule. Asian Americans' judgments were in between those of the other two groups.

Logical versus Dialectical and Intuitive Reasoning

East Asians are less likely than Westerners to decontextualize propositions and reason about them using formal rules. Furthermore, whereas Westerners reason about contradiction by applying a folk form of formal logic that aims to eliminate contradictions, East Asians reason about contradictions by emphasizing the "middle way" between contradictory propositions, or by tolerating opposites.

Experimental psychologists have found a "belief bias" in deductive reasoning: More plausible conclusions are judged as more logically valid than less plausible ones (Revlin, Leirer, Yop, & Yop, 1980). In one study, Norenzayan, Smith, et al. (2002) presented deductive arguments that were either valid or invalid, and had either plausible or nonplausible conclusions. They found that there was a difference in response bias, such that Americans

Group 1   Group 2

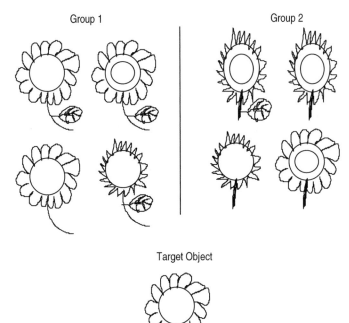

Target Object

FIGURE 23.3. Example of the stimulus sets used in Norenzayan, Smith, et al. (2002, Study 2). Group 1 shares with the target object a strong family resemblance structure, but Group 2 shares with the target object a defining feature, in this case, the stem length (short or long).

overall showed a stronger tendency to judge arguments to be valid. However, regardless of this response bias, there was a culture × conclusion plausibility interaction, such that the belief bias was greater for Koreans than for Americans, but for valid arguments only (see Unsworth & Medin, 2005, for a different interpretation). Importantly, this difference was not due to any difference in abstract logical reasoning ability between the Americans and the Koreans. Koreans' validity judgments were the same as Americans' when the propositions were formal and abstract. Thus, the difference between the two groups apparently resides in the willingness to decontextualize meaningful propositions sufficiently to be able to apply logical rules to their underlying structure.

An important aspect of the Western analytic stance is the belief that talking facilitates thinking. This is not surprising given that analytic thinking is intimately connected to linguistic representation of thoughts. This belief is so culturally ingrained that Western pedagogy takes it for granted that verbalization is a central part of learning. Talking is taken as a near-equivalent to, and direct evidence for, thinking,

as reflected in cultural practices such as debate and disputation in the Socratic method of teaching. In East Asian cultures, where an intuitive orientation is valued, however, talking is discouraged and silence is valued, as reflected in cultural practices such as silent meditation. Given the divergent cultural beliefs about talking, Kim (2002) examined whether the effect of verbalization on thinking is culturally specific. Asian Americans and European Americans thought aloud while solving reasoning problems such as Raven's Progressive Matrices. Talking impaired Asian Americans' performance but not that of European Americans. A follow-up study showed that talking impaired Asian Americans' cognitive performance, but articulatory suppression did not. Conversely, European Americans' cognitive performance was impaired by articulatory suppression but unaffected by talking. These results suggest that the underlying mechanism for the cultural difference is the differential use of internal speech in thinking. The exact relationship of these findings to the cultural differences in analytic versus holistic thinking remain to be examined. Talking recruits linguistic representation of the problem and as a result should facilitate analytic thinking but inhibit holistic thinking. An interesting open question, then, is whether the cultural differences regarding the effect of talking on thinking are generally the same for all modes of thinking, or whether they are especially pronounced for analytic tasks.

Many philosophers of science and ethnographers have pointed to a type of "dialectical" reasoning held to be characteristic of East Asians (S. H. Liu, 1974; Lloyd, 1990; Needham, 1962/1978; Peng & Nisbett, 1999; Spencer-Rodgers & Peng, 2003; Zhang & Chen, 1991). The orientation underlying this approach may be described (in a rather nondialectical fashion) as a set of three principles.

1. *The principle of change*: Reality is a process that is not static, but dynamic and changeable.
2. *The principle of contradiction*: Contradiction is a constant element of life.
3. *The principle of relationship or holism*: Nothing is isolated and independent; instead everything is related to everything else.

Taken together, these principles imply an attitude toward contradiction that is very different from that found in the West. Contradiction is to be expected and is not necessarily resolved. Propositions that appear contradictory on the surface may both contain some truth, and a constant goal is to search for the "middle way" between extremes.

Peng and Nisbett (1999) derived a number of predictions from the previous set of principles. Chinese collections of proverbs were found to have a larger proportion of "dialectical" proverbs containing contradictions ("Too humble is half proud") than do English collections, and Chinese undergraduates were found to like dialectical proverbs more than did American undergraduates. Chinese were more likely than Americans to prefer arguments having a dialectical or holistic character rather than a logical structure. When asked to deal with inter- and intrapersonal conflicts, Chinese were more likely to say that both sides had some merit, whereas Americans were more likely to say that one side or the other was correct.

These different ways of reasoning also emerged in the way persuasive messages were processed. When presented with a plausible proposition, both Chinese and Americans assented to it, but when participants were presented with both the plausible proposition and a less plausible proposition that appeared inconsistent with each other, Chinese and Americans responded in very different ways. Chinese became less confident about the plausible proposition, but Americans became even more convinced of the correctness of the plausible proposition! The Americans' behavior is hard to justify on logical grounds, but it is understandable given Western insistence that a proposition must be true or false. Westerners' arguments against the weaker proposition would serve to strengthen belief in the more plausible proposition. Chinese, in contrast, ended up believing that both propositions were about equally plausible, a tendency that is also hard to defend on logical grounds. This remarkable tendency can be understood as the result of Chinese desire to seek the "middle way" and to find the truth in apparently contradictory propositions.

These different modes of reasoning are also implicated in the ways that self-knowledge is organized. A series of studies revealed that among East Asian participants, self-knowledge is more contextual, flexible, holistic, and dialectical compared to that of European American participants (Spencer-Rodgers & Peng, 2004; Spencer-Rodgers, Peng, Wang, & Hou, 2004). In one study, when presented with either positive or negative feedback that was counterschematic (i.e., inconsistent with prior self-concepts), Chinese were more likely than Americans subsequently to alter their self-beliefs, suggesting the Chinese had self-views that were more dialectical in nature.

The dialectical frame in East Asian cultures has important implications for reasoning about change in events. In a series of studies, Ji, Nisbett, and Su (2001) described various current states and asked whether participants thought the state would continue or change. For example, participants who were told about a man who grew up in a poor family were asked to predict whether he would remain poor in adulthood or grow rich one day. For each of four events, Chinese were more likely than Americans to think that the future would be different from the past. Ji et al. also presented to participants alleged, recent trends in world events about which participants were unlikely to have direct knowledge; for example, participants were told that the world's economy has been growing in the last decade, and they were asked to predict whether this trend would go up, go down, or remain the same. Chinese participants were more likely to predict that the next step would halt or reverse the direction of change, whereas Americans were more likely to predict that the trend would continue in a linear fashion. In one study, Chinese participants were more likely to predict reversals of trends in all but one of 12 cases (Ji et al., 2001).

Recently, Choi, Koo, and Choi (2005) devised a multifaceted self-report tool, the Analysis–Holism Scale (AHS), to measure analytic–holistic thinking style (e.g., "Everything in the universe is somehow related to each other"; "It is more desirable to take the middle ground than to go to extremes"; "It is more important to pay attention to the whole than its parts"). They then demonstrated that it adequately differentiated between-culture groups (Americans vs. Koreans) and within-culture groups (Korean students in Oriental medicine vs. other majors) as expected. Furthermore, the scale predicted analytic versus holistic solutions in tasks that measured attention, categorization, causal reasoning, and perceptions of change. Those with high scores on the AHS paid attention more to the field than to the object, categorized objects more based on similarity than on rules, considered a greater amount of information in causal explanation, and possessed a cyclic view of change more strongly than did those with low scores in the AHS.

Normative Considerations Regarding Culture Differences in Reasoning

So far our discussions of cultural variation in cognition have been descriptive, without addressing the related, important normative issue of how to evaluate the accuracy and practical value of different modes of thought. This is a particular challenge for the universalist position that argues for the "psychic unity" of humankind. If all of humanity shares the same invariant mental processes, how then do we explain cultural differences that are observed? The strong universalist position can offer two possible answers to this challenge. The first universalist answer views cultural differences in terms of a deficit model. In this view, there is a true universal human mind (often implicitly assumed to approximate the Western ideal), and any observed deviation from this ideal mind is evidence for cultural or individual deficit. In this view, cultures may be ordered in terms of having more or less of an inherently desirable thing (e.g., logical rules, the use of probabilistic principles). The second possible answer is that cultural differences are superficial appendages that mask underlying deep similarities.

We find both versions of this universalist position problematic. We disagree with the superficial culture interpretation, and we have presented in this chapter considerable evidence that cultural differences in cognition are real and central to cognitive functioning. Yet we also reject the deficit model of these cultural differences and consider them ethnocentric projections, unless it is established that the same processes are valued across cultures and to the same extent. Instead we favor evaluating modes of thought in terms of the task goals and the very cultural values and practices in which they are embedded.

Consistent with the view that normative judgments themselves vary across cultures, many East Asian scholars have noted that logic in East Asian cultures does not enjoy the normative status that it does in the West. In Japanese culture, for example, "to argue with logical consistency is thus discouraged, and if one does so continuously one may not only be resented but also be regarded as immature" (Nagashima, 1973, p. 96). These normative evaluations may even affect interpersonal judgments. Ji et al. (2001) found that people who see events as changing cyclically (a dialectical pattern of reasoning) are judged to be wise more so by Chinese participants than by Americans. Recently Buchtel and Norenzayan (2005) asked participants to rank the importance of acting in a logical or an intuitive manner in relatively impersonal and interpersonal contexts. Overall, Americans ranked logic higher than intuition, whereas Koreans ranked these two about equally. Moreover, Americans favored "being logical" more than Koreans did, whereas the opposite pattern was found for "being intuitive." In a second study, American and Chinese participants read about a company manager who made a decision either consistent with a procedural rule or consistent with intuition, and were asked a variety of questions that assessed their impressions of the target. Of particular interest, Chinese judged the intuition-following actor to be wiser and more reasonable than the rule-following actor, whereas Americans showed equal preference. These cultural differences were more pronounced in impersonal contexts and were attenuated or disappeared in interpersonal contexts, in which intuition was favored by all. Cultural differences in value judgments about reasoning in some contexts remind us that an important part of cross-cultural research is to remain watchful of inadvertently projecting one's own values and judgments about a cognitive tendency that is not valued as highly in one's own culture, but may be more highly valued in another cultural group (see Cole & Scribner, 1974).

The philosopher Stephen Stich (1990) has addressed the normative status of cultural differences in thinking by arguing that "there are no intrinsic epistemic virtues. . . . Cognitive mechanisms or processes are to be viewed as tools or policies and evaluated in much the same way that we evaluate other tools or policies" (p. 24). According to Stich (see also Resnick, 1994), if there are culturally diverse ways to conduct the business of everyday cognition, and if there are culturally diverse systems of justification that serve the needs of various cognitive communities, then the reasonable philosophical position would be to evaluate thinking in terms of the local standards of justification, as well as the specific task requirements and inferential goals that vary across contexts.

This is not to say that it is always unreasonable to criticize specific inferential practices, even by the standards of another culture, but that criticism must take into account task goals and cultural contexts. And if we decide to apply the normative criteria of formal logic and probability theory to these modes of thought, we find that the analytic and holistic modes of thought generate a medley of normative and non-normative outcomes. For example, in deductive reasoning, analytic thinkers tend to decontextualize more than do holistic thinkers, but in causal attribution, the former more readily commit the fundamental attribution error than the latter. Conversely, holistic thinkers are more accurate in covariation detection (Ji et al., 2000), yet they are more vulnerable to hindsight bias (Choi & Nisbett, 1998). Furthermore, in some of the research reported here, European Americans have been shown to make errors in their efforts to be logically consistent that actually result in *incoherent* judgments in the sense that one judgment actually

follows from the opposite of the other (Peng & Nisbett, 1999). These errors were avoided by East Asian participants, who, however, made logical errors of their own in their attempts to reconcile opposing views. Similarly, Masuda and Nisbett (2005) examined scene perception and found change-blindness in both American and Japanese samples; however, Americans showed more change-blindness for background objects, whereas Japanese showed more change-blindness for focal objects. Thus, neither the analytic nor the holistic mode guarantees accuracy in perception and reasoning as defined by probability theory and formal logical principles.

EXPLAINING CULTURAL DIFFERENCES IN ANALYTIC AND HOLISTIC THOUGHT

What are the origins of these cognitive differences? To answer this complex question it is important to distinguish between *distal* and *proximal* explanations. Distal explanations are historical analyses that involve social, economic, and even geographic factors (Norenzayan & Nisbett, 2000; Nisbett, 2003). Proximal explanations involve individual-level processes, including beliefs, knowledge, social experiences, and psychological orientations, that have been shaped by these historical developments, are identifiable at the individual level, and could be directly implicated in these cognitive differences. The attempt to answer the distal question must, of course, be speculative at this time, because it involves complex sociological and historical issues. Nisbett (2003; Nisbett et al., 2001) has noted considerable parallels between contemporary cognitive differences in holistic and analytic thought, and studies of ancient Chinese and Greek philosophy, mathematics, and science that have influenced modern East Asia and the West, respectively (Becker, 1986; Fung, 1983; S. H. Liu, 1974; Lloyd, 1990; Nakamura, 1964/1985; Needham, 1962/1978; Zhang, 1985). Although these two ancient cultures shared many similarities, their metaphysical belief systems were different. Early Greek and Chinese philosophy, science, and mathematics were quite different in their strengths and weaknesses. Many Greek philosophers looked for universal rules to explain events and were concerned with categorizing objects with precision, and with respect to their "essences." There was a marked distrust of holistic approaches. Chinese philosophers, especially Taoists, were more pragmatic and intuitive, and were distrustful of formal logic and rational distinctions (Fung, 1983; S. H. Liu, 1974; Lloyd, 1990; Nakamura, 1964/1985; Needham, 1962/1978).

Following scholars in several fields (Becker, 1986; Nakamura, 1964/1985), Nisbett and his colleagues (2001) argued that the social and economic systems of the two countries encouraged their respective cognitive orientations. China was an agrarian society with strong obligations and clear role relations specifying how to deal with family, clan, and village, and with tight vertical control of social relations. Action was carried out in the context of many role relations. Harmony with one's fellows was believed to be a primary end of the society (Munro, 1969). In contrast, the economy of Greece owed more to herding, fishing, and trading than to cooperative agriculture.

A goal of harmony would tend to encourage attention to the field as a whole, whereas the individualistic stance might allow for the luxury of attending to the object alone. Attention to the field would encourage finding relationships between events in the field, whereas attention to the object might encourage attending to the attributes of the object to be able to categorize it and apply rules to it. The harmony goal would tend to discourage debate and encourage consensual heuristics, such as *dialecticism*, that seek the "middle way" and the resolution of opposing positions (Lloyd, 1990). The consequence of the practice of debate is an emphasis on logical consistency and the avoidance of contradiction. Not surprisingly, pedagogical practices also reflect these cultural goals: Critical analysis and argumentation is emphasized in Western classrooms, and experience-based learning is emphasized in Chinese classrooms (for a review, see Tweed & Lehman, 2002).

The cognitive differences in reasoning to some degree mirror differences in philosophical traditions. As provocative as this congruence may be, it is difficult to know at this time whether these traditions are directly implicated in such reasoning processes, or whether the influence of these traditions on thinking is mediated through proximal factors.

At this time, the most compelling proximal explanation for the cognitive differences is the differing social orientations of people in East Asia and Western cultures. As discussed earlier, East Asian children are socialized into a tight social network of mutual obligation and role relations, and, as a result, they develop an interdependent orientation of the self. In contrast, Western children from a young age are socialized into a social network of loosely connected, autonomous individuals, and, as a result, develop an independent orientation. An interdependent self-orientation may translate into context-sensitive information processing, whereas an independent self-orientation may encourage an object-focused processing. The cross-cultural evidence is consistent with this hypothesis: An analytic mode of processing is more prevalent in Western cultures, where people are also more independent, whereas a holistic mode of processing is more prevalent in East Asian cultures, where people are also more interdependent. However, research on the direct influence of these orientations on thinking has been sparse. Nevertheless, there is growing experimental evidence that inducing independent versus interdependent self-orientations affects analytic and holistic processing in predictable ways (Kühnen, Hannover, & Schubert, 2001; see also Kühnen & Oyserman, 2002).

A particular way of thinking is also transmitted and fostered through formal education in a society. For example, Koo and Choi (2005) reasoned that Oriental medicine reflects many aspects of East Asian holistic thinking, and hypothesized that the exposure to Oriental medicine training would foster the holistic way of thinking. They tested this idea by comparing the students of Oriental medicine and those of non-Oriental medicine in Korea in some cognitive domains. They found that the students of Oriental medicine believed in a cyclic pattern of change more strongly than did their counterparts. If a certain event had been increasing or decreasing, the students of Oriental medicine expected that the trend would reverse its direction in the future. They also thought that an event was determined by numerous factors, and that a given factor could not be dismissed easily while explaining a certain event. Therefore, they considered a greater number of factors in causal attribution. Importantly, a chronological trend emerged, such that holistic causal beliefs became stronger the longer students were exposed to training in Oriental medicine, and this trend remained after Koo and Choi accounted for age differences.

CAVEATS AND FUTURE DIRECTIONS

The accumulated evidence for cultural variation in cognition and perception is robust and reliable: These differences emerge from a variety of unrelated paradigms and methodologies, with a variety of samples, and many artifactual explanations have been ruled out (see Nisbett et al., 2001; Nisbett & Masuda, 2003). A meta-analytic review of studies comparing East Asians (Chinese, Koreans, Japanese) and North Americans (excluding Asian North Americans) indicated that the effect size for cultural differences is as strong for attentional and perceptual tasks as it is for tasks that involve language-based conceptual processes (Miyamoto, Kitayama, & Talhelm, 2006). Not surprisingly, East Asians tested in East Asian countries diverged more strongly than East Asians tested in North America. Now that there is convincing evidence that cultural differences in basic cognitive processes exist, two major challenges lie ahead for cultural psychologists. First, relatively little research has been done about the underlying proximal social-psychological factors that explain cultural differences in cognition. Second, most of the research has focused narrowly on comparisons of Western and East Asian participants, with relatively little attention given to most of the rest of the world's cultures, including both indigenous and industrialized populations in Africa, Latin America, Eastern Europe, the Mediterranean area, and the Middle East.

What factors encourage a holistic mode of processing in East Asian contexts and an analytic mode of processing in Western contexts? This important question is particularly complex, because multiple processes are likely to converge to produce the cultural differences, and disentangling them in the laboratory is a challenge. The hypothesis that different orientations of the self in these two cultures are causally responsible, as discussed earlier, has already received experimental support (Kühnen, Hannover, & Schubert, 2001). Further research can investigate this hypothesis in greater detail and establish the extent to which the cultural differences originate in different conceptions of the self. Although the use of self-report measures of cultural value orientations or self-construal across cultures are vulnerable to serious methodological problems (see Oyserman, Kemmelmeier, & Coon, 2002; Heine, Lehman, Peng, & Greenholtz, 2002), convergent methods that include valid self-report measures, experimental methods, as well as population-level measures can be used in future cross-cultural research for this purpose. Other factors are only beginning to receive attention: differences in language (Ji et al., 2004; Tardif, 1996); residential mobility (Oishi, 2004); voluntary settlement patterns (Kitayama, Ishii, Imada, Takemura, & Ramaswamy, 2006); the perceptual environment (Miyamoto et al., 2006); exposure to different kinds of formal education within a culture, such as Oriental medicine or Western-style schooling (Koo & Choi, 2005; Scribner, 1977); and within-culture religious beliefs and practices (A. Cohen & Rozin, 2001; Sanchez-Burks, 2002). Greater concerted attention to within-culture analyses of the relationship of social and ecological experiences to cognition will propel cultural psychology into a second stage of inquiry, in which cultural differences in psychology are not only discovered but also explained in terms of the critical variables that produce and sustain cultural variation (Heine & Norenzayan, 2005).

More systematic cross cultural research programs are also needed that examine cultures outside of East Asia and Europe and North America (for an example of a research program on cognition in native American groups in Central America and the United States, see Medin et al., Chapter 25, this volume). Broadening the range of cultures under investigation is important for at least two reasons. First, it facilitates understanding of certain patterns of thought that are highly elaborated in other cultures but not well-represented in the samples currently under investigation. For example, Norenzayan (2005a) recently began exploring fatalistic thinking, characterized by a tendency to see outcomes in life as inevitable and multidetermined, and to attribute these outcomes to powerful agentic external forces, such as fate, destiny, or God. Fatalistic thinking is widespread in some regions of the world, such as in the Mediterranean area, and in many religious traditions. Not surprisingly, little is known about the psychology of this pattern of belief and thought given that it is an uncommon form of reasoning in the highly secular Western and East Asian samples that are the object of investigation in most of current cultural psychology.

Second, inclusion of more of the world's cultures allows greater opportunities to test specific hypotheses regarding the transmission mechanisms underlying cultural variation in thinking. For example, if the differences between East Asians and Westerners in analytic–holistic thinking are explainable in terms of degrees of independence–interdependence, then other cultures where independence versus interdependence are prevalent should encourage analytic versus holistic processing, respectively. Kühnen, Hannover, and Roeder (2001) tested this hypothesis with participants in two individualistic cultures, United States and Germany, and two collectivistic ones, Russia and Malaysia, and found results consistent with this hypothesis in the domain of perceptual processing. Zebian and Denny (2001) compared integrative thinking (similar to holistic thinking) in a group of European Canadians to that in an immigrant Middle Eastern group with varying degrees of Western education, and found that the Middle Eastern group was on average more integrative than the European Canadian group. Furthermore, the authors found that exposure to a Western-style university education resulted in less integrative thinking among the Middle Easterners. Recently, Norenzayan (2005b) tested Canadian, Chinese, and Arab individuals in perceptual processing and deductive reasoning. Although the Chinese, as expected, showed more holistic processing than Canadians, Arabs were even more holistic than the Chinese! Similarly, Henrich (2005) examined classification and perception among the Mapuche, an indigenous group of farmers in southern Chile. Although the Mapuche have had little exposure to the cultural traditions of East Asia, their processing patterns were overwhelmingly holistic. Is it possible that the most interesting cultural divide is not the one between West and East, but between the West versus the rest? Are the cultures of the non-Western world, regardless of their cultural exposure to East Asian traditions, predominantly holistic in their cognitive outlook? Results like these invite more systematic investigation of the specific social and ecological variables that can account for such cultural variation.

CONCLUSIONS: UNIVERSALS AND CULTURAL PARTICULARS IN COGNITION

This chapter has examined how cognitive processes are shaped by the cultural context in which they occur. This is not to deny that basic process primitives appear in the human child at a very early age and may have innate components. People everywhere are likely to possess cognitive strategies implicated in domain-specific reasoning, such as theory of mind, as well as domain-general ones that realize exemplar-based categorization, depth perception, long-term memory, covariation detection, and so forth. In fact, cross-cultural research is one of the principal ways that such process primitives can be uncovered (Norenzayan & Heine, 2005; Norenzayan et al., 2006; see also Cohen, Chapter 8, and Medin et al., Chapter 25, this volume). However, these primitive cognitive structures do not preclude the cultural dependence of human cognition.

A fruitful analogy is to think of the mind as a *toolbox* (Cole, 1996; Resnick, 1994; Stich, 1990; Vygotsky, 1978). Cognitive structures can be thought of as tools for everyday problem solving. Just as the handyman's specialized toolbox is accessed to construct and repair, the mental toolbox is accessed to solve myriad problems of everyday life. But to the extent that the worlds people inhabit are different (or are believed to be so), there emerge different affordances that elicit the use of different tools. In a world joined together by nails, a hammer is a more useful tool than a wrench. In a world held together by nuts and bolts, a wrench is a more useful tool than a hammer.

Based on this reasoning, Norenzayan and Heine (2005) discussed three distinct levels of universals that also encompass three kinds of cultural variation in cognitive processes, giving rise to four types of hierarchically organized classes. From strongest to weakest claims for cross-cultural universality, a cognitive phenomenon can be (1) an *accessibility universal*, if it emerges across cultures and in the same magnitude; (2) a *functional universal*, if it emerges across cultures in the same context but differs in magnitude; (3) an *existential universal*, if it exists in principle in the psychological repertoire of various cultures but is elicited by different contingencies and in different magnitudes; and (4) a *nonuniversal*, if it is absent from the psychological repertoire of some cultures. Below we briefly illustrate these distinctions.

At the shallowest level, there may be cultural differences in the cognitive accessibility of thought processes. Societies differ in the cultural practices they promote, affording differential expertise in the use of a cognitive strategy, or differential knowledge about a domain. The result is that a given cognitive process may be equally available in principle, but differentially accessible in different cultures. As a result, the same phenomenon may emerge across cultures, but with systematically different effect sizes. An example of this is cultural variation in the correspondence bias in the attitude attribution paradigm, which refers to the tendency to attribute behavior to an actor's attitude, even when the actor is operating under social constraints. In most contexts, this bias appears in East Asian samples, but in a much weaker form (Choi et al., 1999).

Differential cultural expertise with a given cognitive process, or differential familiarity with a given domain, may yield an even more dramatic class of cultural variation in reasoning: In principle, people may possess similar cognitive repertoires, yet habitually rely on qualitatively different cognitive strategies in that repertoire to solve the same problems of everyday life. Thus, even if all cultures possessed similar cognitive toolboxes (i.e., existential universals), the tools of choice for the same problem may be different. In many studies reviewed in this chapter, the same problem triggered qualitatively different cognitive responses in the two cultural groups (see Nisbett et al., 2001). For example, confronted with apparently contradictory propositions, East Asians responded by trying to find the middle way, whereas Americans responded by polarizing their judgments. Research on logical reasoning among traditional peoples also reflects this kind of cultural difference. Whereas Western participants approach many kinds of problems by decontextualizing them and applying logical rules, traditional nonliterate folk approach the same problems by reasoning from their knowledge of the argument contents (Cole et al., 1971; Luria, 1931). Different levels of expertise in a domain may also lead to the use of different cognitive strategies to solve the same problem (e.g., Medin & Atran, 2004; Medin et al., Chapter 25, this volume).

Finally, the actual existence of particular cognitive processes may differ across cultures, in that different cultures may construct complex reasoning strategies out of universal primitive ones in feats of cognitive engineering, as suggested by Dennett (1995). The invention of symbolic systems such as calendars, number-naming conventions, pictographic and alphabetic writing, and formal logic provide examples. Beginning in the West in the 17th century, statistical, methodological, and cost–benefit rules having applicability to scientific reasoning, as well as to policy analysis and everyday judgment and decision-making, began to be developed (Hacking, 1975). There is great variation among members of Western society today in understanding and using these rules. Similarly, Chinese philosophy developed the ancient Taoist notions of *yin* and *yang* into sophisticated ways of reasoning about change, moderation, relativism, and the need for multiple viewpoints. A case can be made that complex numerical reasoning that goes beyond one–two–many is contingent on a culturally available counting system (Gordon, 2004; Pica et al., 2004), and in that sense it is a nonuniversal. Quantity estimation, in contrast, appears to be invariant across cultures in magnitude and likely to be an accessibility universal. This framework highlights the fact that universality and cultural variability are not mutually incompatible and, in fact, theories in psychology can gain precision and generality by explicitly articulating both the invariant and culturally variable aspects of cognitive processes.

Human thinking occurs in a cultural context. Yet for most of its history, psychology proceeded as if the study of thinking is unrelated to the cultural environment in which the mind develops and functions. This picture has been changing with the growth of cross-cultural research that investigates the ways cultural experiences are implicated in human thinking. Cross-cultural research is the principal way—perhaps the only way—that legitimate inferences can be made about human universals, as well as about culture-specific patterns in cognition. As a result, the psychology of cognition and perception promises to be on firmer scientific ground to the extent that it encompasses the world's cultural diversity.

ACKNOWLEDGMENTS

The writing of this chapter was supported by a University of British Columbia Hampton Fund Research Grant No. 12R41699 to Ara Norenzayan. We thank the editors, Dov Cohen and Shinobu Kitayama, for their thoughtful comments.

REFERENCES

Atran, S. (1998). Folk biology and the anthropology of science: Cognitive universals and cultural particulars. *Behavioral and Brain Sciences, 21,* 547–609.

Atran, S., Medin, D. L., & Ross, N. O. (2005). The cultural mind: Environmental decision making and cultural modeling within and across populations. *Psychological Review, 112,* 744–776.

Au, T. (1983). Chinese and English counterfactuals: The Sapir–Whorf hypothesis revisited. *Cognition, 15,* 155–187.

Avis, J., & Harris, P. L. (1991). Belief-desire reasoning among Baka children: Evidence for a universal conception of mind. *Child Development, 62,* 460–467.

Baillargeon, R. (1995). Physical reasoning in infancy. In M. S. Gazzaniga (Ed.), *The cognitive neurosciences* (pp. 181–204). Cambridge, MA: MIT Press.

Barkow, J. H., Cosmides, L., & Tooby, J. (Eds.). (1992). *The adapted mind: Evolutionary psychology and the generation of culture.* London: Oxford University Press.

Becker, C. B. (1986). Reasons for the lack of argumentation and debate in the Far East. *International Journal of Intercultural Relations, 10,* 75–92.

Benjamin, L. T. (1988). *A history of psychology: Original sources and contemporary research.* New York: McGraw-Hill.

Berlin, B., Breedlove, D., & Raven, P. (1973). General principles of classification and nomenclature in folk biology. *American Anthropologist, 74,* 214–242.

Berlin, B. O., & Kay, P. D. (1969). *Basic color terms.* Berkeley: University of California Press.

Block, N. (1995). The mind as the software of the brain. In E. E. Smith & D. N. Osherson (Eds.), *Thinking: An invitation to the cognitive science* (pp. 377–425). Cambridge, MA: MIT Press.

Bloom, A. H. (1981). *The linguistic shaping of thought: A study in the impact of language on thinking in China and the West.* Hillsdale, NJ: Erlbaum.

Bond, M. H. (1996). Chinese values. In M. H. Bond (Ed.), *Handbook of Chinese psychology* (pp. 208–226). Hong Kong: Oxford University Press.

Boroditsky, L. (2001). Does language shape thought?: English and Mandarin speakers' conceptions of time. *Cognitive Psychology, 43,* 1–22.

Boroditsky, L. (2003). Linguistic relativity. In L. Nadel (Ed.) *Encyclopedia of Cognitive Science* (pp. 917–921). London: Macmillan.

Buchtel, E., & Norenzayan, A. (2005). *Rule-based and intuitive reasoning: Culture, reasoning style, and values.* Unpublished manuscript, University of British Columbia, Vancouver.

Callaghan, T., Rochat, P., Liilard, A., Claux, M., Odden, H., et al. (2005). Synchrony in the onset of mental state reasoning: Evidence from five cultures. *Psychological Science, 16,* 378–384.

Carey, S. (2004). Bootstrapping and the origins of concepts. *Daedalus,* 59–68.

Carroll, J. B., & Casagrande, J. B. (1958). The function of language classification in behavior. In E. Macoby, T. Newcomb, & E. Hartley (Eds.), *Readings in social psychology* (pp. 18–31). New York: Holt.

Chalfonte, B. L., & Johnson, M. K. (1996). Feature memory and binding in young and older adults. *Memory and Cognition, 24,* 403–416.

Choi, I., Choi, J., & Norenzayan, A. (2004). Culture and decisions. In D. J. Koehler & N. Harvey (Eds.), *Blackwell handbook of judgment and decision making* (pp. 504–524). Oxford, UK: Blackwell.

Choi, I., Dalal, R., Kim-Prieto, C., & Park, H. (2003). Culture and judgment of causal relevance. *Journal of Personality and Social Psychology, 84,* 46–59.

Choi, I., Koo, M., & Choi, J. (2005). *Measuring holistic versus analytic thinking style.* Unpublished manuscript, Seoul National University, Seoul, Korea.

Choi, I., & Nisbett, R. E. (1998). The cultural psychology of surprise: Holistic theories and recognition of contradiction. *Journal of Personality and Social Psychology, 79,* 890–905.

Choi, I., Nisbett, R. E., & Norenzayan, A. (1999). Causal attribution across cultures: Variation and universality. *Psychological Bulletin, 125,* 47–63.

Chua, H. F., Boland, J. E., & Nisbett, R. E. (2005). Cultural variation in eye movements during scene perception. *Proceedings of the National Academy of Sciences USA, 102,* 12629–12633.

Cohen, A., & Rozin, P. (1999). Religion and the morality of mentality. *Journal of Personality and Social Psychology, 81,* 697–710.

Cohen, D. (2001). Cultural variation: Considerations and implications. *Psychological Bulletin, 127,* 451–471.

Cole, M. (1996). *Cultural psychology: A once and future discipline.* Cambridge, MA: Belknap/Harvard University Press.

Cole, M., Gay, J., Glick, J. A., & Sharp, D. W. (1971). *The cultural context of learning and thinking.* New York: Basic Books.

Cole, M., & Scribner, S. (1974). *Culture and thought: A psychological introduction.* New York: Wiley.

Cousins, S. D. (1989). Culture and self-perception in Japan and the United States. *Journal of Personality and Social Psychology, 56,* 124–131.

Dehaene, S. (1997). *The number sense: How the mind creates mathematics.* Oxford, UK: Oxford University Press.

Dennett, D. C. (1995). *Darwin's dangerous idea: Evolution and the meanings of life.* New York: Simon & Schuster.

Edgerton, R. (1971). *The individual in cultural adaptation.* Los Angeles: University of California Press.

Fiske, A. P., Kitayama, S., Markus, H. R., & Nisbett, R. E. (1998). The cultural matrix of social psychology. In D. T. Gilbert, S. T. Fiske, & G. Linzey (Eds.), *Handbook of social psychology* (4th ed., pp. 915–981). Boston: McGraw-Hill.

Foley, R., & Lahr, M. (1997). Mode 3 technologies and the evolution of modern humans. *Cambridge Archaeological Journal, 7,* 3–36.

Fung, Y. (1983). *A history of Chinese philosophy* (D. Bodde, Trans.; Vols. 1–2). Princeton, NJ: Princeton University Press.

Gelman, R., & Gallistel, C. R. (2004). Language and the origin of number concepts. *Science, 306*, 441–443.

Gordon, P. (2004). Numerical cognition without words: Evidence from Amazonia. *Science, 306*, 496–499.

Hacking, I. (1975). *The emergence of probability.* Cambridge, UK: Cambridge University Press.

Hedden, T., Ji, L., Jing, Q., Jiao, S., Yao, C., Nisbett, R. E., et al. (2000). *Culture and age differences in recognition memory for social dimensions.* Paper presented at the Cognitive Aging Conference, Atlanta.

Heider, E. R., & Oliver, C. C. (1972). The structure of the color space in naming and memory for two languages. *Cognitive Psychology, 3*, 337–354.

Heine, S. J., Lehman, D. R., Peng, K., & Greenholtz, J. (2002). What's wrong with cross-cultural comparisons of subjective Likert scales?: The reference-group problem. *Journal of Personality and Social Psychology, 82*, 903–918.

Heine, S. J., & Norenzayan, A. (2006). Towards a psychological science for a cultural species. *Perspectives on Psychological Science, 1*, 251–269.

Henrich, J. (2005). *Perception and reasoning among the Mapuche.* Unpublished manuscript, Emory University, Atlanta, GA.

Henrich, J., & Boyd, R. (1998). The evolution of conformist transmission and between-group differences. *Evolution and Human Behavior, 19*, 215–242.

Hong, Y., Chiu, C., & Kung, T. (1997). Bringing culture out in front: Effects of cultural meaning system activation on social cognition. In K. Leung, Y. Kashima, U. Kim, & S. Yamaguchi (Eds.), *Progress in Asian social psychology* (Vol. 1, pp. 135–146). Singapore: Wiley.

Hunt, E., & Agnoli, F. (1991). The Whorfian hypothesis: A cognitive psychology perspective. *Psychological Review, 98*, 377–389.

Hutchins, E. (1995). *Cognition in the wild.* Cambridge, MA: MIT Press.

Ji, L., Nisbett, R. E., & Su, Y. (2001). Culture, change, and prediction. *Psychological Science, 12*, 450–456.

Ji, L., & Nisbett, R. E., & Zhang, Z. (2004). Is it culture or is it language?: Examination of language effects in cross-cultural research on categorization. *Journal of Personality and Social Psychology, 87*, 57–65.

Ji, L., Peng, K., & Nisbett, R. E. (2000). Culture, control, and perception of relationships in the environment. *Journal of Personality and Social Psychology, 78*, 943–955.

Kim, H. S. (2002). We talk, therefore we think?: A cultural analysis of the effect of talking on thinking. *Journal of Personality and Social Psychology, 83*, 828–842.

Kitayama, S., Duffy, S., Kawamura, T., & Larsen, J. (2003). Perceiving an object and its context in different cultures: A cultural look at New Look. *Psychological Science, 14*, 201–206.

Kitayama, S., Ishii, K., Imada, T., Takemura, K., & Ramaswamy, J. (2006). Voluntary settlement and the spirit of independence: Evidence from Japan's "Northern Frontier." *Journal of Personality and Social Psychology, 91*, 369–384.

Knowles, E. D., Morris, M. W., Chiu, C., & Hong, Y. (2001). Culture and the process of person perception: Evidence for automaticity among East Asians in correcting for situational influences on behavior. *Personality and Social Psychology Bulletin, 27*, 1344–1356.

Koo, M., & Choi, I. (2005). Becoming a holistic thinker: Training effect of Oriental medicine on reasoning. *Personality and Social Psychology Bulletin, 31*, 1264–1272.

Krull, D. S., Loy, M. H.-M., Lin, J., Wang, C.-F., Chen, S., & Zhao, X. (1999). The fundamental attribution error: Correspondence bias in individualist and collectivist cultures. *Personality and Social Psychology Bulletin, 25*, 1208–1219.

Kühnen, U., Hannover, B., & Roeder, U. (2001). Cross-cultural variations in identifying embedded figures: Comparisons from the United States, Germany, Russia, and Malaysia. *Journal of Cross-Cultural Psychology, 32*, 365–371.

Kühnen, U., Hannover, B., Schubert, B. (2001). The semantic–procedural interface model of the self: The role of self-knowledge for context-dependent versus context-independent modes of thinking. *Journal of Personality and Social Psychology, 80*, 397–409.

Kühnen, U., & Oyserman, D. (2002). Thinking about the self influences thinking in general: Cognitive consequences of salient self-concept. *Journal of Experimental Social Psychology, 38*, 492–499.

Lave, J., & Wenger, E. (1991). *Situated learning: Legitimate peripheral participation.* Cambridge, UK: Cambridge University Press.

Lee, F., Hallahan, M., & Herzog, T. (1996). Explaining real life events: How culture and domain shape attributions. *Personality and Social Psychology Bulletin, 22*, 732–741.

Levinson, S. C. (1996). Language and space. *Annual Review of Anthropology, 25*, 353–382.

Levinson, S. C., Kita, S., Haun, D., & Rasch, B. H. (2002). Returning the tables: Language affects spatial reasoning. *Cognition, 84*, 155–188.

Li, P., & Gleitman, L. (2002). Turning the tables: Language and spatial reasoning. *Cognition, 83*, 265–294.

Lillard, A. (1998). Ethnopsychologies: Cultural variations in theories of mind. *Psychological Bulletin, 123*, 3–32.

Liu, L. G. (1985). Reasoning counterfactually in Chinese: Are there any obstacles? *Cognition, 21*, 239–270.

Liu, S. H. (1974). The use of analogy and symbolism in traditional Chinese philosophy. *Journal of Chinese Philosophy, 1*, 313–338.

Lloyd, G. E. R. (1990). *Demystifying mentalities.* New York: Cambridge University Press.

Lucy, J. A. (1997). Linguistic relativity. *Annual Review of Anthropology, 26*, 291–312.

Lucy, J. A., & Gaskins, S. (1997). Grammatical categories and the development of classification preferences: A comparative approach. In S. C. Levinson & M. Bowerman (Eds.), *Language acquisition and conceptual development*. Cambridge, UK: Cambridge University Press.

Lucy, J. A., & Shweder, R. (1979). Whorf and his critics: Linguistic and nonlinguistic influences on color memory. *American Anthropologist, 81,* 581–615.

Luria, A. R. (1931). Psychological expedition to Central Asia. *Science, 74,* 383–384.

Luria, A. R. (1971). Towards the problem of the historical nature of psychological processes. *International Journal of Psychology, 6,* 259–272.

Markus, H. R., & Kitayama, S. (1991). Culture and the self: Implications for cognition, emotion, and motivation. *Psychological Review, 98,* 224–253.

Markus, H. R., Mullally, P. R., & Kitayama, S. (1997). Selfways: Diversity in modes of cultural participation. In U. Neisser & D. Jopling (Eds.), *The conceptual self in context*. Cambridge, UK: Cambridge University Press.

Masuda, T., & Kitayama, S. (2003). Perceiver-induced constraint and attitude attribution in Japan and the U.S.: A case for the cultural dependence of the correspondence bias. *Journal of Experimental Social Psychology, 40,* 409–416.

Masuda, T., & Nisbett, R. E. (2001). Attending holistically versus analytically: Comparing the context sensitivity of Japanese and Americans. *Journal of Personality and Social Psychology, 81,* 922–934.

Masuda, T., & Nisbett, R. E. (2005). *Culture and change blindness*. Unpublished manuscript, Hokkaido University, Sapporo, Japan.

Medin, D. L. & Atran. S. (2004). The native mind: Biological categorization, reasoning and decision making in development across cultures. *Psychological Review, 111,* 960–983.

Miller, J. G. (1984). Culture and the development of everyday social explanation. *Journal of Personality and Social Psychology, 46,* 961–978.

Miller, K. F., & Paredes, D. R. (1996). On the shoulders of giants: Cultural tools and mathematical development. In R. J. Sternberg & T. Ben-Zeev (Eds.), *The nature of mathematical thinking* (pp. 83–117). Mahwah, NJ: Erlbaum.

Miller, K. F., Smith, C. M., Zhu, J., & Zhang, H. (1995). Preschool origins of cross-national differences in mathematical competence: The role of number naming systems. *Psychological Science, 6,* 56–60.

Miller, K. F., & Stigler, J. W. (1987). Counting in Chinese: Cultural variation in basic cognitive skill. *Cognitive Development, 2,* 279–305.

Miyamoto, Y., & Kitayama, S. (2002). Cultural variation in correspondence bias: The critical role of attitude diagnosticity of socially constrained behavior. *Journal of Personality and Social Psychology, 83,* 1239–1248.

Miyamoto, Y., Kitayama, S., & Talhelm, T. (2006, January). *A meta-analytic review of cultural differences in cognitive processes*. Poster presented at the 6th Conference of the Society for Personality and Social Psychology, Palm Springs, CA.

Miyamoto, Y., Nisbett, R. E., & Masuda, T. (2006). Culture and the physical environment: Holistic versus analytic perceptual affordances. *Psychological Science, 17,* 113–119.

Morris, M. W., & Peng, K. (1994). Culture and cause: American and Chinese attributions for social and physical events. *Journal of Personality and Social Psychology, 67,* 949–971.

Munro, D. J. (1969). *The concept of man in early China*. Stanford, CA: Stanford University Press.

Nagashima, N. (1973). A reversed world: Or is it? In R. Horton, & R. Finnegan (Eds.), *Modes of thought: Essays on thinking in Western and non-Western societies* (pp. 92–111). London: Faber & Faber.

Nakamura, H. (1985). *Ways of thinking of Eastern peoples*. Honolulu: University of Hawaii Press. (Original work published 1964)

Needham, J. (1978). *Science and civilisation in China. Vol. 4: Physics and physical technology*. Cambridge, UK: Cambridge University Press. (Original work published 1962)

Needham, J. (1978). *The history of Chinese science and technology*. Chiu-Lung: Chung Hua Shu Chu. (Original work published 1962)

Neisser, U. (1963). The multiplicity of thought. *British Journal of Psychology, 54,* 1–14.

Nisbett, R. E. (2003). *The geography of thought*. New York: Free Press.

Nisbett, R. E., & Masuda, T. (2003). Culture and point of view. *Proceedings of the National Academy of Sciences USA, 100,* 11163–11170.

Nisbett, R. E., & Norenzayan, A. (2002). Culture and cognition. In D. L. Medin (Ed.), *Stevens' handbook of experimental psychology: Cognition* (3rd ed., pp. 561–597). New York: Wiley.

Nisbett, R. E., Peng, K., Choi, I., & Norenzayan, A. (2001). Culture and systems of thought: Holistic vs. analytic cognition. *Psychological Review, 108,* 291–310.

Norenzayan, A. (2005a). *Fatalistic thinking across cultures and religions*. Unpublished raw data, University of British Columbia, Vancouver.

Norenzayan, A. (2005b). *Analytic and holistic thinking in Arabs, Chinese, and Canadians*. Unpublished manuscript, University of British Columbia, Vancouver.

Norenzayan, A., Choi, I., & Nisbett, R. E. (2002). Cultural similarities and differences in social inference: Evidence from behavioral predictions and lay theories of behavior. *Personality and Social Psychology Bulletin, 28,* 109–120.

Norenzayan, A., & Heine, S. J. (2005). Psychological universals across cultures: What are they and how can we know? *Psychological Bulletin, 135,* 763–784.

Norenzayan, A., & Nisbett, R. E. (2000). Culture and causal cognition. *Current Directions in Psychological Science, 9,* 132–135.

Norenzayan, A., Schaller, M., & Heine, S. (2006). Evolution and culture. In M. Schaller, J. Simpson, & D. Kenrick (Eds.), *Evolution and social psychology* (pp. 343–366). New York: Psychology Press.

Norenzayan, A., Smith, E. E., & Kim, B., & Nisbett, R. E. (2002). Cultural preferences for formal versus intuitive reasoning. *Cognitive Science, 26,* 653–684.

Oishi, S. (2004). *The socio-ecological model of the self: The role of residential mobility.* Paper presented at the 1st Cultural Psychology Preconference, Society for Personality and Social Psychology, New Orleans, LA.

Oyserman, D., Kemmelmeier, M., & Coon, H. (2002). Rethinking individualism and collectivism: Evaluation of theoretical assumptions and meta-analyses. *Psychological Bulletin, 128,* 3–72.

Peng, K., & Knowles, E. (2003). Culture, education, and the attribution of physical causality. *Personality and Social Psychology Bulletin, 29,* 1272–1284.

Peng, K., & Nisbett, R. E. (1999). Culture, dialectics, and reasoning about contradiction. *American Psychologist, 54,* 741–754.

Pica, P., Lerner, C., Izard, V., & Dehaene, S. (2004). Exact and approximate arithmetic in an Amazonian indigenous group. *Science, 306,* 499–501.

Pinker, S. (1997). *How the mind works.* New York: Norton.

Rensink, R. A., O'Regan, J. K., & Clark, J. J. (1997). To see or not to see: The need for attention to perceive changes in scenes. *Psychological Science, 8,* 368–373.

Resnick, L. B. (1994). Situated rationalism: Biological and social preparation for learning. In L. A. Hirschfeld & S. A. Gelman (Eds.), *Mapping the mind: Domain specificity in cognition and culture* (pp. 474–494). Cambridge, UK: Cambridge University Press.

Revlin, R., Leirer, V., Yop, H., & Yop, R. (1980). The belief–bias effect in formal reasoning: The influence of knowledge on logic. *Memory and Cognition, 8,* 584–592.

Rhee, E., Uleman, J. S., Lee, H. K., & Roman, R. J. (1996). Spontaneous self-descriptions and ethnic identities in individualistic and collectivistic cultures. *Journal of Personality and Social Psychology, 69,* 142–152.

Richerson, P. J., & Boyd, R. (2005). *Not by genes alone: How culture transformed human evolution.* Chicago: University of Chicago Press.

Roberson, D., Davies, I., & Davidoff, J. (2000). Color categories are not universal: Replications and new evidence from a stone-age culture. *Journal of Experimental Psychology: General, 129,* 369–398.

Rogoff, B. (1990). *Apprenticeship in thinking: Cognitive development in social context.* New York: Oxford University Press.

Sanchez-Burks, J. (2002). Protestant relational ideology and (in)attention to relational cues in work settings. *Journal of Personality and Social Psychology, 83,* 919–929.

Saunders, B. A. C., & van Brakel, J. (1997). Are there non-trivial constraints on color categorization? *Behavioral and Brain Sciences, 20,* 167–178.

Schaller, M. (2001). Unintended influence: Social–evolutionary processes in the construction and change of culturally-shared beliefs. In J. P. Forgas & K. D. Williams (Eds.), *Social influence: Direct and indirect processes* (pp. 77–93). Philadelphia: Psychology Press.

Scribner, S. (1975). Recall of classical syllogisms: A cross-cultural investigation of error on logical problems. In R. Falmagne (Ed.), *Reasoning: Representation and process* (pp. 153–174). Hillsdale, NJ: Erlbaum.

Scribner, S. (1977). Modes of thinking and ways of speaking: Culture and logic reconsidered. In P. N. Johnson-Laird & P. C. Wason (Eds.), *Thinking: Readings in cognitive science* (pp. 483–500). New York: Cambridge University Press.

Segall, M. H., Campbell, D. T., & Herskovits, M. J. (1966). *The influence of culture on visual perception.* New York: Bobbs-Merrill.

Shweder, R. A. (1991). Cultural psychology: What is it? In R. A. Shweder (Ed.), *Thinking through cultures: Expeditions in cultural psychology* (pp. 73–110). Cambridge, MA: Harvard University Press.

Simons, D. J. (2000). Current approaches to change blindness. *Visual Cognition, 7,* 1–15.

Simons, D. J., & Chabris, C. F. (1999). Gorillas in our midst: Sustained inattentional blindness for dynamic events. *Perception, 28,* 1059–1074.

Slobin, D. (1996). From "thought and language" to "thinking for speaking." In J. Gumperz & S. Levinson (Eds.), *Rethinking linguistic relativity* (pp. 70–96). Cambridge, UK: Cambridge University Press.

Sloman, S. (1996). The empirical case for two systems of reasoning. *Psychological Bulletin, 119,* 30–52.

Spelke, E. S. (1990). Principles of object perception. *Cognitive Science, 14,* 29–56.

Spelke, E. S., Phillips, A., & Woodward, A. L. (1995). Infants' knowledge of object motion and human action. In D. Sperber, D. Premack, & A. J. Premack (Eds.), *Causal cognition: A multidisciplinary debate* (pp. 44–78). Oxford, UK: Oxford University Press.

Spencer-Rodgers, J., & Peng, K. (2003). The dialectical self: Contradiction, change, and holism in the East Asian self-concept. In R. M. Sorrentino, D. Cohen, J. M. Olsen, & M. P. Zanna (Eds.), *Culture and social behavior: The Ontario Symposium* (Vol. 10, pp. 227–249). Mahwah, NJ: Erlbaum.

Spencer-Rodgers, J., Peng, K., Wang, L., & Hou, Y. (2003). Dialectical self-esteem and East–West differences in psychological well-being. *Personality and Social Psychology Bulletin, 30,* 1416–1432.

Sperber, D. (1996). *Explaining culture: A naturalistic approach.* Cambridge, MA: Blackwell.

Stich, S. P. (1990). *Fragmentation of reason.* Cambridge, MA: MIT Press.

Stewart van Leeuwen, M. (1973). Tests of the carpentered world hypothesis by race and environment in America and Zambia. *International Journal of Psychology, 8,* 83–94.

Tardif, T. (1996). Nouns are not always learned before verbs: Evidence from Mandarin-speakers early vocabularies. *Developmental Psychology, 32,* 492–504.

Tomasello, M. (1999). *The cultural origins of human cognition.* Cambridge, MA: Harvard University Press.

Tomasello, M., Kruger, A. C., & Ratner, H. H. (1993). Cultural learning. *Behavioral and Brain Sciences, 16,* 495–552.

Triandis, H. C. (1989). The self and social behavior in differing cultural contexts. *Psychological Review, 96,* 269–289.

Triandis, H. C. (1995). *Individualism and collectivism.* Boulder, CO: Westview Press.

Tweed, R. G., & Lehman, D. R. (2002). Learning considered within a cultural context: Confucian and Socratic approaches. *American Psychologist, 57,* 89–99.

Unsworth, S. J., & Medin, D. L. (2005). Cultural differences in belief bias associated with deductive reasoning? *Cognitive Science, 29,* 525–529.

Vygotsky, L. S. (1978). *Mind in society: The development of higher psychological processes.* Cambridge, MA: Harvard University Press.

Wellman, H. M., Cross, D., & Watson, J. (2001). Meta-analysis of theory-of-mind development: The truth about false belief. *Child Development, 72,* 655–684.

Whorf, B. L. (1956). *Language, thought and reality.* New York: Wiley.

Witkin, H. A., & Berry, J. W. (1975). Psychological differentiation in cross-cultural perspective. *Journal of Cross Cultural Psychology, 6,* 4–87.

Witkin, H. A., Dyk, R. B., Faterson, H. F., Goodenough, D. R., & Karp, S. A. (1974). *Psychological differentiation.* Potomac, MD: Erlbaum.

Witkin, H. A., Lewis, H. B., Hertzman, M., Machover, K., Meissner, P. B., & Karp, S. A. (1954). *Personality through perception.* New York: Harper.

Wundt, W. (1916). *Elements of folk psychology: Outlines of a psychological history of the development of mankind.* London: Allen & Unwin/Macmillan.

Zebian, S., & Denny, J. P. (2001). Integrative cognitive style in Middle Eastern and Western groups. *Journal of Cross-Cultural Psychology, 32,* 58–75.

Zhang, D. L. (1985). The concept of "Tian Ren He Yi" in Chinese philosophy. *Beijing University Journal, 1,* 8.

Zhang, D. L., & Chen, Z. Y. (1991). *Zhongguo Siwei Pianxiang* [The orientation of Chinese thinking]. Beijing: Social Science Press.

CHAPTER 24

Narrative Reverberations

How Participation in Narrative Practices Co-Creates Persons and Cultures

PEGGY J. MILLER
HEIDI FUNG
MICHELE KOVEN

In *The Girl with the Brown Crayon: How Children Use Stories to Shape Their Lives*, Vivian Gussin Paley (1997) tells the story of a small black girl's passion for the books of Leo Lionni, a passion that transforms the kindergarten class and Paley's final year of teaching. The student, Reeny, is hooked first by *Frederick*, the story of a brown mouse whom she recognizes to be a kindred spirit. The students read and reread each book until they have memorized it. They discuss, ponder, and dramatize the story, and create posters that depict characters and scenes. Surprising things happen: Characters from different books turn out to be friends, Frederick shows up in a classmate's closely guarded fantasy world, previously inhabited entirely by rabbits. The Leo Lionni stories call forth other stories: epics from India, stories from a one-room schoolhouse in Mississippi, Harriet Tubman's adventures freeing slaves, including Reeny's great-great-grandmother. Paley notes that stories "proceed as if nothing else is going on" (p. viii).

In the process, they bring disparate people, places, and times into their orbit. By the end of the school year Reeny, the natural-born leader, innovator, and practitioner of the introspective life, is ready for first grade. Her teacher, contemplating an uncertain identity outside the classroom, faces many questions and a new beginning, but one in which the story of Reeny and Leo Lionni's stories will play a part.

We begin with this example because it dramatizes especially well how narrative reverberates through the lives of individuals, connecting them to other people, other stories, and other activities, and teaching them who they are or might become. Our goal in this chapter is to explain how narrative practices, such as those in Paley's classroom, are implicated in the co-creation of persons and cultures across the lifespan and across a variety of cultural contexts. Although the co-creation of person and culture is widely recognized to be a fundamental problem in cultural psychology, the mechanisms of this process have remained mysterious. We argue that everyday narrative practices can be fruitfully examined as one key site for how and where the co-creation of persons and cultures is accomplished.

The chapter is organized in the following manner: We first define practice approaches to narrative and identify some of the intellectual currents that have contributed to this perspective. We then engage the problem of the co-creation of person and culture at two disparate moments in the life course: early childhood and late adulthood. Growing literature shows that very young children participate in oral narrative, and that these "primary" stories are culturally differentiated from the beginning. At this very early moment stories are already implicated in the socialization process, drawing children into local systems of meaning and launching them along pathways toward particular versions of personhood. Without claiming to be exhaustive, we review work in this area, underscore important insights, and point to promising questions for future work. We then turn our attention to the other end of the life course. This literature is much more sparse, raising a host of questions. We use two examples of ethnographic work—Basso's (1996) study of Western Apache narrative practices and Fung's (2003) study of a Taiwanese grandmother's story of her two marriages—to illustrate the cumulative consequences of decades of participation in narrative practices. At both ends of the life course narrative serves as a medium of both socialization, reproducing meanings and anchoring identities, and innovation and transformation, enabling people to alter their experience and reenvision their lives.

PRACTICE APPROACHES TO NARRATIVE

If meaning making lies at the heart of cultural psychology and narrative is a universal tool of meaning making, then the study of narrative is critical to furthering the most basic aims of cultural psychology. The process of negotiating and renegotiating meanings via narrative has been called "one of the crowning achievements of human development" (Bruner, 1990, p. 67). But what types of "meaning" does the analyst investigate? Cultural psychologists and scholars from allied disciplines have argued that the power of narrative cannot be fully appreciated without recognizing that it is a social practice, not just a form of representation. In other words, the role of stories can be most fruitfully studied not only by examining the content and structure of stories but also by seeing narratives as embedded activities (e.g., Bauman, 1986; Miller, 1994; Wortham, 2001).

So, following the Reeny example, we could examine the referential meaning of the Lionni books, their themes and plots, to discern how the characters and actions are represented. Such an analysis might help us to understand part of why Reeny found these books so appealing. But it would leave out a great deal. It would leave out how Reeny and her classmates *used* these stories to make sense of themselves, one another, and the world. It would leave out the intensity and the varied modes of their engagement: listening silently with the whole body, memorizing, questioning, rewriting, disagreeing, dramatizing, and painting. It would leave out how friendships grew, faltered, and revived through and around these stories, and how the whole class cohered around a common frame of reference and an evolving set of narrative practices. And it would leave out the temporal trajectory of these stories: the history of how these children and teachers immersed themselves day after day in the Lionni stories, decontextualizing and recontextualizing them again and again (Bauman & Briggs, 1990).

A practice or sociopragmatic approach to narrative also raises questions that reach beyond the classroom itself. What did the various participants contribute to this emerging narrative community from their own cultural experiences? Apparently, Reeny's avid interest and confident engagement in stories predated her arrival at kindergarten. When her mother, father, and grandmother make successive guest appearances at school, we hear the oral stories that are Reeny's birthright. No wonder Reeny recognizes Frederick: "That brown mouse seem to be just like me!" (Paley, 1997, p. 5). Similarly, the Lionni stories remind Paley's coteacher, who grew up in India, of the stories of the monkey prince that her mother and grandmother told her at bedtime, prompting her to share these stories with the children. Although the Lionni stories are fresh, new, and mind-expanding, they carry the children and teachers back to other stories, forming a narrative circle between home and school. Paley's description illustrates that narrative cannot be sealed off from the rest of social life, a basic premise of practice approaches to narrative.

Premises of Practice Approaches to Narrative

The turn toward a practice approach to narrative is part of a larger trend toward practice-centered conceptions of language in cultural psychology and allied disciplines (e.g., Bauman & Briggs, 1990; Duranti & Goodwin, 1992; Goodnow, Miller, & Kessel, 1995; Ochs & Schieffelin, 1984; Shweder et al., 2006). These conceptions rest on the premise that to speak is to act—to create, perform, and transform social realities. A number of intellectual currents have fed into such practice-centered views of language, including scholarship that addresses the pragmatic features of talk—what people "do" with words (Austin, 1975) and sociocultural theory, with its focus on semiotically mediated activity (Cole, 1996; Wertsch, 1991). These perspectives converge on a conception of language that privileges the analysis of speech events in context (Bauman & Briggs, 1990; Bauman & Sherzer, 1989; Duranti & Goodwin, 1992; Hanks, 1996; Hymes, 1974; Jakobson, 1960). Hanks (1996) describes speech as "a form of engagement in the world. . . . To speak is to occupy the world, not only to represent it, and this occupancy entails various modes of expression, of which propositional meaning is only one" (p. 236). Terms such as "talk," "speaking praxis," "language use," and "communicative practices" are therefore used to signal a contrast with the narrowly referential conception of language that holds sway in most research on human development and cross-cultural psychology. Instead of reducing language to a representational system or repository of knowledge, this approach recognizes the functional inseparability of talk and nonverbal action, and attends to how speech forms implicitly index or point to dimensions of interactional and sociocultural context (Silverstein, 1976/1995).

This approach enriches cultural psychology by expanding the toolbox of analytic techniques that scholars can use to examine talk as a cultural phenomenon. It allows the analyst to look at what participants "do" with each other in interaction—how, through talk, they position themselves relative to each other, and to broader sociocultural values and types of people.

Furthermore, because a practice approach assumes that words cannot be sealed off from silence or from gaze, posture, gesture, and other practices of the body, it allows the analyst to treat talk (including narrative) as multimodal, inviting questions about how silence is patterned, and how verbal and nonverbal systems are choreographed and integrated.

In addition, a practice approach recognizes that speaking is organized beyond the sentence level into dialogues and genres (including a multitude of narrative genres). These larger communicative events and stretches of discourse, while serving as units of analysis, are themselves multiply embedded in larger sociocultural contexts and networks of cultural practices. In contrast to approaches that take the disembodied word, sentence, or text as the unit of analysis, this approach permits a deeper cultural analysis, for it recognizes that cultural principles are expressed not only in the content of talk but also in the way that discourse is organized internally and in relation to larger events and sequences of talk.

Creating Persons through Repeated Participation in Narrative

We said earlier that sociocultural theory is one of the intellectual currents contributing to a practice approach to narrative. Scholars working out of this tradition emphasize the routine or recurring nature of cultural practices, including narrative practices, in everyday life (e.g., Miller & Goodnow, 1995; Scribner & Cole, 1981). From this perspective, one way that cultural principles are expressed is in terms of the types of narrative practiced routinely. Several scholars have applied ideas from Vygotskian theory in an effort to understand the role that narrative plays in childhood socialization (e.g., Fivush, 1993; Nelson, 1989, 1996; Sperry & Sperry, 2000). For example, following Vygotsky's account of the acquisition of scientific concepts, Miller (1994) proposed a discourse model of socialization in which institutions are organized to bring novices and members together recurrently for particular activities mediated by particular forms of discourse that lead to particular social and psychological consequences for the participants. As applied to the family, the institution in which early socialization occurs, the model posits that young children are socialized into systems of meaning through recurring interactions with family members that are mediated by narrative and other discursive practices. This approach to socialization has specific implications for empirical work, requiring that researchers identify the kinds of narrative practices that young children routinely encounter in their everyday lives and the kinds of participant roles that are available to them.

Establishing the recurrent nature of narrative practices is especially important from the standpoint of the co-creation of person and culture. The power that narrative has to create certain kinds of persons rests in part on the frequency with which children participate in narrative. In the next section of this chapter, "Narrative in Early Childhood," we return to this issue. For now, we underscore two points. First, most research on children's narratives relies on elicited narratives; thus it cannot address the question of which narratives occur routinely in the child's life. Although elicited narratives can inform us about many important questions, observational and ethnographic studies are needed to address this question. Second, an important trend in research on the consequences of children's participation in narrative (and other cultural practices) is toward an expanded view of those consequences. Scholars argue that children not only acquire cognitive skills, such as the ability to tell stories to themselves and to other people, but they also develop selves and identities, affective stances, forms of moral agency, and ways of being (e.g., Fung, Miller, & Lin, 2004; Goodnow et al., 1995; Lave & Wenger, 1990; Miller, Fung, & Mintz, 1996; Rogoff, 1990; Wenger, 1998).

Creating Persons by Representing and Enacting Selves in Narrative

In addition to sociocultural theory, a variety of other theoretical traditions have treated narrative as a particularly rich type of discursive practice. This work, some of it familiar to cultural psychologists, draws from research on discourse in sociolinguistics that examines narrative "evaluation" (Labov, 1972; Labov & Waletzky, 1967), linguistic anthropology that examines "voicing" or "footing" (Bakhtin, 1981; Bauman, 1986; Goffman, 1979; M. H. Goodwin, 1990; Hill, 1995; Koven, 2002; Ochs & Capps, 2001; Voloshinov, 1973; Wortham, 2001) and conversation analysis (M. H. Goodwin, 1990; Jefferson, 1978, 1984; Mandelbaum, 1987, 1989; Sacks, 1974) that addresses the participant frameworks out of which stories emerge and which they transform. (See Koven, 2002, for discussion of these

several approaches.) Across these traditions, scholars investigate the "meaning" of stories not for their themes or plots but for the social actions participants accomplish. In such work, with its focus on "meaning" as interactional accomplishment, scholars have sometimes resisted addressing the psychological import of stories, out of a reluctance to see meaning as situated in and produced by the individual. However, with the stance that psychological meaning is deeply intertwined with social activity, such sociocentric accounts are perfectly compatible with current visions of cultural psychology.

More specifically, scholars taking a sociopragmatic approach have investigated how participation in narrative practices can construct participants' selves or identities (e.g., Bruner, 1990; Hill, 1995; Holland, Lachicotte, Skinner, & Cain, 1998; Miller, 1994; Ochs & Capps, 1996; Schiffrin, 1996; Urban, 1989). According to Wortham (2001), for example, narratives construct participants' identities insofar as narratives allow people simultaneously to enact and represent themselves in particular ways. Wortham argues that most attempts to understand how autobiographical narrative constructs and transforms the self are inadequate, because they analyze narrative only at the representational or content level. In other words, autobiographical narratives function not only to represent the self-protagonist in past events but also to position the narrator in relation to his or her audience in the here-and-now event of storytelling. He analyzes one woman's telling of her life story, showing how her description of herself as a character was mirrored by the stance she took toward her interviewer. While describing herself in the story as repeatedly moving from a passive to an active self over the course of her life, she simultaneously alternated positioning herself first as passive and vulnerable and then as active and assertive vis-à-vis the interviewer over the course of the interview. Wortham argues that such parallels, or "doubling," across representational and interactional levels of analysis constitute especially potent moments of self-creation and re-creation. Attention to the content of stories alone would miss how participants' selves are constructed in and through the storytelling interaction itself.

In keeping with this perspective, in a later section of this chapter, "Narratives in Late

Adulthood," we discuss a Taiwanese grandmother's narrative of her two marriages, which she had never shared with anyone, including her grown children. These intimate and intensely emotional events were tellable only to the ethnographer, precisely because she was an outsider to the family. We argue that the meanings that Mrs. Lin constructed about herself can be most fully appreciated by taking into account not only her narrative representations of her marriages but also the social circumstances that disallowed the telling of these stories to anyone but herself in the course of her everyday life.

NARRATIVE IN EARLY CHILDHOOD

In the Beginning, Personal Storytelling Abounds

By the time she entered kindergarten, Reeny was a veteran of narrative, steeped in oral stories about herself and her family. Surrounded as she was by gifted storytellers, we can surmise that she was exposed to stories from birth. Indeed, it is now well established that children from many cultural backgrounds within and beyond the United States begin to tell stories of personal experience in conversation during the second or third year of life (e.g., see reviews by Miller, Cho, & Bracey, 2005; Ochs & Capps, 2001; Shweder et al., 2006). At this early age, children step into the narrative practices of family and community, thereby laying claim to a vitally important cultural resource (Bruner, 1990). Even linguistically isolated deaf children, whose parents choose not to expose them to a conventional sign system, are able to create gestured narratives (Van Deusen-Phillips, Goldin-Meadow, & Miller, 2001). These stories carry hints of culture-specific meaning, suggesting that conversational narrative is a remarkably robust medium of socialization.

Young children's stories of personal experience tend to be simple, invoking small departures from the baseline of their ordinary, expectable experience: A child gets a shot; shares, unprompted, with a sibling; goes to a birthday party; helps to cook a meal; writes on the bedroom wall; defends herself against a cousin's aggression. Small events such as these have emotional or moral significance to the child and her family and are thus "reportable." Consider the following example, in which the child Amy fell down and hurt herself, an unexpected event with obvious emotional import. This story was initiated by Amy's mother: "She pulled a little sneaky the other day, went out the back door and fell down the back steps and busted her back all up. . . . Didn't you? Went out there and fell." Amy nodded her head, then said, "Me big fall down," lifting up her dress to show the damage. Her mother replied, "You fell down, yeah [smiles]. You hit your back." Although Amy was only 19 months old, she was able to contribute to this story of her own mishap, echoing her mother's account, and adding a nonverbal embellishment (Miller & Sperry, 1988). Another child, age 3 years, launched a story about a memorable encounter during a recent family visit to the zoo: "Remember the walrus? . . . This is what he said '[makes spitting noises].' " Her mother replied, "Yeah, at the zoo. You went to the zoo again." The child then repeated the walrus's noise and enacted his surprising antics (Burger & Miller, 1999).

These stories may seem unremarkable, so mundane as to be negligible. From the standpoint of socialization, however, they are anything but negligible. Their power lies partly in their sheer abundance. Ethnographic observations of young children in the contexts of everyday family life show that telling stories of personal experience is a *recurring practice* in a wide variety of communities. For example, stories involving 2½-year-olds occurred at average rates of three to four per hour in both middle-class Taiwanese families in Taipei and middle-class European American families in Chicago (Miller, Wiley, Fung, & Liang, 1997). In a follow-up study of the same children at 3, 3½, and 4 years of age, stories of personal experience continued at similar rates (Chen, Lin, Miller, & Fung, 2005). Narratives accounted for one-fourth of 2-year-olds' naturally occurring talk in working-class African American families in the Black Belt of Alabama (Sperry & Sperry, 1995, 1996). In working-class European American families in Chicago, 3-year-olds participated in conarrations at an average rate of six times per hour (Burger & Miller, 1999). These and other studies suggest that the early years of life are a period of intense initiation into narrative. In interaction after interaction, personal storytelling gets woven, densely but almost invisibly, into the fabric of young children's social experience. Before long, telling and listening to stories become second nature to them.

Early Storytelling Is Culturally Differentiated

Regardless of where they occur, these small, mundane stories are saturated with value and replete with culturally patterned messages. Personal stories vary within and across cultures along a variety of parameters that encompass how the genre is defined and practiced (Miller et al., 2005; Miller & Moore, 1989; Ochs & Capps, 2001).

For example, in her classic ethnographic study of neighboring, working-class communities in the Piedmont Carolinas, Heath (1983) found that members of Roadville, a European American community, adhered to a criterion of literal truth when narrating their personal experiences, a pattern that also occurred in the working-class communities of South Baltimore and Daly Park (Miller, Hengst, Alexander, & Sperry, 2000). This contrasted with the African American community of Trackton, where a "story" was not a story if it lacked fictional embellishment. Roadville and Trackton also enacted opposing norms toward denigration versus aggrandizement in their portrayals of the self-protagonist. Roadville children's stories occurred in response to adult invitations and focused on each child's own weakness or foolishness. Trackton children created bold, self-expressive, and triumphant self-protagonists, and asserted their right to tell stories by adroitly working their way into multiparty talk, commanding the floor and receiving approbation for their verbal artistry.

In their study of an African American community in rural Alabama, Sperry and Sperry (1995, 1996, 2000) found that 2-year-olds produced more fantasy stories than factual stories of past experience. "Both caregivers and children enjoyed telling stories of escaping from 'Nicoudini,' the 'Boogabear,' 'Werewolf,' or the spectral deer who entered their home one misty evening. Families told such stories easily and frequently, and children gathered around to be thrilled by the imagined terror and to practice creating it themselves" (Sperry & Sperry, 1996, p. 462). Caregivers actively discouraged girls' fantasy stories but were more accepting of boys' fantasy stories, a finding that may help to explain how men in this community get to be so good at "tall-bragging." Hypothetical stories, that is, stories about what could happen, were a relatively late development.

Another dimension of cultural variability in early storytelling has to do with the didactic use of stories. Several studies show that Chinese parents treat personal storytelling as an explicitly didactic medium (e.g., Van Deusen-Phillips et al., 2001; Q. Wang, 2004; Q. Wang & Leichtman, 2000; Q. Wang, Leichtman, & Davies, 2000; X. Wang, Bernas, & Eberhard, 2005). For example, Miller, Fung, and their colleagues conducted a series of comparisons of middle-class Taiwanese families in Taipei and middle-class European American families in Chicago, and found that the Taiwanese families were much more likely to tell stories in which they cast the 2½-year-old child-protagonist as a transgressor (Miller et al., 1996, 1997). In keeping with local beliefs that parents should take every opportunity to correct young children through concrete exemplars (Fung, 1999), many of these stories occurred immediately after the child had committed a misdeed in the here and now. In conarrated stories, and in stories told about the child in the child's presence, families repeatedly invoked moral and social rules, structured their stories so as to establish the child's misdeed as the point of the story, and concluded their stories with didactic codas.

By contrast, the European American families rarely told stories about young children's past transgressions. Even in those rare instances when a European American child's transgression was narrated, a qualitatively different interpretation was constructed, one that downplayed the misdeed or framed it as humorous (Miller et al., 1996). Thus, whereas Taiwanese families were more likely to use personal storytelling as a didactic resource for correcting young children and conveying moral and social standards, European American families were more likely to use personal storytelling as a medium of entertainment and self-affirmation. This contrast was also evident in parents' beliefs about storytelling (Miller, Sandel, Liang, & Fung, 2001) and in pretend play (Haight, Wang, Fung, Williams, & Mintz, 1999).

Moreover, the contrasting versions of personal storytelling practiced by the European American and Taiwanese families reflect and reinforce larger systems of cultural meaning in each cultural case. The self-favorability bias enacted by the European American families has been linked to discourses that valorize self-esteem (Miller et al., 1997, 2001); the didactic bias enacted by the Taiwanese families has been linked to Confucian discourses that valorize teaching, listening, and self-improvement, discourses that continue to circulate in the complex mix of local and global influences that are reshaping child rearing and education in contemporary Taiwan (Fung et al., 2004).

In summary, studies of children's early storytelling in families and communities demonstrate that this narrative genre is culturally differentiated from the beginning. Wherever personal storytelling is practiced with young children, it takes on local color, absorbing values, affective stances, and moral orientations. As they participate routinely in personal storytelling, children not only imbibe values and acquire narrative skills but also begin to carve out different versions of personal experience. Personal storytelling thus highlights—and is implicated in—an early developmental moment in the co-creation of person and culture. Particular frameworks of evaluation and interpretation, linked to larger currents of cultural meaning, operate again and again in oral stories as narrators and listeners create and respond to here-and-now social contingencies. Each story conarrated with the child, each story told to a family member in the child's presence, provides another opportunity for the child to hear which experiences are reportable and how these experiences should be assessed. In this way, interpretive frameworks are not only reproduced but also repeatedly instantiated in personally relevant terms.

To return to the comparisons between European Americans and Taiwanese, we catch a glimpse of how culturally distinct selves might originate. One of the most intriguing findings of cultural psychology is that adult selves are culturally variable. For example, comparative studies challenge the assumption that the need for positive self-regard is universal, demonstrating instead that it is specific to North American culture, with its distinctive ideologies and philosophical traditions (Heine & Lehman, 2003; Heine, Lehman, Markus, & Kitayama, 1999). By contrast, Japanese selves have a more critical focus (Heine & Lehman, 2003; Heine et al., 1999), and the Chinese concept of personhood is rooted in the Confucian emphasis on a lifetime commitment to the continuously broadening and deepening process of self-cultivation, self-perfection, and self-transformation (Li, 2004a, 2004b; Tu, 1985,

1994; Q. Wang & Li, 2003). These findings about adults raise a critical developmental question: How do such culturally diverse selves come about? We propose that a need for positive self-regard is rooted, in part, in storytelling that is systematically biased toward self-favorability, whereas an inclination to self-improvement is rooted, in part, in the narration of misdeeds and the explicit invocation of moral standards. In the next section, we take a closer look at the roots of self-improvement, focusing on one Taiwanese child.

Co-Creating Persons and Cultures through Personal Storytelling

In the studies conducted by Fung, Miller, and their colleagues, youngsters from Taipei were exposed to one transgression story per hour on average (Miller et al., 1997). In the following lengthy example, described more fully by Fung et al. (2004), Yoyo (2½ years old) and his grandmother, Mrs. Lin, conarrated an incident that occurred earlier in the day, in which Yoyo committed two interlinked misdeeds: He knocked down a screen that divided the living room from the dining area, then protested when his mother spanked him. His grandmother initiated this story by saying, "Oh, yes, this morning, when Mom was spanking you, what did you say?" as she pulled Yoyo close and held him in her arms. Yoyo replied quietly, "[I] won't push the screen down [again]," while his grandmother lowered her head and leaned toward him to listen. In the ensuing 12 turns, she continued to review the incident with him, focusing her didactic efforts on his incorrect response—he had said, "Don't hit me!"— when his mother spanked him for knocking down the screen. His grandmother patiently pointed out where he went wrong and rehearsed in a hypothetical scenario what Yoyo should have said. Eventually, apparently satisfied that Yoyo now understood how he should behave when his mother corrects him, his grandmother explained to him that in the future he would be able to choose how to act: "Next time when Mom is going to spank you, which sentence is better for you to say to her?" Yoyo replied, "Hmm. Hmm. Say, 'I won't, I won't push the screen down.' " His grandmother replied, "Oh, yes, now you have choices. You say, 'Mom, I won't push the screen down.' In that way, Mom won't spank you. So next time when Mom is spanking you, you shouldn't say, 'You don't hit me [raises her voice and stamps on the floor with her right foot in imitation of YoYo's incorrect behavior]. You don't hit me [raises her voice and stamps on the floor again].' You shouldn't talk that way. . . . Instead, [if] you say to Mom, 'I won't push the screen down,' what would Mom do to you?" Yoyo then replied, "[She will give me] a tender touch." His grandmother repeated, "A tender touch," laughed loudly, picked him up, and held him tightly.

This conarration involved true–false questions, either–or options, repeated rehearsals, and a lesson that moved rapidly from the past, to the hypothetical, to the future. Without ever explicitly directing Yoyo to listen, his grandmother seemed to assume that even though he was only 2½ years old, he could follow a complex line of moral reasoning and learn from his past mistakes. And she seemed to trust that having learned, he would exercise sounder moral judgment in the future.

For his part, Yoyo was highly attentive to his grandmother throughout this protracted lesson. Most of his responses were of two sorts: he repeated words, preselected for him by his grandmother, or he assented verbally or nonverbally to her guidance. This pattern of responding might suggest that he was merely parroting what his grandmother said. Toward the end of the episode, however, he came up with his own novel response, one that surprised and delighted his grandmother. When Yoyo forecast that his mother would give him "a tender touch," he conveyed his faith that next time he would make the right choice, and that the right choice would restore him to his mother's good graces. In other words, as his grandmother expected, Yoyo not only listened and comprehended but also joined her to reflect upon his own behavior and project a better self.

Another important feature of this example is that it is the last in a series of five thematically linked retellings of the "same" events. These retellings unfolded over the course of an hour and a half and, at times, included Yoyo's older brother as conarrator, along with Yoyo and his grandmother (see Fung et al., 2004).

Thus, when this conarration is examined in the context of ongoing narrative activity, it is striking how much time and energy this family spent reviewing Yoyo's misdeeds. Equally striking, Yoyo accepted these critiques with patient forbearance, even when his older brother joined in. Yoyo listened attentively, admitted to his wrongdoing, rehearsed rules for appropriate conduct, and imagined doing better in the future. The retellings of these misdeeds varied in subtle ways, highlighting different facets of the past events, making links to other events, and developing slightly different moral implications. This is typical of the way that children's transgressions are narrated in the Taiwanese families, but there was nothing remotely like Yoyo's narratives in our corpus of narratives from the European American families in Longwood; instead young children's misdeeds were edited out of the narrative record entirely, downplayed, or laughed about (Miller et al., 1996, 1997).

The narrative practices in Taipei, which are part and parcel of the child's daily experience, bring together again and again the ingredients of self-improvement, thereby helping to explain how children like Yoyo come to be self-improving persons—keen listeners and morally discerning agents, with strong attachments to caregivers and high standards of self-evaluation. Yoyo's family not only repeatedly narrated his past transgressions, constantly updating the currently relevant misdeeds requiring his attention but also zeroed in on particular lapses, subjecting them to intense moral scrutiny. These practices continued when Yoyo was 3, 3½, and 4 years old (Chen et al., 2005).

In her influential account of Inuit socializing "dramas," J. Briggs (1998) characterized the provocative questions posed by family members as "magnets" that drew the child's attention to any events that might provide clues to their meaning. Similarly, we argue that Yoyo's own misdeeds became magnets for his attention and imagination. Within this set of recurring practices—practices that were simultaneously narrative, moral, social, affective, and self-relevant—Yoyo over time became a more active participant (Chen et al., 2005). At 3½ and 4 years of age, he not only continued to listen carefully to his caregivers but he also initiated stories about his own and others' misdeeds, disagreed with others' accounts of his behavior, and engaged in complex moral reasoning about his past and future actions. In short, our argument is that the narrative practices described here constitute an early route toward self-improvement. Yoyo's habitual participation in these practices from such a young age not only naturalizes the project of self-improvement but also provides a distinct developmental pathway.

The Dynamics of Narrative Practices

When narratives are treated as situated practices, rather than disembodied texts, it becomes apparent that storytelling is a dynamic process, emerging from particular circumstances, shaped by the interests of narrating participants, recurring in different combinations, and affording children a range of participant roles. Children participate repeatedly with family members in networks of narrative practices characterized by systematic variability and crosscutting redundancies. In story after story they reproduce cultural frameworks and instantiate them in personally relevant terms. However, narrative is also a medium of innovation, a means by which individuals transform their experiences and identities (Holland et al., 1998; Wortham, 2001).

The dynamic nature of narrative practices is most apparent when narrators tell the "same" story repeatedly, as happened with the story in which Yoyo knocked down the screen, then protested when punished. In that example, other family members took the lead in reinvoking this story for Yoyo's edification, expanding with each retelling the set of relevant associations. In the example presented at the beginning of this chapter, 5-year-old Reeny developed a passionate and infectious attachment to a written story. Children as young as 2 years of age develop similar passions—prolonged and intense attachments to particular stories, which they revisit again and again for weeks, months, and even years (e.g., Alexander, Miller, & Hengst, 2001; Engel, 1995; Miller, Hoogstra, Mintz, Fung, & Williams, 1993; Nelson, 1989; Wolf & Heath, 1992). The middle-class European American children in these studies treated their special stories as resources for discussion and pretense, and used them to ponder problems and to manage emotions, activities that were tolerated and supported by parents. These studies suggest that from the time young children enter into narrative sense making, they have the capacity to respond differentially to the ordinary narrative flow, seizing certain stories for especially active and intense engagement.

Most germane to the current point, however, are findings about how children's repeated engagements with their special stories change over time. Some children use their stories to manage emotions, seeking out their special stories at moments of distress or conquering fear

evoked by the story itself through incremental, child-controlled engagement with the scary parts (Alexander et al., 2001). In one example, a child was initially so frightened by several incidents in a videotaped story that she hid in the corner of the room; some days later, she no longer hid but covered her eyes; eventually she watched intently the formerly scary segments, commented on them, and enacted them with her sister.

Miller et al. (1993) described a child's attachment to "The Tale of Peter Rabbit" by Beatrix Potter. During the period from 23 to 24 months of age, Kurt produced six spontaneous retellings of the Peter Rabbit story. These retellings were not "copies" of the original story; rather, he incorporated stories of his own experience into the retellings, creating in effect a hybrid genre. Micro-level analysis of the content and plot of the successive retellings were conducted and revealed dramatic changes over time: Kurt successively appropriated and resolved conflicts posed by the written story, conflicts that paralleled concurrent experiences in his life. While retaining many elements of the Peter Rabbit story, he systematically transformed its plot, restoring harmony among the characters and canonical order to *his* world. Like the child who subdued her fear of the scary videotaped story, this child used his special story, in conjunction with stories of personal experience, as a tool of emotion regulation.

In addition to showing that very young children can transform their own experience through narrative, these studies also draw attention to three other important points. First, very few studies trace the "natural history" of stories over time; especially rare are studies that examine how stories operate over the long term in children's lives. A compelling exception with older children is Cindy Dell Clark's (2003) study of 5- to 8-year-olds with diabetes or severe asthma. One way that these children coped with chronic illness and frightening medical procedures was by imagining that a superhero from a favorite TV show kept them company. The superhero used his powers to protect the child during recurring moments of vulnerability. Second, these studies remind us that personal storytelling is not the only narrative genre that young children encounter; many youngsters inhabit worlds that are densely populated by written stories, stories from television and videotapes, and/or other genres of oral narrative. We still know very little about the narrative repertoires of young children (but see Hicks, 1991; Kamberelis, 1993; Preece, 1987; Sperry & Sperry, 1995).

Third, the practice perspective on narrative that we outlined earlier draws attention to the many ways stories are embedded in, blended with, or otherwise keep company with other stories, other genres, and other activities. This emphasis on pervasive intertextuality is usually associated with Mikhail Bakhtin (1981), the Russian literary scholar and philosopher of language. From a Bakhtinian perspective, stories of personal experience qualify as a "primary" genre, in that they are simple and combine readily to form "secondary" genres (Miller et al., 2000; Ochs & Capps, 2001). In other words, the stories of personal experience that we described earlier not only provide young children from diverse communities and cultures, with readily available and culturally hued resources for making sense of their own experience, but they also become a mediating tool by which children forge personal connections to other stories. The example of Kurt interweaving stories of personal experience with stories of Peter Rabbit illustrates this especially well: He inserted himself into Peter Rabbit's world and brought Peter Rabbit into his. As researchers apply Bakhtinian constructs to the analysis of children's discourse, it is becoming clear that narrative sense making involves juxtaposing and interweaving multiple narrative genres and multiple, even conflicting voices and ideological perspectives, and that every community affords such heterogeneity (e.g., Cazden, 1993; Dyson, 1993; Hicks, 1994; Kamberelis & Scott, 1992; Miller et al., 2000; Taylor, 1995; Tobin, 2000; Wertsch, 1991; Wortham, 2001).

NARRATIVE IN LATE ADULTHOOD

Cultural psychologists and scholars from related fields have paid less attention to narrative at the other end of the life course. Because we have less information about the kinds of narrative practices in which older adults routinely engage or how these practices are culturally differentiated, this section of the chapter is necessarily more speculative. It does appear, however, that there are some parallels with early childhood. For example, the "primary" genre of personal storytelling, which emerges so early

in many groups, continues to be practiced by older adults. Although none of the studies of early narrative cited previously focused on older adults, stories of personal experience told by grandparents and other older adults formed part of the narrative environment that these youngsters inhabited (e.g., Miller et al., 2005). Another practice that extends into older adulthood is the use of stories of personal experience to mediate or personalize other stories, such as religious texts, histories of the group, or stories of ancestors (e.g., Basso, 1996; Hudley, Haight, & Miller, 2003). And just as very young children may become "attached" to certain stories, revisiting, savoring, or revising them again and again, adults may be haunted, baffled, or sustained for decades by stories from their own or others' lives (e.g., Bruner, 1990; Coles, 1989; Fung, 2003; Gone, 1999, 2005; Hudley et al., 2003; Logan, 1989; Steedman, 1986). As the person tells the story repeatedly to self and others, it accrues layer upon layer of meaning and may be used to reinforce favored interpretations, to make sense or fail to make sense of events, to rationalize actions, or to construct new interpretations and craft new identities. Repeated tellings and reinterpretations of personal experience are institutionalized in psychotherapy, in religious conversion, and in Alcoholics Anonymous meetings (Holland et al., 1998; Spence, 1984; Stromberg, 1993).

Against this backdrop of continuity, there are obviously many differences between these disparate periods of life. Some older adults become narrative virtuosos (e.g., Bauman, 1986; Hudley et al., 2003), and in some cultural groups, people weave their stories of personal experience into overarching life stories, that is, oral stories of their lives over the long term (e.g., Linde, 1993; Peacock & Holland, 1993). In a recent collection of studies about narrative across the lifespan, Pratt and Fiese (2004) concluded that older adults' stories are often "epochal," embodying an appreciation of the sweep of history and of their own place in a generational trajectory, and that they use stories to ponder the meaning of their lives for themselves and for their offspring.

Western Apache Narratives and the Attainment of Wisdom

Older adults may use stories to socialize the young, as Yoyo's grandmother did via stories of personal experience, and as Reeny's teacher did via written stories. In such cases older adults use stories to introduce cultural novices to valued ways of being and acting. But stories matter to older adults not just for their generativity; older adults may use narratives as tools of lifelong meaning making, plumbing the subtle meanings of stories, anchoring and reorienting themselves and other adults in a moral universe, remaking themselves if necessary. This process is exemplified in Basso's (1996) classic account of Western Apache narrative practices. Basso discovered that the Western Apache exploited two symbolic resources—land and narrative—for maintaining the moral order. Stories about the early history of the group were known to have happened at particular locations in the natural landscape. As people went about their daily business, they moved through a landscape that was saturated with moral tales, tales that "make you live right," as one informant put it (p. 38), and they developed enduring ties to the stories and to the places where the stories had occurred. As a consequence of these bonds, people who behaved improperly were moved to reflect on and correct their misconduct. At times a member of the community might find it necessary to "aim" a story at an offender. If taken to heart, the story and the place with which it was associated would "stalk" the offender and promote beneficial change.

According to Basso (1996), a profound understanding of narrative was essential to the attainment of wisdom, as understood by the Western Apache. Because the path to wisdom was long and arduous, only a few individuals were able to persist and become truly wise. Wise men and women were highly respected and often lived to be very old. Wise people committed to memory a whole repertory of cautionary tales and reflected upon them at deeper and deeper levels. When a crisis arose, the wise person consulted these stories, determined which story fit the current situation, and used that story as a guide. "This is accomplished by picturing in one's mind the exact location where the narrated events unfolded and imagining oneself as actually taking part in them, always in the role of a story character who is known to be wise" (p. 140). If a strong sense of identification occurred, this confirmed that the narrative would be helpful in the current situation; if not, another story was selected. Wise men and women were able to consult dozens of cautionary stories very quickly.

Once the appropriate story was identified, the wise person was able to see in his or her mind what needed to be done to resolve the current situation, thereby mending a quarrel or averting a disaster. Sometimes survival itself depended on the narrative interventions of wise people.

Basso's (1996) compelling account of Western Apache practices harkens back to a point made earlier in this chapter, namely, that narrative derives its constitutive power in part from the routinization of narrative practices in everyday life. Because stories permeate the land itself, stories are inescapable to community members, and wise people accumulate many years of experience engaging with these practices at ever deeper levels. This account also underscores that narrative practices are simultaneously public and private, interpersonal and intrapersonal. Stories mediate social relations and infiltrate people's hearts and minds. The internal mental landscape of wise people becomes just as densely populated with stories as the natural world in which they dwell.

This account is thus strongly resonant with Vygotsky's understanding of language and other semiotic resources as tools that are both publicly shared and privately utilized (Berk, 2001; Vygotsky, 1978, 1934/1987; Wertsch, 1985). According to Vygotsky, these resources originate in relationships between people, but eventually children are able to use them to communicate with others and with themselves. In a similar vein, Nelson (1996) concluded that language is more than a vehicle of enculturation: To a large extent "language and the surrounding culture take over the human mind" (p. 325), profoundly changing the nature of cognition and communication. The Western Apache case illustrates that this process continues through adulthood and may not reach its apogee until late in the life course.

Yoyo's Grandmother's Secret Stories

The extraordinary narrative achievements of Western Apache wise people are manifest both interpersonally and intrapersonally. But what about "secret" stories, stories that can only be told to oneself, that is, intrapersonally? In this section, we present and analyze an elderly Taiwanese widow's stories of her two marriages, stories that she could not share with significant others in her life. From a Vygotskian perspective, such stories are no less social than stories told to a relative or friend; both involve social interactions—one with an actual person, the other with an imagined other. Moreover, complex social judgments are involved in the narrator's assessment that certain stories dare not be shared with others.

Untellability: A Preface to Mrs. Lin's Stories

The issue of tellability—or rather *untellability*—has received relatively little attention in scholarship on narrative (see Ochs & Capps, 2001). An untellable story is one that cannot be told to others without the risk of censure. In this section we take up an example of a story that raises the issue of the moral constraints on the tellability of a story. Narrators strive not only to be seen as good storytellers (Labov & Waletzky, 1967) but also as good persons. When people have personally challenging experiences that are potentially socially problematic, they may be compelled to keep such narratable events to themselves. That these events cannot be readily shared does not make them any less important. Indeed, their nonsharability may motivate the individual to keep these events alive through various forms of "private" narration.

The secret stories that caught our attention are the result of ethnographic serendipity, involving the same Taiwanese grandmother we quoted in the earlier example of Yoyo's narrated misdeeds. These stories were clearly of great, long-standing personal salience to Mrs. Lin, but were shared for the first time with another when told to the ethnographer. In this case, we see how participants may make use of the ethnographic encounter to narrate and enact stories in ways that would be considered taboo or inappropriate in their everyday lives. This highlights the importance of the socially untellable and people's creative use of novel speech events.

In the ensuing analysis, an important methodological issue emerges, one that is closely related to the conceptual issue of tellability. Typically, scholars of discourse analyze narratives that are told aloud and can be recorded. How can analysts study untellable stories, stories that are ordinarily told only to oneself in private, internal conversation? In the example at hand, we draw upon several sources of evidence: Mrs. Lin's narration of these stories to the ethnographer, her explicit admission that she had never before shared these stories with

another person, general background information about Taiwanese women's lives in Mrs. Lin's generation, and specific information about Mrs. Lin and her family.

Mrs. Lin's Stories: Untellable Except to the Ethnographer

Heidi Fung had known Mrs. Lin for 2 years when she asked to interview her about her child-rearing beliefs and practices. *A-ma* (a Taiwanese term for addressing elderly women, especially grandmothers) was in mourning over the loss of her second husband. Her daughter, Yoyo's mother, suggested that Fung take her to a restaurant and interview her there as a way to cheer her up. The researcher, therefore, conducted the interview with Mrs. Lin outside her home and away from her family. During that lunch, instead of answering Fung's questions, Mrs. Lin steered the interview in her own direction and insisted on telling stories about her two marriages. Fung found these stories to be so fascinating—so riveting, intimate, and emotionally powerful—that she met with Mrs. Lin on three later occasions over the course of a decade to talk with her further about her marriages (see Fung, 2003, for a detailed account).

What stood out in *A-ma*'s stories was a series of dreams about her first husband, Mr. Lin, all of which occurred after his untimely death at the age of 29. She reported that this was the first time that she had ever told anyone else about these dreams. She related that during the 30 days immediately following his death, he appeared to her every night in a dream. Even more remarkably, in the succeeding decades, he continued to appear in her dreams at key moments in her life (described later), up to the time of Fung's final interview, which occurred 45 years after his death. Each time Fung visited, *A-ma* was ready to share the dreams with her. Not only were the same dreams repeatedly narrated within the same session and across sessions, but there were always new dreams to tell. While the telling and sharing of her stories emerged out of the mutual trust that Fung and *A-ma* had built over the years, their relationship was also fostered by Fung's sympathetic listening and keen interest in Mrs. Lin's stories. *A-ma* had not found such responses in other contexts in her life, giving Fung privileged access to these previously private experiences. *A-ma* positioned Fung not only as an ethnographer but also as a woman with sufficient maturity and marital experience to appreciate her dilemma. Because Fung was divorced, *A-ma* may also have recognized Fung as someone who had made a difficult decision in *her* life as a woman.

A-ma was 19 when she married for the first time. She deeply loved and admired Mr. Lin, a talented man who grew up in the same village with her and became a primary school teacher. She had resisted her family's efforts to arrange a marriage for her and was proud that hers was a "love marriage." With three children arriving in quick succession, life was a mixture of sweetness and strain. After 6 years of marriage, Mr. Lin passed away. *A-ma* was 25 years old. At the funeral, she vowed to him in Japanese,[1] "All our children, count on me (*wo chengdan le*)." She said, "Although I had always been a frail woman (*ruoruo de nyuren*), at that very moment, I suddenly became a man, I become a full man (*wanwan quanquan de nanxing*)." For the sake of their children, she transformed herself into a strong person to undertake the roles and responsibilities of both father and mother.

At age 38, after 13 years of widowhood, *A-ma* faced the daunting financial challenge of paying for the higher education of her eldest daughter, with two younger sons following close behind. One of her first husband's former students noticed her adversity and introduced her to Mr. Wang, a retired KMT military officer. The prospect of remarrying posed a painful moral dilemma for Mrs. Lin: Declining to remarry would preserve her fidelity to her beloved husband but imperil their children's education; agreeing to remarry would betray her husband but honor her vow to raise and educate their children. A devout Christian, *A-ma* made a deal with God, "If my daughter is going to be admitted to the [subsidized] normal college, I won't even give a thought to this matter [of remarrying]. This is how a mark had been made [between God and me]." When her daughter was admitted to a private college, *A-ma* was deeply disappointed but followed God's will. She married Mr. Wang.

On their wedding night something unexpected happened: Her first husband appeared to her in a dream. Subsequently, whenever *A-ma* moved or traveled afar, on the first night in the new locale, Mr. Lin would reappear. In these dream visitations, Mr. Lin simply stood in front of her bed looking at her without saying a word, leaving her to sob her heart out. Mrs. Lin interpreted these experiences to mean

that Mr. Lin followed her wherever she went, making his presence known to her at important moments in her life. It was his way of showing his continuing love for her and of reassuring her that he did not blame her for remarrying.[2] Consequently, Mrs. Lin believed that she did not need to feel guilty or ashamed in relation to her first husband.

However, Mr. Lin's dream visitations had profound and lasting consequences for *A-ma*'s life with her second husband. Over the 24 years of her marriage to Mr. Wang, which ended with his death, *A-ma* tried hard to decline a sexual relationship with him, and the tension between them was not released until Mr. Wang gradually lost interest in sex in his later years. In her conversations with Fung, *A-ma* described her remarriage as "selling her soul" for the sake of her children. Indeed, although Mr. Wang loved her dearly and helped bring up and provide the best education for her children, and although she was deeply grateful to him, she could never give him the kind of affection that she had given to her first husband. In other words, although on the surface, *A-ma* betrayed her faithfulness to her first husband, in reality, she stood firm in remaining loyal to him—spiritually, mentally, and physically.

Why Mrs. Lin's Stories Were Untellable

The foregoing reprise is a severely truncated description of the narrated events (Mrs. Lin's two marriages) and of the events of narration (Mrs. Lin's tellings of these events to the researcher in the successive "interviews") that a practice approach would require to do justice to Mrs. Lin's remarkable narrative of her two marriages. One would have to examine the transcripts of *A-ma*'s meetings with Fung for more details of the developing relationship between Fung and *A-ma*, and of the complex relationship between *A-ma*'s narration and the events narrated. However, this example does offer an opportunity to illustrate how attention to both levels of analysis can help to penetrate the meanings of such a complex story.

Over the course of the four tellings, Mrs. Lin became more forthcoming in what she revealed to the ethnographer. Although her children knew that she sometimes dreamed about their father, she did not tell them or anyone else about Mr. Lin's dream visitations or other intimate details of her marriages. These profoundly meaningful and emotionally powerful experiences—the intense mutual love between Mrs. Lin and her first husband, the dreams surrounding his early death, and his continuing felt presence in her life, enduring through and beyond her second marriage—were not narratable in the contexts that she ordinarily inhabited. Thus, a defining feature of Mrs. Lin's everyday narrative practice was that she could not, or would not, narrate these experiences to the significant others in her life.

Why was this the case? And why did she make an exception for the ethnographer? Mrs. Lin herself said explicitly that she could only share her story with an outsider (*wairen*), someone who was not a member of her family. Perhaps the story—particularly the sexual details, which only gradually emerged across the several tellings—was too intimate to be shared with her own children. In addition, although Mrs. Lin treasured her first husband's visitations, she regarded them as mysterious and noted that her sister-in-law, widowed after 50 years of marriage, did not have similar experiences. Perhaps she wondered whether her highly educated, "modern" children would regard the visitations as bizarre and unsettling. We believe, however, that the most important reason for her reluctance to share her stories with her children was her conviction that her children would not be able to comprehend her unconventional actions. How could she make them understand that she "betrayed" their father to better *their* lives, and that she remained loyal to him and received his full support on her decision to remarry?

Mrs. Lin had good reason to fear that her children would not accept her version of events. Her children, especially her eldest son, had complex feelings about their stepfather, Mr. Wang. The eldest son refused to invite him to his wedding, a very disrespectful act that broke Mr. Wang's heart. Apparently, he felt that Mr. Wang had no place at a formal occasion that honored and furthered the Lin family line. According to the younger son, his older brother felt guilty because he had been unable to care for his mother and siblings for the Lin family. If he had fulfilled his responsibilities as eldest son, his mother would not have had to remarry. This implies some disapproval of Mrs. Lin's decision to remarry on the grounds that she dishonored the Lin family, echoing the traditional Chinese precept that "good" widows, no matter how young, should not remarry (Holmgren, 1985; Mann, 1987; Sommer,

1996; Waltner, 1981). Political currents also may have colored the children's feelings toward Mr. Wang. Unlike Mr. Lin, who was born and grew up in the same fishing village as Mrs. Lin, Mr. Wang came from mainland China and spoke a different dialect of Chinese. Whereas Mr. Lin was a literati and schoolteacher, Mr. Wang had been a member of the KMT army that retreated to Taiwan with Chiang Kai-shek in the late 1940s. His very different background and perhaps different political inclination likely aggravated the children's complex feelings about their mother's remarriage. In summary, we surmise that *A-ma*'s marital life was a touchy topic within the family, leading her to doubt that her children would welcome or appreciate her story about her two marriages.

The ethnographer, on other hand, was not a member of the family, and *A-ma* first related her story to Fung outside the family context. Furthermore, Fung did not have complex feelings about Mrs. Lin's decision to remarry. Indeed, she admired *A-ma* for having the courage to take an anomalous path, forging a life of emotional truth and integrity as a woman. To have someone from the younger generation take such a strong and sympathetic interest in her narrative must have been gratifying to *A-ma*, affording her a context that she creatively appropriated to narrate the previously unsharable. Here is an instance of the "doubling" across representational and interactional levels of analysis (Wortham, 2001) that we discussed earlier. In the ethnographic encounter, Mrs. Lin found a recipient for her story, that is, a context that transcended the normative constraints on tellability that governed her everyday life. The singularity of this context paralleled the singularity of her story, a story that transcended the normative constraints on a married woman's life.

Thus, the analysis of the communicative events in which Mrs. Lin told, or refrained from telling, the story of her two marriages helps us to appreciate more fully the gravity of the moral dilemma—whether or not to remarry—that she recounted in the narrated event. We can now see that there were lasting consequences of her decision to marry Mr. Wang. As she had hoped, Mr. Wang helped her to secure a future for her children. But those opportunities came at a cost in peace of mind and family harmony: her guilt toward Mr. Wang, her eldest son's rejection of Mr. Wang, and Mr. Wang's hurt feelings. Perhaps the most poignant consequence was that Mrs. Lin was not able to share with her children the story of her deep love and loyalty to their father.

With this analysis in place, we can now return to the earlier point about private narration. We argue that A-ma's eternal bond to her first husband was sustained not only by his dream visitations but also by her private narrations of these visitations and of the events of their brief marriage. The level of detail with which she narrated the most temporally distant of these events to Fung supports this interpretation, implying a great deal of rehearsal. Mrs. Lin may have experienced these internal narratives as a form of private speech to herself and/or as conversations with Mr. Lin, as internal interlocutor. What is certain, however, according to her own testimony, is that the nature of her subjective experience changed during the many years that she abided with him after his premature death. In exactly the same wording each time, A-ma repeatedly declared to Fung: "It's not that he occupies my mind [as he did when he first passed away], it's that he actually lives in my mind. Although the person is dead, his soul stays alive." In this astonishing refrain, Mrs. Lin told the ethnographer that her first husband was now alive in her; they had been reunited. Apparently, this transformation in Mrs. Lin's understanding of herself in relation to her husband—from someone who could not stop thinking about him to someone who could not be separated from him—was accomplished through her repeated private narrations.

In summary, although the empirical record is slim when it comes to the narrative practices of older adults, the Western Apache case, and the example of Mrs. Lin suggest that more attention to this phase of life would be worthwhile for cultural psychology. When compared with the narrative practices of young children, the practices of Mrs. Lin and of Western Apache wise men and women are breathtakingly complex. Here are cultural traditions in their most fully realized form, the fruition of a lifetime of repeated practice, in counterpoint to the hints of culture-specific meaning in the stories of young children. These narratives from late adulthood also illustrate the range and diversity of culture-specific subjectivities and social relationships that can be created through decades of narrative practice: wise people with the capacious memory and moral discernment to repair the social fabric; and a woman who charts an unconventional and largely undisclosed life, and whose marital bond transcends her husband's death.

CONCLUSION

Narrative is a canonical topic in cultural psychology, subsuming many important problems. Our task in this chapter was to address a single, fundamental problem—the role of narrative in the co-creation of person and culture. Drawing upon stories from a variety of cultural traditions, we have argued that practice approaches to narrative can help cultural psychologists to gain purchase on this problem. When narrative is examined as a practice, not just a form of representation, it becomes possible to see how stories reverberate across time and space, connecting people to other people, other stories, and other activities, and infiltrating their hearts and minds.

At both ends of the life course, stories keep happening, just as they do in this chapter. This fundamental characteristic of narrative as an everyday practice endows narrative with constitutive power that goes beyond the capacity of narrative to invoke realities beyond those of the here and now of the telling. Different stories occur in combination with other stories and other activities, and certain stories get repeated like musical themes with variation. All of these practices are saturated with cultural meaning at two levels—how the past event is represented, and how the story is told in the here and now. Regardless of the age of the narrating participants—whether tiny child or older adult—each is helping to keep the practices alive. At the same time, each is getting transformed or retransformed into certain kinds of persons. Because some narrative practices are so frequent and begin so early, it is likely that they become naturalized and taken for granted over the life course, and that the transformations they bring about are beyond the conscious awareness of the participants. Concurrent with this naturalizing trajectory is apparently another trajectory in which participants consciously appropriate shared narrative resources for their own purposes—to manage their emotions, to embark on the journey toward wisdom, or to chart a life path that transcends the conventional terms within which a woman's life could be imagined.

Throughout this chapter we have identified specific questions and phenomena that deserve further inquiry, including the affective–cognitive capacity to become attached to some stories rather than others and the history of stories in people's lives, ranging from fleeting to lifelong. In conclusion we underscore three methodological implications of practice approaches to narrative. Most research on narrative trains the spotlight on a specific narrative or corpus of narratives, leaving prior, adjacent, or concurrent discursive practices in the shadows. Yet a central premise of practice approaches is that stories do not exist in a vacuum; they coexist with other practices, both narrative and nonnarrative. In their closely observed and provocative study of early narrative practices in a rural African American community, Sperry and Sperry (2000) found that very young children's precocious facility with fantasy narrative could not be explained by caregivers' "direct" socialization. Caregivers denied that they encouraged fantasy narratives, and close examination of the fantasy narratives revealed that the children themselves introduced most of the fantasy themes; relatively few were introduced by caregivers. But caregivers did routinely threaten young children with visits from fearsome creatures as a way of socializing right and wrong. Children imported these affectively charged threats and imaginary creatures from prior disciplinary episodes into their narrations. Sperry and Sperry argue that these affectively significant ideas support the production of fantasy much as objects support children's pretend play. In other words, the very early privileging of fantasy narrations over literal stories—which distinguishes early narrative development in this community—could only be understood by looking beyond narrative itself to examine the conjunction between specific narrative practices and specific disciplinary practices.

In addition to widening the angle of vision beyond narrative to encompass the other practices with which narrative keeps company, practice approaches to narrative invite a closer look at narrative as a multimodal performance (C. Goodwin, 1984; Hanks, 1996; Ochs & Capps, 1996). Van Deusen-Philips et al. (2001) found that linguistically isolated deaf children whose parents chose not to expose them to a conventional sign system produced culturally appropriate narrations despite their lack of a language model, suggesting that these cultural messages were available through nonverbal channels. They argued that the universality of narrative as a socializing medium rests not only on its capacity for ordering and valuing experience according to many different cultural systems but also on its versatility as a form of enactment. Narrators gesture, adopt postures, display facial expressions, laugh (Jefferson, 1978, 1984), cry (Hill, 1989, 1995), and perform "voices" with more than their mouths. And listeners listen with their eyes and their bodies, not just their ears. It is likely that Yoyo heard A-ma's corrections of his past misdeeds differently when she was holding him in her arms than when she was not. Thus, cultural psychologists who seek to understand the cultural constitution of persons will do well to seek a more balanced approach, one that recognizes that narrative is not only a verbal practice but also a practice of the body.

Finally, and most fundamentally, practice approaches have implications for how researchers position themselves to hear and see narratives in the first place. Each research tool—participant observation, interviews, elicitations—entails some kind of engagement between researcher and participant, and that engagement is part of what has to be documented and analyzed to understand the stories that emerge (or fail to emerge). In other words, the theoretical perspective adopted in this chapter recognizes that the ethnographic encounter is a communicative event, and that findings are intelligible and culturally valid only if the ethnographer is able to adapt his or her research practices to local communicative norms (C. L. Briggs, 1986; Hymes, 1974; Miller, Hengst, & Wang, 2003; Ochs, 1988). Many of the studies cited in this chapter rest on this kind of creative adaptability. But such flexibility is not limited to the ethnographer, as is amply demonstrated by Mrs. Lin. A-ma did not accede to the constraints of the researcher-researched relationship or of the initial interview. She appropriated the interview, casting Fung as the recipient of her secret stories and foregrounding Fung's identity as a certain kind of woman. A-ma overlaid the ethnographer encounter with her own purposes. The larger point is this: When the research encounter is regarded as a site in which the ethnographer and participant enter into and reinvent a set of practices, both parties may be surprised by the stories that come to light.

NOTES

1. When Mrs. Lin was young, Taiwan was a colony of Japan (from 1895 to 1945). Although most Taiwanese people spoke *Holo* (also known as *Tai-gi* or Taiwanese) at home, Japanese was the official language used in governmental institutions and schools during that period. When the Kuo-min-tang (KMT; Chinese Nationalist Party) government reclaimed sovereignty over Taiwan in 1945, Japanese was banned. Due to the nostalgic sentiment held by the generation of Taiwanese who grew up in the colonial period, Japanese somehow gradually changed from a generally public language to a language of affection and emotion in private communication. Thus, one possible explanation why Mrs. Lin vowed to her deceased husband in Japanese could be that she experienced Japanese to be more appropriate than *Holo*, her native tongue, for expressing the intensity of her inner feelings for him.

2. It is interesting that Mrs. Lin regarded her first husband's dream visitations so positively. An alternative interpretation might be that Mr. Lin's dream visitations were acts of surveillance, signifying his disapproval of her second marriage. Such an interpretation would be compatible with Mrs. Lin's own strong wish not to remarry. Unfortunately, we have no way of knowing how she interpreted Mr. Lin's dream visitations when they first occurred many years earlier, or whether her interpretations changed over time, culminating in her conviction late in life that Mr. Lin's dream visitations signified his continuing love and support for her.

REFERENCES

Alexander, K. J., Miller, P. J., & Hengst, J. A. (2001). Young children's emotional attachments to stories. *Social Development, 10,* 374–398.

Austin, J. L. (1975). *How to do things with words.* Cambridge, MA: Harvard University Press.

Bakhtin, M. M. (1981). *The dialogic imagination.* Austin: University of Texas Press.

Basso, K. (1996). *Wisdom sits in places: Landscape and language among the Western Apache.* Albuquerque: University of New Mexico Press.

Bauman, R. (1986). *Story, performance, and event: Contextual studies of oral narrative.* New York: Cambridge University Press.

Bauman, R., & Briggs, C. L. (1990). Poetics and performance as critical perspectives on language and social life. *Annual Review of Anthropology, 19,* 59–88.

Bauman, R., & Sherzer, J. (Eds.). (1989). *Explorations in the ethnography of speaking.* Cambridge, UK: Cambridge University Press.

Berk, L. E. (2001). *Awakening children's minds.* New York: Oxford University Press.

Briggs, C. L. (1986). *Learning how to ask: A sociolinguistic appraisal of the role of the interview in social science research.* Cambridge, UK: Cambridge University Press.

Briggs, J. L. (1998). *Inuit morality play: The emotional education of a three-year-old.* New Haven, CT: Yale University Press.

Bruner, J. S. (1990). *Acts of meaning.* Cambridge, MA: Harvard University Press.

Burger, L. K., & Miller, P. J. (1999). Early talk about the past revisited: Affect in working-class and middle-class children's co-narrations. *Journal of Child Language, 26,* 133–162.

Cazden, C. B. (1993). Vygotsky, Hymes, and Bakhtin: From word to utterance and voice. In E. A. Forman, N. Minick, & C. A. Stone (Eds.), *Contexts for learning: Sociocultural dynamics in children's development* (pp. 197–212). New York: Oxford University Press.

Chen, E. C. H., Lin, S. M., Miller, P., & Fung, H. (2005, April). *Storytelling as a medium of socialization for preschoolers: A follow-up study of narrative practices in Taiwanese and Euro-American families.* Poster presented at the biennial meeting of the Society for Research in Child Development (SRCD), Atlanta, GA.

Clark, C. D. (2003). *In sickness and in play: Children coping with chronic illness.* New Brunswick, NJ: Rutgers University Press.

Cole, M. (1996). *Cultural psychology: A once and future discipline.* Cambridge, MA: Harvard University Press.

Coles, R. (1989). *The call of stories.* Boston: Houghton Mifflin.

Duranti, A., & Goodwin, C. (1992). *Rethinking context: Language as an interactive phenomenon.* New York: Cambridge University Press.

Dyson, A. H. (1993). *Social worlds of children learning to write in an urban primary school.* New York: Teachers College Press.

Engel, S. (1995). *The stories children tell: Making sense of the narratives of childhood.* New York: Freeman.

Fivush, R. (1993). Emotional content of parent–child conversations about the past. In C. A. Nelson (Ed.), *Memory and affect in development: Minnesota Symposia on Child Psychology* (Vol. 26, pp. 39–77). Hillsdale, NJ: Erlbaum.

Fung, H. (1999). Becoming a moral child: The socialization of shame among young Chinese children. *Ethos, 27,* 180–209.

Fung, H. (2003). When culture meets psyche: Understanding the contextualized self through the life and dreams of an elderly Taiwanese woman. *Taiwan Journal of Anthropology, 1,* 149–175.

Fung, H., Miller, P. J., & Lin, L. C. (2004). Listening is active: Lessons from the narrative practices of Taiwanese families. In M. W. Pratt & B. E. Fiese (Eds.), *Family stories and the life course: Across time and generations* (pp. 303–323). Mahwah, NJ: Erlbaum.

Goffman, E. (1979). Footing. *Semiotica, 25,* 1–29.

Gone, J. P. (1999). "We were through as keepers of it":

The "missing pipe narrative" and Gros Ventre cultural identity. *Ethos, 27,* 415–440.

Gone, J. P. (2005, June). *"I came to tell you of my life": Narrative expositions of "mental health" in an American Indian community.* Paper presented at a Festschrift honoring Julian Rappaport, Urbana, IL.

Goodnow, J. J., Miller, P. J., & Kessel, F. (Eds.). (1995). *Cultural practices as context for development.* San Francisco: Jossey-Bass.

Goodwin, C. (1984). Notes on story structure and the organization of participation. In M. Atkinson & J. Heritage (Eds.), *Structures of social action* (pp. 225–246). Cambridge, UK: Cambridge University Press.

Goodwin, M. H. (1990). *He-said-she-said: Talk as social organization among black children.* Bloomington: Indiana University Press.

Haight, W., Wang, X., Fung, H., Williams, K., & Mintz, J. (1999). Universal, developmental and variable aspects of young children's play: A cross-cultural comparison of pretending at home. *Child Development, 70,* 1477–1488.

Hanks, W. F. (1996). *Language and communicative practices.* Boulder, CO: Westview Press.

Heath, S. B. (1983). *Ways with words: Language, life, and work in communities and classrooms.* Cambridge, UK: Cambridge University Press.

Heine, S. J., & Lehman, D. R. (2003). Move the body, change the self: Acculturative effects on the self-concept. In M. Schaller & C. Crandall (Eds.), *Psychological foundations of culture* (pp. 305–331). Mahwah, NJ: Erlbaum.

Heine, S. J., Lehman, D. R., Markus, H. R., & Kitayama, S. (1999). Is there a universal need for positive self-regard? *Psychological Review, 106,* 766–794.

Hicks, D. A. (1991). Kinds of narrative: Genre skills among first graders from two communities. In A. McCabe & C. Peterson (Eds.), *Developing narrative structure* (pp. 55–87). Hillsdale, NJ: Erlbaum.

Hicks, D. A. (1994). Individual and social meanings in the classroom: Narrative discourse as a boundary phenomenon. *Journal of Narrative and Life History, 4,* 215–240.

Hill, J. H. (1989). Weeping as a meta-signal in a Mexicano woman's narrative. *Journal of Folklore Research, 27,* 29–47.

Hill, J. H. (1995). The voices of Don Gabriel: Responsibility and self in a modern Mexicano narrative. In D. Tedlock & B. Mannheim (Eds.), *The dialogic emergence of culture* (pp. 97–147). Chicago: University of Illinois Press.

Holland, D., Lachicotte, W., Skinner, D., & Cain, C. (1998). *Identity and agency in cultural worlds.* Cambridge, MA: Harvard University Press.

Holmgren, J. (1985). The economic foundations of virtue: Widow-remarriage in early and modern China. *Australian Journal of Chinese Affairs, 13,* 1–27.

Hudley, E. V. P., Haight, W., & Miller, P. J. (2003). *"Raise up a child": Human development in an African-American family.* Chicago: Lyceum.

Hymes, D. (1974). *Foundations in sociolinguistics: An ethnographic approach.* Philadelphia: University of Pennsylvania Press.

Jakobson, R. (1960). Closing statement: Linguistics and poetics. In T. A. Sebeok (Ed.), *Style in language* (pp. 350–377). Cambridge, MA: MIT Press.

Jefferson, G. (1978). Sequential aspects of storytelling in conversation. In J. Shenkein (Ed.), *Studies in the organization of conversational interaction* (pp. 219–248). New York: Academic Press.

Jefferson, G. (1984). On the organization of laughter in talk about troubles. In J. M. Atkinson & J. Heritage (Eds.), *Structures of social action: Studies in conversation analysis* (pp. 346–369). New York: Cambridge University Press.

Kamberelis, G. (1993). Tropes are for kids: Young children's developing understanding of narrative, poetic, and expository written discourse genres. *Dissertation Abstracts International, 54*(12), 4379A. (UMI No. 9409724)

Kamberelis, G., & Scott, K. D. (1992). Other people's voices: The coarticulation of texts and subjectivities. *Linguistics and Education, 4,* 359–403.

Koven, M. (2002). An analysis of speaker role inhabitance in narratives of personal experience. *Journal of Pragmatics, 34,* 167–217.

Labov, W. (1972). *Language in the inner city: Studies in the Black English vernacular.* Philadelphia: University of Pennsylvania Press.

Labov, W., & Waletsky, J. (1967). Narrative analysis: Oral versions of personal experiences. In J. Helm (Ed.), *Essays on the verbal and visual arts* (pp. 12–44). Seattle: University of Washington Press.

Lave, J., & Wenger, E. (1990). *Situated learning: Legitimate peripheral participation.* Cambridge, UK: Cambridge University Press.

Li, J. (2004a). "I learn and I grow big": Chinese preschoolers' purposes for learning. *International Journal of Behavioral Development, 28,* 116–128.

Li, J. (2004b). Learning as a task or a virtue: U.S. and Chinese preschoolers explain learning. *Developmental Psychology, 40,* 595–605.

Linde, C. (1993). *Life stories: The creation of coherence.* New York: Oxford University Press.

Logan, O. L. (1989). *Motherwit: An Alabama midwife's story.* New York: Penguin.

Mandelbuam, J. (1987). Couples sharing stories. *Communication Quarterly, 35,* 144–170.

Mandelbaum, J. (1989). Interpersonal activities in conversational storytelling. *Western Journal of Speech Communication, 53,* 114–126.

Mandelbaum, J. (1993). Assigning responsibility in conversational storytelling: The interactional construction of reality, *Text, 13,* 247–266.

Mann, S. (1987). Widows in the kinship, class, and community structure of Qing dynasty China. *Journal of Asian Studies, 46,* 37–55.

Miller, P. J. (1994). Narrative practices: Their role in socialization and self-construction. In U. Neisser & R. Fivush (Eds.), *The remembering self: Construction and accuracy in the self-narrative* (pp. 158–179). New York: Cambridge University Press.

Miller, P. J., Cho, G. E., & Bracey, J. R. (2005). Working-class children's experience through the prism of personal storytelling. *Human Development, 43*, 115–135.

Miller, P. J., Fung, H., & Mintz, J. (1996). Self-construction through narrative practices: A Chinese and American comparison of early socialization. *Ethos, 24*(2), 237–280.

Miller, P. J., & Goodnow, J. J. (1995). Cultural practices: Toward an integration of culture and development. In J. J. Goodnow, P. J. Miller, & F. Kessel (Eds.), *Cultural practices as contexts for development: New directions for child development* (Vol. 67, pp. 5–16). San Francisco: Jossey-Bass.

Miller, P. J., Hengst, J. A., Alexander, K. A., & Sperry, L. L. (2000). Narrative genres: Tools for creating alternate realities. In K. Rosengren, C. Johnson, & P. Harris (Eds.), *Imagining the impossible: The development of magical, scientific, and religious thinking in contemporary society* (pp. 212–246). New York: Cambridge University Press.

Miller, P. J., Hengst, J. A., & Wang, S.-H. (2003). Ethnographic methods: Applications from developmental cultural psychology. In P. Camic, J. Rhodes, & L. Yardley (Eds.), *Qualitative research in psychology: Expanding perspectives in methodology and design* (pp. 219–242). Washington DC: American Psychological Association.

Miller, P. J., Hoogstra, L., Mintz, J., Fung, H., & Williams, K. (1993). Troubles in the garden and how they get resolved: A young child's transformation of his favorite story. In C. A. Nelson (Ed.), *The Minnesota Symposia on Child Psychology: Vol. 26. Memory and affect in development* (pp. 87–114). Hillsdale, NJ: Erlbaum.

Miller, P. J., & Moore, B. B. (1989). Narrative conjunctions of caregiver and child: A comparative perspective on socialization through stories. *Ethos, 17*, 428–449.

Miller, P. J., Sandel, T., Liang, C. H., & Fung, H. (2001). Narrating transgressions in Longwood: The discourses, meanings, and paradoxes of an American socializing practice. *Ethos, 29*, 159–186.

Miller, P. J., & Sperry, L. L. (1988). Early talk about the past: The origins of conversational stories of personal experience. *Journal of Child Language, 15*, 293–315.

Miller, P. J., Wiley, A., Fung, H., & Liang, C. H. (1997). Personal storytelling as a medium of socialization in Chinese and American families. *Child Development, 68*, 557–568.

Nelson, K. (Ed.). (1989). *Narratives from the crib.* Cambridge, MA: Harvard University Press.

Nelson, K. (1996). *Language in cognitive development: The emergence of the mediated mind.* New York: Cambridge University Press.

Ochs, E. (1988). *Culture and language development: Language acquisition and language socialization in a Samoan village.* Cambridge, UK: Cambridge University Press.

Ochs, E., & Capps, L. (1996). Narrating the self. *Annual Review of Anthropology, 25*, 19–43.

Ochs, E., & Capps, L. (2001). *Living narrative: Creating lives in everyday storytelling.* Cambridge, MA: Harvard University Press.

Ochs, E., & Schieffelin, B. B. (1984). Language acquisition and socialization: Three developmental stories and their implications. In R. A. Shweder & R. A. LeVine (Eds.), *Culture theory: Essays on mind, self, and emotion* (pp. 276–320). Cambridge, UK: Cambridge University Press.

Paley, V. G. (1997). *The girl with the brown crayon: How children use stories to shape their lives.* Cambridge, MA: Harvard University Press.

Peacock, J., & Holland, D. (1993). The narrated self. *Ethos, 21*, 367–383.

Pratt, M. W., & Fiese, B. E. (Eds.). (2004). *Family stories and the life course: Across time and generations.* Mahwah, NJ: Erlbaum.

Preece, A. (1987). The range of narrative forms conversationally produced by young children. *Journal of Child Language, 14*, 353–373.

Rogoff, B. (1990). *Apprenticeship in thinking.* New York: Oxford University Press.

Sacks, H. (1974). An analysis of the course of a joke's telling in conversation. In R. Bauman & J. Sherzer (Eds.), *Explorations in the ethnography of speaking* (pp. 337–353). New York: Cambridge University Press.

Schiffrin, D. (1996). Narrative as self-portrait: Sociolinguistic constructions of identity. *Language in Society, 25*, 167–203.

Scribner, S., & Cole, M. (1981) *The psychology of literacy.* Cambridge, MA: Harvard University Press.

Shweder, R. A., Goodnow, J., Hatano, G., LeVine, R. A., Markus, H., & Miller, P. J. (2006). The cultural psychology of development: One mind, many mentalities. In W. Damon (Series Ed.) & R. M. Lerner (Vol. Ed.), *Handbook of child psychology: Vol. 1. Theoretical models of human development* (6th ed., pp. 716–792). New York: Wiley.

Silverstein, M. (1995). Shifters, linguistic categories, and cultural description. In B. Blount (Ed.), *Language, culture, and society: A book of readings* (pp. 187–221). Long Grove, IL: Waveland Press. (Original work published 1976)

Sommer, M. (1996). The uses of chastity: Sex, law, and the property of widows in Qing China. *Late Imperial China, 17*, 77–130.

Spence, P. (1984). *Narrative truth and historical truth.* New York: Norton.

Sperry, L. L., & Sperry, D. E. (1995). Young children's presentation of self in conversational narration. In L. L. Sperry & P. A. Smiley (Eds.), *Exploring young children's concepts of self and other through conversation: New directions for child development* (Vol. 69, pp. 47–60). San Francisco: Jossey-Bass.

Sperry, L. L., & Sperry, D. E. (1996). Early development

of narrative skills. *Cognitive Development, 11*, 443–465.

Sperry, L. L., & Sperry, D. E. (2000). Verbal and nonverbal contributions to early representation: Evidence from African-American toddlers. In N. Budwig, I. C. Uzgiris, & J. V. Wertsch (Eds.), *Communication: An arena of development* (pp. 143–165). Norwood, NJ: Ablex.

Steedman, C. K. (1986). *Landscape for a good woman: A story of two lives.* New Brunswick, NJ: Rutgers University Press.

Stromberg, P. G. (1993). *Language and self-transformation: A study of the Christian conversion narrative.* Cambridge, UK: Cambridge University Press.

Taylor, C. E. (1995). "You think it was a fight?": Co-constructing (the struggle for) meaning, face, and family in everyday narrative activity. *Research on Language and Social Interaction, 28*, 283–317.

Tobin, J. (2000). *Good guys don't wear hats.* New York: Teachers College Press.

Tu, W. M. (1985). Selfhood and otherness in Confucian thought. In A. J. Marsella, G. Devos, & F. L. K. Hsu (Eds.), *Culture and self: Asian and Western perspectives* (pp. 231–251). New York: Tavistock.

Tu, W. M. (1994). Embodying the universe: A note on Confucian self-realization. In R. T. Ames, W. Dissanayake, & T. P. Kasulis (Eds.), *Self as person in Asian theory and practice* (pp. 177–186). Albany: State University of New York Press.

Urban, G. (1989). The "I" of discourse in Shokleng. In B. Lee & G. Urban (Eds.), *Semiotics, self, and society* (pp. 27–51). Berlin: Mouton de Gruyter.

Van Deusen-Phillips, S. B., Goldin-Meadow, S., & Miller, P. J. (2001). Watching stories, seeing worlds: Similarities and differences in the cross-cultural narrative development of linguistically isolated deaf children. *Human Development, 44*, 311–336.

Voloshinov, V. N. (1973). *Marxism and the philosophy of language.* New York: Seminar Press.

Vygotsky, L. (1978). *Mind in society.* Cambridge, MA: Harvard University Press.

Vygotsky, L. (1987). *Thinking and speech* (N. Minick, Trans.). New York: Plenum Press. (Original work published 1934)

Waltner, A. (1981). Widow and remarriage in Ming and early Qing China. In R. W. Guisso & S. Johannesen (Eds.), *Women in China: Current directions in historical scholarship* (pp. 129–146). Youngstown, NY: Philo Press.

Wang, Q. (2004). The emergence of cultural self-constructs: Autobiographical memory and self-description in European American and Chinese children. *Developmental Psychology, 40*, 3–15.

Wang, Q., & Leichtman, M. D. (2000). Same beginnings, different stories: A comparison of American and Chinese children's narratives. *Child Development, 71*, 1329–1346.

Wang, Q., Leichtman, M. D., & Davies, K. I. (2000). Sharing memories and telling stories: American and Chinese mothers and their 3-year-olds. *Memory, 8*, 159–178.

Wang, Q., & Li, J. (2003). Chinese children's self-concepts in the domains of learning and social relations. *Psychology in the School, 40*, 85–101.

Wang, X., Bernas, R., & Eberhard, P. (2005, April). *Responding to children's everyday transgressions in Chinese working-class families: A snapshot of Lianhua workers' village.* Poster presented at the biennial meeting of the Society for Research in Child Development (SRCD), Atlanta, GA.

Wenger, E. (1998). *Communities of practice: Learning, meaning, and identity.* New York: Cambridge University Press.

Wertsch, J. (1985). *Vygotsky and the social formation of mind.* Cambridge, MA: Harvard University Press.

Wertsch, J. (1991). *Voices of the mind.* Cambridge, MA: Harvard University Press.

Wolf, S. A., & Heath, S. B. (1992). *The braid of literature: Children's worlds of reading.* Cambridge, MA: Harvard University Press.

Wortham, S. E. F. (2001). *Narratives in action: A strategy for research and analysis.* New York: Teachers College Press.

CHAPTER 25

Culture, Categorization, and Reasoning

DOUGLAS L. MEDIN
SARA J. UNSWORTH
LAWRENCE HIRSCHFELD

Do people from different cultures have different categories and concepts? What aspects of the way a person thinks depend on the culture in which one grew up? In this chapter we review research on concepts and reasoning from a cultural perspective. It is tempting to plunge right into the literature, without saying much about the notion of culture itself, because, as many people believe, everyone has a pretty good idea about what culture is. To the contrary, we believe that a great deal hinges on how one conceptualizes culture, including challenging methodological and interpretive issues, and deep commitments to research strategies. Therefore, we plunge right away into different approaches to studying culture.

What is at stake is not so much determining which approaches to culture are correct and which are incorrect but rather what their strengths and weaknesses might be relative to the questions and issues one would like to address. First, there is an issue on which everyone who studies culture can agree. Given that much of the history of cognitive and social psychology has focused nearly exclusively on college students at major research universities, we really need to know the generalizability of these findings. Both the presence and absence of gen-erality are informative. We think that *the* scandal of cognitive and social psychology is its narrow empirical base—it reflects either immense optimism with respect to universality or is too pessimistic about being taken seriously. In short, psychology needs cultural research to be legitimate.

The challenges arise when cultural differences are observed. Aside from jarring us out of our complacency, what more can we say? A central problem is that culture is not an independent variable, and cultural comparisons provide very little by way of experimental control. This is where different approaches to culture part company, strategically speaking. We now take a closer look, starting with intuitive approaches to culture.

APPROACHES TO STUDYING CULTURE

We begin with an important distinction: The question of how cultures should be studied is separable from the question of how to define cultures. Intuitively, one might define "culture" as the shared knowledge, values, beliefs, and practices among a group of people, typically living in geographical proximity, who share a history, a language, and cultural identification. Although we think a definition of a culture in terms of history, proximity, language, and identification is useful and (if not too rigidly applied) perhaps even necessary, it does not follow that the cultural content of interest must be shared ideas and beliefs.

We see three problems with the intuitive view of culture and its focus on shared content. First, it prejudges the issue of what constitutes cultural content. If culture is shared and we encounter a tradition in which a diversity of ideas, values, and practices compete, are we to conclude that the tradition is not cultural because it is not consensual? Second, this view of culture is static, in that either cultural change is not a relevant object of study or is treated as (cultural) loss, or in some cases, extinction. Third, this approach may implicitly essentialize culture by conceptualizing it as an entity with systematic, law-like properties.

In this section we look at a number of approaches that in different ways endorse or reject this agenda for cultural research.

Culture as Norms and Rules

It is very natural to think that the cultural contents of interest must be shared to qualify as "cultural." Note, however, that this commitment undercuts the dynamic side of cultural processes. There might well be distinctive values, beliefs, and knowledge within a culture that nonetheless are not consensual. For example, a culture may have a set of beliefs and practices known only to a privileged group of people (e.g., healers, elders, ruling elite).

Some influential models of culture formation and evolution in biology and anthropology take a somewhat more liberal view of consensus. Based on group-level traits, they assume that cultures are integrated systems consisting of widely shared social "norms" ("rules," "theories," "grammars," "codes," "systems," "models," "worldviews," etc.) that maintain inheritable variation (Rappaport, 1999; Laland, Olding-Smee, & Feldman, 2000; Wilson, 2002). Some political scientists also tend to view cultures as socially "inherited habits" (Fukuyama, 1995), that is, as socially transmitted bundles of normative traits (Huntington, 1996; Axelrod, 1997).

The interest in inheritable variation loosens the restrictions on consensus and raises questions about the basis for variation. But here

cognitive scientists are likely to be disappointed by the implicit assumption that the gist of cultural learning is the (automatic) absorption of norms and values from the surrounding culture (by processes no more complicated than imitation). We believe that these assumptions do not pay sufficient attention to the sorts of inferential and developmental cognitive processes that allow human beings to build and participate in cultural life.

Cultural Psychology

Studies in the area of "cultural psychology" have made important contributions to human understanding by showing that knowledge systems and associated ways of thinking previously assumed to be universal actually vary widely across the world (for a review, see Cohen, 2001). The lesson drawn is that "psychologists who choose not to do cross-cultural psychology may have chosen to be ethnographers instead" (Nisbett, Peng, Choi, & Norenzayan, 2001, p. 307). In brief, cultural psychology is succeeding in divesting academic psychology of implicit and ingrained ethnocentric biases.

Cultural psychology differs from the "norms and rules" approach in at least two distinct ways: (1) Cultural psychology has tended to focus on reducing cultural differences to differences in values along a small set of dimensions; and (2) cultural psychologists have claimed that these differences also mediate differences in cognitive processes. In short, culture affects not only what people think about but also how they think.

The area draws much of its inspiration from researchers such as Hofstede (1980) and Triandis (1995), who sought to characterize cultural differences in terms of a small number of relevant dimensions. The project is successful if converging evidence points to the same small set of dimensions. Examples of such dimensions that have received a lot of attention are individualism versus collectivism and egalitarian versus hierarchical social structure. Other researchers, such as Nisbett (2003), have used socio-historical analysis to analytically derive differences in worldviews or preferred modes of thought. Examples of these differences are analytic versus holistic and logic versus dialecticism. In short, Nisbett and his associates (2001) are suggesting that what they call cultural studies must include not only contents per se but also thinking processes that themselves may be differentially distributed across cultures.

The recent interest in cultural psychology (for a review and critique, see Oyserman et al., 2002, and associated commentaries) has produced a considerable array of intriguing findings. In our view, however, the field risks being inherently self-limiting, because it tends to focus on very abstract, superordinate-level contrasts. It is difficult to argue with success, but it is equally difficult to overcome the impression that the picture is somewhat oversimplified. Here is an analogy. Suppose we were trying to understand the object concepts associated with a language and culture. It would be possible to take a large sample of such concepts, develop some measure of similarity, and then do multidimensional scaling (MDS). We would probably be able to recover meaningful dimensions of similarity such as size, animacy, and affective valence. But knowing object concepts as we do, we would likely have the feeling that a great deal was missing. In the 1950s Osgood, Suci, and Tannenbaum (1957) undertook a project of this sort (using the so-called "semantic differential technique") and uncovered several abstract dimensions, such as valence (pleasantness vs. unpleasantness) and potency (active vs. passive). Although dimensions such as positive versus negative evaluation have been of some use in subsequent research (Niedenthal, Halberstadt, & Innes-Ker, 1999), no one would mistake this dimensional analysis with a theory of semantics and overall, the MDS approach has fallen into neglect.

A second limitation of cultural psychology is that when a hypothesized cultural difference is reported, it is not clear how explanation or interpretation can be extended beyond simple description. In some cases researchers have been able to exert some experimental control by priming tendencies to act individualistically versus collectively (e.g., Gardner, Gabriel, & Lee, 1999; Briley, Morris, & Simonson, 2000). These sorts of studies reinforce the dimensional analysis and potentially extend its scope (Oyserman & Lee, Chapter 10, this volume). There is always the risk, however, of circularity in analysis. If priming does not affect some candidate task measuring individualism versus collectivism, then perhaps the prime is ineffective or the task does not entail individualism and collectivism.

Perhaps we are guilty of prejudging the initial phase of a two-step project. A focus on within-culture variations in modes of thought might illuminate how different cultural institutions shape ways of thinking and vice versa (see Kitayama, Duffy, & Uchida, Chapter 6, this volume; Kitayama, Ishii, Imada, Takemura, & Ramaswamy, 2006).

Context and Situated Cognition

Alternative views of "cultural psychology" call into question the use of standard forms of experimental procedure as flawed on the grounds that they are biased in their focus on the individual mind/brain in isolation. Instead of considering cognitions to be embedded exclusively in individual minds, with "culture" as just one component of individual cognition, these theorists maintain that human cognitions should be properly situated in a cultural–historical context and "practical activity" (Cole, 1996; cf. Vygotsky, 1978). A related concern is that cultural cognitions may be better understood as "distributed cognitions" that cannot be described exclusively in terms of individual thought processes, but only as "emergent structures" that arise from irreducible levels of interactional complexity involving differential linking of individual minds in a given population (Hutchins, 1995). Cole (1996) argues that subjects and objects are not only directly connected but also indirectly connected through a medium comprising artifacts, which are simultaneously material and conceptual. One consequence of this view is an emphasis on studying cognition in context, where cognitive labor may be distributed across both individuals and artifacts (e.g., plumb lines or computers). Because context includes people's conceptions of artifacts, it is inherently relational.

We share some of these concerns raised by the situated view, such as difficulties with standard experimental procedures, including 2 × 2 designs with culture, in effect, treated as an independent variable (Atran, Medin, & Ross, 2005) and lack of concern with differential distributions of cognitions among minds within populations. We also agree that cultural notions are intimately tied to the study of development, and that one excellent research avenue involves looking at how cognition plays out in particular contexts.

But we find other aspects of the situated view somewhat problematic. First, it is not always clear when a proposal is to be read as a metaphor and when it is to be taken literally, for example, the idea that cognition is "distributed" or even "stretched across mind, body, activity and setting" (Lave, 1988, p. 1). The focus on practical activity can be very useful, but to make activity the primary, or in some cases the sole unit of analysis, is to ignore individual cognitions.

The situated view and cultural psychology represent two end points on a continuum of scope and specificity. Cultural psychology aims to identify a small set of cognitive processes that (are thought to) operate very widely. In contrast, situationists are more impressed with the lack of transfer of cognitive skills across settings (e.g., Lave, 1988). The final view we discuss falls in the middle of this continuum.

Cultural Epidemiology

We endorse looking at cultures in terms of mental representations (and attendant behaviors) that are distributed across individuals in a population—what Sperber and others have called "cultural epidemiology."[1] This view focuses on the stabilizing role of cognitive structures in production and transmission of ideas (and attendant behaviors) that achieve widespread cultural distribution. These are not exclusively or even mainly shared as nearly identical mental representations across individual minds (Atran, 2001; Sperber, 1996). For example, imitation has strong limits: Given the multiple mappings between acts and mental representations of them (including their meaning), there is no guarantee of any sort of fidelity. Rather, much of the cultural transmission and stabilization of ideas (artifacts and behaviors) involves the communication of fragmentary bits of information that manage to trigger prior, rich inferential structures (Sperber & Hirschfeld, 2004).

We see two main limitations of the distributional view of culture: (1) Its focus on ideas may not give appropriate weight to the role of institutions, artifacts, and contexts; and (2) the notion of "idea" is underspecified in much the same way that the notion of a feature is underspecified in models of similarity (Murphy & Medin, 1985). Both limitations reflect the fact that the distributional view is stated at a fairly abstract level, so they are probably the same symptom. For instance, in an attempt to concretize the notion of "idea," one will likely find that ideas are not only influenced by institutions, artifacts, and contexts but also include

key features of these phenomena in their representational makeup.

At the same time, the distributed view of culture has several important strengths. First, it directs attention to within-culture variation and processes of cultural transmission. Second, cultural differences are a beginning point for analyses, not an end point. Third, this view requires that cultural consensus be empirically demonstrated rather than simply presumed. Consequently, cultures are seen as a dynamic system in which different perspectives and ideas may be in competition. All of these factors are relevant to the methodological considerations to which we turn next.

METHODOLOGY FOR CULTURAL RESEARCH

It is our view that cultures can be effectively studied as causally distributed patterns of mental representations, their public expressions, and the resultant behaviors in given ecological contexts. We say "distributed" to emphasize that the distribution of ideas may be highly variable, and "causally" to make the point that whether and how representations are formed, transmitted, or transformed depends on particular contexts, as we elaborate below. People's mental representations interact with other people's mental representations to the extent that those representations can be physically transmitted in a public medium (language, dance, signs, artifacts, etc.). These public representations in turn are sequenced and channeled by ecological features of the external environment (including the social environment) that constrain psychophysical interactions between individuals (Sperber, 1996).

A significant departure from a culture as "shared norms and rules" perspective is that the variable distribution of ideas, which are themselves objects of study, and disagreement across observers, is treated as signal, not as noise. The distribution view avoids the limitations of considering "culture" a well-bounded system or cluster of practices and beliefs (see Brumann, 1999, and commentaries for examples), in favor of using a set of techniques for assessing groupwide patterns that statistically demonstrate cultural consensus or lack thereof. This proposal has the advantage that it avoids trying to define culture, focusing attention instead on the distribution of cultural representations.

In our work we have relied extensively on the cultural consensus model (CCM) of Romney, Weller, and Batchelder (1986), an important tool for analyzing commonalities and differences within and across cultural groups. The CCM has been an effective tool for cognitive anthropologists (e.g., Moore, Romney, Hsia, & Rush, 2000; Romney & Batchhelder, 1999; Romney, Brewer, & Batchelder, 1996). Consensus modeling permits recovery of graded patterns of variation within and between populations (down to the level of the individual and up to the level of combining cultural patterns to show "metacultural" interaction and consensus). Rather than locating "cultural analysis" at any one level, one can explore the existence of agreement patterns, linking them to environmental (social and physical) processes and phenomena.

Other researchers (e.g., Eid & Diener, 2001) have employed latent class analysis to identify subgroups. A limitation of latent class analysis not shared by the CCM is that fairly large sample sizes are needed to identify subgroups.

Accordingly, it is less useful to try to estimate population parameters for such norms and associated behaviors (especially when cultural studies consist of cross-national samples of college students) than to establish the pathways that determine how ideas (in our case, categories and concepts) affect reasoning and behaviors. For example, in some of our work we have identified cultural differences in approaches to nature but then have been able to link within-group variation in mental models with corresponding within-group variation in cross-group stereotyping (Medin, Ross, Cox, & Atran, 2006).This means that trying to establish a truly random sample may be much less useful than selecting a sample that is most likely to reveal some cultural processes of interest (this contrasting strategy is known as *purposive sampling*).

The Cultural Consensus Model

The CCM assumes that widely shared information is reflected by a high concordance among individuals. Estimation of individual competencies is derived from the pattern of interinformant agreement on the first factor of a principal component analysis (essentially factor analysis). A cultural consensus is found to the extent that the data overall conform to a single factor solution (the first latent root is

large in relation to all other latent roots), and individual scores on the first factor are strongly positive. These competency scores should not be mistaken for scores of expertise. The cultural model provides a measure for culturally shared knowledge; hence, the levels of competencies measure the extent to which an individual shares what everyone else agrees upon. The CCM is not a theory of culture or of the cultural transmission of information, any more than analysis of variance is a theory of cognition. It is only a tool that can be used to evaluate such theories.

Of course, general agreement may be coupled with systematic disagreement, and the CCM is an effective tool for uncovering both shared and unshared knowledge. After the consensus parameters are estimated for each individual, the expected agreement between each pair of informants is generated (as the product of their respective consensus parameters). Next, the expected agreement matrix is subtracted from the raw agreement matrix to yield a matrix of deviations from expected agreement (cf. Hubert & Golledge, 1981). If raw and residual agreement are significantly associated, then a significant portion of residual agreement consists of deviations from the consensus. One can then explore other factors (e.g., cultural subgroups, social network distance) that might predict or explain the residual agreement. For example, Medin, Lynch, Coley, and Atran (1997) asked tree experts to sort local species of trees into groups and found a clear overall consensus, coupled with reliable residual agreement. They then examined second-factor scores and found that they correlated strongly with occupation (e.g., parks maintenance worker, taxonomist, landscaper). Subsequent comparisons revealed systematic differences in the basis for sorting across groups.

Logic and Strategy in Cross-Cultural Comparison

One reason that comparative research has been unpopular is that it is not always clear how to do it successfully. When one compares two groups and finds clear differences, interpretive problems quickly emerge. Which of the many ways in which the two groups differ are crucial? For example, López, Atran, Coley, Medin, and Smith (1997) found that U.S. undergraduates and Itza' Maya of Guatemala showed different patterns of responding on a category-based inductive reasoning task involving mammals. Although this undermines the universality of the particular reasoning phenomenon, the two groups differed in myriad ways (age, education, literacy, livelihood, language, cosmology, etc.). Which of these differences matters? Practically speaking, it may be impossible to disentangle these various factors. Suppose we could control for age, education, literacy, and the like in comparing Itza' Maya and undergraduates. How do we decide which variables represent "culture" and should therefore not be controlled, and which variables do not, and should be controlled? The Itza' Maya practice agroforestry and also hunt and collect plants in the forest. Should these factors be controlled or are they part of Maya culture?

Now suppose that we control for every variable we can think of and still find differences. In this case, it seems that one is more or less forced to reify or essentialize culture; that is, the only explanation of the cultural difference involves appealing to some abstract notion of "culture." In short, it seems that we may be caught between two equally undesirable possibilities: (1) to end up with a notion of culture that solely has recourse to circular explanations of differences ("The Itza' are different because they are Itza' "); (2) to conclude that cultural comparisons just represent confounded experiments, and the notion of culture is not needed once proper experimental control is achieved.

Triangulation as a Research Strategy

There is no theoretically neutral way to define culture (see Atran et al., 2005). We have just suggested that the idea that culture is whatever is left when all potentially confounding variables are controlled is self-defeating. Granted, it is useful to control for variables that are clearly irrelevant to culture. But one must bear in mind that decisions about what is irrelevant are necessarily theory-based and commit one to a particular notion of culture.

Because (cultural) groups cannot be found that represent orthogonal combinations of variables, it may be impossible in principle to disentangle the various sources of variation among groups. The general idea of triangulation is to use observations from a third group to get at least modest leverage for understanding initial group differences. The third group should resemble the first group in some potentially important ways and the second group in other ways. If the third group performs like one of the groups and differently from the other group, then the variables shared by the third group and the group it mimics become candidates for critical variables.

To illustrate this strategy, consider again the findings of López et al. (1997). In that study, we compared Itza' Maya elders and University of Michigan undergraduates on categorization and reasoning involving local mammals (local to Petén and to Guatemala and Michigan, respectively). We told informants of a new disease that we know affects *coyotes* and *wolves*, and another new disease that affects *coyotes* and *cows*. Then we asked which disease is more likely to affect all mammals.

University of Michigan undergraduates overwhelmingly said the disease that coyotes and cows get is more likely to affect all mammals. They justified their answers by appealing to the dissimilarity of the two premises, or *diversity*; that is, they said that if some disease affects mammals as different as coyotes and cows, it is likely to affect all mammals. This reasoning strategy seems straightforward, and the Osherson, Smith, Wilkie, Lopez, and Shafir (1990) model for category-based reasoning predicts that people will prefer more diverse premises in drawing inductions to a category. What is surprising is that the Itza' Maya did not show a diversity effect. In some cases they were reliably *below* chance in picking the more diverse premises on these kinds of tests.

Why did the Itza' not use a diversity-based reasoning strategy? Obviously, there are any number of hypotheses one could conjure up. Perhaps the question was not asked quite the same way in Itza' Maya (back translation is no guarantee of equivalence), or perhaps formal education is a prerequisite for this form of abstract thought, or perhaps the Itza' have a very different conceptualization of disease. The answer just is not clear.

Here is where our triangulation strategy proved to be effective. In this case, the third group was U.S. tree experts who were asked to reason about novel tree diseases. They resembled both the Michigan undergraduates in many respects (language, formal education, etc.) and the Itza' with respect to having considerable domain knowledge. A typical diversity probe might be as follows: "White pine and weeping willows get one new disease and river birch and paper birch get another. Which is more likely to affect all trees?" Using these kinds of probes, Proffitt, Coley, and Medin (2000) found that parks workers, like the Itza', showed reliably below chance diversity responding. As we elaborate later, both groups were employing a reasoning strategy that is sensible and coherent—it just does not show up in undergraduate reasoning, for reasons that we will soon make clear. For now, we simply note that the triangulation strategy pinpoints domain knowledge as a key variable in diversity responding (though, as we will see, this is not the whole story).

At first glance, it might appear that the triangulation strategy is just a 2×2 design with one cell missing. In our example, one factor might be *cultural group* and the other, *expertise*, with the missing cell being the Itza' Maya, who lack knowledge of biological kinds. But a 2×2 design presumes what the triangulation strategy is intended to discover, namely, which factors are crucial to group differences. So, in our case, *expertise* seems to be the main factor and the factor of *culture* is just a stand-in for the many ways the groups might differ, which may or may not be relevant for some specific task. The logic of triangulation implies compression of any number of possible 2×2 designs that together entail a host of possible explanations for group differences. Instead of 2^N controlled designs, each of which allows inference to a single factor, a carefully chosen third group deliberately confounds a number of variables. By carefully choosing a third group, C, that resembles both the first group, A, in a number of ways and the second group, B, in a number of other ways, one can assess the relative importance of the set of culturally confounded variables by which C differs from A versus C differs from B.

OVERVIEW OF CONCEPTS AND CATEGORIES

It is not easy to organize this review, because (mainstream) psychology has a different history and perspective than anthropology. Our compromise is to come at it both ways, noting the frequent parallels. We begin our overview with theories of concepts and categories that have arisen out of mainstream cognitive psychology, which has been more concerned with mental representations and abstract structural properties of categories than has anthropology. We then review research emanating from both anthropology and psychology that has investi-

gated concepts and categorization across cultures.

In what follows, we use *concept* to refer to a mental representation, and *category* to refer to the set of entities or examples picked out by the concept. It is generally accepted that instances of a concept are organized into categories (Smith & Medin, 1981). Almost all theories about the structure of categories assume that, roughly speaking, similar things tend to belong to the same category and dissimilar things tend to be in different categories. For example, robins and sparrows both belong to the category *bird* and are more similar to each other than they are to squirrels or pumpkins. "Similarity" is a pretty vague term, but it is most commonly defined in terms of shared properties or attributes. Although alternative theories assume that concepts are structured in terms of shared properties, theories differ greatly in their organizational principles. The *classical view* assumes that concepts have defining features that act like criteria or rules for determining category membership. For example, a triangle is a closed geometric, three-sided form, with the sum of the interior angles equaling 180°. Each of these properties is necessary for an entity to be a triangle, and these properties together are sufficient to define a "triangle."

A fair amount of research has examined people's knowledge about object categories such as *bird*, *chair*, and *furniture*, and this evidence goes against the classical view. People not only fail to come up with defining features but also they do not necessarily agree with each other (or even with themselves when asked at different times) on whether something is an example of a category (Bellezza, 1984; McCloskey & Glucksberg, 1978). Philosophers and scientists also have worried about whether naturally occurring things such as plants and animals (so-called "natural kinds") have defining features. The current consensus is that most natural concepts do not fit the classical view.

The major alternative to the classical view, the *probabilistic view* (see Smith & Medin, 1981), argues that concepts are organized around properties that are characteristic or typical of category members, but, crucially, they need not be true of all members; that is, the features are only *probable*. For example, most people's concept of bird may include the properties of building nests, flying, and having hollow bones, even though not all birds have these properties (e.g., ostriches, penguins).The probabilistic view has major implications for how we think about categories. First, if categories are organized around characteristic properties, some members may have more of these properties than other members. In this sense, some members may be better examples or more typical of a concept than others. For example, Rosch and Mervis (1975) found that the more frequently a category member's properties appeared within a category, the higher its rated *typicality* for that category. For instance, robins were rated to be very typical birds and penguins were rated as very atypical birds. A second implication is that category boundaries may be fuzzy. Nonmembers of a category may have almost as many characteristic properties of a category as do certain members. For example, whales have a lot of the characteristic properties of fish, yet they are mammals. Third, learning about a category cannot be equated with determining its defining features, because there may not be any (see, Murphy, 2002, for a general review).

Is typicality based only on central tendency? Although typicality effects are robust (and problematic for the classical view), other research shows that the underlying basis for typicality effects may vary with both the kind of category and the population being studied. Barsalou (1985) reported that the internal structure of taxonomic categories is based primarily on the central tendency (or the average member) of a category. In contrast, the internal structure of goal-derived categories, such as "things to wear in the snow," is determined by some ideal (or the best possible member) associated with the category. The best example of snow clothing, a down jacket, was not the example most like other category members; instead it was the example with the maximum value of the goal-related dimension of providing warmth.

One might think that ideals will only come into play when the category of interest lacks the natural similarity structure that characterizes common taxonomic categories, such as *bird*, *fish*, and *tree*. However, recent evidence undermines this idea. Lynch, Coley, and Medin (2000) found that, for tree experts (people who know a lot about trees, e.g., landscapers, parks workers and taxonomists), the internal structure of the category *tree* was organized around the positive ideal of height and the negative ideal of weediness. The best examples of *tree* were not trees of average height but trees of extraordinary height (and free of "weedy" char-

acteristics, e.g., having weak limbs, growing where they are not wanted, and being susceptible to disease).

Other research is consistent with the idea that people who have considerable knowledge in a domain tend to base typicality judgments on ideals, and not on the number of typical features (Johnson, 2001). For instance, for Itza' Maya adults living in the rain forests of Guatemala the best example of bird is the wild turkey, which is culturally significant, prized for its meat, and strikingly beautiful (Bailenson, Shum, Atran, Medin, & Coley, 2002). The Lynch et al. (2000) finding that U.S. tree experts based typicality on ideals suggests that it is not just that the Itza' have a different notion of what typicality means. Burnett, Medin, Ross, and Blok (2005) also found that Native American and European American fishermen's typicality judgments were based on ideals, though those ideals differed somewhat across groups.

If categories are not represented in terms of definitions, what form do our mental representations take? One suggestion about how concepts are represented is known as the "family resemblance principle." The general idea is that category members resemble each other in the way that family members do. A simple summary representation for such a family resemblance structure would be an example that possessed all the characteristic features of a category. The best example is referred to as the *prototype*.

In a prototype model of categorization, a new example is classified by comparing the new item to the prototype. If the candidate example is similar enough to the prototype for a category, it is classified as a member of that category. More detailed analyses, however, show problems with prototypes as mental representations. Prototype theory implies that the only information abstracted from categories is the central tendency. A prototype representation discards information concerning category size, the variability of the examples, and correlations among attributes. The evidence suggests that people can use all three of these types of information (Estes, 1986; Flannagan, Fried, & Holyoak, 1986; Fried & Holyoak, 1984; Medin, Altom, Edelson, & Freko, 1982).

An alternative approach, which is also consistent with the probabilistic view, assumes that much more information about specific examples is preserved. This approach appropriately falls under the general heading of *exemplar theories.* Exemplar models assume that people initially learn some examples of different concepts, then classify a new instance on the basis of how similar it is to the previously learned examples. The idea is that a new example reminds the person of similar, old examples and he or she assumes that similar items will belong to the same category. For example, suppose you are asked whether large birds are more or less likely to fly than small birds. You probably will answer "less likely," based on retrieving examples from memory and noting that the only nonflying birds you can think of are large (e.g., penguin, ostrich).

Quite a few experiments have contrasted the predictions of exemplar and prototype models. In head-to-head competition, exemplar models have been substantially more successful than prototype models (see Estes, 1994; Lamberts, 1995; Medin & Coley, 1998; Nosofsky, 1992; Nosofsky & Palmeri, 1997; Storms, De Boeck, & Ruts, 2000; Verbeeman, Vanoverberghe, Storms, & Ruts, 2001; Smits, Storms, Rosseel, & De Boeck, 2002; but for opposing views see Homa, 1984; Smith & Minda, 1998, 2000).

Why should exemplar models fare better than prototype models? One of the main functions of classification is to allow one to make inferences and predictions on the basis of partial information (see Anderson, 1990a, 1990b). Relative to prototype models, exemplar models tend to be conservative about discarding information that facilitates predictions. For instance, sensitivity to correlations of properties within a category enables finer predictions: From noting that a bird is large, one can predict that it cannot sing. In short, exemplar models support predictions and inferences better than do prototype models.

A number of researchers have argued that the organization of concepts is knowledge-based (rather than similarity-based) and driven by intuitive theories about the world (for a general review, see Carey, 1985; Keil, 1989; Murphy & Medin, 1985; Murphy, 2002). The idea that concepts might be knowledge- rather than similarity-based suggests a natural way in which concepts may change, namely, through the addition of new knowledge and theoretical principles. There is also good evidence that these theories help determine that abstract and observable features to which learners pay attention (Spalding & Ross, 2000; Wisniewski & Medin, 1994). The set of categories for mental disorders now differs from that 100 years ago,

in part because our knowledge base has become more refined. Often knowledge of diseases develops from information about patterns of symptoms to a specification of underlying causes. For example, the advanced stages of syphilis were treated as a mental disorder until the causes and consequences of this venereal disease were better understood. Kim and Ahn (2002) have shown that clinical psychologists organize their knowledge of mental disorders in terms of the rich causal theories (and not the atheoretical diagnostic manual they are supposed to use) that guide their diagnostic classification and reasoning.

FOLKBIOLOGY AND NATURAL KINDS ACROSS CULTURES

Perhaps one of the most natural questions to ask about concepts is whether people in different cultures have different ones. Concepts are the building blocks of thought, and at the heart of this question is whether people in different cultures think differently. Usually this question is tied up with the question of whether and how language influences thought (see Gentner & Goldin-Meadow, 2003, for a series of reviews and comments on this issue, which we do not cover separately here). Of course, if thought processes of two cultural groups were radically incommensurable, one would quickly realize there dramatic differences but be at something of a loss to explain them. The fact that one part of learning a foreign language involves finding out what term or word is used to refer to *bird*, *fish*, *chair*, *Tuesday*, or *mother* suggests that comparable concepts and categories are in play.

Folkbiology

Research in the domain of living kinds has allowed a natural comparison of concepts across cultures. Perhaps the most striking result is the strong cross-cultural agreement in categorizing plants and animals. Consider an ethnobiologist undertaking the study of folkbiology in some new culture. The project could hardly get under way before he or she asks what living kinds are found in that culture, what terms exist in the language referring to living kinds, and what the relation is between those terms and what is there (the issue of reference). How does one describe what living kinds exist in some cultural context? A reasonable starting point is to use scientific taxonomy as a reference or standard. For example, one might ask whether every kind that science recognizes as a distinct species has a distinct name (Diamond & Bishop, 1999). Upon finding that many kinds do not have distinct names, it is natural for one to ask what principles determine whether or not a species has a distinct name (Berlin, 1992). For example, naming could be driven by relevance to humans (utility), perceptual discontinuities, or even size (Hunn, 1999).

Scientific taxonomy is, of course, a hierarchical taxonomy and, as such, provides both a standard and a heuristic for asking other questions about universal aspects of folktaxonomies. Two important analytic points are involved here: First, although the particular kinds of plants and animals to be found may vary across cultures, the abstract structure in terms of species, genus, family, order, class, division, and kingdom will be represented. Consequently, scientific taxonomy provides something of a conceptual grid for cross-cultural comparisons. The second, related point is that scientific taxonomy allows one to establish corresponding ranks, such that it becomes meaningful to state that *oak* is at the same level or rank as *trout*. This does not mean that they are psychologically at the same rank, but it does provide a basis for asking questions, such as whether some culture differentiates mammals more than fish. As it turns out, ethnobiologists have found that folk ranks and folktaxonomies only roughly approximate scientific taxonomies (Hunn, 1975). By *roughly*, we mean that the correlation between scientific taxonomic distance of species (i.e., the number of nodes that must be traversed to connect species x and species y) and folktaxonomic distance is about .75. On the one hand, this may be seen as quite high but on the other, this accounts for only about 50% of the variance.

Folkbiology is a field blessed with many intriguing and important issues that lend themselves to an analysis in terms of culture and cognition. Let us turn to a few of them.

Are Folkbiological Categories Recognized or Constructed?:
Egghead versus Utilitarian Perspectives

A basic issue within ethnobiology concerns whether categories are recognized or constructed (see Malt, 1995; Brown, 1995). One view—known within ethnobiology as the "intellectualist view"—is that the structure of kinds in nature comprises "chunks" that more or less impose themselves on minds (at least on minds with a perceptual system like ours). This position is reinforced by the finding that folk categories often correspond to scientific species or genera and by quite strong cross-cultural agreement in folktaxonomic systems (e.g., Atran, 1990; Berlin, 1992; though Atran interprets agreement in terms of universal properties of mind rather than the structure of nature alone).

The alternative, or "utilitarian," view is that folktaxonomic systems are influenced by goals, theories, and belief systems, and that they may be culture-dependent constructions (Hunn, 1982; Ellen, 1993). For instance, Hunn (1982) noted that the Tzeltal peoples do not differentiate as finely among butterflies as they do among butterfly larvae, because the larvae are important for food and are also crop pests. Berlin (1978) found that Aguaruna and Tzeltal peoples formed generic categories for plants that were of no utility to them, yet further division into more specific categories was made for plants that were considered useful. In short, the role of utility seems to vary with taxonomic rank. The intellectualist view appears to be fairly accurate at the rank of folk generics (e.g., dog, pine, trout), and the utilitarian view holds more sway at the level of folk species (e.g., poodle, white pine, brook trout) and variety (e.g., toy poodle, Western white pine).

Other, intermediate positions hold that the intellectualist and utilitarian views are not necessarily mutually exclusive. For example, their relative influence may depend on factors such as rank in the hierarchy (Bulmer, 1970): Cultures may differ more in the structure and use of categories such as *tree* or *bird* (corresponding roughly to class in scientific taxonomy) than they do for *oak* or *robin* (corresponding roughly to the generic or species level).

A final twist on this issue arises from studies that have included informants from groups with less intimate contact with nature. Consider the research conducted by López et al. (1997). When comparing folkbiological taxonomies, López et al. found that Americans and Itza' were more or less equally competent in their classification of mammals, as judged by the correlation between sorting distance and formal taxonomic distance. Furthermore, classification in both groups was largely based on the morphology and behaviors of the mammals. However, relative to the American undergraduates, the Itza' were more likely to differentiate among smaller mammals, were less likely to group mammals together in large groups, gave greater weight to ecological considerations, and gave less weight to size and domesticity. Indeed, for the undergraduates, most of the variance in sorting could be accounted for on the basis of size alone. In other words the undergraduates had a somewhat impoverished knowledge of mammals relative to that of the Itza'.

In related work, Bailenson et al. (2002) asked U.S. experts, U.S. novices (college students) and Itza' Maya to sort pictures of U.S. and Guatemalan birds into groups. They found that the Itza' sorting correlation with scientific taxonomy for U.S. birds was actually higher than the correlation of the U.S. novice sorting for U.S. birds, again suggesting that the U.S. college students had somewhat impoverished knowledge of birds (for more data and discussion of the cognitive consequences of impoverished contact with the biological world, see Johnson & Mervis, 1998; Medin & Atran, 2004).

Does Nature Have Joints?

THE BASIC LEVEL

An important observation about categories is that people are not confused about which label to use when asked about an object. For example, a person looking at a four-legged furry animal that had just fetched a ball would more likely call it a *dog* than an *animal* or a *poodle*. This intermediate level of abstraction, which seems to provide the label that we would use as a default, is called the *basic level*, and it appears to be especially salient and psychologically privileged. For example, basic-level concepts are the first to be learned, the natural level at which objects are named, and the highest level in which the instances all share the same parts and overall shape (Rosch, Mervis, Gray, Johnson, & Boyes-Braem, 1976). The basic level resides at a middle level of abstraction. More abstract categories (e.g., animal) are called *superordinates*, and more specific categories (e.g., golden retriever) are called *subordinates*. Berlin (1992) found that among traditional societies, the basic level for plant and animal categories seems to correspond to the folk-generic level (e.g., *maple*, *trout*). Berlin calls these categories "beacons on the landscape of biological reality" (p. 53). Consistent with this claim, the genus level is the rank

where cross-cultural agreement in categorization is maximized.

Although traditional ethnobiological studies point to the folk-generic level as privileged, Rosch et al. (1976) found that for American undergraduates, the basic level seemed to correspond to the more abstract life-form level (e.g., *tree*, *fish*). One way of reconciling these two claims is to again argue that American undergraduates do not have the requisite experience with biological kinds to develop what would otherwise be a universal appreciation of the genus level. Some cross-cultural studies have directly addressed this issue.

Coley, Medin, and Atran (1997) have examined whether the cultural differences in the privileged or basic level in taxonomic classification correspond to cultural differences in the privileged level for folkbiological induction. A level is defined as privileged if inferences to this level are significantly stronger than inferences to the immediate superordinate level, but no stronger than inferences to a subordinate level (if there is a subordinate level). The former task may measure consequences of experience, and the latter may assess expectations rather than knowledge about categories. Coley et al. told American undergraduates and the Itza' elders that an unfamiliar property was characteristic of all members of a particular category, and asked how likely this was to be true of members of a more general category. If the basic level is the level above which information is lost, and below which little information is gained (Rosch et al., 1976), then the privileged level for induction should be the basic level. Based on Berlin's (1992) and Rosch et al.'s (1976) research, Coley et al. (1997) predicted that the privileged level for induction should be the folk-generic level for the Itza' and the life-form level for the American undergraduates.

Coley et al. (1997) found that the privileged level for inductive inferences was the folk-generic level for both groups of participants; that is, the strongest inductions were made from the folk-generic level to the life-form level, relative to all other inductions. Thus, there is a dissociation of knowledge and expectations in Americans' folkbiological categories. In spite of the fact that undergraduates may have little specific knowledge about the sparrow, trout, or oak, expectations about the informativeness of categories serve to maximize inductive inferences at the folk-generic taxonomic level. Indeed, Coley, Hayes, Lawson, and Maloney (2004) found that for living kinds, inductions are influenced more by expected informativeness (measured by collecting ratings of perceived similarity among category members at different levels) than by specific knowledge of the concepts themselves (measured by asking participants to list known features for concepts at different hierarchical levels).

CULTURE VERSUS EXPERTISE

There is evidence that as one becomes more expert in an area, what was previously the subordinate level becomes the basic level. For example, *dog* might be a basic-level category for most people, but *poodle* might be a basic-level category for dog trainers (Tanaka & Taylor, 1991; see also Johnson & Mervis, 1997, 1998). This difference in expertise accounts for some of the discrepancies between Berlin's (1992) findings and those of Rosch et al. (1976). One might argue, however, that expertise and culture are not totally dissociable, because as López et al. (1997) argued, knowledge is part of culture (see also Wolff, Medin, & Pankratz, 1999). Furthermore, differences in expertise do not preclude the potentiality for other "cultural" influences to play a role in categorization and reasoning.

An example in which group differences could be attributed to differences in culture, over and above differences in expertise, comes from research by Medin, Ross, Atran, Burnett, and Blok (2002). They examined categorization of freshwater fish among the Menominee and majority-culture European Americans in north-central Wisconsin. Both groups live in an area of Wisconsin with many rivers, lakes, and streams, and both groups have extensive knowledge about the fish that live in those waters. In addition, both groups fish similar species and use similar practices (e.g., fly-fishing, ice fishing). Given these similarities, it is possible to predict that these two groups would share similar conceptualizations of fish.

However, Medin et al. (2002) found differences between Menominee and majority-culture fishermen in categorization of freshwater fish. Importantly, these individuals had high levels of expertise about fish, and expertise did not differ between groups. Nevertheless, these groups exhibited differences in certain tasks. For instance, Medin et al. asked majority-culture and Menominee fish experts to sort name cards of 44 species of local fish into categories, then examined cross-group similarities and differences. Although a combined analysis showed an overall consensus, Menominee participants exhibited higher within-group than between-group consensus. Majority-culture fish experts showed no greater within- than across-group residual agreement. This analysis suggests that the two groups share a common model but that Menominee experts have an additional basis of organization.

Other analyses reinforce these group differences. Multidimensional scaling of majority-culture sorts yield two-dimensional solutions that correlate with size and desirability. Menominee sorting required an additional dimension corresponding to ecological relations (shared habitat). Majority-culture fishermen were more likely than the Menominee fishermen to give taxonomic or morphological justifications for their sortings (62 vs. 33%, respectively), and the Menominee fishermen were more likely than the majority-culture fishermen to give ecological justifications for their sortings (40 vs. 6%, respectively). These data indicate that levels of expertise (knowledge of a domain) and kinds of experience (practice and goals) cannot fully account for how individuals categorize living things. Later experiments showed that these cultural differences were differences in knowledge organization rather than knowledge per se. For example, a speeded fish–fish interaction task showed large cultural differences (Menominee experts reported more relations, more reciprocal relations, and more relations involving immature fish) that disappeared when the pace of the task was relaxed.

The same difference in cultural orientation was obtained for a group of less expert Menominee and majority-culture fishermen. Based on these findings, Medin et al. (2002) suggested that both experts and nonexperts exhibit a high degree of consensus with respect to fish in their area, but that these groups diverge in a culture-specific way: a difference in the salience of ecological relations as a basis for knowledge organization.

What Do We Know about Categorization as a Basis for Folkbiological Reasoning?

INDUCTIVE REASONING

One primary function of concepts is that they support *reasoning*. One does not need to store every fact and possibility if inferences can be derived from information that is stored. From the knowledge that all animals breathe, that reptiles are animals, and that rattlesnakes are reptiles, one may reason (deductively) that rattlesnakes must also breathe, even though one may never have directly stored that fact. Indeed, Medin et al. (1997) found that for parks personnel and tree taxonomists who sorted based on morphological properties, the sorting data were a good predictor of performance on reasoning tasks. And as mentioned earlier, López et al. (1997), who investigated taxonomic classification of mammals and similarity, typicality, and diversity effects among Itza' and U.S. college participants, found that although both the Itza' and the U.S. students exhibited similarity and typicality effects when making inductions, only the U.S. students exhibited a diversity effect.

Why are the Itza' not showing taxonomic diversity effects in reasoning? The short answer appears to be that "diversity" is an abstract reasoning strategy that tends to be used by experts only when more concrete causal/ecological reasoning fails. Other work shows that Itza' Maya, U.S. bird experts, most U.S. tree experts, and European American and Native American fish experts do not show diversity effects in reasoning (Bailenson et al., 2002; Burnett et al., 2005; Proffitt et al., 2000). Instead, causal/ecological reasoning dominates. What knowledge seems to provide is flexibility, in the form of a variety of strategies that allow the reasoner to project different properties in different ways. In evidence of this flexibility, Shafto and Coley (2003) found that whereas fishermen projected diseases according to food chain relations among marine animals, they projected more abstract or ambiguous properties like "a property called sarca" among the same animals according to similarity or taxonomic relatedness, as did domain novices.

There is also suggestive evidence of cultural differences among college students in reasoning. For example, Choi, Smith, and Nisbett (1999) found that diversity effects involving specific conclusions (rather than a superordinate category) were weaker among Korean college students than among U.S. college students, at least for biological stimuli. Choi et al. attributed this effect to U.S. students' tendency to think more in terms of categories. They suggested that the fact that both groups show specific diversity effects for social categories reflects the interdependent social orientation of Korean students.

SUMMARY

The results on inductive reasoning echo the findings on categories and concepts: Performance is strongly influenced by domain knowledge, and results with U.S. undergraduates do not generalize very well to other populations.

Is Reasoning from Folkbiological Categories Similarity Based or Theory Based?

Especially within cognitive psychology, folkbiology is an appealing domain from the contending standpoints of both similarity- and theory-based views of categorization and category-based reasoning. On the one hand, our perceptual system is surely an adaptation to the natural world, and if similarity-based models are going to succeed anywhere, it should be here. On the other hand, the biological world is apparently a world of fairly stable clusters of complex features, whose remarkable endurance in the face of constant change presumably owes to naturally occurring causal patterns. Understanding causal patterns in the world is a primary goal of theory-driven knowledge in science, and the history of science is coterminous with trying to understand biological causality in particular. If theory-based knowledge were to develop anywhere outside of science—in other cultures, or in everyday thinking—it should be here.

From the perspective of similarity, there are evident patterns of covariation for biologically related attributes (e.g., toothless, two-legged beings generally have wings, feathers, and can fly). Perhaps most people in the world are aware of these covariations without necessarily understanding their causal origins or interrelations, such as the role of feathers in flight. In other words, there could be quite a bit of biologically relevant data stored but not theoretically assimilated.

Nevertheless, people in different cultures acknowledge, and often try to better understand, at least some of the causal interrelations among covariant biological attributes (Gelman, 2003). These include irreversible patterns of biological growth (maturation) the apparent constancy of covariant morphological, anatomical, and behavioral patterns across generations (reproduction and inheritance); the success of mutually constraining actions of interrelated attributes in maintaining life (bodily function); and the breakdown of interrelated bodily functions (illness and death).

Suppose, as ethnobiologists generally agree, that people everywhere witness certain covariant biological patterns (roughly corresponding to perceptually salient species or genera) but interpret the causal relationships underlying these patterns in different ways. This might suggest that similarity based reasoning precedes theoretically based reasoning, at least in the biological domain. This was a message of developmental studies in the 1980s (Carey, 1985; Inagaki & Sugiyama, 1988; Keil & Batterman, 1984). More recent studies have lowered the age at which children are thought to reason causally about biological kinds. But the origins of causal reasoning in folkbiology remain a matter of controversy.

This controversy hinges on two related questions: (1) What is the earliest age at which children can be said to have a theory of biology? and (2) Does biological thought constitute a distinct domain? Not surprisingly, the answer to these questions depends on how one defines the terms.

THEORY AND DOMAIN

A number of researchers have argued that even very young children's categorization and reasoning is guided by certain skeletal principles (Gelman, 2002) or a framework theory and a unifying concept of an underlying essence that makes things the sorts of things that they are (Gelman, 2003; Gelman & Hirschfield, 1999; Hirschfeld & Gelman, 1994; Medin & Atran, 2004).

FRAMEWORK THEORIES

Susan Carey (1982, 1985) has shown that children's biological theories guide their conceptual development. In one study, 6-year-old children rated a toy monkey as more similar to people than to a worm, but they also judged the worm to be more likely than the toy monkey to have a spleen (a spleen was described as "a green thing inside people"). Although worms may be less similar to people than are toy monkeys, they are more similar in some respects, namely, common biological functions. And Carey's work shows that children's biological theories help them determine which respects are relevant. Thus, the 6-year-old children's rudimentary biological knowledge influences the structure of their concept of animal (see also Au & Romo, 1999; Coley, 1995; Keil, 1989; Simons & Keil, 1995;

for other studies on the development of biological knowledge, see Hatano and Inagaki, 1999; Inagaki & Hatano, 2002; see Gelman, 2003, for comprehensive reviews).

DOMAIN SPECIFICITY

A number of researchers, especially in the area of cognitive development, have suggested that cognition is organized in terms of distinct domains, each characterized by (usually) innate constraints or skeletal principles of development. For example, naive psychology (theories about people), naive biology (theories about livings things), and naive physics (theories about the physical world) may constitute distinct domains with somewhat different principles of conceptual development (see Hirschfeld & Gelman, 1994, for examples).

Although is it difficult to define a domain precisely, the notion of domain specificity has served to organize a great deal of research on conceptual development. For example, there has been a strong focus on the question of whether and when young children distinguish between psychology and biology. Carey (1985) argued that young children understand biological concepts in terms of a naive psychology in which human beings are the prototypical psychological entity. She suggested that only later on do children reorganize their knowledge into a less anthropocentric, biological form in which human beings are simply one animal among many. It is possible, however, that these results were driven by the relatively impoverished experience that children from large cities may have with nature. Rural European American and rural Native American children do not show this anthropocentric pattern (Ross, Medin, Coley, & Atran, 2003). In any event Carey's (1985) claims have sparked a great deal of research, and the current consensus is that young children do have biologically specific theories, though they may differ in content and degree of elaboration from those of adults (for extensive reviews, see Gelman, 2003; Inagaki & Hatano, 2002; Keil, 1989). Some of this research involves children's understanding of *essences*, a topic to which we next turn.

PSYCHOLOGICAL ESSENTIALISM

One way of integrating similarity and explanation is through psychological essentialism (Gelman, Coley, & Gottfried, 1994; Keil,

1989; Medin & Ortony, 1989). The main ideas are as follows: People act as if things (e.g., objects) have essences or underlying natures that make them the thing that they are. Essentialism is an idea present in many cultures (e.g., Atran, 1990; Walker, 1992). For biological categories in our culture, people often identify essence with genetic structure. The essence constrains or generates properties of organisms that may vary in their centrality. For example, people in our culture believe that the categories *male* and *female* are genetically determined, but to pick out someone as male or female we rely on characteristics such as hair length, height, facial hair, and clothing that represent a mixture of secondary sexual characteristics and cultural conventions. Although these characteristics are less reliable than genetic evidence, they are far from arbitrary. Not only do they have some validity in a statistical sense but also they are tied to our biological and cultural conceptions of male and female.

Why should people act as if things have essences? Possibly the reason is that it may be a good strategy for learning about the world; that is, our perceptual and conceptual systems appear to have evolved such that the essentialist heuristic is very often correct (Atran, 1990; Medin & Wattenmaker, 1987; Shepard, 1987). Classifying on the basis of similarity will be relatively effective much of the time, but that similarity will yield to knowledge of deeper principles. Gelman and Wellman (1991) showed that even young children seem to use notions of essence in reasoning about biological kinds (see also Gelman & Hirschfeld, 1999). Susan Gelman has systematically traced the development of essentialism and its role in conceptual and linguistic development (see Gelman, 2003, for a review).

The third experiment by Gelman and Wellman (1991) provides an example of a method for examining children's beliefs about nature versus nurture in biology. Children were told a story about a baby who, shortly after birth, was taken away from the birth parent to live with animals of a different species (a between-species manipulation). Importantly, the children were told that the baby never saw another animal of its mother's species again. Once children heard the story, they were asked whether the baby would have a particular property possessed by the birth parent or a particular property possessed by the adoptive parent when it was all grown up. Some of the properties were behavioral (e.g., a horse's neigh and a tiger's roar) and some of the properties were physical (e.g., kangaroos have a pouch and goats do not have a pouch). All of the properties were "known" in that they were category-typical properties about which the children would already have had some knowledge. Results showed that 4- and 5-year-old children exhibited a birth bias (i.e., they were more likely to say that the baby had the same property as the birth parent rather than the adoptive parent) for both behavioral and physical properties.

This initial study has sparked a number of other investigations, some driven by methodological issues and others aimed at testing the cross-cultural universality of a birth bias in children's reasoning. The upshot is quite strong support for a widespread birth bias in young children, even though adults' patterns of reasoning diverge across studies (e.g., Astuti, Solomon, Carey, Ingold, & Miller, 2004; Atran et al., 2001; Sousa, Atran, & Medin, 2002; Waxman, Medin, & Ross, in press).

We have presented only one theory and one interpretation of the data from the adoption properties paradigm. It would be misleading to imply that there is any strong consensus on essentialism. For example, as some researchers argue the key is that people are sensitive to causal relations, and that the notion of an essence is not needed (e.g., Rehder & Hastie, 2001; Rips, 2001; Strevens, 2000; see Ahn et al., 2001, for counterarguments).

Summary

Although it is hard to summarize across vast literatures, our impression is that the more categories are grounded by real-world contingencies, the greater the cross-cultural agreement in categorization. For example, in the domain of biology, the most relevant and informative rank corresponds to the scientific level of genus (and in most local contexts to species), and cross-cultural agreement is also the most unequivocal at this level (e.g., Berlin, 1992; Malt, 1995).

Cross-cultural studies of people's biology have influenced cognitive theories of concept and categories in at least two distinct ways. One is that undergraduates at major U.S. universities are often the "odd group out," and "standard" results do not hold up well to cross-cultural scrutiny (see Medin & Atran,

2004, for a summary). The other is that extensive experience with the same biological kinds (involving the same activities and goals) does not guarantee convergence with respect to conceptions of living kinds. In particular it appears that cultural groups differ substantially in their understandings of relations among kinds or, in other words, in their folkecology.

Another way to state this generalization is to note that shared categories need not imply shared meanings. For example, Atran et al. (2002) studied Itza' Maya and Ladino agro-culturalists in Guatemala and noted that the Ladino term for the forest (*tierra agarrada de nadie*) translates into "the land guarded by no one," contrasting sharply with the Itza' Maya tendency to refer to the forest as *ki-wotoch*, which translates as "our home." Guess which group has more sustainable practices? The point is that a major source of cultural differences is not in fixing reference but rather in meanings, which may guide attitudes and behaviors. We now turn to a second critically important domain, social reasoning.

SOCIAL CATEGORIES AND CULTURE

The ability to categorize individuals into social categories is fundamental to interpreting and predicting the behavior of others. Indeed, given the complexity of human cultural life, the competencies underlying social categorization are among the most important human reasoning capacities. Therefore, it is not surprising that these competencies are grounded in our species' evolutionary past and are among the earliest discriminations human infants make. Many species, including most nonhuman primates, inhabit complex social environments in which the capacity to identify and classify conspecifics is paramount. Chimpanzee social relationships, for example, require the capacity to distinguish other chimps with respect to sex, age grade, kin relation, residential group, as well as position in status hierarchies (de Waal, 1998). Given how deeply rooted these distinctions are in human natural history, we should not be surprised to find that human *infants* display precocious sensitivity to the age (Brooks & Lewis, 1976), gender (Miller, 1983), language spoken (Mehler et al., 1988), and even race (Kelly, Quinn, & Slater, 2005) of other humans in their environment.

Intriguingly, despite the evident universal dimensions of the capacity for social discrimination and ultimately categorization, the degree to which social categories are contingent aspects of culture is striking. Anthropologists, comparative sociologists, and historians have documented extraordinary differences in the way peoples partition and reason about the social world. Even those classifications that otherwise seem grounded in natural "fact" vary dramatically across cultures. Consider the classification of kinfolk. On the one hand, as anyone who has witnessed a young child acquire language knows, kinterms such as *Mama* and *Papa* are invariably among the first words produced and understood (Hirschfeld, 1989). On the other hand, and perhaps less familiar to many readers, the classification of kin, at least to the anthropologist, is the preternaturally varying system of cultural categorization. Particularly for speakers of English, kinship categories represent the cultural recognition of relations of procreation and affiliation, and more or less accurately map them linguistically (Goodenough, 1955). All "full" siblings are biologically equally close relations, first cousins are somewhat less so, second cousins, even less so, and so on. Yet the thrust of kinship studies—which *was* largely what anthropologists studied during much of the 20th century—has been the demonstration that understanding consanguinity requires an understanding of the specificities of cultural tradition, not the universals of human procreation (Schneider, 1980).

As an illustration, consider the system of kin classification of the Batak of highland Sumatra, with whom one of us (LH) worked. Kin categories not only identify relations of consanguinity but also specify what these relations *mean*. In the case of the Batak system, kin categories pick out proscriptive marriage partners (in fact, this system, found throughout much of southeast Asia, has figured in one of anthropology's most influential debates [Leach, 1970; Lévi-Strauss, 1949]). In contrast to the American system, in which marriage between first cousins is generally avoided, among the Batak, kin classified as parallel cousins (the child of a parent's same-sex sibling; e.g., the father's brother's child) are in the same category as one's siblings. Accordingly, marriage between them is prohibited. On the other hand, cross-cousins (the child of a parent's opposite-sex sibling; e.g., the mother's brother's daughter) are *preferred* marriage partners. Blatantly, these contrasting classifications do not reflect relations of biological proximity; parallel and cross cousins are equally close biologically.

The classification of kinfolk, of course, is not the only system of "natural" categories that vary across cultures. Even "givens" such as "sex" (*not* gender) vary intriguingly across cultural traditions, as Laqueur (1990) demonstrated in his history of the shift from a one-sex system to the modern two-sex system. The notion of *child*, on the one hand, is evidently a universal (e.g., infants are able to discriminate between children and adults, *and* to distinguish both from midgets), but it is also widely recognized as a cultural construction (Ariès famously [1962] argued that children were not recognized as a distinct category of being prior to the 15th century). As with most categories, a particular pattern of partitioning a domain is linked to a particular pattern of reasoning about the domain as well. In contemporary U.S. society, for example, children are typically not considered capable to cross a busy street without supervision, whereas 8-year-olds are preferred caregivers for infants in much of the world (Morelli, Rogoff, & Angelillo, 2003).

As with many systems of categorization, the study of social categories therefore involves a tension between attention to their universal psychological bases and to the considerable cultural variation that mark them. Our goal in this section is to address this tension directly, and in doing so, we take an approach that is distinct from many other chapters in this volume. Among other things, we do not pretend to present a balanced or comprehensive review of existing work on culture and social categorization. Rather we suggest, following Sperber (1996), that much cultural variation in cognition is best explained by identifying the factors that shape the distribution of cognitive representations within a given population. This approach does not assume, or even favor, identifying either the boundaries or key features (symbols, meanings, propositions, regimes of truth, etc.) of a particular culture. Sperber's epidemiological theory does not oblige us to distinguish between cultural and other forms of knowledge but simply requires that we identify the factors underlying the (more or less) stable, recurring distribution of representation in a particular population. Nor, in this view, is it assumed that all linked cultural phenomena can be mapped on the same population (i.e., have

identical distributions) or that the same factors underlie the distribution of different cultural phenomena within the same cultural tradition. In brief, culture is more or less a sort of thing, not a unique level of variation.

Sperber's (1996) approach does not discount cultural variation. Rather, it holds that cultural variation can in significant measure be explained as the outcome of the operation of invariant cognitive processes. Specifically, Sperber argues that variation in the distribution of many cultural phenomena is governed by evolved and modular, domain-specific cognitive competencies that render some representations "catchier"—hence, more widely and stably distributed—than others. It is not that these cognitive competencies are dedicated to producing cultural phenomena—that they were evolved to output cultural phenomena. Rather, culturally varying representations are produced by these competencies and are exploited for cultural purposes. Sperber gives as an example the widely varying and culturally important elaborations of human faces found in virtually all cultures. Ranging from special-purpose makeup to sculpture to masks to gargoyles, the ubiquity *and* variation in the cultural elaboration of faces rest on an evolved and robust capacity to identify and remember human faces, even from degraded and/or programmatic representations (e.g., a circle with two dot and a dash). Plausibly evolved to track individual persons and their actions, the special *psychological* salience of human faces makes them excellent objects of cultural variation, if *excellent* in this context means "widely and stably distributed."

We propose that parallel, domain-specific processes underlie cultural variation in some social categories. Humans, we suggest, are endowed with a psychological module—elsewhere Hirschfeld (1996) has referred to it as "naive sociology"—that governs the development of the capacity to reason about others' actions by virtue of their membership in social groups. Although the competency for naive sociology may be innately prepared, elaborations of its output vary substantially across cultures. Indeed, our proposal is that social categories are central to virtually all systems that regulate and organize human behavior *precisely because* these systems are so easy to learn and remember, and they are so easy to learn and remember because they are grounded in a universal, cognitive competency.

To understand better the nature and scope of the modular competence for naive sociology, it is useful to identify and contrast it with another evolved, domain-specific capacity for understanding the behavior of others. In addition to reasoning about people with respect to memberships in groups, humans readily account for the actions of others as a function of other unseen mental states and dispositions. In previous research, the two capacities have typically been studied independently, giving the impression that they may represent distinct phenomena. But as Hamilton and his colleagues argue, group-based reasoning in fact relies on the same cognitive mechanisms and processes as person perception (Crawford, Sherman, & Hamilton, 2002; Hamilton & Sherman, 1996). To the contrary, we argue that each of these capacities is based in a distinct evolved, modular device. Theory of mind (ToM)—the capacity to interpret and predict another's actions on the basis of unseen mental states—appears to be a species-specific capacity (Povinelli & Bering, 2002; Tomasello, Call, & Hare, 2003). Frith and Frith (2003; Gallagher & Frith, 2003) provide evidence that ToM involves a special-purpose neurocognitive module. Although culture is likely to elaborate, highlight, or place them in the background, clearly these attributions of intentional states have an innate basis.

Reasoning about individual persons involves both attributions of transient mental states (Johnny stole a cookie from the cookie jar because he *believed* that cookies were in the cookie jar, and he *believed* that consuming them would satisfy his *desire* to sate his hunger) or enduring dispositions and traits (Johnny stole a cookie from the cookie jar because he is an intrinsically *dishonest* person). Conventional psychological wisdom about both transient mental states, particularly emotions, and dispositions and traits has been challenged during the last two decades (as several chapters in this volume attest) by anthropologists (Lutz, 1988) and cultural psychologists (Markus & Kityama, 1991). It is important to distinguish, at least in this context, between how peoples *talk* about motivation to act and how such motivation is actually psychologically achieved. Johnny may say that he believes in ghosts, when in fact he does not believe that sentient creatures can pass through solid objects (Atran, 2002; Barrett & Keil, 1996; Boyer, 2001), and at the group level, Johnny might say that the Nuer believe in ghosts. But the Nuer do not actually believe anything, only individual Nuer form beliefs—in particular, Johnny-the-Nuer's beliefs about what the Nuer supposedly believe (Sperber, 1996).

Even though cultures vary widely in the degree to which attributions of mental states and attributions of dispositions and traits are engaged, the cognitive processes that make such attributions possible vary little across cultures. Experience also does not significantly alter the individual's capacity to make either kind of attribution. For example, living in a cultural environment that disprefers attributions of dispositions and traits in favor of more interdependent representations of self does not reduce the individual's *capacity* for such attributions (Nisbett, 2003). Similarly, being reared in a more communal cultural environment does not reduce the individual's capacity, if not proclivity, to interpret behavior in terms of private, individually experienced mental states (Avis & Harris, 1991).

Our concern here is the human capacity to use group membership in interpreting and predicting the actions of others (Berreby, 2005; Furth, 1996; Hirschfeld, 1989; Jackendoff, 1992). Membership in social groups serves to identify both the *kind* of person an individual is and the *roles* the individual may assume. It also *explains* behavior as a function of group affiliation. The hypothesis that this sort of explanation is the result of the operation of a modular cognitive competency is supported by several lines of research. The first concerns the range of variation in *types* of social categories encountered. Despite considerable variation in their elaborations, surprisingly few dimensions of social difference predominate in all cultures and across all historical epochs: sex/gender, age, kinship, language spoken, and race/ethnicity. Each of these social dimensions, across a broad range of cultures, is seen as having a particular essence that governs the development and behavior of the organism (Gelman, 2003; Haslam, Rothchild, & Ernst, 2000; Hirschfeld, 1996; Mahalingham, 1998). As we observed earlier, the ability to classify people over these types of categories emerges quite early, in some important respects during infancy (for gender, see Miller, 1983; for age, see Brooks & Lewis, 1976; for language spoken, see Mehler et al., 1988). This kind of robust development, in which cultural experience appears to have limited effect, is a hallmark of a modular competence.

A second line of supporting evidence comes from considerable research on stereotyping. A number of studies have now demonstrated that many stereotypes are based in nonconscious, automatic processes (e.g., similarity judgments, categorization formation, within- and between-category biases [Greenwald & Banaji, 1995; Hilton & von Hippel, 1996], among other strategies of category-based reasoning under uncertainty). Relevant to this discussion is work demonstrating that even quite young children are subject to subtle social biases. Children, like adults, show ingroup favoritism even when membership is based on trivial commonalities (Nesdale & Flesser, 2001). Recent studies have demonstrated the early emergence of a susceptibility to stereotype threat (Ambady, Shih, & Kim, 2001), strikingly at an age when racial and ethnic stereotypes play virtually no role in shaping children's behavior. Imaging studies suggest that the perception of and reasoning about race and racial stereotypes may involve unique patterns of neural activation (Eberhardt, 2005; Hart et al., 2000; Phelps et al., 2000; Richeson et al., 2003; Wheeler & Fiske, 2005).

These findings aside, most work on stereotypes in social psychology would not be thought to support the domain-specific competency hypothesis we propose. Indeed, according to a long-standing view in social psychology, social categorization differs from other object categories only to the degree that social categories are object categories whose target stimuli are people (Hamilton & Trolier, 1986). A developmental corollary is the widely held claim that stereotypes arise through a process of social learning: Children are exposed to stereotypes, particularly those expressed by important adult models such as parents and teachers, and as a result, come to hold them (e.g., Powslishta, Sen, Serbin, Poulin-Dubois, & Eichstedt, 2001).

Social learning presupposes social modeling, particularly modeling of attitudes and practices by parents, teachers, and other significant persons in the child's environment. "As the twig is bent, so grows the tree" goes the old saw. Yet several studies show that children's racial and ethnic biases are not reliably associated with the beliefs and attitudes of parents or peers. This is the case even when children believe that their attitudes correspond to those of parents and peers, and even when parents intervene to shape directly their children's racial and ethnic

attitudes (Aboud & Doyle, 1996). These findings are inconsistent with the view of social development, according to which young children's early understanding of social categories is tethered to surface differences in appearance. Young children, according to this view, grasp neither racial nor gender constancy, instead believing that superficial and reversible changes in skin color actually change an individual's racial identity or that superficial aspects of appearance such as hair length or gendered clothing determine one's gender. Finally, according to this model, it is only as children mature that their understanding becomes more adult-like (e.g., grasping the notions of racial and gender constant, and eventually coming to understand both as functions of a person's biological constitution/heritage). For example, Aboud and Skerry (1983) found that when Canadian 5-year-olds were shown pictures of a familiar Anglo child dressed in traditional Eskimo clothing, most agreed that the child had become Eskimo. Semaj (1980) found a similar pattern of reasoning when he asked young children whether a child's race would change if he wore a blond wig and light makeup; they also judged that the child's race would change.

Our proposal predicts a different pattern of development: Even early representations of social groups are theory-like and untethered to perceptual appearance. Thus, like the modular competencies for folkbiology, ToM, naive physics, and numerosity, a competence for naive sociology predicts that children develop largely on their own more adult-like knowledge of social groups, and form more adult-like representations of them. Hirschfeld (1996) speculated that children may have found Aboud and Skerry's (1983) and Semaj's (1980) transformation tasks difficult, because the changes were both implausibly abrupt and difficult to integrate with gradual changes typical of biological processes. To rule out this possibility, Hirschfeld (1996) asked preschoolers whether racial and other corporeal properties could change in the familiar context of transformations that occur over one's lifespan and over generations. When asked which property would remain unchanged as a person grew up (hair and skin color vs. clothing style and color), even 3-year-olds judged that racial properties were more constant than sartorial ones. More strikingly, when asked which property would remain unchanged as a person grew up (hair and skin color vs. body build), 4-year-olds judged that racial properties were more constant than body build. The same pattern of judgment was obtained when Hirschfeld asked which properties would remain constant between a parent and his or her child (i.e., if a heavyset parent was black he was more likely to have a thin, black child than a heavyset white one).

Similar results were found when Hirschfeld (1996) asked preschoolers whether a child would develop racial properties matching her birth parents or those of her adopted parents. Hirschfeld's studied the judgments of North American and Northern European children; however, the same theory-like understanding of race has been documented by Giménez and Harris (2002) among Spanish preschoolers, by Astuti et al. (2004) in their work with 6-year-olds in Madagascar, and by Mahalingham (1998) in his study of South Asian preadolescents.

Modular competencies also appear to channel children's attention to specific kinds of things (e.g., with folkbiology, nonhuman living organisms, or with naive physics, the relationship between the movements of objects). In domains, such as naive sociology, in which cultural input evidently plays a significant role, the modular competence specifies that membership in essentialized groups is particularly informative, it does not specify whether the essentialized group is a race, as in contemporary North America, or caste, as in contemporary South Asia; the relevant entities are inferred from cultural information rather than given by the environment. A crucial task for the child is to determine which sources of cultural knowledge are likely to provide the most relevant information. In conventional social learning theory, it is assumed that parents and teachers are the best sources of information. As observed earlier, however, this does not appear to be the case with racial information. On reflection, this is hardly surprising: If children are to develop culturally meaningful understanding, they should look to culturally meaningful sources of information. Relying on very local sources—say, a particular family tradition or a particular teacher's image of the world—risks forming beliefs that may be marginal to the dominant cultural traditions. If, however, the child attends to representations in the larger community, then her knowledge is more likely in line with the broader contours of the cultural tradition in which she participates. The issue is essentially one of sampling. In the case of the young child, it means attending to—privileging—less frequently encountered sources over more frequently encountered, local ones.

As an illustration, consider the development of accent. Young children of non-native speakers do not develop the accents of their parents. They develop normative speech patterns, often not well modeled by their parent (Harris, 1998; Hirschfeld, 1996). Presumably this occurs because the local source of linguistic information is discounted relative to less local, and less frequently encountered, sources. Somehow the child knows to sample the broader speech community in language learning. If our proposal is correct, then we would expect to find examples of this sampling bias in the development of social categories, particularly in reasoning based on social category membership. In support of this claim, Hirschfeld (1996) conducted a study examining the development of the "one drop of blood rule," the culturally specific expectation that a person with any traceable black ancestor is black. Children's interpretation of racial admixture was not found to be shaped by race, as social learning theory would predict. By age 12, children living in a predominantly white city judged that a child with one black parent would have phenotypically black features. Black 12-year-olds living in a community with a large minority population, in contrast, judged that a child with one black and one white parent would look mixed. The crucial case was the white children living in the community with a large minority population. Like black 12-year-olds from the same community, the white children judged that the mixed-race couple would have a child that looked mixed. In short, children's reasoning about race was more influenced by community—the cultural environment—in which they lived than by their race/ethnicity.

In summary, social reasoning makes use of a variety of skills and competencies, but there is emerging evidence that key competencies are invariant across cultures and are likely to be in part innate. In the domain of reasoning about individual persons, attributions of mental states and traits are likely to be grounded in one innate module, whereas in the domain of reasoning about individual persons as members of groups, there seems to be an innate preparedness to detect group memberships and use them as the basis for social inference. Cultures are likely to exploit such innate competencies, advantaging cultural representations whose stability and recurrence are enhanced by them. Cultural variation and universal psychological processes are not opposing explanations but are instead functions of the same human cognitive architecture.

OTHER ISSUES TO CONSIDER

The following section addresses additional methodological issues that should be considered when conducting research on culture, categorization, and reasoning. Included in the discussion of these issues is a brief introduction to other kinds of concepts (e.g., non-natural kinds, emotions) not covered earlier in this chapter. Reference to these kinds of concepts is included in this chapter for completeness, but readers interested in a more comprehensive review should refer to the literature cited in this section and beyond.

Task Sensitivity

When searching for cultural differences, it is important to consider whether the task being used is sensitive enough or appropriate for finding cultural differences. For instance, replicating earlier work by Chiu (1972) and Nisbett and colleagues (2001), Unsworth, Sears, and Pexman (2005) found that Chinese adults are more likely to group both natural and non-natural kinds together if they share a relationship (e.g., a car and a tire), and that Canadian adults might be more likely to group natural and non-natural kinds together if they belong to the same category (e.g., a car and a bus). However, cultural differences in categorization were not observed in a timed categorization task, although differences in response latencies were analogous with the differences in categorization found in the previous experiment. The authors interpreted the results as suggesting that differences in categorization styles are associated with differences in semantic activation, but, importantly, they noted that the results also suggest that the nature of the categorization task may determine the extent to which these cultural differences are observed. Interestingly, Medin et al. (2002) found the opposite pattern to that found by Unsworth et al. (2005), such that cultural differences were observed in a speeded task but disappeared in an unspeeded task (this study is described in more detail in an

earlier section of this chapter). Medin et al. (2002) suggested that the cultural differences observed were due to differences in "habits of the mind" that are more easily observed in a speeded task. If such an explanation is correct, then it is unclear why the opposite pattern was found by Unsworth et al. (2005). This inconsistency would be interesting to follow up in future research. Importantly, though, both studies reveal the importance of considering whether the task is sensitive enough to detect cultural differences. Such considerations could impact the kinds of conclusions drawn about the variability of particular aspects of cognition across cultural communities.

Elaboration of Concepts

Yet another issue to bear in mind is whether an investigation of cultural differences is "deep enough," that is, whether the myriad ways in which concepts can differ across communities have been explored. Two areas of research that could benefit from further analysis include the studies of emotion concepts and of artifact concepts.

A number of researchers have investigated the extent to which emotion concepts vary across cultural communities (e.g., Boster, 2005; Ekman, 1972; Izard & Buechler, 1980; Johnstone & Scherer, 2000; Kim & Hupka, 2002; Lutz, 1988; Markus & Kitayama, 1991; Páez & Vergara, 1995; Romney, Moore, & Rusch, 1997; Rosaldo, 1984; Russell, 1991; Scherer & Wallbott, 1994; P. B. Smith & Bond, 1993; Wierzbicka, 1992).

Research about emotion concepts and culture has primarily focused on the extent to which emotions are biologically determined, and therefore universal (e.g., Ekman, 1972; Izard & Buechlar, 1980), or socially constructed, and therefore culturally relative (e.g., Lutz, 1985, 1987, 1988; Rosaldo, 1980, 1984). Although some researchers argue in favor of one or the other of these two extremes, most researchers adopt a kind of hybrid theory, in which they believe that some components of emotions, such as certain physiological responses (e.g., facial expressions, the release of particular hormones) may be experienced universally, but that the way particular emotions are displayed and the kinds of emotion categories people form may be culturally specific.

The kinds of similarities and differences researchers might examine include (1) whether an emotion is lexicalized or not; (2) the degree of correspondence of lexicalized emotion terms across cultures; and (3) whether there are differences in rules about expressions of emotions and conceptualizations about whether the resulting behaviors are voluntary or not (e.g., running amok).

It is well-known that there is substantial cultural variability in lexicons of emotion. Thus, many cultures have at least several emotion words that correspond to basic emotions such as joy, anger, sadness, fear, and disgust, but some cultures have only a few words for these emotions (Russell, 1991). Nevertheless, when words for basic emotions are present, there is an impressive cross-cultural similarity in the meanings of these words. For example, Scherer and Wallbott (1994) asked participants in 37 countries across five continents to complete questionnaires about seven different emotions (joy, anger, fear, sadness, disgust, shame, and guilt). Participants first recalled experiences in which they felt each emotion and were then asked specific questions about those emotional experiences. Results revealed that the seven emotions differed substantially from each other, and that geographical and sociocultural differences were observed, but such differences were much smaller than the overall differences between the emotions themselves. A similar conclusion was obtained by Kim and Hupka (2002), who compared Koreans and Americans, and Romney et al. (1997), who tested perceived similarities of English and Japanese emotion terms.

However, Boster (2005) has pointed out that such research often involves an attempt to match semantic meanings of emotion terms using methods such as back-translation, and that such methodology can be problematic in assessing cross-cultural variation. In particular, translation methods often occur before data collection, so it is not surprising to see cross-cultural agreement elicited by terms that have been chosen specifically because they correspond to each other across languages. Furthermore, although other research may not rely on translation as a first step (see Russell, 1983, 1989), such research often involves similarity judgments on only a couple of shallow dimensions (e.g., evaluation [positive, negative], arousal) that may not capture deep semantic structure and might therefore fail to capture important semantic variations across cultures. To examine emotion concepts at a deeper level

of analysis, future research might include an investigation into whether some cultural groups elaborate a subset of emotional concepts (e.g., those associated with guilt in Japan) more than others, or whether expressions of particular emotions vary with respect to social roles in some cultural groups more than in others. One useful approach for future research might be to conduct ethnographic studies to generate further predictions about where cultural differences might exist and to obtain a more comprehensive understanding about the nature of particular cultural differences.

Studies examining culture and the concepts of artifacts have led to conclusions similar to those made for cultural differences in emotion concepts, namely, that differences in naming practices can sometimes be much more pronounced than conceptual differences. For instance, Malt, Sloman, Gennari, Shi, and Wang (1999) asked English-, Chinese-, and Spanish-speaking adults to categorize nonnatural kinds (60 different bottles and jars) explicitly on the basis of different kinds of similarity, and after several types of analyses, concluded that there were no cultural differences in these similarity-based sorts. Importantly, Malt et al. noted that there is little agreement about the most relevant features for artifact categorization, so separate sorts were based on similarity of physical qualities (e.g., what it looks like, what it is made of), similarity of function (e.g., how it is used), and "overall" similarity. None of these sorts produced cultural differences. However, Malt et al. did find substantial differences in naming patterns for these objects (whether the item is named a bottle, a jar, or a container, etc.), suggesting that the relationship between similarity and naming of these artifacts is not very straightforward. Further research should examine whether cultural differences in categorizing the objects emerge if categorization is based on other dimensions (contextual relevance of particular bottles, etc.; conceptual elaboration of particular bottles) and whether these different types of sorts map more directly onto naming patterns in the different communities. Again, ethnography would be a useful tool in this regard.

Attribution of Differences

Once cultural differences have been found, it is important to consider whether the differences can really be attributed to differences in the concept or process of interest, or whether there is an alternative explanation for the results. For example, Norenzayan, Smith, Jun Kim, and Nisbett (2002) argued that East Asians were less likely than European Americans to abandon intuitive reasoning (i.e., reasoning based on experience and information from the senses) in favor of formal reasoning (i.e., reasoning based on rules and formal logic), and although some of their findings are compelling, other results must be considered with caution. In Experiments 1 and 2 they found cross-cultural differences in categorization and conceptual structure, and in Experiments 3 and 4, cross-cultural differences in deductive reasoning. However, the cultural differences observed in Experiment 4 are not attributable to differences in deductive reasoning or even to intuitive or formal reasoning more generally. We shall soon see why.

In the fourth experiment, Norenzayan et al. (2002) examined cultural differences in deductive reasoning by giving Korean and U.S. college students valid and invalid arguments that were either abstract or concrete; for the concrete problems, the conclusions were either believable (consistent with real-world knowledge) or unbelievable (inconsistent with real-world knowledge). The groups did not differ on the abstract problems, but Norenzayan et al. found that Koreans were less likely than were U.S. college students to endorse concrete arguments with unbelievable conclusions. They concluded that the Koreans' reliance on intuitive reasoning led to less accurate responses in this task.

The Norenzayan et al. (2002) results are not unambiguous, in that they do not separate response biases (i.e., the tendency to be more or less liberal when deciding to accept an argument as valid) from the ability to distinguish between valid and invalid arguments. In fact, Unsworth and Medin (2005) showed that Korean participants overall were much less likely to accept an argument as valid, and that cultural differences in reasoning disappeared when response biases were taken into consideration. The reason for the cultural difference in response bias or criterion setting is unclear, and this particular finding would be interesting to examine more closely in its own right. Furthermore, future research specific to deductive reasoning might profit by narrowing the examination to a domain in which specific cultural differences might be expected (e.g., Meno-

minee deductive reasoning in the domain of biology, or Chinese deductive reasoning in the domain of social relationships).

SUMMARY AND CONCLUSIONS

We are very much in the position of describing a moving target. The intersection of culture, categorization, and reasoning currently is receiving a great deal of attention, and new empirical findings appear almost daily. This field of research has largely overcome its ugly beginnings, in which cognitive tasks developed in Western countries were transported wholesale to other cultures, and contexts and any differences noted were interpreted as deficits (see Cole & Scribner, 1974, for a review). We say "largely" because cultural research needs to be constantly vigilant about "home court assumptions" that get in the way of our understanding other cultures. We see room for both broad contrasts based on a few dimensions of difference and very specific examinations of single cultural groups. But to yield powerful generalizations, the broad contrasts will have to be coupled with careful ethnography and sociohistorical analyses. We have tried to show that a serious concern with the fine-grained, typically narrative specificity of ethnographic and historical investigations does not mean abandoning psychology's powerful theories and methods, honed in laboratory studies. Social scientists have long been skeptical of the "anthropological veto," the claim that since it does not happen like that in Pago Pago, one has got it wrong (see Bloch, Solomon, & Carey, 2001, for a nice example of the tension between experimental probes and ethnographic observation). It is uncontroversial that cognition, no matter how widely a *task* may be distributed, is something that happens in individual minds. It is no more controversial that individual minds inhabit complex cultural environments—indeed, that the mind's evolution was profoundly shaped by complex cultural circumstances. Categorization and reasoning simply cannot be understood without taking into account both the mind and the environment that supports it.

In the same vein, we believe that it is impossible for studies of single cultures to be theoretically neutral. Therefore, the promise for this field lies on middle ground, where both within- and between-culture similarities and differences are recruited in the service of understanding how culture affects thought. As we have seen, triangulation can be an effective strategy for understanding both within-culture differences and across-cultural similarities. In addition, the CCM has proven to be a useful tool in the service understanding variation. In ongoing work in Guatemala and among cultural groups in Wisconsin, we are collecting social network data along with cognitive measures to see whether similarities in values and beliefs can be linked to social network proximities. If so, we may be in a position to observe cultural processes at work.

Finally, it is also worth pointing out that attending to complex cultural environments does not require *cross*-cultural research. In other words, research that is sensitive to cultural processes does not necessarily require observations of *differences* or comparisons *between* cultural communities to be meaningful and interesting. Simply directing attention towards any community not typically represented in psychological research will help to inform our understanding of cognitive and psychosocial phenomena in new and exciting ways. Given the overwhelming focus of cognitive research on U.S. college students, it behooves us to do meaningful ethnography, apply consensus analysis, and employ converging measures, with the goal of understanding the nature and dynamics of their culture.

NOTE

1. The notion of "cultural epidemiology" has two distinct traditions: one focused on the relatively high-fidelity "reproduction" and patterning of cultural (including psychological) traits within and across human populations, and the other focused on the ways cognitive structures "generate" and chain together ideas, artifacts, and behaviors within and across human populations. Jacques Monod (1971), the Nobel Prize–winning biologist, was the first to use the concept of "culture as contagion"—although more as metaphor than theory. Cavalli-Sforza and Feldman (1981) were pioneers in working out a theory in which culture is conceptualized as distributed through a population; however, no microscale cognitive processes or structures were modeled or considered, only macroscale social psychological traits. Lumsden and Wilson (1981) explicitly advocated a theory of culture as distributed mental representations, but the combination of a high degree of mathematical sophistication and a rudimentary awareness of basic conceptual structures failed to spawn any further serious research along their lines.

Two more fully developed epidemiological approaches soon emerged. Boyd and Richerson (1985) were able to show how biases in transmission, such as prestige or conformism, could help to explain the spread and stabilization of macrosocial psychological traits among populations. Sperber (1985) provided the first theoretical blueprint for how individual-level microcognitive structures (as opposed to invocation of imitation or other cultural reproduction processes) could account for cultural transmission and stabilization. Until now, there has been little fruitful interaction between these two traditions (see Laland & Brown, 2002; Henrich & Boyd, 2002). We believe that these two "epidemiological" traditions are compatible, and our empirical example suggests that they can be mutually informative.

REFERENCES

Aboud, F. E., & Doyle, A.-B. (1996). Parental and peer influences on children's racial attitudes [Special Issue]. *International Journal of Intercultural Relations, 20*(3–4), 371–383.

Aboud, F. E., & Skerry, S. A. (1983). Self and ethnic concepts in relation to ethnic constancy. *Canadian Journal of Behavioural Science, 15*, 14–26.

Ahn, W., Kalish, C., Gelman, S. A., Medin, D. L., Luhmann, C., Atran, S., et al. (2001). Why essences are essential in the psychology of concepts. *Cognition, 82*, 59–69.

Ambady, N., Shih, M., & Kim, A. (2001). Stereotype susceptibility in children: Effects of identity activation on quantitative performance. *Psychological Science, 12*(5), 385–390.

Anderson, J. R. (1990a). *Cognitive psychology and its implications* (3rd ed.). New York: Freeman.

Anderson, J. R. (1990b). *The adaptive character of thought.* Hillsdale, NJ: Erlbaum.

Ariès, P. (1962). Centuries of childhood: A social history of family life. New York: Knopf.

Astuti, R., Solomon, G. A., & Carey, S. (2004). Constraints on conceptual development: A case study of the acquisition of folkbiological and folksociological knowledge in Madagascar. In W. A. Collins (Ed.), *Monographs of the Society for Research in Child Development* (pp. 1–135). Oxford, UK: Blackwell.

Astuti, R., Solomon, G. E. A., Carey, S., Ingold, T., & Miller, P. H. (2004). Constraints on conceptual development: A case study of the acquisition of folkbiological and folksociological knowledge in Madagascar. Boston, MA: Blackwell.

Atran, S. (1990). *Cognitive foundations of natural history.* Cambridge, UK: Cambridge University Press.

Atran, S. (2001). The trouble with memes: Inference versus imitation in cultural evolution. *Human Nature, 12*, 351–381.

Atran, S. (2002). In gods we trust: The evolutionary landscape of religion. Oxford, UK: Oxford University Press.

Atran, S., Medin, D., Lynch, E., Vapnarsky, V., Ucan Ek', E., & Sousa, P. (2001). Folkbiology doesn't come from folkpsychology: Evidence from Yukatek Maya in cross-cultural perspective. *Journal of Cognition and Culture, 1*, 3–42.

Atran, S., Medin, D., & Ross, N. (2005). The cultural mind: Environmental decision making and cultural modeling within and across populations. *Psychological Review, 112*, 744–776.

Atran, S., Medin, D., Ross, N., Lynch, E., Vapnarsky, V., Ucan Ek', E., et al. (2002). Folkecology, cultural epidemiology, and the spirit of the commons: A garden experiment in that Maya Lowlands, 1991–2001. *Current Anthropology, 43*, 421–450.

Au, T. K., & Romo, L. F. (1999). Mechanical causality in children's "folkbiology." In D. L. Medin & S. Atran (Eds.), *Folkbiology* (pp. 355–401). Cambridge, MA: MIT Press.

Avis, J., & Harris, P. L. (1991). Belief–desire reasoning among Baka children: Evidence for a universal conception of mind. *Child Development, 62*(3), 460–467.

Au, T. K., Romo, L. F., & DeWitt, J. E. (1999). Considering children's folkbiology in health education. In M. Siegal & C. Peterson (Eds.), *Children's understanding of biology and health* (pp. 209–234). London: Cambridge University Press.

Axelrod, R. (1997). Advancing the art of simulation. *Complexity, 3*, 193–199.

Bailenson, J., Shum, M., Atran, S., Medin, D., & Coley, J. (2002). A bird's eye view: Biological categorization and reasoning within and across cultures. *Cognition, 84*, 1–53.

Barrett, J. L., & Keil, F. C. (1996). Conceptualizing a nonnatural entity: Anthropomorphism in God concepts. *Cognitive Psychology, 31*(3), 219–247.

Barsalou, L. W. (1985). Ideals, central tendency, and frequency of instantiation as determinants of graded structure in categories. *Journal of Experimental Psychology: Learning, Memory, and Cognition, 11*, 629–654.

Bellezza, F. S. (1984). Reliability of retrieval from semantic memory: Noun meanings. *Bulletin of the Psychonomic Society, 22*, 377–380.

Berlin, B. (1978). Ethnobiological classification. In E. Rosch & B. B. Lloyd (Eds.), *Cognition and categorization* (pp. 9–26). Hillsdale, NJ: Erlbaum.

Berlin, B. (1992). *Ethnobiological classification*. Princeton, NJ: Princeton University Press.

Berreby, D. (2005). *Us and them: Understanding your tribal mind*. New York: Little, Brown.

Bloch, M., Solomon, G., & Carey, S. (2001). Zafimaniry: An understanding of what is passed on from parents to children. A cross-cultural investigation. *Journal of Cognition and Culture, 1*(1), 43–68.

Boster, J. (2005). Emotion categories across languages. In H. Cohen & C. Lefebvre (Eds.), *Handbook of categorization in cognitive science* (pp. 188–223). London: Elsevier Science.

Boyd, R., & Richerson, P. J. (1985). *Culture and the evolutionary process*. Chicago: The University of Chicago Press.

Boyer, P. (2001). *Religion explained: The human instincts that fashion gods, spirits and ancestors*. London: Heinemann.

Briley, D., Morris, M., & Simonson, I. (2000). Reasons as carriers of culture: Dynamic versus dispositional models of cultural influence on decision making. *Journal of Consumer Research, 27*, 157–178.

Brooks, J., & Lewis, M. (1976). Infants' responses to strangers: Midget, adult, and child. *Child Development, 47*(2), 323–332.

Brown, C. (1995). Lexical acculturation and ethnobiology: Utilitarianism and intellectualism. *Journal of Linguistic Anthropology 5*, 51–64.

Brumann, C. (1999). Why a successful concept should not be discarded. *Current Anthropology, 40*, S1–S14.

Bulmer, R. (1970). Which came first, the chicken or the egg-head? In J. Pouillon & P. Maranda (Eds.), *Echanges et communications: Mèlanges offerts [daggerdbl] Claude Lèvi-Strauss*. The Hague: Mouton.

Bulmer, R. (1974). Folk biology in the New Guinea Highlands. *Social Science Information, 13*, 9–28.

Burnett, R., Medin, D., Ross, N., & Blok, S. (2005). Ideal is typical. *Canadian Journal of Psychology, 59*, 3–10.

Burnett, R., Medin, D., Ross, N. O., & Block S. V. (2005). Ideal is typical. *Canadian Journal of Psychology, 59*, 3–10.

Carey, S. (1982). Semantic development: The state of the art. In E. Wanner & L. R. Gleitman (Eds.), *Language acquisition: The state of the art*. Cambridge, UK: Cambridge University Press.

Carey, S. (1985). *Conceptual change in childhood*. Cambridge, MA: Bradford Books.

Cavalli-Sforza, L. L., & Feldman, M. W. (1981). *Cultural transmission and evolution: A quantitative approach*. Princeton, NJ: Princeton University Press.

Chiu, L. (1972). A cross-cultural comparison of cognitive styles in Chinese and American children. *International Journal of Psychology, 7*, 235–242.

Choi, I., Nisbett, R., & Smith, E. (1999). Culture, category salience, and inductive reasoning. *Cognition, 65*, 15–32.

Cohen, D. (2001). Cultural variation: Considerations and implications. *Psychological Bulletin, 127*, 451–471.

Cole, M. (1996). *Cultural psychology*. Cambridge, MA: Harvard University Press.

Cole, M., & Scribner, S. (1974). *Culture and thought: A psychological introduction*. New York: Wiley.

Coley, J. D. (1995). Emerging differentiation of folkbiology and folkpsychology: Attributions of biological and psychological properties to living things. *Child Development, 66*, 1856–1874.

Coley, J. D., Hayes, B., Lawson, C., & Moloney, M. (2004). Knowledge, expectations, and inductive inferences within conceptual hierarchies. *Cognition, 90*, 217–253.

Coley, J., Medin, D., & Atran, S. (1997). Does rank have its privilege?: Inductive inferences in folk-biological taxonomies. *Cognition, 64*, 73–112.

Crawford, M. T., Sherman, S. J., & Hamilton, D. L. (2002). Perceived entitativity, stereotype formation, and the interchangeability of group members. *Journal of Personality and Social Psychology, 83*, 1076–1094.

de Waal, F. B. M. (1998). *Chimpanzee politics: Power and sex among apes* (Rev. ed.). Baltimore: Johns Hopkins University Press.

Diamond, J., & Bishop, K. (1999). Ethno-ornithology of the Ketengban people. In D. L. Medin & S. Atran (Eds.), *Folkbiology* (pp. 17–46). Cambridge, MA: MIT Press.

Eberhardt, J. L. (2005). Imaging race. *American Psychologist, 60*(2), 181–190.

Eid, M., & Diener, E. (2001). Norms for experiencing emotions in different cultures: Inter- and intranational differences. *Journal of Personality and Social Psychology, 81*, 869–885.

Ekman, P. (1972). Universals and cultural differences in facial expressions of emotion. In J. Cole (Ed.), *Nebraska Symposium on Motivation 1971* (Vol. 19, pp. 207–283). Lincoln: University of Nebraska Press.

Ellen, R. (1993). *The cultural relations of classification.* Cambridge, UK: Cambridge University Press.

Estes, W. K. (1986). Array models for category learning. *Cognitive Psychology, 18*, 500–549.

Estes, W. K. (1994). *Classification and cognition.* New York: Oxford University Press.

Flannagan, M. J., Fried, L. S., & Holyoak, K. J. (1986). Distributional expectations and the induction of category structure. *Journal of Experimental Psychology: Learning, Memory, and Cognition, 12*, 241–256.

Fried, L. S., & Holyoak, K. J. (1984). Induction of category distributions: A framework for classification learning. *Journal of Experimental Psychology: Learning, Memory and Cognition, 10*, 234–257.

Frith, U., & Frith, C. (2003). Development and neurphysiology of mentalizing. *Philosophical Transactions of the Royal Society of London, 358*, 459–473.

Fukuyama, F. (1995). *Trust.* New York: Free Press.

Furth, H. (1996). *Desire for society: Children's knowledge as social imagination.* New York: Plenum Press.

Gardner, W., Gabriel, S., & Lee, A. (1999). "I" value freedom but "we" value relationships: Self-construal priming mirrors cultural differences in judgment. *Psychological Science, 10*, 321–326.

Gallagher, H. L., & Frith, C. D. (2003). Functional imagine of "theory of mind." *Trends in Cognitive Sciences, 7*(2), 77–83.

Gelman, R. (2002). Cognitive development. In H. Pashler & D. L. Medin (Eds.), *Stevens' handbook of experimental psychology, third edition* (Vol. 2, pp. 533–559). New York: Wiley.

Gelman, S. A. (2003). *The essential child: Origins of essentialism in everyday thought.* Oxford, UK: Oxford University Press.

Gelman, S. A., Coley, J. D., & Gottfried, G. M. (1994). Essentialist beliefs in children: The acquisition of concepts and theories. In L. A. Hirschfeld & S. A. Gelman (Eds.), *Mapping the mind* (pp. 341–367). Cambridge, UK: Cambridge University Press.

Gelman, S., & Hirschfeld, L. (1999). How biological is essentialism? In D. Medin & S. Atran (Eds.), *Folkbiology* (pp. 403–446). Cambridge, MA: MIT Press.

Gelman, S., & Wellman, H. (1991). Insides and essences. *Cognition, 38*, 213–244.

Gentner, D., & Goldin-Meadow, S. (Eds.). (2003). *Language in mind: Advances in the study of language and thought.* Cambridge, MA: MIT Press.

Giménez, M., & Harris, P. L. (2002). Understanding constraints on inheritance: Evidence for biological thinking in early childhood. *British Journal of Developmental Psychology, 20*(3), 307–324.

Goodenough, W. (1955) Componential analysis and the study of meaning. *Language, 32*, 185–216.

Greenwald, A. G., & Banaji, M. R. (1995). Implicit social cognition: Attitudes, self-esteem, and stereotypes. *Psychological Review, 102*, 4–27.

Hamilton, D. L., & Sherman, S. J. (1996). Perceiving persons and groups. *Psychological Review, 103*, 336–355.

Hamilton, D. L., & Trolier, T. K. (1986). Stereotypes and stereotyping: An overview of the cognitive approach. In J. Dovidio & S. Gaertner (Eds.), *Prejudice, discrimination, and racism* (pp. 127–163). Orlando, FL: Academic Press.

Harris, J. R. (1998). *The nurture assumption: Why children turn out the way they do.* New York: Free Press.

Hart, A. J., Whalen, P. J., Shin, L. M., McInerney, S. C., Fischer, H., & Rauch, S. L. (2000). Differential response in the human amygdala to racial outgroup vs. ingroup face stimuli. *Neuroreport, 11*, 2351–2355.

Haslam, N., Rothschild, L., & Ernst, D. (2000). Essentialist beliefs about social categories. *British Journal of Social Psychology, 39*(1), 113–127.

Hatano, G., & Inagaki, K. (1999). A developmental perspective on informal biology. In D. L. Medin & S. Atran (Eds.), *Folkbiology* (pp. 321–354). Cambridge, MA: MIT Press.

Henrich, J., & Boyd, R. (2002). On modeling cognition and culture: Why replicators are not necessary for cultural evolution. *Journal of Cognition and Culture, 2*, 87–112.

Heyman, G. D., & Gelman, S. A. (2000). Preschool children's use of trait labels to make inductive inferences. *Journal of Experimental Child Psychology, 77*(1), 1–19.

Heyman, G. D., & Gelman, S. A. (2000). Beliefs about the origins of human psychological traits. *Developmental Psychology, 36*(5), 663–678.

Hilton, J. L., & von Hippel, W. (1996). Stereotypes. *Annual Review of Psychology, 47*, 237–271.

Hirschfeld, L. A. (1989). Rethinking the acquisition of kinship terms. *International Journal of Behavioral Development, 12*, 541–568.

Hirschfeld, L. A. (1995). Do children have a theory of race? *Cognition, 54,* 209–252.

Hirschfeld, L. A. (1996). *Race in the making.* Cambridge, MA: MIT Press.

Hirschfeld, L. A., & Gelman, S. A. (Eds.). (1994). *Mapping the mind: Domain specificity in cognition and culture.* New York: Cambridge University Press.

Hofstede, G. (1980). *Culture's consequences: International differences in work-related values.* Beverly Hills, CA: Sage.

Homa, D. (1984). On the nature of categories. In G. H. Bower (Ed.), *The psychology of learning and motivation: Advances in research and theory* (Vol. 18, pp. 49–94). San Diego, CA: Academic Press.

Hubert, L., & Golledge, R. (1981). A heuristic method for the comparison of related structures. *Journal of Mathematical Psychology, 23,* 214–226.

Hunn, E. S. (1975). A measure of the degree of correspondence of folk to scientific biological classification. *American Ethnologist, 2,* 309–327.

Hunn, E. S. (1982). The utilitarian factor in folk biological classification. *American Anthropologist, 84,* 830–847.

Hunn, E. S. (1999). Size as limiting the recognition of biodiversity in folkbiological classifications: One of four factors governing the cultural recognition of biological taxa. In D. L. Medin & S. Atran (Eds.), *Folkbiology* (pp. 47–70). Cambridge, MA: MIT Press.

Huntington, S. (1996). *The clash of civilizations and the remaking of the world order.* New York: Simon & Schuster.

Hutchins, E. (1995). *Cognition in the wild.* Cambridge, MA: MIT Press.

Inagaki, K., & Hatano, G. (2002). *Young children's naive thinking about the biological world.* New York: Psychology Press.

Inagaki, K., & Sugiyama, K. (1988). Attributing human characteristics: Developmental changes in over- and under-attribution. *Cognitive Development, 3,* 55–70.

Izard, C. E., & Buechler, S. (1980). Aspects of consciousness and personality in terms of differential emotions theory. In R. Plutchik & H. Kellerman (Eds.), *Emotion, theory, research, and experience: Vol. I. Theories of emotion* (pp. 165–181). New York: Academic Press.

Jackendoff, R. (1992). *Language of the mind: Essays on mental representation.* Cambridge, MA: MIT Press.

Johnson, K. E. (2001). Determinants of typicality throughout the continuum of expertise. *Memory and Cognition, 29,* 1036–1050.

Johnson, K., & Mervis, C. (1997). Effects of varying levels of expertise on the basic level of categorization. *Journal of Experimental Psychology: General, 126,* 248–277.

Johnson, K. E., & Mervis, C. B. (1998). Impact of intuitive theories on feature recruitment throughout the continuum of expertise. *Memory and Cognition, 26,* 382–401.

Johnstone, T., & Scherer, K. R. (2000). Vocal communication of emotion. In M. Lewis & J. M. Haviland-Jones (Eds.), *Handbook of emotions* (pp. 220–235). New York: Guilford Press.

Keil, F. (1989). *Concepts, kinds, and cognitive development.* Cambridge MA: MIT Press.

Keil, F. C., & Batterman, N. (1984). A characteristic-to-defining shift in the development of word meaning. *Journal of Verbal Learning and Verbal Behavior, 23,* 221–236.

Kelly, Quinn, & Slater (2005). Three-month-olds, but not newborns, prefer own-race faces. *Developmental Science, 8*(6), F31–F36.

Kim, H. J., & Hupka, R. B. (2002). Comparison of associative meaning of the concepts of anger, envy, fear, and jealousy between English and Korean. *Cross-Cultural Research, 36,* 229–255.

Kim, N. S., & Ahn, W. (2002). Clinical psychologists' theory-based representations of mental disorders predict their diagnostic reasoning and memory. *Journal of Experimental Psychology: General, 131,* 451–476.

Kitayama, S., Ishii, K., Imada, T., Takemura, K., & Ramaswamy, J. (2006). Voluntary settlement and the spirit of independence: Evidence from Japan's "Northern Frontier." *Journal of Personality and Social Psychology, 91,* 369–384.

Laland, K. N., & Brown, G. R. (2002). *Sense and nonsense: Evolutionary perspectives on human behavior.* Oxford, UK: Oxford University Press.

Laland, K., Olding-Smee, F. J., & Feldman, M. (2000). Niche construction, biological evolution and cultural change. *Behavioral and Brain Sciences, 23,* 131–146.

Laqueur, T. (1990). *Making sex: Body and gender from the Greeks to Freud.* Cambridge, MA: Harvard University Press.

Lamberts, K. (1995). Categorization under time pressure. *Journal of Experimental Psychology: General, 124,* 161–180.

Lave, J. (1988). *Cognition in practice.* Cambridge, UK: Cambridge University Press.

Leach, E. R. (1970). *Political systems of Highland Burma: A study of Kachin social structure.* London: Athlone Press.

Lèvi-Strauss, C. (1949). *Les structures elementaires de la parenté.* Paris: Presses Universitaires de France.

López, A., Atran, S., Coley, J., Medin, D., & Smith, E. (1997). The tree of life: Universals of folk-biological taxonomies and inductions. *Cognitive Psychology, 32,* 251–295.

Lumsden, C. J., & Wilson, E. O. (1981). *Genes, mind, and culture: The coevolutionary process.* Cambridge, MA: Harvard University Press.

Lutz, C. (1985). Ethnopsychology compared to what? Explaining behavior and consciousness among the Ifaluk. In G. White & J. Kirkpatrick (Eds.), *Person, self, and experience: Exploring Pacific ethnopsychologies* (pp. 35–79). Berkeley: University of California Press.

Lutz, C. (1987). Goals, events, and understanding in Ifaluk emotion theory. In D. Holland & N. Quinn

(Eds.), *Cultural models in language and thought* (pp. 290–312). Cambridge, UK: Cambridge University Press.

Lutz, C. (1988). *Unnatural emotions: Everyday sentiments on a Micronesian atoll and their challenge to Western theory*. Chicago: University of Chicago Press.

Lynch, E., Coley, J., & Medin, D. (2000). Tall is typical: Central tendency, ideal dimensions and graded category structure among tree experts and novices. *Memory and Cognition, 28*, 41–50.

Mahalingam, R. (1998). Essentialism, power and representation of caste: A developmental study. *Dissertation Abstracts International, 60*(2-B).

Malt, B. (1995). Category coherence in cross-cultural perspective. *Cognitive Psychology, 29*, 85–148.

Malt, B. C., Sloman, S. A., Gennari, S., Shi, M., & Wang, Y. (1999). Knowing versus naming: Similarity and the linguistic categorization of artifacts. *Journal of Memory and Language, 40*, 230–262.

Markus, H., & Kitayama, S. (1991). Culture and the self: Implications for cognition, emotion, and motivation. *Psychological Review, 98*, 224–253.

McCloskey, M., & Glucksberg, S. (1978). Natural categories: Well-defined or fuzzy-sets? *Memory and Cognition, 6*, 462—472.

Medin, D., & Atran, S. (2004). The native mind: Biological categorization and reasoning in development and across cultures. *Psychological Review, 111*, 960–983.

Medin, D., Lynch, E., Coley, J., & Atran, S. (1997). Categorization and reasoning among tree experts: Do all roads lead to Rome? *Cognitive Psychology, 32*, 49–96.

Medin, D., & Ortony, A. (1989). Psychological essentialism. In S. Vosniadou & A. Ortony (Eds.), *Similarity and analogical reasoning* (pp. 179–195). New York: Cambridge University Press.

Medin, D., Ross, N., Atran, S., Burnett, R., & Blok, S. (2002). Categorization and reasoning in relation to culture and expertise. In B. Ross (Ed.), *The psychology of learning and motivation: Advances in research and theory* (Vol. 41, pp. 1–38). New York: Academic Press.

Medin, D. L., Altom, M. W., Edelson, S. M., & Freko, D. (1982). Correlated symptoms and simulated medical classification. *Journal of Experimental Psychology: Learning, Memory, and Cognition, 8*, 37–50.

Medin, D. L., & Coley, J. D. (1998). Concepts and categorization. In J. Hochberg & J. E. Cutting (Eds.), *Handbook of perception and cognition: Perception and cognition at century's end* (2nd ed., pp. 403–440). San Diego: Academic Press.

Medin, D. L., Ross, N. O., Cox, D. G., & Atran, S. (in press). Why folkbiology matters: Resource conflict despite shared goals and values. *Human Ecology*.

Medin, D. L., & Wattenmaker, W. D. (1987). Family resemblance, conceptual cohesiveness and category construction. *Cognitive Psychology, 19*, 242–279.

Mehler, J., Jusczyk, P., Lambertz, G., Halsted, N.,

Bertoncini, J., & Amiel-Tison, C. (1988). A precursor of language acquisition in young infants. *Cognition, 29*, 143–178.

Miller, C. L. (1983). Developmental changes in male/female voice classification by infants. *Infant Behavior and Development, 6*(3), 313–330.

Monod, J. (1971). *Chance and necessity: An essay on the natural philosophy of modern biology*. New York: Knopf.

Moore, C., Romney, A. K., Hsia, T., & Rush, C. (2000). The universality of the semantic structure of emotion terms. *American Anthropologist, 101*, 530–546.

Morelli, G. A., Rogoff, B., & Angelillo, C. (2003). Cultural variation in young children's access to work or involvement in specialised child-focused activities. *International Journal of Behavioral Development, 27*(3), 264–274.

Murphy, G. L. (2002). *The big book of concepts*. Cambridge, MA: MIT Press.

Murphy, G. L., & Medin, D. L. (1985). The role of theories in conceptual coherence. *Psychological Review, 92*, 289–316.

Nesdale, D., & Flesser, D. (2001). Social identity and the development of children's group attitudes. *Child Development, 72*(2), 506–517.

Niedenthal, P. M., Halberstadt, J. B., & Innes-Ker, A. H. (1999). Emotional response categorization. *Psychological Review, 106*, 337–361.

Nisbett, R., Peng, K., Choi, I., & Norenzayan, A. (2001). Culture and systems of thought: Holistic versus analytic cognition. *Psychological Review, 108*, 291–310.

Nisbett, R. E. (2003). *The geography of thought: How Asians and westerners think differently—and why*. New York: Free Press.

Norenzayan, A., Smith, E. E., Kim, B. J., & Nisbett, R. E. (2002). Cultural preferences for formal versus intuitive reasoning. *Cognitive Science, 26*, 653–684.

Nosofsky, R. M. (1992). Exemplar-based approach to relating categorization, identification, and recognition. In F. G. Ashby (Ed.), *Multidimensional models of perception and cognition* (pp. 363–393). Hillsdale, NJ: Erlbaum.

Nosofsky, R. M., & Palmeri, T. J. (1997). An exemplar-based random walk model of speeded classification. *Psychological Review, 104*, 266–300.

Ocherson, D. N., Smith, E. E., Wilkie, O., Lopez, A., & Shafir, E. (1990). Category-based induction. *Psychological Review, 97*, 185–200.

Osgood, C. E., Suci, G. J., Tannenbaum, P. H. (1957). *The measurement of meaning*. Urbana: University of Illinois Press.

Oyserman, D., Coon, H. M., & Kemmelmeier, M. (2002). Rethinking individualism and collectivism: Evaluation of theoretical assumptions and meta-analyses. *Psychological Bulletin, 128*(1), 3–72.

Páez, D., & Vergara, A. (1995). Cultural differences in emotional knowledge. In J. A. Russell, J. M. Fernandez-Dols, A. S. R. Manstead, & J. C. Wellencamp (Eds.), *Everyday conceptions of emotion: An introduction to the psychology, anthropology, and linguistics of emotion (pp. 415–434). Boston: Kluwer.

Phelps, E. A., O'Connor, K. J., Cunningham, W. A., Funayama, E. S., Gatenby, J. C., Gore, J. C., et al. (2000). Performance on indirect measures of race evaluation predicts amygdala activation. *Journal of Cognitive Neuroscience, 12*, 729–738.

Povinelli, D. J., & Bering, J. M. (2002). The mentality of apes revisited. *Current Directions in Psychological Science, 11*(4), 115–119.

Powlishta, K. K., Sen, M. G., Serbin, L. A., Poulin-Dubois, D., & Eichstedt, J. A. (2001). From infancy to middle childhood: The role of cognitive and social factors in becoming gendered. In R. K. Unger (Ed.), *Handbook of the psychology of women and gender* (pp. 116–132). New York: Wiley.

Proffitt, J., Coley, J., & Medin, D. (2000). Expertise and category-based induction. *Journal of Experimental Psychology: Learning, Memory, and Cognition, 26,* 811–828.

Rappaport, R. (1999). *Ritual and religion in the making of humanity.* Cambridge, UK: Cambridge University Press.

Rehder, B., & Hastie, R. (2001). Causal knowledge and categories: The effects of causal beliefs on categorization, induction, and similarity. *Journal of Experimental Psychology: General, 130,* 323–360.

Richeson, J. A., Baird, A. A., Gordon, H. L., Heatherton, T. F., Wyland, C. L., Trawalter, S., et al. (2003). An fMRI investigation of the impact of interracial contact on executive function. *Nature Neuroscience, 6,* 1323–1328.

Rips, L. (2001). Necessity and natural categories. *Psychological Bulletin, 127,* 827–852.

Romney, A. K., & Batchelder, W. (1999). Cultural consensus theory. In R. Wilson & F. Keil (Eds.), *The MIT encyclopedia of the cognitive sciences* (pp. 208–209). Cambridge, MA: MIT Press.

Romney, A. K., Brewer, D. D., & Batchelder, W. H. (1996). The relation between typicality and semantic similarity structure. *Journal of Quantitative Anthropology, 6,* 1–14.

Romney, A. K., Moore, C. C., & Rusch, C. D. (1997). Cultural universals: Measuring the semantic structure of emotion terms in English and Japanese. *Proceedings of the National Academy of Sciences USA, 94,* 5489–5494.

Romney, A. K., Weller, S., & Batchelder, W. (1986). Culture as consensus: A theory of culture and informant accuracy. *American Anthropologist, 88,* 313–338.

Rosaldo, M. (1980). *Knowledge and passion: Ilongot notions of self and social life.* Cambridge, UK: Cambridge University Press.

Rosaldo, R. (1984). Grief and a headhunter's rage: On the cultural force of emotions. In E. Brunner & S. Plattner (Eds.), *Text, play, and story: The construction and reconstruction of the self and society* (pp. 178–195). Washington, DC: American Ethnological Society.

Rosch, E., & Mervis, C. B. (1975). Family resemblance: Studies in the internal structure of categories. *Cognitive Psychology, 7,* 573–605.

Rosch, E., Mervis, C., Grey, W., Johnson, D., & Boyes-Braem, P. (1976). Basic objects in natural categories. *Cognitive Psychology, 8,* 382–439.

Ross, N., Medin, D., Coley, J. D., & Atran, S. (2002). Cultural and experiential differences in the development of folkbiological induction. *Cognitive Development, 18,* 25–47.

Russell, J. A. (1983). Pancultural aspects of the human conceptual organization of emotions. *Journal of Personality and Social Psychology, 45,* 1281–1288.

Russell, J. A. (1989). Measures of emotion. In R. Plutchik & H. Kellerman (Eds.), *Emotion: Theory, research, and experience* (Vol. 4, pp. 83–111). New York: Academic Press.

Russell, J. A. (1991). Culture and the categorization of emotion. *Psychological Bulletin, 110,* 426–450.

Scheffler, H. W., & Lounsbury, F. G. (1971). A study in structural semantics: The Siriono kinship system. Englewood Cliffs, NJ: Prentice Hall.

Scherer, K. R., & Wallbott, H. G. (1994). Evidence for universality and cultural variation of differential emotion response patterning. *Journal of Personality and Social Psychology, 66,* 310–328.

Schneider, D. (1980). *American kinship: A cultural account.* Chicago: University of Chicago Press.

Semaj, M. B. (1980). The development of racial evaluation and preference: A cognitive approach. *Journal of Black Psychology, 6,* 59–79.

Shafto, P., & Coley, J. D. (2003). Development of categorization and reasoning in the natural world: Novices to experts, naive similarity to ecological knowledge. *Journal of Experimental Psychology: Learning, Memory, and Cognition, 29,* 641–649.

Shepard, R. N. (1987). Toward a universal law of generalization for psychological science. *Science, 237,* 1317–1323.

Simons, D. J., & Keil, F. C. (1995). An abstract to concrete shift in the development of biological thought: The insides story. *Cognition, 56,* 129–163.

Smith, E., & Medin, D. (1981). *Categories and concepts.* Cambridge, MA: Harvard University Press.

Smith, J. D., & Minda, J. P. (1998). Prototypes in the mist: The early epochs of category learning. *Journal of Experimental Psychology: Learning, Memory, and Cognition, 24,* 1411–1436.

Smith, J. D., & Minda, J. P. (2000). Thirty categorization results in search of a model. *Journal of Experimental Psychology: Learning, Memory, and Cognition, 26,* 3–27.

Smith, P. B., & Bond, M. H. (1993). *Social psychology across cultures.* New York: Harvester Wheatsheaf.

Smits, T., Storms, G., Rosseel, Y., & De Boeck, P. (2002). Fruits and vegetables categorized: An application of the generalized context model. *Psychonomic Bulletin and Review, 9,* 836–844.

Sousa, P., Atran, S., & Medin, D. (2002). Essentialism and folkbiology: Further evidence from Brazil. *Journal of Cognition and Culture, 2*, 195–223.

Spalding, T. L., & Ross, B. H. (2000). Concept learning and feature interpretation. *Memory and Cognition, 28*, 439–451.

Sperber, D. (1985). Anthropology and psychology: Toward and epidemiology of representations. *Man, 20*, 73–89.

Sperber, D. (1996). *Explaining culture.* Oxford, UK: Blackwell.

Sperber, D., & Hirschfeld, L. (2004). The cognitive foundations of cultural stability and diversity. *Trends in Cognitive Sciences, 8*(1), 40–46.

Storms, G., De Boeck, P., & Ruts, W. (2000). Prototype and exemplar based information in natural language categories. *Journal of Memory and Language, 42*, 51–73.

Strevens, M. (2000). The naive aspect of essentialist theories. *Cognition, 74*, 149–175.

Tanaka, J., & Taylor, M. (1991). Object categories and expertise: Is the basic level in the eye of the beholder? *Cognitive Psychology, 23*, 457–482.

Tomasello, M., Call, J., & Hare, B. (2003). Chimpanzees understand psychological states—the question is which ones and to what extent. *Trends in Cognitive Sciences, 7*(4), 153–156.

Triandis, H. (1995). *Individualism and collectivism.* Boulder, CO: Westview Press.

Unsworth, S. J., & Medin, D. L. (2005). Cross-cultural differences in belief bias with deductive reasoning? *Cognitive Science, 29*, 525–529.

Unsworth, S. J., Sears, C. R., & Pexman, P. M. (2005). Cultural influences on categorization processes. *Journal of Cross-Cultural Psychology, 36*, 662–688.

Verbeemen, T., Vanoverberghe, V., Storms, G., & Ruts, W. (2001). Contrast categories in natural language concepts. *Journal of Memory and Language, 44*, 1–26.

Vygotsky, L. (1978). *Mind in society.* Cambridge, MA: Harvard University Press.

Walker, S. J. (1992). Supernatural beliefs, natural kinds and conceptual structure. *Memory and Cognition, 20*, 655–662.

Waxman, S. R., Medin, D. L., & Ross, N. (in press). Folkbiological reasoning from a cross-cultural developmental perspective: Early essentialist notions are shaped by cultural beliefs. *Developmental Psychology.*

Wheeler, M. E., & Fiske, S. T. (2005). Controlling racial prejudice and stereotyping: Social cognitive goals affect amygdala and stereotype activation. *Psychological Science, 16*, 56–63.

Wierzbicka, A. (1992). *Semantics, culture, and cognition: Universal human concepts in culture-specific configurations.* Oxford, UK: Oxford University Press.

Wilson, D. S. (2002). *Darwin's cathedral.* Chicago: University of Chicago Press.

Wisniewski, E., & Medin, D. (1994). On the interaction of theory and data in concept learning. *Cognitive Science, 18*, 221–281.

Wolff, P., Medin, D., & Pankratz, C. (1999). Evolution and devolution of folkbiological knowledge. *Cognition, 73*, 177–204.

CHAPTER 26

Culture and Memory

QI WANG
MICHAEL ROSS

Every introductory psychology text has a chapter on memory. Students learn that Hermann Ebbinghaus, a philosopher, began the scientific study of memory in the late 19th century by testing his own recall for thousands of letter strings. They learn that the memory system has different components, including shorter and longer term memory storages. They learn about different forms of memory, such as semantic, episodic, source, declarative, and implicit memory, and that these different kinds of memory appear to be encoded in different parts of the brain. Students learn that even information that is encoded in the brain can be forgotten and misremembered for various reasons, that some, but not all, types of memory decline with normal aging. They learn that brain injuries, traumas, and diseases can have highly selective effects on memory, destroying particular forms of memory while leaving other types intact. Students learn all of this and much more—including that some of the claims in this paragraph are controversial. Students typically do not learn, however, that social psychological and cultural factors influence memory.

Just as memory researchers disregard social psychology, social psychologists tend to neglect memory. In describing topics that social psy-

chologists study, the website for the Society for Personality and Social Psychology states: "By exploring forces within the person (such as traits, attitudes, and goals) as well as forces within the situation (such as social norms and incentives), personality and social psychologists seek to unravel the mysteries of individual and social life in areas as wide-ranging as prejudice, romantic attraction, persuasion, friendship, helping, aggression, conformity, and group interaction." One searches in vain for any mention of memory.

Such reciprocal neglect is understandable. Memory seems to encompass basic cognitive and neurological processes that transcend social context and culture. To be consciously remembered, information has to be noticed and encoded in memory, and that is presumably true whether a person lives in Beijing, Bombay, or Boston. Nevertheless, Frederic Bartlett (1932), a pioneer in the study of memory, entitled his classic book, *Remembering: A Study in Experimental and Social Psychology.* Unlike many of his peers who studied university students' recollections of Ebbinghaus's letter strings, Bartlett investigated recall of meaningful material in different social contexts. First, he discovered that people's perceptions, understanding, and memory of new information are strongly influenced by their prior knowledge, or in Bartlett's own term, schemas. Second, Bartlett insisted that memory is often an active construction rather than the simple recovery of information stored in the brain: "What is said to be reproduced is, far more generally than is commonly admitted, really a construction, serving to justify whatever impression may have been left by the original. It is this 'impression,' rarely defined with much exactitude, which most readily persists" (p. 176). Thirty-five years later, Neisser (1967) made a similar point, arguing that only fragments of an episode are stored in memory. He suggested that people reconstruct an event from these bits of memory, just as a paleontologist reconstructs a dinosaur from a few bones. Building upon this framework, we examine in this chapter the impact of culture on schemas, and how prior information in the form of shared knowledge shapes the constructive process of memory.

If cultural and social factors are often neglected in the study of memory, then the reader might well suppose that this chapter will be very brief. Well, do not get your hopes up. In recent years the number of relevant studies has increased dramatically, reflecting psychologists' increased interest in culture. A simple search using PsycINFO and the key words *culture* and *memory* indicates that studies assess-

ing culture and memory were rare until the 1980s, with a dramatic rise in the early 1990s (Figure 26.1). We begin our analysis of this literature by explaining what we mean by the term "culture."

Concurring with Bartlett and others (e.g., Bruner, 1990; D'Andrade, 1992; Holland & Quinn, 1987; Valsiner, 2000; Vygotsky, 1978; Wang & Brockmeier, 2002), we view culture as both a system (values, schemas, scripts, models, metaphors, and artifacts) and a process (rituals, daily routines, and practices) of symbolic mediation. By operating on social institutions (e.g., the family) as well as on the actions, thoughts, emotions, and moral values of individuals, culture regulates both intrapersonal and interpersonal psychological functions. Through socialization, individuals acquire knowledge and competencies that serve culturally prescribed goals. Similar to other abilities, memory is useful to the extent that it helps people achieve their objectives. We assess whether culture affects why people remember, how people remember, when people remember, what people remember, and whether they judge remembering to be necessary at all.

We focus on a particular type of memory, autobiographical recall. Autobiographical memory refers to memory for personal experiences. Autobiographical memories often include de-

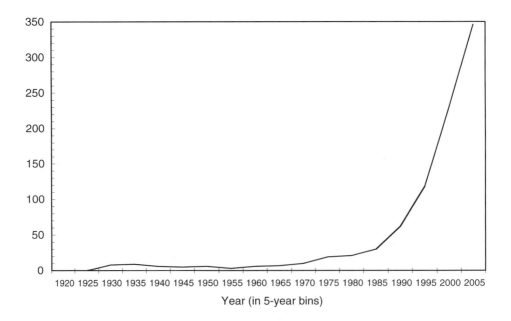

FIGURE 26.1. Number of publications in 5-year time bins of articles with any mention of culture and memory (from the PsycINFO database).

tails of what happened, who was involved, and where and when the episodes occurred (Tulving, 2002). A great deal of research on memory and culture concerns autobiographical memory. Our discussion reflects this reality. We adopt a functional approach to examine cultural emphases on different goals and functions of autobiographical remembering. We show that such cultural differences have important consequences for the content, style, emergence, and general accessibility of autobiographical memories.

FUNCTIONS OF REMEMBERING

According to Neisser (1982), the primary task of memory researchers is to understand "how people use their own past experiences in meeting the present and the future," a task that has to be carried out in different settings "because changes in the social and cultural environment can change the uses of the past" (p. 12). Throughout human history, an accurate memory probably has provided an evolutionary advantage. At a basic survival level, a good memory could help individuals find food and avoid danger. Furthermore, ecological factors often encourage the development of particular memory skills. For instance, Australian Aboriginal children and adolescents of the desert regions develop extraordinary visual–spatial memory that enables them to navigate in their physical surroundings (Kearins, 1981, 1986). Social factors also play an important role. In New Zealand, Maori adults, who grew up in a culture with a strong oral tradition, develop an enhanced ability to remember events from the remote past (MacDonald, Uesiliana, & Hayne, 2000). More generally, people become skilled at remembering information important to their everyday activities.

In all cultures, verbatim or precisely accurate memory is necessary in some contexts. In Western classrooms, children memorize both poems and the multiplication tables. Eight times eight is precisely 64. Sixty-three and 65 are wrong, despite their proximity to 64. Similarly, religious texts are often memorized by their devotees. In most contexts, however, children and adults are not required to produce a verbatim memory. Daily remembering typically involves recalling the meaningful gist of episodes rather than exquisite detail. For example, if a friend asks about your lunch, you might report eating a hamburger and salad at the local diner. Your friend is probably not interested in knowing the exact contents of your salad; whether the hamburger bun had seeds; other items on the menu and what they cost; the precise time at which you ate; the specific booth you occupied; the number of other customers and what they had for lunch; the name, height, and weight of your server; the number of restaurant personnel and their genders; the location of the cash register and safe; and so forth. Even if your friend were interested in such details you would probably not be able to provide all of them. For example, we seldom pay sufficient attention to our servers to be able to distinguish them from other servers in a restaurant.

What constitutes meaningful gist, however, is highly dependent on a person's goals (Conway & Pleydell-Pearce, 2000). Suppose that your primary goal on entering the restaurant was to case the joint to plan a robbery with your friend. You would then notice and recall quite different information (Anderson & Pichert, 1978), including perhaps the number and genders of the personnel, and the location of the cash register and safe. People's goals and memories vary with their personal concerns. More important from this perspective, people's goals and memories vary in response to their social context and culture.

Different cultures champion different views of the very concept of memory. The Indian Buddhist conception of memory (*Smriti*) includes factors of apperception or awareness of object (*Phassa*), perception (*Sanna*), insight (*Panna*), and mindfulness (*Sati*) (Deshpande, 1996). This Buddhist perspective is different from both classical and more modern Western views of memory. Discussions of memory in classical and medieval Western writings focus on image, impression, storehouse, and recollection; modern empirical approaches emphasize encoding, recall, and recognition (Carruthers, 1990). According to Buddhism, memory during waking states (*Abhavita-Smar-tavya*) is the creation of God. Also, certain mental states, such as that achieved during meditation, enable individuals to remember everything, including events from previous lives. Whereas modern psychologists tend to ascribe the loss of memory to encoding and retrieval failures or to neurological dysfunction, Indian Buddhist scriptures attribute forgetting to daytime naps or too much alcohol. A person who sleeps during the day or consumes alcohol suffers from increased *Kafa* and *Pitta* and "cannot obtain any clear knowledge, philosophical [or] otherwise" (Deshpande, 1996, p. 63). To improve memory, Indian Buddhist thinking advocates that individuals free themselves from lust, anger, delusion, and egoism. In contrast, Western models of memory emphasize the use of memorial strategies to improve recall. Differing cultural beliefs about memory are likely to affect how and when people use memory. We focus on a number of different intrapersonal (self-defining, directive, self-enhancing, and emotional expression) and interpersonal (e.g., relationship maintenance) functions of autobiographical memory, and discuss findings for other types of memory for which relevant data are available.

INTRAPERSONAL FUNCTIONS OF AUTOBIOGRAPHICAL MEMORY

Self-Definition

According to Western intellectual tradition, self-definition is perhaps the most important intrapersonal function of autobiographical memory. Memory is assigned a central role in the development, maintenance, and expression of an enduring self-concept (Bruner, 1990; Brockmeier & Carbaugh, 2001; Hume, 1739/1882; James, 1890/1950; McAdams, 1993; Nelson, 1996; Pillemer, 1998; Ross, 1989; Singer & Salovey, 1993). In a *Treatise on Human Nature*, Hume (1739/1882, p. 542) proclaimed the importance of autobiographical memory: "Had we no memory, we never should have any notion . . . of that chain of causes and effects, which constitute our self or person." From this perspective, people establish the meaning, purpose, and value of their existence by recollecting and identifying with their past selves (Antze, 1996; Herman, 1992; Lowenthal, 1985). They mine their pasts to establish both who they are and who they are not. For example, a mathematician who is confident of her own intellectual attainment might remember the thrill of past successes, such as winning competitions and receiving awards. She may also remember a few disconfirming episodes, such as failing a high school algebra class. She might rationalize such incidents by attributing poor performances to immaturity, and thereby maintain her current (mature) identity as an accomplished mathematician (Wilson & Ross, 2001). To some extent, "the

sureness of 'I was' is a necessary component of the sureness of 'I am' " (Wyatt, 1963, p. 319).

This emphasis on using personal memory to define one's self-identity may be intimately linked to the Western conception of selfhood, which focuses on autonomy and independence. The self is a unique collection of inner attributes, qualities, dispositions, and opinions (Fiske, Kitayama, Markus, & Nisbett, 1998; Geertz, 1973; Kağitçibaşi, 1996; Markus & Kitayama, 1991; Shweder et al., 1998; Triandis, 1989). By helping individuals to distinguish themselves from others, memories of distinctive personal experiences serve as an important and even necessary component of an independent self-construal. To a Western reader, this emphasis on the importance of autobiographical memory for self-identity might seem to be an obvious truism. Otherwise how could you "know" yourself?

Yet in many other cultures, such as those in East Asia, autobiographical memory is not central to self-identity. In these cultures, an interdependent or relational self-construal is defined largely by an individual's place within his or her network of relationships (Fiske et al., 1998; Kağitçibaşi, 1996; Markus & Kitayama, 1991; Shweder et al., 1998; Triandis, 1989). Social status and roles, such as memberships in the family, the workplace, religious groups, or the nation, are crucial constituents of self and identity. In this context, autobiographical memories seem not to be particularly important to individuals. Wang and Conway (2004) reported that European American middle-aged adults rated their autobiographical memories as more personally important to them than did Chinese, regardless of the life period in which the events occurred. Sankaranarayanan and Leichtman (2000) observed that their rural Indian informants had great difficulty when asked to report memories of childhood experiences. They often appeared puzzled and even annoyed, asking, "Why would one want to remember such things?" In an even more striking case, anthropologist Röttger-Rössler (1993) was unable to collect autobiographical stories in a rural Indonesian community: "Not one villager was willing to speak about his or her own life, not even some episodes of it" (p. 366). Despite their close relationship with the researcher, villagers felt uncomfortable and embarrassed when asked to talk about themselves. When they spoke about personal experiences in everyday conversations, their accounts were "event-centered." According to Röttger-Rössler, "it is almost impossible to learn something about the feelings and emotions of the narrator" (p. 366). In contrast, Western respondents often seem happy to provide self-revealing accounts of their own lives.

The varied cultural emphases on the self-defining value of autobiographical memories are reflected in people's ability to recall very long-term memories, such as their earliest childhood experiences (MacDonald et al., 2000; Mullen, 1994; Wang, 2001a). Although adults from all cultures are typically unable to recall events from their first years of life (Pillemer & White, 1989), there are cultural differences in the accessibility of early memories. In general, when people are asked to relate their earliest childhood memory, the earliest events recalled by adults of European descent originally took place, on average, at about 3½ years of age; in contrast, the earliest childhood events recalled by participants of Asian heritage occurred between 6 and 17 months later (MacDonald et al., 2000; Mullen, 1994; Wang, 2001a). In a recent study, researchers examined adults' general ability to access memories of early childhood in the United States (all European Americans), England, and China (Wang, Conway, & Hou, 2004). Participants were asked to recall as many events occurring before the age of 5 years as they could within 5 minutes. U.S. participants recalled the greatest number of childhood memories ($M = 12.24$), followed by British participants ($M = 9.83$), and then Chinese ($M = 5.68$). Consistent with other studies, the earliest childhood memories of Chinese participants were approximately 6 months later than their Western counterparts. Although it is possible that participants' memories of early childhood events are affected by photos they have seen or stories they have heard, researchers studying early memories attempt to focus on events participants remember independently of external sources.

What are the bases of these early memory differences? Conceivably, cultural conceptions of selfhood guide remembering (Mullen, 1994; Wang, 2001a; Wang et al., 2004). An autonomous self-view might motivate individuals to attend to, encode, ruminate, and talk about significant personal experiences. These experiences should help individuals to distinguish themselves from others and reaffirm their independence and unique identity. Consequently, individuals' cognitive resources may be chan-

neled into the early development of an organized, articulated, and durable autobiographical memory system. In contrast, the relational self-view associated with many Asian cultures might instead promote the retention of knowledge critical for social harmony and collective solidarity. The development of a structured autobiographical memory system may not be accentuated in this context.

It is obviously an overgeneralization to presume that all Westerners have an autonomous view of self and all Easterners have a relational view of self. Regardless of culture, most people will perceive themselves as possessing both relational and personal aspects. In Eastern cultures, relational qualities should predominate on average, but the degree to which this is the case will vary across individuals and circumstances (I. Choi, Nisbett, & Norenzayan, 1999; Hong, Morris, Chiu, & Benet-Martinez, 2000; Mascolo & Li, 2004; Voronov & Singer, 2002). Similarly in Western cultures, personal traits should predominate on average, but the balance of personal and relational traits in self-views will vary across individuals. To test the association between the autonomous–relational dimension of the self and autobiographical memory, Wang and colleagues (Wang, 2001a; Wang, Leichtman, & White, 1998) examined self-descriptions and earliest childhood memories in European American and Chinese young adults. In both cultures, participants who focused on personal unique attributes in their self-descriptions tended to report earlier and more detailed childhood memories than did participants who focused on social roles and categories in their self-descriptions.

If individuals view themselves as possessing both personal and relational aspects, it ought to be possible to prompt them to focus temporarily on either their relatively unique personal self or their relational self (Trafimow, Silverman, Fan, & Law, 1997). Wang and Ross (2005) showed that such shifts in attention can affect the accessibility of early memories. European and Asian American participants were asked to describe themselves as either a unique individual (personal prime) or as a member of various social groups (relational prime) prior to recalling their earliest childhood memory. The personal prime increased the accessibility of earlier first memories among Asians, such that they reported their earliest childhood memories from approximately 3½ years of age, just as European Americans did. European Americans were unaffected by the prime, presumably because they had accessed the earliest memories possible in this experimental paradigm (Mullen, 1994; Pillemer & White, 1989; Wang, 2006).

Previous findings that first memories of Asians are later than the first memories of Westerners would seem to reflect a stable cultural difference: Asians cannot retrieve earlier memories because they do not have such recollections in their memory store. However, the Wang and Ross (2005) priming study suggests the intriguing possibility that cultural disparities reflect differences in memory *accessibility* rather than memory availability. In general, childhood memories recalled from an early age tend to focus more on the self and less on others than do those from an older age (Wang, 2001a). Consequently, it makes sense that a personal prime provides a cue that enables Asians to access earlier first memories than they normally would. It would be making too much of a single study, however, to argue that cultural differences in the age of earliest recall are *entirely* due to memory accessibility rather than availability. More research along these lines is needed.

The impact of culture on memory goes far beyond the age of earliest memories. The divergent modes of self are associated with different genres of autobiographical remembering, as reflected in the style and content of memory recall. One intriguing cultural difference in autobiographical remembering concerns whether people report specific (e.g., "the time I fell in a pond") or generic memories (e.g., "often playing with other kids in the woods"). Differences in the specificity of autobiographical memories may reflect cultural variation in the nature of self and identity. Specific episodes are often personal experiences that could promote a unique, autonomous sense of self. Generic memories might imply the importance of social conventions, as well as emphasize an individual's relation to significant others and the community. As a result, generic memories could contribute to a relational sense of self.

Studies of children's autobiographical memories reveal cultural differences in the specificity of recall. American preschoolers reported a greater proportion of specific autobiographical memories than did their same-age Korean and Chinese counterparts (Han, Leichtman, & Wang, 1998; Wang, 2004a). Minami and McCabe (1991) interviewed Japanese and American children ages 6 to 9 years about past injuries. Japanese children tended to speak of collections of experiences rather than focusing on any one particular injury, despite being repeatedly prompted to talk about a single episode. In contrast, North American children tended to talk about one specific injury at great length. Cultural differences in memory specificity, evident in the preschool years, persist into adulthood. Both Western and Asian adults produce specific memories, but the tendency to do so is consistently stronger among Westerners (Wang & Conway, 2004; Wang, 2006).

Different cultural views of the self are even related to individuals' memory imagery. Asian Canadians are more likely than European Canadians to adopt a third-person (as opposed to a first-person) perspective on themselves when recalling events in which they were the focus of other people's attention (Cohen & Gunz, 2002). In a third-person perspective, individuals see themselves in the scene, as if viewing themselves through the eyes of a bystander (e.g., they see themselves talking in front of an audience). Conceivably, recalling personal events from the perspective of an audience serves as a reminder that one should behave properly and conform to group standards. Such norms are clearly defined and emphasized in Asian cultures, where the self is regarded as fundamentally interconnected to significant others rather than as an autonomous entity.

In a related vein, memory *content* also appears to vary with culture. From an information-processing point of view, an autonomous, independent self-construal may lead individuals to attend to event information relevant to their own roles, actions, feelings, and predilections. Such information is likely to be well represented in memory and highly accessible during recall. In contrast, an interdependent self-construal might enhance attentiveness to collective activities and significant others, with the result that such relational information is readily accessible during recall. Consistent with this analysis, researchers have reported systematic cross-cultural differences in the content of autobiographical memories (Mullen, 1994; Wang, 2001a, 2006; Wang & Conway, 2004; Wang & Ross, 2005). European Americans often provide memories of unique personal experiences (successes, failures, fears, nightmares, etc.), with frequent descriptions of emotions, personal opinions, and self-determination. Conversely, native Chinese and Asian Americans often report memory events that are focused on group actions and interpersonal relations (school activities, family outings, disputes with neighbors, etc.). Such differences are also observed among preschool-age children. European American youngsters tend to report more detailed, emotional, and self-focused accounts of personal experiences than do their Asian peers (Han et al., 1998; Wang, 2004a; Wang & Leichtman, 2000).

The impact of an autonomous versus relational sense of self on memory extends to remembering lists of words. Wagar and Cohen (2003) asked university students to relate words in a list to the self ("Does the word describe you?") or to a friend ("Does the word describe your best friend?"). The words either represented personal qualities (happy, generous, etc.) or social roles (brother, roommate, etc.). Later, participants were shown a list of words, including some words from the previous list and some new words. Participants were asked to identify the words correctly as new or old. Asian Canadians identified collective traits encoded in relation to the self most quickly and personal traits encoded in relation to the self most slowly. Wagar and Cohen suggested that these results indicate that the self-concept of Asian Canadians consists chiefly of social role traits: "When collective traits were encoded into a schematically rich collective, long-term self, strong memory traces were formed" (p. 472). European Canadians showed a standard self-reference effect (Rogers, Kuiper, & Kirker, 1977). They more quickly recognized words originally encoded in relation to self than in relation to their best friend, regardless of trait type.

Autobiographies provide an example of how cultural views of self influence memory content. Traditional Chinese autobiography imitated biography almost "slavishly" (Wu, 1990). Authors usually reported public and official events, and seldom disclosed their inner emotions or motives. Even when writing about unique personal experiences, such as adventures in foreign lands, autobiographers focused on facts about the places they visited rather than on their own "inner life," such as their thoughts and feelings. Wu suggested that using the format of biography to tell a personal story might protect the autobiographer "from the censure of egomania, of doing something unconventional" (p. 3). It is also possible that

Chinese autobiographers fail to report personal details because they are less accessible: Research on cultural differences in autobiographical memory suggests that the recollections of Chinese autobiographers would be less self-focused than the memories of Western autobiographers, even if the memory reports were private and confidential (as is the case in psychological research). Although autobiography has evolved as an independent literature genre in China, contemporary Chinese autobiographical writings still lack self-focus in comparison to their European and American counterparts (Pillemer, 1998).

The commitment to a unique individual self is highlighted in the first modern (Western) autobiography—Rousseau's *Confessions* (1782/ 2000, p. 5):

> I am resolved on an undertaking that has no model and will have no imitator. I want to show my fellow-men a man in all the truth of nature; and this man is to be myself. Myself alone. I feel my heart and I know men. I am not made like any that I have seen; I venture to believe that I was not made like any that exists. If I am not more deserving, at least I am different. As to whether nature did well or ill to break the mould in which I was cast, that is something no one can judge until after they have read me.

Baumeister (1987) provided another perspective on the relation between self-views and autobiography. He reviewed the scholarly literature on changes in Western beliefs about the self from the 11th through the 20th centuries. The Western notion of an inner self that is distinguishable from appearances and public actions did not emerge as a widespread belief until about the 16th century. Moreover, it was only in the 19th century that "personality (rather than social rank and roles) came to be increasingly regarded as a, even *the*, central aspect of the self" (p. 166). Most interesting for this analysis, this 19th century shift in views of the self is accompanied and evidenced by trends in autobiographical writing, which began to highlight personal information. In addition to supporting the association between self-views and autobiography, Baumeister's review indicates that self-knowledge reflects the relation of the individual to society. When societies change, self-views change, and so does autobiography.

In related research, Dekker (2000) examined transformations in "egodocuments," including diaries, autobiographies, and other forms of personal records, from the Golden Age to Romanticism (17th–19th centuries) in Holland. Before 1800, a standard personal record contained extensive descriptions of family background. The individual was depicted primarily as a link in a family tree. A new type of record emerged around 1800. Authors began to dwell on their childhood, and the self became the center of their text. Egodocuments also came to be an important outlet for expressing personal feelings. These changes reflect the growing individualism during this historical era in Holland, and the shifts in social conventions with regard to emotions and ideas about children.

Psychologists do not tend to study history, but they can use the tools of experimental psychology to produce individual shifts in autobiographical remembering that might take generations or even centuries to occur at a societal level. If historical and cultural variations in autobiographical memory are due to differing self-views, then people who regard themselves primarily in terms of personal traits should exhibit a more Western style of autobiographical memory regardless of their culture: Their autobiographical memories should be detailed, specific (rather than generic), and self-focused. In the Wang and Ross (2005) priming study described earlier, the personal prime elicited memories that focused more on the rememberer and less on social interactions than did the relational prime, regardless of culture. Psychologists also study individual differences in self-views within a culture. Regardless of cultural group, children and adults who dwell more on personal attributes and predilections when describing themselves are also more likely to provide self-focused, specific memories compared to those who dwell more on social roles and group memberships when describing themselves (Wang, 2001a, 2004a).

It is important to keep in mind that cultural variations in memory may reflect different processes at every stage of remembering, from perception and meaning analysis to retention and recall. Compared to European Americans, East Asians attend to, perceive, and retain more contextual information and relationships in their environment (Masuda & Nisbett, 2001). They also refer more to the context or the group when explaining physical and social phenomena (Chiu, Morris, Hong, & Menon, 2000; I. Choi et al., 1999). Not all information that people notice is preserved in long-term memory, however, as anyone who has studied for an examination can testify. Information is more likely to be retained if it is consolidated with preexisting cognitive frameworks, such as views of self (Anderson & Pichert, 1978; Bartlett, 1932; Rogers et al., 1977). Finally, people's goals and beliefs at the time of retrieval, including their culturally shared beliefs and self-views, influence which elements of the retained information they access, as well as how they build on that information to construct an autobiographical memory (Bartlett, 1932; Neisser, 1967; Ross, 1989).

Directive Function

Regardless of culture, people rely on autobiographical memory to guide many of their everyday decisions. In selecting a toy from a bin, a book from a shelf, or a favorite food from a menu, children and adults may refer to memories of their previous experiences. In addition to guiding mundane actions, memories play a major role in Eastern and Western moral and religious traditions. According to Confucian ethics, people should engage in daily recollections of their actions, examining their behavior on three dimensions: Have I done my best for others? Have I been trustworthy in my dealings with friends? Have I failed to revisit what the Master has taught me? This practice of autobiographical reflection (zi-xing, 自省) is considered essential for an individual to achieve the Confucian fundamental value, ren (仁), the supreme virtues of benevolence, moral vitality, and a sensitive concern for others.

Memory plays a directive role in Western religious traditions as well. In his *Confessions*, St. Augustine analyzed memory to achieve a greater understanding of himself and God. Also, by documenting and publicizing how he changed from a wayward youth to a wise man of God, he hoped to inspire others to do the same. More directly comparable to Confucian self-examination is the Examen, a centuries-old feature of Catholic spirituality that involves a retrospective analysis of one's thoughts and actions on a daily basis. During the Examen, individuals review their entire day in detail, recalling what happened and how they acted. When and why did they act badly (e.g., become cross with someone)? When and why did they behave correctly (e.g., aid an elderly person)? They apologize to God for their faults, thank God for their virtues, and pray that God will guide them in the right direction in the future (Catholic Update, March 2003).

Along the same lines, Jewish tradition dictates that, during the "Days of Repentance" that conclude with Yom Kippur, Jews recall their misdeeds of the previous year, identifying sins that they have committed against the laws of God and sins against persons. They can appease God through prayer, confessing their sins and asking for forgiveness. To atone for sins against another person, they must first seek reconciliation with that person. Individuals who succeed in repenting their sins are granted a good and happy new year.

There are similarities and differences between the directive functions of autobiographical memory in Eastern and Western moral and religious traditions. In each case, self-improvement is an important goal. The major cultural difference concerns the focus of the improvement. Confucian ethics, adopted by many Eastern traditions, emphasize the importance of interdependence and maintaining good relationships with other people. A focus on relationships with others is also important in Western religious traditions, but an even greater concern is people's individual relationship with their God and the implications of this relationship for their own well-being.

Although autobiographical memory serves a directive function in Western cultures, it might play a greater role in Eastern cultures. Wang and Conway (2004) found that when recalling personal experiences across the lifespan, Chinese middle-aged adults were more likely than their European American counterparts (48% vs. 9%) spontaneously to generate mores, worldviews, and behavioral lessons from the memory events. Examples include "Since then, I have realized that there are more nice people than bad ones in this world," and "I learned that perfection takes practice."

In the Confucian intellectual tradition, "learning implies full knowledge of the precedents of a past age" (Nakamura, 1964, p. 205). This emphasis on the accumulation of knowledge to understand the world produces a positive and trusting attitude toward the past, as exemplified in the often-observed tendency to take ancient wisdom for granted (Lin, 1939). This acceptance is in direct contrast to the Western tradition that encourages independent thinking. Existing ideas and theories are questioned, developed, and overturned rather than memorized exactly (Tweed & Lehman, 2002).

An intriguing illustration of this cultural difference concerns the practices of magicians in China and North America. In a documentary broadcast on Canadian television in 2001, American magicians Penn and Teller visited China to observe and exchange tricks with local magicians. Penn and Teller were surprised to discover that Chinese magicians pride themselves on learning to reproduce tricks exactly as their masters have shown them. In contrast, North American magicians favor putting a new spin on an old trick (Bienstock, Grogan, & Smith, 2003). Thus, the different intellectual values assigned to the past can affect how individuals in diverse cultures use memories to direct their activities.

Individuals in Western cultures do report using their memories to guide their behaviors in some contexts. Pillemer (1998) analyzed an 8-year-old child's memory of being kidnapped at gunpoint and the horrifying lessons the memory contained about which situations are dangerous and to be avoided. Memories of more common life episodes can also contain guidelines for current and future actions. For example, a college student reported that she learned an important lesson about planning after a miserable trip; a football captain reported using memories of previous losses to motivate his team members; and individuals often described past advice offered by parents or teachers (Pillemer, 2003). Webster and colleagues (Webster, 1993, 1997; Webster & Cappeliez, 1993) developed a 43-item Reminiscence Functions Scale, in which participants indicate on a 6-point scale how often they reminisce with a particular function in mind. On the basis of responses to this scale, the researchers identified two autobiographical memory uses closely related to directive functions: problem solving (remembering past problem-solving strategies for the present purpose) and teach/inform (using reminiscence to relay instructional information to others).

It is unclear whether people's subjective reports about the functions of memory reveal how they actually use their memories in everyday life. For example, people's answers on the Reminiscence Functions Scale might reflect their understanding of how memory *should* be used in their culture. Similarly people might claim to remember and respect the advice of their parents—but do they act on the advice? To study whether people actually use their autobiographical memories as a guide, researchers need to examine directly whether people draw on their recollections while making judgments and decisions.

In one relevant set of studies, researchers examined people's estimates of when they would finish a project (e.g., a school assignment or household renovation). It seems obvious that autobiographical memory could be useful in predicting task completion times. If people want to estimate how long it will take to renovate a kitchen, they should try to recall their own or others' past renovations. Yet individuals in Western cultures often neglect information about past experiences when predicting task completion times (Buehler, Griffin, & Ross, 1994, 2002; Kahneman & Tversky, 1979). People frequently base their predictions on their intentions and hopes rather than on their own or others' previous experiences. As a consequence, they are too optimistic, a phenomenon that Kahneman and Tversky labeled "the planning fallacy."

Do East Asians exhibit a similar disdain for memories of past experiences while estimating task completion times? The answer is apparently "yes." Buehler and his colleagues (Buehler, Otsubo, Lehman, Heine, & Griffin, 2004) found that Japanese participants were as likely as their Canadian counterparts to underestimate their task completion times and to ignore past experiences when making predictions. At least in this context, there is no evidence that East Asian university students make more use of the past to guide their predictions than do Canadian university students.

Prediction is about the future and may orient people away from the past. It seems likely that research in other decision-making domains will provide more convincing evidence of the directive function of autobiographical memory. Regardless, the prediction research suggests the value of studying directly how people use memory to guide their judgments and decisions. Until there is more research of this sort, whether or to what degree there are cultural differences in the directive functions of memory is still an open question.

Self-Enhancement

A great deal of social-psychological research on Western participants supports the idea that individuals are often motivated to think favorably about themselves. Wilson and Ross (2001) have shown that people can use autobiograph-

ical memories to support positive self-conceptions. In one set of studies, people evaluated their current selves (what they are like now) more favorably than they evaluated their past selves (what they were like several years earlier). While not denying that people can improve, Wilson and Ross observed that the retrospective criticism of past selves was often overly harsh and seemed to be motivated by a desire to enhance the current self. Individuals can be relatively pleased with their present selves, if they regard it as superior to their former selves. Even when they do not judge themselves to be perfect now, they can derive self-satisfaction by presuming that they are more mature, hardworking, and socially skilled now than they used to be.

Several studies have provided evidence that retrospective self-criticism is motivated by concerns for self-enhancement and does not simply reflect actual self-improvement (Wilson & Ross, 2001). For example, derogation of past selves is especially evident on important traits, occurs for self-appraisals but not for ratings of acquaintances, is more pronounced among high than among low self-esteem individuals, and occurs even when concurrent ratings imply that no actual improvement has transpired.

Ross and Wilson (2002) described a second way in which people use autobiographical memory to maintain or enhance positive self-regard. They asked participants to remember past incidents that reflected either favorably or poorly on themselves. They then asked participants to report how far away in time the incidents felt (e.g., *feels like yesterday* vs. *feels far away*). Participants reported feeling farther away in time from earlier experiences with unfavorable implications for their current self-views than from equally distant experiences with flattering implications. For example, participants who performed poorly in a course felt more distant from the course than did participants who performed well. This asymmetry in subjective time estimates occurs even when participants are first reminded of the exact date of the episode. According to Ross and Wilson, the asymmetry reflects the motivation to maintain favorable self-regard. By subjectively distancing an unflattering episode, individuals can attribute it to an inferior, earlier self and dissociate their current self from blame. In contrast, people can continue to claim credit for former accomplishments by feeling temporally close to such episodes.

The Wilson and Ross studies were conducted on Western participants. The use of memory to facilitate favorable self-appraisals contradicts a primary purpose of remembering in Confucian cultures. East Asians are exhorted to use memory as a means of attaining self-criticism and self-reflection (Wang & Conway, 2004). From this cultural perspective, individuals should use memory to attain actual self-improvement rather than the more illusory self-enhancement that seems to gratify Western participants. Therefore, East Asians should not derogate past selves to feel good about their current selves; nor should they feel farther away in time from unflattering episodes than from equally distant pleasing episodes. Recently, researchers obtained these very results (Ross, Heine, Wilson, & Sugimori, 2005) when they replicated the two memorial biases in Canadian samples but found these same biases to be absent in Japanese samples.

Just as people can use memory to support favorable views of themselves, they can also use it to maintain favorable views of their relationships and, consequently, their relational self. Karney and his associates (Karney & Coombs, 2000; Karney & Frye, 2002) found that Western participants' retrospective evaluations of their marriages followed a pattern that echoed the findings of Wilson and Ross for individual recall. Spouses remembered their earlier marital satisfaction as lower than their present satisfaction, even when it was actually higher (as evidenced by their actual ratings at the earlier time period). By underestimating their former satisfaction levels, individuals can create the illusion of marital improvement in the face of decline.

Other memory biases also help people maintain favorable evaluations of current relationships. Research on Western participants reveals that dating partners interpret past conflicts in a relationship-enhancing fashion. In a recent study, dating couples were asked to recall a conflict in which one partner was the perpetrator and the other was the victim (Cameron, Ross, & Holmes, 2002). Transgressions committed against intimates threaten a perpetrator's self-regard, as well as the happiness and security of a relationship. Consequently perpetrators should be particularly motivated to downplay the negative consequences of their actions. Relative to their victims, perpetrators described their actions as more justifiable and perceived greater improvement (in themselves, their victims, and the relationship) since the time of the transgression. Perpetrators were also more optimistic about the future of their relationship. Ironically, perpetrators were more confident that their relationship would persist than were control participants who were not asked to recall any transgression.

The studies by Karney, Cameron, and their respective associates were conducted with North American participants. We are unaware of any similar studies of participants from non-Western cultures. If the studies of intrapersonal memory biases serve as a reliable guide, then we should expect studies of East Asian participants to reveal less evidence of relation-enhancing memory biases. Relative to Western participants, East Asians should be more interested in learning from past problems and achieving genuine rather than illusory relationship improvement. Alternatively, given their cultural emphasis on interpersonal harmony and a relational self-construal, East Asians might exhibit similar or even greater memorial biases to enhance their significant relationships.

Emotional Expression and Memory

There is an extensive literature on similarities and differences across cultures in the experience, expression, and determinants of emotion (e.g., Kitayama & Markus, 1994; Oishi, 2002). Our purpose, rather than to review this research, is to examine the role of memory. Much of the research on emotion is retrospective in nature. For example, people are asked how frequently they felt various emotions in the last month (e.g., Eid & Diener, 2001). Such reports are retrospective constructions that can provide valuable information about people's beliefs and schemas. However, such constructions might or might not accurately characterize the original emotional experiences. Perhaps it is not surprising, then, that retrospective reports have been shown to be both accurate, in the sense that recollections are correlated with earlier online reports of mood (e.g., Feldman Barrett, 1997), and also biased by the rememberer's personality and beliefs about emotional experiences (Christensen, Wood, & Feldman Barrett, 2003; Feldman Barrett, 1997; Robinson & Clore, 2002).

Doubts about the accuracy of recalled emotions are particularly significant when researchers use recall as the basis for claiming cross-cultural differences in emotional experience. When asked to remember their past emotional experiences, European American and Canadian participants recall experiencing many more positive (e.g., happy) than negative emotions (e.g., sad) in their everyday lives. In contrast, samples of East Asian Americans and Canadians, as well as participants living in Japan, report experiencing about the same number of positive and negative emotions (Markus & Kitayama, 1994; Oishi, 2002; Ross, Xun, & Wilson, 2002). The cultural discrepancy appears to be especially strong for positive emotions: European Americans and Canadians recall experiencing positive emotions more frequently than do Asians. Along the same lines, surveys indicate that Japanese respondents report being less satisfied with their lives as a whole than do their counterparts in North America and Western Europe (e.g., Diener, Diener, & Diener, 1995; Kitayama, Markus, & Kurokawa, 2000; Veenhoven, 1993).

These research findings can be interpreted as indicating that Westerners experience a greater frequency of positive emotions on a daily basis than do their East Asian counterparts. Alternatively, perhaps Western and East Asian individuals experience about the same number of pleasant and unpleasant episodes, but Westerners recall a greater number of their pleasant experiences. Such a recall bias in Western cultures could reflect a cultural schema that happiness is important and common (Oishi, 2002). If this positive outlook is less evident in East Asia, then Westerners and East Asians might recruit memories that support their differing beliefs, with the result that Westerners recall more happy experiences.

Oishi (2002) compared retrospective accounts of emotion to daily diary and online reports of emotional experiences. He found that European and Asians Americans did not differ in daily diary reports of the quality of their day, or in online reports of current positive (e.g., pleasant, calm, happy) and negative moods (e.g., unpleasant, sad, worried). Interestingly, cultural differences clearly emerged at the end of the week, when participants were asked how good or bad the week was, or how often they had experienced different positive and negative moods. European Americans retrospectively reported greater satisfaction with the week and a higher frequency of positive emotions. Note that Asian Americans did not report a higher frequency of negative moods than did European Americans. Asians do not appear to accentuate the negative; they simply dwell less on their positive experiences than do their Western counterparts when recalling the past.

Oishi's (2002) data also raise a more profound question. Are East Asians truly less happy than their Western counterparts? The answer to this question depends on whether one focuses on current or retrospective reports. Certainly a good case could be made for the importance of memory: A current emotional experience is fleeting, whereas memory can be more enduring. As Oishi observed, "Retrospective judgments seem to be as important as actual experiences in understanding subjective experiences of well-being. . . . Online and global reports capture different but equally important aspects of well-being" (p. 1405).

Oishi's (2002) study is unlikely to be the final word on whether cross-cultural differences in emotional experience reflect retrospective biases or online differences in emotional experience. Other researchers using different samples and procedures might well find evidence of online differences. From our own perspective, the Oishi study is important for two reasons. First, it reminds us yet again that recall should never be assumed to be an exact replica of earlier experience—recall is a reconstruction of the past. Second, Oishi showed that retrospective reports can be psychologically significant even when they do not mirror online reports. As well, retrospective reports provide valuable information about cultural similarities and differences in people's beliefs and feelings.

INTERPERSONAL FUNCTIONS OF AUTOBIOGRAPHICAL MEMORY

Remembering is a private experience. Only rememberers can directly know their own thoughts and feelings. However, individuals often share reminiscences with each other, so remembering can be a social exchange as well. In conversations, people may invoke their memories of past occurrences to achieve a host of goals, including education, entertainment, mutual understanding, improved social bonds, and emotional regulation (Bluck, 2003; Pasupathi, 2001; Robinson & Swanson, 1990; Ross & Holmberg, 1990; Webster, 1997). Although the nature and frequency of conversations reflect the general norms of discourse in a culture, variations in sharing memory may also reveal how people interpret and remember events. As well, conversations about the past can further shape people's subsequent memories of the episodes.

Cross-cultural researchers have tended to focus on parent–child memory conversations (S. H. Choi, 1992; Miller, Fung, & Mintz, 1996; Miller, Wiley, Fung, & Liang, 1997; Minami & McCabe, 1995; Mullen & Yi, 1995; Wang, 2001b). This research is of particular interest, because theorists have argued that memory conversations between parents and children play a critical role in the development of autobiographical memory (see Nelson & Fivush, 2004). We begin our discussion of memory conversations by focusing on cultural variations in the interpersonal functions of memory and the associated differences in conversational styles and content. We then discuss memory conversations and their developmental implications for children's own memory operations.

Relationship Maintenance

Memory conversations permit individuals to sustain and enhance their relationships in a relatively effective and effortless manner. Sharing personal memories with others can elicit empathic and emotional responses that can serve to deepen intimacy between the conversational partners. As a result, such conversations are considered a valuable social practice in Western cultures (Fivush, 1994; Nelson, 1993; Pasupathi, 2001; Pillemer, 1998). This interpersonal function of memory seems to take a different form in East Asian cultures. Relationships among individuals are defined primarily by existing social orders and are thus less voluntary (Bond, 1991; Markus & Kitayama, 1991; Shweder et al., 1998; Triandis, 1989). Memory conversations in Eastern cultures tend to define and reinforce an individual's duties, obligations, and appropriate behavior, as well as to establish his or her position in a relational hierarchy.

The use of memory sharing to maintain positive relationships in Western cultures is illustrated in this European American mother's account of when and why she usually shared memories with her 4-year-old son (Wang, 2006, unpublished raw data):

> Every night at the dinner table, we talk about what happened during the day. We ask what happened during the day, whom he played with, what was the best thing about the day. Also I ask if anything made him sad during the day. Sometimes, about once a week, at bedtime I tell Jake memories about when he was a baby, things he did. He loves that. Jake always also loves to hear about memories of what my husband & I did when we were young. About once a month we get out videotapes of family trips that we've taken, that Jake has been on. That seems to be boring for the kids; they prefer talking about the vacation and remembering that way instead. We talk about happy memories usually. Sad or bad memories we normally only talk about if we're trying to say, "this happened last time, we don't want to have it happen again," like having to leave a restaurant for bad behavior. I share good memories, memories of times that I know Jake enjoyed, to see him smile, to share a happy moment remembering, to think of happy experiences that we might want to do again.

Accordingly, empirical studies have revealed that compared with Asian parents, European American parents are often more eager to engage their children in conversations about the past and focus more on the children's own feeling states during the conversations (Fivush & Wang, 2005; Martini, 1996; Minami & McCabe, 1995; Mullen & Yi, 1995; Wang, 2001b). During a 1-day observation of European American and Korean mother–child conversations, Mullen and Yi (1995) found that American mothers talked with their 3-year-olds about past events three times as often as Korean mothers did. Martini (1996) observed that during evening meals at home, European American parents were twice as likely as Japanese American parents to ask their children to talk about past events.

In a related series of studies, researchers have examined mother–child conversations about emotional events (Fivush & Wang, 2005; Wang, 2001b; Wang & Fivush, 2005). When European American and Chinese mothers were asked to nominate positive events to discuss with their children, they chose similar types of occurrences. In both groups, the majority of events (U.S. parents, 81%, Chinese parents, 83%) concerned family activities, parties, vacations, and holiday events (Wang & Fivush, 2005). The memory conversations were similar in length, and mothers in both cultures spoke more than their children. Nevertheless, compared with Chinese mothers and children, European American mothers and children engaged in more interactive conversations about these happy episodes, whereby mother and child frequently took turns in participating in the conversation (Wang, 2001b; Wang & Fivush, 2005).

When discussing negative emotional experiences, European American mother–child dyads were also more interactive than were Chinese dyads. Furthermore, the negative events most frequently selected by American mothers concerned child injuries/illnesses (26%), and frightening events and objects such as thunderstorms and monsters (26%). After the conversation, American mothers often reassured their children that everything was all right (e.g., "It's really nothing to be scared about in the pool. Daddy was there, and you've got a big floater"). A focus on the child's emotions and the mother's corresponding sympathetic responses conceivably helps to reinforce the intimacy of a conversational exchange. Chinese mothers, however, most frequently selected social conflicts between their children and significant others, such as parents and peers (58%). The significant other was frequently a third party that was not present during the memory conversation. Chinese mothers often tried to restore the harmonious relationship between the child and the individual who caused the negative emotion in the child (e.g., "Dad didn't let you play with that bottle because it's dangerous to little children. He loves you"). They also taught children "moral lessons" about the inappropriateness of their negative emotional experience or behavior (e.g., "Isn't it wrong for you to get mad at Papa?"). Chinese mothers seem to use memory conversations to resolve conflicts between the child and significant others, and to establish the child's proper place in his or her social world (Wang, 2004b).

Emotional Regulation

In Western cultures, most scientific researchers and advice columnists emphasize the harmful effects of bottling up emotions, as well as the benefits of discussing stressful experiences with others, including therapists (for reviews, see Pennebaker, Zech, & Rimé, 2001; Rimé, Corsini, & Herbette, 2002; see van Emmerik, Kamphuis, Hulsbosch, & Emmelkamp, 2002, for a dissenting opinion). In traditional Chinese medicine there are indications of Western-like talk therapies. However, Chinese patients often expect an "authoritative" physician to detect their emotional problems from nonverbal cues

and are reluctant to provide elaborate accounts. Professional psychotherapy and counseling services appear to be more recent trends in China (Cheung, 1986).

The use of memory talk for therapeutic emotional regulation is further shaped by different cultural beliefs concerning emotion and emotion sharing, which are often mirrored in divergent socialization goals and practices. Studies with Western families indicate that early family emotional discourse, including references to feeling states and causal explanations, helps children to understand and to regulate their emotions (Bretherton, Fritz, Zahn-Waxler, & Ridgeway, 1986; Denham & Kochanoff, 2002; Denham, Zoller, & Couchoud, 1994; Dunn, Brown, & Beardsall, 1991; Fivush, Berlin, Sales, Mennuti-Washburn, & Cassidy, 2003). In memory conversations about positive or negative emotional experiences with their 3-year-old children, European American mothers often employed a "cognitive approach" to emotional regulation (Wang, 2001b; Wang & Fivush, 2005). The mothers frequently talked with their children about the causes and consequences of feeling states and provided elaborate explanations as to why and how an emotion was experienced. Such emotional discourse highlights the personal importance of emotion and facilitates the development of children's emotional understanding and regulation. The following conversational excerpt of an American mother and her 3-year-old daughter is illustrative (Wang & Fivush, 2005):

MOTHER: . . . Do you remember doing some crying?

CHILD: Why did I cry?

MOTHER: I'm not quite sure why you cried. But do you remember where you were?

CHILD: I cried because I had any, no any balloon.

MOTHER: They had no balloons. But then, were you also crying because, did you not want to go home?

CHILD: Yeah.

MOTHER: Where were you?

CHILD: At Stewart Park!

MOTHER: (*Laughs.*) You did cry a lot at Stewart Park, but, um, this was in Joe's parking lot. Do you remember Joe's Restaurant parking lot? Do you remember standing by the door and crying?

CHILD: Yeah.

MOTHER: You do?

CHILD: Yeah.

MOTHER: What were you crying about?

CHILD: 'Cause I didn't wanted to leave yet; it was because I wanted to eat.

MOTHER: Oh, you wanted to eat some more (*laughs*). Is that why?

CHILD: Yeah.

MOTHER: Hmm. I remember Mommy tried to pick you up and you put up a little bit of a fight. You were crying real hard. Maybe it was 'cause of the balloon and maybe it was 'cause you were hungry. But we knew that you could get another balloon, right?

CHILD: Yep.

In contrast, Chinese mothers tended to use a "behavioral approach" to emotional regulation that focused on proper behavior and provided few causal explanations for the emotion itself. Although mothers attributed emotions to the child and other people involved in the memory event, they rarely went further to discuss the causes and consequences of the emotions. Emotion, particularly negative affect, was often depicted as a result of the child's past wrongdoing. Mothers led their children to the understanding that they should behave properly in the future to avoid negative emotion. The following conversational excerpt between a Chinese mother and her 3-year-old son is illustrative (Wang & Fivush, 2005):

MOTHER: Do you remember why Dad spanked you last time?

CHILD: Chess!

MOTHER: Why chess? What did you do with chess?

CHILD: Not obedient!

MOTHER: How were you not being obedient?

CHILD: I threw the pieces on the floor.

MOTHER: All over the floor, right? And did you do it on purpose?

CHILD: Umm. I'll be careful next time!

MOTHER: Right! That's why Dad spanked your bottom, right? . . . Did you cry then?

CHILD: I cried.

MOTHER: Did it hurt?

CHILD: It hurt.

MOTHER: It hurt? It doesn't hurt anymore, right?

CHILD: Right. I'll be careful next time.

MOTHER: Umm, be careful.

Studies of adults have suggested cultural variation with regard to how, when, with whom, and to what extent emotions are shared in memory conversations (Rimé et al., 2001, 2002). Koreans reported that 20% of their emotional experiences were never shared; for U.S. participants, the comparable figure was only 5%. French and U.S. respondents also claimed to have repetitively shared a single emotional episode with others more frequently (about five times) than did Korean, Singapore, and Japanese respondents (two or three times). In addition, Westerners reported sharing the emotional event sooner after its occurrence (a delay of 1 or 2 days) than did Asians (4–5 days in the case of Singaporeans). Although people in both Western and Asian cultures reported sharing emotions most frequently with best friends and rarely with strangers, French and U.S. participants were more inclined to share emotions with their family members (spouse, parents, siblings, and grandparents) than were Asians (see Rimé et al., 2002). These findings should be treated with caution, because they depend on the accuracy of people's retrospective reports of frequency and dates, which can be quite unreliable (e.g., Tanur, 1992). Nonetheless, the findings again suggest varied cultural views of the social sharing of emotional experiences and the functions such memory conversations may serve.

Memory Conversations and the Development of Autobiographical Memory

Early parent–child memory sharing appears to be critical to the emergence and development of autobiographical memory (Nelson & Fivush, 2004). Parents play a guiding role as they discuss shared experiences and encourage their children's active participation in the conversations. These exchanges show children how to represent memory information verbally and provide them with a framework for organizing and structuring their personal memories (Harley & Reese, 1999; Leichtman, Pillemer, Wang, Koreishi, & Han, 2000; McCabe & Peterson, 1991; Fivush, 1994). By modeling par-

ents' conversational styles and ways of thinking and talking about the past, children further
learn to evaluate, remember, and share past experiences in a culturally acceptable fashion
(e.g., Minami & McCabe, 1995; Wang &
Brockmeier, 2002). Culture-specific ways of
memory sharing may thus have important consequences for children's developing autobiographical memory.

Memory conversations differ across cultures
in content and in the degree of elaboration and
support that mothers provide to their young
children (S. H. Choi, 1992; Martini, 1996;
Minami & McCabe, 1995; Mullen & Yi, 1995;
Wang, 2001b; Wang & Fivush, 2005; Wang,
Leichtman, & Davies, 2000). Western mothers
often engage their children in elaborate memory
conversations, in which they provide detailed information and feedback to maintain children's
active participation. Moreover, Western mothers frequently focus discussions on their children's roles and predilections, asking them what
they want, what they think, and how they feel.
Such conversations provide a model of autobiographical memory that highlights the child's role
as an autonomous being with distinctive and
unique characteristics. Asian mothers, in contrast, often play a directive role when sharing
memories with their children. They tend to initiate test-like conversations, provide less elaboration or help to engage the child, and place past
events in a relational context by focusing on
group actions. Consistent with a cultural emphasis on the moral value of the past, Asian parents often include teaching and moralizing in
their conversations with their children (Miller et
al., 1996, 1997; Mullen & Yi, 1995; Wang,
2001b, 2004b; Wang et al., 2000). Such conversations direct children to pay attention to the
roles of significant others and to monitor their
own behavioral conduct when remembering
past experiences.

The stylistic and content differences in early
parent–child reminiscing are mirrored in children's independent memory reports (Han et al.,
1998; Wang, 2004a; Wang & Leichtman,
2000). When recounting their personal experiences with a researcher, European American
preschool and grade school children often provide elaborate and detailed memory narratives,
and frequently comment on their own feelings,
preferences, and opinions. In comparison,
Asian children often provide "bare-bones" accounts of the past, speak frequently of significant others and social interactions, and show a
concern for moral correctness and authority.

Although Asian parents generally provide
less support than Western parents to encourage
their children to give detailed recollections during memory conversations, some mothers in
both cultures are more elaborative than others.
For instance, within a culture, mothers differ in
the degree to which they use elaborative questions during memory conversations with their
young children (e.g., "Do you remember what
we did at the party?"). Differences in maternal
reminiscing style appear to have both immediate and long-term influences on children's remembering. Western children whose mothers
are highly elaborative provide more detailed
memories to their mothers during the memory
conversations. Moreover, these same children
independently provide more detailed personal
memories weeks and even years later (e.g.,
Harley & Reese, 1999; McCabe & Peterson,
1991). In a recent longitudinal study with native Chinese families in China, immigrant Chinese families in the United States, and European American families, Wang (2005, in press)
found the same pattern of results. Maternal
reminiscing styles had immediate and long-
term effects on children's shared and independent recall. More important from the current
perspective, mothers' use of elaborations was
positively associated with their value orientation toward independence and an autonomous
self-construal.

This research suggests that early parent–
child memory conversations lead children to
remember and talk about their personal experiences in culturally acceptable ways. As Pillemer
(1998) noted, "Parents' implicit or explicit
communicative goals influence which functions
will assume center stage in the child's own
memory operations" (p. 129).

LANGUAGE AND MEMORY

If parent–child memory conversations are critical to the development of autobiographical
memory, then it would seem that language is
also important to the development of autobiographical memory. However, language is not
essential for remembering. Dogs recognize people and remember how to respond to verbal
and physical commands. Young infants remember faces, voices, pictures, and actions long before they acquire language (Bauer, 2002). Although language is not essential for memory, it
probably is necessary for autobiographical
memory (Nelson & Fivush, 2004). It is unlikely

that dogs or young infants possess autobiographical memory, which would include details such as where, when, and why they acquired their knowledge.

Language plays a role in a young child's developing memory skills by providing both a communicative and a representational tool for remembering (Nelson & Fivush, 2004). Through narrative practices and language socialization in general (e.g., Ochs, 1996), language serves as an important vehicle for cultural messages about what to remember, how to remember, and why to remember it. Some theorists argue that the social-cognitive shift associated with the acquisition of language helps to explain people's inability to remember events from their first years of life (Neisser, 1962; Schachtel, 1947). Schachtel attributed early memory loss to the shift from preverbal to language-based cognitive schemas. According to Schachtel, this shift produces new modes of social-cognitive activity that cannot be fully integrated with earlier representations; as a result, very few early memories are preserved. A study by Simcock and Hayne (2002) provides support for Schachtel's proposal that children cannot translate prelinguistic experience into language. Young children participated in a unique event, and their memories were assessed 6 months or 1 year later. Children demonstrated both verbal and nonverbal memory of the event. Yet children *never* recalled any information about the event in words if they could not talk about that information when the event first occurred, even though they had acquired the language skills to do so by the time of recall.

Researchers have also studied the effects of acquiring a second language on recall. Cultural practices and meanings are so deeply embedded in language that the acquisition of a second language often entails the establishment of a new cognitive system—schemas, mental models or representations—that reflects new ways of construing the social and physical world (Kim, 2002; Ochs, 1996; Schrauf, 2000; Valsiner, 2001). As a result, bilingual individuals may possess separate knowledge structures that are activated by the associated language. Ross and colleagues (2002) surveyed Chinese-born bilingual students living in Canada. The survey was conducted in either Chinese or English. Those who participated in Chinese described themselves in more collective terms and endorsed traditional Chinese values more strongly than did those surveyed in English. Indeed, the responses of the bilingual group interviewed in English were barely distinguishable from the responses of European Canadians.

In a related experiment, Hoffman, Lau, and Johnson (1986) had Chinese–English bilinguals read character descriptions written in either English or Chinese and respond to questions using the language of the descriptions. Some of the descriptions reflected a personality type, with an economical label or schema available in English but not in Chinese (liberal type, artistic type). Some of the descriptions reflected a personality type with an economical label available in Chinese but not in English. For example the Chinese term *shi-gu* applies to a person who has traveled a lot, has varied job experiences, is devoted to his family, and has good interpersonal skills. Although each of these attributes is familiar to English speakers, there is no English personality term or schema that readily captures the complete set of attributes. After reading the passages, participants were tested for their ability to recognize statements from the descriptions. Those participating in Chinese showed better recognition for statements from descriptions that had economical Chinese labels. Those writing in English showed better recognition for statements from descriptions that had economical English labels. In short, memory was better if participants could link the material to preexisting, language-specific cognitive schemas.

The association between cognitive frameworks and language further implies that people should remember events better in the language in which they originally encoded them. Marian and Neisser (2000) tested this hypothesis on Russian–English bilinguals and found language-dependent recall. Participants retrieved more memories from the Russian-speaking period of their lives when interviewed in Russian, and more memories from the English-speaking period of their lives when interviewed in English. In addition, memories recalled in English tended to be more self-focused, whereas memories recalled in Russian were more other-oriented (Marian & Kaushanskaya, 2004), suggesting that language at retrieval can bring memory in line with cultural value systems. Schrauf and his colleagues have also shown that bilingual immigrants can recall childhood events (occurring in the country of origin) better in their mother tongue than in their adopted language (Larsen, Schrauf, Fromholt, & Rubin, 2002; Schrauf, 2000; Schrauf & Rubin, 2000). Moreover, people's internal language of retrieval is consistent with the language at encoding. For instance, Hispanic bilingual immigrants in the United States report retrieving autobiographical memories in Spanish for events occurring in their country of origin, and in English for events occurring in the United States (Schrauf & Rubin, 2000). These findings suggest that memory information is specific to the semantic and lexical systems of the language at encoding and is more accessible when congruent systems are activated at retrieval (Marian & Neisser, 2000; Schrauf, 2000).

AGING, MEMORY, AND CULTURE

In contrast to the rather extensive cross-cultural literature on children's memory, there is relatively little cross-cultural research being conducted at the opposite end of the age spectrum. Psychological research on Western participants reveals age-related declines in memory (Craik, 2000). Is the memory decline in later adulthood a cultural artifact due to negative stereotypes about aging? Levy and Langer (1994) reported a study that seemed to support this view. They hypothesized that in cultures such as China, where attitudes toward the elderly are more favorable than in the West, age-related declines in memory should be less apparent. Levy and Langer provided nonverbal memory tests to younger and older mainland Chinese and to Americans. Older Chinese performed better than their American counterparts, and not significantly worse than younger Chinese. As is typically the case on these types of memory tests, younger Americans outperformed older Americans.

Yoon, Hasher, Feinberg, and Rahhal (2000) noted several problems with the Levy and Langer (1994) study, ranging from low sample sizes to the possibility that the memory test might have been biased in favor of the Chinese. Yoon and colleagues (2000) studied older and younger Chinese Canadians who had lived in Canada for less than 5 years, as well as older and younger Anglophone Canadians. Their main finding was that, regardless of culture, younger adults outperformed older adults on a variety of memory tests. On two memory tests that might be biased in favor of Chinese participants (as a result of differing cognitive processing abilities engaged by written Chinese and English), older Chinese outperformed the

older Anglophone Canadians, but still did not perform as well as their younger Chinese counterparts. At this point in time, there does not seem to be strong evidence of cultural differences in age-related memory decline.

LOOKING AHEAD

We have shown that culture contributes to how, when, what people remember, and whether they judge remembering to be important at all. We have also shown that cultural influences take place in the larger context of setting the goals and purposes of remembering, in the interpersonal sphere of daily mnemonic practices and exchanges, and at the individual level of shaping cognitive schemas and memory strategies. As both a system and a process of symbolic mediation, culture manifests itself in memory construction via multiple pathways (e.g., Cohen & Gunz, 2002; Kearins, 1981; Ross et al., 2005; Wang, Hutt, Kulkofsky, McDermott, & Wei, 2006).

In recent decades, Western countries have opened their borders to increasing numbers of immigrants from Asian cultures, and psychologists are now shifting their focus from international comparisons of cognition and behavior to an examination of Asian immigrants. Many of these immigrants lead a bicultural life, switching cultural frames and identities across situations and languages (Benet-Martinez, Leu, Lee, & Morris, 2002; Perunovic, Ross, & Wilson, 2005). In this multicultural context, experimental and longitudinal studies of development will be needed to reveal how cultural influences are transmitted to and internalized by individuals, and further manifested in their memory operations. Future research should also go beyond the East–West dichotomy and examine other cultures, as well as heterogeneity within a culture, such as differences in demographic patterns, economic progress, and educational facilities.

Finally, a historical perspective will further our understanding of the influence of culture and cultural transformation on the workings and functions of memory. The changing nature of autobiography illustrates the potential value of historical analyses. Since its emergence, autobiography has been undergoing continuous changes in accordance with the cultural and technological changes in contemporary societies. In recent years, the tendency toward public self-revelation and autobiographical accounting has perhaps reached new heights in the form of blogs posted for all interested viewers on the Internet. The postings are selective and idiosyncratic, but then so are most autobiographies. Researchers interested in autobiographical memory will no doubt avail themselves of this rich Internet resource that has the potential to transcend many linguistic and cultural boundaries.

At the outset, we noted that the subject of memory in general, and autobiographical memory in particular, has received increasing attention in recent years. The extensive theories and empirical findings we have discussed in this chapter further elucidate an exciting field of scientific inquiry. Still greater efforts are required from memory researchers in different fields of psychology, in collaboration with those in anthropology, sociology, education, ethnography, linguistics, philosophy, and literature, to take a multidisciplinary approach and draw on diverse theoretical perspectives to address the central role of culture in remembering. Only then can we reach a genuine understanding of human difference, experience, and complexity in the processes and functions of memory.

REFERENCES

Anderson, R. C., & Pichert, J. W. (1978). Recall of previously unrecallable information following a shift in perspective. *Journal of Verbal Learning and Verbal Behavior, 17*, 1–12.

Antze, P. (1996). Telling stories, making selves: Memory and identity in multiple personality disorder. In P. Antze & M. Lambek (Eds.), *Tense past: Cultural essays in trauma and memory* (pp. 3–24). New York: Routledge.

Bartlett, F. C. (1932). *Remembering: A study in experimental and social psychology.* New York: Cambridge University Press.

Bauer, P. J. (2002). Early memory development. In U. Goswami (Ed.), *Blackwell handbook of childhood cognitive development* (pp. 127–146). Oxford, UK: Blackwell.

Baumeister, R. F. (1987). How the self became a problem: A psychological review of historical research. *Journal of Personality and Social Psychology, 52*, 163–176.

Benet-Martinez, V., Leu, J., Lee, F., & Morris, M. W. (2002). Negotiating biculturalism: Cultural frame switching in biculturals with oppositional versus compatible identities. *Journal of Cross-Cultural Psychology, 33*, 492–516.

Bienstock, R. E., Grogan, M., & Smith, H. (Producers). (2003, September). *Penn & Teller's magic and mystery tour* [Television broadcast]. CBC Documentary Special.

Bluck, S. (2003). Autobiographical memory: Exploring its functions in everyday life. *Memory, 11*, 165–178.

Bond, M. H. (1991). *Beyond the Chinese face.* Hong Kong: Oxford University Press.

Bretherton, I., Fritz, J., Zahn-Waxler, C., & Ridgeway, D. (1986). Learning to talk about emotions: A functionalist perspective. *Child Development, 57*, 529–548.

Brockmeier, J., & Carbaugh, D. (Eds.). (2001). *Narrative and identity: Studies in autobiography, self and culture.* Amsterdam: Benjamins.

Bruner, J. (1990). *Acts of meaning.* Cambridge, MA: Harvard University Press.

Buehler, R., Griffin, D., & Ross, M. (1994). Exploring the "planning fallacy": Why people underestimate their task completion times. *Journal of Personality and Social Psychology, 67*, 366–381.

Buehler, R., Griffin, D., & Ross, M. (2002). Inside the planning fallacy: The causes and consequences of optimistic time predictions. In G. Thomas, D. Griffin, & D. Kahneman (Eds.), *Heuristics and biases: The psychology of intuitive judgement* (pp. 250–270). New York: Cambridge University Press.

Buehler, R., Otsubo, Y., Lehman, D. R., Heine, S. T., & Griffin, D. (2004). *Culture and optimism: The planning fallacy in Japan and North America.* Unpublished manuscript, Wilfrid Laurier University, Waterloo, Ontario, Canada.

Cameron, J. J., Ross, M., & Holmes, J. G. (2002). Loving the one you hurt: Positive effects of recounting a transgression against an intimate partner. *Journal of Experimental Social Psychology, 38*, 307–314.

Carruthers, M. J. (1990). *The book of memory: A study of memory in Medieval culture.* New York: Cambridge University Press.

Catholic Update. (2003, March). Available online at www.americancatholic.org/Newsletters/CU.asp

Cheung, F. M. C. (1986). Psychopathology among Chinese people. In M. H. Bond (Ed.), *The psychology of the Chinese people* (pp. 171–212). Hong Kong: Oxford University Press.

Chiu, C. Y., Morris, M. W., Hong, Y. Y., & Menon, T. (2000). Motivated cultural cognition: The impact of implicit cultural theories on dispositional attribution varies as a function of need for closure. *Journal of Personality and Social Psychology, 78*, 247–259.

Choi, I., Nisbett, R. E., & Norenzayan, A. (1999). Causal attribution across cultures: Variation and universality. *Psychological Bulletin, 125*, 47–63.

Choi, S. H. (1992). Communicative socialization processes: Korea and Canada. In S. Iwasaki, Y. Kashima, & K. Leung (Eds.), *Innovations in cross-cultural psychology* (pp. 103–122). Amsterdam: Swets & Zeitlinger.

Christensen, T. C., Wood, J. V., & Feldman Barrett, L. (2003). Remembering everyday experience through the prism of self-esteem. *Personality and Social Psychology Bulletin, 29,* 51–62.

Cohen, D., & Gunz, A. (2002). As seen by the other . . .: Perspectives on the self in the memories and emotional perceptions of Easterners and Westerners. *Psychological Science, 13,* 55–59.

Conway, M., & Pleydell-Pearce, C. W. (2000). The construction of autobiographical memories in the self-memory system. *Psychological Review, 107,* 261–288.

Craik, F. I. M. (2000). Age-related changes in human memory. In D. C. Park & N. Schwarz (Eds.), *Cognitive aging: A primer* (pp. 75–92). Philadelphia: Psychology Press.

D'Andrade, R. G. (1992). Schemas and motivation. In R. G. D'Andrade & C. Strauss (Eds.), *Human motives and cultural models* (pp. 23–44). New York: Cambridge University Press.

Dekker, R. (2000). *Childhood, memory and autobiography in Holland: From the Golden Age to Romanticism.* New York: St. Martin's Press.

Denham, S. A., & Kochanoff, A.T. (2002). Parental contributions to preschoolers' understanding of emotion. *Marriage and Family Review, 34,* 311–343.

Denham, S. A., Zoller, D., & Couchoud, E. A. (1994). Socialization of preschoolers' emotion understanding. *Developmental Psychology, 30,* 928–936.

Deshpande, C. G. (1996). Memory as depicted in Eastern and Western thoughts. *Psycho-Lingua, 26*(2), 57–65.

Diener, E., Diener, M., & Diener, C. (1995). Factors predicting the subjective well-being of nations. *Journal of Personality and Social Psychology, 69,* 851–864.

Dunn, J., Brown, J., & Beardsall, L. (1991). Family talk about feeling states and children's later understanding of others' emotions. *Developmental Psychology, 27,* 448–455.

Eid, M., & Diener, E. (2001). Norms for experiencing emotions in different cultures: Inter- and intranational differences. *Journal of Personality and Social Psychology, 81,* 869–885.

Feldman Barrett, L. (1997). The relationships among momentary emotion experiences, personality descriptions, and retrospective ratings of emotion. *Personality and Social Psychology Bulletin, 23,* 1100–1110.

Fiske, A. P., Kitayama, S., Markus, H. R., & Nisbett, R. E. (1998). The cultural matrix of social psychology. In D. T. Gilbert, S. T. Fiske, & G. Lindzey (Eds.), *The handbook of social psychology* (Vol. 2, 4th ed., pp. 915–981). Boston: McGraw-Hill.

Fivush, R. (1994). Constructing narrative, emotions, and self in parent–child conversations about the past. In U. Neisser & R. Fivush (Eds.), *The remembering self: Construction and accuracy in the self-narrative* (pp. 136–157). New York: Cambridge University Press.

Fivush, R., Berlin, L. J., Sales, J. M., Mennuti-Washburn, J., & Cassidy, J. (2003). Functions of parent–child reminiscing about emotionally negative events. *Memory, 11,* 179–192.

Fivush, R., & Wang, Q. (2005). Emotion talk in mother–child conversations of the shared past: The effects of culture, gender, and event valence. *Journal of Cognition and Development, 6*(4), 489–506.

Geertz, C. (1973). *The interpretation of cultures.* New York: Basic Books.

Han, J. J., Leichtman, M. D., & Wang, Q. (1998). Autobiographical memory in Korean, Chinese, and American children. *Developmental Psychology, 34,* 701–713.

Harley, K., & Reese, E. (1999). Origins of autobiographical memory. *Developmental Psychology, 35,* 1338–1348.

Herman, J. (1992). *Trauma and recovery: The aftermath of violence—from domestic abuse to political terror.* New York: Basic Books.

Hoffman, C. Lau, I., & Johnson, D. R. (1986). The linguistic relativity of person cognition: An English–Chinese comparison. *Journal of Personality and Social Psychology, 51*(6), 1097–1105.

Holland, D., & Quinn, N. (Eds.). (1987). *Cultural models in language and thought.* New York: Cambridge University Press.

Hong, Y. Y., Morris, M. W., Chiu, C. Y., & Benet-Martinez, V. (2000). Multicultural minds: A dynamic constructivist approach to culture and cognition. *American Psychologist, 55,* 709–720.

Hume, D. (1882). *A treatise of human nature* (Vol. 1). London: Longmans Green. (Original work published 1739)

Kağitçibaşi, Ç. (1996). *Family and human development across cultures: A view from the other side.* Hillsdale, NJ: Erlbaum.

Kahneman, D., & Tversky, A. (1979). On the interpretation of intuitive probability: A reply to Jonathan Cohen. *Cognition, 7,* 409–411.

Karney, B. R., & Coombs, R. H. (2000). Memory bias in long-term close relationships: Consistency or improvement? *Personality and Social Psychology Bulletin, 26,* 959–970.

Karney, B. R., & Frye, N. E. (2002). "But we've been getting better lately": Comparing prospective and retrospective views of relationship development. *Journal of Personality and Social Psychology, 82,* 222–238.

James, W. (1950). *Principles of psychology.* New York: Dover. (Original work published 1890)

Kearins, J. M. (1981). Visual spatial memory in Australian aboriginal children of the desert regions. *Cognitive Psychology, 13,* 434–460.

Kearins, J. M. (1986). Visual spatial memory in Aboriginal and White Australian children. *Australian Journal of Psychology, 38,* 203–214.

Kim, H. S. (2002). We talk therefore we think?: A cultural analysis of the effect of talking on thinking. *Journal of Personality and Social Psychology, 4,* 828–842.

Kitayama, S., & Markus, H. R. (Eds.). (1994). *Emotion and culture.* Washington, DC: American Psychological Association.

Kitayama, S., Markus, H. R., & Kurokawa, M. (2000). Culture, emotion, and well-being: Good feelings in Japan and the United States. *Cognition and Emotion, 14*, 93–124.

Larsen, S. F., Schrauf, R. W., Fromholt, P., & Rubin, D. C. (2002). Inner speech and bilingual autobiographical memory: A Polish–Danish cross-cultural study. *Memory, 10*, 45–54.

Leichtman, M. D., Pillemer, D. B., Wang, Q., Koreishi, A., & Han, J. J. (2000). When Baby Maisy came to school: Mothers' interview styles and preschoolers' event memories. *Cognitive Development, 15*, 1–16.

Levy, B., & Langer, E. (1994). Aging free from negative stereotypes: Successful memory in China and among the American deaf. *Journal of Personality and Social Psychology, 66*(6), 989–997.

Lin, Y. T. (1939). *My country and my people.* New York: John Day.

Lowenthal, D. (1985). *The past is a foreign country.* New York: Cambridge University Press.

MacDonald, S., Uesiliana, K., & Hayne, H. (2000). Cross-cultural and gender differences in childhood amnesia. *Memory, 8*, 365–376.

Marian, V., & Kaushanskaya, M. (2004). Self-construal and emotion in bicultural bilinguals. *Journal of Memory and Language, 51*, 190–201.

Marian, V., & Neisser, U. (2000). Language-dependent recall of autobiographical memories. *Journal of Experimental Psychology: General, 129*, 361–368.

Markus, H. R., & Kitayama, S. (1991). Culture and the self: Implications for cognition, emotion, and motivation. *Psychological Review, 98*, 224–253.

Markus, H. R., & Kitayama, S. (1994). The cultural construction of self and emotion: Implications for social behavior. In S. Kitayama & H. R. Markus (Eds.), *Emotion and culture: Empirical studies of mutual influence* (pp. 89–130). Washington, DC: American Psychological Association.

Martini, M. (1996). "What's new?" at the dinner table: Family dynamics during mealtimes in two cultural groups in Hawaii. *Early Development and Parenting, 5*, 23–34.

Mascolo, M. F., & Li, J. (Eds.). (2004). *Culture and developing selves: Beyond dichotomization.* San Francisco: Jossey-Bass.

Masuda, T., & Nisbett, R. E. (2001) Attending holistically versus analytically: Comparing the context sensitivity of Japanese and Americans. *Journal of Personality and Social Psychology, 81*, 922–934.

McAdams, D. P. (1993). *The stories we live by: Personal myths and the making of the self.* New York: Morrow.

McCabe, A., & Peterson, C. (1991). Getting the story: A longitudinal study of parental styles in eliciting narratives and developing narrative skill. In A. McCabe & C. Peterson (Eds.), *Developing narrative structure* (pp. 217–253). Hillsdale, NJ: Erlbaum.

Miller, P. J., Fung, H., & Mintz, J. (1996). Self-construction through narrative practices: A Chinese and American comparison of early socialization. *Ethos, 24*, 237–280.

Miller, P. J., Wiley, A. R., Fung, H., & Liang, C. H. (1997). Personal storytelling as a medium of socialization in Chinese and American families. *Child Development, 68*, 557–568.

Minami, M., & McCabe, A. (1991). *Haiku* as a discourse regulation device: A stanza analysis of Japanese children's personal narratives. *Language in Society, 20*, 577–599.

Minami, M., & McCabe, A. (1995). Rice balls and bear hunts: Japanese and North American family narrative patterns. *Journal of Child Language, 22*, 423–445.

Mullen, M. K. (1994). Earliest recollections of childhood: A demographic analysis. *Cognition, 52*, 55–79.

Mullen, M. K., & Yi, S. (1995). The cultural context of talk about the past: Implications for the development of autobiographical memory. *Cognitive Development, 10*, 407–419.

Nakamura, H. (1964). *Ways of thinking of Eastern peoples: India, China, Tibet, and Japan.* Honolulu: East–West Center Press.

Nelson, K. (1993). Explaining the emergence of autobiographical memory in early childhood. In A. F. Collins, S. E. Gathercole, M. A., Conway, & P. E. Morris (Eds.), *Theories of memory* (pp. 355–385). Hillsdale, NJ: Erlbaum.

Nelson, K. (1996). *Language in cognitive development: The emergence of the mediated mind.* New York: Cambridge University Press.

Nelson, K., & Fivush, R. (2004). The emergence of autobiographical memory: A social cultural developmental theory. *Psychological Review, 111*, 486–511.

Neisser, U. (1962). Cultural and cognitive discontinuity. In T. E. Gladwin & W. C. Sturtevant (Eds.), *Anthropology and human behavior* (pp. 54–71). Washington, DC: Anthropological Society of Washington.

Neisser, U. (1967). *Cognitive psychology.* East Norwalk, CT: Appleton–Century–Crofts.

Neisser, U. (1982). Memory: What are the important questions? In U. Neisser (Ed.), *Memory observed* (pp. 3–19). San Francisco: Freeman.

Ochs, E. (1996). Linguistic resources for socialising humanity. In J. Gumperz & S. Levinson (Eds.), *Rethinking linguistic reality* (pp. 407–437). Cambridge, UK: Cambridge University Press.

Oishi, S. (2002). The experiencing and remembering of well-being: A cross-cultural analysis. *Personality and Social Psychology Bulletin, 28*, 1398–1406.

Pasupathi, M. (2001). The social construction of the personal past and its implications for adult development. *Psychological Bulletin, 127*, 651–672.

Pennebaker, J. W., Zech, E., & Rimé, B. (2001). Disclosing and sharing emotion: Psychological, social, and health consequences. In R. O. Hansson & M. S. Stroebe (Eds.), *Handbook of bereavement research: Consequences, coping, and care* (pp. 517–543). Washington, DC: American Psychological Association.

Perunovic, W. Q. E., Ross, M., & Wilson, A. E. (2005).

Language, culture, and conceptions of the self. In R. M. Sorrentino, D. Cohen, J. M. Olson, & M. P. Zanna (Eds.), *Cultural and social behavior: The Ontario Symposium* (Vol. 10, pp. 165–180). Mahwah, NJ: Erlbaum.

Pillemer, D. B. (1998). *Momentous events, vivid memories.* Cambridge, MA: Harvard University Press.

Pillemer, D. B. (2003). Directive functions of autobiographical memory: The guiding power of the specific episode. *Memory, 11,* 193–202.

Pillemer, D. B., & White, S. H. (1989). Childhood events recalled by children and adults. In H. W. Reese (Ed.), *Advances in child development and behavior* (Vol. 21, pp. 297–340). New York: Academic Press.

Rimé, B., Corsini, S., & Herbette, G. (2002). Emotion, verbal expression, and the social sharing of emotion. In S. R. Fussell (Ed.), *The verbal communication of emotions: Interdisciplinary perspectives* (pp. 185–208). Mahwah, NJ: Erlbaum.

Rimé, B., Finkenauer, C., Mesquita, B., Pennebaker, J. W., Singh-Manoux, A., & Yogo, M. (2001, July). The social sharing of emotion: An overview of cross-cultural data. In Q. Wang & M. A. Conway (Cochairs), *Memory and culture.* Symposium conducted at the third International Conference on Memory, Valencia, Spain.

Robinson, J. A., & Swanson, K. L. (1990). Autobiographical memory: The next phase. *Applied Cognitive Psychology, 4,* 321–335.

Robinson, M. D., & Clore, G. L. (2002). Belief and feeling: Evidence for an accessibility model of emotional self-report. *Psychological Bulletin, 128,* 934–960.

Rogers, T. B., Kuiper, N. A., & Kirker, W. S. (1977). Self-reference and the encoding of personal information. *Journal of Personality and Social Psychology, 35,* 677–688.

Ross, M. (1989). Relation of implicit theories to the construction of personal histories. *Psychological Review, 96,* 341–357.

Ross, M., Heine, S. J., Wilson, A. E., & Sugimori, S. (2005). Cross-cultural discrepancies in self-appraisals. *Personality and Social Psychology Bulletin, 31,* 1175–1188.

Ross, M., & Holmberg, D. (1990). Recounting the past: Gender differences in the recall of events in the history of a close relationship.. In J. M. Olson & M. P. Zanna (Eds.), *Self-inference processes: The Ontario Symposium* (Vol. 6, pp. 135–152). Hillsdale, NJ: Erlbaum.

Ross, M., & Wilson, A. E. (2002). It feels like yesterday: Self-esteem, valence of personal past experiences, and judgments of subjective distance. *Journal of Personality and Social Psychology, 82,* 792–803.

Ross, M., Xun, E., & Wilson, A. E. (2002). Language and the bicultural self. *Personality and Social Psychology Bulletin, 28,* 1040–1050.

Röttger-Rössler, B. (1993). Autobiography in question: On self presentation and life description in an Indonesian society. *Anthropos, 88,* 365–373.

Rousseau, J. J. (2000). *Confessions.* New York: Oxford University Press. (Original work published 1782)

Sankaranarayanan, A., & Leichtman, M. D. (2000). *Adults' recollections of childhood in urban and rural India and the United States.* Unpublished raw data.

Schachtel, E. G. (1947). On memory and childhood amnesia. *Psychiatry, 10,* 1–26.

Schrauf, R. W. (2000). Bilingual autobiographical memory: Experimental studies and clinical cases. *Culture and Psychology, 6,* 387–417.

Schrauf, R. W., & Rubin, D. C. (2000). Internal languages of retrieval: The bilingual encoding of memories for the personal past. *Memory and Cognition, 28,* 616–623.

Shweder, R. A., Goodnow, J., Hatano, G., LeVine, R. A., Markus, H. R., & Miller, P. J. (1998). The cultural psychology of development: One mind, many mentalities. In W. Damon (Series Ed.) & R. M. Lerner (Vol. Ed.), *Handbook of child psychology: Vol. 1. Theoretical models of human development* (5th ed., pp. 865–937). New York: Wiley.

Simcock, G., & Hayne, H. (2002). Breaking the barrier?: Children fail to translate their preverbal memories into language. *Psychological Science, 13,* 225–231.

Singer, J. A., & Salovey, P. (1993). *The remembered self: Emotion and memory in personality.* New York: Free Press.

St. Augustine. (1991). *Confessions.* New York: Oxford University Press.

Tanur, J. M. (Ed.). (1992). *Questions about questions: Inquiries into the cognitive bases of surveys.* New York: Russell Sage Foundation.

Trafimow, D., Silverman, E. S., Fan, R. M., & Law, J. S. F. (1997). The effects of language and priming on the relative accessibility of the private self and the collective self. *Journal of Cross-Cultural Psychology, 28,* 107–123.

Triandis, H. C. (1989). The self and social behavior in differing cultural contexts. *Psychological Review, 96,* 506–520.

Tulving, E. (2002). Episodic memory: From mind to brain. *Annual Review of Psychology, 53,* 1–25.

Tweed, R. G., & Lehman, D. R. (2002). Learning considered within a cultural context: Confucian and Socratic approaches. *American Psychologist, 57,* 89–99.

Valsiner, J. (2000). *Culture and human development.* London: Sage.

Valsiner, J. (2001). Process structure of semiotic mediation in human development. *Human Development, 44,* 84–97.

van Emmerik, A. A. P., Kamphuis, J. H., Hulsbosch, A. M., & Emmelkamp, P. M. G. (2002). Single session debriefing after psychological trauma: A meta-analysis. *Lancet, 360,* 766–771.

Veenhoven, R. (1993). Bibliography of happiness: 2,472 contemporary studies on subjective appreciation of life. Rotterdam, the Netherlands: Erasmus University.

Voronov, M., & Singer, J. A. (2002). The myth of individualism–collectivism: A critical review. *Journal of Social Psychology, 142,* 461–480.

Vygotsky, L. (1978). *Mind in society.* Cambridge, MA: Harvard University Press.

Wagar, B. M., & Cohen, D. (2003). Culture, memory, and the self: An analysis of the personal and collective self in long-term memory. *Journal of Experimental Social Psychology, 39*, 468–475.

Wang, Q. (2001a). Cultural effects on adults' earliest childhood recollection and self-description: Implications for the relation between memory and the self. *Journal of Personality and Social Psychology, 81*, 220–233.

Wang, Q. (2001b). "Did you have fun?": American and Chinese mother–child conversations about shared emotional experiences. *Cognitive Development, 16*, 693–715.

Wang, Q. (2004a). The emergence of cultural self-construct: Autobiographical memory and self-description in American and Chinese children. *Developmental Psychology, 40*, 3–15.

Wang, Q. (2004b). The cultural context of parent–child reminiscing: A functional analysis. In M. W. Pratt & B. Fiese (Eds.), *Family stories and the life course: Across time and generations* (pp. 279–301). Mahwah, NJ: Erlbaum.

Wang, Q. (2005, April). *The socialization of self in Chinese and immigrant Chinese families*. In R. Chao & H. Fung (Co-chairs), Cultural perspectives of Chinese socialization. Invited symposium at the biennial meeting of the Society for Research in Child Development (SRCD), Atlanta, GA.

Wang, Q. (2006). Earliest recollections of self and others in European American and Taiwanese young adults. *Psychological Science, 17*(8), 708–714.

Wang, Q. (in press). "Remember when you got the big, big bulldozer?": Mother–child reminiscing over time and across cultures. *Social Cognition*.

Wang, Q., & Brockmeier, J. (2002). Autobiographical remembering as cultural practice: Understanding the interplay between memory, self and culture. *Culture and Psychology, 8*, 45–64.

Wang, Q., & Conway, M. A. (2004). The stories we keep: Autobiographical memory in American and Chinese middle-aged adults. *Journal of Personality, 72*, 911–938.

Wang, Q., Conway, M. A., & Hou, Y. (2004). Infantile amnesia: A cross-cultural investigation. *Cognitive Sciences, 1*, 123–135.

Wang, Q., & Fivush, R. (2005). Mother–child conversations of emotionally salient events: Exploring the functions of emotional reminiscing in European American and Chinese Families. *Social Development, 14*(3), 473–495.

Wang, Q., Hutt, R., Kulkofsky, S., McDermott, M., & Wei, R. (2006). Emotion situation knowledge and autobiographical memory in Chinese, immigrant Chinese, and European American 3-year-olds. *Journal of Cognition and Development, 7*(1), 95–118.

Wang, Q., & Leichtman, M. D. (2000). Same beginnings, different stories: A comparison of American and Chinese children's narratives. *Child Development, 71*, 1329–1346.

Wang, Q., Leichtman, M. D., & Davies, K. (2000). Sharing memories and telling stories: American and Chinese mothers and their 3-year-olds. *Memory, 8*, 159–177.

Wang, Q., Leichtman, M. D., & White, S. H. (1998). Childhood memory and self-description in young Chinese adults: The impact of growing up an only child. *Cognition, 69*(1), 73–103.

Wang, Q., & Ross, M. (2005). What we remember and what we tell: The effects of culture and self-priming on memory representations and narratives. *Memory, 13*(6), 594–606.

Webster, J. D. (1993). Construction and validation of the Reminiscence Functions Scale. *Journals of Gerontology: Series A, Psychological Sciences and Social Sciences, 48*, 256–262.

Webster, J. D. (1997). The Reminiscence Functions Scale: A replication. *International Journal of Aging and Human Development, 44*, 137–148.

Webster, J. D., & Cappeliez, P. (1993). Reminiscence and autobiographical memory: Complementary contexts for cognitive aging research. *Developmental Review, 13*, 54–91.

Wilson, A. E., & Ross, M. (2001). From chump to champ: People's appraisals of their earlier and present selves. *Journal of Personality and Social Psychology, 80*(4), 572–584.

Wu, P.-Y. (1990). *The Confucian's progress: Autobiographical writings in traditional China*. Princeton, NJ: Princeton University Press.

Wyatt, F. (1963). The reconstruction of the individual and of the collective past. In R. H. White (Ed.), *The study of lives* (pp. 304–320). New York: Atherton Press.

Yoon, C., Hasher, L., Feinberg, F., & Rahhal, T. A. (2000). Cross-cultural differences in memory: The role of culture-based stereotypes about aging. *Psychology and Aging, 15*, 694–704.

CHAPTER 27

Language, Cognition, and Culture
Beyond the Whorfian Hypothesis

CHI-YUE CHIU
ANGELA K-Y. LEUNG
LETTY KWAN

The idea that every distinctive language would give rise to a distinctive culture stayed at the center of American anthropology throughout much of the 20th century. According to Benjamin Whorf (1956), who had written most enthusiastically on the linguistic shaping of thoughts and culture, "Users of markedly different languages are pointed by their grammars toward different types of observations, and hence are not equivalent as observers but must arrive at somewhat different views of the world" (p. 252). In other words, the grammar of a language constrains the way its speakers perceive the world and mentally represent what they perceive. As a result, there is an isomorphic relation between the structure of a language and the mental processes of the people who speak it. This idea is often referred to as *linguistic relativity.*

Whorf also held that in the coevolution of language and culture, "the nature of the language is the factor that limits free plasticity and rigidifies channels of development [of culture] in the more autocratic way" (Whorf, 1956, p. 156). Thus, the grammar of a language is

taken to be the cause of the speakers' cognitions. This assumption is often referred to as *linguistic determinism* (Chiu, Krauss, & Lee, 1999).

The original form of linguistic determinism consists of six propositions:

1. There is no inherent structure in people's experiences; perceptual order emerges when people organize their experiences with mental categories.
2. Language is a major cognitive tool people use to categorize their experiences.
3. As a language evolves, it develops a coherent internal logic.
4. The internal logic of a language embodies a metaphysics or naive conception of the reality; as such, the internal logic of a language stands in isomorphic relation to that of its associated culture.
5. Markedly different languages evoke in the mind of its speakers different mental representations of similar linguistic referents.
6. Language constrains the development of nonlinguistic cultural norms.

Taken together, these propositions imply that the structural properties of a language have general effects on cognition that extend beyond the immediate context of language use.

Whorf's writings have inspired a search for the linguistic foundation of human sociality in social psychology. However, the original form of linguistic determinism, inspiring as it is, lacks the empirical support needed to sustain the early enthusiasm for it (Brown, 1976; Glucksberg, 1988). The demise of the Whorfian hypothesis has led to a decline in interest in the linguistic foundation of culture in social psychology, and to an overriding concern with language universals in linguistics. As Chomsky (1992) puts it, "The computational system of language that determines the forms and relations of linguistic expressions may indeed be invariant; in this sense, there is only one human language, as a rational Martian observing humans would have assumed" (p. 50).

Language is a polysemous word, with both a generic sense (as in "Language pervades our social life") and a specific sense (as in "English is a language spoken by most Americans"). These two senses are related but not synonymous. Whorf (1956) clearly intended the specific sense of *language*, and the empirical support for Whorf's formulation of linguistic determinism is tenuous (Glucksberg, 1988). Despite this, there is considerable evidence that language (in its generic sense) can, under some circumstances, affect the way we think, remember, and perceive. Advances in the cognitive and linguistic sciences have provided much new knowledge about the mechanisms of cognition and their relations to various aspects of language. These developments lead to alternative views of how language may be implicated in cognitive processes such as memory, categorization, thinking, and problem solving (e.g., see Hoosain, 1991; Hunt & Agnoli, 1991). They also suggest some of the conditions and mechanisms for such cognitive effects of language (Hunt & Banaji, 1988).

In this chapter, instead of questioning whether we should accept or reject the Whorfian hypothesis, we focus on how language may be implicated in human cognitions. We posit that the availability of certain structural properties in a language is *important but not sufficient* for it to affect cognitions. Instead, we suggest that the vocabulary of a language provides its speakers with some *linguistic tools* for encoding experiences and expressing thoughts, and that these tools may influence cognitions *only when they are used*. Furthermore, when used in a communication context, because of the interactive nature of communication, aside from being a tool for expressing thoughts and ideas, language is also a tool for negotiating shared meanings in the context.

As an illustration of these arguments, consider a hypothetical scenario in which a person with no knowledge of Chinese characters is asked to describe Figure 27.1a. The description is likely to be rather lengthy, with plenty of details of the figure's components (e.g., the flattened oval on the top, the cross below it, the curved arms that extend to both sides, and the tail pointing to the left). In contrast, a person who has good command of the Chinese language may refer to this figure simply as "the ancient form of the character zi" (child; see Figure 27.1b for the modern form the character). This example illustrates how the availability of a linguistic code (zi) in a language (Chinese) for encoding a stimulus affords an economical referring expression of the stimulus.

When language is used to characterize a state of affairs, a linguistic representation of that state of affairs is created or evoked. For example, an English speaker may use the color term *blue* to describe a greenish-blue chromatic light that has the wavelength of 490 μm. As a result, the light is linguistically represented as "a blue light." Linguistic representations may then compete with and overshadow the perceptual representations of that state of affairs. In the previous example, the linguistic representation (*blue light*) may compete with and overshadow the original visual representation of the light (a greenish-blue light of 490 μm). Consequently, the speaker may visualize and remember the

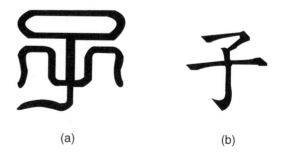

(a)   (b)

FIGURE 27.1. Ancient (a) and modern (b) forms of the Chinese character zi (child).

light as being bluer than it is (Thomas & DeCapito, 1966).

Members of a speech community share not only the formal rules of a language but also the ground rules and assumptions that underlie language usage. According to Grice (1975), communication is a collaborative activity. In a conversation, the speakers are expected to make their contribution "as informative as is required, at the stage at which it occurs, by the accepted purpose or direction of the talk exchange" (p. 45). The speaker is expected to be aware of these rules and adhere to them. Back to the example of describing the old form of the Chinese character zi, when the Chinese speaker describes it to someone who knows nothing about Chinese characters, it is unlikely that she would refer to it simply as "the old form of the Chinese character zi," because she expects her addressee not to possess the knowledge necessary to identify the referent from this expression. Instead, she may say something like "This is the old form of the Chinese character zi; it has a flattened oval on the top and a cross below it" (Lau, Chiu, & Hong, 2001).

A grounding process is implicated in interpersonal communication. At the beginning of the conversation, the speaker's utterance represents his or her hypothesis about what the addressee will understand, and the addressee has a hypothesis about what the speaker means by the utterance (Clark & Brennan, 1991). Furthermore, as the conversation proceeds, the participants use each other's response as evidence to test and revise their hypotheses. They acquire common ground and eventually establish consensus on the referential meanings of the stimulus. An indication of this grounding process is that the referring expression would become much shorter and more efficient after the speaker has described the same referent to the same speaker several times (Krauss & Glucksberg, 1977). In this example, the referring expression of Figure 27.1a becomes shorter ("the old form of zi") after the Chinese speaker has described it to the same addressee several times. Eventually, both participants agree to refer to it as "the old form of zi." In short, language is not merely a tool for expressing thoughts and ideas; it is also a tool for negotiating meanings: Through the use of language in communication, private cognitions are rendered public and directed toward a shared representation of the referent (Schegloff, 1991).

In summary, like Whorf, we hold that language has important influences on human cognitions. However, unlike Whorf, we submit that the structural properties of a language do not rigidly determine thoughts. Instead, grammar and vocabulary limit the tools that are available to speakers of the language for constructing and negotiating meanings. The emergent properties of the communication context constrain the likelihood and the manner that certain expressions or ways of expressions in a language will be evoked and applied in the context. These processes may in turn direct the development of shared cognitions in the speech community. In the sections that follow, we review the evidence for these ideas.

LANGUAGE AND MIND: THE EMPIRICAL EVIDENCE

To recap, we posit that (1) the availability of certain structural properties in a language is *important but not enough* for language to impact cognitions; (2) the characteristic ways of referring to a state of affairs in a language are *linguistic tools* speakers of the language can use to encode experiences and express thoughts; (3) these tools influence cognitions only when they are used; (4) when language is used to characterize a state of affairs, a linguistic representation of that state of affairs is created or evoked, which may compete with and overshadow the perceptual representation of that state of affairs; and (5) individuals who participate in communication acquire common ground and eventually establish consensus on the referential meanings of the stimulus through communication. In this section, we review the empirical evidence for these five propositions.

Grammar and Thought

The original form of the Whorfian hypothesis focuses on the relationship between a language's grammar and the language users' cognitions. According to Whorf (1956), "It is not words mumbled, but *rapport* between words, which enables them to work together at all to any semantic result" (p. 67; emphasis in original). "Words and speech are not the same thing. . . . The patterns of sentence structure that guide words are more important than the words" (p. 253). In his view, an integrated "fashion of speaking" shapes the linguistic aspects of thoughts. Whorf used the term *cryptotype* to refer to "a submerged, subtle, and elusive meaning, corresponding to no actual word, yet shown by linguistic analysis to be functionally important in the grammar" (p. 70). An example of cryptotype is the inanimate object class in Navaho (a Native American language). Navaho classifies inanimate objects into "round objects" and "long objects," and a different verb stem is required for a "round" or a "long" subject (or object) in a sentence. Whorf believed that an analysis of *cryptotypes* is needed to reveal the linguistic aspects of thinking.

Research inspired by Whorf's ideas has provided some support for the idea that the grammar of a language encodes a cultural worldview (the linguistic relativity hypothesis). However, the idea that the cognitive effects of a language's grammar extend beyond the immediate context of language use (the linguistic determinism hypothesis) has received little support.

Grammar Encodes a Cultural Worldview

Whorf and his followers assumed that the grammatical structure of every language embodies a cultural worldview. There is some evidence for this assumption. For example, the system of pronouns in a language reflects the conceptions of the social self in the culture. The use of a pronoun sustains attention on its referent, bringing the person out from the conversational background. In some languages (e.g., English), the use of a pronoun is grammatically obligatory. In other languages (e.g., Spanish), the subject pronoun can be dropped, because the referent can be recovered from the verb inflections. In some languages (e.g., Chinese), the subject pronoun can be dropped even though there is no verb inflection, or the subject–verb agreement rule. The grammatical obligatory use of the first-person pronoun maximally distinguishes the speaker's self. Similarly, obligatory use of the second-person pronoun maximally distinguishes the addressee(s). The omission of either or both of the two classes of pronouns deemphasizes the salience of their corresponding referent(s).

Consistent with the idea that language encodes cultural conceptions of the self, groups whose language allows pronoun drop tend to stress the importance of being interdependent with the social world, maintaining good rela-

tionship and fitting in, whereas groups whose language disallows pronoun drop tend to stress the desirability of being independent from people around them and expression of the inner set of attributes and abilities (E. Kashima & Kashima, 1998; Y. Kashima & Kashima, 2003).

How individuals process verbal and coverbal information may also reflect their cultural worldview. Listeners tend to extract different information from an utterance's verbal contents and coverbal cues (e.g., vocal tone, gesture, gaze pattern); they extract the utterance's intended meanings from its verbal contents, and infer contextual information (e.g., the speaker's status, personality characteristics, and emotional states) from coverbal cues (Krauss & Chiu, 1988). Consistent with the view that American societies are low-context societies, in which people tend to have many connections but of shorter duration, or for some specific reason, knowledge is codified, public, external, and accessible, and cultural beliefs and expectations are spelled out explicitly, and Japanese societies are high-context societies, in which people have long-term relationships, knowledge is situational and relational, and verbally explicit communications are infrequent (see Hall, 1990), European Americans respond automatically to the verbal contents of a message, and Japanese respond automatically to the vocal tone (Ishii, Reyes, & Kitayama, 2003). In short, a language's grammar and the way language is processed may reflect the implicit organization of knowledge in the language community.

Linguistic Determinism: A Strong Claim in Search of Evidence

In the original formulation of the Whorfian hypothesis, the *structural aspects* of a language are assumed to *shape* the way its speakers *habitually* represent the reality. For example, time is a continuum. However, in standard average European (SAE) languages, no formal markers distinguish real plurals (e.g., seven dogs) from imaginary plurals (e.g., seven days). According to Whorf, because of this linguistic property, speakers of SAE languages may habitually assume that time can be dissected into discrete units (e.g., days, weeks). Whorf also believed that the three-tense (past, present, and future) system in SAE verbs predisposes speakers of SAE languages to the perception of time as a straight line extending from the past to the present, and the future. In short, in Whorf's view, speakers of languages with markedly different grammars are linguistically predisposed to different perceptions and representations of otherwise identical experience (e.g., time).

As noted, there is consistent evidence that the grammar of a language may embody a certain cultural worldview. However, support for the idea that the cognitive effects of a language's grammar extend beyond the immediate context of language use is tenuous. Research that directly tested the linguistic determinism hypothesis has examined the cognitive effects of grammatical markers of shapes, counterfactual ideas and entification, gender, and false beliefs. As described below, no conclusive evidence for linguistic determinism was found in this research.

GRAMMATICAL MARKERS OF SHAPES

In an early study, Carroll and Casagrande (1958) presented to Navaho-speaking children, English-speaking Navaho children, and white middle class children in Boston two objects that differed in color and shape. Next, they showed a third object similar to the first two objects either in color or in shape, and had the participants indicate which of the first two objects went best with the third one. The results are equivocal. Consistent with the linguistic determinism hypothesis, when compared to the English-speaking Navaho children, Navaho-speaking children were more inclined to group objects with a similar shape together. However, contrary to the linguistic determinism hypothesis, when compared to the English-speaking Boston children, Navaho-speaking children made *fewer* shape-based choices.

COUNTERFACTUAL REASONING AND ENTIFICATION

Unlike English, Chinese lacks formal grammatical markers for counterfactuals. Also, unlike English, Chinese does not have a formal way to express a condition or event as an entity (entification). Bloom (1981a) posits that these two grammatical features hinder Chinese speakers' development of conceptual schemas for abstract, theoretical thinking. He further argues that the Chinese way of speaking shapes Chinese speakers' moral outlook, orienting them toward pragmatic moral beliefs, and

away from a formalized theoretical approach to morality (Bloom, 1981b).

Findings from several studies seemed to support Bloom's views. In one study, Chinese speakers and English speakers read a passage that contained counterfactual statements in their respective native languages. Later in the study, their comprehension of the passage was tested. English speakers did much better than Chinese speakers on the test. Moreover, Chinese–English bilinguals performed much better on the English version of the test than on the Chinese translation of it (Bloom, 1981a). Bloom believes that the lack of formal markers for counterfactuals in the Chinese language hinders its speakers' counterfactual reasoning ability.

However, Bloom's findings are difficult to interpret, because the English passages in his studies were written in idiomatic English, but the Chinese passages were not written in idiomatic Chinese (Au, 1983, 1984, 2004). Thus, the two versions of the passages are not equally comprehensible. Indeed, when the Chinese version was rewritten in idiomatic Chinese, Chinese and English speakers performed equally well on the comprehension test. Moreover, when English speakers were presented with English passages written in nonidiomatic English, they made a considerable amount of comprehension errors (Au, 1983). Furthermore, Chinese grade-school children who have almost no knowledge of English subjunctive understand counterfactual statements (Au, 1983; Liu, 1985). Finally, among Chinese-speaking children with little exposure to the English language, the ability to understand counterfactual statements increases with age. By age 11, almost all Chinese children who know little English can solve counterfactual problems (Liu, 1985). In short, it seems that counterfactual reasoning ability increases with cognitive maturity and is not related to the language one speaks.

Does the lack of formal entification markers in the Chinese language hinder its speakers' formal reasoning ability? To answer this question, Bloom (1981a) developed another comprehension test. The test passage contained factual information about the relationships of different events. To answer the comprehension question correctly, these events need to be transformed into entities and placed into a theoretical framework. As Bloom expected, Chinese speakers performed more poorly on this test than did English speakers.

However, to Bloom's embarrassment, Takano (1989) pointed out that the designated correct answer in Bloom's comprehension test was actually an incorrect answer. Moreover, among the undergraduates who had taken Bloom's test, those with more formal training in scientific reasoning were *less* likely to choose the designated correct answer. Furthermore, those who challenged the validity of Bloom's comprehension question were able to provide better explanations of the functional relationships among the variables described in the passage than those who chose the "correct" answer.

GRAMMATICAL GENDER

Grammatical gender research provides another opportunity to test the effects of grammar on cognitive representations. Languages differ in whether they assign a gender to all nouns that refer to animates (e.g., *psychologist*) or to nouns that refer to inanimates (e.g., *moon*). Some languages (e.g., Spanish, Italian, French, German, Arabic, and Hebrew) mark gender with morphological information carried by pronouns, determiners, nouns, and adjectives, and others (e.g., English) do not. It is often assumed that, at least in most European languages, the basis of grammatical gender assignments to inanimate objects is arbitrary. For example, in French, the word for "the moon" is feminine (*la lune*) and the word for "the sun" is masculine (*le soleil*). However, in German, "the moon" is masculine (*der Mond*) and "the sun" is feminine (*die Sonne*).

Some studies suggest that users of a language with a grammatical gender system tend to infer psychological gender properties from gender inflections of nouns. For example, French speakers conceptualize the moon in more psychologically feminine ways and the sun in more psychologically masculine ways than do German speakers. In a classic study, Ervin (1962) taught native speakers of Italian nonsense words that possessed either the masculine Italian affix (*-o*) or the feminine one (*-a*). In this study, the participants rated the nonsense words with masculine endings as more like men than those with feminine endings, and vice versa. Similar results have been obtained in speakers of Arabic (Clarke, Losoff,

McCracken, & Rood, 1984; Clarke, Losoff, McCracken, & Still, 1981). However, because participants in these studies were asked to judge the gender connotations of words, it is unclear whether these judgments reveal participants' knowledge of grammatical gender or the effects of grammatical gender on categorization (see Sera et al., 2002). Nonetheless, other studies have used more sophisticated tests of categorization to assess the effects of grammatical gender. For example, participants were shown pictures (vs. words) of objects and asked to assign either a man's voice or a woman's voice to the objects. Using these methods, researchers have obtained robust effects of grammatical gender on object categorization in Spanish (Martinez & Shatz, 1996; Sera, Berge, & del Castillio Pintado, 1994; Sera et al., 2002) and French speakers (Sera et al., 2002). These findings seem to support the linguistic determinism hypothesis.

However, two problems undermine the validity of this conclusion. First, the effects of grammatical gender on object categorization are not uniform across languages with a grammatical gender system. For example, the cognitive effects of grammatical gender are absent in Finnish speakers (Clarke et al., 1981, 1984) and German speakers (Sera et al., 2002). Second, although assignments of gender to objects are mostly arbitrary in some languages (e.g., German), this is not the case in other languages (e.g., Spanish). For example, in Spanish, a female gender is often attributed to an object that is used by women, natural, round, or light. Likewise, a male gender is often attributed to an object that is used by men, artificial, angular, or heavy. Moreover, native speakers of English (a language without a grammatical gender system) tend to assign male or female voices to pictured objects corresponding to Spanish gender. Thus, Spanish grammatical gender seems to be highly correlated with natural gender. In a series of computer and experimental simulation studies, Sera et al. (2002) found that generalization of masculine and feminine traits to inanimate objects is likely to occur when the grammatical gender system has only two gender categories, and when there is a high correlation between grammatical and natural gender. The result of this simulation study is consistent with the empirical observation that grammatical gender effect is found among Spanish speakers but not among German speakers. In short, the weight of the evidence to date is in favor of the conclusion that object categorization by gender may stem from the natural gender associations of objects. Natural and grammatical gender may or may not correspond. Grammatical gender effects are likely to be found only when they do.

FALSE BELIEFS

Puerto Rican (PR) Spanish and Turkish have formal verb forms for marking false belief states explicitly. For example, PR Spanish uses *creer* to denote that the speaker is neutral on whether the grammatical subject in the sentence holds a true belief or not, and adds a reflexive clitic to the verb phrase (*creer-se*) to denote that the speaker is sure that the grammatical subject holds a false belief. English and Brazilian (BR) Portuguese have no such specific forms. Shatz, Diesendruck, Martinez-Beck, and Akar (2003) compared the performance on a false belief understanding task of PR Spanish-speaking preschoolers and Turkish-speaking preschoolers with their English-speaking and BR Portuguese-speaking counterparts. In this study, Experimenter 1 showed the preschooler in the presence of Experimenter 2 a crayon box and a blue box. Then, after Experimenter 2 left the room to get some paper, Experimenter 1 opened both boxes, remarked that the crayon box was empty and the blue box contained crayons, and asked the preschooler, "Where does [Experimenter 2] think the crayons are?" and "Where is [Experimenter 2] going to look for the crayons when [he or she] returns to draw?" In the two languages with formal markers for false beliefs, the verb *think* in the first question provided an explicit linguistic cue of the false belief state. The critical question is: Does the presence of formal markers for false belief states in a language facilitate understanding of these states (e.g., Experimenter 2 would expect to find the crayons in the crayon box)? Furthermore, is it necessary for the explicit marker to be present in the immediate language use context for it to improve understanding of false belief states? According to the original version of the Whorfian hypothesis, the grammar of a language predisposes its users to a certain pattern of cognition irrespective of whether the grammatical feature is present in the immediate communication context.

If having formal grammatical markers for false beliefs in one's own language improves understanding of false belief states, Turkish and PR Spanish speakers and Turkish speakers should do better than BR Portuguese speakers and English speakers on the comprehension task. In addition, if false belief markers help by improving children's general ability to understand false belief states, irrespective of the language used in any particular case, Turkish and PR Spanish speakers should do better than BR Portuguese speakers and English speakers on the general question about false beliefs ("Where is [Experimenter 2] going to look for the crayons?"), as well as the explicitly marked question ("Where does [Experimenter 2] think the crayons are?"). However, if the grammatical markers for false belief states help only locally, without influencing reasoning in a more general way, the Turkish and PR Spanish speakers should outperform the BR Portuguese speakers and English speakers only when the explicitly marked question was asked. In this study, only a local effect of explicit grammatical markers was found.

The results indicate that the presence of a formal grammatical marker of false belief states in one's language facilitates false belief understanding. Specifically, only 37% of the BR Portuguese- or English-speaking children (children who spoke unmarked languages) answered most of the false belief comprehension questions correctly. In contrast, 71% of the Turkish- and PR Spanish-speaking children (children who spoke marked languages) answered most of the false belief questions correctly when they responded to the *marked* (*think*) questions.

The results also show that marking for false belief in a language has a local rather than a general effect. When the Turkish- and PR Spanish-speaking children heard the unmarked (*look*) questions, only 32% answered most of the false belief questions correctly.

CONCLUSION

Consistent with the linguistic relativity hypothesis, there is evidence that some grammatical properties of a language embody a distinctive cultural worldview. However, the strong claim that the grammar of a language *shapes* its speakers' thought processes lacks empirical support. The lack of clear support for the linguistic determinism hypothesis highlights the need to explore alternative ways of conceptualizing the relationship of language, cognition, and culture.

Effects of Linguistic Encoding

The linguistic determinism hypothesis is not the only way to formulate the relation of language and thought. Whorf's primary concern was how *structural differences among languages* (independent of cultural experiences) predispose users of different languages to highly patterned, systematic, and distinctive thought processes. It is conceivable that the Whorfian hypothesis (1956) is incorrect, and that language (in its generic sense) importantly affects cognition. Indeed, there is considerable evidence that language use influences (1) problem solving (how an object is labeled can affect the way it is used in a problem-solving task; e.g., Ranken, 1963), (2) decision making (the verbal framing of a formally identical decision problem can result in different decisions; e.g., Kahneman & Tversky, 1984), and (3) memory performance (describing a human face may distort accuracy in a delayed recognition test; e.g., Schooler & Engstler-Schooler, 1990).

What is distinctive and interesting about the studies that show clear effects of language on some cognitive process is that, in one way or another, they all involve effects resulting from *the use of language to represent a state of affairs*. This critical commonality leads to an alternative formulation of the relation of language and cognition: Languages with different structural properties afford different tools for characterizing a state of affairs. A language has important cognitive consequences only when its structural features or referring expressions are applied in the immediate language use context (Chiu et al., 1999; Krauss & Chiu, 1998). The result of the false beliefs study reviewed earlier is consistent with this formulation: Among Turkish- and PR Spanish-speaking children, comprehension of false belief states improved only when the comprehension question included an explicit linguistic marker of false belief states.

Recoding interference may explain the effects of linguistic encoding on how a state of affairs is perceived, experienced, and remembered. Schooler and Engstler-Schooler (1990) proposed a recoding interference hypothesis to

account for the memory effects of linguistic encoding. According to this hypothesis, the same state of affairs can be encoded in both verbal and visual representational formats. For example, an eyewitness in a crime scene may visualize the face of a suspect or describe it.

The use of a particular referring expression may evoke an online linguistic representation of the referent that colors the immediate perception of the referent. When it is difficult to verbalize a state of affairs, representations in the verbal and visual formats may contain different information. In the previous example, the verbal description of the face and the visual image of it may contain different information. Under such circumstances, competition may occur between the two forms of representations, and subsequent memory representation of the referent may be assimilated into its linguistic representation (Chiu, Krauss, & Lau, 1998).

In a series of experiments that tested this hypothesis, Schooler and his associates (Schooler & Engstler-Schooler, 1990; Fallshore & Schooler, 1995) had participants either describe or simply visualize a face they had seen. Participants who described the face were *less* able to recognize the face in a delayed recognition test compared to those who had seen the face and visualized it. Featural information about faces is easier to verbalize than configural information (Fallshore & Schooler, 1995). Thus, it is possible that describing a face evoked relatively feature-based representations, whereas perceptually processing the same face created representations that were relatively configuration-based. When the participants recalled the face in a delayed memory task, the verbal representation may have competed with the visual representation and lowered recognition accuracy (Schooler & Engstler-Schooler, 1990).

Recoding interference may also account for some variations between language groups in referent perception and memory. Language is a system of representational symbols; humans use language to represent both immediate events (e.g., "I am hungry now") and nonimmediate events (e.g., "Dov and Dre gave birth to happy Ilana in the summer of 2004") (D'Andrade, 2002). As a representation system, language possesses an important property: Speakers of a language can use different referring expressions to indicate the same referent (people with low IQs may be referred to as *mentally retarded* or *intellectually challenged*). Some referring expressions (e.g., *a license* or *a permit*) are semantically identical and evoke similar representations of the referent, whereas others carry very different connotations (e.g., *a failure* vs. *a setback*). Because languages vary in their vocabulary for referring to the same referent, using different languages to characterize the same referent may evoke or create different linguistic and memory representations of the same referent. In the following subsections, we illustrate this argument with three research examples: color codability and color memory, person memory, and figurative encoding of time.

Color Codability and Color Cognition

Color codability refers to the availability of a linguistic code in a language that allows a color to be expressed easily, rapidly, briefly, and uniformly. The effects of color codability meet the criteria thought to be necessary to test the Whorfian hypothesis (see Rosch, 1987). First, variations in color vocabulary can be readily found in natural languages. Second, investigators can measure the physical units of colors (e.g., wavelength) independent of how colors are coded in different languages. Third, members in different language communities should have more or less equivalent experiences with colors. Thus, difference in color memory across people in different language communities should be attributed not to their difference in experience with colors but to the variations in color codability across languages. Finally, nonlinguistic measures of color cognition—color perception, color memory—are available.

Our review of the research literature on the perceptual and memory effects of color codability leads to the following conclusions. First, the properties of the visual system may limit the range of language's effects on color categorization. For example, no language has color categories that include two color spaces (e.g., yellow and blue) and exclude the connecting color space (e.g., green) (Davidoff, 2001). Second, within the constraints imposed by the visual system and the structure of the color space, different languages partition the color space differently (Roberson, Davies, & Davidoff, 2000, Experiment 1a). Third, when a color term is used to label a color, a linguistic representation of the color is created, which may bias the immediate perception and subse-

quent memory of the color. Fourth, variations in the availability of basic color terms across languages may produce different perceptions and memories of the color. Finally, although speakers of two languages with markedly different color vocabularies may see and remember the same colors differently, the differences in color perception or memory between these two language groups would disappear when linguistic encoding of colors is prohibited.

As a reaction to the linguistic determinism hypothesis, some researchers have sought to demonstrate the presence of a universal perceptual order, independent of language. Findings from the early studies seemed to support a view of the "universal evolution" of color terminology (Berlin & Kay, 1969) that can be mapped onto the neurophysiological substrate of color perception (Kay & McDaniel, 1978). Other studies (e.g., Heider, 1972) conducted at about the same time showed that speakers of different languages have better memory for focal colors (paradigm exemplars of basic colors) than for nonfocal colors, and language has no effect on color memory. In a study of 24 languages, Heider found that focal colors, compared to nonfocal colors, are named more rapidly and given shorter names, indicating that focal colors are more codable than nonfocal ones. Heider also found that although there are only two color terms in Dugum Dani (the language of a Stone Age tribe in Irian Jaya), Dugum Dani–speakers have better recognition memory for focal colors than for nonfocal colors. Based on these results, Heider (1972; Rosch, 1973) concluded that the availability of an explicit linguistic code in one's language has no effect on color memory. Instead, some universal perceptual–cognitive processes underlying the internal structure of color categories mediate both color naming and color memory.

The presence of a universal perceptual order leaves no room for any color codability effects on color perception and memory. However, later studies showed that although the properties of the human visual system may limit the range of cognitive effects of color codability, the evidence for the presence of a universal perceptual order is not convincing. Other researchers also found that speakers of different languages partition the color spectrum slightly differently, and that the way the spectrum is partitioned in a language seems to have some important cognitive consequences on color perception and memory.

In reaction to Heider's claim (1972) that focal colors are remembered better than nonfocal ones in all language groups, Lucy and Shweder (1979) argued that the focal colors used in Heider's experiments had higher perceptual salience than did the nonfocal colors. The inherent perceptual salience of focal colors might have given focal colors certain perceptual advantage over the nonfocal colors in the memory test. In the experiments conducted by Lucy and Shweder (1979; see also Garro, 1986; Lucy & Shweder, 1988), after controlling for perceptual salience, focal and nonfocal colors had the same level of recognition accuracy.

Roberson et al. (2000) also suspect that in Heider's (1972) study, the memory advantage of focal colors for Dugum Dani speakers was due to the participants' tendency to choose a focal color in error for a nonfocal color. When monolingual Berinmo speakers were tested, there was also a memory advantage for focal over nonfocal colors. However, when the aforementioned response bias was corrected, the memory advantage disappeared (Roberson et al., 2000, Experiment 2a). In addition, Berinmo speakers learned to associate a nonfocal color with a picture just as fast as they associated a focal color to a picture (Roberson et al., 2000, Experiment 3b). These findings question whether color focality completely determines color memory in all language groups.

To show that the color vocabulary in a language can influence color memory, researchers have sought to establish the correspondence between how similarly two colors are named in a language, and how likely speakers of the language would confuse the two colors in a delayed recognition memory test. If color vocabulary affects color perception, speakers of the language would find it harder to differentiate between two colors if they were named the same way in the language than if they were named differently.

Although the early findings showed that variations in the way the color space is partitioned in a language seem to have little effect on color memory, subsequent studies revealed some effects of linguistic encoding on color perception and color memory. In the first cross-language study of color codability effect, Heider and Olivier (1972) asked their informants in two language groups (English-speaking Americans, and Dugum Dani) to perform a color-naming task and a color-recognition task. American English has 11 ba-

sic color terms, and Dugum Dani has only two achromatic terms for color. A similarity matrix for color naming and a similarity matrix for color recognition were constructed for each language group. The color-naming matrices were constructed from how often the informants gave different colors the same name, and the color recognition matrices were constructed from how frequently the informants confused one color with another in the recognition task. Multidimensional scaling performed on the four similarity matrices revealed marked differences between the two naming matrices, indicating that the stimulus colors are represented *very differently* in the two languages. However, the two memory matrices were almost identical, indicating that the two language groups have *very similar* memory representations of the stimulus colors.

However, a recent replication of the Heider and Olivier (1972) study found some effects of color codability on color memory. The participants in this study (Roberson et al., 2000, Experiment 1a) were native English speakers and monolingual Berinmo speakers from three villages in Papua, New Guinea. There are five basic color terms in Berinmo, which do not map directly onto the basic color terms in English. The investigators used multidimensional scaling to estimate the probabilities that each pair of different colors in the stimulus array would be confused in Berinmo naming, Berinmo memory, English naming, and English memory. If two colors were likely to be confused in Berinmo naming, they were also likely to be confused in Berinmo memory ($r = .54$). However, the correspondence between Berinmo memory and English memory patterns was also significant: If two colors were likely to be confused in Berinmo memory, then they were also likely to be confused in English memory ($r = .44$). More importantly, the correlation of .54 was reliably higher than the correlation of .44, indicating that the Berinmo patterns of naming and memory were more closely matched than were Berinmo memory and English memory patterns.

Another cross-language study also provided evidence for the effect of color codability on color perception. In this study, Kay and Kempton (1984, Study 1) presented three color chips at a time to native speakers of English and speakers of Tarahumara (a Uto-Aztecan language of northern Mexico), and had them judge the similarity or difference of the three colors. Unlike English, Tarahumara lacks the lexical distinction between the color categories of "green" and "blue." When the participants' judgments were compared to the physical distance of the stimuli in terms of their wavelengths, the English-speaking participants, but not Tarahumara-speaking ones, systematically overestimated the distance between two colors when the green–blue color boundary passed between them.

However, Kay and Kempton (1984) believe that the English-speaking participants might have used a naming strategy when they were performing the judgment task. For instance, they might have labeled the color left of the green–blue lexical category boundary "green" and the two colors to the right of the boundary "blue." Due to recoding interference, they overestimated the perceptual distance between the first color and other colors. However, the Tarahumara-speaking participants could not use this naming strategy, because their language lacks the lexical distinction between the color categories of "green" and "blue."

Kay and Kempton's (1984) reasoning is consistent with the findings from an earlier study of linguistic encoding and color experience. In this study, Thomas and DeCapito (1966) trained their participants to emit a finger-lift response to greenish-blue light with the wavelength of 490 μm and later tested their generalization gradient. Participants in the named condition were led to label the 490 μm chromatic light either as "green" or as "blue" when it was presented, whereas participants in the control condition were not. Participants who had labeled the colored light "green" showed stronger generalization responses to wavelengths greater than 495 μm (the wavelengths of greenish light) compared to the participants who had labeled it "blue." They also exhibited weaker generalization responses to wavelengths shorter than 485 μm (wavelengths of bluish light). Participants in the control condition yielded a generalization gradient intermediate between the two groups.

To test their idea directly, Kay and Kempton (1984, Study 2) induced English-speaking participants to use both verbal labels ("blue" and "green") to encode the same color. First, the participants saw the target color with a greener color, and they spontaneously encoded the target color as the "bluer" color. Next, they saw the same target color with a bluer color, and spontaneously encoded the target color as the "greener" color. Following this, the participants evaluated the perceptual distances between the target color, the greener color, and the bluer color. Because the target color was encoded both as a bluer color (when it was paired with the greener color) and a greener color (when it was paired with the bluer color), the effects of the two encodings cancelled out each other. Under this circumstance, the English-speaking participants' judgments were similar to those of the Tarahumara speakers, and corresponded closely with the physical distance of the colors.

Roberson et al. (2000) reported similar findings in a conceptual replication of the Kay and Kempton (1984) experiments. The participants in the Roberson et al.'s experiments were English speakers and Berinmo speakers. Like Tarahumara, Berinmo makes no lexical distinction between "blue" and "green" colors. However, English lacks linguistic labels that refer to *nol* and *wor* colors in Tarahumara. When asked to judge the perceptual similarity between pairs of colors, English speakers judged two colors across the green–blue boundary as more dissimilar to the two colors within the green or blue category. However, they did not show such categorical perception for colors across the *nol–wor* boundary. The reverse was true for the Berinmo speakers. Similar results were obtained among both English speakers and Berinmo speakers in color category learning and color memory. More important, in a subsequent color memory study, Roberson and Davidoff (2000) tested the effect of articulation suppression on color memory. The research participants were Berinmo speakers. In this study, when a verbal interference procedure was introduced to prevent subvocal encoding of the stimuli, the cross-category advantage in color memory was removed.

In short, variations in the availability of basic color terms across languages may produce different perceptions and memories of color. Thus, speakers of two languages with markedly different color vocabularies may see and remember the same colors differently. However, such cognitive differences seem to be mediated by recoding interference, and would disappear when linguistic encoding of colors is prohibited.

Person Memory

Analogous language effects have been found in studies of social memory. In one study,

Hoffman, Lau, and Johnson (1986) presented to their Chinese–English bilingual participants and native English-speaking participants personality descriptions about several target persons. Some descriptions had high Chinese codability: The targets could be coded in a brief Chinese personality term (*shi gu*) that has no equivalent translations in English, or in more clumsy English expressions. The remaining ones had high English codability: The targets could be coded in a brief English personality term ("liberal") that has no equivalent Chinese translations, or in more clumsy Chinese expressions. The Chinese–English bilinguals either read a Chinese version of the personality descriptions and were encouraged to think in Chinese, or read an English version of the same descriptions and were encouraged to think in English. The English-speaking participants read the English version of the descriptions. Five days later, all participants returned for the second session to make further inferences about the targets in the character descriptions. In response to descriptions of high Chinese codability, the Chinese–English bilinguals using Chinese, compared to the Chinese–English bilinguals using English and the English speakers, made more inferences that were congruent with the brief Chinese personality terms. They also made fewer inferences that were congruent with the brief English personality terms in response to the descriptions with high English codability.

In short, people use economical terms in their language to encode person information. The lexical term used to characterize person information may influence how the information is represented subsequently.

Figurative Speech

Members of each culture have certain characteristic ways of describing events. The use of widely shared figurative descriptions of universal experiences (e.g., the experience of time) offers a good illustration of the social-cognitive processes implicated in the relationship of language use and cognition. Recall that Whorf (1956) believed that some grammatical features in SAE languages (such as the three-tense system of verbs and the absence of formal grammatical markers for real and imaginary plurals) predispose speakers of SAE languages to represent time as a linear continuum that can be conveniently dissected into discrete units (years, days, minutes, or milliseconds). Instead of focusing on the cognitive consequences of the grammatical features of a language, some researchers have investigated *what* the most coherent figurative expressions of time are in a particular language, and *how* they affect the language group's experience of time. This research shows that different linguistic groups have developed different characteristic figurative expressions for encoding time. When a figurative expression is used to characterize time, it evokes a linguistic representation that embodies the figurative meanings in the expression. This representation may in turn color the way the speaker experiences time.

Cultures differ in how time is represented metaphorically. In a cross-linguistic study, Zhou (2004) found that the most coherent cluster of time metaphors in the English language represents time as a moving object, and that the one in the Chinese language represents time as a container. She collected 140 Chinese and 131 English time metaphors from native Chinese and English speakers, and from several dictionaries of quotations in the two languages. Next, she had Chinese and English speakers judge the appropriateness of the metaphors in their language. Factor analyses performed on the appropriateness ratings showed that in the English language, metaphors representing time as bounded objects traveling speedily in space (e.g., winged chariot) accounted for 13.7% of the variance in the appropriateness ratings. These metaphorical representations render the perception of time as something that is meant to be caught, yet difficult to catch. Other clusters of time metaphors each accounted for less than 5% of the variance.

In the Chinese language, metaphors that represent time as a boundless bearer of undefined or ill-defined objects, memories, and emotions (e.g., container, ocean) accounted for 13.5% of the variance of the appropriateness ratings (other clusters of time each accounted for less than 6% of the variance). These metaphors render the perception of time as a boundless container that extends in space, with an unlimited capacity for carrying human memories, experiences, and emotions.

English and Chinese speakers also use different directional metaphors to talk about time. For example, English speakers prefer using front–back terms when they talk about time (e.g., ahead of time, behind schedule). In contrast, Chinese speakers prefer using up–down terms to describe time, referring to yesterday as *one day up* and tomorrow as *one day down*, for example (Boroditsky, 2001).

Research has shown that individuals can process the metaphorical meaning conveyed in a figurative expression at least as efficiently as they process the meaning conveyed in a literal expression (Glucksberg, 2001). In one experiment, Glucksberg had participants make speeded judgments of whether utterances such as "Some lawyers are sharks" are true or false. Participants who answered "no" responded to the utterances' literal meanings and those who answered "yes" responded to the utterances' figurative meanings. Affirmative responses were faster than negative ones, indicating that the figurative meanings were processed more efficiently than were the literal meanings.

Moreover, encoding an object with a figurative (vs. literal) expression may lead to memory distortion of the object in the direction of the figurative expression (Lau, Chiu, & Lee, 2001). For example, when a triangle is presented, individuals who have been led to describe it figuratively ("It looks like a mountain") are less able to recognize the figure in a delayed memory test, compared to those who have been led to describe it literally ("It is a triangle").

Similarly, encoding time with a figurative expression may also influence how time is experienced. In a series of experiments, Boroditsky (2001) demonstrates how activating time metaphors in a language may influence its speakers' experience of time. In one experiment, English and Chinese speakers answered a true–false question about time (e.g., March comes earlier than April) after they were primed with the front–back relation (the vehicle of the dominant directional metaphor for time in English) or the up–down relation (the vehicle of the dominant directional metaphor for time in Chinese). The front–back and the up–down primes consisted of two different sets of true–false questions (e.g., "The black worm is ahead of the white worm" vs. "The black ball is above the white ball"). As expected, for the English speakers, the front–back primes produced faster response to the time question than did the up–down primes, and the reverse was true for the Chinese speakers. Furthermore, in the same series of experiments, after native English speakers had been trained to use the up–down metaphor for time, their response pattern looked like that of Chinese speakers. Appar-

ently, the dominant metaphor for time in a language community allows its members to process temporal information efficiently. When the metaphor is activated, people use it as a tool to process temporal information.

Conclusion

The research findings are consistent with the propositions mentioned earlier in this chapter. First, speakers use the characteristic ways of referring to a state of affairs in their language as linguistic tools to encode experiences and express thoughts. When (and only when) these tools are used to characterize certain state of affairs, they influence cognitions by evoking or creating a linguistic representation that competes with and overshadows the perceptual representation of that state of affairs.

Communication and Cognition

Language is not just a collection of words and rules. It is a *communal tool kit* that individuals in a speech community use to construct meanings (Bruner, 1990; Semin, 1998). A speech community shares not only the rules of a language but also common understandings of its use and interpretation (Brenneis, 2002). When individuals translate a thought into external speech, they must cast it in a form that is appropriate for linguistic operations and pertinent to the communication function (Langacker, 1976). The lexical terms in a language limit the ways a thought can be expressed verbally, and so do the contexts of language use, which include the ground rules and assumptions that govern usage, audience design, and the immediate, ongoing, and emerging properties of the communication situation (Krauss & Chiu, 1998).

The cognitive consequences of communication received some attention in early color memory studies. Lantz and Strefflre (1964) argued that color codability predicts color memory only when color codability reflects how easy it is to describe the color accurately to an intended audience. To test this idea, they asked a group of participants (the encoders) to name an array of colors. Next, another group of participants (the decoders) were asked to identify the color associated with each of the color names generated by the first group of participants. From the decoders' performance, the investigators derived a communicability score for each color. Finally, they measured the memorability of each color by administrating a recognition memory task to a third group of participants. Colors that were more communicable were easier to recognize.

In another study, communication accuracy and recognizability data were collected for the Farnsworth–Munsell color chips from native Spanish speakers and native speakers of Yucatec, a Mayan language (Stefflre, Vales, & Morley, 1966). The correlation between communication accuracy and recognition accuracy was .45 in the Yucatec-speaking sample and .59 in the Spanish-speaking sample. Both correlations were statistically reliable. However, communication accuracy in Spanish and communication accuracy in Yucatec were uncorrelated, indicating colors that are easy to communicate in one language community are not necessarily so in another. This finding also eliminates the alternative explanation that communicable colors are focal colors. Other studies also found that easily communicated colors in one language community are also easy to remember in that community (see also Garro, 1986; Lucy & Shweder, 1979, 1988).

How frequently different colors are mentioned in communication may explain the positive correlation of color communicability and recognizability. There may be high consensus in the language community on the referring expressions for colors that are frequently referenced in communication. The established referential communication norms for these colors may render them more communicable than other colors. Meanwhile, people may have better memory for the colors that they frequently encounter and talk about (Lau, Lee, & Chiu, 2004).

Construction of Shared Reality

Sperber (1996) suggests that the best way to study how culture spreads and evolves is by examining how shared representations "are cognized by individuals and how they are communicated within a group" (p. 97). If any state of affairs can be described differently, how do people collaboratively establish its referring expression and consensual meaning?

Some researchers have examined how shared reality arises as communicators tune their message to the assumed beliefs and attitudes of the addressee. This research reveals that speakers estimate their addressee's knowledge about a referent when they formulate referring expressions (Clark & Carlson, 1982; Clark & Marshall, 1981; Clark & Murphy, 1982; Clark, Schreuder, & Buttrick, 1983; Krauss & Fussell, 1991, 1996; Krauss, Fussell, & Chen, 1995). Expressions tend to be briefer when the addressee is estimated to be knowledgeable about the referent, and vice versa (Fussell & Krauss, 1991, 1992; Lau, Chiu, & Hong, 2001). In addition, speakers tend to include in their communicative message expressions that are part of the established common ground (Fussell & Krauss, 1989a, 1989b; Krauss & Glucksberg, 1977; Krauss, Vivekananthan, & Weinheimer, 1968). Furthermore, when speakers learn that their addressee has a positive or negative attitude toward a target person, they would tune their descriptions of the target person in the direction of the addressee's attitude toward the target person. Moreover, the speakers' subsequent impressions of the target person become evaluatively consistent with the addressee's attitudes (Higgins & McCann, 1984; Higgins, McCann, & Fondacaro, 1982; McCann, Higgins, & Fondacaro, 1991).

The processes through which dyadic communication produces shared representations between two individuals may mediate the emergence of spatial distributions of shared representations in a collective, which in turn may lead to formation of complex systems of social representations, often referred to as cultures. According to the dynamic social impact theory (Latané, 1996), physical proximity increases the opportunity to communicate: People are more likely to communicate with people in the same neighborhood or workplace than with people living far away. When people communicate with others, shared representations are established. As communication continues, there is a tendency for sets of beliefs, values, and practices to become spatially differentiated (or clustered). At the same time, within a particular clustered location, previously unrelated beliefs, values, or practices become associated (or correlated) and relatively homogeneous (or consolidated; Brauer, Judd, & Jacquelin, 2001). Although consolidation could ultimately result in complete amalgamation, clustering protects minorities from majority influence, thus ensuring continuing diversity.

To simulate the hypothesized processes of culture formation, Latané and his colleagues (Latané & Bourgeois, 1996; Latané & L'Herrou, 1996) organized participants into e-mail groups and informed them of the majority opinions. Each participant was allowed to communicate by e-mail with only a fixed number of individuals (approximating physical constraints in real life). Over a number of electronic sessions, opinions began to cluster together. Thus, within each communication group, opinions became more homogenous, and previously uncorrelated issues became correlated. However, at the end of the studies, even with incentives to agree with the opinions of the majority, there still remained pockets of minority opinions.

Similar results were obtained in a 3-year longitudinal study of political socialization of business and social science students (Guimond & Palmer, 1985). In this study, over time, social sciences students developed a shared, coherent perspective about social problems. They became more likely than business students to attribute poverty and unemployment to systemic factors. Furthermore, previously uncorrelated beliefs about the causes of poverty became related in the third year.

Summary

Language is not just a collection of symbols and formal rules; it is a framework for action in a language community. The use of language in human communication plays an important role in the development of shared cognitive styles and shared cognitions, which are core elements of culture. Language enables culture, but it does not determine the course of its development (Bruner, 1990).

The role of language use in cultural processes can be summarized as follows:

1. Language encodes cultural meanings. The characteristic expressions in a language afford economical ways of characterizing experiences and expressing thoughts. These expressions are likely to be used in everyday communication.
2. Using language to characterize a state of affairs may evoke or create linguistic representations that compete with and overshadow the perceptual representations of that state of affairs.
3. A speech community shares the formal rules of a language, as well as the ground rules and assumptions that underlie language usage. The contexts of language use (e.g., audience design) influence the forms linguistic

representations of certain state of affairs will take. Through communication, private cognitions are made public and directed toward a shared representation of the referent (Schegloff, 1991).

CONCLUSIONS AND FUTURE DIRECTIONS

The preceding analysis of the relationship of language and culture embodies a constructivist view of culture (see Chiu & Chen, 2004; Ng, Chiu, & Candlin, 2004). In this view, through the use of language as discourse, the shared reality expresses itself in communicative actions; that is, language plays a pivotal role in constituting the existing social reality by providing a set of shared symbols for constructing shared meanings.

In a review, Lehman, Chiu, and Schaller (2004) discerned a lopsided emphasis in the psychology literature on cultural differences. Their review reminds researchers of the need for a body of psychological knowledge that explains how discursive practices maintain the stability of a culture, and the role of language use in culture change.

Although cultural psychologists have not done much to uncover language's role in the reproduction and transformation of culture, some investigators have begun to examine how shared ideas are reproduced and propagate through interpersonal communication. The four aspects of this process that have received relatively more research attention are (1) reproduction of conventional cultural knowledge through communication, (2) institutionalization of cultural knowledge in communication practices, (3) language as a carrier of cultural meanings, and (4) language as a marker of cultural identities.

Language Use and Reproduction of Culture

Communication and Reproduction of Conventional Cultural Ideas

Successful reproduction of cultures requires reproduction of shared meanings in communication (Sperber, 1996). In series of experiments, Lyons and Kashima (2001, 2003) found that conventional ideas are more likely to be reproduced in dyadic communication compared to unconventional ones. These findings provide important leads into the discursive foundation of culture. If conventional ideas are more likely than unconventional ones to be included in communications, they should be more inheritable in cultural transmission. As Sperber (1996, p. 83) puts it, cultural ideas that are "repeatedly communicated and minimally transformed in the process will end up belonging to the culture."

Institutionalization of Cultural Knowledge

Shared cognitions that emerge from communication are often instituted in communicative practices. For instance, compared to East Asians, European Americans focus their attention more on the object (vs. object–context relation; Masuda & Nisbett, 2001). This cultural difference is instituted in adult–child communication. English-speaking American children use more nouns (which reference objects or abstract entities) and fewer verbs (which describe how the grammatical subject acts upon the external environment or internal state) than do Mandarin-speaking children in China (Tardif, 1996; Tardif, Gelman, & Xu, 1999). Moreover, English-speaking caregivers also emphasize nouns over verbs when they talk to children, whereas Mandarin-speaking caregivers have the reverse trend (Tardif, Shatz, & Naigles, 1998). As another example, the Confucian tradition in Chinese culture emphasizes moral and social standards, and Chinese families often reference such standards in personal storytelling, whereas American families typically use personal storytelling as a medium of entertainment and affirmation (Miller, Wiley, Fung, & Liang, 1997).

Language Activates Cultural Meanings

Because of the close association of language use and culture, the presence of a language may evoke its associated cultural meanings. Earle (1969) reported the first experimental demonstration of language priming effect and found that bilingual Hong Kong Chinese students are less dogmatic when they respond to the Dogmatism Scale (Rokeach, 1960) in English than when they answer the same questionnaire translated into Chinese. Earle proposes that Hong Kong bilinguals, who have learned Chinese and English in distinct settings, can maintain two somewhat differently structured belief systems, reflecting the contexts in which they acquired the two languages and, more gener-

ally, the two language cultures. As such, the Chinese version of the questionnaire activates the more dogmatic Chinese language culture, and the English version activates the less dogmatic English language culture. Similar language-priming effects have been reported among Hong Kong Chinese, Chinese Canadians, and Greek–Dutch bilinguals on spontaneous self-concept, self-esteem, and causal attribution (Bond, 1983; Ross, Xun, & Wilson, 2002; Trafimow, Silverman, Fan, & Law, 1997; Verkuyten & Pouliasi, 2002).

Language as a Marker of Cultural Identity

Language can also be a marker of cultural identity. There is consistent evidence that the language one speaks is an important dimension for both self- and social categorization (Bourhis, Giles, & Tajfel, 1973). Giles, Taylor and their associates compared the relative contributions of language, cultural background, and geographical residence to self- and social categorization in five groups: Welsh bilinguals from South Wales (Giles, Taylor, & Bourhis, 1977), English Canadians, French Canadians (Taylor, Bassili, & Aboud, 1973), Anglo Americans and Franco Americans (Giles, Taylor, Lambert, & Albert, 1976). They found that for all groups, the language spoken was the most salient dimension of self- and ethnic identities.

In addition, listeners' attitudes toward speakers of certain languages or dialects reflect their evaluations of the relative status of the speakers' ethnolinguistic group (Brennan & Brennan, 1981; Callan, Gallois, & Forbes, 1983; Genesee & Holobow, 1989; Lyczak, Fu, & Ho, 1976; Mazurkewich, Fister-Stoga, Mawle, Somers, & Thibaudeau, 1986; Sebastian & Ryan, 1985; Tong, Hong, Lee, & Chiu, 1999). Furthermore, although people's speech styles tend to converge (i.e., to become more like those of their partners), speakers may react to identity-threatening circumstances by accentuating speech and nonverbal differences between themselves and members of the other group (Bourhis et al., 1973; Bourhis & Giles, 1977; Bourhis, Giles, Leyens, & Tajfel, 1979; Taylor & Royer, 1980). Likewise, the presence of the language of an unfriendly out-group may also lead one to affirm the cultural values of one's own group (Bond & Cheung, 1984; Bond & Yang, 1982; Yang & Bond, 1980).

Finally, speakers tend to describe in-group and out-group behaviors differently. For example, speakers spontaneously use more abstract verb phrases (e.g., hate) and fewer concrete verb phrases (e.g., hit) when they describe behaviors of a stereotyped ethnocultural group than when they describe the behaviors of their own group (Hamilton, Gibbons, Stroessner, & Sherman, 1992). Encoding a behavior with an abstract verb implies that the behavior is stable and consistent across situations, whereas encoding a behavior with a concrete verb limits the generality of the behavior to a concrete situation (Semin & Fiedler, 1988, 1991). Thus, this finding suggests that behaviors of stereotyped groups are likely to be linguistically encoded as reflecting abstract qualities of the group members. However, the tendencies to describe the behaviors of out-group members in abstract verb types are not uniform across different types of behavior. Undesirable out-group behaviors tend to be described with abstract verb types, whereas desirable out-group behaviors tend to be described with concrete verb types (Fiedler, Semin, & Finkenauer, 1993; Maass, Milesi, Zabbini, & Stahlberg, 1995; Maass, Salvi, Arcuri, & Semin, 1989). In short, the ways people use language may reinforce cultural stereotypes, as well as the boundary separating their own group from other ethnic groups.

Language and Culture Change

In a relatively impermeable culture, or a culture that has few contacts with other cultures, the communicative mechanisms described in the previous paragraph give rise to a relatively stable cultural tradition. However, even in such relatively closed cultures, changes in the mode and means of production, technology, political system, and interdependence structure may present a need to open negotiation of meanings in public discourse. In a multicultural society, exposure to knowledge from different cultures highlights cultural contrasts and triggers a meaningful negotiation process that fuels culture change (Ota, 2004). The tracking of communicative messages in settings where intercultural contacts are frequent and intense may reveal how language and culture coevolve. For example, as tourists participate in international travel, they are socialized into the reality represented in travel magazines, newspaper travelogues, and televised holiday programs. The language and rhetoric used in these media provide the semiotic materials for analyzing how the culture and identity of global citizens evolve (Jaworski & Thurlow, 2004).

Indeed, as the speed of globalization accelerates, communicative acts may function like a barometer of culture change. For instance, China has undergone rapid economic and social transformation in the last two decades. How might this transformation change the collectivist values in China? Zhang and Shavitt (2003), who analyzed the values promoted in Chinese advertising, found that both modernity and individualism predominate in current Chinese advertising. In addition, individualism and modern values are more pervasive in magazine advertisements (which target young consumers) than in television commercials (which target older consumers). All these changes suggest that after half a century of psychological research and intense debates on language's role in cognitive and cultural processes, the field is still open, with exciting territories that remain to be discovered and explored.

REFERENCES

Au, T. (1983). Chinese and English counterfactuals: The Sapir–Whorf hypothesis revisited. *Cognition, 15,* 155–187.

Au, T. (1984). Counterfactuals: In reply to Alfred Bloom. *Cognition, 17,* 289–302.

Au, T. (2004). Making sense of differences: Language, culture, and social reality. In S.-h. Ng, C. Candlin, & C.-y. Chiu (Eds.), *Language matters: Communication, culture, and social identity* (pp. 139–153). Hong Kong: City University of Hong Kong Press.

Berlin, B., & Kay, P. (1969). *Basic color terms: Their universality and evolution.* Berkeley: University of California Press.

Bloom, A. H. (1981a). *The linguistic shaping of thought: A study in the impact of language on thinking in China and the West.* Hillsdale, NJ: Erlbaum.

Bloom, A. H. (1981b). Language and theoretical vs. reality centered morality. In R. W. Wilson, S. L. Greenblatt, & A. A. Wilson (Eds.), *Moral behavior in Chinese society* (pp. 21–37). New York: Praeger.

Bond, M. H. (1983). How language variation affects inter-cultural differentiation of values by Hong Kong bilinguals. *Journal of Language and Social Psychology, 2,* 57–66.

Bond, M. H., & Cheung, M.-k. (1984). Experimenter language choice and ethnic affirmation by Chinese trilinguals in Hong Kong. *International Journal of Intercultural Relations, 8,* 347–356.

Bond, M. H., & Yang, K. S. (1982). Ethnic affirmation versus cross-cultural accommodation: The variable impact of questionnaire language on Chinese bilinguals from Hong Kong. *Journal of Cross-Cultural Psychology, 13*, 169–185.

Boroditsky, L. (2001). Does language shape thought? *Cognitive Psychology, 42*, 1–22.

Bourhis, R. Y., & Giles, H. (1977). The language of intergroup distinctiveness. In H. Giles (Ed.), *Language, ethnicity and intergroup relations* (pp. 119–135). London: Academic Press.

Bourhis, R. Y., Giles, H., & Tajfel, H. (1973). Language as a determinant of Welsh identity. *European Journal of Social Psychology, 3*, 447–460.

Bourhis, R. Y., Giles, H., Leyens, J.-P., & Tajfel, H. (1979). Psycholinguistic distinctiveness: Language divergence in Beligum. In H. Giles & R. S. Clair (Eds.), *Language and social psychology* (pp. 158–185). Oxford, UK: Blackwell.

Brauer, M., Judd, C. M., & Jacquelin, V. (2001). The communication of social stereotypes: The effects of group discussion and information distribution on stereotypic appraisals. *Journal of Personality and Social Psychology, 81*, 463–475.

Brennan, E. M., & Brennan, J. S. (1981). Accent scaling and language attitudes: Reactions to Mexican American English speech. *Language and Speech, 24*, 207–221.

Brenneis, D. (2002). Some cases for culture. *Human Development, 45*, 264–269.

Brown, R. (1976). Reference: In memorial tribute to Eric Lenneberg. *Cognition, 4*, 125–153.

Bruner, J. (1990). *Acts of meaning.* Cambridge, MA: Harvard University Press.

Callan, V. J., Gallois, C., & Forbes, P. A. (1983). Evaluative reactions to accented English: Ethnicity, sex role, and context. *Journal of Cross-Cultural Psychology, 14*, 407–426.

Carroll, J. B., & Casagrande, J. B. (1958). The function of language classification in behavior. In E. E. Maccoby, T. R. Newcomb, & E. L. Hartley (Eds.), *Readings in social psychology* (3rd ed., pp. 18–31). New York: Holt, Rinehart & Winston.

Chiu, C.-y., & Chen, J. (2004). Symbols and interactions: Application of the CCC model to culture, language, and social identity. In S.-h. Ng, C. Candlin, & C.-y. Chiu (Eds.), *Language matters: Communication, culture, and social identity* (pp. 155–182). Hong Kong: City University of Hong Kong Press.

Chiu, C.-y., Krauss, R. M., & Lau, I. (1998). Some cognitive consequences of communication. In S. R. Fussell & R. J. Kreuz (Eds.), *Social and cognitive approaches to interpersonal communication* (pp. 259–276). Mahwah, NJ: Erlbaum.

Chiu, C.-y., Krauss, K. M., & Lee, S. (1999). Communication and social cognition: A post-Whorfian approach. In T. Sugiman, M. Karasawa, J. Liu, & C. Ward (Eds.), *Progress in Asian social psychology* (Vol. 2, pp. 127–143). Map-Ku, Korea: Kyoyook-Kwahak-Sa.

Chomsky, N. (1992). *Language and thought.* Wakefield, RI: Moyer Bell.

Clark, H. H., & Brennan, S. E. (1991). Grounding in communication. In L. B. Resnick, J. Levine, & S. D. Teasley (Eds.), *Perspectives on socially shared cognition* (pp. 127–149). Washington, DC: American Psychological Association.

Clark, H. H., & Carlson, T. B. (1982). Speech acts and hearers' beliefs. In N. V. Smith (Ed.), *Mutual knowledge* (pp. 1–59). New York: Academic Press.

Clark, H. H., & Marshall, C. E. (1981). Definite reference and mutual knowledge. In A. K. Joshi, I. Sag, & B. Webber (Eds.), *Elements of discourse understanding* (pp. 10–63). Cambridge, UK: Cambridge University Press.

Clark, H. H., & Murphy, G. L. (1982). Audience design in meaning and reference. In J.-F. L. Ny & W. Kintsch (Eds.), *Language and comprehension* (pp. 287–296). New York: North Holland.

Clark, H. H., Schreuder, R., & Buttrick, S. (1983). Common ground and the understanding of demonstrative reference. *Journal of Verbal Learning and Verbal Behavior, 22*, 245–258.

Clarke, M., Losoff, A., McCracken, M. D., & Rood, D. (1984). Linguistic relativity and sex/gender studies: Epistemological and methodological considerations. *Language Learning, 34*, 47–67.

Clarke, M., Losoff, A., McCracken, M. D., & Still, J. (1981). Gender perception in Arabic and English. *Language Learning, 31*, 159–169.

D'Andrade, R. (2002). Cultural Darwinism and language. *American Anthropologist, 104*, 223–232.

Davidoff, J. (2001). Language and perceptual categorization. *Trends in Cognitive Sciences, 5*, 382–387.

Earle, M. (1969). A cross-cultural and cross-language comparison of dogmatism scores. *Journal of Social Psychology, 79*, 19–24.

Ervin, S. M. (1962). The connotations of gender. *Word, 18*, 249–261.

Fallshore, M., & Schooler, J. W. (1995). The verbal vulnerability of perceptual expertise. *Journal of Experimental Psychology: Learning, Memory, and Cognition, 21*, 1608–1623.

Fiedler, K., Semin, G. R., & Finkenauer, C. (1993). The battle of words between gender groups: A language-based approach to intergroup processes. *Human Communication Research, 19*, 409–441.

Fussell, S. R., & Krauss, R. M. (1989a). The effects of intended audience on message production and comprehension: Reference in a common ground framework. *Journal of Experimental Social Psychology, 25*, 203–219.

Fussell, S. R., & Krauss, R. M. (1989b). Understanding friends and strangers: The effects of audience design on message comprehension. *European Journal of Social Psychology, 19*, 509–525.

Fussell, S. R., & Krauss, R. M. (1991). Accuracy and bias in estimates of others' knowledge. *European Journal of Social Psychology, 21*, 445–454.

Fussell, S. R., & Krauss, R. M. (1992). Coordination of knowledge in communication: Effects of speakers' assumptions about others' knowledge. *Journal of Personality and Social Psychology, 62*, 378–391.

Garro, L. (1986). Language, memory, and focality: A re-examination. *American Anthropologist, 88,* 128–136.

Genesee, F., & Holobow, N. E. (1989). Change and stability in intergroup perceptions. *Journal of Language and Social Psychology, 8,* 17–38.

Giles, H., Taylor, D. M., & Bourhis, R. Y. (1977). Dimensions of Welsh identity. *European Journal of Social Psychology, 7,* 165–174.

Giles, H., Taylor, D. M., Lambert, W. E., & Albert, G. (1976). Dimensions of ethnic identity: An example from Northern Maine. *Journal of Social Psychology, 100,* 11–19.

Glucksberg, S. (1988). Language and thought. In R. S. Sternberg & E. E. Smith (Eds.), *The psychology of human thought* (pp. 214–241). New York: Cambridge University Press.

Glucksberg, S. (2001). *Understanding figurative language: From metaphor to idioms.* Oxford, UK: Oxford University Press.

Grice, H. P. (1975). Logic and conversation. In P. Cole & J. Morgan (Eds.), *Syntax and semantics: Vol. 3. Speech acts* (pp. 43–58). New York: Academic Press.

Guimond, S., & Palmer, D. L. (1985). The political socialization of commerce and social science students: Epistemic authority and attitude change. *Journal of Applied Social Psychology, 26,* 1985–2013.

Hall, E. T. (1990). *Understanding cultural differences.* Yarmouth, ME: Intercultural Press.

Hamilton, D. L., Gibbons, P. A., Stroessner, S. J., & Sherman, J. W. (1992). Stereotype and language use. In G. R. Semin & K. Fiedler (Eds.), *Language, interaction and social cognition* (pp. 102–128). London: Sage.

Heider, E. R. (1972). Universals in color naming and memory. *Journal of Experimental Psychology, 93,* 10–20.

Heider, E. R., & Olivier, D. C. (1972). The structure of the color space in naming and memory for two languages. *Cognitive Psychology, 3,* 337–354.

Higgins, E. T., & McCann, C. D. (1984). Social encoding and subsequent attitudes, impressions and memory: "Context-driven" and motivational aspects of processing. *Journal of Personality and Social Psychology, 47,* 26–39.

Higgins, E. T., McCann, C. D., & Fondacaro, R. (1982). The "communication game": Goal-directed encoding and cognitive consequences. *Social Cognition, 1,* 21–37.

Hoffman, C., Lau, I., & Johnson, D. R. (1986). The linguistic relativity of person cognition: An English–Chinese comparison. *Journal of Personality and Social Psychology, 51,* 1097–1105.

Hoosain, R. (1991). *Psycholinguistic implications for linguistic relatively: A case study of Chinese.* Hillsdale, NJ: Erlbaum.

Hunt, E., & Agnoli, F. (1991). The Whorfian hypothesis: A cognitive psychology perspective. *Psychological Review, 98,* 377–389.

Hunt, E., & Banaji, M. R. (1988). The Whorfian hypothesis revisited: A cognitive science view of linguistic and cultural effects on thought. In J. W. Berry, S. H. Irvine, & E. B. Hunt (Eds.), *Indigenous cognition: Functioning in cultural context* (pp. 57–84). Dordrecht, the Netherlands: Martinus Nijhoff.

Ishii, K., Reyes, J. A., & Kitayama, S. (2003). Spontaneous attention to word content versus emotional tone: Differences among three cultures. *Psychological Science, 14,* 39–46.

Jaworski, A., & Thurlow, C. (2004). Language, tourism and globalization: Mapping new international identities. In S.-h. Ng, C. Candlin, & C.-y. Chiu (Eds.), *Language matters: Communication, culture, and social identity* (pp. 297–321). Hong Kong: City University of Hong Kong Press.

Kahneman, D., & Tversky, A. (1984). Choices, values, and frames. *American Psychologist, 39,* 341–350.

Kashima, E. S., & Kashima, Y. (1998). Culture and language: The case of cultural dimensions and personal pronoun use. *Journal of Cross-Cultural Psychology, 29,* 461–486.

Kashima, Y., & Kashima, E. (2003). Individualism, GNP, climate, and pronoun drop: Is individualism determined by affluence and climate, or does language use play a role. *Journal of Cross-Cultural Psychology, 34,* 125–134.

Kay, P., & Kempton, W. (1984). What is the Sapir–Whorf hypothesis? *American Anthroplogist, 86,* 65–79.

Kay, P., & McDaniel, C. K. (1978). The linguistic significance of the meanings of basic color terms. *Language, 54,* 610–646.

Krauss, R. M., & Chiu, C.-y. (1998). Language and social behavior. In D. T. Gilbert, S. T. Fiske, & G. Lindzey (Eds.), *The handbook of social psychology* (4th ed., Vol. 2, pp. 41–88). New York: McGraw-Hill.

Krauss, R. M., & Fussell, S. R. (1991). Perspective-taking in communication: Representations of others' knowledge in reference. *Social Cognition, 9,* 2–24.

Krauss, R. M., & Fussell, S. R. (1996). Social psychological approaches to the study of communication. In E. T. Higgins & A. Kruglanski (Eds.), *Social psychology: Handbook of basic principles* (pp. 655–701). New York: Guilford Press.

Krauss, R. M., Fussell, S. R., & Chen, Y. (1995). Coordination of perspective in dialogue: Intrapersonal and interpersonal processes. In I. Markova, C. G. Graumann, & K. Foppa (Eds.), *Mutualities in dialogue* (pp. 124–145). Cambridge, UK: Cambridge University Press.

Krauss, R. M., & Glucksberg, S. (1977). Social and nonsocial speech. *Scientific American, 236,* 100–105.

Krauss, R. M., Vivekananthan, P. S., & Weinheimer, S. (1968). "Inner speech" and "external speech." *Journal of Personality and Social Psychology, 9,* 295–300.

Langacker, R. W. (1976). Semantic representations and the linguistic relativity hypothesis. *Foundations of Language, 14,* 307–357.

Lantz, D., & Stefflre, V. (1964). Language and cognition revisited. *Journal of Abnormal and Social Psychology, 69,* 472–481.

Latané, B. (1996). Dynamic social impact: The creation of culture by communication. *Journal of Communication, 46,* 13–25.

Latané, B., & Bourgeois, M. J. (1996). Experimental evidence for dynamic social impact: The emergence of subcultures in electronic groups. *Journal of Communication, 46,* 35–47.

Latané, B., & L'Herrou, T. (1996). Spatial clustering in the conformity game: Dynamic social impact in electronic groups. *Journal of Personality and Social Psychology, 70,* 1218–1230.

Lau, I. Y.-M., Chiu, C.-y., & Hong, Y. (2001). I know what you know: Assumptions about others' knowledge and their effects on message construction. *Social Cognition, 19,* 587–600.

Lau, I. Y.-M., Chiu, C.-y., & Lee, S.-L. (2001). Communication and shared reality: Implications for the psychological foundations of culture. *Social Cognition, 19,* 350–371.

Lau, I. Y.-M., Lee, S.-L., & Chiu, C.-y. (2004). Language, cognition and reality: Constructing shared meanings through communication. In M. Schaller & C. Crandall (Eds.), *The psychological foundations of culture* (pp. 77–100). Mahwah, NJ: Erlbaum.

Lehman, D., Chiu, C.-y., & Schaller, M. (2004). Culture and psychology. *Annual Review of Psychology, 55,* 689–714.

Liu, L. G. (1985). Reasoning counterfactually in Chinese: Are there any obstacles? *Cognition, 21,* 239–270.

Lucy, J. A., & Shweder, R. A. (1979). Whorf and his critics: Linguistic and nonlinguistic influences on color memory. *American Anthropologist, 81,* 581–615.

Lucy, J. A., & Shweder, R. A. (1988). The effect of incidental conversation on memory for focal colors. *American Anthropologist, 90,* 923–931.

Lyczak, R., Fu, G. S., & Ho, A. (1976). Attitudes of Hong Kong bilinguals toward English and Chinese speakers. *Journal of Cross-Cultural Psychology, 7,* 425–438.

Lyons, A., & Kashima, Y. (2001). The reproduction of culture: Communication processes tend to maintain cultural stereotypes. *Social Cognition, 19,* 372–394.

Lyons, A., & Kashima, Y. (2003). How are stereotypes maintained through communication?: The influence of stereotype sharedness. *Personality and Social Psychology Bulletin, 85,* 989–1005.

Maass, A., Milesi, A., Zabbini, S., & Stahlberg, D. (1995). Linguistic intergroup bias: Differential expectancies or in-group protection? *Journal of Personality and Social Psychology, 68,* 116–126.

Maass, A., Salvi, D., Arcuri, L., & Semin, G. R. (1989). Language use in intergroup contexts: The linguistic intergroup bias. *Journal of Personality and Social Psychology, 38,* 689–703.

Masuda, T., & Nisbett, R. E. (2001). Attending holistically versus analytically: Comparing the context sensitivity of Japanese and Americans. *Journal of Personality and Social Psychology, 81,* 922–934.

Mazurkewich, I., & Fista-Stoga, F., Mawle, D., Somers, M., & Thibaudeau, S. (1986). A new look at language attitudes in Montreal. *Genetic, Social, and General Psychology Monographs, 112,* 201–217.

McCann, C. D., Higgins, E. T., & Fondacaro, R. A. (1991). Primacy and recency in communication and self-persuasion: How successive audiences and multiple encodings influence subsequent judgments. *Social Cognition, 9,* 47–66.

Miller, P., Wiley, A. R., Fung, H., & Liang, C.-h. (1997). Personal storytelling as a medium of socialization in Chinese and American families. *Child Development, 68,* 557–568.

Ng, S.-h., Chiu, C.-y., & Candlin, C. (2004). Communication, culture, and identity: Overview and synthesis. In S.-h. Ng, C. Candlin, & C.-y. Chiu (Eds.), *Language matters: Communication, culture, and social identity* (pp. 1–23). Hong Kong: City University of Hong Kong Press.

Ota, H. (2004). Culture and intergenerational communication: Implications of cultures for communication across age groups. In S.-h. Ng, C. Candlin, & C.-y. Chiu (Eds.), *Language matters: Communication, culture, and social identity* (pp. 183–201). Hong Kong: City University of Hong Kong Press.

Ranken, H. B. (1963). Language and thinking: Positive and negative effects of naming. *Science, 141,* 48–50.

Roberson, D., & Davidoff, J. (2000). The "categorical perception" of colors and facial expressions: The effect of verbal interference. *Memory and Cognition, 28,* 977–986.

Roberson, D., Davies, I., & Davidoff, J. (2000). Color categories are not universal: Replications and new evidence from a stone-age culture. *Journal of Experimental Psychology: General, 129,* 369–398.

Rokeach, M. (1960). *The open and closed mind: Investigations into the nature of belief systems and personality systems.* New York: Basic Books.

Rosch, E. H. (1973). On the internal structure of perceptual and semantic categories. In T. E. Moore (Ed.), *Cognitive development and the acquisition of language* (pp. 254–279). New York: Academic Press.

Rosch, E. H. (1987). Linguistic relativity. *Et cetera, 44,* 254–279.

Ross, M., Xun, W. Q. E., & Wilson, A. E. (2002). Language and the bicultural self. *Personality and Social Psychology Bulletin, 28,* 1040–1050.

Schegloff, E. A. (1991). Conversation analysis and socially shared cognition. In L. B. Resnick, J. M. Levine, & S. D. Teasley (Eds.), *Perspectives on socially shared cognition* (pp. 150–171). Washington, DC: American Psychological Association.

Schooler, J. W., & Engstler-Schooler, T. Y. (1990). Visual overshadowing of visual memories: Some things are better left unsaid. *Cognitive Psychology, 22,* 36–71.

Sebastian, R. J., & Ryan, E. B. (1985). Speech cues and social evaluations: Markers of ethnicity, social class and age. In H. Giles & R. N. S. Clair (Eds.), *Recent advances in language, communication and social psychology* (pp. 112–143). Hillsdale, NJ: Erlbaum.

Semin, G. R. (1998). Cognition, language, and communication. In S. R. Fussell & R. J. Kreuz (Eds.), *Social and cognitive approaches to interpersonal communication* (pp. 229–257). Mahwah, NJ: Erlbaum.

Semin, G. R., & Fiedler, K. (1988). The cognitive functions of linguistic categories in describing persons: Social cognition and language. *Journal of Personality and Social Psychology, 54,* 558–568.

Semin, G. R., & Fiedler, K. (1991). The linguistic category model, its bases, application and range. In W. Stroebe & M. Hewstone (Eds.), *European review of social psychology.* (Vol. 2, pp. 1–30). New York: Wiley.

Sera, M. D., Berge, D., & del Castillio Pintado, J. (1994). Grammatical and conceptual forces in the attribution of gender by English and Spanish speakers. *Child Development, 68,* 820–831.

Sera, M. D., Elieff, C., Forbes, J., Burch, M. C., Rodriguez, W., & Dubois, D. P. (2002). When language affects cognition and when it does not: An analysis of grammatical gender and classification. *Journal of Experimental Psychology: General, 131,* 377–397.

Shatz, M., Diesendruck, G., Martinez-Beck, I., & Akar, D. (2003). The influence of language and socioeconomic status on children's understanding of false belief. *Developmental Psychology, 39,* 717–729.

Sperber, D. (1996). *Explaining culture: A naturalistic approach.* Cambridge, MA: Blackwell.

Stefflre, V., Vales, V. C., & Morley, L. (1966). Language and cognition in Yucatan: A cross-cultural replication. *Journal of Personality and Social Psychology, 4,* 112–115.

Takano, Y. (1989). Methodological problems in cross-cultural studies of linguistic relativity. *Cognition, 31,* 141–162.

Tardif, T. (1996). Nouns are not always learned before verbs: Evidence from Mandarin speakers' early vocabularies. *Developmental Psychology, 32,* 492–504.

Tardif, T., Gelman, S. A., & Xu, F. (1999). Putting the "noun bias" in context: A comparison of English and Mandarin. *Child Development, 70,* 620–635.

Tardif, T., Shatz, M., & Naigles, L. (1998). Caregiver speech and children's use of nouns versus verbs: A comparison of English, Italian, and Mandarin. *Journal of Child Language, 24,* 535–565.

Taylor, D. M., Bassili, J. N., & Aboud, F. E. (1973). Dimensions of ethnic identity: An example for Quebec. *Journal of Social Psychology, 89,* 185–192.

Taylor, D. M., & Royer, L. (1980). Group processes affecting anticipated language choice in intergroup relations. In H. Giles, W. P. Robinson, & P. Smith (Eds.), *Language: Social psychological perspectives* (pp. 185–192). Oxford, UK: Pergamon.

Thomas, D. R., & DeCapito, A. (1966). Role of stimulus labeling in stimulus generalization. *Journal of Experimental Psychology, 71,* 913–915.

Tong, Y., Hong, Y.-y., Lee, S.-l., & Chiu, C.-y. (1999). Language as a carrier of social identity. *International Journal of Intercultural Relations, 23,* 281–296.

Trafimow, D., Silverman, E. S., Fan, R. M.-T., & Law, J. S. F. (1997). The effects of language and priming on the relative accessibility of the private self and the collective self. *Journal of Cross-Cultural Psychology, 28,* 107–123.

Verkuyten, M., & Pouliasi, K. (2002). Biculturalism among older children: Cultural frame switching, attributions, self-identification, and attitudes. *Journal of Cross-Cultural Psychology, 33,* 596–609.

Whorf, B. L. (1956). *Language, thought, and reality: Selected writings of Benjamin Lee Whorf.* New York: Wiley.

Yang, K. S., & Bond, M. H. (1980). Ethnic affirmation by Chinese bilinguals. *Journal of Cross-Cultural Psychology, 11,* 411–425.

Zhang, J., & Shavitt, S. (2003). Cultural values in advertisements to the Chinese X-generation. *Journal Advertising, 32,* 23–33.

Zhou, R. (2004). A comparative study of Chinese and English metaphorical representation of time. In S.-h. Ng, C. Candlin, & C.-y. Chiu (Eds.), *Language matters: Communication, culture, and social identity* (pp. 203–218). Hong Kong: City University of Hong Kong Press.

PART VI

EMOTION AND MOTIVATION

CHAPTER 28

Culture and Subjective Well-Being

WILLIAM TOV
ED DIENER

With great perseverance
He meditates, seeking
Freedom and happiness.
—THE BUDDHA, Chapter 2, *The Dhammapada*

Over 2,000 years ago, the Buddha perceived suffering to be the nature of existence. But for him, the attainment of nirvana was not simply a break from this cycle of suffering, it was also a return to true bliss. Although it was not the direct purpose of meditation, happiness was certainly an important consequence, and a critical topic in Buddhist philosophy (Gaskins, 1999). Across time and cultures, generations of people have in their own way reflected upon the question of happiness. As long as it has been pondered, it may come as a surprise that the scientific study of happiness, or subjective well-being (SWB; E. Diener, 1984) has advanced only recently.

One of the challenges has been defining happiness in a way that enables it to be measured. Given that conceptions of happiness may vary across different societies, a number of questions arise regarding *how* culture influences the idea and experience of happiness. Do the structure and content of SWB differ? Do certain cultures emphasize some components more than others? Are the correlates and causes of happiness similar across cultures? Do people react differently to the experience of well-being (e.g., when they feel pleasant affect)?

As it has been studied over the past two decades, SWB involves frequent pleasant emotion, infrequent unpleasant emotion, and life satisfaction (LS). The first two components are affective; the last is a cognitive evaluation. These three components are not the only elements of SWB. Happiness also can be said to consist of other dimensions, such as meaning and purpose in life. However, in this review we focus on LS, pleasant affect, and unpleasant affect, in part because these constructs have been researched more frequently across cultures. Furthermore, these components of SWB are major focal points that allow for a certain degree of precision in measuring the fuzzier, folk concept of happiness.

WHY STUDY SWB ACROSS CULTURES?

The cross-cultural study of SWB is one indicator of the quality of life in a society. It was once considered taboo to suggest that societies could be evaluated at all (Shweder, 2000). To appraise *any* aspect of a culture was to ignore its worth and integrity. However, this extreme form of cultural relativism has given way to the view that though one must be careful in comparing and evaluating, societies may differ in variables such as health and satisfaction that are desirable in most cultures. It is true that some indicators of life quality may impose values about the good life that are not shared by all people. However, even if SWB is internally framed with respect to each culture, societies could still be evaluated in terms of how well they succeed according to these internal criteria.

Culture and SWB research can also shed light on basic emotional processes. In measuring SWB across various societies, researchers have confronted issues regarding the universality of emotions, and how the representation of emotions in memory is influenced by cultural norms. The field can also add to our understanding of culture. For example, how do cultures differ in their socialization of pleasant and unpleasant affect, and how do emotions contribute to the reinforcement of cultural values and practices? These questions reflect a cultural-psychological perspective. Thus, the topic is of both applied and theoretical importance.

HISTORY OF THIS FIELD OF INQUIRY

Anthropologists adopted cultural relativity as a way of avoiding a Western, ethnocentric bias in observing other cultures. They made the important observation that values and practices might vary across cultures, but this need not imply that some cultures are necessarily better than others. In particular, we should avoid judging other cultures by the standards of our own. However, taken to extremes, cultural relativism would prevent one from saying that Nazi Germany, or Cambodia under the Khmer Rouge, were in many respects undesirable cultures (Edgerton, 1992). This level of extreme value relativity would make cultural psychology irrelevant to public discourse. According to Edgerton, not all practices in a culture are adaptive; some may even be harmful. He defined "maladaptive cultures" as those in which there is rampant dissatisfaction or impaired physical and mental health. Thus, there are certain criteria by which we can judge the success of a culture. As one such criterion, SWB is important because a society functions poorly when a majority of its people are discontent and depressed.

It should be noted that very little quantitative work has examined the well-being of small cultures (e.g., Biswas-Diener, Vittersø, & Diener, 2005), although a number of international surveys of SWB in modern nations have been conducted (e.g., Cantril, 1965; Inglehart, 1990; see Table 28.1). Only recently has research examined the structure and causes of SWB in different cultures. In 1995, for example, E. Diener and M. L. Diener found that self-esteem correlated more strongly with LS in individualist than in collectivist cultures, and that financial satisfaction more strongly predicted LS in poor than in rich nations. Since then, there has been a rapid growth in the field of culture and well-being, and both universal and unique correlates of SWB have been documented. We foresee further growth in this research area in the decade to come.

GENERAL APPROACHES
TO CROSS-CULTURAL COMPARISONS OF SWB

The comparisons that researchers make across cultures are guided by their assumptions about the interplay between culture and SWB. We review some of these approaches here.

TABLE 28.1. LS in Various Nations (1999–2002)

Nation	Year	LS	SD	Nation	Year	LS	SD
Puerto Rico	2001	8.49	1.97	Vietnam	2001	6.52	2.06
Denmark	1999	8.24	1.82	Japan	2000	6.48	1.97
Malta	1999	8.21	1.62	Peru	2001	6.44	2.40
Ireland	1999	8.20	1.83	Iran	2000	6.38	2.41
Mexico	2000	8.14	2.35	South Africa	2001	6.31	2.69
Iceland	1999	8.05	1.59	South Korea	2001	6.21	2.32
Austria	1999	8.03	1.92	Poland	1999	6.20	2.53
Northern Ireland	1999	8.00	1.75	Morocco	2001	6.06	2.54
Finland	2000	7.87	1.65	Slovakia	1999	6.03	2.22
Netherlands	1999	7.85	1.34	Estonia	1999	5.93	2.18
Canada	2000	7.85	1.88	Hungary	1999	5.80	2.42
Luxembourg	1999	7.81	1.87	Bosnia-Herzegovina	2001	5.77	2.39
USA	1999	7.66	1.82	Bangladesh	2002	5.77	2.18
Sweden	1999	7.64	1.86	Algeria	2002	5.67	2.86
Venezuela	2000	7.52	2.50	Uganda	2001	5.65	2.47
El Salvador	1999	7.50	2.43	Montenegro	2001	5.64	2.38
Belgium	1999	7.43	2.13	Turkey	2000	5.62	2.79
Germany	1999	7.42	1.96	Serbia	2001	5.62	2.47
Great Britain	1999	7.40	1.94	Jordan	2001	5.60	2.50
Argentina	1999	7.30	2.26	Bulgaria	1999	5.50	2.65
Singapore	2002	7.24	1.80	Egypt	2000	5.36	3.35
Italy	1999	7.17	2.11	Latvia	1999	5.27	2.39
Chile	2000	7.12	2.16	Romania	1999	5.23	2.77
Spain	1999	7.09	1.92	Lithuania	1999	5.20	2.66
Czech Republic	1999	7.06	1.97	Albania	2002	5.17	2.25
Portugal	1999	7.04	1.96	India	2001	5.14	2.23
Israel	2001	7.03	2.17	Macedonia	2001	5.12	2.72
France	1999	7.01	1.99	Pakistan	2001	4.85	1.46
Indonesia	2001	6.96	2.06	Belarus	2000	4.81	2.21
Nigeria	2000	6.87	2.32	Russia	1999	4.56	2.57
Croatia	1999	6.68	2.30	Ukraine	1999	4.56	2.59
Greece	1999	6.67	2.19	Moldova	2000	4.56	2.32
Philippines	2001	6.65	2.53	Zimbabwe	2001	3.95	2.79
China	2001	6.53	2.47	Tanzania	2001	3.87	3.22

Note. LS scores are based on responses to the question, "All things considered, how satisfied are you with your life as a whole now?" on a 10-point scale from 1 (*dissatisfied*) to 10 (*satisfied*). Data from Veenhoven (n.d.).

Dimensional Approach

Some theorists hold that the causes of well-being are fundamentally the same for all people. Ryff and Singer (1998) posited that purpose in life, quality relationships, self-regard, and a sense of mastery are universal features of well-being. Self-determination theorists (Deci & Ryan, 1985; Ryan & Deci, 2000) maintain that well-being hinges on the fulfillment of *innate* psychological needs such as autonomy, competence, and relatedness. If these sources of well-being are universal, they provide dimensions along which we can compare societies. Cultures should differ in SWB to the extent that they provide people with different levels autonomy, meaning, and relationships.

A related perspective is the universalist position on emotions. Drawing on diverse findings, some researchers propose that there are discrete, basic emotions that appear in all cultures (Ekman & Friesen, 1971; Izard & Malatesta, 1987; Plutchik, 1980; Tomkins, 1962, 1963). For example, facial expressions of anger, sadness, and joy appear early in infancy (Izard & Malatesta, 1987) and are easily recognized in many different cultures (Ekman & Friesen, 1971; Ekman et al., 1987). Facial expressions of laughing and crying among congenitally blind infants (Thompson, 1941) suggest that there may be genetic programs directing the expression of emotions. The possibility of biologically based, basic emotions is important, for it implies that we can compare people across societies on these emotions (however, see Ortony & Turner, 1990, for a critique of the basic emotions concept).

Uniqueness Approach

In contrast to the universalist approach, some ethnographers emphasize emotions as social constructions. According to these researchers, the very concept of emotion may differ across cultures. Lutz (1988) noted that Western ethnopsychologies often view emotions as hidden and private. In contrast, her work in Micronesia revealed that Ifalukian concepts of emotions are more public and relational. Cultures may also differ in their labeling of specific feelings. For example, according to Wierzbicka (1986) there is no word for "disgust" in Polish. Extreme versions of the uniqueness approach hold that emotions are purely a Western idea, and that internal experiences can be represented in countless ways across cultures. More moderate formulations, on the other hand, maintain that biologically based emotions may be universal, but that culture can significantly alter their development and labeling. Thus, although sadness is often considered a basic emotion with recognizable antecedents, the Tahitians do not appear to have such a label for it (Levy, 1982). Instead, they often refer to feelings of sickness or exhaustion, for which the causes are nonspecific. Although the uniqueness approach does not preclude the possibility of making comparisons across cultures (e.g., Wierzbicka, 1986), it takes as its starting point the culturally patterned subtleties of emotional experience.

Identity Approach

Another perspective on universality is that regardless of the specific elements, all cultures enjoy *identical levels* of SWB. Cultures may differ in their values and in the needs they fulfill, but people eventually adapt, leading all societies to be relatively happy. The identity approach likens well-being to a "hedonic treadmill" upon which people run but never change position. Only in cultures that are severely disrupted or experiencing trauma (e.g., warfare or famine) is adaptation impossible, resulting in widespread unhappiness. The identity perspective may sound absurd, but in Table 28.2, diverse groups appear to enjoy somewhat comparable levels of LS. For instance, the Amish, Inughuit,

TABLE 28.2. LS of Selected Groups

Positive groups	LS
Forbes richest Americans[a]	5.8
Pennsylvania Amish[b]	5.8
Inughuit (Inuit group from Northern Greenland)[c]	5.8
East African Maasai[c]	5.4
International college students (47 nations)[b]	4.9
Calcutta slum dwellers[d]	4.6
Neutral point of scale = 4.0	
Groups below neutral	LS
Calcutta sex workers[d]	3.6
Calcutta homeless[d]	3.2
California homeless[b]	2.9

Note. LS scores are based on responses to the statement "You are satisfied with your life," on a 7-point scale from 1 (*strongly disagree*) to 7 (*strongly agree*). [a] E. Diener, Horwitz, and Emmons (1985); [b] E. Diener and Seligman (2004); [c] Biswas-Diener et al. (2004); [d] Biswas-Diener and Diener (2001).

and Maasai all report LS that is not significantly different from the richest Americans, suggesting that material luxury is not necessary for well-being. All these groups may be meeting needs, such as for social relationships, that are critical for SWB. Thus, important conditions for happiness may be met in nonindustrial societies such as the Maasai. In contrast, the LS of the homeless indicates that not all groups are happy, and that people do not fully adapt to all conditions.

The Middle Path

In this chapter, we take a middle path. We argue that there are some universals, such as the tendency for people to be *slightly* happy, unless they are exposed to harsh conditions. Some variables, such as temperament and positive relationships, influence SWB in all cultures. There may also be common goals, such as the need for respect, that characterize people in all cultures. Furthermore, because cultural influences often permeate national boundaries, cultures are not completely independent of one another. However, each culture also retains unique qualities and should not be compared with others in a careless way. Not all comparisons of SWB are meaningful, because the value placed on certain subjective states, and the labels for them, often differ. The patterning of well-being may also vary across cultures, making it dangerous to compare variables at a high level of abstraction. Thus, although comparisons are possible, they should only be made with due care to take into account the unique factors present in various societies.

Cultural differences in SWB can be likened to differences between individuals. People can be compared on certain universal features such as height and weight. They can also be compared on factors such as health, but health is made up of many lower-order concepts that may relate to each other differently across individuals. Although societies can be compared in terms of individuals' longevity, patterns of illness differ across cultures. In a similar way, cultures can be compared on SWB, but there are also unique facets of well-being in each society that are best captured by specific descriptions of the local culture.

In the sections that follow, we cover several major topics in culture and SWB research. We begin with the issue of patterning and structure, examining how the elements of SWB cohere across societies. Next, we consider whether cultures differ in mean levels of SWB where the structures can be compared, and what factors might contribute to these differences. We then review various correlates and causes of SWB, showing both similarities and differences in cultural recipes for happiness. Following this discussion, we ask whether SWB leads to the same outcomes in different cultures, or whether there are unique effects that depend on the role of emotions in a culture. Finally, we assess the various challenges involved in measuring SWB across cultures, and the impact that measurement artifacts may have on the findings.

PATTERNING AND STRUCTURE

The validity of cross-cultural comparisons of SWB depends on how it is structured in different societies. If there are both universal and culture-specific emotions, do aggregates such as pleasant and unpleasant affect apply to all cultures? Is the concept of LS understood by people in all societies? Also, do the three components of SWB relate to each other similarly across cultures? We review the research bearing on these issues below.

Levels of Analyses

As discussed earlier, the existence of universal emotions has been debated for some time. Researchers have used a number of methodologies to answer the question of universality, including ethnography, facial expression recognition, and emotion taxonomies. After conducting cross-cultural research on facial expression recognition, Ekman and Friesen (1971; Ekman et al., 1987) suggested that happiness, anger, fear, sadness, and disgust are universal. However, there are also emotions that appear in some cultures but not others. Some appear to be labeling of specific situation–outcome pairings in relation to feelings. In Japan, for example, the term *kanashii* refers specifically to sadness arising from personal loss (Mesquita & Fridja, 1992). Other indigenous emotions seem to be complex blends, such as *aviman* in India, which has been described as "prideful, loving anger" (Scollon, Diener, Oishi, & Biswas-Diener, 2004).

According to Mesquita, Fridja, and Scherer (1997), the debate over universality has hindered culture and emotion research by focusing on the mere presence of certain emotions in a culture rather than on how emotions are "practiced." They argue that emotional experience is a process that includes appraisal of a situation, physiological reactions, overt behaviors, and other components. What distinguishes one emotion from another is the *pattern* of components. At a general level, universal patterns of emotional experience may exist due to innate, neurophysiological programs. For example, joy may inherently feel pleasant and evoke the urge to laugh or smile. However, at the level of specific components, cultural differences may abound. The *type* of events that elicit joy, or attempts to regulate it, may vary across societies.

The perspective provided by Mesquita et al. (1997) resonates with several lines of research on well-being. In assessing the cross-cultural applicability of pleasant and unpleasant affect, SWB researchers have not only been interested in *which* emotions are present, but also in how frequently they are experienced, how they are patterned, and how norms can shape the structure and composition of pleasant and unpleasant affect. In short, the field of culture and SWB has been concerned as much with the ecology, or practice, of emotions (Mesquita et al., 1997) as with the comparability of SWB across cultures. We see that the distinction between pleasant and unpleasant affect can be made at a general level, and that there are both similarities and differences in the specific aspects of these emotions.

Structural Evidence

In an early study, Watson, Clark, and Tellegen (1984) found that the mood structure of Japanese participants formed two factors, identifiable as positive and negative affect. This two-factor structure was very similar to that of American participants. Hierarchical cluster analyses of emotion words from the United States, Italy, and China also revealed superordinate groupings of positive and negative emotions (Shaver, Wu, & Schwartz, 1992). Pleasant and unpleasant emotion clusters were also observed in experience sampling data provided by Japanese, Indian, and two American samples (Scollon et al., 2004). Moreover, indigenous emotions that were included in the Japanese and Indian samples did not form separate clusters, but grouped together with the pleasant and unpleasant emotions.

M. L. Diener, Fujita, Kim-Prieto, and E. Diener (2004) studied the frequency of 12 emotions and found that they formed positive and negative clusters in seven regions of the world (Africa, Latin America, East Asia, Southeast Asia, West Asia, Eastern Europe, and Western Europe). Moreover, in virtually all of these regions, a core group of emotions consistently loaded onto either positive or negative clusters; that is, positive emotions included *pleasant*, *cheerful*, and *happy*, whereas negative emotions included *unpleasant*, *sad*, and *angry*. Similarly, Shaver et al. (1992) found that one positive (*joy*) and three negative emotions (*anger*, *sadness*, and *fear*) formed basic-level categories in all three cultures they studied. Thus, when speaking of emotion aggregates, there is compelling evidence that pleasant and unpleasant affect are perceived in all cultures. There is also support for the universality of particular emotions such as joy, anger, and sadness. However, cultural differences may arise regarding more specific emotions. For instance, outside of the core emotions, M. L. Diener et al. (2004) observed differences in how other emotions clustered. *Pride* clustered with positive emotions in Latin America, Western Europe, and East Asia, but with negative emotions in Africa, Southeast Asia, Eastern Europe, and West Asia. *Pride* also aligned with negative emotions among smaller

samples in India and Italy (Scollon et al., 2004; Shaver et al., 1992). These findings should be interpreted cautiously. The simple fact that pride clusters with negative emotions in a culture does not necessarily mean that it is experienced as a negative emotion. In the case of M. L. Diener et al.'s data, the cluster analyses were based on the frequency of experience and included weights for means, standard deviations, and correlations—any of which could have affected how emotion terms clustered. In those regions where *pride* was experienced less frequently, it clustered with the negative emotions, which were generally experienced less often than positive emotions. In contrast, *worry* and *stress* clustered with the positive emotions in Western Europe and East Asia, primarily because they were frequently experienced in those areas. Thus, emotional experience may be universal in some ways but culturally varied in others. Recently, Kuppens, Ceulemans, Timmerman, Diener, and Kim-Prieto (2006) found that although positive and negative affect emerged as strong universal intracultural dimensions, there were also smaller, but significant, nation-level dimensions of emotional experience on which nations could be discriminated.

Differences in the frequency of emotions may be related to cultural norms. For example, cultural norms might make some situations more common than others. Thus, the American cultural environment might afford more opportunities for self-enhancement (and the experience of pride), whereas the Japanese cultural environment might be more conducive to self-criticism (Kitayama, Markus, Matsumoto, & Norasakkunkit, 1997). According to Markus and Kitayama (1994), normative social behavior and cultural models of the self might also shape the desirability of certain emotions. In individualist cultures, pride is an enjoyable emotion that highlights individual achievement, as well as success in meeting the cultural goals of autonomy and independence. However, in collectivist cultures, emotions resulting from sympathy and humility may feel good because they are consistent with the cultural goals of interdependence. Emotions that conflict with these norms may be deemphasized and less frequently experienced. Thus, pride may not be as valued in some collectivist Asian cultures because it is self-focusing and separates the individual from the group (Kitayama & Markus, 2000; Markus & Kitayama, 1994;

Scollon et al., 2004). In a similar way, the Oriyas in India devalue anger, because it is regarded as socially destructive (Menon & Shweder, 1994). On the other hand, shame[1] is viewed as a good emotion for *women* to have, because it is integral to sustaining the patriarchal order of society.

The Oriya case draws attention to *intracultural* variation in emotion norms; that is, norms may not apply or be uniformly perceived across all individuals within a culture. Eid and Diener (2001) investigated this issue by examining the desirability and appropriateness of pleasant and unpleasant affect in the United States, Australia, China, and Taiwan. They found that norms for pleasant emotions (e.g., joy, affection, pride, and contentment) were more heterogeneous in China and Taiwan than in the United States and Australia. For instance, the vast majority (83%) of Australians and Americans regarded all four pleasant emotions as appropriate. In contrast, only 9% of Chinese and 32% of Taiwanese felt this way. A majority of the Taiwanese (57%) had mixed feelings about pride, although joy, affection, and contentment were appropriate. A plurality of the Chinese (32%) felt that joy and affection were appropriate, but that pride was clearly inappropriate. Another class of individuals found only among the Chinese (16%) regarded all pleasant emotions as *inappropriate*. These findings suggest that culture may influence emotion norms in two ways. First, cultures may foster unique normative patterns, as observed in the Chinese sample. Second, some patterns may be pancultural, but their relative frequency within cultures may differ. All pleasant emotions are clearly favored in the United States and Australia. The ambivalence toward pride in China and Taiwan is consistent with previous research on collectivist Asian cultures.

However, the relation between emotion norms and emotional experience may not always be direct. Recent work by Tsai, Knutson, and Fung (2006) suggests that the emotions people value (ideal affect) are not necessarily the ones they experience most frequently (real affect), although the correlations are moderate. These researchers found that although cultural values predicted the *preference* for high- versus low-arousal pleasant emotions, the reported *frequency* of these emotions was better predicted by personality traits. Furthermore, norms may influence some emotions more than others. M. L. Diener et al. (2004) found that

the correlation between the appropriateness and frequency of an emotion was larger for "secondary" emotions such as pride, guilt, gratitude, and jealousy, than for the core emotions; that is, norms appear to predict more strongly the experience of secondary emotions than the experience of core emotions. Indeed, the main cultural differences in structure were due to how the secondary emotions clustered, and the various geopolitical regions diverged most in the frequency of these emotions. For example, people from Southeast Asia more frequently reported experiences of guilt and shame, whereas people from Latin America registered more pride than people from other areas. Also, norms for pride and guilt were more variable across cultures than norms for other emotions (Eid & Diener, 2001). Differences in the experience of peripheral emotions, such as pride, may reflect cultural ideologies regarding attribution styles, such as whether success should be attributed to the self or to the situation (Heine, Lehman, Markus, & Kitayama, 1999). In contrast, a core emotion such as happiness is much broader and may tend to follow from a range of outcomes that are considered good in each culture, so that valuing general happiness is likely to be more common across cultures.

In addition to emotions, there is also support for similarity in the structure of LS across cultures. Vittersø, Røysamb, and Diener (2002) carried out confirmatory factor analyses on the five items of the Satisfaction with Life Scale (SWLS; E. Diener, Emmons, Larsen, & Griffin, 1985) and found that a one-factor model fit the data reasonably well in 41 nations. In all nations, the comparative fit index was above .90. This finding suggests that the SWLS measures a single construct, and that the concept of "life satisfaction" may be similarly understood across a wide range of cultures. That is not to say that the *criteria* for LS are universal; rather, people in a number of diverse cultures appear to react to queries about LS in a consistent way.

The Relation between Emotions and LS

Although the structure of emotions is somewhat consistent across cultures, and the items of the SWLS also seem to cohere reliably, the relation between emotions and LS may vary across cultures (Schimmack, Radhakrishnan, Oishi, Dzokoto, & Ahadi, 2002; Suh, Diener, Oishi, & Triandis, 1998). Suh et al. examined the relation between LS and affect balance (the difference in frequency of pleasant and unpleasant affect). They found that LS and affect balance correlated positively across 40 nations; thus, experiencing more pleasant than unpleasant affect predicted greater LS across cultures. However, the correlations were stronger in more individualist countries. Suh et al. (Study 2) also assessed cultural norms for LS by asking participants what they perceived to be the ideal level of LS in their culture. When LS was predicted from both emotions and perceived norms for LS, the former was highly predictive among individualist cultures, accounting for 76% of the variance in LS. In contrast, norms and emotions were equally predictive of LS in collectivist cultures, accounting for 39% and 40% of the variance, respectively. A possible explanation is that in individualist cultures, where personal goals and preferences are emphasized, emotions may be important because one's own feelings are often a relevant factor in one's judgments. However, in collectivist cultures, there may be a greater tendency to use norms as a guide for one's attitudes and behavior, and not be the "nail that stands out." Thus, when judging their LS, people from collectivist cultures might weigh norms at least as much as their own emotions. This raises the possibility that collectivists are simply responding in a normatively appropriate manner. Though it is difficult to rule out this alternative explanation, other data suggest that this is not invariably the case. For example, perceived norms for negative emotions were not reliably related to self-reported frequency of these emotions among Chinese and Taiwanese respondents (Eid & Diener, 2001; we discuss further methodological issues later in the chapter).

Conclusion

There are universals in the structure of SWB that make some comparisons possible. Pleasant affect, unpleasant affect, and LS are not unfamiliar concepts to most of the world's people. Nevertheless, to some degree, cultural norms shape which emotions are pleasant and unpleasant to feel. Therefore, when using aggregates such as pleasant and unpleasant affect, one must be careful, because specific emotions may cohere differently within the larger aggregate. The comparison of emotion aggregates should only be made with emotions that cohere similarly in each culture. Finally, emotions may

be more relevant to global LS in individualist cultures, where internal experience is highly valued. This difference highlights the importance of measuring emotions and LS as separate components of SWB; that is affective and cognitive evaluations of well-being reflect different aspects of the superordinate construct of SWB.

COMPARING THE MEAN LEVELS OF SWB OF CULTURES

In discussing the happiness of societies, it may seem surprising that a majority of people in the world report being happy. That is not to say that all of humanity is in a state of elation or jubilance, or that there is no variation across cultures in overall levels of well-being. A wide range of economic, sociocultural, and biological factors may affect the mean level of subjective well-being in a society, but in most cultures, the mean level is above neutral.

Most People Are Happy

A study involving 31 nations ($N = 13,118$) revealed that 63% of men and 70% of women reported positive levels of LS (E. Diener & Diener, 1995). These findings may be limited, in that many of the nations studied were fairly industrialized, and most of the participants were college students. However, E. Diener and Diener (1996) plotted the distribution of mean SWB responses from nationally representative samples from 43 nations and found that 86% were above the neutral point (see Table 28.1 for more data based on representative probability samples). Furthermore, positive levels of well-being appear to be fairly stable over time. National levels of SWB in the United States, Japan, and France fluctuated over a 46-year period but never dipped below neutral (Veenhoven, 1993). Positive levels of well-being have also been observed among smaller, nonindustrialized societies such as the Maasai in Kenya, the Inughuit in Greenland, and the Amish in the United States (Biswas-Diener et al., 2005).

The claim that "most people are happy" is not meant to deny that there remains significant ill-being and suffering in the world. It is important to note that data from the poorest nations of the world (e.g., Rwanda, Mozambique, and Afghanistan) are often lacking (see Table 28.1). Moreover, although most people report levels of SWB above the midpoint, very few report being extremely happy. Only 4% of E. Diener and Diener's (1995) sample were at the top of the LS scale. Similarly, although the Maasai, Inughuit, and Amish were all significantly above neutral on several measures of SWB, a very small minority reported perfect LS, or *always* experiencing pleasant affect (Biswas-Diener et al., 2005). Thus, the skew in well-being seems to reflect a moderate form of happiness. Although measurement artifacts are an important concern (see "Methodological Issues"), the replicability of these findings across numerous societies and over a number of different methods is impressive.

Perhaps it should not seem so shocking that most people are at least mildly happy with their lives. Some researchers argue that a disposition toward pleasant affect facilitates exploratory behavior, which could have conferred evolutionary advantages (E. Diener & Diener, 1996; Fredrickson, 1998; Ito & Cacioppo, 1999). According to Ito and Cacioppo, the motivational system is slightly biased toward approach behavior, even in the absence of stimuli—a phenomenon called "positivity offset." Such a bias would be more advantageous than a purely neutral disposition, because, in the absence of danger, it would help humans learn more about their environment. As a consequence of broadening behavioral and attentional foci, positive emotions might also have helped humans to build social relationships and other resources important for survival (Fredrickson, 1998). The connection between pleasant affect and approach tendencies receives some support from a 27-nation study by Wallbott and Scherer (1988). With few cultural differences, participants reported that "moving toward" was an action tendency most characteristic of joy, whereas "withdrawing" was more typical of unpleasant emotions.

In light of this research, it becomes important to ask when and why a society falls below the midpoint of SWB. One observed trend is that people living in severe destitution often report being unhappy. Prostitutes and homeless people living in Calcutta, India, reported negative levels of LS (Biswas-Diener & Diener, 2001). The LS of Malaysian farmers living below the poverty line also fell below the midpoint (Howell, Howell, & Schwabe, 2006). Difficulty in meeting basic needs or other circumstances, such as lack of respect, might have decreased the well-being of these groups. In the next section, we consider how economic factors might influence the SWB of a society.

Economic Development and Related Variables

The wealth of a nation frequently correlates with its level of SWB. Depending on whether one looks at purchasing power or per capita gross domestic product (GDP), the correlation between economic wealth and the SWB of a nation ranges from .58 to .84 (E. Diener, Diener, & Diener, 1995; Inglehart & Klingemann, 2000; Veenhoven, 1991). As robust as this finding is, the exact process by which economic development increases happiness remains unclear.

Wealthier societies are better able to meet the basic needs of their citizens, and this contributes to SWB (E. Diener, Diener, et al., 1995). We consider the role of basic needs fulfillment in a later section. For now, it is also worth noting that economic development is often associated with many other social conditions. For example, wealth correlates with greater human rights, as well as greater equality (in income, access to education, and between the sexes; E. Diener, Diener, et al., 1995). Rights and equality also correlate with each other. Moreover, people in wealthier nations are often more satisfied with friends and home life (E. Diener & Suh, 1999). A possible explanation proposed by Ahuvia (2002) is that rising wealth alters the cultural environment by freeing the individual from economic dependence on his or her family. This independence could attenuate norms for reciprocity while facilitating the pursuit of individual happiness (e.g., by allowing one more choice in friends and lifestyle). Thus, several mechanisms are possible, and the various correlates of wealth make it difficult to isolate the unique contribution of wealth to SWB. The relation between economic development and SWB is thus entangled in a causal web of several factors, and future researchers need to separate their causal influences on SWB.

Aside from economic development, Inglehart and Klingemann (2000) suggested that national levels of SWB might also reflect historical factors. In 1997, the former communist states of Eastern Europe and the U.S.S.R. had among the lowest levels of well-being—lower than nations with less wealth, but without a history of communism. Even after controlling for wealth, rights, and other variables, the number of years under communist rule negatively predicted a nation's mean level of SWB. However, Inglehart and Klingemann warn against hasty praise for capitalistic or democratic societies. Although the collapse of communism in the Soviet Union was preceded by relatively low levels of SWB, it was followed by *even lower* levels of SWB (see also Veenhoven, 2001). Political instability and economic decline after the fall of communism may have created conditions inimical to SWB. These ideas require further research, especially as conditions change in the region.

Norms for Emotions

As mentioned earlier, the experience of well-being can be shaped by cultural norms regarding the desirability of LS or certain emotions (M. L. Diener et al., 2004; Suh et al., 1998). Desirable emotions might be experienced more frequently than those that are seen as inappropriate (M. L. Diener et al., 2004) or they may correlate more with general happiness (Markus & Kitayama, 1994). Norms for emotions may explain why Asian—especially East Asian—samples often report lower SWB than those from Europe and the Americas (E. Diener & Diener, 1995; Kang, Shaver, Sue, Min, & Jing, 2003; Sheldon et al., 2004; Suh, 2002). Economic development may be a factor, but it cannot completely account for the lower SWB of East Asians. For example, Japan has greater purchasing power than many Latin American nations (E. Diener, Diener, et al., 1995), yet it reports lower SWB than do the latter (E. Diener & Suh, 1999; E. Diener & Oishi, 2000). This could be because Japanese and other Asians show a greater acceptance of unpleasant emotions than do people in the Americas (E. Diener & Suh, 1999). Moreover, East Asians may also value low activation positive affect (e.g., serenity) more than high activation positive affect (e.g., excitement) because the former emotions facilitate collectivist goals of attending to the social context (Tsai et al., 2006).

How might emotion norms translate into experience? One pathway is through the socialization of emotions in children (M. L. Diener & Lucas, 2004) and the willingness to report specific emotions, or through recall of which emotions are experienced (Oishi, 2002). Wirtz (2004) asked participants to report how they felt about past events, both currently and at the time of the event. Whether the emotions were pleasant or unpleasant, Japanese participants'

current feelings were less intense than their remembered feelings from the past. In contrast, European Americans reported significant decay for unpleasant but not pleasant emotions. Thus, cultural norms might also shape the relation between recalled emotions and current feelings, which might also influence judgments about current LS.

Schimmack, Oishi, and Diener (2002) suggested that East Asian views of pleasant and unpleasant emotions might be rooted in the dialecticism of Asian philosophies (e.g., Buddhism and Daoism) that have historically shaped these cultures. For example, in Chinese folk wisdom, both sides of a contradiction are equally likely, and a compromise between the two is preferable (Peng & Nisbett, 1999). East Asian emotion norms may be dialectical in the sense that a middle way between extreme pleasant and extreme unpleasant affect is considered desirable. In contrast, many Western European and Latin American cultures prefer pleasant over unpleasant affect. These cultural differences are reflected in emotion reports. Among participants from Western Europe and the Americas, the frequency of pleasant affect was inversely related to the frequency of unpleasant affect (Schimmack et al., 2002). Among Asian participants, however, this negative correlation was weak (see also Bagozzi, Wong, & Yi, 1999). Kitayama, Markus, and Kurokawa (2000) actually observed a *positive* correlation between pleasant and unpleasant affect in Japan. Finally, over a 1-week period of experience sampling, Scollon et al. (2004) found that European Americans and Hispanic Americans experienced more pleasant affect than Asians and Asian Americans. Moreover, there were no differences in unpleasant emotions. Asians and Asian Americans did not experience as much pleasant affect as the other groups, but they were not biased in the direction of greater unpleasant affect either.

Are East Asians simply unhappy at worst and apathetic at best? Caution must be taken not to equate lower levels of well-being as *ill-being*. First, the SWB of East Asians is lower *in comparison to* Latin Americans and Western Europeans. Although mean levels of SWB are often lower among Asian samples, they are rarely below the neutral midpoint. Second, Kitayama and Markus (2000) note that balance and moderation are central to East Asian concepts of health. A preference for low- rather than high-activation positive affect may be consistent with this perspective (Tsai et al., 2006).

Another source of cultural variation in emotion norms may be religious doctrine. Across 40 nations, Kim-Prieto and Diener (2004) found that Christians reported a greater frequency of happiness and less shame than Muslims, even after controlling for the effect of nations. A subsequent comparison of the emotion content of religious texts revealed that joy and love were more frequently mentioned in the New Testament, whereas shame and guilt were more frequently mentioned in the Quran. Thus, differences in norms or the socialization of emotions may be rooted in religious doctrine. An important implication of these findings is that the cultural forces that impinge on SWB may extend beyond ethnic and geographic delineations.

Genetic Differences

Might cultural differences in well-being be due to genetic differences between groups? Although much more research is needed, some individual differences in SWB may be related to genetics. Polymorphisms in the serotonin-related *5-HTT* gene have been linked to individual differences in anxiety (Lesch et al., 1996), as well as susceptibility to depression (Caspi et al., 2003). Lykken and Tellegen (1996) maintain that roughly half of the individual variance in SWB is related to genetic variation.

A limitation of this research is that it has been carried out within single societies, and effects *within* a sample may not necessarily be driven by the same causal forces as those *between* samples. Although there are ethnic and cultural differences in gene frequencies (Cavalli-Sforza, 1991), direct links between such differences and SWB have not yet been made. However, studies of infant temperament reinforce the possibility of genetic effects. Freedman and Freedman (1969) found ethnic differences in infants less than 4 days old. Compared to European American infants, Chinese American infants were calmer and less reactive to a cloth placed on their face. Similarly, 4-month-old infants in China exhibited less behavioral arousal than did European American and Irish infants (Kagan et al., 1994). Nevertheless, the role of socialization practices cannot be overlooked. In contrast to these findings, Ahadi, Rothbart, and Ye (1993) found that 6-year-old Chinese children exhibited relatively more negative affectivity than did their European American peers. The authors suggested that strict Chinese socialization practices might foster a greater sensitivity to punishment, leading to more frequent negative affect. Thus, genetic influences do not rule out the impact of life circumstances on the various components of SWB. Recently, Diener and colleagues (E. Diener, Lucas, & Scollon, 2006; Fujita & Diener, 2005) argued for a "soft set point" conception of SWB. People can adapt to many situations, and genes may account for some of the stability in SWB. However, life events and social conditions (e.g., widowhood or poverty) can still have a substantial impact on happiness at both individual and group levels. Much more research on culture, genetics, and SWB is required before firm conclusions can be made.

Conclusion

In many societies, a majority of the people report being happy, but very few report extreme happiness. Although there are biological and evolutionary accounts for why this is so, other factors are likely to influence mean levels of well-being. These factors include economic development and cultural norms for emotions. However, much more research is needed before we can understand exactly how and why societal levels of SWB differ across cultures. Specifically, the exact process underlying the relation between economic development and SWB remains unclear, as does how such development affects cultural values related to well-being.

CORRELATES AND CAUSES OF SWB

Cultures might differ in not only the type and frequency of emotions people experience but also in the causes of SWB. Often the evidence is in terms of cross-sectional correlations, however, so we mostly review what covaries with pleasant and unpleasant affect, and LS in different cultures. Furthermore, Kitayama and Markus (2000) suggested that SWB is not only personal happiness but also includes one's relations with others. Thus, happiness might take different forms across cultures, with different factors causing it.

The Self and SWB

To the extent that self-concepts vary across cultures (Markus & Kitayama, 1991), one might expect the relation between self and SWB to vary as well. For instance, although self-esteem is often a strong correlate of LS, Heine et al. (1999) questioned the need for positive self-views in collectivist cultures. In Japan, where interdependence is emphasized, a self-critical tendency may be valued as a way of improving one's ability to meet social obligations (but see Brown & Kobayashi [2002, 2003] for evidence of self-enhancement in Japan, and Heine's [2003] response). Miller, Wang, Sandel, and Cho (2002) found that rural Taiwanese mothers also place little emphasis on developing their children's self-esteem, and some worried that high self-esteem would impair their child's capacity to take criticism. Thus, in collectivist cultures, self-esteem may be viewed as unimportant, or even *undesirable*, for achieving cultural goals. In contrast, a primary concern for European American mothers was to help their children develop and maintain a strong sense of self-esteem (Miller et al., 2002).

If high self-esteem is deemphasized in collectivist cultures, then one might expect self-esteem to relate less strongly to LS than it would in more individualist cultures. This is exactly what a number of researchers have found (E. Diener & Diener, 1995; Oishi, Diener, Lucas, & Suh, 1999; Park & Huebner, 2005). Although self-esteem correlated with LS across most countries, the strength of association could be predicted by the individualism of a country. For example, self-esteem and LS correlated .60 in the United States, but only .08 among women in more collectivist India (E. Diener & Diener, 1995). Similarly, Park and Huebner (2005) found that satisfaction with self was a much stronger predictor of LS for U.S. adolescents than for Korean adolescents. As with emotions (Suh et al., 1998), people in collectivist cultures may be guided by norms downplaying the importance of self-esteem when they make LS judgments. Alternatively, people with high self-esteem may be frowned upon in collectivist cultures for holding or expressing attitudes that violate norms. Of course, norms should also influence the factors that *do* correlate with LS. For example, Park and Huebner (2005) suggested that the heavy emphasis on academic achievement in Korea might explain why school satisfaction predicted LS for Korean adolescents but not for American adolescents.

Another characteristic that may be less socially valued in collectivist cultures and less important for SWB is identity consistency. In traditional Western psychology, self-consistency across situations implies a coherent self-identity and good mental health. However, in East Asian cultures, where individuals are expected to adjust themselves to the social situation, identity consistency might be taken as a sign of immaturity. Suh (2002) found that Americans evinced greater consistency than Koreans across social roles. For example, if Americans were talkative with their friends, they were also more likely to be talkative with parents, siblings, and strangers than were Koreans. Furthermore, identity consistency was a much stronger predictor of SWB for Americans than for Koreans. Not only were self-consistent individuals happier in the American sample, but they were also rated by informants as more likable and socially skilled than less consistent individuals. In contrast, Korean informants showed no such preference for consistent targets (Suh, 2002).

Culture may also affect the relation between personality and LS. On the one hand, research suggests that the influence of personality on emotional experience may be pancultural (Lucas, Diener, Grob, Suh, & Shao, 2000; Tsai et al., 2006). In five countries, Schimmack et al. (2002) found that extraversion correlated positively with affect balance, whereas neuroticism was negatively correlated. Moreover, the relation between personality and LS was mediated by affect balance. Thus, extraverts enjoy greater LS in part because they experience frequent pleasant affect. However, because the relation between *emotions* and LS is stronger in individualist cultures (see "Patterning and Structure"), the relation between personality and LS is also moderated by culture. Thus, extraversion and neuroticism are more predictive of LS in individualist cultures (Germany and the United States) than in collectivist cultures (Ghana, Japan, and Mexico). Extraverts everywhere may experience more pleasant affect than neurotics, but how much this contributes to LS may depend on the cultural value of emotional experience. Alternatively, Benet-Martínez and Karakitapoglu-Aygun (2003) proposed that cultures favor the development of some personality traits over others. They found that individualism predicted both extraversion and neuroticism, and that the relationship between personality and LS was mediated by self-esteem and friendship satisfaction.

An important issue concerns the role of autonomy in SWB. Self-determination theory (SDT; Deci & Ryan, 1985; Ryan & Deci, 2000) contends that autonomy is a basic human need that, if not fulfilled, will lead to lower levels of well-being. One source of the debate may be the very definition of autonomy. For example, Oishi (2000) operationalized autonomy as horizontal individualism (i.e., an emphasis on independence and individual self-worth). He found that the positive association between autonomy and LS is stronger in more individualist nations such as Australia and Denmark, than in more collectivist nations such as China, Korea, and Bahrain. However, Chirkov, Ryan, Kim, and Kaplan (2003) argued that the construct of autonomy must be distinguished from independence and individualism (see also Ryan & Deci, 2000). In the framework of SDT, autonomy is the sense that one has willingly engaged in and fully endorses an act. Individuals may be dependent on others and still experience autonomy, if they find value in that dependence and engage in it of their own volition. What is of importance is the *internalization* of the values that one is exercising. Thus, although Koreans viewed their culture as more collectivist and less individualist than Americans viewed their own culture, the internalization of *both* types of values predicted SWB in both countries, as well as in Russia and Turkey (Chirkov et al., 2003). Using a similar definition of autonomy, Sheldon et al. (2004) found that self-concordant individuals (i.e., those who pursued goals they perceived as freely chosen) tend to report higher levels of SWB in the United States, South Korea, Taiwan, and China. Thus, autonomy as independence is not universal, whereas autonomy as feeling that one's behavior is freely chosen and not coerced may be universal.

These views are not contrary to the goal-as-moderator model advanced by Oishi (2000). This model posits that the relation between culture and SWB is moderated by personal goals. Culture may influence one's goals, but individuals do not always pursue culturally endorsed goals. For example, a Chinese student who values personal success may be happier studying alone than offering help to his fellow classmates, although the latter better reflects the cultural goal of interdependence. However, although attaining personal goals may bring emotional well-being, it may not always yield a sense of meaning in life. Ideally, personal goals that are aligned with cultural values lead to both happiness and meaning (Oishi, 2000). Thus, the role of personal goals is similar to the importance of internalization proposed by SDT. Although independence from others might not predict happiness equally across cultures, acting from one's volition is predicted by both SDT and Oishi's theory to lead to happiness universally.

Both perspectives suggest that the distinction between personal and collective goals may often be blurred. For example, the SWB of Asians and Asian Americans is better predicted by satisfaction with goals involving family and friends than with goals concerned mainly with the self (Oishi & Diener, 2001; Radhakrishnan & Chan, 1997). However, among collectivist cultures, the goals of one's group may also be experienced as one's own (Markus & Kitayama, 1994), making them both collective and personal. In contrast, only personal goals were predictive of the SWB of European Americans (Oishi & Diener, 2001; Radhakrishnan & Chan, 1997). Taken together, the findings suggest that some motives may correlate universally with well-being, whereas other motives or goals are culture-specific correlates of well-being.

Relationships with Others and SWB

The preceding research implies that social relationships may influence SWB differently across cultures. For instance, although emotional experience is often considered private and internal, Kitayama and Markus (2000) suggested that the Japanese may experience good feelings *intersubjectively*, as features of an interpersonal situation that dissipate once the individual is out of that context. Consistent with this idea, Oishi, Diener, Scollon, and Biswas-Diener (2003) found that Japanese reported less pleasant affect when alone than did Americans. Furthermore, although both groups experienced more pleasant affect when with friends than when alone, the effect was greater for the Japanese (as well as for Hispanic Americans; Oishi et al., 2003).

In general, East Asians may be more other-focused in their emotional experience than North Americans (Cohen & Gunz, 2002;

Kitayama et al., 2000). Kitayama et al. compared how *engaged* (relationship focused) and *disengaged* (self-focused) emotions relate to general good feelings (e.g., happiness) among Japanese and American participants. For Japanese participants, positive engaged emotions (e.g., friendly feelings) correlated more strongly with general good feelings than did positive disengaged emotions (e.g., pride). The reverse was true for American participants. However, a recent priming study by No and Hong (2004) suggests that the influence of culture on emotional experience is dynamic. Compared to baseline, Korean American biculturals primed with Korean cultural icons became more relational and less egocentric in their projection of emotions onto others. Similar effects may be observed in the experience of SWB; that is, what makes an individual happy may shift as the salience of cultural frames shifts, such as when living in another culture for an extended period of time.

The relative importance of relationships across cultures also influences LS. Among Hong Kong Chinese, for example, relationship harmony was just as important as self-esteem in predicting LS (Kwan, Bond, & Singelis, 1997). In contrast, self-esteem was a stronger predictor of LS for Americans. Interestingly, relationship quality may have both direct and indirect effects on LS. Kang et al. (2003) not only replicated Kwan et al.'s (1997) findings in the United States, Korea, and mainland China, but they also showed that relationship quality was positively associated with self-esteem in the latter two groups. Relationship quality was also predictive of Asian Americans' self-esteem, but *not* of European Americans' self-esteem (Kang et al., 2003).

A relationship of particular relevance to SWB is marriage. Across 42 societies, married people reported more pleasant and less unpleasant affect than the divorced (E. Diener, Gohm, Suh, & Oishi, 2000). However, small cultural effects were observed. Divorce seems to reduce pleasant affect to a lesser extent in collectivist than in individualist cultures. Gohm, Oishi, Darlington, and Diener (1998) found that in collectivist cultures, the offspring of divorced parents reported greater LS than those whose parents remained in high-conflict marriages. These groups did not differ in individualist cultures. Both findings could be related to greater social support in collectivist cultures, which would help to sustain well-be-

ing after divorce. Alternatively, the pressure to stay together may be greater in these societies, so that couples divorce only after severe marital conflict. In this case, the decision to divorce might offer greater relief to spouses and their offspring. More research is needed to test these hypotheses.

Income and SWB

According to Veenhoven (1991), income contributes to SWB only insofar as it allows one to fulfill basic needs. Beyond the level needed to satisfy physical needs, income has less of an impact on SWB. Veenhoven's theory resembles that of Maslow (1954), which posits that lower-order needs (e.g., physical and security needs) must be gratified before higher-order needs (i.e., belongingness, esteem, and self-actualization) become salient. However, some scholars have questioned whether the fulfillment of needs follows a linear hierarchy (Yang, 2003). Moreover, diminishing returns on the effects of material goods do not always imply that higher-order needs have been prioritized. An implication drawn from both theories, however, is that income has a greater impact on SWB in poor societies, because physical needs such as having adequate food, water, and housing are highly salient, and the effects of income on meeting these needs are direct. Indeed, researchers have found that financial satisfaction predicts LS more strongly in poorer than in wealthier countries (E. Diener & Diener, 1995; Oishi et al., 1999).

Although the relation between income and happiness is reduced among the wealthier nations, it is worth noting that income still contributes to SWB *beyond* the basic subsistence level (Diener, Diener, et al., 1995; E. Diener, Sandvik, Seidlitz, & Diener, 1993). Perhaps greater amounts of income facilitate the pursuit of other goals (e.g., relationships or philanthropy) that add to one's level of SWB, though little is known about *how* money is spent across cultures.

Although Maslow's needs hierarchy provides some understanding of the link between income and SWB, it is important to consider recent revisions of and critiques on the cross-cultural applicability of this model. Yang (2003) argued that Maslow's higher-order needs (belongingness, esteem, and self-actualization) are framed within an individualist context. He suggested that in collectivist societies, these needs are framed in ways that reaffirm social relationships and group identity. Moreover, he proposed (after Yu, 1992, cited in Yang, 2003) that bearing and rearing children be considered needs that are present in all societies, because they ensure the transmission of genes to the next generation. Unlike the strictly hierarchical nature of Maslow's model, Yang suggested that needs can be experienced and fulfilled simultaneously. For example, raising children may fulfill both belongingness and esteem needs. Furthermore, individuals may emphasize or deemphasize transmission needs throughout the life course. The relative importance of child-rearing versus esteem needs might also differ across cultures, and the role that income plays in satisfying these needs could likewise vary.

Conclusion

A number of correlates of SWB are strikingly different across cultures, yet some correlates appear to be universal. Variations in the cognitive and affective experience of happiness correspond with cultural differences in self-definition and the importance of social relationships. Income also contributes to SWB, though the relation is stronger among poorer than among wealthier societies. Thus, cultural-psychological differences are rooted not only in values but also in the material world. However, because culture is dynamic, what makes people happy may change across generations, as well as within the individual, as different aspects of a culture become salient. Nevertheless, there may be some universal correlates of SWB even in the face of cultural variations, such as autonomous internalization of cultural values.

OUTCOMES OF SWB

Research on SWB has traditionally been a search for the who, what, and how of happiness—that is, who is happy, what makes people happy, and how the various components of happiness relate to each other. Because happiness has historically been thought of as an end in itself, these were the first questions to be asked, and the field of SWB advanced greatly as these issues began to be studied more rigorously. However, the question of *why* happiness is important has only recently received more serious attention.

Lyubomirsky, King, and Diener (2005) propose that although success may produce happiness, it may also be the case that happiness leads to success. They reviewed several experimental and longitudinal studies suggesting that many outcomes of pleasant affect are desirable (e.g., prosocial behavior, self-esteem, likability, creativity, and longevity). These characteristics in turn lead to success in many life domains, such as marriage, work, and health. The framework developed by Lyubomirsky et al. is an intriguing area that requires much more research. Not only does the direction of causality await further clarification in some domains but also the benefits and *costs* of pleasant affect must be investigated in a wider range of cultures.

The studies reviewed by Lyubomirsky et al. (2005) were conducted primarily in North America, Europe, and Australia. Whether pleasant affect is similarly beneficial in, for example, East Asia is certainly open for analyses. Would pleasant emotions produce similar outcomes in Japan, where self-criticism and self-improvement are seen as important for success (Heine et al., 1999)? Heine et al. (2001) observed that North Americans are more likely to persist on a task after receiving success feedback, whereas Japanese are motivated to persist if they receive failure feedback. The facilitative effect of pleasant affect among Westerners may be related to the general desirability of these emotions in their cultures (Eid & Diener, 2001). However, East Asian cultures do not devalue all pleasant emotions (e.g., Tsai et al., 2006). An important topic for future investigation is whether specific pleasant emotions are beneficial, whereas others (e.g., pride; Eid & Diener, 2001; Scollon et al., 2004) are detrimental for success in certain cultures.

At a societal level, Inglehart and Klingemann (2000) suggested that rising levels of SWB might help legitimize and stabilize newly formed governments. They pointed out that major political changes in Belgium and the former U.S.S.R. in the early 1990s were *preceded* by decreasing levels of SWB. Furthermore, although many democratic societies had high levels of well-being, democracy did not predict SWB after controlling for gross national product (GNP; Inglehart & Klingemann, 2000). Thus democratic institutions may increase SWB through rising wealth, but greater SWB might also help to sustain these institutions. These propositions are preliminary, and more research is required to understand the causal process. Measuring national levels of SWB consistently and over a broad period of time could shed light on how fluctuations in well-being relate to sociopolitical developments.

METHODOLOGICAL ISSUES

A critical question is whether measures of SWB are valid and reliable across cultures. Even within cultures, Schwarz and Strack (1999) pointed out several potential threats to the validity of self-reported SWB. They warned that self-reports are vulnerable to contextual factors (e.g., question wording and order effects) that can change the standards by which people evaluate their lives. However, Schimmack, Diener, and Oishi (2002; Oishi, Schimmack, & Colcombe, 2003) showed that the information people use to make LS judgments is largely systematic and personally relevant. Thus, although self-reports of SWB may be subject to momentary influences, more often than not, they convey meaningful information about an individual's evaluation of his or her life.

Nevertheless, there are additional challenges when SWB research is conducted across cultures. A basic issue is the adequate translation of written materials. Poor translations can alter the intended meaning of SWB measures, leading to spurious cultural differences. A number of studies, however, suggest that translation effects are unlikely to explain the substantial cultural differences that have been observed. For example, bilingual Chinese reported lower life satisfaction than bilingual European Americans, whether they completed the SWLS in Chinese or in English (Shao, 1993). Similarly, M. L. Diener et al. (2004) gathered reports of emotional experience from multiple locations in China, Singapore, and India. Within the same country, some subsamples completed the survey in the local language, whereas others completed an English version. Results indicated that subsamples *within* a nation were more similar in emotional experience, regardless of the language used. Cultural differences obtained with translated measures of SWB have also been substantiated by *non*-self-report measures (Balatsky & Diener, 1993; Biswas-Diener et al., 2005). For instance, not only did Russians report lower SWB than Americans, they also recalled proportionately less positive events than did the latter (Balatsky & Diener, 1993).

Another issue is whether the use of numbers, or unfamiliarity with Likert scales could affect findings. In the slums of Calcutta, Biswas-Diener and Diener (2001) supplemented their 7-point Likert scales with a gradient of frowning and smiling faces. Some respondents were still confused by the task, forcing the researchers to reduce their measures to a 3-point scale. Despite these initial difficulties, they obtained an alpha coefficient of .80 for the SWLS. Still, when conducting research in certain cultures, the novelty of psychological testing can result in lower reliabilities (e.g., Biswas-Diener et al., 2005). Moreover, the reliability of the SWLS was found to correlate positively with the GNP of a nation (Vitterso et al., 2002). Higher reliabilities do not completely account for the greater LS found in wealthier nations, but they do appear to influence results and may be due to greater familiarity with psychological testing in those countries. Nevertheless, measures of LS and happiness are predictive of social integration and elderly suicide rates across nations (Wu & Bond, 2006), providing some evidence that these measures are capturing important aspects of people's life experiences.

Different response styles have occasionally been proposed as an explanation for cultural differences in well-being, especially with regard to the lower SWB among Asian samples. One hypothesis is that due to humility norms, Asian respondents tend toward neutrality by overselecting responses at the midpoint of the scale. E. Diener, Suh, Smith, and Shao (1995) examined this possibility among Chinese, Japanese, Korean, and American samples but did not find such a tendency. East Asians showed as much variation as Americans in their satisfaction with various domains. The former even reported a greater range of emotional intensity than the latter. Similarly, Veenhoven (2001) showed that negative response tendencies are unlikely to explain the lower levels of SWB among Russians. Interestingly, the lower scores on SWB run counter to the finding that acquiescence bias (the tendency to respond in agreement with items) tends to be higher in collectivistic nations (Johnson, Kulesa, Cho, & Shavitt, 2005; Smith, 2004). If acquiescence influences responses on SWB measures, one would expect to see higher means in East Asia, but this is clearly not the case.

On the other hand, social desirability may underlie some differences in reported SWB. In cultures where LS and pleasant affect are considered desirable, there may be a tendency to project higher SWB. People in some cultures appear to have a "positivity bias," in which satisfaction with global domains (e.g., education) are high even though satisfaction with more specific domains (e.g., textbooks, professors, and lectures) are *lower* on average (E. Diener, Scollon, Oishi, Dzokoto, & Suh, 2000). E. Diener, Scollon, et al. found that this positivity bias predicted LS beyond objective measures such as income, and that it correlated positively with norms for LS. This finding may explain the discrepant relation between wealth and happiness in Japan and Latin America. Latin Americans exhibited high desirability for LS, as well as a strong positivity bias. In contrast, Japanese and other East Asians reported lower desirability for LS and a corresponding *negativity* bias, such that global satisfaction was lower than would be expected from specific domain satisfactions (E. Diener, Scollon, et al., 2000). These biases could be considered artifacts, but they may also represent interesting cultural phenomena in and of themselves. Furthermore, it is worth reiterating that cultural differences in satisfaction judgments and emotional experience have been observed using other methodologies. For instance, a 1-week daily diary study showed that European Americans' global past-week satisfaction was more positive than their average satisfaction for *each day* of that week (Oishi, 2002). In contrast, Asian American participants did not exhibit a significant bias in global versus daily satisfaction ratings. Similarly, Kim-Prieto (2005) found that European Americans and Asians were similar in happiness reported "now," but Asians reporting feeling less during the past year and "in general." Finally, the recall of *pleasant*, but not unpleasant emotions during a vacation predicted the desire of European Americans to repeat the trip, whereas for Asian Americans the reverse was true (Wirtz, 2004). Interestingly, experience-sampling data revealed that the two groups did not differ in their *online* experience of pleasant and unpleasant emotions. Thus, the global judgment, and not the specific reports, influenced participants' decisions. Instead of dismissing global judgments altogether, E. Diener, Scollon, et al. (2000) suggested that global and domain-specific judgments are both distinctly informative aspects of SWB. Nevertheless, cross-cultural researchers should continue to use

multiple methods (memory measures, informant reports, etc.) whenever possible.

Perhaps a fundamental concern is whether it is appropriate to use nations as a proxy for studying culture. Researchers often define groups by their countries of origin and attribute any differences among these groups to culture. However, culture is not necessarily confined to geopolitical boundaries (Hermans & Kempen, 1998; Hong & Chiu, 2001). By equating entire nations with single cultures, we risk overlooking important differences within nations, as well as similarities that extend beyond national borders. In the case of emotion norms, many different norm patterns for pleasant and unpleasant affect may coexist within a nation (Eid & Diener, 2001). At the same time, however, nations within a certain *region* (e.g., East Asia or Latin America) appear to have similar patterns of emotional experience (M. L. Diener et al., 2004).

It is not entirely meaningless to group samples by nation. People living within a country are likely to have shared experiences and common histories, which are crucial in the formation of a common culture. Still, cultural entities may be defined at different levels, in any number of ways. It is important to realize the trade-offs inherent at a given level of analysis. Speaking of "regional cultures" allows us to make generalizations, but at the sacrifice of specificity. A focus on subcultural grouping may provide rich, nuanced data, but at the cost of generalizability. A further point is that culture is dynamic. The penetration of Western media and popular culture into other parts of the world can stimulate cultural change, leading to generational differences within nations. Thus, different age groups within a nation might differ in their attitudes and experience of SWB. More longitudinal research is needed to disentangle cohort effects from developmental effects.

Finally, group differences in SWB might be related to socioeconomic status (SES), not just to cultural beliefs and values per se. Income and education levels can determine the quality of life for people in a society, which in turn could lower or raise SWB. However, SES may sometimes be confounded with cultural groupings, especially when a history of discrimination has prevented certain groups from attaining higher status (Betancourt & López, 1993). Apart from discrimination, people from high versus low SES groups may face different realities and prioritize different values and beliefs (e.g., Snibbe & Markus, 2005). In either case, controlling for SES would result in a removal of cultural effects as well. Thus, separating SES from culture may not always be a straightforward task. On the other hand, cultural effects that persist even after controlling for socioeconomic variables pose interesting questions for future research and theory (see Rice & Steele, 2004) concerning the nature of culture and how it should be operationalized.

FUTURE DIRECTIONS

Although cultural variations in SWB have been replicated across self-report and memory measures, an important agenda for future research is to determine the extent to which these differences are reflected in the actual experience of well-being. More frequent applications of the experience-sampling method across cultures will provide further clarification of such differences. In one of the few such studies, Scollon et al. (2004) found that cultural differences in reports of past emotional experience do have some basis in online experience, but they also reflect aspects of the self-concept that independently influence the recall of emotions. These findings are provocative, but they must be replicated across more cultures. Other methods of assessing SWB, such as Kim's (2004) implicit association measure of LS, have only recently been developed and could provide further insights. Also critical will be the further development and integration of biological markers of well-being. For example, a predisposition toward positive affectivity has been linked to individual differences in chronic left-brain activation (Ito & Cacioppo, 1999). The immune system and neurotransmitter systems (e.g., serotonin and dopamine) may also play a role in well-being. These and other types of measures will help us know whether differences in SWB lie in actual experience or only in self-reports.

There is also a continuing need for theory on the functioning of SWB in culture—how it is defined in each culture, how it supports culture, and the types of outcomes associated with SWB in various societies. SWB is an important criterion for evaluating the success of a society, but by itself it is insufficient. To be happy in the face of starvation or inequality would seem preposterous to most people. Happiness and cultural conceptions of the good life are often tied to the sociomoral fabric of a society. As Markus and Kitayama (1994) suggested, being a competent member of one's culture typically "feels good" or "right." Thus, in some ways, LS may involve an implicit moral judgment on one's life, or on oneself as a person. Future studies of indigenous concepts of well-being, as well as the relation of SWB to the moral structures of a society, will help researchers further contextualize their interpretations of SWB.

Finally, viewing culture dynamically will enhance our understanding of cultural variation in SWB. Dynamic constructionists (e.g., Hong & Chiu, 2001) suggest that the influence of culture is not rigid and sweeping, but that it can fluctuate with the social context. Particularly among immigrants and other individuals who have been exposed to multiple cultures, *which* culture is influential may depend on cues in the environment (e.g., at home vs. at school) that activate different sets of cultural knowledge. An intriguing issue is how such cultural frame switching might moderate the relation between LS and correlates such as self-esteem. How bicultural individuals feel about and integrate their cultural identities (Haritatos & Benet-Martínez, 2002; Kim, Sarason, & Sarason, 2006) might also influence their well-being as they navigate between different cultural contexts. A related topic is how the causes of SWB change across the lifespan, or across different cohorts within the same culture. Thus, dynamic cultural perspectives contribute to a more fluid notion of SWB, raising new questions about the structure of well-being and its outcomes.

CONCLUSIONS

We have learned that comparisons of well-being are possible for some variables, and that there are probably some universal causes of well-being and ill-being. At the same time, we have learned that fascinating differences exist between cultures in the patterning and content of SWB variables, as well as in the causes and correlates of SWB. These differences should guide us in our attempts to make valid comparisons. For instance, some emotions may be understood similarly across cultures, whereas others have different connotative meanings. Direct comparisons, then, should be made with the former and not the latter. Even where SWB components are different, we could compare cultures according to their own criteria by measuring the attainment of culturally valued goals and experiences. Such an approach to well-being still allows us to assess success in different cultural contexts.

The effect size of culture on well-being can vary depending on the specific component of SWB under study. Cultures perhaps vary more in frequency and perceived norms for pleasant emotions than for unpleasant emotions (Eid & Diener, 2001; Scollon et al., 2004). In the case of unpleasant emotions, there is a stronger trend toward much larger differences within than between cultures. The uneven effects of culture on SWB not only resonate with dynamic views of culture but also call for circumspection in the type of inferences we draw from societal levels of SWB.

Much has been learned in the past decade of research in culture and SWB. Researchers began by making simple comparisons of nations on life satisfaction and happiness. Next they began to ask questions about the validity of measures across cultures, and about the causes and correlates of SWB in different societies. The field continues to advance, with more sharply focused research questions concerning *when* cultural influences come into play, *which* aspects of well-being are affected, and *what* the outcomes of SWB are across cultures. We are also entering an era in which research will treat culture as more dynamic, and individuals as bearers of more than one cultural tradition. These issues will continue to require multimeasure strategies and, we hope, stimulate the development of new methodologies. In this regard, progress in the various areas of cultural psychology and SWB, as well as more interdisciplinary work with the other social and biological sciences, will benefit both perspectives greatly.

ACKNOWLEDGMENTS

We would like to thank Sumie Okazaki for her helpful and insightful comments on an earlier draft of this chapter. This work was supported by a National Science Foundation Graduate Fellowship awarded to William Tov.

NOTE

1. The Oriya emotion *lajya* or *lajja* was translated by Menon and Shweder (1994) as shame. However, a less negative, alternative translation is "feeling shy." These two emotions are related but not the same. We thank Vijay Kumar Shrotriya for this observation. Our point is simply that the meaning of an emotion (hence, its value) can shift in different cultural contexts in ways that are not obvious from its valence alone.

REFERENCES

Ahadi, S. A., Rothbart, M. K., & Ye, R. (1993). Children's temperament in the US and China: Similarities and differences. *European Journal of Personality, 7,* 359–377.

Ahuvia, A. C. (2002). Individualism/collectivism and cultures of happiness: A theoretical conjecture on the relationship between consumption, culture and subjective well-being at the national level. *Journal of Happiness Studies, 3,* 23–36.

Bagozzi, R. P., Wong, N., & Yi, Y. (1999). The role of culture and gender in the relationship between positive and negative affect. *Cognition and Emotion, 13,* 641–672.

Balatsky, G., & Diener, E. (1993). Subjective well-being among Russian students. *Social Indicators Research, 28,* 225–243.

Benet-Martínez, V., & Karakitapoglu-Aygun, Z. (2003). The interplay of cultural syndromes and personality in predicting life satisfaction: Comparing Asian Americans and European Americans. *Journal of Cross-Cultural Psychology, 34,* 38–60.

Betancourt, H., & López, S. R. (1993). The study of culture, ethnicity, and race in American psychology. *American Psychologist, 48,* 629–637.

Biswas-Diener, R., & Diener, E. (2001). Making the best of a bad situation: Satisfaction in the slums of Calcutta. *Social Indicators Research, 55,* 329–352.

Biswas-Diener, R., Vittersø, J., & Diener, E. (2005). Most people are pretty happy, but there is cultural variation: The Inughuit, the Amish, and the Maasai. *Journal of Happiness Studies, 6,* 205–226.

Brown, J. D., & Kobayashi, C. (2002). Self-enhancement in Japan and America. *Asian Journal of Social Psychology, 5,* 145–168.

Brown, J. D., & Kobayashi, C. (2003). Motivation and manifestation: Cross-cultural expression of the self-enhancement motive. *Asian Journal of Social Psychology, 6,* 85–88.

Cantril, H. (1965). *The pattern of human concerns.* New Brunswick, NJ: Rutgers University Press.

Caspi, A., Sugden, K., Moffitt, T. E., Taylor, A., Craig, I. W., Harrington, H., et al. (2003). Influence of life stress on depression: Moderation by a polymorphism in the 5-HTT gene. *Science, 301,* 386–389.

Cavalli-Sforza, L. L. (1991). Genes, peoples, and languages. *Scientific American, 256*(5), 104–110.

Chirkov, V., Ryan, R. M., Kim, Y., & Kaplan, U. (2003). Differentiating autonomy from individualism and independence: A self-determination theory perspective on internalization of cultural orientations and well-being. *Journal of Personality and Social Psychology,* *84,* 97–110.

Cohen, D., & Gunz, A. (2002). As seen by the other: Perspective on the self in the memories and emotional perceptions of Easterners and Westerners. *Psychological Science, 13,* 55–59.

Deci, E. L., & Ryan, R. M. (1985). *Intrinsic motivation and self-determination in human behavior.* New York: Plenum.

The Dhammapada: The sayings of the Buddha (T. Byron, Trans.). (1976). New York: Random House.

Diener, E. (1984). Subjective well-being. *Psychological Bulletin, 95,* 542–575.

Diener, E., & Diener, C. (1996). Most people are happy. *Psychological Science, 7,* 181–185.

Diener, E., & Diener, M. (1995). Cross-cultural correlates of life satisfaction and self-esteem. *Journal of Personality and Social Psychology, 68,* 653–663.

Diener, E., Diener, M., & Diener, C. (1995). Factors predicting the subjective well-being of nations. *Journal of Personality and Social Psychology, 69,* 851–864.

Diener, E., Emmons, R. A., Larsen, R. J., & Griffin, S. (1985). The Satisfaction with Life Scale. *Journal of Personality Assessment, 49,* 71–75.

Diener, E., Gohm, C. L., Suh, E., & Oishi, S. (2000). Similarity of the relations between marital status and subjective well-being across cultures. *Journal of Cross-Cultural Psychology, 31,* 419–436.

Diener, E., Horwitz, J., & Emmons, R. (1985). Happiness of the very wealthy. *Social Indicators Research, 16,* 263–274.

Diener, E., Lucas, R. E., & Scollon, C. N. (2006). Beyond the hedonic treadmill: Revising the adaptation theory of well-being. *American Psychologist, 61,* 305–314.

Diener, E., & Oishi, S. (2000). Money and happiness. In E. Diener & E.M. Suh (Eds.), *Culture and subjective well-being* (pp. 185–218). Cambridge, MA: MIT Press.

Diener, E., Sandvik, E., Seidlitz, L., & Diener, M. (1993). The relationship between income and subjective well-being: Relative or absolute? *Social Indicators Research, 28,* 195–223.

Diener, E., Scollon, C. K. N., Oishi, S., Dzokoto, V., & Suh, E. M. (2000). Positivity and the construction of life satisfaction judgments: Global happiness is not the sum of its parts. *Journal of Happiness Studies, 1,* 159–176.

Diener, E., & Seligman, M. E. P. (2004). Beyond money: Toward an economy of well-being. *Psychological Science in the Public Interest, 5,* 1–31.

Diener, E., & Suh, E. M. (1999). National differences in subjective well-being. In D. Kahneman, E. Diener, & N. Schwarz (Eds.), *Well-being: The foundations of hedonic psychology* (pp. 434–450). New York: Russell Sage Foundation.

Diener, E., Suh, E. M., Smith, H., & Shao, L. (1995). National differences in reported subjective well-being: Why do they occur? *Social Indicators Research, 34,* 7–32.

Diener, M. L., Fujita, F., Kim-Prieto, C., & Diener, E. (2004). *Culture and emotional experience.* Unpublished manuscript, University of Utah.

Diener, M. L., & Lucas, R. E. (2004). Adult's desires for children's emotions across 48 countries: Associations with individual and national characteristics. *Journal of Cross-Cultural Psychology, 35,* 525–547.

Edgerton, R. B. (1992). *Sick societies: Challenging the myth of primitive harmony.* New York: Free Press.

Eid, M., & Diener, E. (2001). Norms for experiencing emotions in different cultures: Inter- and intranational differences. *Journal of Social and Personality Psychology, 81,* 869–885.

Ekman, P., & Friesen, W. V. (1971). Constants across cultures in the face and emotion. *Journal of Social and Personality Psychology, 17,* 124–129.

Ekman, P., Friesen, W. V., O'Sullivan, M., Chan, A., Diacoyanni-Tarlatzis, I., Heider, K., et al. (1987). Universals and cultural differences in the judgments of facial expressions of emotion. *Journal of Social and Personality Psychology, 53,* 712–717.

Fredrickson, B. L. (1998). What good are positive emotions? *Review of General Psychology, 2,* 300–319.

Freedman, D. G., & Freedman, N. C. (1969). Behavioural differences between Chinese-American and European-American newborns. *Nature, 224,* 1227.

Fujita, F., & Diener, E. (2005). Life satisfaction set point: Stability and change. *Journal of Personality and Social Psychology, 88,* 158–164.

Gaskins, R. W. (1999). "Adding legs to a snake": A reanalysis of motivation and the pursuit of happiness from a Zen Buddhist perspective. *Journal of Educational Psychology, 91,* 204–215.

Gohm, C. L., Oishi, S., Darlington, J., & Diener, E. (1998). Culture, parental conflict, parental marital status, and the subjective well-being of young adults. *Journal of Marriage and the Family, 60,* 319–334.

Haritatos, J., & Benet-Martínez, V. (2002). Bicultural identities: The interface of cultural, personality, and socio-cognitive processes. *Journal of Research in Personality, 36,* 598–606.

Heine, S. J. (2003). Self-enhancement in Japan?: A reply to Brown and Kobayashi. *Asian Journal of Social Psychology, 6,* 75–84.

Heine, S. J., Kitayama, S., Lehman, D. R., Takata, T., Ide, E., Leung, C., et al. (2001). Divergent consequences of success and failure in Japan and North America: An investigation of self-improving motivations and malleable selves. *Journal of Personality and Social Psychology, 81,* 599–615.

Heine, S. J., Lehman, D. R., Markus, H. R., & Kitayama, S. (1999). Is there a universal need for positive self-regard? *Psychological Review, 106,* 766–794.

Hermans, H. J. M., & Kempen, H. J. G. (1998). Moving cultures: The perilous problems of cultural dichotomies in a globalizing society. *American Psychologist, 53,* 1111–1120.

Hong, Y., & Chiu, C. (2001). Toward a paradigm shift: From cross-cultural differences in social cognition to social-cognitive mediation of cultural differences. *Social Cognition, 19*, 181–196.

Howell, C. J., Howell, R. T., & Schwabe, K. A. (2006). Does wealth enhance life satisfaction for people who are materially deprived?: Exploring the association among the *Orang Asli* of Peninsular Malaysia. *Social Indicators Research, 76*, 499–524.

Inglehart, R. (1990). *Culture shift in advanced industrial society.* Princeton, NJ: Princeton University Press.

Inglehart, R., & Klingemann, H.-D. (2000). Genes, culture, democracy, and happiness. In E. Diener & E. M. Suh (Eds.), *Culture and subjective well-being* (pp. 185–218). Cambridge, MA: MIT Press.

Ito, T. A., & Cacioppo, J. T. (1999). The psychophysiology of utility appraisals. In D. Kahneman, E. Diener, & N. Schwartz (Eds.), *Well-being: The foundations of hedonic psychology* (pp. 470–488). New York: Russell Sage Foundation.

Izard, C. E., & Malatesta, C. Z. (1987). Perspectives on emotional development I: Differential emotions theory of early emotional development. In J. D. Osofsky (Ed.), *Handbook of infant development* (2nd ed., pp. 494–554). New York: Wiley.

Johnson, T., Kulesa, P., Cho, Y. I., & Shavitt, S. (2005). The relation between culture and response styles: Evidence from 19 countries. *Journal of Cross-Cultural Psychology, 36*, 264–277.

Kagan, J., Arcus, D., Snidman, N., Feng, W. Y., Hendler, J., & Greene, S. (1994). Reactivity in infants: A cross-national comparison. *Developmental Psychology, 30*, 342–345.

Kang, S.-M., Shaver, P. R., Sue, S., Min, K.-H., & Jing, H. (2003). Culture-specific patterns in the prediction of life satisfaction: Roles of emotion, relationship quality, and self-esteem. *Personality and Social Psychology Bulletin, 29*, 1596–1608.

Kim, D.-Y. (2004). The implicit life satisfaction measure. *Asian Journal of Social Psychology, 7*, 236–262.

Kim, D.-Y., Sarason, B., & Sarason, I. G. (2006). Implicit social cognition and culture: Explicit and implicit psychological acculturation, and distress of Korean-American young adults. *Journal of Social and Clinical Psychology, 25*, 1–32.

Kim-Prieto, C. Y. (2005). *Culture's influence on experienced and remembered emotions.* Unpublished doctoral dissertation, University of Illinois, Urbana–Champaign.

Kim-Prieto, C., & Diener, E. (2004). *Religion's role in cultural differences in emotional experiences.* Unpublished manuscript, University of Illinois, Urbana–Champaign.

Kitayama, S., & Markus, H. R. (2000). The pursuit of happiness and the realization of sympathy: Cultural patterns of self, social relations, and well-being. In E. Diener & E. M. Suh (Eds.), *Culture and subjective well-being* (pp. 113–161). Cambridge, MA: MIT Press.

Kitayama, S., Markus, H. R., & Kurokawa, M. (2000).

Culture, emotion, and well-being: Good feelings in Japan and the United States. *Cognition and Emotion, 14*, 93–124.

Kitayama, S., Markus, H. R., Matsumoto, H., & Norasakkunkit, V. (1997). Individual and collective processes in the construction of the self: Self-enhancement in the United States and self-criticism in Japan. *Journal of Personality and Social Psychology, 72*, 1245–1267.

Kuppens, P., Ceulemans, E., Timmerman, M. E., Diener, E., & Kim-Prieto, C. (2006). Universal intracultural and intercultural dimensions of the recalled frequency of emotional experience. *Journal of Cross-Cultural Psychology, 37*, 491–515.

Kwan, V. S. Y., Bond, M. H., & Singelis, T. M. (1997). Pancultural explanations for life satisfaction: Adding relationship harmony to self-esteem. *Journal of Personality and Social Psychology, 73*, 1038–1051.

Lesch, K.-P., Bengel, D., Heils, A., Sabol, S. Z., Greenberg, B. D., Petri, S., et al. (1996). Association of anxiety-related traits with a polymorphism in the serotonin transporter gene regulatory region. *Science, 274*, 1527–1531.

Levy, R. I. (1982). On the nature and functions of the emotions: An anthropological perspective. *Social Science Information, 21*, 511–528.

Lucas, R. E., Diener, E., Grob, A., Suh, E. M., & Shao, L. (2000). Cross-cultural evidence for the fundamental features of extraversion. *Journal of Personality and Social Psychology, 79*, 452–468.

Lutz, C. A. (1988). *Unnatural emotions: Everyday sentiments on a Micronesian atoll and their challenge to Western theory.* Chicago: University of Chicago Press.

Lykken, D., & Tellegen, A. (1996). Happiness is a stochastic phenomenon. *Psychological Science, 7*, 186–188.

Lyubomirsky, S., King, L., & Diener, E. (2005). The benefits of frequent positive affect: Does happiness lead to success? *Psychological Bulletin, 131*, 803–855.

Markus, H. R., & Kitayama, S. (1991). Culture and the self: Implications for cognition, emotion, and motivation. *Psychological Review, 98*, 224–253.

Markus, H. R., & Kitayama, S. (1994). The cultural construction of self and emotion: Implications for social behavior. In S. Kitayama & H. R. Markus (Eds.), *Emotion and culture: Empirical studies of mutual influence* (pp. 89–130). Washington, DC: American Psychological Association.

Maslow, A. H. (1954). *Motivation and personality.* New York: Harper & Row.

Menon, U., & Shweder, R. A. (1994). Kali's tongue: Cultural psychology and the power of shame in Orissa, India. In S. Kitayama & H. R. Markus (Eds.), *Emotion and culture: Empirical studies of mutual influence* (pp. 241–284). Washington, DC: American Psychological Association.

Mesquita, B., & Frijda, N. H. (1992). Cultural variations in emotions: A review. *Psychological Bulletin, 112*, 179–204.

Mesquita, B., Fridja, N. H., & Scherer, K. R. (1997). Culture and emotion. In J. W. Berry, P. R. Dasen, & T. S. Saraswathi (Eds.), *Handbook of cross-cultural psychology* (2nd ed., Vol. 2, pp. 255–297). Boston: Allyn & Bacon.

Miller, P. J., Wang, S., Sandel, T., & Cho, G. E. (2002). Self-esteem as folk theory: A comparison of European American and Taiwanese mother's beliefs. *Parenting: Science and Practice*, 2, 209–239.

No, S., & Hong, Y.-Y. (2004, January). *Negotiating bicultural identity: Contrast and assimilation effects in cultural frame switching.* Poster presented at the annual meeting of the Society for Personality and Social Psychology, Austin, TX.

Oishi, S. (2000). Goals as cornerstones of subjective well-being. In E. Diener & E. M. Suh (Eds.), *Culture and subjective well-being* (pp. 87–112). Cambridge, MA: MIT Press.

Oishi, S. (2002). The experience and remembering of well-being: A cross-cultural analysis. *Personality and Social Psychology Bulletin*, 28, 1398–1406.

Oishi, S., & Diener, E. (2001). Goals, culture, and subjective well-being. *Personality and Social Psychology Bulletin*, 27, 1674–1682.

Oishi, S., Diener, E. F., Lucas, R. E., & Suh, E. M. (1999). Cross-cultural variations in predictors of life satisfaction: Perspectives from needs and values. *Personality and Social Psychology Bulletin*, 25, 980–990.

Oishi, S., Diener, E., Scollon, C. N., & Biswas-Diener, R. (2003). Cross-situational consistency of affective experiences across cultures. *Journal of Personality and Social Psychology*, 86, 460–472.

Oishi, S., Schimmack, U., & Colcombe, S. J. (2003). The contextual and systematic nature of life satisfaction judgments. *Journal of Experimental Social Psychology*, 39, 232–247.

Ortony, A., & Turner, T. J. (1990). What's basic about basic emotions? *Psychological Review*, 97, 315–331.

Park, N., & Huebner, E. S. (2005). A cross-cultural study of the levels and correlates of life satisfaction among adolescents. *Journal of Cross-Cultural Psychology*, 36, 444–456.

Peng, K., & Nisbett, R. E. (1999). Culture, dialectics, and reasoning about contradiction. *American Psychologist*, 54, 741–754.

Plutchik, R. (1980). *Emotion: A psychoevolutionary synthesis.* New York: Harper & Row.

Radhakrishnan, P., & Chan, D. K.-S. (1997). Cultural differences in the relation between self-discrepancy and life satisfaction. *International Journal of Psychology*, 32, 387–398.

Rice, T. W., & Steele, B. J. (2004). Subjective well-being and culture across time and space. *Journal of Cross-Cultural Psychology*, 35, 633–647.

Ryan, R. M., & Deci, E. L. (2000). Self-determination theory and the facilitation of intrinsic motivation, social development, and well-being. *American Psychologist*, 55, 68–78.

Ryff, C. D., & Singer, B. (1998). The contours of positive human health. *Psychological Inquiry*, 9, 1–28.

Schimmack, U., Diener, E., & Oishi, S. (2002). Life-satisfaction is a momentary judgment and a stable personality characteristic: The use of chronically accessible and stable sources. *Journal of Personality*, 70, p. 345–384.

Schimmack, U., Oishi, S., & Diener, E. (2002). Cultural influences on the relation between pleasant emotions and unpleasant emotions: Asian dialectic philosophies or individualism–collectivism? *Cognition and Emotion*, 16, 705–719.

Schimmack, U., Radhakrishnan, P., Oishi, S., Dzokoto, V., & Ahadi, S. (2002). Culture, personality, and subjective well-being: Integrating process models of life satisfaction. *Journal of Personality and Social Psychology*, 82, 582–593.

Schwarz, N., & Strack, F. (1999). Reports of subjective well-being: Judgmental processes and their methodological implications. In D. Kahneman, E. Diener, & N. Schwarz (Eds.), *Well-being: The foundations of hedonic psychology* (pp. 61–84). New York: Russell Sage Foundation.

Scollon, C. N., Diener, E., Oishi, S., Biswas-Diener, R. (2004). Emotions across cultures and methods. *Journal of Cross-Cultural Psychology*, 35, 304–326.

Shao, L. (1993). *Multilanguage comparability of life satisfaction and happiness measures in mainland Chinese and American students.* Unpublished master's thesis, University of Illinois, Urbana–Champaign.

Shaver, P. R., Wu, S., & Schwartz, J. C. (1992). Cross-cultural similarities and differences in emotion and its representation: A prototype approach. *Review of Personality and Social Psychology*, 13, 175–212.

Sheldon, K. M., Elliot, A. J., Ryan, R. M., Chirkov, V., Kim, Y., Wu, C., et al. (2004). Self-concordance and subjective well-being in four cultures. *Journal of Cross-Cultural Psychology*, 35, 209–223.

Shweder, R. A. (2000). Moral maps, "First World" conceits, and the new evangelists. In L. E. Harrison & S. P. Huntington (Eds.), *Culture matters: How values shape human progress* (pp. 158–172). New York: Basic Books.

Smith, P. B. (2004). Acquiescent response bias as an aspect of cultural communication style. *Journal of Cross-Cultural Psychology*, 35, 50–61.

Snibbe, A. C., & Markus, H. R. (2005). You can't always get what you want: Educational attainment, agency, and choice. *Journal of Personality and Social Psychology*, 88, 703–720.

Suh, E., Diener, E., Oishi, S., & Triandis, H. C. (1998). The shifting basis of life satisfaction judgments across cultures: Emotions versus norms. *Journal of Personality and Social Psychology*, 74, 482–493.

Suh, E. M. (2002). Culture, identity consistency, and subjective well-being. *Journal of Personality and Social Psychology*, 83, 1378–1391.

Thompson, J. (1941). Development of facial expression

of emotion in blind and seeing children. *Archives of Psychology*, (No. 264).

Tomkins, S. S. (1962). *Affect, imagery, and consciousness: Vol. 1. The positive affects*. New York: Springer.

Tomkins, S. S. (1963). *Affect, imagery, and consciousness: Vol. 2. The negative affects*. New York: Springer.

Tsai, J., Knutson, B., & Fung, H. H. (2006). Cultural variation in affect valuation. *Journal of Personality and Social Psychology*, *90*, 288–307

Veenhoven, R. (n.d.). Distributional findings in nations. In *World database of happiness*. Retrieved September 5, 2004, from *www.eur.nl/fsw/research/happiness*

Veenhoven, R. (1991). Is happiness relative? *Social Indicators Research*, *24*, 1–34.

Veenhoven, R. (1993). *Happiness in nations*. Rotterdam, the Netherlands: Risbo.

Veenhoven, R. (2001). Are the Russians as unhappy as they say they are?: Comparability of self-reports across nations. *Journal of Happiness Studies*, *2*, 111–136.

Vittersø, J., Røysamb, E., & Diener, E. (2002). The concept of life satisfaction across cultures: Exploring its diverse meaning and relation to economic wealth. In E. Gullone & R. A. Cummins (Eds.), *The universality of subjective well-being indicators* (pp. 81–103). Dordrecht, the Netherlands: Kluwer Academic.

Wallbott, H. G., & Scherer, K. (1988). How universal and specific is emotional experience?: Evidence from 27 countries on five continents. In K. R. Scherer (Ed.), *Facets of emotion: Recent research* (pp. 31–56). Hillsdale, NJ: Erlbaum.

Watson, D., Clark, L. A., & Tellegen, A. (1984). Cross-cultural convergence in the structure of mood: A Japanese replication and a comparison with U.S. findings. *Journal of Social and Personality Psychology*, *47*, 127–144.

Wierzbicka, A. (1986). Human emotions: Universal or culture-specific? *American Anthropologist*, *88*, 584–594.

Wirtz, D. (2004). *Focusing on the good versus focusing on the bad: An analysis of East–West differences in subjective well-being*. Unpublished doctoral dissertation, University of Illinois, Urbana–Champaign.

Wu, W. C. H., & Bond, M. H. (2006). National differences in predictors of suicide among young and elderly citizens: Linking societal predictors to psychological factors. *Archives of Suicide Research*, *10*, 45–60.

Yang, K. S. (2003). Beyond Maslow's culture-bound linear theory: A preliminary statement of the double-Y model of basic human needs. In V. Murphy-Berman & J. J. Berman (Eds.), *Nebraska Symposium on Motivation: Vol. 49. Cross-cultural differences in perspectives on the self* (pp. 176–255). Lincoln: University of Nebraska Press.

CHAPTER 29

Culture and Motivation

What Motivates People to Act in the Ways That They Do?

STEVEN J. HEINE

What motivates people to act in the ways that they do? It is difficult to conceive of a more fundamental question in psychology. Many key social-psychological theories regarding topics such as cognitive dissonance, conformity, agency, approach–avoidance, self-enhancement, and achievement are grounded in an understanding of the forces that impel human behavior.

Although questions regarding motivation have been central to psychology since the earliest days of the field, not until recently was focused consideration directed at the ways that culture might be implicated in human motivations. On the one hand, it is not obvious that people from divergent cultures would be motivated differently. After all, humans are all of the same species, and we should expect a great deal of similarity in their motivations, regardless of cultural background. Indeed, a variety of key psychological motivations are likely common across all human cultures. For example, people everywhere want things that improve the quality of their lives, such as getting access to nice material rewards, having stimu-

lating relationships, and earning the respect of their peers (for a review, see Kenrick, Li, & Butner, 2003).

On the other hand, humans are unlike all other species in the extent to which they depend on cultural learning to survive (e.g., Tomasello, 1999). Because of this, human motivations cannot be understood solely in terms of biological predispositions interacting with the constraints and affordances provided by physical environments. Rather, those biological predispositions are expressed in the context of particular cultural environments that shape the ways motivations are made manifest. For example, the ways that people get access to material rewards, the kinds of relationships that they might find stimulating, and the ways they secure the respect of their peers are not identical across all contexts. They are rooted in people's values, their beliefs about what can be easily accomplished, their expectations of the consequences associated with their actions, and the ways that they understand their behaviors—all of which are importantly shaped by cultural context. In other words, human motivations are grounded in cultural meaning systems (Bruner, 1990; Shweder, 1990). As such, we should expect motivations to be expressed differently across cultures to the extent that cultures vary in the ways that particular behaviors are rendered meaningful. Here I review the literature on recent efforts to investigate how cultures differ in the ways that motivations are shaped and expressed.

RELIGION AND ACHIEVEMENT MOTIVATION

One of the earliest cultural-psychological theories regarding motivation, and perhaps the most profound, was proposed by a sociologist. In 1904–1905 Max Weber published a highly influential and controversial series of essays entitled *The Protestant Ethic and the Spirit of Capitalism* (1904/1992). Weber recognized a fundamental tenet of cultural psychology that, in contrast to most events in the natural world, human behavior is necessarily interwoven with meaning. Events do not simply impinge themselves upon people; it is people's interpretation of what those events mean that motivates them to respond accordingly.

Weber's theory was developed and explored largely outside of a psychological context; however, specific psychological hypotheses have since been proposed and tested (e.g., McClelland, 1961; Sanchez-Burks, 2002). Given its nonpsychological roots, the theory may be somewhat unfamiliar to many psychologists and warrants some background description. Weber was interested in the question of how the revolutionary doctrine of capitalism was able to emerge out of the traditional economies of the medieval era. At the time that Weber published his ideas, the dominant theory in the social sciences was Marxism, which proposed that capitalism emerged as the result of structural changes in the economy. Specifically, Marx maintained that as industries developed technologies that increased the productivity of workers, the surplus value of workers' efforts accumulated and was reinvested into production. Capitalism was thus seen to follow from industrialization, and, indeed, was viewed as an inevitable consequence of it. In contrast to the economic determinism of Marxism, Weber viewed capitalism as the product of people deriving meaning from a particular cultural context. He proposed that capitalism was built on the foundation of a number of cultural beliefs

that emerged alongside the Protestant Reformation.

Protestantism initially emerged as a reaction to some corruption in the medieval Catholic Church, but Weber maintained that it contained ideas that shaped much more than the spiritual lives of its followers. One idea to emerge from Protestantism was the notion that individuals were able to communicate with God directly, and were not dependent upon the Church as an intermediary. This individualized relation between each person and God has been argued to be central to the blossoming of individualism that emerged during the Reformation and continues to influence much of Western society today (e.g., Baumeister, 1987; McClelland, 1961).

A second idea to emerge was related to this belief in an individualized relation between God and each person. Martin Luther proposed that each individual had a "calling"; that is, each person had a unique, God-given purpose to fulfill during his or her mortal existence. The idea was that people are all God's servants in the world, and that each individual was given a specific duty or job to take care of while he or she tended the planet. God gave individuals unique skills and capabilities to enable them to fulfill their calling, and it was incumbent upon them to discover that calling. People's highest moral duty was to serve God well by working hard at their calling. Weber argued that by developing this notion of a calling, Luther was able to imbue daily labor with a spiritual significance that had traditionally been reserved for religious activities such as prayer and ritual. With the Protestant Reformation, work had thus become a moral obligation rather than something necessary for subsistence. As such, people's attitudes shifted from work as *a means to survive* to work as an *inherently meaningful activity* in itself. This shift in attitudes, Weber maintains, had an enormous impact on the economic development of Protestant nations.

The early Puritan sects of Protestantism (e.g., Calvinism, Methodism, Pietism, and Baptism) also proposed the radical idea of predestination, that is, the belief that it was already determined before one was born whether one was of the fortunate "Elect" who was destined for Heaven, or was one of the wretched many who was doomed to burn in Hell forever. Which fate was one's own was a distinction that no doubt mattered a great deal to the Puritans. Weber submitted the counterintuitive proposition that this belief in predestination played a key role in the development of capitalism. One might expect that if people's fates were predetermined, then they might respond by deciding to enjoy their lives, because there was nothing that they could do to change their fates. They might as well live it up while the living was good. However, this interpretation was apparently rarely seized upon; rather, the notion of predestination brought with it "a feeling of unprecedented inner loneliness" (Weber, 1904/1992, p. 104), and individuals were highly motivated to escape it by convincing themselves that they were among the privileged Elect. Because people did not know their fate for certain, they had to make inferences based on available cues. The primary cue that one was among the Elect was possessing absolute certainty about this fact, and evidence for this certainty could be seen in the products of one's efforts to fulfill this calling. It was believed that God would not reward those who were doomed to burn in Hell, so any sign of material success was perceived as evidence that one was among the Elect. Furthermore, because one's time on earth was to be spent serving God through one's calling rather than enjoying the fruits of one's labor, any accumulated wealth was to be reinvested to further one's efforts, and to accumulate even more wealth and evidence of one's chosen status. Modern capitalism, as Weber viewed it, was thus concerned with the accumulation of wealth for its own sake, and not for the sake of the material pleasures that it brought. Weber proposed that the combination of beliefs in an individualized relation with God, a calling, and predestination provided the cultural foundation for capitalism.

Weber's thesis has been highly controversial since it was first published. Giddens (1992) described the many ways that people were offended by this theory: Weber's characterizations of Catholicism as having a retarding influence upon modern economic development alienated most Catholics; his description of Puritan life as being bound up in an ecclesiastical straitjacket was not appreciated by Protestants; people of other religious backgrounds felt ignored (there is clear evidence of a moralized work ethic among people of Confucian and Jewish backgrounds, for example, something which Weber (1951, 1952) emphasized in some of his other works); and Weber's contention that religious ideas can transform economies

perturbed the Marxists and most economists. It seems that some were so incensed by Weber's thesis that they were willing to offer some rather far-fetched alternative accounts for the greater economic success Weber identified among Protestants compared to Catholics. For example, Huntington (1915) argued that the relative success of Protestant nations was due to their more temperate climate (with no account offered for the relative lack of success among the more temperate Catholic nations). Fanfani (1935) went so far as to propose, without any supporting data, that people in Protestant nations tend to have longer heads than people in Catholic ones, which somehow allowed Protestants to be more successful.

Despite the continuing controversy, much evidence is consistent with Weber's thesis. Some evidence comes from economists and historians, who note that power and wealth moved in Europe from places such as Spain and northern Italy before the Protestant Reformation began in 1517, to Northern European Protestant centers in Germany, the Netherlands, and England, until its most colossal bloom in the 20th-century United States (e.g., Landes, 1999). A consideration of per capita income among countries of the world revealed that largely Protestant nations earned more than mixed Protestant and Catholic nations, and that these earned more than predominantly Catholic nations (Furnham, 1990). Jackson, Fox, and Crockett (1970) found that Protestants in the United States were more likely to enter high-status, nonmanual occupations than Catholics of the same occupational origin, controlling for a variety of other societal variables. McClelland (1961) found that Protestant nations were far more industrialized than their Catholic counterparts.

There is also much psychological evidence supporting Weber's thesis. McClelland (1961) recognized that Weber's proposal was inherently a theory about motivation, and that one could derive testable hypotheses regarding a greater need for achievement among those raised Protestant than among those raised Catholic. For example, he found that, compared with Catholic parents, Protestant parents expected their children to become self-reliant at an earlier age. Likewise, he compared the stories written by young boys and found that those written by German Protestants had higher need for achievement scores than those written by German Catholics (McClelland,

1961). Various other lines of research have followed McClelland's pioneering efforts. Giorgi and Marsh (1990) found pronounced differences between Western European Catholics and mainstream Protestants in the embracing of an intrinsic work ethic (interestingly, the relation was clear both when contrasting individuals of different religions *within* countries, and when comparing countries) as evidenced in a measure of work values. Furthermore, this relation was identifiable regardless of individuals' level of religiosity, suggesting that the work ethic had become secularized. The Protestant ethic has also been associated with negative attitudes toward laziness and being overweight (Quinn & Crocker, 1999), and a concern with self-esteem and self-deception (which I elaborate on later; Baumeister, 1987; Crocker & Park, 2004).

Sanchez-Burks and colleagues (Sanchez-Burks, 2002; Sanchez-Burks et al., 2003; Sanchez-Burks, Nisbett, & Ybarra, 2000) investigated Weber's thesis in the laboratory. Sanchez-Burks (2002) was interested in exploring an aspect of Protestant ideology emphasized by Calvinism; that is, when Protestants are engaged in their morally sanctioned work, they should be entirely focused on their work, thus maintaining a rather impassive attitude toward potential distractions, such as other people (Bendix, 1977; Hampden-Turner & Trompenaars, 1993). Protestants should maintain a relational style toward others that is relatively detached while they are working; however, in contexts where there are no work obligations, they should switch back into a more attentive relational style (Weber, 1947). Sanchez-Burks (2002) sought to test this hypothesis by comparing Protestants and non-Protestants in two different settings. The participants in his experiment were all European American students raised either as Protestants (specifically Presbyterians and Methodists, the two Protestant sects influenced by Calvinist ideology that were most represented among the student body) or as non-Protestants (Catholics, atheists, and other religious backgrounds). These participants were assigned to engage either in a task in a work environment or a casual nonwork setting. Participants in the two conditions worked together with a confederate of the experimenter who was kept blind to participants' religious background. The confederates were instructed to nervously shake their feet the entire time they were talking with the

participants. The primary dependent variable was a measure of unconscious mimicry (Bargh, Chen, & Burrows, 1996; Chartrand & Bargh, 1999): specifically, how much more the participants shook their own feet when they were with the confederates compared with time when they were alone. Male participants revealed a pattern precisely in line with predictions derived from Weber's thesis (women, Sanchez-Burks argued, tend to maintain more of a relational focus regardless of circumstance); that is, male non-Protestants were just as likely to mimic the confederate's foot shaking in a casual setting as in a work setting. In stark contrast, the Protestant males showed very little evidence of mimicry in the work setting but considerable mimicry in the casual setting. It appears that when Protestant males are focused on a work task they are able to shut out relational concerns, something which neither Protestant women nor non-Protestants seem to do. When Protestant men are actually working, they do not seem to have much interest in anything else.

Fueling the controversy in Weber's thesis, however, are some cross-cultural studies comparing Likert scale means on various self-report measures of the Protestant work ethic that do not appear to be consistent with Weber's thesis. Indeed, studies that have compared the means on these scales reveal either no cultural difference in the Protestant work ethic or a weaker work ethic among nations of a largely Protestant background (e.g., the United States, Australia, and Britain) than among people from countries with little exposure to Protestant ideology (e.g., India, Malaysia, Mexico, Sri Lanka, Uganda, and Zimbabwe; Baguma & Furnham, 1993; Furnham, Bond, & Heaven, 1993; Furnham & Muhiudeen, 1984; Isonio & Garza, 1987; Niles, 1994); that is, the evidence for an association between Protestantism and achievement motivation is far more consistent in laboratory studies (e.g., Sanchez-Burks, 2002), and studies that measure various cultural products associated with the Protestant work ethic (e.g., McClelland, 1961) than in studies that utilize cross-cultural comparisons of means from self-report measures. This is consistent with a growing body of evidence that comparisons of means of subjective Likert scale measures across cultures can be compromised by various response artifacts, such as reference-group effects, and yield results of dubious validity (Heine, Kitayama,

Lehman, Takata, et al., 2001; Heine, Lehman, Peng, & Greenholtz, 2002; Peng, Nisbett, & Wong, 1997).

In summary, to the extent that Max Weber was correct a century ago, we can understand some of people's achievement motivations to be derived from religious ideas that they encounter in their cultures. Weber's thesis remains controversial, however; a great deal of evidence in support of it has been marshaled from a variety of different disciplines. Laboratory investigations of Protestant ideology are relatively new to psychology, and there will surely be further challenges and validations of Weber's thesis in the future.

MOTIVATIONS FOR CONSISTENCY

One of the most central themes in Western social psychology derives from the notion that people are motivated to be consistent. Dating back to Heider (1958) and Festinger (1957), researchers have emphasized the importance that people place on viewing themselves and their behaviors in a way that coheres in a consistent and sensible manner. This motivation can be identified in a number of diverse research paradigms, including cognitive dissonance, self-verification theory, autobiographical memories, and the "foot-in-the-door" paradigm, and is a fundamental assumption underlying personality theory (Mischel, 1973). When people encounter inconsistency, so the theorizing goes, they encounter a problem that needs to be rectified. As the 2004 U.S. presidential election highlighted, it was a costly liability for John Kerry to be perceived as someone who changed his opinions, in contrast to the determined and steadfast George W. Bush. Consistency is a desired end state that people are motivated to achieve.

Although the Western research demonstrates that a motivation for consistency is an extremely powerful drive, it is less clear how well this motivation generalizes to other cultural contexts. In particular, there is a growing body of evidence that consistency motivations are weaker among East Asians. For example, consider the results of a study by Kanagawa, Cross, and Markus (2001). They sought to investigate how much people's context affects the ways that they view themselves. College students from Japan and the United States were asked to complete the Twenty Statements Test;

however, the students' context at the time of the study was varied. Some participants completed the questionnaire in a professor's office; other participants sat next to a fellow student; still others sat in a large group of about 20–50 people, and some students completed the questionnaire alone. Kanagawa et al. calculated the ratio of positive statements that students made about themselves compared to the number of negative statements. They found that the American responses looked quite similar across the four conditions. Their selves were described in pretty much the same way regardless of situation. In contrast, the Japanese responses varied considerably across situations. They were considerably less self-critical when they were by themselves than when they were with others, especially when they were with a professor. The general positivity of Japanese individuals' attitudes toward themselves appeared quite different depending on who was in the room with them. Likewise, other research with the Twenty Statements Test reveals that East Asians tended not to describe themselves by abstracting features across situations, in contrast to American's tendencies to view themselves more in terms of pure psychological attributes (M. H. Bond & Cheung, 1983; Cousins, 1989). Thus, East Asians appear to be more willing than Westerners to describe themselves in divergent ways across different contexts (also see Suh, 2002).

One reason why East Asians appear to be more accepting of inconsistency can be traced to a predilection for what Peng and Nisbett (1999) referred to as "naive dialecticism." In contrast to Western formal reasoning traditions that require that contradictions be resolved, principles of Chinese reasoning recognize contradiction as natural and as something to be accepted. When presented with two apparently contradictory arguments, Westerners appear to accept just one of them, whereas Chinese accept the merits of both (Peng & Nisbett, 1999). This tolerance for contradiction among East Asians generalizes to their self-concepts. Spencer-Rodgers, Peng, Wang, and Hou (2004) found that East Asians are more likely than Westerners to have ambivalent views of themselves, agreeing with statements about themselves that would appear to be contradictory. These contradictory views also generalize to East Asians' personality traits, implicit theories, and attitudes (Hamamura, Heine, & Paulhus, 2007; Spencer-Rodgers, Boucher,

Mori, Wang, & Peng, 2007). Furthermore, when East Asians encountered new, contradictory information about themselves, they were more likely than Americans to accept it and to adjust their self-views (Spencer-Rodgers et al., 2007). In summary, inconsistent beliefs are tolerated more among East Asians than among Westerners.

This cultural difference in a motivation for consistency is not isolated to how people describe themselves and their beliefs. Indeed, social psychology's favorite theory, cognitive dissonance, also reveals pronounced cultural variation. Heine and Lehman (1997) found that whereas North Americans show pronounced dissonance reduction strategies, Japanese showed no tendency to rationalize their decisions after they made them, even when they were confronted with threatening feedback. This absence of a motivation for dissonance among East Asians in standard dissonance paradigms appears to be reliable (also see Hiniker, 1969; Hoshino-Browne et al., 2005; Kitayama, Snibbe, & Markus, 2004). However, East Asians do appear to show some interesting variants on the dissonance reduction process. Hoshino-Browne et al. (2005) found that although East Asians did not rationalize their own decisions, they would rationalize the decisions that they made for other people. Kitayama et al. (2004) found that even though Japanese individuals would not rationalize their decisions in a standard dissonance condition, they showed pronounced dissonance when placed in a subtly activated interpersonal context. It appears that motivations for consistency among East Asians emerge in rather different forms than they do for Westerners. Whereas North Americans appear to aspire for consistency within themselves, East Asians are concerned with being consistent with their behavior in the context of others (also see Cialdini, Wosinska, & Barrett, 1999, for comparable cultural differences between Americans and Poles). Hence, there is a similarity across cultures in motivations to keep something consistent; however, what people endeavor to keep consistent varies importantly across cultures.

As much research has demonstrated, then, North Americans are motivated to be consistent across situations. In general, it is often a useful starting point to assume that traits and practices become common within a culture because they are functional (although there are many clear instances of maladaptive cultural

traits and practices; see Richerson & Boyd, 2005). To the extent that the consistency of self-views serves a function, we should expect that consistency has more favorable outcomes for North Americans than for East Asians.

Suh (2002) tested this hypothesis by exploring the correlates of self-consistency among Koreans and Americans. He found that, for Americans, there were strong positive correlations between consistency and subjective well-being, peer-rated likability, and evaluations of social skills. Apparently, Americans feel better about themselves if they see themselves as consistent, and other people view consistent individuals to be especially socially skilled and likable. In contrast, the correlations with the Koreans were much smaller. Being consistent in Korea was not associated as strongly with feeling good about oneself (see Campbell et al., 1996, for similar findings with Japanese), and it was not associated as much with being perceived as especially socially skilled or likable. Koreans are likely less consistent across situations compared to Americans, because there are fewer benefits in Korea for viewing oneself consistently in this way. The benefits of self-consistency do not appear to be constant across cultures.

MOTIVATIONS FOR SELF-ENHANCEMENT AND SELF-ESTEEM

The motivation that has probably been researched the most across cultures is the motivation to *self-enhance*, that is, a desire to view oneself positively. A great deal of research from a diverse array of methodologies reveals that Westerners apparently have a strong need to view themselves in positive terms. For example, measures of self-esteem reveal that the vast majority of North Americans score in the top half of their scale (Baumeister, Tice, & Hutton, 1989). Indeed, individuals with low self-esteem, operationalized as those with scores below the theoretical midpoint of the scale, are relatively rare in North American cultural contexts (less than 7% of a large European Canadian sample; Heine & Lehman, 2004). In addition, evidence for the positivity of Westerner's self-views can be seen in the common finding that people often exaggerate the positivity of their evaluations; that is, they show self-enhancing biases. Reviews of this literature (e.g., Greenwald, 1980; D. T. Miller & Ross,

1975; Taylor & Brown, 1988) indicate that North Americans' self-perceptions tend to be systematically biased toward an overly positive view of the self. Moreover, the ever-growing body of research on self-evaluation maintenance provides further testimony to the strong motivations that Westerners have for positive self-views. This literature documents the variety of compensatory self-protective responses that are elicited when people encounter threats to their self-esteem. Such strategies include self-evaluation maintenance (e.g., Tesser, 1988), self-affirmation (e.g., Steele, 1988), compensatory self-enhancement (e.g., Baumeister & Jones, 1978), downward social comparison (e.g., Wills, 1981), motivated reasoning (e.g., Kunda, 1990), and self-handicapping (e.g., Tice, 1991). That such a wide variety of self-esteem maintenance tactics exists highlights the importance of maintaining a positive self-evaluation, at least within North American culture, where the majority of this research has been conducted.

This research reveals quite clearly that motivations for positive self-views are powerful and pervasive among Westerners. However, Westerners' tendency to endorse more independent views of self (Markus & Kitayama, 1991a), and much research identifying a pronounced positive relationship between independent self-construals and positive self-views within a variety of different cultures (correlations range between .33 and .51; e.g., Heine, 2003; Oyserman, Coon, & Kemmelmeier, 2002; Singelis, Bond, Lai, & Sharkey, 1999) raises the possibility that such positive self-views would be more elusive in cultural contexts that are less characterized by independence.

Much research has investigated motivations for positive self-views in more collectivist cultures, particularly in East Asian cultures. Overall, the evidence suggests that these motivations are far weaker among East Asians. For example, East Asians score significantly lower than Westerners on various different measures of self-esteem (e.g., Chan, 2000; Feather & McKee, 1993; Spencer-Rodgers et al., 2004), and show less evidence for a diverse array of self-enhancing biases (e.g., Heine & Lehman, 1995; Heine & Renshaw, 2002; Kurman, 2001; Markus & Kitayama, 1991b; Norasakkunkit & Kalick, 2002). Evidence for a variety of self-evaluation maintenance strategies is also weaker among East Asians (e.g., Heine, Kitayama, & Lehman, 2001; Heine, Kitayama,

Lehman, Takata, et al., 2001; White & Lehman, 2005). These cultural differences in self-enhancing motivations emerge remarkably consistently and are highly pronounced. Heine and Hamamura (2007) recently conducted a meta-analysis of self-enhancing tendencies among Westerners and East Asians, and found significant cultural differences in every study for 30 of the 31 methodologies used (the one exception being comparisons of self-esteem using the Implicit Associations Test; Greenwald & Farnham, 2000; Kitayama & Uchida, 2003). The average effect size for the cultural differences across all studies was $d = 0.84$. Furthermore, whereas the average effect size for self-enhancing motivations was large ($d = 0.86$) within the Western samples, these motivations were largely absent among the East Asian samples ($d = -0.02$) with Asian Americans falling in between ($d = 0.33$). Apparently, East Asians possess little motivation to self-enhance (Heine, Lehman, Markus, & Kitayama, 1999).

However, it is possible that East Asians really are just as motivated as Westerners to evaluate themselves positively, but that various Western biases in the research methodologies employed have prevented researchers from reliably identifying these motivations. For example, one possibility is that East Asians are more motivated to enhance their group selves rather than their individual selves, and comparisons of people's individual self-enhancing tendencies thus obscure their group self-enhancing motivations. The reasoning behind this alternative hypothesis appears compelling; however, many studies reveal that Westerners show stronger motivations than East Asians to enhance their group selves as well (e.g., Heine, 2003; Snibbe, Markus, Kitayama, & Suzuki, 2003), which challenges this account. Another possibility is that East Asians value a different set of traits than what has been explored in research thus far, and that if they were asked to evaluate themselves on traits they viewed to be especially important, the cultural differences would be reduced. Although some evidence supports this alternative account using the "better-than-average effect" paradigm (e.g., Brown & Kobayashi, 2002; Sedikides, Gaertner, & Vevea, 2005), other methodologies reveal that East Asians are more self-critical for especially important traits (e.g., Heine & Lehman, 1999; Heine, Kitayama, Lehman, Takata, et al., 2001; Kitayama, Markus, Matsumoto, & Norasakkunkit, 1997; for a complete meta-analysis on this topic, see Heine, Kitayama, & Hamamura, in press). Moreover, when a cognitive bias ("Everybody is better than their group's average effect"; Klar & Giladi, 1997) is controlled for in the "better-than-average effect" paradigm, the relation between trait importance and self-enhancement is no longer evident among East Asians (see Heine & Hamamura, 2007), suggesting that this observed relation is largely a cognitive bias as opposed to evidence of self-enhancement. A last alternative account to consider is that East Asians are just feigning modesty in these studies (and perhaps Westerners are feigning bravado; see Kurman, 2003; Suzuki & Yamagishi, 2004), and that their private self-feelings are just as positive as they are for Westerners. However, that these cultural differences are at least as pronounced in anonymous situations that employ hidden behavioral measures (e.g., Takata, 2003; Heine, Kitayama, Lehman, Takata, et al., 2001), renders this account less plausible. One piece of evidence in support of this alternative account is the lack of cultural differences found with the Implicit Associations Test measure of implicit self-esteem (e.g., Kitayama & Uchida, 2003). Although it is not yet clear what implicit self-esteem indicates, I would suggest that it likely taps into an affective feeling toward the self, and that East Asians and Westerners "like" themselves to a comparable extent. To the extent that this is the case, this suggests that self-criticism has fewer negative affective consequences in East Asian contexts than in Western ones (e.g., Heine & Lehman, 1999; Kitayama & Uchida, 2003). Overall, the research provides converging evidence that East Asians do not have as strong a desire as Westerners to view themselves positively.

One question to consider is how might this cultural difference in self-enhancement emerge? A proximal answer could be that these motivations are learned from experiences that individuals have while they are young. One source of evidence in support of this comes from a study by P. J. Miller, Wang, Sandel, and Cho (2002; P. J. Miller, Wiley, Fung, & Liang, 1997), in which parents in Taiwan and the United States were interviewed regarding their attitudes toward child rearing. The researchers found that the stories more often told by European-American parents to their children focused on a past success of the child. In stark contrast, the Taiwanese parents were more likely to tell stories about past transgressions of the child (P. J. Miller et al., 1997). When researchers explicitly asked parents what they thought about self-esteem, answers between the two groups were highly divergent (P. J. Miller et al., 2002). The European American parents viewed self-esteem as central to child rearing and saw it as a positive quality that enhanced children's development, and something that should be cultivated by parents. The Taiwanese parents, in contrast, had little to say about the words that most closely approximated self-esteem (it is perhaps telling that there is no direct translation of *self-esteem* in East Asian languages), and what they did have to say about it was often somewhat negative; for example, in expressing the belief that too much self-esteem could lead to frustration when things were not working out well for the children. Similar to this cultural difference in children's experiences with their families, North American schools are more likely than their East Asian counterparts to make efforts to inculcate self-esteem (e.g., Lewis, 1995; Stevenson & Stigler, 1992). In summary, cultural environments in North America and East Asia provide different opportunities for learning ideas regarding whether positive self-views are desirable.

However, a more distal answer to the question of the origins of cultural differences is also needed, because the data I have presented do not address how parents and schools in the different cultures arrived at their respective views. One way to consider how these cultures came to differ in their predilections for self-enhancement is to look at the emergence of motivations for positive self-views over history. Baumeister (1987) explored Western literature across the centuries and submitted that the notion of individual selves was not evident in the texts until the 12th century, when the Christian concept of the last judgment changed from being an issue of salvation of collectives to the salvation of individual souls. It was not until the 16th century and the birth of the Protestant Reformation, however, that something akin to self-enhancing motivations first became clearly evident in literature. The Calvinist doctrine of predestination burdened people with a great deal of psychic anxiety at not knowing whether they were doomed to spend the rest of eternity burning in Hell. With such an enormous, and ultimately unknowable, threat lurking in the back of their minds, people were motivated to grasp at any shred of evidence suggesting that they might be among the Elect, and motivations for self-deception and self-enhancement grew accordingly (Pye, 2000; Weintraub, 1978).

More recently, there is evidence for growing motivations for self-enhancement within the United States. Twenge and Campbell (2001) conducted a meta-analysis of studies that measured self-esteem among American college students using the Rosenberg Self-Esteem Scale (Rosenberg, 1965). Over a 30-year period, college students' self-esteem consistently rose to the point that participants in the most recent studies had self-esteem scores that were larger than those in the earlier studies by an effect size of approximately $d = 0.60$. Given the relation between independent self-views and self-esteem, discussed earlier, this might be further evidence that the United States has become more individualistic since the end of World War II (e.g., Putnam, 2000; Rosen, 1998). Historical research is relatively new to psychology, and much remains unknown about the reasons underlying changes in self-enhancement motivations over time; however, this is an important avenue to explore in understanding the origin of cultural differences.

MOTIVATIONS FOR FACE AND SELF-IMPROVEMENT

Another way to address the question of why motivations for positive self-views vary across cultures is to consider the different kinds of positive views that one might desire. One way of having a positive self-view is to have high self-esteem; that is, the individual views him or herself positively. Another way of having a positive self-view is to have a good deal of "face," which is an interesting concept that is of considerable importance in much of the world, although it receives much less attention among Westerners. Indeed, the expression "to lose face" did not enter the English language until the late 19th century as a direct translation from Chinese (*Oxford English Dictionary*, 1989). Face has been defined as the amount of social value that others grant you if you live up to the standards associated with your position (e.g., Ho, 1976). In hierarchical collectivist societies, such as the kinds found in East Asia, face takes on special importance (H. C. Chang & Holt, 1994). What is prioritized is not how positively people think of themselves, but

whether significant others think they are doing well. If others grant an individual face, he or she will enjoy all the benefits that come with the enhanced status and power. In such a cultural context, people can become highly motivated to maintain and enhance their face (Heine, 2005).

An important characteristic of face is that it is more easily lost than it is gained. Because the amount of face that people have access to is determined by their position, they cannot readily increase their face, unless they are promoted to a higher position. This renders face as something that is difficult to enhance. However, face is lost whenever an individual is perceived to fail to live up to the standards of his or her role (Ho, 1976). One is therefore always vulnerable in public situations, and because others determine one's face, one must count on the goodwill of others to be able to maintain face. Given that face is so easily lost, it seems that a good strategy would be to adopt a very cautious approach and try to ensure that one is not acting in a way that might lead to rejection by others (Heine, 2005). If one can attend to any potential weaknesses and work toward correcting them by improving oneself, this should decrease the chance that others would view one as having lost face (Heine, Kitayama, Lehman, Takata, et al., 2001).

This kind of defensive, cautious approach to not losing a resource is consistent with a prevention focus, that is, an orientation toward avoiding negative outcomes. This is in contrast to a concern with enhancing the positivity of one's self-view, which is consistent with a promotion focus, that is, a concern with achieving positive outcomes (Higgins, 1996). If a concern with face leads to a prevention orientation, and East Asians are more concerned with face, then we should expect to see greater evidence of prevention orientations among them. Much research has confirmed this pattern (e.g., Elliot, Chirkov, Kim, & Sheldon, 2001; Ip & Chiu, 2002; Lockwood, Marshall, & Sadler, 2005). For example, A. Y. Lee, Aaker, and Gardner (2000) asked Hong Kong Chinese and Americans to rate the importance of some tennis games. The Chinese saw games that were framed as opportunities to avoid a loss as more important than those framed as opportunities to win, and the Americans showed the opposite pattern.

If one has a promotion focus, one should focus efforts on things one is good at, because these will provide more opportunities for success. Things that one is not good at, in contrast, should be avoided, because they are not likely to lead to success. In contrast, if one has a prevention focus, one should focus efforts on things that one does badly, because correcting shortcomings will help one to avoid future failures. This suggests that East Asians should respond quite differently than Westerners to successes and failures. Heine, Kitayama, Lehman, Takata, et al. (2001) had Japanese and Canadian participants come into the laboratory, where they received private feedback that they had done poorly on a creativity test. Participants were left alone in a room with another set of creativity items, and how long they persisted on this task was timed. The Canadians persisted significantly longer after success than after failure, a finding that replicates much of the work on persistence research in the West (e.g., Feather, 1966; Pyszczynski & Greenberg, 1983). In stark contrast, the Japanese persisted significantly longer after failure than after success. Apparently, the Canadians were more interested in working on what they were good at, what would more likely provide them with opportunities to view themselves positively. The Japanese, in contrast, were more interested in working on the things they did badly, apparently so that they could improve themselves and be less likely to fail in the future. This *self-improvement* motivation, a desire to seek out potential weaknesses and work on correcting them, is a strong motivation in East Asian contexts (e.g., Hoshino-Browne & Spencer, 2000; Kitayama et al., 1997). Interestingly, this cultural difference has even been shown to influence people's choice of leisure activities. Oishi and Diener (2003) found that when given a choice to play either basketball or darts, European Americans tend to choose the activity they are good at, whereas Asian Americans do not. Whether one is primarily concerned with focusing on positive aspects of the self or focusing on areas of the self that need improving affects the kinds of choices people make in their lives.

AGENCY AND CONTROL

All organisms have needs and desires, and must work within the constraints and affordances of their environments to achieve them. Unlike other organisms, humans live in cultural environments, which has significant consequences for how they strive to achieve their needs and desires. People have theories about how they can exert control within particular contexts, and those theories are shaped importantly by cultural learning. People strive to achieve their needs and desires in ways that are consistent with their theories for exerting agency in specific ways.

One theory that people possess, which is relevant to their experiences of control, is whether they perceive their selves to be easily malleable and changeable or stable and fixed. Dweck, Hong, and Chiu (1993; Dweck & Leggett, 1988) term these two implicit theories *incremental* and *entity* theories of self, respectively. In addition to the implicit theories that people possess about the malleability of the self, they also have implicit theories about the malleability of the world. For example, people can see the world as something fixed and beyond their control to change (an entity theory of the world), or they can think of the world as flexible and responsive to their efforts to change (an incremental theory of the world). To the extent that people from different cultures perceive selves and their social worlds to be more or less fluid and malleable, they will possess different theories about how individuals can, should, and do act.

Su et al. (1999) offer a nice metaphor to capture the potential ways that people's selves and social worlds can be malleable: Imagine that someone is building a stone wall. There are a couple of different approaches that they could attempt. One is to emphasize the integrity of the wall at the expense of the individual stones; that is, people could have a clear plan of the shape of the wall that they want to maintain and choose stones of approximately the correct size, then carve them down so that they fit perfectly into the wall. The stones would change to accommodate the wall. An alternative way to build the wall would be to allow the wall to take on the shape of the individual stones. People could choose stones of roughly of the right size and shape and assemble them into a wall. The wall would change in shape to reflect the nature of the individual stones. The enterprise of stone wall building will vary a great deal depending on whether one views the individual stones or the resultant wall as flexible and capable of being changed.

As in this metaphor, there are occasions in which there are clear social constraints to which individuals must adjust themselves, and there are occasions in which social relationships and organizations change to adjust themselves to the nature of their individual members. Although it would seem to be the case that everyone must sometimes view their individual selves as more flexible than their social worlds, and sometimes see their social worlds as more malleable than themselves, the extent to which these beliefs are embraced can vary importantly across cultures.

Primary and Secondary Control

Rothbaum, Weisz, and Snyder (1982) proposed that there are at least two ways that people can gain control in their lives. People achieve a sense of *primary control* by striving to shape existing realities to fit their perceptions, goals, or wishes. This construct captures how most researchers studying control have operationalized it. Much less studied is *secondary control*, which people achieve when they attempt to align themselves with existing realities, leaving the realities unchanged but exerting control over their psychological impact.

Although everyone experiences primary and secondary control on occasion, cultures differ in the extent to which people engage in these two strategies. In hierarchical, collectivist cultures, such as in East Asia, the social world remains somewhat impervious to efforts by a lone individual to change things (e.g., Chiu, Dweck, Tong, & Fu, 1997). Power and agency tend to be concentrated in groups or as mandated by the role that an individual occupies; thus, there are many domains in which people are unable to exert much direct influence. Likewise, East Asians are more likely to have a flexible and incremental view of themselves (Norenzayan, Choi, & Nisbett, 2002), although the evidence for this is more consistent with experimental manipulations and measures of concrete responses than with comparisons of means on Likert score measures (Heine, Kitayama, Lehman, Takata, et al., 2001). When the self is perceived to be more mutable than the social world, it follows that people would be quite willing to adjust themselves to fit in better with the demands of their social worlds.

In contrast, people from Western cultures tend to stress the malleability of the world relative to the self (Su et al., 1999). God told Adam that he would have dominion over all the earth;

the world was there for humans to change and use to their liking. This belief persists in the West, manifest in the view that the individual has potential control in shaping the world to fit his or her own desires. When people view individuals to be the center of experience and action, they accordingly look to individuals as a source of control. Moreover, the independent self is experienced as relatively immutable and consistent (Heine, Kitayama, Lehman, Takata, et al., 2001; Suh, 2002). This view that the self is an immutable entity, working within the context of a mutable world, sustains a perception of primary control.

Weisz, Rothbaum, and Blackburn (1984) make the case that many socializing experiences in Japan lead Japanese people to be more comfortable with engaging in secondary control strategies. For example, Japanese infants spend much more time in contact with their mothers; thus, they learn to adjust themselves to what their mothers are doing. Japanese workers change jobs far less frequently than their Western counterparts, and it was not uncommon for workers to be promised lifetime employment—a system which ensures that employees learn to adjust themselves to whatever demands the company places on them. Weisz and colleagues propose that these and other socialization experiences lead people to seek strategies of control that are most likely to lead to beneficial consequences within the constraints of their respective cultural environments.

Morling, Kitayama, and Miyamoto (2002) investigated whether control strategies differed between Japanese and Americans in line with the hypotheses of Weisz and colleagues. In one study, participants were asked to list occasions when they had tried either to influence people or objects that surrounded them (i.e., primary control experiences) or to adjust themselves to these people or objects (i.e., secondary control experiences). Americans were better able to recall influencing situations than adjusting ones, whereas Japanese remembered more adjusting situations than influencing ones. In this respect, the term "secondary control" might be somewhat of a misnomer in Japan, because this type of control may be more common there than "primary control." Furthermore, although both Japanese and Americans evaluated influencing situations to have felt more powerful than adjusting ones, suggesting that primary control might universally be experienced as powerful, Japanese reported feeling more powerful about their adjusting situations than did the Americans. This cultural difference was evident in the way that participants described their adjusting experiences. For example, Americans were more likely than Japanese to report feeling that they were compelled to adjust, as though it was against their will. They often described their experiences as something that they "had to do," for example, "I had to adjust last school year when my roommate's boyfriend moved into our house." In contrast, the Japanese rarely indicated that they felt compelled to adjust, or that the adjustment experience was negative. In summary, experiences of primary control seem to be more frequent among people from Western than from Eastern cultural backgrounds, and a variety of other studies yield comparable findings (e.g., M. H. Bond & Tornatzky, 1973; W. C. Chang, Chua, & Toh, 1997; Seginer, Trommsdorff, & Essau, 1993).

Being part of a group can mean that an individual must sometimes go along with others as a means to get along well. Secondary control strategies are effective ways to manage one's successful functioning in group contexts. However, if people spend a great deal of time thinking about how they are members of groups, and thinking of others in terms of the groups to which they belong, they might also come to think of control in a different way; that is, they might start to perceive groups as agents, as entities that can make decisions and exert control. Do people in collectivistic cultures see groups as agents in similar ways that people in individualistic cultures see individuals as agents?

This question was investigated by Menon, Morris, Chiu, and Hong (1999). One way that they considered the role of group agency was to see how newspapers in different countries referred to the agents in scandals involving rogue traders. For example, the British stock trader Nick Leeson was convicted in 1995 of fraud when he was involved in a scandal that resulted in the loss of over $1 billion and the ultimate collapse of his employer, Baring's Bank. Menon and colleagues were interested in how newspapers in the United States and Japan (specifically, the *New York Times* and *Asahi Shinbun*) reported on this and various other rogue trader scandals in the news. Did the reporters describe the problem as ultimately lying within an individual, such as Nick Leeson, or did they describe the problem as being due to the management of an organization, such as Baring's Bank? The articles written about the scandals were analyzed with respect to the frequency with which they addressed the individuals involved or the organizations that employed them. The *New York Times* was more likely to explore the scandals in terms of the problems with the individual trader. In stark contrast, however, the *Asahi Shinbun* focused its reporting on the problems inherent in the organizations that could allow this scandal to occur. Apparently, Japanese are more likely to see events in the world as occurring due to the behaviors and decisions of groups, whereas Americans tend to understand events in terms of the individuals involved. Menon and colleagues further demonstrated how robust this cultural difference was by showing in another study that cultures differed in their explanations of not only human behaviors but also of animal behaviors. They found that Americans were more prone to explain a rancher's accident in terms of the behavior of a rogue cow, whereas Chinese preferred to explain the same accident in terms of the unruly behaviors of the entire herd (however, note that Ishii & Kitayama, 2005, provide evidence that dispositional inferences for group behavior are similar among Americans and East Asians). The same event can be understood quite differently depending on one's view of agency.

Making Choices

One way that people can exercise control over their worlds is by making choices. People make countless choices every day and in doing so they structure their lives to match up to their desires. Making choices is perhaps the most direct way that people engage in primary control strategies.

Choice is something that is surely valued everywhere; however, the extent to which people value choice, and exercise it, is influenced by the contexts in which people find themselves. People in individualist societies are less dependent on the actions of others than those in collectivist ones. People in collectivist societies should, on average, be more concerned with the goals of their groups, and, as such, be more willing to adjust their behaviors (and reduce their choices), so that they can coordinate the actions of the group toward those goals. One stark example of this cultural difference is that in many collectivist cultures today (and perhaps in nearly all cultures several centuries ago), critical life decisions, such as who one would marry or what job one would pursue, have been made by families rather than by the individuals themselves (e.g., G. R. Lee & Stone, 1980).

Iyengar and Lepper (1999) explored how children from different cultural backgrounds would respond to situations in which they made choices on their own or had the choices made by someone else. They recruited fifth-grade students of European and Asian ancestry from two elementary schools in the San Francisco Bay area, and randomly assigned the students to play a computerized math game in one of three conditions. In a "personal choice" condition, students were allowed to make a number of choices that were all irrelevant to their success in the game. For example, they could choose which of four icons would represent their spaceship, and which of four names they would give to their spaceship. In an "outgroup choice" condition, students saw the same four options for the spaceship icons and possible names; however, they were told that the choices had already been made for them by students from another school. Last, students in an "ingroup choice" condition were shown the same options and were told that they were assigned to a particular spaceship, because that was what most of their classmates had wanted. All the students then had the opportunity to play the game, and their persistence was assessed. The students of European background attempted the most games when they got to choose their own space ships. They played significantly fewer games when either the students from the other school or their classmates made their choices for them. In contrast, Asian American students attempted the most games when their classmates chose their space ships for them. However, like the European Americans, they were not very motivated when an outgroup member made their choices for them. Apparently, Asian Americans viewed the situation of their ingroups making choices for them as opportunities to promote harmony and a sense of belongingness with other group members. European Americans seemed to view the same situation as something that stripped them of their freedom to choose. Thus, how people feel when close others make choices for them varies a great deal across cultures.

There is also evidence of cultural variation in perceptions of control within individualist cultures. The vast majority of psychological research is conducted with a limited sample that is not only largely restricted to participants from Western cultural backgrounds but also usually further limited to college students from those same cultural backgrounds (Sears, 1986). College students are not necessarily representative of humankind. For example, they differ from the rest of the population in that they are more likely to be from upper-middle-class backgrounds and are more likely themselves to raise their own families in an upper-middle-class environment compared with non-college-educated people.

How might we expect people of upper-middle-class backgrounds to differ in their perceptions of control than those from working-class backgrounds? One obvious way is that working-class people earn less money and, because of that, have fewer choices available. Working-class people also have different kinds of relationships compared with upper-middle-class people (they tend to have fewer friends, to live closer to them, to have more frequent contact with kin, and to rely more on kin for material assistance; Allan, 1979; Markus, Ryff, Curhan, & Palmerscheim, 2004). Working-class adults participate in a different cultural world compared with upper-middle-class adults, and they are more likely to face hardships in their lives, and to have less control over these hardships than do upper-middle-class adults.

Snibbe and Markus (2005) explored differences in control experiences by comparing working-class and upper-middle-class Americans. In one study, they asked people at a shopping mall to complete a questionnaire, for which they were offered a pen as compensation. In a "free choice" condition, the experimenter let participants choose any pen they wanted. In a "usurped choice" condition, participants were allowed to choose a pen; however, after making their choice, the experimenter said, "I'm sorry. You can't have that pen. It's the last one of its kind that I have. Here, take this one." The experimenter then replaced their chosen pen with the same kind of pen that the previous participant in the "free choice" condition had chosen. At the end of the questionnaire, participants were asked to evaluate the pen that they had received. The working-class participants in the usurped choice condition were almost as satisfied as they were with the pen that they received in the free choice condition. In contrast, however, the upper-middle-class participants were significantly less satisfied when their choice had been taken away from them. Snibbe and Markus argue that upper-middle-class Americans are raised to favor choices, and to express themselves through their choices. As such, they learn to respond quite negatively whenever they perceive that they do not have any choice in a situation. In contrast, working-class Americans grow up learning that much of what they encounter in life is beyond their control, and that a good way to maintain their independence is to emphasize their integrity and resilience during tough times. This orientation leads to an outlook to accept and cope with occasions where they do not end up with what they wanted. Several other studies conducted by Snibbe and Markus further support their case. Even within an individualized culture, we can see clear differences in people's perceptions of choice and control.

MOTIVATIONS TO FIT IN OR TO STICK OUT

In many occasions when people are deciding how to behave in a group of others, they can decide to go either of two ways. First, they can strive to act in a way that fits in well with others, thereby increasing group harmony at the expense of their own individual distinctiveness. Alternatively, they can decide to act in such a way that they stick out from others, highlighting their uniqueness at the potential risk of not getting along so well with others. People are often in the position to make such a decision, and the way they reach their decisions is influenced by their cultures.

Perhaps the most dramatic explorations of how people make decisions on whether they should fit in or stick out were conducted by Solomon Asch (1956), using his famous conformity paradigm. Participants were faced with a decision of either stating what they saw, and thereby contradicting a unanimous group of confederates who had already expressed a discrepant view, or of going along with the group and ignoring what they had seen with their own eyes. In his studies, Asch found that most Americans would conform at least once in the context of this paradigm.

Asch argued that people conformed in this experimental design because of a desire to be accepted by others, reflecting the normative in-

fluence of conformity. People tend to fare better when others do not view them negatively and reject them. The social costs of dissenting would seem to be considerably greater in collectivist societies, in which people have more obligations with their ingroup members and a stronger motivation to achieve a sense of belongingness. The Asch conformity paradigm has been immensely influential, and it has been replicated well over 100 times in 17 different countries. A meta-analysis of these studies revealed one clear trend: Although Americans show a great deal of conformity in this paradigm, people from more collectivist cultures conform even more (R. Bond & Smith, 1996). Conformity was particularly pronounced among people from collectivist cultures when people were conforming with decisions made by their ingroups. Motivations to fit in are stronger in cultural contexts that encourage people to maintain strong relationships with others (although it is possible that there are weaker cultural differences for informational conformity).

In contrast to a motivation to conform, we can also consider people's motivations to stick out and to be unique. People with independent views of self see their identity as ultimately grounded in their individual qualities. Their identity is not so much shared with others and is perceived to be fundamentally unique. Maintaining a view of oneself that is consistent with cultural values of independence, then, should be aided by striving to view oneself as a unique and special individual. Thinking of oneself as unique highlights that one really is separate from others.

In contrast, people with interdependent views of self see their identity as ultimately grounded in their relationships with significant others. Identity is experienced as shared; thus, there should be less motivation to view oneself as separate and distinct from those important others. Aspiring for a view of self that emphasizes one's interdependence should be aided when individuals do not view themselves as especially different. Being different suggests that one might not be fitting in as well. As such, we should expect to find that people with interdependent views of self would be less motivated to see themselves as unique compared with those with independent views of self.

Kim and Markus (1999) investigated this hypothesis with a clever study. Participants of European and Asian descent were recruited at an airport and asked to complete a questionnaire. In return for their time, they were offered a pen. The experimenter had a bag full of red and green pens, and would reach down and pull out a handful (five) of them, and ask the participant to take a pen of his or her choice. This ensured that all participants had to make a choice between pens of two different colors, and that they also had to choose between pens that were either of a majority color (three or four pens of the same color) or of a minority color (one or two pens of the same color). The findings revealed that the European Americans were much more likely to choose the pen of the minority color. In stark contrast, East Asians were more likely to choose the pen of the majority color. Apparently, the European Americans maintain a desire to express their uniqueness by making what they think are unique choices, whereas East Asians maintain a desire to express their belongingness by making what they think are common choices. Other analyses, and other studies that Kim and Markus conducted, corroborated that this is why the people made these divergent choices (also see Kim & Drolet, 2003).

Motivations for uniqueness are therefore quite different between these two cultural groups. An important question to consider is how these particular motivations, and cultural ideas more generally, came to be so widespread within cultures, yet so different between cultures. Kim and Markus (1999) were interested in this question when studying cultural differences in motivations for uniqueness. They felt that one way to observe these different motivations being communicated would be to look at messages in advertisements. The kind of message that would be most persuasive would reflect ideas widely shared within a culture. Kim and Markus investigated the commonness of themes that expressed either uniqueness or conformity in magazine advertisements in Korea and the United States. They looked at several categories of magazines (business magazines, women's magazines, etc.) from each country and took note of each advertisement they encountered. They coded each ad with respect to whether it contained a theme for conformity (e.g., "Seven out of 10 people are using this product") or a theme for uniqueness (e.g., "Ditch the Joneses"). They found that uniqueness themes were more common in American ads than in Korean ones, and that conformity themes were more common in Korean ads than

in American ones. This suggests that the kinds of cultural messages that people encounter on a day-to-day basis are helping to reinforce the different views of self in the two cultures.

CONCLUSION

To have a rich understanding of how people are motivated it is necessary to understand the cultural contexts that afford and constrain the kinds of things that people will pursue. Although all of the motivations discussed in this chapter are likely understood and experienced by people from all cultures (i.e., they are all existential, if not functional, universals; Norenzayan & Heine, 2005), the degree that they are emphasized, and whether they are prioritized, varies considerably, as the previously discussed research demonstrates. People from different cultures vary in their motivations, because they have become attuned to the different contingencies associated with those motivations. For example, when individuals are participating in a context in which the benefits of fitting in far outweigh the costs, they will likely become especially motivated to fit in when in that context. To the extent that individuals usually find themselves in such contexts, and rarely find themselves in contexts in which greater benefits can be derived from sticking out, an orientation toward seeking ways to fit in should become routinized and prioritized for them. Furthermore, if individuals are continually surrounded by others who are also habitually attending to fitting in, because they too more often find themselves in contexts where such an orientation is facilitated, an emphasis on fitting in will likely become a norm that serves to guide how individuals value fitting in more generally. Because cultures differ precisely in the kinds of situations they provide their members, people in different cultures come to be motivated in importantly divergent ways. In these ways, culture and psyche come to make each other up (Shweder, 1990).

REFERENCES

Allan, G. A. (1979). *A sociology of friendship and kinship*. London: Allen & Unwin.

Asch, S. (1956). Studies of independence and conformity: A minority of one against a unanimous majority. *Psychological Monographs, 70*(No. 416).

Baguma, P., & Furnham, A. (1993). The Protestant work ethic in Great Britain and Uganda. *Journal of Cross-Cultural Psychology, 24,* 495–507.

Bargh, J. A., Chen, M., & Burrows, L. (1996). Automaticity of social behavior: Direct effects of trait construct and stereotype activation on action. *Journal of Personality and Social Psychology, 71,* 230–244.

Baumeister, R. F. (1987). How the self became a problem: A psychological review of historical research. *Journal of Personality and Social Psychology, 52,* 163–176.

Baumeister, R. F., & Jones, E. E. (1978). When self-presentation is constrained by the target's knowledge: Consistency and compensation. *Journal of Personality and Social Psychology, 36,* 608–618.

Baumeister, R. F., Tice, D. M., & Hutton, D. G. (1989). Self-presentational motivations and personality differences in self-esteem. *Journal of Personality, 57,* 547–579.

Bendix, R. (1977). *Max Weber: An intellectual portrait.* Berkeley: University of California Press.

Bond, M. H., & Cheung, T. (1983). College students spontaneous self-concept. *Journal of Cross-Cultural Psychology, 14,* 153–171.

Bond, M. H., & Tornatzky, L. G. (1973). Locus of control in students from Japan and the United States: Dimensions and levels of response. *Psychologia, 16,* 209–213.

Bond, R., & Smith, P. B. (1996). Culture and conformity: A meta-analysis of studies using Asch's (1952b, 1956) line judgment task. *Psychological Bulletin, 119,* 111–137.

Brown, J. D., & Kobayashi, C. (2002). Self-enhancement in Japan and America. *Asian Journal of Social Psychology, 5,* 145–168.

Bruner, J. (1990). *Acts of meaning.* Cambridge, MA: Harvard University Press.

Campbell, J. D., Trapnell, P., Heine, S. J., Katz, I. M., Lavallee, L. F., & Lehman, D. R. (1996). Self-concept clarity: Measurement, personality correlates, and cultural boundaries. *Journal of Personality and Social Psychology, 70,* 141–156.

Chan, Y. M. (2000). Self-esteem: A cross-cultural comparison of British-Chinese, White British, and Hong Kong Chinese children. *Educational Psychology, 20,* 59–74.

Chang, H.-C., & Holt, G. R. (1994). A Chinese perspective on face as inter-relational concern. In S. Ting-Toomey (Ed.), *The challenge of facework: Cross-cultural and interpersonal issues* (pp. 95–132). Albany: State University of New York Press.

Chang, W. C., Chua, W. L., & Toh, Y. (1997). The concept of psychological control in the Asian context. In K. Leung, U. Kim, S. Yamaguchi, & Y. Kashima (Eds.), *Progress in Asian social psychology* (pp. 95–117). Singapore: Wiley.

Chartrand, T. L., & Bargh, J. A. (1999). The chameleon effect: The perception–behavior link and social interaction. *Journal of Personality and Social Psychology, 76,* 893–910.

Chiu, C., Dweck, C. S., Tong, J. U., & Fu, J. H. (1997). Implicit theories and conceptions of morality. *Journal of Personality and Social Psychology, 73,* 923–940.

Cialdini, R. B., Wosinska, W., & Barrett, D. W. (1999). Compliance with a request in two cultures: The differential influence of social proof and commitment/consistency on collectivists and individualists. *Personality and Social Psychology Bulletin, 25,* 1242–1253.

Cousins, S. D. (1989). Culture and selfhood in Japan and the U.S. *Journal of Personality and Social Psychology, 56,* 124–131.

Crocker, J., & Park, L. E. (2004). The costly pursuit of self-esteem. *Psychological Bulletin, 130,* 392–414.

Dweck, C. S., Hong, Y., & Chiu, C. (1993). Implicit theories: Individual differences in the likelihood and meaning of dispositional inference. *Personality and Social Psychology Bulletin, 19,* 644–656.

Dweck, C. S., & Leggett, E. L. (1988). A social-cognitive approach to motivation and personality. *Psychological Review, 95,* 256–273.

Elliot, A. J., Chirkov, V. I., Kim, Y., & Sheldon, K. M. (2001). A cross-cultural analysis of avoidance (relative to approach) personal goals. *Psychological Science, 12,* 505–510.

Fanfani, A. (1935). *Catholicism, Protestantism and capitalism.* New York: Sheed & Ward.

Feather, N. (1966). Effects of prior success and failure on expectations of success and subsequent performance. *Journal of Personality and Social Psychology, 3,* 287–298.

Feather, N. T., & McKee, I. R. (1993). Global self-esteem and attitudes toward the high achiever for Australian and Japanese students. *Social Psychology Quarterly, 56,* 65–76.

Festinger, L. (1957). *A theory of cognitive dissonance.* Stanford, CA: Stanford University Press.

Furnham, A. (1990). *The Protestant work ethic: The psychology of work-related beliefs and behaviors.* London: Routledge.

Furnham, A., Bond, M. H., & Heaven, P. (1993). A comparison of Protestant work ethic beliefs in thirteen nations. *Journal of Social Psychology, 133,* 185–197.

Furnham, A., & Muhiudeen, C. (1984). The Protestant work ethic in Britain and Malaysia. *Journal of Social Psychology, 122,* 157–161.

Giddens, A. (1992). Introduction. In M. Weber, *The Protestant ethic and the spirit of capitalism.* London: Routledge.

Giorgi, L., & Marsh, C. (1990). The Protestant work ethic as a cultural phenomenon. *European Journal of Social Psychology, 20,* 499–517.

Greenwald, A. G. (1980). The totalitarian ego: Fabrication and revision of personal history. *American Psychologist, 35,* 603–618.

Greenwald, A. G., & Farnham, S. D. (2000). Using the Implicit Association Test to measure self-esteem and self-concept. *Journal of Personality and Social Psychology, 79,* 1022–1038.

Hamamura, T., Heine, S. J., & Paulhus, D. L. (2007). *Cultural differences in response styles: The role of dialectical thinking.* Unpublished manuscript, University of British Columbia.

Hampden-Turner, C., & Trompenaars, A. (1993). *The seven cultures of capitalism: Value systems for creating wealth in the United States, Japan, Germany, France, Britain, Sweden, and the Netherlands.* New York: Doubleday.

Heider, F. (1958). *The psychology of interpersonal relations.* New York: Wiley.

Heine, S. J. (2003). An exploration of cultural variation in self-enhancing and self-improving motivations. In V. Murphy-Berman & J. J. Berman (Eds.), *Nebraska Symposium on Motivation: Vol. 49. Cross-cultural differences in perspectives on the self* (pp. 101–128). Lincoln: University of Nebraska Press.

Heine, S. J. (2005). Constructing good selves in Japan and North America. In R. M. Sorrentino, D. Cohen, J. M. Olson, & M. P. Zanna (Eds.), *Culture and social behavior: The Tenth Ontario Symposium* (pp. 115–143). Hillsdale, NJ: Erlbaum.

Heine, S. J., & Hamamura, T. (2007). In search of East Asian self-enhancement. *Personality and Social Psychology Review, 11,* 1–24.

Heine, S. J., Kitayama, S., & Hamamura, T. (in press). The inclusion of additional studies yield different conclusions: A comment on Sedikides, Gaertner, & Vevea (2005). *Asian Journal of Social Psychology.*

Heine, S. J., Kitayama, S., & Lehman, D. R. (2001). Cultural differences in self-evaluation: Japanese readily accept negative self-relevant information. *Journal of Cross-Cultural Psychology, 32,* 434–443.

Heine, S. J., Kitayama, S., Lehman, D. R., Takata, T., Ide, E., Leung, C., et al. (2001). Divergent consequences of success and failure in Japan and North America: An investigation of self-improving motivations and malleable selves. *Journal of Personality and Social Psychology, 81,* 599–615.

Heine, S. J., & Lehman, D. R. (1995). Cultural variation in unrealistic optimism: Does the West feel more invulnerable than the East? *Journal of Personality and Social Psychology, 68,* 595–607.

Heine, S. J., & Lehman, D. R. (1997). Culture, dissonance, and self-affirmation. *Personality and Social Psychology Bulletin, 23,* 389–400.

Heine, S. J., & Lehman, D. R. (1999). Culture, self-discrepancies, and self-satisfaction. *Personality and Social Psychology Bulletin, 25,* 915–925.

Heine, S. J., & Lehman, D. R. (2004). Move the body, change the self: Acculturative effects on the self-concept. In M. Schaller & C. Crandall (Eds.), *Psychological foundations of culture* (pp. 305–331). Mahwah, NJ: Erlbaum.

Heine, S. J., Lehman, D. R., Markus, H. R., & Kitayama, S. (1999). Is there a universal need for positive self-regard? *Psychological Review, 106,* 766–794.

Heine, S. J., Lehman, D. R., Peng, K., & Greenholtz, J. (2002). What's wrong with cross-cultural comparisons of subjective Likert scales?: The reference-group problem. *Journal of Personality and Social Psychology, 82,* 903–918.

Heine, S. J., & Renshaw, K. (2002). Interjudge agreement, self-enhancement, and liking: Cross-cultural divergences. *Personality and Social Psychology Bulletin, 28,* 578–587.

Higgins, E. T. (1996). The "self-digest": Self-knowledge serving self-regulatory functions. *Journal of Personality and Social Psychology, 71,* 1062–1083.

Hiniker, P. J. (1969). Chinese reactions to forced compliance: Dissonance reduction or national character. *Journal of Social Psychology, 77,* 157–176.

Ho, D. Y. F. (1976). On the concept of face. *American Journal of Sociology, 81,* 867–884.

Hoshino-Browne, E., & Spencer, S. J. (2000, February). *Cross-cultural differences in attribution and perseverance.* Poster presented at the 1st Convention of the Society for Personality and Social Psychology, Nashville, TN.

Hoshino-Browne, E., Zanna, A. S., Spencer, S. J., Zanna, M. P., Kitayama, S., & Lackenbauer, S. (2005). On the cultural guises of cognitive dissonance: The case of Easterners and Westerners. *Journal of Personality and Social Psychology, 89,* 294–310.

Huntington, E. (1915). *Civilization and climate.* New Haven, CT: Yale University Press.

Ip, G. W., & Chiu, C. (2002, June). *Assessing prevention pride and promotion pride in Chinese and American cultures: Validity of the regulatory focus questionnaire.* Paper presented at the conference on Culture and Social Behavior: The Tenth Ontario Symposium, London, Ontario, Canada.

Ishii, K., & Kitayama, S. (2005, January 20). *Group agency bias in Japan and the US.* Paper presented at the Cultural Psychology Preconference, New Orleans, LA.

Isonio, S. A., & Garza, R. T. (1987). Protestant work ethic endorsement among Anglo Americans, Chicanos, and Mexicans: A comparison of factor structures. *Hispanic Journal of Behavioral Sciences, 9,* 413–425.

Iyengar, S. S., & Lepper, M. R. (1999). Rethinking the value of choice: A cultural perspective on intrinsic motivation. *Journal of Personality and Social Psychology, 76,* 349–366.

Jackson, E. F., Fox, W. S., & Crockett, H. J. (1970). Religion and occupational achievement. *American Sociological Review, 35,* 48–63.

Kanagawa, C., Cross, S. E., & Markus, H. R. (2001). "Who am I?": The cultural psychology of the conceptual self. *Personality and Social Psychology Bulletin, 27,* 90–103.

Kenrick, D. T., Li, N. P., & Butner, J. (2003). Dynamical evolutionary psychology: Individual decision-rules and emergent social norms. *Psychological Review, 1,* 3–28.

Kim, H. S., & Drolet, A. (2003). Choice and self-expression: A cultural analysis of variety seeking.

Journal of Personality and Social Psychology, 85, 373–382.

Kim, H. S., & Markus, H. R. (1999). Deviance or uniqueness, harmony or conformity?: A cultural analysis. *Journal of Personality and Social Psychology, 77,* 785–800.

Kitayama, S., Markus, H. R., Matsumoto, H., & Norasakkunkit, V. (1997). Individual and collective processes in the construction of the self: Self-enhancement in the United States and self-criticism in Japan. *Journal of Personality and Social Psychology, 72,* 1245–1267.

Kitayama, S., Snibbe, A. C., & Markus, H. R. (2004). Is there any "free" choice?: Self and dissonance in two cultures. *Psychological Science, 15,* 527–533.

Kitayama, S., & Uchida, Y. (2003). Explicit self-criticism and implicit self-regard: Evaluating self and friend in two cultures. *Journal of Experimental Social Psychology, 39,* 476–482.

Klar, Y., & Giladi, E. E. (1997). "No one in my group can be below the group's average": A robust positivity bias in favor of anonymous peers. *Journal of Personality and Social Psychology, 73,* 885–901.

Kunda, Z. (1990). The case for motivated reasoning. *Psychological Bulletin, 108,* 480–498.

Kurman, J. (2001). Self-enhancement: Is it restricted to individualistic cultures? *Personality and Social Psychology Bulletin, 12,* 1705–1716.

Kurman, J. (2003). Why is self-enhancement low in certain collectivist cultures?: An investigation of two competing explanations. *Journal of Cross-Cultural Psychology, 34,* 496–510.

Landes, D. S. (1999). *The wealth and poverty of nations.* New York: Norton.

Lee, A. Y., Aaker, J. L., & Gardner, W. L. (2000). The pleasures and pains of distinct self-construals: The role of interdependence in regulatory focus. *Journal of Personality and Social Psychology, 78,* 1122–1134.

Lee, G. R., & Stone, L. H. (1980). Mate-selection systems and criteria: Variation according to family structure. *Journal of Marriage and the Family, 42,* 319–326.

Lewis, C. C. (1995). *Educating hearts and minds.* New York: Cambridge University Press.

Lockwood, P., Marshall, T. C., & Sadler, P. (2005). Promoting success or preventing failure: Cultural differences in motivation by positive and negative role models. *Personality and Social Psychology Bulletin, 31,* 379–392.

Markus, H. R., & Kitayama, S. (1991a). Culture and the self: Implications for cognition, emotion, and motivation. *Psychological Review, 98,* 224–253.

Markus, H. R., & Kitayama, S. (1991b). Cultural variation in the self-concept. In G. R. Goethals & J. Strauss (Eds.), *Multidisciplinary perspectives on the self* (pp. 18–48). New York: Springer-Verlag.

Markus, H. R., Ryff, C. D., Curhan, K. B., & Palmerscheim, K. A. (2004). In their own words: Well-being at midlife among high school and college-educated adults. In C.D. Ryff & R.C. Kessler (Eds.), *A portrait of midlife in the U.S.* (pp. 273–319). Chicago: University of Chicago Press.

McClelland, D. (1961). *The achieving society.* Princeton, NJ: Van Nostrand.

Menon, T., Morris, M. W., Chiu, C., & Hong, Y. (1999). Culture and the construal of agency: Attribution to individual versus group dispositions. *Journal of Personality and Social Psychology, 76,* 701–717.

Miller, D. T., & Ross, M. (1975). Self-serving biases in the attribution of causality: Fact or fiction? *Psychological Bulletin, 82,* 213–225.

Miller, P. J., Wang, S., Sandel, T., & Cho, G. E. (2002). Self-esteem as folk theory: A comparison of European American and Taiwanese mothers' beliefs. *Parenting: Science and Practice, 2,* 209–239.

Miller, P. J., Wiley, A. R., Fung, H., & Liang, C. (1997). Personal storytelling as a medium of socialization in Chinese and American families. *Child Development, 68,* 557–568.

Mischel, W. (1973). Toward a cognitive social learning reconceptualization of personality. *Psychological Review, 80,* 252–253.

Morling, B., Kitayama, S., & Miyamoto, Y. (2002). Cultural practices emphasize influence in the United States and adjustment in Japan. *Personality and Social Psychology Bulletin, 28,* 311–323.

Niles, F. S. (1994). The work ethic in Australia and Sri Lanka. *Journal of Social Psychology, 134,* 55–59.

Norasakkunkit, V., & Kalick, M. S. (2002). Culture, ethnicity, and emotional distress measures: The role of self-construal and self-enhancement. *Journal of Cross-Cultural Psychology, 33,* 56–70.

Norenzayan, A., Choi, I., & Nisbett, R. E. (2002). Cultural similarities and differences in social inference: Evidence from behavioral predictions and lay theories of behavior. *Personality and Social Psychology Bulletin, 28,* 109–120.

Norenzayan, A., & Heine, S. J. (2005). Psychological universals: What are they and how can we know? *Psychological Bulletin, 131,* 763–784.

Oishi, S., & Diener, E. (2003). Culture and well-being: The cycle of action, evaluation, and decision. *Personality and Social Psychology Bulletin, 29,* 939–949.

Oxford English Dictionary (2nd ed.). (1989). New York: Oxford University Press.

Oyserman, D., Coon, H. M., & Kemmelmeier, M. (2002). Rethinking individualism and collectivism: Evaluation of theoretical assumptions and meta-analyses. *Psychological Bulletin, 128,* 3–72.

Peng, K., & Nisbett, R. E. (1999). Culture, dialectics, and reasoning about contradiction. *American Psychologist, 54,* 741–754.

Peng, K., Nisbett, R. E., & Wong, N. Y. C. (1997). Validity problems comparing values across cultures and possible solutions. *Psychological Methods, 2,* 329–344.

Putnam, R. D. (2000). *Bowling alone: The collapse and revival of American community.* New York: Simon & Schuster.

Pye, L. W. (2000). "Asian values": From dynamos to dominoes? In L. E. Harrison & S. P. Huntington (Eds.), *Culture matters* (pp. 244–255). New York: Basic Books.

Pyszczynski, T., & Greenberg, J. (1983). Determinants of reduction in intended effort as a strategy for coping with anticipated failure. *Journal of Research in Personality, 17,* 412–422.

Quinn, D. M., & Crocker, J. (1999). When ideology hurts: Effects of belief in the Protestant ethic and feeling overweight on the psychological well-being of women. *Journal of Personality and Social Psychology, 77,* 402–414.

Richerson, P. J., & Boyd, R. (2005). *Not by genes alone.* Chicago: University of Chicago Press.

Rosen, B. C. (1998). *Winners and losers of the information revolution: Psychosocial change and its discontents.* Westport, CT: Praeger.

Rosenberg, M. (1965). *Society and the adolescent self-image.* Princeton, NJ: Princeton University Press.

Rothbaum, F., Weisz, J. R., & Snyder, S. S. (1982). Changing the world and changing the self: A two-process model of perceived control. *Journal of Personality and Social Psychology, 42,* 5–37.

Sanchez-Burks, J. (2002). Protestant relational ideology and (in)attention to relational work settings. *Journal of Personality and Social Psychology, 83,* 919–929.

Sanchez-Burks, J., Lee, F., Choi, I., Nisbett, R., Zhao, S., & Koo, J. (2003). Conversing across cultures: East–West communication styles in work and nonwork contexts. *Journal of Personality and Social Psychology, 85,* 363–372.

Sanchez-Burks, J., Nisbett, R. E., & Ybarra, O. (2000). Cultural styles, relational schemas and prejudice against outgroups. *Journal of Personality and Social Psychology, 79,* 174–189.

Sears, D. (1986). College sophomores in the laboratory: Influences of a narrow data base on social psychology's view of human nature. *Journal of Personality and Social Psychology, 51,* 515–530.

Sedikides, C., Gaertner, L., & Vevea, J. (2005). Pancultural self-enhancement reloaded: A meta-analytic reply to Heine (2005). *Journal of Personality and Social Psychology, 89,* 539–551.

Seginer, R., Trommsdorff, G., & Essau, C. (1993). Adolescent control beliefs: Cross-cultural variations of primary and secondary orientations. *International Journal of Behavioral Development, 16,* 243–260.

Shweder, R. A. (1990). Cultural psychology: What is it? In J. W. Stigler, R. A. Shweder, & G. Herdt (Eds.), *Cultural psychology: Essays on comparative human development* (pp. 1–43). Cambridge, UK: Cambridge University Press.

Singelis, T. M., Bond, M. H., Lai, S. Y., & Sharkey, W. F. (1999). Unpackaging culture's influence on self-esteem and embarrassability: The role of self-construals. *Journal of Cross-Cultural Psychology, 30,* 315–331.

Snibbe, A. C., & Markus, H. R. (2005). You can't always get what you want: Social class, agency, and choice. *Journal of Personality and Social Psychology, 88,* 703–720.

Snibbe, A. C., Markus, H. R., Kitayama, S., & Suzuki, T. (2003). "They saw a game": Self and group enhancement in Japan and the U.S. *Journal of Cross-Cultural Psychology, 34,* 581–595.

Spencer-Rodgers, J., Boucher, H. C., Mori, S. C., Wang, L., & Peng, K. (2005). *Culture and self-perception: Naive dialecticism and East Asian conceptual selves.* Unpublished manuscript, Berkeley, University of California.

Spencer-Rodgers, J., Peng, K., Wang, L., & Hou, Y. (2004). Dialectical self-esteem and East–West differences in psychological well-being. *Personality and Social Psychology Bulletin, 30,* 1416–1432.

Steele, C. M. (1988). The psychology of self-affirmation: Sustaining the integrity of the self. In L. Berkowitz (Ed.), *Advances in experimental social psychology* (Vol. 21, pp. 261–302). San Diego: Academic Press.

Stevenson, H. W., & Stigler, J. W. (1992). *The learning gap: Why our schools are failing and what we can learn from Japanese and Chinese education.* New York: Summit Books.

Su, S. K., Chiu, C.-Y., Hong, Y.-Y., Leung, K., Peng, K., & Morris, M. W. (1999). Self organization and social organization: American and Chinese constructions. In T. R. Tyler, R. Kramer, & O. John (Eds.), *The psychology of the social self* (pp. 193–222). Mahwah, NJ: Erlbaum.

Suh, E. M. (2002). Culture, identity consistency, and subjective well-being. *Journal of Personality and Social Psychology, 83,* 1378–1391.

Suzuki, N., & Yamagishi, T. (2004). An experimental study of self-effacement and self-enhancement among the Japanese. *Japanese Journal of Social Psychology, 20,* 17–25.

Takata, T. (2003). Self-enhancement and self-criticism in Japanese culture: An experimental analysis. *Journal of Cross-Cultural Psychology, 34,* 542–551.

Taylor, S. E., & Brown, J. D. (1988). Illusion and well-being: A social psychological perspective on mental health. *Psychological Bulletin, 103,* 193–210.

Tesser, A. (1988). Toward a self-evaluation maintenance model of social behavior. In L. Berkowitz (Ed.), *Advances in experimental social psychology* (Vol. 21, pp. 181–227). San Diego: Academic Press.

Tice, D. M. (1991). Esteem protection or enhancement?: Self-handicapping motives and attributions differ by trait self-esteem. *Journal of Personality and Social Psychology, 60,* 711–725.

Tomasello, M. (1999). *The cultural origins of human cognition.* Cambridge, MA: Harvard University Press.

Twenge, J. M., & Campbell, W. K. (2001). Age and birth cohort differences in self-esteem: A cross-temporal meta-analysis. *Personality and Social Psychology Review, 5,* 321–344.

Weber, M. (1992). *The Protestant ethic and the spirit of capitalism*. London: Routledge. (Original work published 1904)

Weber, M. (1947). *The theory of social and economic organization* (T. Parsons, Trans.). New York: Free Press.

Weber, M. (1951). *The religion of China: Confucianism and Taoism* (H. H. Gerth, Transl. & ed.). Glencoe, IL: Free Press.

Weber, M. (1952). *Ancient Judaism* (Transl. & ed., H. H. Gerth & D. Martindale). Glencoe, IL: Free Press.

Weintraub, K. J. (1978). *The value of the individual: Self and circumstance in autobiography*. Chicago: University of Chicago Press.

Weisz, J. R., Rothbaum, F. M., & Blackburn, T. C. (1984). Standing out and standing in: The psychology of control in America and Japan. *American Psychologist, 39*, 955–969.

White, K., & Lehman, D. R. (2005). Culture and social comparison seeking: The role of self-motives. *Personality and Social Psychology Bulletin, 31*, 232–242.

Wills, T. A. (1981). Downward comparison principles in social psychology. *Psychological Bulletin, 90*, 245–271.

CHAPTER 30

The Cultural Psychology of Emotion

BATJA MESQUITA
JANXIN LEU

Since Darwin's time, many scholars have seen emotions as a functional adaptation to social living (Ekman, 1992; Oatley & Jenkins, 1992; Tooby & Cosmides, 1990, 1992). Emotions signal the occurrence of pressing social problems or opportunities and provide heuristics for successful behavior (Oatley & Jenkins, 1996). One of the prime reasons that emotions have likely evolved is to monitor and negotiate our social relations.

These social relations vary across cultural contexts. Human beings do not live in uniform worlds. Therefore, their emotions are not, or not most of the time, responses to universal emotional events. Human emotional behavior is not aimed at achieving general, universal goals. Rather, human beings always live in specific environments. As the anthropologist C. Geertz puts it:

> People who are independent of time, place, and circumstance do not now and have not ever existed, and by the very nature of things could not exist. . . . Becoming human is becoming individual, and one becomes individual under the guidance of cultural patterns and historically created systems of meaning in terms of which we give form, order, point, and direction to our lives. (1973, p. 49)

In other words, human beings always function in a specific cultural space, and emotions help navigating this cultural space.

Both the particular relationship arrangements and the meanings that animate and justify these arrangements vary across cultures. Successfully navigating the cultural space means specifically engaging in relationships with other people. Therefore, emotions have to signal culturally relevant relational opportunities and problems, and motivate a culturally appropriate and effective course of action. For example, an emotion signals a *particular* threat that derives its meaning from the cultural relational arrangements and their meanings—the threat of losing honor, for example—rather than merely danger in general. Similarly, the action motivated by this threat is the type of escape or preventive behavior that, given the particular cultural practices of relating, makes sense and has a good chance for success—avoiding contact with men, for example, when you are a Bedouin woman (Abu-Lughod, 1986). The behavior is not escape in general. In summary, the functionality of emotions within a sociocultural context requires that they be coordinated with the specific cultural meanings and practices.

We conceptualize emotions as multifaceted, open phenomena that are shaped to be effective in the sociocultural context in which they occur. The primary facets of emotion are emotional experience, which, among others, is constituted by the appraisal of the situation and action readiness, expressive behavior, autonomic and central nervous system changes, and behavior. Our conceptualization of emotions is markedly different from the commonly held view that emotions are invariant states that, when triggered, manifest themselves in preprogrammed ways. By considering the fit of emotions into their cultural environment, we take a socioculturally functional view.[1] This chapter reviews the evidence for systematic cross-cultural differences in emotional experience as they are mutually constitutive with the cultural meanings and practices in which they occur.

CULTURAL MODELS

The central thesis of this chapter is that emotions within a sociocultural context must accommodate the specific meanings and practices (Bruner, 2003), particularly those of self and relationships. We describe these meanings and practices as *cultural models* (for similar constructs Bruner, 1986, 1990; D'Andrade, 1984; D'Andrade & Strauss, 1992; Holland, Lachicotte, Skinner, & Cain, 1998; Holland & Quinn, 1987; Markus, Mullally, & Kitayama, 1997; Shweder & Haidt, 2000).

Cultural models are not so much verbal propositions as ways that reality, including the psychological reality, is defined. These models reflect and foster the types of personhood and relationships that are sanctioned and condoned. They are manifest in everyday social interaction, the language, the public messages as conveyed by the media, books and educational policies (Markus et al., 1997) and, as we argue in this chapter, in emotions. In each of these reality-constituting practices, certain ways of being and certain types of relating to others are afforded, expected, or shaped. A cultural model is decisive for what a person's world is like (Bruner, 1986), because it constitutes the means by which people make sense of and coordinate their feelings and actions alone and in concert with one another. Although cultural models are typically invisible to those that engage or

enact them, they can be made more explicit in comparing different cultural models.

Throughout the chapter we describe specific cultural models as they become manifest in emotional experience. Most research compares emotion in North American and Japanese contexts. North American independent models highlight the boundaries of each individual, whereas interdependent Japanese models assume the mutual interdependence of people in relationships (Markus & Kitayama, 2003; Triandis, 1995). Consistently, emotions in independent, American contexts seem to highlight the individual as bounded, autonomous, and self-sufficient, and often entail influencing relationships in ways that reinforce the individual's autonomy. On the other hand, emotions in interdependent, Japanese contexts highlight and express the relatedness between people, and further action that leads to a strengthening of interpersonal bonds (Kitayama, Mesquita, & Karasawa, 2006; Markus & Kitayama, 1994; Mesquita et al., 2005).

The comparison of independent North American and interdependent Japanese contexts has revealed that the patterns of emotional experience and behavior are subject to substantial variance. Thus, this comparison has demonstrated the plasticity of emotions, and has made a substantial contribution. It would be wrong to assume, on the basis of this research, that there are two ways of having emotions, an independent and an interdependent way. The scant evidence on emotions in non–East Asian interdependent cultures suggests that emotions in different interdependent cultures can be experienced in very different ways, and the same might be true for independent contexts other than mainstream North America. For example, research conducted among Mexicans, both those living inside and outside of the United States, suggests that emotions in Mexican interdependent contexts differ dramatically from those in Japanese interdependent contexts (discussed later in the chapter). Therefore, understanding the cultural shaping of emotion requires moving beyond the dimensions of independence (individualism) and interdependence (collectivism) to the more detailed cultural models of self and relating. A detailed analysis of the functional role of emotions in specific social contexts is necessary.

Importantly, we postulate that cultural models of self and relating afford and constraint emotional experience and behavior (Miller, 1997). In contrast to what some authors have suggested (Matsumoto & Yoo, 2006), this is not the same as claiming that emotion representations are caused by culture or, in this case, by cultural models of self and relating. We do not conceive of culture as the independent variable and emotion as the dependent variable. Culture is not an entity, and it cannot, in that sense, be responsible for another entity, emotion. Rather, we see patterns of emotion as phenomena that constitute culture (Adams & Markus, 2004). The prevalent patterns of emotion differ across sociocultural contexts that may be demarcated by not only national boundaries but also age, religion, class, or gender. This way of viewing culture as *constituted by the prevalent emotion patterns* does not imply a strict homogeneity between the people within a cultural context.

EMOTION AND EMOTIONAL EXPERIENCE

Emotions are central to social life (Frijda & Mesquita, 1994; Keltner & Haidt, 1999). Among other functions, they reflect the meaning a given social context has to an individual, and they are heuristics for action, predisposing an individual toward action that promotes certain end goals. Thus, emotions can be seen as links between the person and his or her environment. We postulated earlier that emotions must reflect the cultural models in which they occur, because the personal and social meaning of social episodes and the desired personal and social end states are implicated in the cultural models of self and relating.

Cultural shaping of emotions does not necessarily imply that everything about the emotion is culturally learned. It is possible and likely that the potential for particular aspects of emotion, such as certain configurations of the face, or certain physiological responses, is hardwired. The extent to which this is the case has yet to be empirically established in full. However, the existence of hardwired responses in no way negates the cultural constitution of emotions. The combinations, rates of occurrence, and meanings of hardwired responses, and "what it is like to have an emotion," should be expected to vary widely, in ways that are consistent with the cultural model.

We would expect that cultural models shape responses at every level of the emotion: the appraisal of the event, action readiness, bodily changes, expressive and instrumental behavior, and conscious regulatory processes. Our view is different, therefore, from the one proposed by Levenson Soto, and Pole (Chapter 32, this volume). We would predict that cultural differences emerge in each of the components, provided—and this is an important and often overlooked clause—that emotions are studied in contexts that are *relevant* to the cultural models, that is, in contexts that are personally and relationally relevant. Thus, we would predict cultural differences not only in experience (appraisal of the situation, action readiness) but also in expressive behavior, autonomic and central nervous system changes, and instrumental or relational behavior. Toward the end of this chapter, we argue that, so far, comparative cultural research on these latter aspects of emotion has largely failed to appreciate the ways in which cultural models materialize in emotions due to a lack of consideration of the relevant cultural contexts. Thus, the research paradigms used to study cross-cultural variation in behavior and nervous system activity were not designed to find cultural differences. Because culture-sensitive research can primarily be found in the domain of *emotional experience*, this is the prime topic of this chapter.

Constituents of Emotional Experience

First, consistent with many current theories of emotions, we treat emotional experience as having content that can be meaningfully analyzed (Barrett, 2006; Barrett, Mesquita, Ochsner, & Gross, 2007; Ellsworth & Scherer, 2003; Frijda, 1986, 2006; Frijda, Kuipers, & Terschure, 1989; Scherer, 1984). In this chapter, the focus is on those aspects of emotional experience that most directly implicate the relationship of an individual with his or her context: appraisals of the situation and action readiness. We thus assume that the meaning represented by these facets of emotion constitutes the core of emotional experience (for similar views see Barrett, 2006; Clore & Ortony, 2000; Frijda, 2006). Importantly, the meaning of the situation and the projected action and goal fulfillment (i.e., action readiness) are considered central parts of the emotional experience itself. This is in contrast to many other theories of emotion that consider them peripheral to the actual emotion (e.g., Levenson et al., Chapter 32, this volume).

Focal, Normative, or Ideal Representations of Emotions

Emotional life in a culture is more than the added emotional responses that may be observed or reported. People in many cultures show unique regularities in the frequencies of certain responses that are better understood when one considers the focal, normative, and ideal representations of emotions in those cultures. The unique shapes of people's emotional lives in different cultures are, among other factors, motivated by the central themes of cultural models (Mesquita & Ellsworth, 2001; Mesquita & Frijda, 1992), ideal affect (Tsai, Knutson, & Fung, 2006), and what anthropologists have referred to as emotional style (Middleton, 1989) or *ethos* (Schieffelin, 1985, pp. 172–173):

> Ethos refers to the dominant emotional emphases, attitudes, and modes of expression of a culture as a whole. . . . The concept of ethos has generally been used as a descriptive ethnographic characterization. However, to the extent that individuals regularly exhibit attitudes and moods characterized by the ethos, that ethos can be considered expressively normative. That is, it is culturally expected that a person feel a certain way and adopt a certain affective posture and expressive style in relation to particular events. . . . A culture's ethos is thus not only a characterization of a style of feeling and behavior but also a model for it.

Our second mission in this chapter is to describe how focal, normative, and ideal emotional representations are parts of the cultural models.

OVERVIEW OF THE REST OF THE CHAPTER

Our approach builds on the notion that emotional experience is always saturated with meaning, and that meaning is cultural (Bruner, 1986). Though emotions may and often do involve hardwired processes, the meanings at the core of emotions are particularized to culture.

In the sections that follow, we first aim to render the cultural shaping of emotion constituents transparent, indicating how emotional constituents themselves fit and contribute to the cultural models. We then focus on systematic cultural differences in the focal, normative, and ideal representations of emotions, and what seem to be resultant regularities in emotional patterns.

CULTURAL DIFFERENCES IN THE CONSTITUENTS OF EMOTIONAL EXPERIENCE

When people in different cultures say they feel "angry," they may refer to quite different experiences. In this section, we start from the assumption that emotional experience can be described as an aggregate of the constituent meanings (Barrett et al., 2007; Frijda, 2006). We furthermore assume that the culturally most prevalent emotional experiences systematically reflect the cultural models of self and relating, and can thus be studied in a theory driven and meaningful way (Mesquita, 2003; Mesquita & Markus, 2004). In the following sections we discuss cultural differences in appraisal and in action readiness changes.

Appraisal

Appraisals are "psychological representations of emotional significance" (Clore & Ortony, 2000, p. 32). Cultural models transpire in appraisals. Thus, independent appraisals consist of the perceived impact of the situation for individual goals, whereas interdependent appraisals likely specify the impact of the situation on relational goals. Naturally, cultural models vary on more than just the dimension of individual versus relational meaning. More intricate descriptions of cultural models tend to provide better contexts for understanding the cultural specificity of appraisals.

What Is the Emotional Situation?

The appraisal of an emotional situation is rooted in what the relevant stimulus is judged to be. Some have called this the appraisal dimension of "interest": What is the situation that might be relevant for me (Ellsworth, personal communication, 2004; Frijda, 1986)? There is some evidence that the parsing of reality is characterized by the pertinent cultural model.

An experience sampling study by Oishi, Diener, Scollon, and Biswas-Diener (2004) found that whereas the social context affected emotional experience in interdependent cultures, it did not do so in independent cultural contexts. Thus, according to this study, emotions were experienced no differently in situations with or without others in independent contexts, but emotional experiences in interdependent contexts were different depending on the presence of certain others. The way reality was parsed appeared to be different.

In this study, American college students in the Midwest (mostly European Americans), Hispanic students living in California, Japanese college students in Japan, and Indian college students in India completed a mood questionnaire five times a day. The mood questionnaires consisted of a positive and a negative affect scale. Each time students filled out the mood questionnaire, they also indicated the nature of the situation in terms of six options: whether they were alone, with a friend, with a classmate/coworker, with a romantic partner, with a stranger, or with family. Though cross-situational consistency of both positive and negative affect was prevalent across all four cultures, affect was more dependent on the type of situation in interdependent (Hispanic, Japanese) than in independent (non-Hispanic American) cultures.[2] More specifically, in the Hispanic and Japanese groups, the mean level of positive affect experienced in a family context was not significantly correlated with positive affect in a number of other social situations. In contrast, positive affect among European Americans was consistent across all six emotional situations. For negative affect, Hispanics were the only group to report different mean levels of affect in family contexts than for the other social situations; negative affect in the other three cultural groups was consistent across situations. Oishi et al. (2004) concluded that, particularly in the case of positive affect, the precise nature of the social context was more consequential for the feelings of the interdependent cultural groups in this study than for the independent group.

Oishi and colleagues (2004) also calculated differences in the degree of *overall* within-person variability in affective experiences across situations by computing a standard deviation of mean positive and negative affect across six situations for each individual. In general, the standard deviation was larger for positive than for negative affect, meaning that the influence of the type of situation was larger for positive than for negative emotion. Furthermore, there were clear cultural differences in the direction one would expect. For positive emotions, the mean within-individual cross-situational variation was higher among Japanese and Hispanic respondents than among Americans, whereas for negative emotions, all

three interdependent cultural groups had a higher mean within-individual cross-situational variation than Americans. Therefore, within individuals the level of positive and negative emotion was more affected by the specific social situations in interdependent than in independent culture, consistent with the relational orientation prevalent in interdependent cultures. It should be noted that these differences in *within*-person cross-situational variation were found against the backdrop of robust universal *between*-person effects. The similarity in between-person effects meant that across cultures, a person's mean affect was predictive of his or her affect in different situations.

A study on emotional perception supports the idea that the parsing of reality varies according to the different cultural models. In this study, respondents reported on someone else's emotional experience rather than their own. Japanese and European American individuals were presented with cartoon stimuli depicting a central person who expressed anger, sadness, or happiness, surrounded by four other people whose facial expressions varied independently from that of the central person (Masuda, Ellsworth, Mesquita, Leu, & Veerdonk, 2005). Respondents were asked to rate the central person's emotional experience. The results strongly suggest that the situation of interest is constructed as the relationship among the Japanese, but not among European Americans. Consistent with an independent model, Americans judged the central person's emotional experience by his expression alone, disregarding the emotions of the surrounding people. Consistent with an interdependent model, however, the Japanese participants considered the emotions of all the people in the picture.

Therefore, when assessing the central person's emotional experience, Japanese participants were affected by the emotional expressions of others in the situation, not just by the expression of the central person. For example, anger ratings of an angry person were up if other people in the situation were angry as well, compared to a situation in which the other people were not angry. In the Japanese group, the emotions of the people in the background influenced what emotion was perceived in the central person. Japanese respondents recognized more happiness in an angry central person, when he was surrounded by happy people. Therefore, the meaning of the situation in a Japanese interdependent context is to be found in what is going on with *everybody* in the social interaction.

In a subsequent experiment, Masuda and his colleagues (2005) measured eye movement during the same emotion judgment task, and found that whereas Americans attended mostly to the central person, Japanese started to divide their attention between the central person and the surrounding people after the first second. Thus, the reality perceived or attended to seemed to differ very early on in the task. Independent models are associated with perception of a bounded individual, whereas interdependent models guide and afford a relational perception.

Similar results were obtained by Tsang and Wu (2005), who had Taiwanese students rate the happiness of schematic representations of either smiley or sad faces. The central face was surrounded by four other faces that were also either smiley or sad, and varied independently of the expression of the central face. Consistent with interdependent Taiwanese models, the central face was rated higher on happiness when surrounded by happy than by sad faces. Tsang and Wu used two different shapes for the surrounding faces. These faces were either round like the central face, or egg-shaped to differ slightly from the central face. The effect of the emotion of the surrounding faces on the judgment of the central face was moderated by the degree of similarity between the central and the surrounding faces. Surrounding faces that were similar to the central face had a significantly larger effect on happiness ratings than surrounding faces that were different. On the basis of these results one might infer that in interdependent contexts, other people become part of the emotion stimulus to the extent that they are seen as related to the individual or belonging to the same group.

Cultural models thus afford certain perceptions of emotional stimuli. Whereas interdependent emotional experience is focused on the group, independent emotional experience is associated with attention to the individual. These different perceptions of reality are the basis of different types of emotional experience. Future research should explore the divergent implications of these types of emotional experience in terms of their cognitive and behavioral consequences. Cognitive and behavioral implications would also provide stronger validation of the position taken here.

What Is the Perspective on the Situation?

Cultural models appear to be reflected in the emotional experience in yet another way, namely, by the perspective taken on emotional events. Whereas people in independent contexts view emotional situations mainly from their own perspective (called an inside-out perspective; Hamaguchi, 1985), people in interdependent contexts assess the emotional meaning from the perspective of other people, either particular other people or a generalized other (cf. Mead, 1934). The latter perspective has been called outside-in (Hamaguchi, 1985).

Several studies suggest that the perspective of others is experienced as part of the situational appraisal in interdependent contexts, but much less so in independent contexts. For example, Mesquita (2001) compared emotions in independent and interdependent cultural contexts in the Netherlands. Respondents reported three types of emotional events from their past: positive, offensive, and immoral situations. Surinamese and Turkish minorities in the Netherlands, the interdependent cultural groups, reported more awareness of how the situation would be perceived by others than did respondents from the Dutch independent majority group. The Turkish and Surinamese groups regarded the emotional meanings of the situation as more "obvious" than did the Dutch; they assumed that others would interpret, feel, and act in a similar manner in the target situation. The meaning of emotional situations in interdependent contexts was perceived to be a feature of the world that could only be perceived similarly by others, whereas the meaning in the independent context was construed inside-out. To the extent that people perceived the appraisal of an event or a person to be shared by others, it was more likely to turn into a long-term belief (Mesquita, 1993). For example, in the Surinamese and Turkish groups, more often than in the Dutch group, an offense by a friend led to the lasting belief that the friend was unworthy of one's friendship. Others' perspectives were experienced as convergent with one's own, and provided the appraisal with some force and justification.

Similarly, in a study comparing American and Japanese respondents, both university students and a community sample, the interdependent Japanese respondents reported more appraisals that reflected an awareness of the meaning of the situation to others than did the American respondents (Mesquita et al., 2005). However, in contrast to the interdependent groups in the Netherlands, Japanese respondents represented the perspective of others as different from their own. Respondents in this study reported their emotional experience and behavior in three types of situations from their past—offense, humiliation, or being valued. Respondents' emotion narratives were recorded and later coded. In the negative situations in particular, Japanese respondents considered the meaning of the events for other people as it differed from their own. For example, more than 40% of the Japanese, versus none of the Americans, explained the situation from the perspective of a third person or a generalized other, an appraisal that can be seen to reflect an outside-in perspective. The Japanese consideration of the divergent perspective of others may be responsible for the fact that the most frequently reported response to offense was doing nothing, as opposed to the assertiveness and aggression reported by European Americans. The awareness of the perspective of another person may make one less likely to act against the offender.

Evidence for an outside-in perspective in interdependent cultures and an inside-out perspective in independent cultures also emerges from a study among Canadians of Western and Eastern descent on the attribution of emotional experience to others (Cohen & Gunz, 2002). Respondents recalled an emotional event from the past that had induced a given emotion. Emotions were selected to form relational pairs, such that when one person has one emotion, a relating person may be expected to have the complementary emotion (e.g., sympathy–sadness). After one emotion was primed, respondents rated a set of ambiguous emotional faces. Because it is important in interdependent contexts to see one's own emotions from the perspective of another person, Easterners were expected to recognize more of the complementary emotion in the faces presented. Westerners, lacking the perspective of a complementary emotion, were expected to rely on their own experience when reading other people's ambiguous faces. The results confirmed these predictions. For example, when sympathy was primed, Easterners perceived higher levels of the complementary emotion of sadness. On the other hand, Westerners perceived the faces as more similar to the emotions they had just de-

scribed. When primed with sympathy, Westerners perceived more sympathy in the faces. Canadian respondents of Eastern descent (interdependent cultural model) showed an implicit awareness of others' perspective on the respondents' emotions, whereas Westerners lacked such perspective.

Relational Appraisal

The social and relational implications of emotional events are more readily emphasized in interdependent than in independent cultural contexts. First, the status of relationships with others tends to be more central in interdependent than in independent appraisal. Kitayama and his colleagues demonstrated that emotional appraisals of the situation as one of interpersonal engagement were more prevalent in Japanese than in North American student populations (Kitayama, Markus, & Kurokawa, 2000; Kitayama et al., 2006). In a pilot study, Kitayama and Markus added indigenous Japanese words "that presuppose the presence of others" (cited in Markus & Kitayama, 1991, p. 238) to the standard list of English emotion words, and gave the compiled list of emotions to Japanese students, who provided similarity ratings of all possible pairs of emotions. In addition to the pleasantness and arousal dimensions commonly found in similarity rating studies using standard Western emotion words, the Japanese ratings yielded a dimension of interpersonal engagement, ranging from socially disengaged emotions such as pride and anger at one pole, to socially engaged emotions such as shame and feelings of connection with someone (*fureai*) at the other pole.

In subsequent experience sampling studies, both positive and negative engaged emotions were more frequent than disengaged emotions in Japanese contexts, whereas the reverse was true in independent European American contexts (Kitayama et al., 2006). In these studies, Japanese and European American students rated both engaged and disengaged emotions in a daily experience sampling study, and in response to 22 very diverse emotional events. The largest differences appeared for the disengaged emotions. Whereas Japanese and European American students similarly appraised situations with regard to their implications for relational engagement, European American students reported significantly higher levels of disengaged emotions for both the positive and the negative situations. These differences in disengaged emotions thus resulted in a relatively stronger role for engaged appraisals in the Japanese context.

Convergent evidence comes from another experience sampling study with European American and two groups of Japanese college students, one in the United States, and the other living in Japan (Mesquita & Karasawa, 2002). In this study, respondents reported their most recent emotion every 3 hours throughout the week and rated the eliciting situation with respect to pleasantness, as well as a number of appraisal dimensions that represented independent appraisals (such as self-esteem and control) and interdependent appraisals (such as closeness and face loss), and indicated how pleasant or unpleasant the situation was. Pleasantness in the two Japanese groups was better predicted by the interdependent than by the independent appraisals. In the European American group, pleasantness was predicted no less by independent than by interdependent appraisals.

That pleasantness was predicted no better by independent than by interdependent appraisals should perhaps not be surprising. In European American contexts "good feelings are associated with participating in some form of mutually approving relationship" (Kitayama & Markus, 2000, p. 135). Thus, relational appraisals may be highest when the relationship contributes to feelings of self-efficacy and self-esteem. Consistently, independent and interdependent appraisals in the experience sampling study just described were highly correlated.

On the other hand, independent appraisals in the Japanese groups were uncorrelated with interdependent appraisals. In the Japanese groups, feeling good about the independent aspects of self is unrelated to having a positive bond with others, and the latter, rather than the former, predicts whether one is feeling good (Kitayama & Markus, 2000).

Respect and status were salient social dimensions for the Surinamese and Turkish respondents in the Dutch study reported earlier (Mesquita, 2001). Positive events were described in the interdependent contexts as raising one's status and respectability, and that of one's family or ingroup, whereas negative events were described as threatening or detrimental to status and respectability; this was hardly the case for the Dutch independent context. Thus, the interdependent focus on the implications of an emotional event for one's social worth was suggested by this study as well, despite the fact that it included very different cultural groups.

An emphasis on the social consequences of emotional events can also be found in cultures where many events derive meaning from their relevance to honor. Honor in this sense is based on a person's strength and power over others. Honor situates people socially and determines their right to precedence (Abu-Lughod, 1986; Cohen, 1996; Cohen & Nisbett, 1994, 1997; Cohen, Nisbett, Bowdle, & Schwarz, 1996; Peristiany, 1966). Thus, emotional appraisals in honor-based cultures tend to be fully grounded in a consideration of the social position and social relationships of the individual. Social position is sometimes negotiable (Cohen et al., 1996), but it can also be perceived a result of the natural order of things, such as the lower status (and thus higher vulnerability) of women compared to men (Abu-Lughod, 1986).

More evidence for the different concerns that are central in emotional experience comes from a priming study (Chentsova-Dutton & Tsai, 2005). Asian American and European American college students were randomly assigned to either the individual self-focus condition, in which they wrote "about themselves and the conditions in their own life," or the relational self-focus condition, in which they wrote "about family members and events in their life." After the writing task, respondents watched either a sad film clip or an amusing one. European American respondents watching the amusing clip reported higher-intensity positive emotions and smiled more after the individual focus than respondents in the relational self-focus condition. Conversely, Asian American respondents reported and showed more positive feelings after the relational focus condition than after the individual self-focus condition. One interpretation of this finding is that emotional experience is commonly associated with independent concerns in independent contexts, and with interdependent, relational concerns in interdependent cultural contexts. Once the relevant concerns are activated, the emotions become more intense. A caveat to strong interpretations of this finding is the lack of significant interaction between culture and focus of condition after respondents watched sad film clips.

Control Appraisal

Evidence for the unique shaping of appraisals in independent contexts comes from the research on agency and personal control (Ellsworth & Scherer, 2003; Frijda et al., 1989; Weiner, 1982, 1986). Whereas the tendency to explain outcomes appears to be universal, the tendency to attribute important outcomes to one's own individual agency seems to more specific to independent contexts. This type of agency is a key aspect of independent cultural models, American ones in particular, where success through independent, personal accomplishment is central (Markus & Kitayama, 1991).

Participants in a number of questionnaire studies were asked to remember an instance of a given emotion, describe the situation, then rate the situation on a number of appraisal scales provided by the researchers (Mesquita & Ellsworth, 2001). These appraisal studies yielded impressive evidence for cross-cultural similarities in appraisal, but agency was one of the dimensions on which appraisal profiles tended to vary across cultures. Whereas individual agency was an important dimension of appraisal in the original studies with Western samples (Frijda et al., 1989; Scherer, 1984; Smith & Ellsworth, 1985), it was much less so for non-Western samples (Matsumoto, Kudoh, Scherer, & Wallbott, 1988; Mauro, Sato, & Tucker, 1992; Scherer, 1997). For example, Matsumoto and colleagues (1988), comparing Japanese and American students, found that agency—an important descriptive dimension of emotion for American students—was often considered "not applicable" by Japanese respondents.

Furthermore, agency appears to be an important predictor of pleasantness or well-being in independent but not in interdependent contexts. In American contexts, emotions of agency, such as pride, were found to predict general feelings of well-being. In contrast, emotions of relatedness rather than emotions of agency predicted well-being in Japanese contexts (Kitayama et al., 2000, 2006; Mesquita & Karasawa, 2002). These results may be related to the cross-cultural finding outside the emotion literature, demonstrating that European American children were most motivated in a task they had selected for themselves, whereas Asian American children preferred tasks chosen by their mother or their friends

(Iyengar & Lepper, 1999). The positive connotation of individual agency may thus be specific to independent cultural models.

The differences in salient appraisals reflect different cultural models. Salient independent appraisals consist of individual agency and control; conversely, interdependent appraisals are about a number of different relational meanings of the situation.

Action Readiness and Behavior

Emotions tend to involve behavior, or at least the intention of behavior, aimed at changing the relationship between the self and others. We distinguish conceptually between behavioral goals (action readiness) and behavioral means (the actual behavior), despite the fuzzy empirical distinction. Behavioral goals—or inclinations to behavior—have been termed as *action readiness* (Frijda, 1986), which is related to appraisal in that it constitutes the tendency or preparedness to deal with the emotional issues as construed; actual behavior is the executed effort to do the same. Action readiness and behavior, importantly, are afforded and shaped by the meaning of the event as constructed, and in this way reflect the cultural model.

Action readiness and behavior themselves represent the normative and descriptive relationships between an individual and his or her social context. Both the actual and the most desirable behavioral means to reach the normative relationships between an individual and others constitute the cultural models.

Action Readiness

The few cross-cultural studies that explicitly address cultural differences in action readiness suggest that, in addition to some universal themes in action readiness, there are many cultural differences. A study by Frijda, Markam, Sato, and Wiers (1995) compared the action readiness modes reported by Dutch, Indonesian, and Japanese participants after recalling a given emotional experience. All respondents rated these self-reported instances of emotions on the same action readiness items. Use of stimulus emotion words was the most frequent in recall studies with Dutch and Indonesian respondents. The Japanese words were translations of those concepts.

For each culture, factor analyses on the action readiness items suggested that five (of the six to nine) factors in each of the three cultural groups were similar: *moving away, moving toward, moving against, want help,* and *submission.* These factors can be interpreted as general themes of behavior and explain a substantial part of the differentiation between emotion words. Right away, it should be noted that not *all* factors were universal, and that some of the culture-specific factors were easily understood from the specific cultural models. Consistent with the independent motive of control, for example, *in command* was a unique factor of behavior in the Dutch group. And consistent with the concern for avoidance of disruption, one factor in the Japanese group consisted of disengagement (*apathy, disinterest*), an accepted way to give expression to negative feelings in this culture (Karasawa, personal communication, July 2004).

Moreover, the relative importance of the five shared themes of action readiness differed across cultures. Cultural models of the three groups offer plausible explanations for these variations across cultures. The dimensions of *moving away* and *moving against* were more important in discriminating between emotion words in Dutch than in either of the other languages. Thus, *moving away* and *moving against* were defining elements of Dutch emotional experience. The Dutch cultural model of seeking independence, if necessary through opposition (as a way of expressing oneself; Stephenson, 1989; Van der Horst, 1996), may explain the significance of the action readiness modes of *moving away* and *moving against* in the Dutch emotional experience. On the other hand, the dimensions of *moving toward* and *submission* allowed more differentiation between different emotional experiences in Indonesian and Japanese than in the Dutch contexts. These dimensions fit with the goals of relational harmony in the cultural models of these Asian groups (Markus et al., 1997); moving toward others may reduce social distance, and submitting may make one acceptable to another person.

Different behavioral goals can sometimes be inferred, if cultural differences in the rate of behavior are meaningful within different cultural models. For example, several studies have yielded cultural differences in the rate of general bodily or somatic activity, which can be conceived as a way to occupy space in the relationship. In questionnaire research, Japanese respondents reported many fewer hand and arm gestures and whole-body activity than did Americans in situations of anger, sadness, fear, and happiness (Scherer, Matsumoto, Wallbott, & Kudoh, 1988). The difference can be understood as fitting an emphasis on the relationship among the Japanese, and on the individual among American respondents. Especially interesting is that the cultures did not differ in the reported control of these emotions. The lower frequency of active somatic behaviors among the Japanese is more likely the result of a lower level of initially generated activity than of post hoc regulation.

These self-report data converge with actual measurements of general somatic behavior, or the amount of movement in any direction. Tsai and Levenson (1997) found that Chinese American couples who discussed a conflict area in their relationship displayed less general somatic activity than did European American couples. General somatic activity was one of the few physical response measures on which the two cultural groups differed.

There is some indication that the expression of high-activation happiness, another emotion accompanied by expansive behavior, is more common in independent cultures. Tsai, Chentsova-Dutton, Friere-Bebeau, and Przymus (2002) asked European Americans and Hmong Americans to relive high-intensity emotional episodes of a number of emotions, including happiness. The main difference in recorded facial behavior and physiological reactivity was that European Americans had many more social smiles during their recall of intense happy events than did Hmong Americans. This was the case despite the fact that the reported emotional feeling and physiological activity did not differ between cultural groups. Furthermore, highly acculturated Hmong Americans showed significantly more social smiles than less acculturated Hmong Americans, suggesting that adoption of American culture is associated with a higher frequency of social smiles during happiness. European Americans (and, by extension, highly acculturated Hmong Americans) may use their social smiles to convey to others that they experience the socially desirable emotion of happiness, which portrays the individual as independent and successful.

On the other hand, high-activation happiness expressions seem to be rarer in cultures that place an emphasis on harmony in relationships (Lutz, 1987). Expressions of elated happiness are seen as potentially disruptive, because they may painfully contrast with the emotional state of others or may be seen to indicate the plausibility of an individual challenging social obligations and evading responsibilities (Lutz, 1987; Karasawa, personal communication, July 2004). Happiness may have had that same connotation for the Hmong Americans in the study by Tsai and colleagues (2002).

Emotional Behavior Consistent with Situational Meaning

Differences in behavioral intent can sometimes be understood from the differences in appraisal or the meaning of the eliciting event. For example, the behavioral goals of shame differ according to different constructions of the shame stimulus (Mesquita & Karasawa, 2004). Whereas shame in independent Western contexts tends to be linked to withdrawal or the desire to disappear from view (Frijda et al., 1989), shame in interdependent East Asian contexts is associated with attempts to restore relationships. In the latter contexts, it is often accompanied by declarations of shame, public apologies, and public weeping to parents or the nation, and by both public and private declarations of intention to change one's unworthy actions and identity (Mascolo, Fischer, & Li, 2003).

The differences in the behavioral concomitants of shame can be understood from the meanings associated with shame. Shame in independent Western contexts has been associated with an appraisal that the event is incongruent with one's identity goals, and that it is caused by discrepancy with one's own stable characteristics (Tracy & Robins, 2004). Thus, shame occurs when an event conflicts with who one wants to be, as is the case when a student fails an exam, attributing it to lack of ability. On the other hand, shame in interdependent East Asian cultures appears to be the assessment that what happens is incongruent with *relationship goals*—one's obligations to others, to one's parents, to the nation, and so forth—and that it brings dishonor on the people or groups to which one belongs. Of course, even in a Western context the failure to meet one's identity goals derives its significance from the potential for social rejection (Baldwin & Baccus, 2004), which ultimately is a relational concern. Yet the relationship that elicits this type of shame is between relatively autono-

mous individuals, each responsible for his or her own success. It is very different from the focus of the relationship itself that appears to be at the center of shame in East Asian contexts. Consistently, whereas shame in Western cultures focuses on internal flaws, shame in East Asian cultures seems to be centered primarily on negative social outcomes, regardless of whether the individual was responsible for those outcomes (Crystal, Parrott, Okazaki, & Watanabe, 2001).

Shame in East Asian cultures is thus an attempt to repair the relational harm done rather than the expression of ultimate failure it is in the West. The answers to East Asian shame are self-improvement and the public sharing of shame, both ways to reassert oneself as a member of the social group to which one belongs. These behavioral goals are completely different from the common, Western action readiness of shame, wanting to disappear from others' view, which is in turn an appropriate response to ultimate, unchangeable failure and the high potential for rejection.

Similar differences in shame reactions were indeed found in a questionnaire study on shame among salespersons in the Netherlands and the Philippines (Bagozzi, Verbeke, & Gavino, 2003). Salespeople in both cultures rated how they would respond in situations in which statements or actions by customers caused them to feel shame. Salespeople in a Dutch independent context were expected to interpret the shaming by a customer as a sign that their independent self-goals were negatively evaluated, and that they were thus denigrated and ridiculed. Philippine salespeople, on the other hand, were predicted to be concerned about their social identity and the relationship with the customer. Consistent with their projected construal of the situation as harmful to the personal self, Dutch salespeople reported that their shame would lead them to protect themselves from further denigration (i.e., withdraw). On the other hand, Philippine shame was not associated with protective action.

These culturally different responses associated with shame in turn predicted differential performance outcomes, again, as reported. For the Dutch salespeople, protective action—highly related to shame—was *negatively* associated with sales volume, communication effectiveness, and relationship building. Thus, within the Dutch sales business, shame is a counterproductive emotion. On the other hand, shame in the Philippine sales business was positively associated with "adaptive resources," comprising relationship building, civic virtue, and courtesy, apparently in an attempt to fix the relationship with the customer. For Philippine salespeople, shame appears to be a productive emotion.[3]

Another study illustrating the way behavioral goals rest on the cultural understanding of emotional situations compared the behaviors of Northern and Southern men in the United States in an experimental setting in which they were offended (Cohen, Vandello, Puente, & Rantilla, 1999). Offense in Southern cultural settings challenges one's honor, especially when it is intentional, but in Northern cultural settings, it does not (Cohen et al., 1996). For this reason, Southerners avoid any perception of offense by following an elaborate system of politeness rules. This leaves Southerners inexperienced with subtle hostility when it occurs. In contrast, Northern discourse prepares Northerners well for these small hostilities and rudeness. Consistently, Southerners took longer than Northerners to respond angrily (as measured by ratings of facial expressions and the risk of physical or verbal confrontation) to an annoying confederate in an experiment who interfered with task completion. On the other hand, once the annoying behavior had angered the Southerners, they expressed more intense anger and were judged more ready to engage in physical or verbal confrontation. One interpretation of these findings is that once the offense is taken seriously, Southerners *must* reciprocate to defend their honor and even the score.

In the experiment just discussed, the confederate offered his apologies at the end of his annoyances. Apologies were more readily accepted by Northerners who had remained calm, and by Southerners who had become angry than by angry Northerners and calm Southerners. Thus, for Northerners it was easier to forgive when they had not worked themselves up first, but for Southerners it was easier to forgive when the score was even. Finally, 6 months after the experiment was over, Southerners who had remained calm and Northerners who had become angry were much better at recognizing the confederate's picture than were Southerners who had been angry and Northerners who had remained calm. The emotional experience was apparently more memorable for Southerners who had not evened the score

and for Northerners who had violated their cultural script of remaining calm. Both the behaviors observed and the consequences of these behaviors could be understood and predicted from the meaning of the eliciting situation.

Emotional Behavior Tailored to the Cultural Context

There is also some evidence for cultural differences in the specific behaviors people use to realize similar behavioral goals. The questionnaire study of action readiness among Dutch, Indonesian, and Japanese groups is a case in point. For example, the behavioral goal of submission was instantiated by *comply*, *depend*, and *apathy* modes in the Dutch group. In the Indonesian group, it was instantiated by those same three action readiness modes, plus modes that reflected a lack of control over one's actions (*inhibited*, *helpless*, *blocked*, and, negatively, *in command*). In Japan, submission comprised action readiness modes of dependence (*depend* and *comply*), lack of control (*blocked*, *helpless*), and social engagement (*make up for it*, *tenderness*). The specific action readiness modes serving the overarching behavioral goal—submission, in this case—appear to be cross-culturally different in ways consistent with cultural models. In the independent Dutch context, submission is restricted to those contexts in which one is dependent, or without the energy to resist. In interdependent cultures, not taking control may be a sufficient condition for others to take the lead. Therefore, to feel blocked or helpless may automatically mean to submit. Furthermore, consistent with the Japanese model of relationship (e.g., Lebra, 1994), social engagement in Japan may in fact mean being able and willing to yield to other people.

More evidence that behavioral goals fit the meaning of emotional situations comes from the narrative study with North Americans and Japanese, reported earlier (Mesquita et al., 2005). Cultural differences in behavioral goals fit with the models of self and relating. The most prevalent response categories reported by European American respondents were to be *assertive* or *aggressive*, both behaviors that underline the boundaries between different people. On the other hand, the most frequent action readiness or behavior reported in the Japanese group, *doing nothing*, serves to maintain the relationship, or at least not disturb it in any obvious way. These results are unlikely to be produced by differences in the American and Japanese concrete offense situations, because similar results for appraisal and action readiness differences were obtained in a controlled study that used vignettes (Mesquita et al., 2005, Study 2).

Similarly, in comparative work with Dutch, Surinamese, and Turkish respondents in the Netherlands, Mesquita (1993) found that aggressive goals tend to be sought after in ways that make sense within the unique cultural models. For example, Surinamese and Turkish respondents reported a higher tendency to show indifference in situations in which they had been harmed by another person. The high value attached to relatedness in those cultures compared to that among the Dutch turns "indifference"—the denial of engagement—into an effective act of aggression.

Ethnographic work suggests that culture-specific behaviors sometimes are chosen to serve emotional goals in a way that is not disruptive of the cultural models (Mesquita & Frijda, 1992). For example, according to the ethnographers, the Balinese reaction to frightening events is to fall asleep (Bateson & Mead, 1942). This behavior can be understood as a culture-specific instantiation of a more general goal of fear: avoidance. Falling asleep satisfies—at least subjectively—the goal of reducing one's exposure to the threat, while avoiding the emotional disruption that other fear responses are felt to cause. Therefore, falling asleep can be considered a culturally effective way to accomplish the goal of avoidance (or *moving away*).

Withdrawal may have different meanings depending on the specific cultural and situational context. *Satru* in Javanese contexts refers to an institutionalized pattern of avoidance, in which individuals in conflict refuse to speak or interact with one another (H. Geertz, 1961). Given the Javanese ideal of social harmony (*rukun*) that requires the concealment of all dissonant aspects, *satru* "is an excellent mechanism for the adjustment of hostility in a society that plays down violence and the expression of real feelings, since it allows for the avoidance of an outbreak of rage while still permitting significant expression of it" (pp. 117–118). In this case, therefore, withdrawal serves feelings of hostility in a context that does not allow for straightforward hostility.

In summary, the meaning, and, therefore, the appropriateness and effectiveness of certain behaviors in specific contexts differ according to cultural models. Note that a relational or interdependent orientation does not always lead to reaching out and being sociable. Shame in East Asian cultures has been described as leading more often to approach than has shame in Western contexts. However, the Balinese and Javanese examples suggest that the direction of emotional behavior in situations of potential conflict tends to be just the opposite, namely, withdrawal. Conversely, shame in Western contexts tends to be associated with withdrawal, whereas hostility is paired to antagonistic behavior. Thus, the type of emotional behavior in independent and interdependent contexts, rather than being consistently in one direction, follows from the meaning of the behavior, given a certain cultural context.

Evaluating the Importance of Cultural Differences in Meaning

How important are the differences in emotions? Are they superficial variations on a universal theme, or are they essential to emotional experience? We contend that *if* one wants to understand or predict what people in different cultures feel and do during emotional episodes, the culture-specific meanings of emotions are indispensable. It might often be possible to make the cultural differences in emotion dissipate by describing the phenomena at a sufficiently high level of abstraction (Mesquita, Frijda, & Scherer, 1997), but doing so takes away from the understanding of the psychological phenomena (Mesquita & Frijda, 1992; Mesquita et al., 1997). It is possible, for example, to describe the prevalence of relational appraisals in interdependent cultures as an alternative route to positive self-feelings? People in interdependent cultures might determine whether they feel good about themselves by keeping tabs on their social value, in the same way that people in independent cultural contexts monitor their personal value or self-esteem. Conversely, one could argue that self-esteem is the Western manifestation of the universal need to belong (Leary & Baumeister, 2000) and, given this, people across cultures appraise their chances of being accepted or rejected by others. How precisely one's social value is computed—whether by self-esteem, honor, or level of fitting in—may be different across cultures. However, the appraisal of social value can be deemed universal.

We do not deny that it is possible in many

cases to read these universal themes into the observed cultural differences, and to do so may be useful, depending on the research question of interest. However, an accurate representation of the actual emotional experience in different cultures requires understanding of the culturally embedded meanings of emotion-eliciting events (Mesquita et al., 1997). Cultural models constitute the content of feelings, and render emotional acts comprehensible and predictable.

For example, it is important to understand that insults are conceived of as honor violations in the South of the United States. This interpretation explains why, in response to insults, Southerners show more anger and aggressive responses than do Northerners, who do not have an honor culture. This interpretation also explains why Southerners are likely to bear less resentment than Northerners after they have expressed their anger (the score is evened; strength is being exhibited; Cohen et al., 1999). To understand the emotional experience and emotional responses, it is thus important to consider the cultural models that lend meaning to the antecedent event.

Similarly, it is important to know that Westerners are more likely to attribute personal agency to emotional events, because agency appraisals have important correlates in the course and experience of emotions. For example, blaming someone else for an offense—the prevalent American anger appraisal—rather than assuming that these things happen or that another person probably had a good reason—the common Japanese appraisal—has very different implications both for emotional experience and behavior (Mesquita et al., 2005). Blaming the other person tends to result in assertion and aggression. Sympathizing with the offender, on the other hand, leads to decreased emotionality and, in many cases, to doing nothing at all.

The question here is not whether it is *possible* to describe behavior without reference to culturally rich meanings, but whether such description is relevant given the question of interest. We contend that in most cases highly abstract descriptions of people's behavior would capture neither the precise intentions of the behavior nor their subjective experience. If one is to predict or understand what people will do, or want to do, in actual emotional contexts, one has to take into account the meaning that these behaviors have in these contexts, beyond just moving in a certain direction. It is impor-

tant to know whether moving away is an expression of hostility, as is the case for Javanese (H. Geertz, 1961), or an escape from the exposure to others, as is the case in Western shame (Bagozzi et al., 2003; Frijda et al., 1989). The resulting social and behavioral consequences, as well as the experience of this behavior, are likely to be very different depending on its meanings.

NORMATIVE OR IDEAL REPRESENTATIONS OF EMOTION

Emotional life in a culture is more than the sum of single emotional responses, such as those described in the previous section. Different patterns of emotion can be described in terms of the frequency of individual emotional responses, but they become easier to understand when considering the focal, normative, and ideal representations of emotions in those cultures. This discussion turns to an examination of prevalent or prescribed emotion norms and goals, because they affect the evaluation of certain emotional states as "good" or "bad," and also determine what people seek out or avoid.

Focal Emotions and Emotion Regulation

Cultures have emotions they "admire and despise" (Mesquita & Ellsworth, 2001). These so-called focal emotions are central in social discourse. Admired emotions tend to be those reinforcing the cultural model, whereas despised emotions violate the model (Mesquita, 2003). Focal emotions, whether positive or negative, are importantly motivating. In ways that we illustrate shortly, admired emotions are sought out and occur frequently, and despised emotions are avoided and occur rarely (cf. Eid & Diener, 2001; Fessler, 2004; Mesquita & Frijda, 1992).

An example of an admired, therefore focal, emotion is happiness in American contexts. Excited happiness seems to be sought out and cherished in many different ways (D'Andrade, 1984). First, many occasions are created that bring about happiness, such as compliments, celebrations, and awards (Kitayama, Karasawa, Heine, Lehman, & Markus, 1999, cited in Heine, Lehman, Markus, & Kitayama, 1999; Miller, Fung, & Mintz, 1996). Second, Americans tend to seek out those occasions that make them feel unique and, therefore, happy (Elliott, Chirkov, Kim, & Sheldon, 2001; Kim, 2001). Third, when encountering positive events, Americans appear to feel better and appraise the event as contributing more to self-esteem than do people from some other cultural contexts, such as the Japanese (Kitayama, Markus, Matsumoto, & Norasakkunkit, 1997; Leu et al., 2007). Fourth, there is some evidence that Americans express their happiness more, or at least signal to others that they are happy (Tsai et al., 2002; Wierzbicka, 1994). Thus, excited happiness, the ultimate emotional goal in the American independent cultural model, motivates and regulates (1) social production of events, (2) individual selection of events, (3) emotional appraisals typical of happiness, and (4) the expression of emotion.

An example of a despised, and thus focal, emotion is anger in many cultures that value harmony and equilibrium of mind, such as the Utku Inuits in Canada (Briggs, 1970). Anger, a very central topic of discourse among the Utku, is always discussed in association with the dangers attached to it. In-group anger is avoided at all cost. Like approach, avoidance of a focal emotion is accomplished at different levels of the generative process of the emotion (Mesquita & Albert, 2007). First, events that would elicit anger are avoided. For example, the aim of normative behavior is to avoid frustrating others or blocking their goals. Second, anger is mostly avoided and discouraged by others, who disapprove of it, show fear, or incite shame. It is unlikely for this reason too that anger would be sought out. Third, Utku Inuits seem to be reluctant to blame another person for a negative event, because blame is an appraisal that is conditional to anger. Blame does not fit the Utku worldview of resignation and acceptance (Solomon, 1978). Finally, Utku Inuits regulate anger expressions, as is clear from the display rules they convey to children. Thus, the focality of anger, the ultimate threat to social harmony which is so central in the Utku cultural model, can be inferred from (1) the suppression of social events that would elicit anger, (2) the relative absence of blame appraisals, and (3) the near-absence of anger expressions.

Ideal Affect

Even when emotions are not focal in this strong sense, the average person's ideal emotions may differ from one culture to the next. Tsai and colleagues (2006) distinguished between actual and ideal affect, and found cultural differences in ideal affect. Whereas actual affect was measured as the feelings one *typically* feels, ideal affect was measured as the feelings one would *ideally* like to feel (Tsai et al., 2006). Not surprisingly, European Americans, Chinese Americans, and Chinese in Hong Kong in the Tsai et al. study indicated that, ideally, they would like to have more positive and less negative emotions than they actually experienced. For our current purpose, only the findings on ideal affect are discussed.

However, cultural differences were found in the type of ideal affect, such that European Americans and Chinese Americans valued high-activation positive emotions more than did the Chinese. Conversely, Chinese and Chinese Americans valued low-activation positive emotions more than did European Americans. Tsai et al. (2006) propose a link between ideal affect and the preferred type of environmental control. Westerners prefer *influence*, and Easterners prefer adjustment. According to the authors,

> to successfully influence or change the physical or social environment, a person must be able to *mobilize* resources. Because high activation states facilitate mobilization of resources, people with influence goals should value *high activation positive states*; in contrast, low activation states promote attention to environmental stimuli, people with *adjustment* goals should value low activation states. (p. 290; emphasis added)

Emotion Norms

Positive emotions are not necessarily evaluated as positive, nor are negative emotions necessarily negative. Eid and Diener (2001) compared the emotion norms in four countries: two with independent (United States, Australia) and two with interdependent (China, Taiwan) cultural models. They expected that people in cultures with an independent model would tend to focus on positive information about the self; thus, they would value self-conscious emotions such as pride, signaling that personal goals have been accomplished, but would negatively evaluate emotions such as guilt, signaling negative self-information.

Interdependent models, on the other hand, were expected to further a focus on negative information about the self, because this information is important to prevent one from violating social norms; thus, these people were expected to value guilt positively. In these interdependent contexts, pride would make an individual stand out, thus being seen as inappropriate and undesirable. Interdependent models were predicted to lend positive meaning to this negative emotion, and negative meaning to the positive, self-conscious emotion.

In fact, in this study (Eid & Diener, 2001), pride was largely desirable and guilt largely undesirable, in countries with independent models.[4] Furthermore, the majority of people living in independent cultural contexts valued all positive emotions (joy, affection, pride, contentment) positively and all negative emotions (anger, fear, sadness, guilt) negatively. The emotion norms in the interdependent contexts were both different and more numerous. For example, two patterns of positive emotion norms were found about equally often in China. By both Chinese patterns of norms, pride and contentment were assessed as somewhat negative. Taiwanese tended to evaluate joy, affection, and contentment as positive, but pride as neutral or negative. Thus, as expected by the authors, people in interdependent contexts tended to consider some positive emotions as undesirable or inappropriate.

The opposite was found for the negative emotion norms as well. The emotion norms among Australians and Americans, as well as among some Taiwanese, assessed all negative emotions (anger, fear, sadness, and guilt) as undesirable or inappropriate.[5] A good percentage of Chinese, and a somewhat smaller part of Taiwanese, however, evaluated guilt as a positive or neutral emotion; guilt was definitely deemed more undesirable in independent contexts.

Overall, the norm patterns for negative emotions were less clear, and all cultures had more heterogeneous norms for negative emotions than for positive. As Eid and Diener (2001) acknowledge, a better picture of the emotion norms in a culture may be obtained when examining specific situational norms.

Emotion Norms and Ideals Shape Emotional Experience

Ideal and normative affect are more than statements of preference. Tsai and her colleagues (2006) powerfully demonstrated that culturally ideal emotions are important predictors of depression (as measured by the Center for Epidemiologic Studies—Depression Scale [CES-D]). Depression in the European American group was accounted for by the discrepancy between actual and ideal high-activation positive emotion (HAP), and only marginally by low-activation positive emotion (LAP). In the Chinese group, on the other hand, depression was accounted for by the discrepancy between actual and ideal LAP, and not by HAP. This is consistent with the Chinese focus on adjustment.

Interestingly, the only group for which the discrepancies between actual and ideal affect for both HAP and LAP predicted depression was the Chinese American group, which also reported high levels of both HAP and LAP as ideal emotions. Therefore, the ideal emotions in a culture are not only statements about emotions, but, importantly, they also constitute the emotional experience.

That emotion norms shape emotional experience was also suggested in the study by Eid and Diener (2001), discussed earlier. For each of the four countries (China, Taiwan, United States, and Australia), low- to medium-sized correlations were found between positive emotion norms and emotional experience for both the frequency and the intensity of emotional experience. Thus, the cultural norms and ideals for positive emotion shape the patterns of emotional experience. The correlations between negative emotion norms and emotional experience were less strong.

Regulation Goals

Cultural models appear to influence the goals of emotional regulation. Whereas American independent models appear to promote happiness and deemphasize unhappiness, the importance of experiencing both good and bad feelings, and moderating both, is stressed in East Asian contexts (Lu, 2001; Minami, 1971; Ng, Ho, & Smith, 2003). Striving for emotional balance is normative in the latter contexts (Heine et al., 1999), because it signals maturity and role fulfillment.

The evidence for cultural differences in regulatory goals is only indirect. Cultural differences in regulation are inferred from the following findings: (1) Over time, Americans report more positive than negative emotions, and East Asians report a balance between the two; and (2) in experimental tasks, Americans seek out events that are likely to elicit positive affect, whereas East Asians prioritize tasks that prepare them to meet social standards over tasks that are likely to produce positive affect.

Prevalence of Positive Affect or Emotional Balance?

The relative prevalence of positive emotions in North American as compared to Asian cultures has been established both in online measurements of emotion (Mesquita & Karasawa, 2002; Scollon, Diener, Oishi, & Biswas-Diener, 2004; Tsai & Levenson, 1997) and in retrospective reports (Oishi, 2002). For example, in a large experience-sampling study, Mesquita and colleagues sampled the emotions of American, Japanese, and Taiwanese students for 1 week (Mesquita & Karasawa, 2002; Mesquita, Karasawa, & Chu, 2007). Four times a day, students were asked to recall the last emotion they had experienced during the preceding 3-hour interval. Using a bidimensional scale of pleasantness–unpleasantness, Mesquita and colleagues found that American students, on average, appraised the emotional situations in their lives as better than neutral, whereas Japanese and Taiwanese students evaluated their lives on average as neither positive nor negative.

Other studies with different methodologies have established convergent results. Dating European American couples, who watched a tape of their just-completed discussion, reported more positive than negative emotions, whereas Asian American couples reported similar ratios of positive and negative affect (Tsai & Levenson, 1997). Respondents provided the continuous reports of their emotions while watching the videotaped interaction. The experience-sampling studies, as well as the online couple study, were designed to reduce retrospective bias by having respondents report emotions very close to their actual experience. Thus, the emphasis on positive emotions appears to be present in online experiences.

In addition to having more positive experiences, European Americans tend to remember events more positively than do Asians, even if the two groups initially appraised situations as equally positive. In several experiments, European Americans retrospectively rated their satisfaction with a task significantly higher than did Asian Americans, despite the lack of cultural differences in the ratings at the time of that task (Oishi, 2002). Thus, European Amer-

icans tend to remember and represent their emotional lives as more positive than did Asian Americans, in part because they remember their feelings as more positive than they actually were at the moment.

The positive memory bias does not always replicate for European Americans. In one experience-sampling study, Scollon and her colleagues (2004) found that all five cultural groups in the study, European Americans included, underestimated the frequency of their positive emotions in retrospective reports compared to online reports of the same emotions.

The same experience-sampling study provided evidence for balanced emotional styles in East Asian cultures (Scollon, Diener, Oishi, & Biswas-Diener, 2005). Respondents in this study rated their emotions seven times a day for 1 week. The number of positive emotions East Asians (Japanese, Indians, and Asian Americans) reported was positively associated with the number of negative emotions reported. In the two other cultural contexts (European Americans, Hispanics in the United States), there was no significant relationship between positive and negative emotions. The results suggest that, over time, positive emotions in East Asian contexts seem to be moderated or balanced out by negative emotions, whereas this is not the case in the U.S. contexts.

The experience-sampling study also clarifies that East Asian groups did not experience positive and negative emotions at the same moment. This suggests that previous findings that people who experience more positive emotions in those cultures also experience more negative emotions (Bagozzi, Wong, & Youjae, 1999; Kitayama et al., 2000) can best be interpreted as reports over time. Similarly, studies that suggest no relationship between experiencing positive and negative emotions in East Asian context (Schimmack, Oishi, & Diener, 2002) may best be interpreted as reports over time. The two styles of regulation associated with East Asian contexts contrast with the North American experience of positive emotions at the cost of negative emotions.

There is some evidence that the cultural differences in regulatory style are driven by positive rather than negative events. Leu and her colleagues (2007) provided Chinese, Japanese, and American respondents with standardized events in the form of a diary. The diary episodes included both positive and negative events. In the North American group, there was clear evidence for the emphasis on positive emotions at the expense of negative emotions in response to the positive events. Whereas Japanese and Chinese moderated their positive emotions with negative emotions (e.g., citing both happiness and fear of being too happy), European Americans reported positive emotions, almost to the exclusion of negative emotions. In the negative situations, however, no cultural differences in the relationship between positive and negative emotions were found. Thus, when something bad happens, individuals in all three cultures try to see the positive side of it, and to feel some positive affect as well; however, when something good happens, only the Chinese and Japanese try to see the negative side of it. This appears to represent the larger emphasis on maximizing positive feelings and minimizing negative feelings among European Americans, in contrast to a focus on moderating positive and negative emotions among East Asians.

Good Feelings Are Not a Universal Motive

Very important in much of the foregoing discussion is that maximizing positive affect to the exclusion of negative affect is not a universal motive. A number of recent experimental studies comparing task motivation between European American and either Japanese or Asian American respondents (Heine et al., 2001; Oishi & Diener, 2001, 2003) suggest this too. In these studies, North Americans sought out events that they liked, but Japanese (Asian Americans) did not. In one experiment (Heine et al., 2001), respondents received either failure or success feedback on a particular task (e.g., a word association test). All respondents were then given the opportunity to spend more time on the task. Though Japanese and European American respondents both *liked* the success feedback better than the failure feedback, Japanese respondents were motivated to work on a task after failure feedback, whereas European Americans were motivated by success feedback. Apparently, a task that proves pleasurable is not universally motivating.

In another study, Asians and European Americans solved anagrams and rated their enjoyment of the task and its difficulty right after finishing (Oishi & Diener, 2003). About 1 month later, participants were asked either to perform the same task again, or to do a comparable, new task. The more European Americans enjoyed the task the first time, the more likely they were to select it a month later; for the Asian participants, there was no relation between enjoyment and task selection. Thus, positive affect was not a motive for Asian participants.

Based on these studies, we postulate that pursuing positive affect is normative when feeling good about oneself is the goal, as appears to be the case in European American cultural contexts. However, when meeting social standards is the goal, self-improvement takes precedence over feeling good. The latter seems to happen in Japanese and Asian American contexts.

In Conclusion

Cultures, as well as individuals within those cultures, have different representations of the emotions that are desirable or normative. The study of ideal and normative representations brings out an important way in which emotional lives can be different across cultures and, moreover, illustrates that differences in emotion ideals and norms importantly and differentially inform emotional experience and behavior. At the same time, the work on normative and ideal emotions is underdeveloped. The concepts are both insufficiently demarcated and related to each other (but see Tsai et al., 2006). It is not clear, for example, whether people are capable of reporting norms regarding the focal emotions in their culture, or to what extent a person's ideal emotions are derived from culturally endorsed emotion norms. Finally, the mechanisms by which focal, normative, and ideal emotions shape the emotional experience are virtually unexplored.

Beyond Independent and Interdependent Models

The majority of the research reviewed here contrasts the emotions in North American and East Asian contexts. These studies have contributed greatly to an understanding of how culture influences emotion. However, there is a need to move beyond characterizations of cultures as either independent or interdependent, and to address emotions in other cultural contexts. The little evidence collected on emotions in other cultural contexts suggests that we have to consider cultural models of self and relating in more detail than is currently the case.

A study by Schimmack et al. (2002) makes this point. In this study, the zero correlation between positive and negative emotions was shown to be exclusive to East Asian cultures rather than characteristic of collectivist cultures generally. When Schimmack et al. controlled for the East Asian philosophical tradition of a country, collectivism did not contribute any variance to this emotional pattern. Thus, the study shows that our understanding of emotional experience in different cultures is furthered by an understanding of different kinds of interdependent models.

Other studies also demonstrate that the distinction between independent and interdependent cultural models does not suffice for a comprehensive understanding of cultural differences in emotional experience. For instance, there is now ample evidence to suggest that some non-Asian groups from interdependent cultural contexts have high positive affect, higher even than that of European Americans. Thus, in an experience-sampling study, Scollon et al. (2004) found that Hispanic students in California scored significantly higher than European American university students on positive emotions, followed by Asian students both in the United States and in Asia. The elevated positive ratings for Hispanics were found with respect to online ratings, global ratings, and retrospective ratings of positive affect. Furthermore, Hispanics and European American respondents reported somewhat lower negative emotion than did the Asian groups. Hispanics and Asians, both engaging in interdependent models, could not have been more different with respect to their emotions.

Albert and Mesquita (2005) had similar results with low-acculturation and low-education Mexicans in North Carolina. Compared to European Americans who were matched in education, Mexican immigrants reported feeling more positive and less negative emotions on an emotion scale (Barrett & Russell, 1998).

Not much is known about Mexican interdependent models, but it is clear that this kind of interdependence has radically different implications for emotional experience. Whereas East Asians (Japanese in particular) have been described as moderating their positive feelings to fit in with others and fulfill their roles, Mexican contexts do not prescribe this type of emotion regulation. Rather, happiness in Mexican contexts is intertwined with interdependence

and seems to be culturally encouraged. Emotional expressivity is valued (Klein, 2001). Happiness and happy events are seen as assets rather than obstacles for role fulfillment and social adjustment. Happiness is explicitly associated with interdependence in relationships.

At the same time, negative events appear to be downplayed in Mexican cultural contexts, which emphasize that one's individual problems are less important than fulfilling one's roles in social life (Valdes, 1996). Difficulties should be accepted (Diaz-Gerrero, 1967). Acceptance and resignation, rather than self-criticism, appear to be required for role fulfillment. One is supposed to deal with the difficulties the best that one can, without dwelling on them (Valdes, 1996). Though this is far from a comprehensive description of Mexican cultural models, the outlines make it clear that interdependence, and therefore the emotions in different interdependent contexts, can take very different forms.

DISCUSSION

A Cultural Perspective on Emotions

Examining culturally particularized emotions yields some important insights into the nature of emotion generally. These insights would not have been obtained without careful examination of the way emotions fit with the cultural models in which they occur.

Emotions as Social, Relational Phenomena

First, emotions are social phenomena. They are about the relationships between people rather than being strictly personal phenomena within the heart or the head of an individual. Even in cultures that stress the relative independence of different individuals in relationships, as is the case in North American culture (Rothbaum, Pott, Azuma, Miyake, & Weisz, 2000), emotions tend to contribute to the normative type of relationship. Emotions in North American contexts tend to underline the autonomy of people in relationships (Mesquita et al., 2005; Rothbaum, Weisz, Pott, Miyake, & Morelli, 2000), which is the condoned relationship format in this context. On the other hand, emotions in interdependent contexts underline and realize the interdependent relationships in these cultures (Kitayama et al., 2006).

Emotions Are Rooted in Collective Meanings

Second, emotions are not merely subjective individual phenomena. Rather, emotions constitute the cultural models. They are constructions of the emotional situation, based on cultural meanings and practices, and they are goals that make sense only within the parameters of the cultural models.

Collective Representations of Emotions Influence Experience

Third, emotions are not just online experiences that happen to occur. Cultural representations of emotions, especially focal emotions, emotion norms, and ideal affect, motivate the experience of emotions. They do so by facilitating positively valued emotional experiences and inhibiting negative emotional experiences. Emotion representations also are the standards by which the significance of emotions is judged (see Tsai et al., 2006).

The cultural psychology of emotions is not the enterprise of endlessly mapping all possible variations in experience. Rather, a cultural-psychological approach allows for the inference of general principles of emotion through careful descriptive study of the emotional phenomena as they actually occur in their culturally particular forms. The end goal of cultural psychology, like the end goal of all science, is the reduction of rich data to general principles. However, *only* an abstraction that acknowledges the central place of meaning in emotional experience and behavior can really contribute to our understanding of people's actual emotional experience and behavior.

Methods

If culture matters so much, why do so many studies find cross-cultural convergence in emotional phenomena? There are probably two reasons. One has to do with research design and the other, with interpretation of the results.

Research Design

Cross-cultural convergence in emotional phenomena can often be attributed to the use of methods that do not reveal important cultural differences. In a way, one has to be aware of what the differences might be to create paradigms that allow for establishing them. One

has to have a theory of emotional differences to measure them. For example, it would have been impossible to discover that Japanese respondents identify the emotion in a person's face by considering not only that person's facial expression but also the expressions of others in the same environment, had they not been presented a picture displaying several people at once. The traditional paradigm of showing one isolated face without any social context would not have yielded cultural differences in this respect. Similarly, many experimental designs have placed individuals in a situation by themselves (for an exception, see Tsai & Levenson, 1997). It is very unlikely that conditions in which an individual is isolated from his or her social environment will reveal any of the emotional differences associated with differences in the normative relationships between people.

Likewise, many studies are confined to emotions that are salient in Western cultures, and compare these emotions with the translated counterparts in other cultures. It is often not at all clear that these emotions are equally relevant in the cultures of comparison. Certainly, including emotions on the basis of their relevance for another, non-Western culture has been shown to change the results of emotion research. Thus, for example, Kitayama and his colleagues added typical Japanese emotion words to words that are salient in Western cultures, and found a dimension of social engagement that accounted for substantial variance in emotional experience (Kitayama et al., 2000; Kitayama et al., 2006). This dimension could not have been found in cross-cultural research that included only the translations of commonly used English emotion words (Russell, 1983). Importantly, establishing cultural differences in emotions seems to require a theory about the kinds of differences that one might find, as well as the methods that are capable of revealing these differences.[6]

Interpretation of Data

Practices in data interpretation have also contributed to the common conclusion of emotional similarity. As discussed, many studies have described the phenomena at so abstract a level that it would be hard to imagine *not* finding cross-cultural similarities. For example, Scherer and Wallbott (1994) looked at the antecedent events of emotions and found substantial consistency in the antecedent events associated with particular classes of emotions. However, the categories used to code the events were rather abstract. For example, "relationships" constituted one category that was universally the most important elicitor of joy-emotions. This finding seems to be descriptive of a condition of human life—and is interesting in that way—but it does not help to specify the emotional experience in particular cultures. It is questionable, for example, that knowing a positive emotion is elicited by "relationships" will help one to understand or predict the precise appraisals, behavioral goals, and behaviors that are likely to follow.

Another practice in cross-cultural research on emotions is to conclude universality when the percentage of a certain response is higher than chance. However, depending on the number of answers possible, the chance rate of responses can be as low as 18% (for six response options). Although it is important that people associate certain behaviors (Consedine, Strongman, & Magai, 2003), facial expressions (Matsumoto, 1996), and antecedent events (Boucher & Brandt, 1981) significantly more often with the same emotions than would occur by chance, the research does not show that behaviors, facial expressions, and antecedent events are universal. It shows that there is some universal human aspect in these different facets in emotions. The actual emotions may still reveal a lot of cultural specificity.

Differences in Emotion Talk or Emotional Experience?

Much, though certainly not all, of the research that we have reported consists of verbal reports from people in different cultures. Some might comment that whereas the ways people "talk" about their emotions may differ across cultures, the emotions themselves do not (e.g., Ekman, 1992). We maintain that emotional experience itself is different across cultures, and, importantly, that meanings are driving these differences.

There is growing evidence that cultural differences in emotion go beyond the emotion discourse, and that emotional meanings are consequential and affect the kinds of behavior reported. Many behaviors can be explained from the emotional meanings as construed, and this is true for behaviors reported for protagonists in emotional vignettes (e.g., Bagozzi et al., 2003), for self-reported behaviors in past emo-

tional episodes (e.g., Mesquita et al., 2005), and for behaviors such as those observed in ethnographies (e.g., Briggs, 1970).

Cultural construals of emotional situations are also consistent with the results yielded by experimental judgment tasks related to facial expressions. Thus, differences in emotion identification are consistent with the differences between independent and interdependent construals of the situation (Cohen & Gunz, 2002; Masuda et al., 2005). In independent contexts, judgments of facial expressions are based on the emotions of one individual only, whereas judgment of emotions in interdependent cultures is based on the perception that people's emotions are interdependent.

Furthermore, there is clear evidence that the meaning of emotions themselves is consequential. Emotion norms and ideals have been associated with choice behaviors (Oishi & Diener, 2003). Thus, feeling good is an important motive in cultures that value positive emotion, whereas it does not motivate people in cultural contexts that emphasize emotion moderation and role fulfillment. Similarly, cultural evaluations of emotional states are important predictors of depression (Tsai et al., 2006), and of emotional experiences in general (Eid & Diener, 2001). Thus, cultural meanings of emotions themselves are important predictors of both behavior and affective experience.

In summary, understanding the variance in cultural meanings of emotions is an important condition for the understanding of emotional experience itself.

NOTES

1. A functional view does not mean that every instance of emotion fits the cultural goals and practices. It means that, on average, the cultural shaping of emotions renders them more effective in a cultural context than if they were not shaped to fit the cultural model.

2. The Indian students were an exception compared to individuals in the other interdependent cultures.

3. One possible explanation for the difference in types of shame responses is that words representing shame in different cultures simply divide the domain of emotional experience differently. In that case, studies comparing these emotional experiences across cultures by requesting for an experience using the word *shame* would simply prompt different parts of the emotion domain. In support of this hypothesis, Japanese has a single word denoting both shame and embarrassment (Rusch, 2004), and Chinese reportedly has five words for shame alone (Frank, Harvey, & Verdun, 2000). It is

unclear, however, that these differences in vocabulary are solely responsible for the different experiences. First, it is entirely possible that the Japanese do not distinguish sharply between the different uses of the shame word, and that different experiences of this word are experienced as sharing lots of similarities. This would be consistent with findings reported by the anthropologist Daniel Fessler, who studied shame experiences among the inhabitants of a fisher village in the Indonesian province of Bengkulu. Whereas Malay, the language these villagers speak, has only one word that refers to both shame and embarrassment, Fessler concludes that *malu* does not encompass different homonyms. Bengkulu villagers in the Indonesian described the feelings and action tendencies of *malu* as no different when the emotion occurs in classical shame situations compared to embarrassment situations (Fessler, 2004). Second, despite having one rather than five shame words, Americans were perfectly able to distinguish between the five different forms of shame that the Chinese language distinguishes (Frank et al., 2000). Thus, it is not obvious that the differences in shame behaviors are associated with differences in word use.

4. The description of these data is simplified for the purposes of this chapter. In fact, the authors calculate latent classes of people. Some of these latent classes are culturally specific, but most were found across cultures. If a respondent's data fit into a class, this reflects the *likelihood* that this respondent values certain emotions as desirable, undesirable, or neutral. We simplified the data by describing the latent classes to which most respondents in a culture belong and, within each class, the emotion norms that are most likely to be observed.

5. Some Australians and Americans, however, considered anger and sadness as positive emotions.

6. This is, of course, not to deny the cross-cultural similarities in emotions that are found when one studies English emotion terms. There is certainly reason to assume some shared core of emotional experiences based on the research (Oishi et al., 2004; Scherer, 1997; Scherer & Wallbott, 1994; Scollon et al., 2004). The relative importance of these similarities compared to the differences cannot be judged based on the available evidence.

REFERENCES

Abu-Lughod, L. (1986). *Veiled sentiments*. Berkeley: University of California Press.

Adams, G., & Markus, H. R. (2004). Toward a conception of culture suitable for a social psychology of culture. In M. Schaller & C. S. Crandall (Eds.), *The psychological foundations of culture* (pp. 335–360). Mahwah, NJ: Erlbaum.

Albert, D., & Mesquita, B. (2005). *Mexican emotion: A different kind of interdependence?* Unpublished manuscript, Wake Forest University, Winston-Salem, NC.

Bagozzi, R. P., Verbeke, W., & Gavino, J. C. (2003). Culture moderates the self-regulation of shame and its effects on performance: The case of salespersons in the Netherlands and the Philippines. *Journal of Applied Psychology, 88*(2), 219–233.

Bagozzi, R. P., Wong, K. S., & Youjae, Y. (1999). The role of culture and gender in the relationship between positive and negative affect. *Cognition and Emotion, 13*(6), 641–672.

Baldwin, M., & Baccus, J. R. (2004). Maintaining a focus on the social goals underlying self-conscious emotions. *Psychological Inquiry, 15*(2), 139–144.

Barrett, L. F. (2006). Solving the emotion paradox: Categorization and the experience of emotion. *Personality and Social Psychology Review, 10*, 20–46.

Barrett, L. F., Mesquita, B., Ochsner, K., & Gross, J. J. (2007). Emotional experience. *Annual Review of Psychology, 58*(7), 373–403.

Barrett, L. F., & Russell, J. A. (1998). Independence and bipolarity in the structure of current affect. *Journal of Personality and Social Psychology, 74*(4), 967–984.

Bateson, G., & Mead, M. (1942). Balinese character. In *Special publications: New York Academy of Sciences* (pp. 1–47). New York: New York Academy of Sciences.

Boucher, J. D., & Brandt, M. E. (1981). Judgement of emotion: American and Malay antecedents. *Journal of Cross-Cultural Psychology, 12*(3), 272–283.

Briggs, J. L. (1970). *Never in anger: Portrait of an Eskimo family*. Cambridge, MA: Harvard University Press.

Bruner, J. (1986). *Actual minds, possible worlds*. New York: Plenum Press.

Bruner, J. (1990). *Acts of meaning*. Cambridge, MA: Harvard University Press.

Bruner, J. (2003). The narrative construction of reality. In P. Sengers & M. Mateas (Eds.), *Narritive Intelligence* (Vol. 46, pp. 41–62). Amsterdam: Benjamins.

Chentsova-Dutton, Y., & Tsai, J. L. (2005). *Self-focus and emotional responding in European Americans and Asian Americans*. Paper presented at the sixth annual meeting of the Society for Personality and Social Psychology, New Orleans, LA.

Clore, G. L., & Ortony, A. (2000). Cognitive neuroscience of emotion. In R. D. Lane & L. Nadel (Eds.), *Cognitive neuroscience of emotion* (pp. 24–61). New York: Oxford University Press.

Cohen, D. (1996). Law, social policy, and violence: The impact of regional cultures. *Journal of Personality and Social Psychology, 70*(5), 961–978.

Cohen, D., & Gunz, A. (2002). As seen by the other . . .: Perspectives on the self in the memories and emotional perceptions of Easterners and Westerners. *Psychological Science, 13*(1), 55–59.

Cohen, D., & Nisbett, R. E. (1994). Self-protection and the culture of honor: Explaining Southern violence. *Personality and Social Psychology Bulletin, 20*(5), 551–567.

Cohen, D., & Nisbett, R. E. (1997). Field experiments examining the culture of honor: The role of institutions in perpetuating norms about violence. *Personality and Social Psychology Bulletin*, 23(11), 1188–1199.

Cohen, D., Nisbett, R. E., Bowdle, B. F., & Schwarz, N. (1996). Insult, aggression, and the Southern culture of honor: An "experimental ethnography." *Journal of Personality and Social Psychology*, 70(5), 945–960.

Cohen, D., Vandello, J., Puente, S., & Rantilla, A. (1999). "When you call me that, smile!": How norms for politeness, interaction styles, and aggression work together in Southern culture. *Social Psychology Quarterly*, 62(3), 257–275.

Consedine, N., Strongman, K. T., & Magai, C. (2003). Emotions and behaviour: Data from a cross-cultural recognition study. *Cognition and Emotion*, 17, 881–902.

Crystal, D. S., Parrott, W. G., Okazaki, Y., & Watanabe, H. (2001). Examining relations between shame and personality among university students in the United States and Japan: A developmental perspective. *International Journal of Behavioral Development*, 25(2), 113–123.

D'Andrade, R. G. (1984). Culture meaning systems. In R. A. Shweder & R. A. Levine (Eds.), *Culture theory: Essays on mind, self, and emotion* (pp. 88–119). Cambridge, UK: Cambridge University Press.

D'Andrade, R. G., & Strauss, C. (1992). *Human motives and cultural models*. Cambridge, UK: Cambridge University Press.

Diaz-Gerrero, R. (1967). *Psychology of the Mexican: Culture and personality*. Austin: University of Texas Press.

Eid, M., & Diener, E. (2001). Norms for experiencing emotions in different cultures: Inter- and intranational differences. *Journal of Personality and Social Psychology*, 81(5), 869–885.

Ekman, P. (1992). An argument for basic emotions. *Cognition and Emotion*, 6(3/4), 169–200.

Elliott, A., Chirkov, V., Kim, Y., & Sheldon, K. (2001). A cross-cultural analysis of avoidance (relative to approach) personal goals. *Psychological Science*, 12, 505–510.

Ellsworth, P. C., & Scherer, K. R. (2003). Appraisal processes in emotion. In H. Goldsmith & K. R. Scherer (Eds.), *Handbook of affective sciences* (pp. 572–595). New York: Oxford University Press.

Fessler, D. (2004). Shame in two cultures: Implications for evolutionary approaches. *Journal of Cognition and Culture*, 4, 207–262.

Frank, H., Harvey, O. J., & Verdun, K. (2000). American responses to five categories of shame in Chinese cultures: A preliminary cross-cultural construct validation. *Personality and Individual Differences*, 28, 887–896.

Frijda, N. H. (1986). *The emotions*. Cambridge, UK: Cambridge University Press.

Frijda, N. H. (2006). *The laws of emotion*. New York: Erlbaum.

Frijda, N. H., Kuipers, P., & Terschure, E. (1989). Rela-

tions between emotion, appraisal and emotional action readiness. *Journal of Personality and Social Psychology*, 57, 212–228.

Frijda, N. H., Markam, S., Sato, K., & Wiers, R. (1995). Emotion and emotion words. In J. A. Russell (Ed.), *Everyday conceptions of emotion* (pp. 121–143). Dordrecht, the Netherlands: Kluwer Academic.

Frijda, N. H., & Mesquita, B. (1994). The social roles and functions of emotions. In S. Kitayama & H. R. Markus (Eds.), *Emotion and culture: Empirical studies of mutual influence* (pp. 51–88). Washington, DC: American Psychological Association.

Geertz, C. (1973). *The interpretation of cultures*. New York: Basic Books.

Geertz, H. (1961). *The Javanese family*. New York: Free Press.

Hamaguchi, E. (1985). A contextual model of the Japanese: Towards a methodological innovation in Japanese studies. *Journal of Japanese Studies*, 11, 289–321.

Heine, S. J., Kitayama, S., Lehman, D. R., Takata, T., Ide, E., Leung, K., et al. (2001). Divergent consequences of success and failure in Japan and North America: An investigation of self-improving motivations and malleable selves. *Journal of Personality and Social Psychology*, 81(4), 599–615.

Heine, S. J., Lehman, D. R., Markus, H. R., & Kitayama, S. (1999). Is there a universal need for positive self-regard? *Psychological Review*, 106(4), 766–794.

Holland, D., Lachicotte, W., Jr., Skinner, D., & Cain, C. (1998). *Identity and agency in cultural worlds*. Cambridge, MA: Harvard University Press.

Holland, D., & Quinn, N. (1987). *Cultural models in language and thought*. Cambridge, UK: Cambridge University Press.

Iyengar, S. S., & Lepper, M. R. (1999). Rethinking the value of choice: A cultural perspective on intrinsic motivation. *Journal of Personality and Social Psychology*, 76(3), 349–366.

Keltner, D., & Haidt, J. (1999). Social functions of emotions at four levels of analysis. *Cognition and Emotion*, 13(5), 505–521.

Kim, H. (2001). *Deviance: Uniqueness and time in context*. Paper presented at the second annual meeting of the Society for Personality and Social Psychology., San Antonio, TX.

Kitayama, S., & Markus, H. R. (2000). The pursuit of happiness and the realization of sympathy: Cultural patterns of self, social relations, and well-being. In E. Diener & E. Suh (Eds.), *Subjective well-being across cultures* (pp. 113–161). Cambridge, MA: MIT Press.

Kitayama, S., Markus, H. R., & Kurokawa, M. (2000). Culture, emotion, and well-being: Good feelings in Japan and the United States. *Cognition and Emotion*, 14(1), 93–124.

Kitayama, S., Markus, H. R., Matsumoto, D., & Norasakkunkit, V. (1997). Individual and collective processes in the construction of the self: Self-enhancement in the U.S. and self-criticism in Japan. *Journal of Personality and Social Psychology, 72*(6), 1245–1267.

Kitayama, S., Mesquita, B., & Karasawa, M. (2006). Cultural affordances and emotional experience: Socially engaging and disengaging emotions in Japan and the United States. *Journal of Personality and Social Psychology, 91*(5), 890–903.

Klein, A. M. (2001). Tender machos: masculine contrasts in the Mexican baseball league. In A. Yiannakis & M. J. Melnick (Eds.), *Contemporary issues in the sociology of sport* (pp. 291–303). Champaign, IL: Human Kinetics.

Leary, M. R., & Baumeister, R. F. (2000). The nature and function of self-esteem: Sociometer theory. In M. Zanna (Ed.), *Advances in experimental social psychology* (Vol. 32, pp. 1–62). San Diego: Academic Press.

Lebra, T. S. (1994). Mother and child in Japanese socialization: A Japan-U.S. comparison. In P. M. Greenfield & R. R. Cocking (Eds.), *Cross-cultural roots of minority child development* (pp. 259–274). Hillsdale, NJ: Erlbaum.

Leu, J., Mesquita, B., Ellsworth, P., ZhiYong, Z., Huijian, Y., Buchtel, E., et al. (2007). *Understanding dialectical emotions: Emotion representations in East and West.* Unpublished manuscript, University of Washington, Seattle.

Lu, L. (2001). Understanding happiness: A look into Chinese folk psychology. *Journal of Happiness Studies, 2,* 407–432.

Lutz, C. (1987). Goals, events, and understanding in Ifaluk emotion theory. In N. Quinn & D. Holland (Eds.), *Cultural models in language and thought* (pp. 290–312). Cambridge, UK: Cambridge University Press.

Markus, H. R., & Kitayama, S. (1991). Culture and self: Implications for cognition, emotion, and motivation. *Psychological Review, 98*(2), 224–253.

Markus, H. R., & Kitayama, S. (1994). The cultural construction of self and emotion: Implications for social behavior. In S. Kitayama & H. R. Markus (Eds.), *Emotion and culture: Empirical studies of mutual influence* (pp. 89–130). Washington, DC: American Psychological Association.

Markus, H. R., & Kitayama, S. (2003). Models of agency: Sociocultural diversity in the construction of action. In J. J. Berman & V. Murphy-Berman (Eds.), *Cross-cultural differences in perspectives on the self* (Vol. 49, pp. 18–74). Lincoln: University of Nebraska Press.

Markus, H. R., Mullally, P. R., & Kitayama, S. (1997). Selfways: Diversity in modes of cultural participation. In U. Neisser & D. A. Jopling (Eds.), *The conceptual self in context: Culture, experience, self-understanding* (pp. 13–61). Cambridge, UK: Cambridge University Press.

Mascolo, M. F., Fischer, K. W., & Li, J. (2003). Dynamic development of component systems in emotions: Pride, shame and guilt in China and the United States. In R. J. Davidson, K. R. Scherer, & H. H. Goldsmith (Eds.), *Handbook of affective sciences* (pp. 295–408). New York: Oxford University Press.

Masuda, T., Ellsworth, P. C., Mesquita, B., Leu, J., & Veerdonk, E. (2005). *Putting the face in context: Cultural differences in the perception of emotions from facial behavior.* Unpublished manuscript, University of Michigan, Ann Arbor.

Matsumoto, D. (1996). *Unmasking Japan.* Stanford, CA: Stanford University Press.

Matsumoto, D., Kudoh, T., Scherer, K. R., & Wallbott, H. (1988). Antecedents of and reactions to emotions in the United States and Japan. *Journal of Cross-Cultural Psychology, 19*(3), 267–286.

Matsumoto, D., & Yoo, S. H. (2006). The cultural attribution fallacy. *Perspectives on Psychological Science, 1*(3), 234–250.

Mauro, R., Sato, K., & Tucker, J. (1992). The role of appraisal in human emotions: A cross-cultural study. *Journal of Personality and Social Psychology, 62*(2), 301–317.

Mead, G. H. (1934). *Mind, self, and society.* Chicago: University of Chicago Press.

Mesquita, B. (1993). *Cultural variations in emotions. A comparative study of Dutch, Surinamese, and Turkish people in the Netherlands.* Unpublished doctoral dissertation, University of Amsterdam, the Netherlands.

Mesquita, B. (2001). Emotions in collectivist and individualist contexts. *Journal of Personality and Social Psychology, 80*(1), 68–74.

Mesquita, B. (2003). Emotions as dynamic cultural phenomena. In R. Davidson, H. Goldsmith, & K. R. Scherer (Eds.), *The handbook of the affective sciences* (pp. 871–890). New York: Oxford University Press.

Mesquita, B., & Albert, D. (2007). The cultural regulation of emotions. In J. J. Gross (Ed.), *The handbook of emotion regulation* (pp. 486–503). New York: Guilford Press.

Mesquita, B., & Ellsworth, P. C. (2001). The role of culture in appraisal. In K. R. Scherer & A. Schorr (Eds.), *Appraisal processes in emotion: Theory, methods, research* (pp. 233–248). New York: Oxford University Press.

Mesquita, B., & Frijda, N. H. (1992). Cultural variations in emotions: A review. *Psychological Bulletin, 112*(2), 179–204.

Mesquita, B., Frijda, N. H., & Scherer, K. R. (1997). Culture and emotion. In P. Dasen & T. S. Saraswathi (Eds.), *Handbook of cross-cultural psychology* (Vol. 2, pp. 255–297). Boston: Allyn & Bacon.

Mesquita, B., & Karasawa, M. (2002). Different emotional lives. *Cognition and Emotion, 16*(1), 127–141.

Mesquita, B., & Karasawa, M. (2004). Self-conscious emotions as dynamic cultural processes. *Psychological Inquiry, 15,* 161–166.

Mesquita, B., Karasawa, M., & Chu, R. L. (2007). *Predictors of pleasantness in three cultures: A comparison between the United States, Japan, and Taiwan.*

Unpublished manuscript, Wake Forest University, Winston-Salem, NC.

Mesquita, B., Karasawa, M., Haire, A., Izumi, K., Hayashi, A., Idzelis, M., et al. (2005). *What do I feel?: The role of cultural models in emotion representations.* Unpublished manuscript, Wake Forest University, Winston-Salem, NC.

Mesquita, B., & Markus, H. R. (2004). Culture and emotion: Models of agency as sources of cultural variation in emotion. In A. S. R. Manstead, N. H. Frijda, & A. H. Fischer (Eds.), *Feelings and emotions: The Amsterdam symposium* (pp. 341–358). New York: Cambridge University Press.

Middleton, D. R. (1989). Emotional style: The cultural ordering of emotions. *Ethos, 17*(2), 187–201.

Miller, J. G. (1997). Theoretical issues in cultural psychology. In J. Berry, Y. H. Poortinga, & J. Pandey (Eds.), *Handbook of cross-cultural psychology* (Vol. 1, pp. 85–128). Needham Heights, MA: Allyn & Bacon.

Miller, J. G., Fung, H., & Mintz, J. (1996). Self-construction through narrative practices: A Chinese and American comparison of early socialization. *Ethos, 24,* 237–280.

Minami, H. (1971). *Psychology of the Japanese people* (A. Ikoma, Trans.). Toronto: University of Toronto Press.

Ng, A., Ho, S., & Smith, I. (2003). In search of the good life: A cultural odyssey in the East and West. *Genetic, Social, and General Psychology Monographs, 129*(4), 317–363.

Oatley, K., & Jenkins, J. H. (1992). Human emotions: Function and dysfunction. *Annual Review of Psychology, 43,* 55–85.

Oishi, S. (2002). The experiencing and remembering of well-being: A cross-cultural analysis. *Personality and Social Psychology Bulletin, 28,* 1398–1406.

Oishi, S., & Diener, E. (2001). Goals, culture and subjective well-being. *Personality and Social Psychology Bulletin, 27*(12), 463–473.

Oishi, S., & Diener, E. (2003). Culture and well-being: The cycle of action, evaluation, and decision. *Personality and Social Psychology Bulletin, 29,* 939–949.

Oishi, S., Diener, E., Scollon, C. N., & Biswas-Diener, R. (2004). Cross-situational consistency of affective experiences across cultures. *Journal of Personality and Social Psychology, 86,* 460–472.

Peristiany, J. G. (1966). Honour and shame in a Cypriot highland. In J. G. Peristiany (Ed.), *Honour and shame: The values of Mediterranean society* (pp. 171–190). Chicago: University of Chicago Press.

Rothbaum, F., Pott, M., Azuma, H., Miyake, K., & Weisz, J. (2000). The development of close relationships in Japan and the United States: Paths of symbiotic harmony and generative tension. *Child Development, 71*(5), 1121–1142.

Rothbaum, F., Weisz, J., Pott, M., Miyake, K., & Morelli, G. (2000). Attachment and culture: Security in the United States and Japan. *American Psychologist, 55*(10), 1093–1104.

Rusch, C. D. (2004). Cross-cultural variability of the semantic domain of emotion terms: An examination of English *shame* and *embarrassment* with Japanese *Hazukashii. Cross-Cultural Research, 38,* 236–248.

Russell, J. A. (1983). Pancultural aspects of the human conceptual organization of emotions. *Journal of Personality and Social Psychology, 45*(6), 1281–1288.

Scherer, K. R. (1984). Emotion as a multicomponent process: A model and some cross-cultural data. In P. R. Shaver (Ed.), *Review of personality and social psychology* (Vol. 5, pp. 37–63). Beverly Hills, CA: Sage.

Scherer, K. R. (1997). The role of culture in emotion-antecedent appraisal. *Journal of Personality and Social Psychology, 73,* 902–922.

Scherer, K. R., Matsumoto, D., Wallbott, H. G., & Kudoh, T. (1988). Emotional experience in cultural context: A comparison between Europe, Japan, and the U.S. In K. R. Scherer (Ed.), *Facets of emotion* (pp. 5–30). Hillsdale, NJ: Erlbaum.

Scherer, K. R., & Wallbott, H. G. (1994). Evidence for universality and cultural variation of differential emotion response patterning. *Journal of Personality and Social Psychology, 66*(2), 310–328.

Schieffelin, E. L. (1985). Anger, grief, and shame: Toward a Kaluli ehthnopsychology. In G. L. White & J. Kirkpatrick (Eds.), *Person, self, and experience: Exploring Pacific ethnopsychologies* (pp. 168–182). Berkeley: University of California Press.

Schimmack, U., Oishi, S., & Diener, E. (2002). Cultural influences on the relation between pleasant emotions and unpleasant emotions: Asian dialectic philosophies or individualism–collectivism? *Cognition and Emotion, 16*(6), 705–719.

Scollon, C. N., Diener, E., Oishi, S., & Biswas-Diener, R. (2004). Emotions across cultures and methods. *Journal of Cross-Cultural Psychology, 35,* 304–326.

Scollon, C. N., Diener, E., Oishi, S., & Biswas-Diener, R. (2005). An experience sampling and cross-cultural investigation of the relation between pleasant and unpleasant affect. *Cognition and Emotion, 19,* 27–52.

Shweder, R. A., & Haidt, J. (2000). The cultural psychology of emotions: Ancient and new. In M. Lewis & J. M. Haviland-Jones (Eds.), *Handbook of emotions* (2nd ed., pp. 397–414). New York: Guilford Press.

Smith, C. A., & Ellsworth, P. C. (1985). Patterns of cognitive appraisal in emotion. *Journal of Personality and Social Psychology, 48,* 813–838.

Solomon, R. C. (1978). Emotions and anthropology: The logic of emotional world views. *Inquiry, 21,* 181–199.

Stephenson, P. H. (1989). Going to McDonald's in Leiden: Reflections on the concept of self and society in the Netherlands. *Ethos, 17,* 226–247.

Tooby, J., & Cosmides, L. (1990). The past explains the present: Emotional adaptations and the structure of ancestral environments. *Ethology and Sociobiology, 11,* 375–424.

Tooby, J., & Cosmides, L. (1992). The psychological foundations of culture. In J. H. Barkow, L. Cosmides

& J. Tooby (Eds.), *The adapted mind: Evolutionary psychology and the generation of culture* (pp. 19–136). New York: Oxford University Press.

Tracy, J. L., & Robins, R. W. (2004). Putting the self into self-conscious emotions: A theoretical model. *Psychological Inquiry, 15,* 103–125.

Triandis, H. C. (1995). *Individualism and collectivism.* Boulder, CO: Westview Press.

Tsai, J. L., Chentsova-Dutton, Y., Friere-Bebeau, L. H., & Przymus, D. (2002). Emotional expression and physiology in European Americans and Hmong Americans. *Emotion, 2,* 380–397.

Tsai, J. L., Knutson, B., & Fung, H. H. (2006). Cultural variation in affect valuation. *Journal of Personality and Social Psychology, 90*(2), 288–307.

Tsai, J. L., & Levenson, R. W. (1997). Cultural influences on emotional responding: Chinese American and European American dating couples during the interpersonal conflict. *Journal of Cross-Cultural Psychology, 28,* 600–625.

Tsang, S., & Wu, C. (2005). *What constitutes my subjective well-being: Is the subjective well-being of interdependent-self individuals rooted in others' subjective well-being?* Paper presented at the sixth biennial conference of the Asian Association of Social Psychology, Wellington, New Zealand.

Valdes, G. (1996). *Con respeto: Bridging the distances between culturally diverse families and schools: An ethnographic portrait.* New York: Teachers College Press.

Van der Horst, H. (1996). *The low sky: Understanding the Dutch.* The Hague: Scriptum Books.

Weiner, B. (1982). The emotional consequences of casual ascriptions. In M. S. Clark & S. T. Fiske (Eds.), *Affect and cognition* (pp. 185–210). Hillsdale, NJ: Erlbaum.

Weiner, B. (1986). Attribution, emotion and action. In R. M. H. Sorrentino & E. T. Higgins (Eds.), *Handbook of motivation and cognition* (pp. 281–312). New York: Wiley.

CHAPTER 31

Passionate Love and Sexual Desire

ELAINE HATFIELD
RICHARD L. RAPSON
LISE D. MARTEL

Passionate love is a universal emotion experienced by almost all people, in all historical eras, and in all the world's cultures (see Fischer, Shaver, & Carnochan, 1990; Shaver, Morgan, & Wu, 1996). Yet despite its universality, culture has been found to have a profound impact on people's definitions of love and on the way they think, feel, and behave in romantic settings. Cross-cultural studies provide a glimpse into the complex world of emotion and allow us to gain an understanding of the extent to which people's emotional lives are written in their cultural and personal histories, as well as "writ in their genes" and evolutionary history, and in the interaction of the two (Tooby & Cosmides, 1992).

PASSIONATE AND COMPANIONATE LOVE

Defining Love

Poets, novelists, and social commentators have proposed numerous definitions of love. Ahdat Soueif (1999), an Arab novelist, once poetically described the multitude of meanings that "love" possesses in Arabic:

"Hubb" is love, "ishq" is love that entwines two people together, "shaghaf" is love that nests in the chambers of the heart, "hayam" is love that wanders the earth, "teeh" is love in which you lose yourself, "walah" is love that carries sorrow within it, "sababah" is love that exudes from your pores, "hawa" is love that shares its name with "air" and with "falling," "gharm" is love that is willing to pay the price. (pp. 386–387)

Cultural theorists have long been interested in the impact of culture on the meaning that young men and women ascribe to "love." Scholars usually distinguish between two kinds of love: "passionate love" and "companionate love" (Hatfield & Rapson, 1993).

Passionate Love

Passionate love (sometimes called "obsessive love," "infatuation," "lovesickness," or "being in love") is a powerful emotional state. It has been defined as

a state of intense longing for union with another. Passionate love is a complex functional whole including appraisals or appreciations, subjective feelings, expressions, patterned physiological processes, action tendencies, and instrumental behaviors. Reciprocated love (union with the other) is associated with fulfillment and ecstasy. Unrequited love (separation) is associated with feelings of emptiness, anxiety, and despair. (Hatfield & Rapson, 1993, p. 5)

People in all cultures recognize the power of passionate love. In South Indian Tamil families, for example, a person who falls head-over-heels in love with another is said to be suffering from *mayakkam*—dizziness, confusion, intoxication, and delusion. The wild hopes and despairs of love are thought to "mix you up" (Trawick, 1990).

The Passionate Love Scale (PLS) was designed to tap into the cognitive, emotional, and behavioral indicants of such longings (Hatfield & Sprecher, 1986). The PLS has been found to be a useful measure of passionate love with men and women of all ages, in a variety of cultures, and has been found to correlate well with certain well-defined patterns of neural activation (see Bartels & Zeki, 2000, 2004; Doherty, Hatfield, Thompson, & Choo, 1994; Fisher, 2003; Landis & O'Shea, 2000).

Companionate Love

Companionate love is a far less intense emotion. It combines feelings of attachment, commitment, and intimacy (Hatfield & Rapson, 1993). It has been defined as "the affection and tenderness we feel for those with whom our lives are deeply entwined" (p. 9).

Psychologists have used a variety of scales to measure companionate love. Since Sternberg (1988) postulated that companionate relationships require both commitment and intimacy, many researchers have assessed such love by measuring those two components.

Other Definitions of Love

Scientists have proposed a variety of definitions and typologies of love (see Hendrick & Hendrick, 1989; Shaver & Hazan, 1988; Sternberg, 1988). According to Sternberg, for example, types of love are determined by various combinations of passion, intimacy, and commitment. Possible combinations result in romantic love, infatuation, companionate love, liking, fatuous love, empty love, and consummate love.

In this chapter we focus on passionate love; we touch upon other varieties of love only briefly, if at all.

THEORETICAL UNDERSTANDINGS OF PASSIONATE LOVE

Anthropological Perspectives on Passionate Love

Passionate love is as old as humankind. The Sumerian love fable of Inanna and Dumuzi, for example, was spun by tribal storytellers in 2,000 B.C.E (Wolkstein, 1991). Today, most anthropologists argue that passionate love is a universal experience, transcending culture and time (Buss, 1994; Hatfield & Rapson, 1996; Jankowiak, 1995; Tooby & Cosmides, 1992).

Jankowiak and Fischer (1992) drew a sharp distinction between "romantic passion" and "simple lust." They proposed that both passion and lust are universal feelings. Drawing on a sampling of tribal societies from the Standard Cross-Cultural Sample, they found that in almost all of these far-flung societies, young lovers talked about passionate love, recounted tales of love, sang love songs, and spoke of the longings and anguish of infatuation. When passionate affections clashed with parents' or elders' wishes, young couples often eloped.

Social anthropologists have explored folk conceptions of love in such diverse cultures as the People's Republic of China, Indonesia, Turkey, Nigeria, Trinidad, Morocco, the Fulbe of North Cameroun, the Mangrove (an aboriginal Australian community), the Mangaia in the Cook Islands, Palau in Micronesia, and the Taita of Kenya (see Jankowiak, 1995, for a review of this research). In all these studies, people's conceptions of passionate love appear to be surprisingly similar.

Anthropologists have also been interested in the kinds of societies in which our primate ancestors lived. Sommer (1993), for example, asked a challenging question: Did our ancient *Homo sapiens* ancestors live in monogamous, polygamous, polyandrous, or polygynandrous communities? (In monogamy, a man and woman marry—usually for a lifetime. In polygamy, one man may possess many wives; in polyandry, one woman may take several husbands. In polygynandry, or "promiscuous" mating, men and women may mate at will.)

After observing many kinds of primates, Sommer (1993) discovered that it is easy to predict what sort of sexual mating arrangements a primate species will adopt. He needed to know only four facts:

1. In that species, who is bigger—the males or the females?
2. How much do the males' testes weigh?
3. Do females have sexual swellings (which signal sexual receptivity and fertility)?
4. How long does sexual intercourse last?

(The scientists found, for example, that in monogamous species such as gibbons, males and females are generally about the same size. In polygynous species such as orangutans [where successful males must physically dominate their rivals], males are much larger than their mates.)

When Sommer (1993) classified *H. sapiens* on these four characteristics, his calculations led him to conclude that although our human forebears *may* have been monogamous, the odds are that they were polygynous.[1] There is no chance that they were either polyandrous or polygynandrous.

What about our more immediate ancestors? How did they live? On the basis of her calculations, Fisher (1989) concluded that throughout the world, although (in theory) most societies are polygynous, in fact, the overwhelming majority of married men and women are actually in monogamous marriages. Fisher studied the marital arrangements of the 853 societies sampled in the *Ethnographic Atlas* (which contains anthropological information on more than 1,000 representative preindustrial societies throughout the world). She found that although almost all societies (84%) permitted polygyny, men rarely exercised this option. (Only about 10% of men possessed more than one wife. Most possessed just one wife. A few were unmarried.) In 16% of societies, monogamy was prescribed. Polyandry was extremely rare. Only 0.5% of societies permitted polyandry. In recent years, however, theorists such as Wilson and Daly (1992) have observed that in humankind's long evolutionary history, although men and women in theory are "supposed" to be faithful to one partner, in many situations it was of benefit to break the rules and "mate poach." Thus, humans are likely to possess a variety of cognitive structures designed to deal with a multitude of contingencies (for a discussion of the factors that made and make it advantageous (or costly) for men and women to seek a variety of sexual partners,

see Barkow, Cosmides, & Tooby, 1992; Hrdy, 1999; Wilson & Daly, 1992).

Genetic and Biological Perspectives on Love

Recently, social psychologists, neuroscientists, and physiologists have begun to explore the links between love, sexual desire, and sexual behavior.

The first neuroscientists to study passionate love were Birbaumer, Lutzenberger, Elbert, Flor, and Rockstroh (1993). They concluded (on the basis of their EEG [electroencephalogram] assessments) that passionate love is "mental chaos." More recently, Bartels and Zeki (2000, 2004) studied the neural bases of passionate love using fMRI (functional magnetic resonance imaging) techniques. They interviewed young men and women from 11 countries and several ethnic groups who claimed to be "truly, deeply, and madly" in love, and who scored high on the PLS. The authors concluded that passionate love leads to a suppression of activity in the areas of the brain controlling critical thought; they argued that once we get close to someone, there is less need to assess their character and personality in a negative way. Passion also produced increased activity in the brain areas associated with euphoria and reward, and decreased levels of activity in the areas associated with distress and depression. Activity seemed to be restricted to foci in the medial insula and the anterior cingulate cortex and, subcortically, in the caudate nucleus, and the putamen, all bilaterally. Deactivations were observed in the posterior cingulate gyrus and in the amygdala, and were right-lateralized in the prefrontal, parietal, and middle temporal cortices.

What is the conclusion?

> We conclude that human attachment employs a push–pull mechanism that overcomes social distance by deactivating networks used for critical social assessment and negative emotions, while it bonds individuals through the involvement of the reward circuitry, explaining the power of love to motivate and exhilarate. (Bartels & Zeki, 2004, p. 1155)

The authors also found passionate love and sexual arousal to be tightly linked.

Other psychologists who have studied the links between passionate love and sexual desire (using fMRI techniques) have found similar results. Fisher (2003, 2004), for example, investigated the brain chemistry of men and women passionately in love (again using the PLS scale) and found that passionate love markedly increases sexual motivation.

In parallel with this research, a number of social psychologists, neurobiologists, and physiologists have explored the neural and chemical substrates of passionate love, sexual desire, and sexual mating (Carter, 1998; Komisaruk & Whipple, 1998; Marazziti, Akiskal, Rossi, & Cassano, 1999; Marazziti & Canale, 2004).

Scientists interested in the chemistry of passionate love have found that a variety of neurochemicals shape passionate love and sexual desire. According to Fisher (2004), for example, romantic love is associated with the natural stimulant dopamine and perhaps norepinephrine and serotonin. Lust is associated primarily with the hormone testosterone in both men and women. (Estrogen may decrease desire.) Attachment is produced primarily by the hormones oxytocin and vasopressin (see also Hyde, 2005; Marazziti & Canale, 2004; Regan & Berscheid, 1999).

Psychologists' opinions may differ on whether romantic and passionate love are emotions (Aron et al., 2005; Shaver et al., 1996) and whether passionate love, sexual desire, and sexual motivation are closely related constructs (both neurobiologically or physiologically) or very different in nature (Aron et al., 2005; Diamond, 2004; Hatfield & Rapson, 1987). Nonetheless, this pathbreaking research has the potential to answer age-old questions as to the nature of culture, love, and human sexuality.

In spite of the fact that anthropologists, neurobiologists, and physiologists consider passionate love to be a panhuman characteristic (an emotion thought to exist in all cultures and in all historical eras), culture has been found to exert a profound impact on people's romantic and sexual attitudes, emotions, and behaviors.

Historical Perspectives on Love

Any time scholars begin talking glibly about "cultural universals," historians tend to react with skepticism. Historians prefer to emphasize the multiplicity, variability, and mutability of human behavior. They shy away from all single-cause explanations for how cultures and individuals work, and they revel in complexity, movement, and change.

Not surprising, then, when it comes to romance, historians invariably note that passionate attitudes and behaviors have varied dramatically from one culture to another or from one temporal period to the next. Some typical examples include the sage Vatsayana advising men and women to marry for love or the Medieval church condemning such sinful indulgence; early Egyptians practiced birth control, and some Polynesians practiced infanticide; Classical Greeks rewarded couples who were willing to conceive; Eskimos considered it hospitable to share their wives with visitors; Muslims jealousy locked their wives and concubines away in harems; Sumerian and Babylonian temples were staffed by priests, priestesses, and sacred prostitutes; the ancient Hebrews stoned "godless" prostitutes; Hellenes idealized the pure sexual love between older men and young boys; and the Aztecs punished homosexuality by tying men to logs, disemboweling them, covering them with ash, and incinerating them (Tannahill, 1980).

Historians have also documented how profoundly a society's attitudes toward love, sex, and intimacy can alter over time. Consider China, which possesses an ancient culture. Its archeological record begins 5,000 years ago in the *Hongshan* (Red Mountain) dynasty. Its historical record begins 4,000 years ago in the *Xia* (or First Dynasty). The oldest Chinese medical texts on love and sexuality date from 168 B.C.E.

Traditionally, Chinese history is divided into three periods: the Formative Age (prehistory through 206 B.C.E.), the Early Empire (206 B.C.E. to 960 C.E.), and the Later Empire (960–1911 C.E.). The Chinese historian Ruan (1991) argued that during the first 4,000 years of Chinese history, attitudes toward passionate love and sexual desire were generally positive—although hardly uniform and unchanging during these epochs. Medical texts dating back to 168 B.C.E. make it clear that the ancients assumed that love and sexual pleasure were two of the great joys of life. In the Late Empire (1,000 years ago), during the Sung Dynasty, the Neo-Confucianists gained political and religious power, and Chinese attitudes began to alter, gradually becoming more and more negative and repressive concerning sex. Displays of love outside marriage were forbidden, and erotic art and literature were often burned.

When the People's Republic of China was established in 1949, Communist officials imposed even tighter controls on love and "inappropriate" sexual activity. On a visit to Beijing, Money (1977) reported: "I came across a slogan: 'Making love is a mental disease that wastes time and energy' " (p. 543).

Gil (1992) noted:

> A puritanical, if not heavy-handed, sexual "primness" became firmly established. ... This included a denial of romantic love, the affirmation of the absolute role of the collective over the individual as a basic tenet toward which one should direct any affections. The Great Leap Forward demanded, in Communist parlance, the "renunciation of the heart." Party policy deliberately constructed an altruism which sought (for every man and woman) hard work during the day, without being "deflected or confused" by love, sexual desire, or any strivings for private happiness. (p. 571)

Today, of course, in China as throughout much of the rest of the world, the winds of change are wafting. Young people—perhaps as a consequence of globalization (as evidenced in the availability of international cinema, the Web, world travel, and MTV)—are adopting more "liberal" or "worldly" views of passionate love, sexual desire, marriage for love (rather than arranged marriages), and romantic and sexual diversity. In China, then, things appear to have come full circle.

Historical research, then, reminds us that throughout time, people have embraced very different attitudes toward romantic and passionate love, have ascribed very different meanings to "love," have desired very different traits in romantic partners, and have differed markedly in whether such feelings were to be proclaimed to the world or hidden in the deepest recesses of the heart. In the real world, human sexual attitudes and behavior seem forever in flux.

Culture and Passionate Love

Americans are preoccupied with love—or so cross-cultural observers once claimed. In a famous quip, Linton (1936) once mocked Americans for their naive idealization of romantic love and their assumption that romantic love was a prerequisite to marriage:

> All societies recognize that there are occasional violent, emotional attachments between persons of opposite sex, but our present American culture is practically the only one which has attempted to

capitalize these, and make them the basis for marriage. ... The hero of the modern American movie is always a romantic lover, just as the hero of the old Arab epic is always an epileptic. A cynic may suspect that in any ordinary population the percentage of individuals with a capacity for romantic love of the Hollywood type was about as large as that of persons able to throw genuine epileptic fits. (p. 175)

Throughout the world, a spate of commentators have echoed Linton's claim that the idealization of passionate love is a peculiarly Western institution.

A Bit of Background

The world's cultures differ profoundly in the extent to which they emphasize individualism or collectivism (although some cross-cultural researchers focus on related concepts: independence or interdependence, modernism or traditionalism, urbanism or ruralism, affluence or poverty).

Individualistic cultures such as the United States, Britain, Australia, Canada, and the countries of Northern and Western Europe tend to focus on personal goals. Collectivist cultures such as China, many African and Latin American nations, Greece, southern Italy, and the Pacific Islands, on the other hand, press their members to subordinate personal interests to those of the group (Markus & Kitayama, 1991; Triandis, McCusker, & Hui, 1990). Triandis and his colleagues point out that in individualistic cultures, young people are allowed to "do their own thing"; in collectivist cultures, the group comes first.

Hsu (1953, 1985) and Doi (1963, 1973) contend that passionate love is a Western phenomenon, almost unknown in China and Japan—and so incompatible with Asian values and customs that it is unlikely ever to gain a foothold among young Asians. Hsu (1953) writes: "An American asks, 'How does my heart feel?' A Chinese asks, 'What will other people say?' " (p. 50). Hsu points out that the Chinese generally use the term "love" to describe not a respectable, socially sanctioned relationship, but an *illicit* liaison between a man and a woman.

Chu (1985; Chu & Ju, 1993) also argues that, although romantic love and compatibility are of paramount importance in mate selection in America, in China such things matter little.

Traditionally, parents and go-betweens arranged young peoples' marriages. Parents' primary concern is not love and compatibility but *men tang hu tui*. Do the families possess the same social status? Are *they* compatible? Will the marriage bring some social or financial advantage to the two families?

On the basis of such testimony, cross-cultural researchers proposed that romantic love would be common only in modern, industrialized countries. It should be less valued in traditional cultures with strong, extended family ties (Simmons, Vom Kolke, & Shimizu, 1986). It should be more common in modern, industrialized countries than in developing countries (Goode, 1959; Rosenblatt, 1967).

In recent years, cultural researchers have begun to test these provocative hypotheses.

RECENT RESEARCH ON CULTURE AND PASSIONATE LOVE

Recently, cultural researchers have begun to investigate the impact (if any) of culture on people's definitions of love, what they desire in romantic partners, their likelihood of falling in love, the intensity of their passion, and their willingness to acquiesce in arranged marriages versus insisting on marrying for love. From this preliminary research, it appears that although the differences cultural theorists have observed do in fact exist, often cultures turn out to be more similar than one might expect. Let us now turn to this research.

The Meaning of Passionate Love

Shaver, Wu, and Schwartz (1991) interviewed young people in America, Italy, and the People's Republic of China about their emotional experiences. They found that Americans and Italians tended to equate love with happiness, and to assume that both passionate and companionate love were intensely positive experiences. Students in Beijing, China, possessed a darker view of love. In the Chinese language, there are few "happy love" words; love is associated with sadness. Not surprisingly, then, the Chinese men and women interviewed by Shaver and his colleagues tended to associate passionate love with ideographic words such as infatuation, unrequited love, nostalgia, and sorrow love.

Other cultural researchers agree that cultural values may indeed, have a profound impact on the subtle shadings of meaning assigned to the construct of "love" (Cohen, 2001; Kim & Hatfield, 2004; Kitayama, 2002; Luciano, 2003; Nisbett, 2003; Oyserman, Kemmelmeier, & Coon, 2002; Weaver & Ganong, 2004).

There is, however, considerable debate as to how ubiquitous and important such differences are. When social psychologists explored folk conceptions of love in a surprising variety of cultures—including the People's Republic of China, Indonesia, Micronesia, Palau, and Turkey, they found that people in the various cultures possessed surprisingly similar views of love and other "feelings of the heart" (for a review of this research, see K. W. Fischer, Wang, Kennedy, & Cheng, 1998; Jankowiak, 1995; Kim & Hatfield, 2004; Shaver, Murdaya, & Fraley, 2001). In a typical study, for example, Shaver et al. argued that love and "sexual mating, reproduction, parenting, and maintaining relationships with kin and reciprocally altruistic relationships with friends and neighbors are fundamental issues for humans" (pp. 219–220). To test the notion that passionate and companionate love are cultural universals, they conducted a "prototype" study to determine (1) what Indonesian (compared to American) men and women considered to be "basic" emotions, and (2) the meaning they ascribed to these emotions. Starting with 404 Indonesian *perasaan hati* (emotion names or "feelings of the heart") they asked people to sort the words into basic emotion categories. As predicted, the Indonesians came up with the same five emotions that Americans consider to be basic: joy, love, sadness, fear, and anger. Furthermore, when asked about the meanings of "love," Indonesian men and women (like their American counterparts) were able to distinguish passionate love (*asmara*, or sexual desire/arousal) from companionate love (*cinta*, or affection/liking/fondness). There were some differences in the American and Indonesian lexicons, however: "The Indonesian conception of love may place more emphasis on yearning and desire than the American conception, perhaps because the barriers to consummation are more formidable in Indonesia, which is a more traditional and mostly Muslim country" (p. 219).

Much more research needs to be done, of course, before scientists can state this conclusion with any certainty.

Perhaps love is indeed a cultural universal. Or perhaps the times they are "a-changing." One impact of globalization (and the ubiquitous MTV, Hollywood and Bollywoood movies, chat rooms, and foreign travel) may be to ensure that when people speak of "passionate love," they are talking about much the same thing.

What Men and Women Desire in Romantic Partners

Since Darwin's (1871) classic treatise, *The Descent of Man and Selection in Relation to Sex*, evolutionary theorists have been interested in mate preferences. Many evolutionary psychologists contend that there are cultural universals in what men and women desire in a mate.

This contention is supported by a landmark cross-cultural study conducted by Buss (1994), who asked more than 10,000 men and women from 37 countries to indicate what characteristics they sought in potential mates. These people came from a variety of geographic, cultural, political, ethnic, religious, racial, economic, and linguistic groups. Buss found that, overall, the single trait that men and women in all societies valued most was "mutual attraction–love." After that, men and women cared next about finding someone who possessed a dependable character, emotional stability and maturity, and a pleasing disposition. Men tended to care more about the physical appearance and youth of their partners than did women; women tended to be more insistent than men that their mates possess high status and the resources necessary to protect themselves and their children.

Buss was interested in cultural and gender universals; nonetheless, he could not help but be struck by the powerful impact that culture had on other mentioned preferences. In China, India, Indonesia, Iran, Israel (the Palestinian Arabs), and Taiwan, for example, young people were insistent that their mate should be "chaste." In Finland, France, Norway, the Netherlands, Sweden, and West Germany, on the other hand, most judged chastity to be relatively unimportant. A few respondents even jotted notes in the margin of the questionnaire, indicating that, for them, chastity would be a *disadvantage*.

In an alternative analysis of Buss's (1994) data, Wallen (1989) attempted to determine which was most important—culture or gender—in shaping people's mate preferences. He found that for some traits—such as good looks and financial prospects—gender had a great influence on preferences. (Whereas gender accounted for 40–45% of the variance, geographical origin accounted for only 8–17% of the variance.) For other traits, such as chastity, ambition, and preferred age, on the other hand, culture mattered most. (In those instances, gender accounted for only 5–16% of the variance, whereas geographical origin accounted for 38–59% of the variance.) Wallen concluded that, in general, the cultural perspective may well be even more powerful than evolutionary heritage in understanding mate selection.

Cultural researchers provide additional evidence that in different cultural, national, and ethnic groups, people often desire very different things in romantic, sexual, or marital partners. Hatfield and Sprecher (1996), for example, studied three powerful, modern industrial societies—the United States, Russia, and Japan. Men and women in Western, individualistic cultures (e.g., the United States, and to some extent Russia) expected far more from their marriages than did couples in a collectivist culture (e.g., Japan).

As we observed earlier, cultural theorists have predicted that cultural rules should exert a profound impact on the commonness of passionate feelings within a culture, how intensely passion is experienced, and how people attempt to deal with these tumultuous feelings. Alas, the sparse existing data provide only minimal support for this intriguing and plausible-sounding hypothesis.

The Likelihood of Being in Love

Sprecher and her colleagues (1994) interviewed 1,667 men and women in the United States, Russia, and Japan. Based on notions of individualism versus collectivism, the authors predicted that whereas American men and women would be most vulnerable to love, the Japanese would be least likely to be "love besotted." The authors found that they were wrong. In fact, 59% of American college students, 67% of Russians, and 53% of Japanese students said they were in love at the time of the interview. In all three cultures, men were slightly less likely than were women to be in love. There was no evidence, however, that individualistic cultures breed young men and women who are more love struck than do collectivist societies.

Similarly, surveys of Mexican American, Chinese American, and European American students have revealed that in a variety of ethnic groups, young men and women show similarly high rates of "being in love" at the present time (Aron & Rodriguez, 1992; Doherty et al., 1994).

The Intensity of Passionate Love

Cultures also seem to share more similarities than differences in the *intensity* of passionate love that people experience. In one study, Hatfield and Rapson (1996) asked men and women of European, Filipino, and Japanese ancestry to complete the PLS. To their surprise, they found that men and women from the various ethnic groups seemed to love with equal passion.

Their results were confirmed in a study done by Doherty and his colleagues (1994) with European Americans, Chinese Americans, Filipino Americans, Japanese Americans, and Pacific Islanders.

LOVE AND MARRIAGE

In the West, before 1700, no society ever equated *le grand passion* with marriage. In the 12th century, in *The Art of Courtly Love*, for example, Andreas Capellanus (1174/1957) stated:

> Everybody knows that love can have no place between husband and wife. . . . For what is love but an inordinate desire to receive passionately a furtive and hidden embrace? But what embrace between husband and wife can be furtive, I ask you, since they may be said to belong to each other and may satisfy all of each other's desires without fear that anybody will object? (p. 100)

And Capellanus was not even talking about passionate love—just love. To make his argument perfectly clear, he added: "We declare and we hold as firmly established that love cannot exert its powers between two people who are married to each other" (p. 106).

Shakespeare may have written a handful of romantic comedies in which passionately mismatched couples hurtled toward marriage, but his plays were the exception. Until 1500, most courtly love songs, plays, and stories assumed a darker ending—passionate love was either unrequited, unconsummated, or it spun down to family tragedy and the suicide or deaths of the lovers.

As late as 1540, Alessandro Piccolomini could write peremptorily that "love is a reciprocity of soul and has a different end and obeys different laws from marriage. Hence one should not take the loved one to wife" (Hunt, 1959, p. 206). True to his times, Piccolomini, began to change his mind just before he died.

In the great societies of Asia—China, Japan, and India (lands of arranged marriage)—at least since the end of the 17th century (and thousands of *haiku* poems, *Noh* plays, and heroic legends later), the notion that passionate love and sexual desire go together with thwarted hopes for marriage and suicide has been embedded in the Eastern psyche as an Eternal Truth. Classical tales recount the couple's journey together to the chosen place, leaving forever behind them familiar scenes, agonizing mental conflicts, and the last tender farewells (Mace & Mace, 1980).

To today's young individualistic Americans and Europeans, such tales of forbidden romance may seem ridiculous. But to Asian young romantics, who knew that passion had little chance of flowering into marriage, the tales were sublime tragedies.

In traditional cultures, it was the lovers who had to adapt, not society. Individual happiness mattered little; what was important was the well-being of the family and the maintenance of social order. As one modern Chinese woman asserted: "Marriage is not a relation for personal pleasure, but a contract involving the ancestors, the descendants, and the property" (Mace & Mace, 1980, p. 134).

In contemporary societies, however, both East and West, most young men and women do meet, fall in love, feel sexual desire, and live together or marry. In the next section, we will discuss the revolution that is occurring in the ways young men and women (heterosexual and homosexual) currently select their romantic, sexual, and marital partners. We will see that throughout the world, parental power is crumbling, and that arranged marriages are being replaced by the ideal of love marriages.

Arranged Marriages

Throughout history, cultures have varied markedly in who possessed the power to select romantic, sexual, and marital partners.

As we have seen, in the distant past in most societies, parents, kin, and communities usually had the power to arrange things as they chose. Marriage was assumed to be an alliance between two *families* (Dion & Dion, 1993; Lee & Stone, 1980). Families might also consult with religious specialists, oracles, and matchmakers (Rosenblatt & Anderson, 1981). When contemplating a union, parents, kin, and their advisors were generally concerned with a number of background questions. What was the young person's caste, status, family background, religion, and economic position? Did his or her family possess any property? How big was the dowry? Would the individual fit in with the entire family? In Indian families, for example, men and women observed that what their families cared most about in arranging a marriage was religion (whether one was a Hindu, Muslim, Sikh, or Christian), social class, education, and family background (Sprecher & Chandak, 1992). If things looked promising, parents and go-betweens began to talk about the exchange of property, dowries, the young couple's future obligations, and living arrangements.

Some problems were serious enough to rule out any thought of marriage. Sometimes religious advisors would chart the couples' horoscopes. Those born under the wrong sign might be forbidden to marry (Bumroongsook, 1992). Generally, young people were forbidden to marry anyone who was too closely related (say, a brother or sister, or a certain kind of cousin). Sometimes, they were forbidden to marry foreigners. (In Thailand, Thais are often forbidden to marry Chinese, Indian, Japanese, Mons, or Malay suitors [Bumroongsook, 1992].)

Similar assets and liabilities have been found to be important in a variety of countries—such as India (Prakasa & Rao, 1979; Sprecher & Chandak, 1992), Japan (Fukuda, 1991), Morocco (Joseph & Joseph, 1987), and Thailand (Bumroongsook, 1992).

Today, in many parts of the world, parents and matchmakers still arrange their children's marriages. Arranged marriages are common in India, in the Muslim countries, in sub-Saharan Africa, and in cultural enclaves throughout the remainder of the world (Rosenblatt & Anderson, 1981).

Compromising on Love

Cross-cultural surveys document the variety of types of mate selection systems that exist throughout the world (Goode, 1963; Goodwin, 1999; Rosenblatt, 1967; Stephens, 1963). These surveys indicate that currently, in most

of the world, prospective brides and grooms, parents, elders, and the extended family consult with one another before arranging a marriage.

The *Ethnographic Atlas* contains anthropological information on more than 1,000 preindustrial societies throughout the world. When Broude and Green (1983) sampled 186 of these groups, they found that in most societies, parents, kin, and young men and women are supposed to consult with one another in this most important of family decisions. In most societies, men have considerably more power than do women to determine their own fates. In only a minority of societies are men and women allowed complete power in choosing their own mates.

Today, even in the most traditional of societies, parents and husbands are generally forced to balance conflicting interests. The Moroccan tribal world, for example, is definitely a man's world. Men possess absolute authority over their wives and children. They possess the power take several wives. They often promise their sons and daughters to potential allies at very young ages. Yet, in families, things do not always happen as they are "supposed" to; men may in theory possess all the power, but in fact they do not. Joseph and Joseph's (1987) vivid descriptions of Moroccan family life make it clear that even in Morocco, compromise is often required. When "all powerful" Moroccan fathers try to force their children into unappealing marriages, sympathetic family members may employ an avalanche of strategies to thwart them. Young lovers may enlist an army of mothers, uncles, brothers, neighbors, and business partners to plead, threaten, and haggle on their behalf. Mothers may warn prospective brides about their sons' "faults." Young men may complain that an undesirable bride is a witch. Young men and women may threaten to kill themselves. Many young men and women rely on witchcraft or magical charms to get their way. Sometimes these desperate stratagems work; sometimes they do not.

Within a single society, arrangements often vary from ethnic group to ethnic group, class to class, region to region, and family to family (Bumroongsook, 1992).

Marriage for Love

In the West, romantic love has long been considered to be the *sine qua non* of marriage (Kelley et al., 1983; Sprecher et al., 1994).

In the mid-1960s, Kephart (1967) asked more than 1,000 American college students: "If a boy (girl) had all the other qualities you desired, would you marry this person if you were not in love with him (her)?" In that era, men and women were found to possess very different ideas as to the importance of romantic love in a marriage. Men considered passion to be essential (only 35% said they would marry someone they did not love). Women were more practical. They claimed that the absence of love would not necessarily deter them from considering marriage (a full 76% admitted they would be willing to marry someone they did not love). Kephart suggested that whereas men might have the luxury of marrying for love, women did not. A woman's status was dependent on that of her husband; thus, she had to be practical and take a potential mate's family background, professional status, and income into account.

Since the 1960s, sociologists have continued to ask young American men and women about the importance of romantic love. They have found that, year by year, young American men and women increasingly value and demand more and more of love. In the most recent research, 86% of American men and a full 91% of American women answered the question of whether they would wed without love with a resounding "No!" (Allgeier & Wiederman, 1991). Obviously, in the West, romantic love *is* considered to be a prerequisite for marriage. Today, American men and women assume that romantic love is so important, they claim that if they fell out of love, they would not even consider *staying* married (Simpson, Campbell, & Berscheid, 1986)! Some social commentators have suggested that with more experience, these young romantics might find that they are willing to "settle" for less than they think they would, but as of yet there is no evidence to indicate that this is so.

How do young men and women in other countries feel about this issue? Many cultural psychologists have pointed out that cultural values have a profound impact on how people feel about the wisdom of love matches versus arranged marriages.

Throughout the world, arranged marriages are still relatively common. It seems reasonable to argue that in societies such as China (Pimentel, 2000; Xu & Whyte, 1990), India (Sprecher & Chandak, 1992), and Japan (Sprecher et al., 1994), where arranged marriages are fairly typical, they ought to be viewed more positively than in the West, where they are relatively rare.

To test this notion, Sprecher and her colleagues (1994), asked American, Russian, and Japanese students: "If a person had all the other qualities you desired, would you marry him or her if you were not in love?" (Students could answer only "yes" or "no.") The authors assumed that only Americans would demand love *and* marriage; they predicted that both the Russians and the Japanese would be more practical. They were wrong! Both the Americans and the Japanese were romantics. Few of them would consider marrying someone they did not love (only 11% of Americans and 18% of the Japanese said "yes"). The Russians were more practical; 37% said they would accept such a proposal. Russian *men* were only slightly more practical than men in other countries. It was the Russian *women* who were most likely to "settle."

Despite the larger proportion of Russian women willing to enter a loveless marriage, a large majority of individuals in the three cultures would refuse to marry someone they did not love.

Similarly, in a landmark study, Levine, Sato, Hashimoto, and Verma (1995) asked college students in 11 different nations if they would be willing to marry someone they did not love, even if that person had all the other qualities they desired. (Students could answer "yes," "no," or admit that they were "undecided"). In affluent nations such as the United States, Brazil, Australia, Japan, and England, young people were insistent on love as a prerequisite for marriage. Only in traditional, collectivist, undeveloped nations, such as the Philippines, Thailand, India, and Pakistan, were students willing to compromise and marry someone they did not love. In these societies, of course, the extended family is still extremely important and poverty is widespread.

Research suggests that, today, young men and women in many countries throughout the world consider love to be a prerequisite for courtship and marriage. It is primarily in Eastern, collectivist, and poorer countries that passionate love remains a bit of a luxury.

HOW LONG DOES PASSIONATE LOVE LAST?

Passion sometimes burns itself out. Consider this exchange between anthropologist Shostak (1981) and a !Kung (African) tribesman as they observed a young married couple, running after each other:

> As I stood watching, I noticed the young man sitting in the shade of a tree, also watching. I said, "They're very much in love, aren't they?" He answered, "Yes, they are." After a pause, he added, "For now." I asked him to explain, and he said, "When two people are first together, their hearts are on fire and their passion is very great. After a while, the fire cools and that's how it stays." . . . "They continue to love each other, but it's in a different way—warm and dependable." . . . How long did this take? "It varies among couples. A few months, usually; sometimes longer. But it always happens." Was it also true for a lover? "No," he explained, "feelings for a lover stay intense much longer, sometimes for years." (p. 268)

Fisher (2004) argues that the transient nature of passionate love is a cultural universal. She believes that our *Homo sapiens* ancestors experienced passionate love and sexual desire for very practical genetic reasons. Our hominid ancestors were primed to fall ardently, sexually in love for about 4 years. This is precisely the amount of time it takes to conceive a child and take care of it until it is old enough to survive on its own. (In tribal societies, children are relatively self-sufficient by this age. By this time, they generally prefer to spend most of their time playing with other children.) Once our ancestors no longer had a practical reason to remain together, they had every evolutionary reason to fall out of love with their previous partner and to fall in love with someone new. Why were people programmed to engage in such serial pair-bonding? Fisher maintained that such serial monogamy produces maximum genetic diversity, which is an evolutionary advantage. To test her hypothesis that, generally, love is fleeting, Fisher (1989) examined the divorce rates in collecting/hunting, agricultural, pastoral, fishing, and industrial societies, scouring ethnographic records and the *Demographic Yearbooks* of the United Nations. She found that, as predicted, throughout the world, couples most commonly divorced in their fourth year of marriage. She argues that, today, the same evolutionary forces that influenced our ancestors shape the modern cross-cultural pattern of marriage–divorce–remarriage. Fisher's ideas are stimulating, but her exclusion of cultural forces considering their omnipresence in nearly all matters related to love and sex, mandate a certain skepticism on the part of the reader.

THE DARK SIDE OF PASSIONATE LOVE: JEALOUSY

What is jealousy? Social commentators have argued that jealousy consists of two basic components: bruised pride and indignation at the violation of one's property rights.

Anthropologist Mead (1931) contended that jealousy is really little more than wounded pride. The more shaky one's self-esteem, the more vulnerable one is to jealousy's pangs. She observed: "Jealousy is not a barometer by which depth of love can be read. It merely records the degree of the lover's insecurity. . . . It is a negative, miserable state of feeling, having its origin in the sense of insecurity and inferiority" (pp. 120–121). Researchers in the United States, Israel, and the Netherlands have found that people with low self-esteem *are* especially susceptible to jealousy (Bringle & Buunk, 1986; Nadler & Dotan, 1992; White & Mullen, 1989).

The French philosopher René Descartes, writing in the early 17th century, defined jealousy as "a kind of fear related to a desire to preserve a possession (cited in Davis, 1948/1977, p. 129). Researchers in several countries have found that a loss—whether one thinks of one's romantic partner or mate as a beloved person or a mere possession—can stir up jealousy (White & Mullen, 1989). Researchers in Israel (Nadler & Dotan, 1992) and the Netherlands (Bringle & Buunk, 1986) found that individuals experience the most jealousy and the most severe physiological reactions (trembling, increased pulse rate, nausea), when an affair poses a serious threat to their dating or marital relationship.

Berscheid and Fei (1977) provide evidence that both factors (low self-esteem and the fear of loss) are important in fueling jealous passion. They found that the more insecure men and women are, the more dependent they are on their romantic partners and mates, and the more seriously their relationship is threatened, the more fierce their jealousy.

Gender Differences in Jealousy: Evolutionary Theory

What Makes Men and Women Jealous?

Evolutionary psychologists such as Buss (1994), Tooby and Cosmides (1992), and Wilson and Daly (1992) argue that "the specifics of evolutionary biology have a central significance for understanding human thought and action. Evolutionary processes are the "architect" that assembled, detail by detail, our evolved psychological and physiological architecture" (Tooby & Cosmides, 1992, p. 19).

In attempting to understand cultural differences and the factors that predispose cultures to view love and emotional and sexual fidelity as more or less essential, we would do well to look to mankind's evolutionary heritage and the adaptive problems our ancestors attempted to solve by devising jealousy.

For example, according to Buss (1994), in the course of evolution, men and women have been programmed to differ markedly in the kinds of things that incite jealousy. Men can never know for sure whether the children they *think* are theirs (and in which they choose to invest their all), are really their own. Thus, men should find sexual infidelity the most worrying. Women, on the other hand, know that any children they conceive are theirs. Thus, they should care far less about their mates' sexual liaisons. What worries *them* is the possibility that their mates may be forming a *deep, emotional attachment* to a rival and squandering scarce resources on another.

As Wilson and Daly (1992) observed:

> In the case of *Homo sapiens*, parental investments are often substantial, including allocations of time and effort and transfers of resources over the course of decades. Thus a major threat to a man's fitness is the possibility that his mate may become pregnant by another man, especially if the cuckold should fail to detect the fact and invest in the child as his own. If there is a corresponding threat to a woman's fitness . . . it is that her mate will channel resources to other women and their children. It follows that men's and women's proprietary feelings toward their mates are likely to have evolved to be qualitatively different, men being more intensely concerned with sexual infidelity per se and women being more intensely concerned with the allocation of their mates' resources and attentions. (p. 292)

Scientists have also collected sparse evidence that in men, cuckoldry and sexual infidelity incite the most jealousy, while in women, it is their husbands' spending time talking and sharing common interests or resources with other women that is most upsetting (Buss & Schmitt, 1993; Glass & Wright, 1985).

How Do Men and Women React to Jealous Provocations?

Researchers have found that men and women may react in somewhat different ways to jeal-

ous provocation. Israeli psychologists Nadler and Dotan (1992), for example, found that when jealous, men tend to concentrate on shoring up their sagging self-esteem. Jealous women are more likely to try to do something to strengthen the relationship. Bryson (1977) speculated that these gender differences may well be due to the fact that most societies are patriarchal. It is acceptable for men to initiate relationships. Thus, when men are threatened, they can easily go elsewhere. Women do not have the same freedom. Therefore, they devote their energies to keeping the relationship from foundering. Studies in a variety of countries—including Israel (Nadler & Dotan, 1992) and the Netherlands (Buunk, 1982)—have found that these same gender differences exist in many parts of the world.

Alas, when Harris (2003) conducted a "meta-analysis" of more than 100 studies designed to determine whether there were gender differences in what sparked jealousy, she found little support for this contention. Harris reviewed men's and women's self-reports and psychophysiological reactions, as well as data on morbid jealousy, spousal abuse, and jealousy-inspired homicides in a variety of jealousy provoking situations. In summarizing this voluminous research, she was forced to conclude: "The results provide little support for the claim that men and women are innately wired to be differentially upset by emotional and sexual infidelity" (p. 117). Jankowiak (1995) agrees. He argues that men and women in all cultures find both emotional and sexual infidelity extremely upsetting. It is male power, he contends, not innate gender differences, that accounts for differences in men's and women's willingness to express their jealous feelings.

In attempting to explain why there might *not* be a dimorphic sexual jealousy mechanism, Harris (2003) makes two important points: (1) Our ancestral past may have been significantly different from the one envisioned by evolutionary theorists; and (2) even if the adaptive problems were as described, more *general* jealousy mechanisms may have been selected for, rather than the hardwired *specific module* postulated.

Alas, there exists no spaceship that will allow scientists to travel back to the Pleistocene, so we can observe how our hunter–gather forebears lived. In part, we scholars are forced to make up "just so" stories about the past—plausible stories, to be sure, but stories nonetheless. In fact, evolutionary theorists *have* postulated many alternative views of love relationships during the Pleistocene, including the following ideas: (1) That men invested very little in child rearing, versus (2) a significant paternal involvement in childbearing was a key factor in determining the number of viable offspring that lived to reproduce; thus, men were motivated to devote a great deal of time, energy, and resources to child rearing. Harris (2003) lists a number of these possibilities. If the Pleistocene adaptive solutions were different than those we currently envision, then they would, of course, lead to different cognitive structures in today's men and women. Only if cultural and evolutionary theorists work hand in hand will scientists be able to develop compelling theories of human behavior—theories that respect both the "architecture" of the past and the cultural challenges to be met by men and women of the future.

Let us now turn to some of the discoveries of cultural theorists in the area of jealousy.

Cultural Differences in Jealousy

Anthropologists have noted that cultures differ markedly in what sets off jealousy, in how jealous people get, and in whether they have the power to do anything about it (Hupka & Ryan, 1990; Hupka, 1991).

What Sparks Jealousy?

Men and women use a number of clues to tell them that someone they love is drifting away. Hupka (1981) illustrated the point that cultures define very different things as threats to self-esteem, relationships, and property with the following scenario:

> On her return trip from the local watering well, a married woman is asked for a cup of water by a male resident of the village. Her husband, resting on the porch of their dwelling, observes his wife giving the man a cup of water. Subsequently, they approach the husband and the three of them enjoy a lively and friendly conversation into the late evening hours. Eventually the husband puts out the lamp, and the guest has sexual intercourse with the wife. The next morning the husband leaves the house early in order to catch fish for breakfast. Upon his return he finds his wife having sex again with the guest. The husband becomes violently enraged and mortally stabs the guest.
>
> At what point in the vignette may one expect the husband to be jealous? It depends, of course, in which culture we place the husband. A husband

of the Pawnee Indian tribe in the 19th century bewitched any man who dared to request a cup of water from his wife. . . . An Ammassalik Eskimo husband, on the other hand, offered his wife to a guest by means of the culturally sanctioned game of "putting out the lamp." A good host was expected to turn out the lamp at night, as an invitation for the guest to have sexual intercourse with the wife. The Ammassalik, however, became intensely jealous when his wife copulated with a guest in circumstances other than the lamp game or without a mutual agreement between two families to exchange mates, and it was not unusual for the husband to kill the interloper.

> The Toda of Southern India, who were primarily polyandrous at the turn of the century . . . would consider the sequence of events described in the vignette to be perfectly normal. That is to say, the husband would not have been upset to find his wife having sexual relations again in the morning if the man were her *mokhthodvaiol*. The Todas had the custom of *mokhthoditi* which allowed husbands and wives to take on lovers. When, for instance, a man wanted someone else's wife as a lover he sought the consent of the wife and her husband or husbands. If consent was given by all, the men negotiated for the annual fee to be received by the husband(s). The woman then lived with the man just as if she were his real wife. Or more commonly, the man visited the woman at the house of her husband(s).
>
> It is evident from these illustrations that the culture of a society is a more potent variable than characteristics of the individual in predicting which events someone will evaluate as a threat. (pp. 324–325)

Buunk and Hupka (1987) found that there are also cultural differences in the kinds of things that trigger jealousy in modern, industrialized nations. They interviewed 2,079 college students from seven industrialized nations—the United States, Hungary, Ireland, Mexico, the Netherlands, the Soviet Union, and Yugoslavia (the Soviet Union and Yugoslavia no longer exist as nations). Students were asked to take a look at several statements: *flirting* ("It does not bother me when I see my lover flirting with someone else"); *kissing* ("When I see my lover kissing someone else, my stomach knots up"); *dancing* ("When my lover dances with someone else, I feel very uneasy"); *hugging* ("When somebody hugs my lover, I get sick inside"); *sexual relationships* ("It would bother me if my partner frequently had satisfying sexual relations with someone else"); and *sexual fantasy* ("It is entertaining to hear the sexual fantasies my partner has about another person"). They were then asked to indicate to what extent they agreed with each of these statements.

There were some striking cross-national similarities in the kinds of things that people found threatening or nonthreatening. Behaviors such as dancing, hugging, and talking about sexual fantasies were taken in stride. Explicit erotic behavior—flirting, kissing, or having sexual relations with someone else—evoked strong jealousy.

There were some striking cultural differences in *exactly* what people found upsetting, however. United States citizens for example, took "hugging" for granted. They were about average in how upsetting they found the other activities to be. In the Netherlands, kissing, hugging, and dancing evoked less jealousy than in most other countries, but citizens got more upset by the idea of their partner's having sexual fantasies about other people than did others. In Yugoslavia, flirting evoked a more negative emotional response than in any other country, but citizens were least concerned about sexual fantasies or kissing. Hungarians found both hugging and kissing most provoking. Citizens from the Soviet Union were upset by dancing and sexual relations.

The next step, Buunk and Hupka (1987) observed, is to find out why such cultural and cross-national differences exist.

Intensity of Jealousy

Hupka and Ryan (1990; Hupka, 1991) argued that a culture's social structure should have a marked impact on how vulnerable its members are to jealousy. Consider two tribes: the Ammassalik Eskimos (known for their extreme jealousy) and the Toda tribe of India (known for their startling lack of jealousy). The Ammassalik Eskimo family had to be completely self-sufficient (Mirsky, 1937). Each couple had to produce everything that they needed to survive—shelter, clothing, food, and utensils. Loners rarely survived the long, harsh Arctic winters. It is not surprising to discover that the Ammassalik were eager, if not desperate, to find a competent mate. No wonder that those who did had problems with jealousy. A passionate rival was literally a threat to survival.

The Todas of India, on the other hand, had a clan economy (Rivers, 1906). Marriage was a luxury, not a necessity. (The most common form of marriage was fraternal polyandry:

When a woman married, she became the wife of all her husband's brothers.) Not surprisingly, people did not distinguish much between their own children and those of other tribesmen (of course, men had no way of knowing who was the father of "their" children). Companions for friendship and for sex were easy to find. The clan worked together on most tasks and shared everything. The idea of "private" property did not really exist. Not surprisingly, in this society, jealousy was rare.

Hupka and Ryan (1990) argued that there is a simple explanation for such findings. In any culture, the greater the importance of marriage and private property, the more the marital partners are jealous of potential romantic rivals. To test this notion, the authors selected 150 tribal societies from those described in the Human Relations Area Files. The scientists then classified societies' political and economic customs: How important was it to be married? (Was it, for example, necessary for survival?) How easy was it to find sex outside of marriage? How important was private property? (Was everything owned in common? Privately owned? Was theft punished?) How important was it to have children?

Next, the authors coded the extent of jealousy in each society. In some, men generally had little reaction when they heard their mates had been unfaithful. In others, such as the Maori of New Zealand (Mishkin, 1937), husbands demanded money or valuable property from their wives' lovers. If a Bakongo adulterer could not pay the compensation, he had to work the husband's fields, as well as his own. This generally ensured that he would be too exhausted to chase women (White & Mullen, 1989). In other cultures, infidelity was cause for separation or divorce. In some, the adulterous spouse or rival was banished or killed. For example, the ancient Hebrews would stone to death a married woman and her lover if the affair took place in the city. In the country, it was assumed that the woman had been raped but no one had heard her screams; hence, only the man was killed (Murstein, 1974).

The authors found that culture, and the severity of the threat[2] that adultery posed in that culture, had a powerful impact on how men reacted to their wives' adultery. It was culture, not genes, that determined the nature of men's response to news that their wives were having an affair. Would they react with a shrug, with indignation, or with murderous violence? Much depended on the place they called home.

The data also highlighted the importance of power in determining how people respond to jealous provocations. In most tribes, women, who were usually physically weaker than men, had less political and economic power. Although neither men nor women liked infidelity, only the men were in a position to do much about it. In general, women were "supposed" to respond to adultery with only the gentlest forms of aggression. They could express righteous indignation, cry, threaten to walk out, or divorce. The men were allowed to bring out the really big guns: when offended, to banish or murder their mates.

How the Jealous React

Salovey and Rodin (1985) surveyed 25,000 Americans (heterosexual, bisexual, and homosexual) from a variety of ethnic groups. How had they reacted the last time they were jealous? Although men and women differed little, heterosexuals (possibly because of their views of commitment) had a more passionate reaction than did their gay, lesbian, or bisexual peers to provocation. Whatever their gender and orientation, however, jealous lovers described a variety of jealous behaviors: They became obsessed with painful images of their beloved in the arms of their rivals. They sought out confirmation of their worst fears. They searched through their partners' personal belongings for unfamiliar names and telephone numbers. They telephoned their mates unexpectedly, just to see whether they were where they had said they would be. They listened in on their telephone conversations and followed them. They gave their mates the third degree about previous or present romantic relationships.

Anthropologists find that people throughout the world engage in similar kinds of detective work: The Dobuan husband watches his wife while she works the fields and counts her footsteps if she goes into the bush. Too many footsteps mean a possibility of a secret sexual liaison (Mead, 1931). Apache men who leave their encampment generally ask their close blood relatives to spy on their wives (Goodwin, 1942). White and Mullen (1989) found that people try to cope with their jealous feelings, the threats to their self-esteem, and their fears of loss in a variety of ways: Sometimes lovers refuse to see what they do not want to see. Some jealous lovers focus on *themselves*.

"What's wrong with me?" or "What did I do wrong?" they ask. Once they spot "the problem," they set out to try to make themselves more appealing. Other people focus on controlling *their mates*. In Medieval times, British and European nobility locked their wives up in chastity belts while they were off at the Crusades. Other cultures have relied on infibulation (stitching together the labia majora), vaginal plugs, and clitoridectomy (a form of female castration designed to eliminate sexual pleasure), to keep women in check (Daly, Wilson, & Weghorst, 1982). Other lovers focus on eliminating *the rival*.

Eventually, in most societies, most people give up. If the relationship really is over, they recognize it and try to get on with their lives.

Vengeance

Of course, some jealous lovers react more violently. In the 17th century, Burton (1621/1927) wrote in *The Anatomy of Melancholy* that "those which are jealous proceed from suspicion to hatred; from hatred to frenzie; from frenzie to injurie, murder and despair" (p. 428). Historically, since men had the most power, they were allowed to let their "frenzie" lead to murder. Women had to be content with more tepid responses.

Arapaho (Native American) men might beat wives they suspected of having sexual relations with anyone else:

> Occasionally a suspicious man calmly sent his wife away, either to her paramour or to her home. More often he became angry and jealous. Usually he whipped her, and cut off the tip of her nose or her braids, or both. According to Kroeber . . . he also slashed her cheeks. This treatment of an unfaithful wife was conventional and neither her parents nor the tribe did anything about it. (Hilger, 1952, p. 212)

The king of the Plateau tribes of Zimbabwe executed men caught with any of his wives. The wives were grossly mutilated (Gouldsbury & Sheane, 1911). In earlier times, Apache husbands also killed their rivals and mutilated their wives (by cutting off the end of their noses); presumably, that made them less appealing the next time (G. Goodwin, 1942).

In Western cultures, men are far more likely to beat or murder their girlfriends and wives than their rivals (White & Mullen, 1989). Today, in America, family peace centers report that about two-thirds of wives who are forced to seek shelter do so because their husbands' excessive or unwarranted jealousy has led them to repeatedly assault the women (Gayford, 1979). Male jealousy is the leading cause of wife battering and homicide worldwide (Buss, 1994; Daly & Wilson, 1988a, 1988b).

In the West, until recently, such vengeance was approved or treated leniently. The 18th-century English jurist Blackstone commented that killing in a situation where a man or woman is caught in the act "is of the lowest degree of manslaughter; . . . for there could not be a greater provocation" (quoted in Smith & Hogan, 1983, p. 288).

In many countries, the courts have been sympathetic to such "crimes of passion." Traditionally, it was considered to be a man's right to defend his "honor." In Morocco, for example, the law excuses killing one's wife if she is caught in the act of adultery, but a woman would not be excused for killing her husband in the same circumstances (Greenhouse, 1994). In São Paulo (Brazil's most populous city), in 1980–1981, 722 men claimed "defense of honor" for murdering their wives. Brazilian women adopted the slogan "Lovers don't kill," and campaigned against allowing such a defense in murder trials. Once again, we see that, worldwide, the times they are a changing (see Brooke, 1991, for a discussion of the changes globalization has brought to views of "honor" and crimes of violence in one culture—Brazil).

IN CONCLUSION

The preceding studies, then, suggest that the large differences that once existed between Westernized, modern, urban, industrial societies and Eastern, modern, urban industrial societies may be fast disappearing. Those interested in cross-cultural differences may be forced to search for large differences in only the most underdeveloped, developing, and collectivist of societies—such as in Africa or Latin America, in China or the Arab countries (Egypt, Kuwait, Lebanon, Libya, Saudi Arabia, Iraq, or the United Arab Emirates).

However, it may well be that even there, the winds of Westernization, individualism, and social change are blowing. In spite of the censure of their elders, in a variety of traditional cultures, young people are increasingly adopting "Western" patterns—placing a high value on "falling in love," pressing for gender equality in love and sex, and insisting on marrying for love (as opposed to arranged marriages). Such changes have been documented in Finland, Estonia, and Russia (Haavio-Mannila & Kontula, 2003), as well as among Australian aboriginal people of Mangrove and a Copper Inuit Alaskan Indian tribe (see Jankowiak, 1995, for an extensive review of this research).

Naturally, cultural differences still exert a profound influence on young people's attitudes, emotions, and behavior, and such differences are not likely to disappear in our lifetime. In Morocco, for example, marriage was once an alliance between families (as it was in most of the world before the 18th century,) in which children had little or no say. Today, although parents can no longer simply dictate whom their children will marry, parental approval remains critically important. Important though it is, however, young men and women are at least allowed to have their say (see D. A. Davis & Davis, 1995).

Many have observed that, today, two powerful forces—globalization and cultural pride/identification with one's country (what historians call "nationalism")—are contending for men's and women's souls. True, to some extent, the world's citizens may to some extent be becoming "one," but in truth, the delightful and divisive cultural variations that have made our world such an interesting and simultaneously dangerous place, are likely to add spice to that heady brew of love and sexual practices for some time to come. The convergence of cultures around the world may be reducing the differences in the ways passionate love is experienced and expressed in our world, but tradition can be tenacious, and the global future of passionate love cannot be predicted with any certainty.

NOTES

1. Supporting the contention that prehistoric people were monogamous is the fact that today men and women are fairly similar in size. Supporting the contention (more strongly) that our ancestors were polygamous are the following: (1) Men are generally taller and stronger than are women; (2) because selection is based on physical strength and body mass, not sperm competition, men's testes are fairly small; (3) women do not possess sexual swellings; and (4) sexual intercourse can last fairly long, because there are not many rivals competing for access.

2. The authors judged sexual dalliance to be most threatening if in that culture (1) marriage was required for companionship, status, or survival; (2) it was difficult to find sex outside of marriage; (3) property is privately owned; and (4) it was important to have children.

REFERENCES

Allgeier, E. R., & Wiederman, M. W. (1991). Love and mate selection in the 1990s. *Free Inquiry, 11*, 25–27.

Aron, A., Fisher, H. E., Mashek, D. J., Strong, G., Li, H., & Brown, L. L. (2005). Reward, motivation, and emotion systems associated with early-stage intense romantic love. *Journal of Neuropsychology, 94*, 327–337.

Aron, A., & Rodriguez, G. (1992, July 25). *Scenarios of falling in love among Mexican-, Chinese-, and Anglo-Americans.* Paper presented at the Sixth International Conference on Personal Relationships, Orono, ME.

Barkow, J. H., Cosmides, L., & Tooby, J. (Eds.). (1992). *The adapted mind: Evolutionary psychology and the generation of culture.* New York: Oxford University Press.

Bartels, A., & Zeki, S. (2000, November 27). The neural basis of romantic love. *Neuroreport, 11*, 3829–3834.

Bartels, A., & Zeki, S. (2004). The neural correlates of maternal and romantic love. *NeuroImage, 21*, 1155–1166.

Berscheid, E., & Fei, J. (1977). Romantic love and sexual jealousy. In G. Clanton & L. G. Smith (Eds.), *Jealousy* (pp. 101–114). Englewood Cliffs, NJ: Prentice-Hall.

Birbaumer, N., Lutzenberger, W., Elbert, T., Flor, H., & Rockstroh, B. (1993) Imagery and brain processes. In N. Birbaumer & A. Öhman (Eds.), *The structure of emotion* (pp. 132–134). Göttingen, Germany: Hogrefe & Huber.

Bringle, R. G., & Buunk, B. (1986). Examining the causes and consequences of jealousy: Some recent findings and issues. In R. Gilmour & S. Duck (Eds.), *The emerging field of personal relationships* (pp. 225–240). Hillsdale, NJ: Erlbaum.

Brooke, J. (1991, March 29). "Honor" killing of wives is outlawed in Brazil. *The New York Times*, p. B-16.

Broude, G. J., & Green, S. J. (1983). Cross-cultural codes on husband–wife relationships. *Ethology, 22*, 273–274.

Bryson, J. B. (1977, August). Situational determinants of the expression of jealousy. In H. Sigall (Chair), Sexual Jealousy Symposium presented at the 85th meeting of the American Psychological Association, San Francisco, CA.

Bumroongsook, S. (1992). *Conventions of mate selection in twentieth-century central Thailand.* Unpublished Master's thesis, Department of History, University of Hawaii, Honolulu.

Burton, R. (1927). *The anatomy of melancholy.* London: Longman. (Original work published 1621)

Buss, D. M. (1994). *The evolution of desire.* New York: Basic Books.

Buss, D. M., & Schmitt, D. P. (1993). Sexual strategies theory: An evolutionary perspective on human mating. *Psychological Review, 100*, 204–232.

Buunk, B. (1982). Anticipated sexual jealousy: Its relationship to self-esteem, dependency, and reciprocity. *Personality and Social Psychology Bulletin, 8*, 310–316.

Buunk, B., & Hupka, R. B. (1987). Cross-cultural differences in the elicitation of sexual jealousy. *Journal of Sex Research, 23*, 12–22.

Capellanus, A. (1957). *The art of courtly love.* New York: Ungar. (Original work published 1174)

Carter, C. S. (1998). Neuroendocrine perspectives on social attachment and love. *Psychoneuroendocrinology, 23*, 779–818.

Chu, G. C. (1985). The changing concept of self in contemporary China. In A. J. Marsella, G. DeVos, & F. L. K. Hus (Eds.), *Culture and self: Asian and Western perspectives* (pp. 252–277). London: Tavistock.

Chu, G. C., & Ju, Y. (1993). *The great wall in ruins.* Albany: State University of New York Press.

Cohen, D. (2001). Cultural variation: Considerations and implications. *Psychological Bulletin, 127*, 451–471.

Daily, M., & Wilson, M. (1998a). Evolutionary and social psychology and family homicide. *Science, 28*, 519–524.

Daly, M., Wilson, M., & Weghorst, S. J. (1982). Male sexual jealousy. *Ethology and Sociobiology, 3*, 11–27.

Darwin, C. (1871). *The descent of man and selection in relation to sex.* London: Murray.

Davis, D. A., & Davis, S. S. (1995). Possessed by love: gender and romance in Morocco. In William Jankowiak (Ed.), *Romantic passion: A universal experience?* (pp. 219–238). New York: Columbia University Press.

Davis, K. (1977). Jealousy and sexual property. In G. Clanton & L. G. Smith (Eds.), *Jealousy* (pp. 129–135). Englewood Cliffs, NJ: Prentice Hall. (Original work published 1948)

Diamond, L. M. (2004). Emerging perspectives on distinctions between romantic love and sexual desire. *Current Directions in Psychological Science, 13*, 116–119.

Dion, K. K., & Dion, K. L. (1993). Individualistic and collectivistic perspectives on gender and the cultural context of love and intimacy. *Journal of Social Issues, 49*, 53–69.

Doherty, R. W., Hatfield, E., Thompson, K., & Choo, P. (1994). Cultural and ethnic influences on love and attachment. *Personal Relationships, 1*, 391–398.

Doi, L. T. (1963). Some thoughts on helplessness and the desire to be loved. *Psychiatry, 26*, 266–272.

Doi, L. T. (1973). *The anatomy of dependence* (J. Bester, Trans.). Tokyo: Kodansha International.

Fischer, K. W., Shaver, P. R., & Carnochan, P. (1990).

How emotions develop and how they organize development. *Cognition and Emotion, 4,* 81–127.

Fischer, K. W., Wang, L., Kennedy, B., & Cheng, C.-L. (1998). Culture and biology in emotional development: Socioemotional development across cultures. *New Directions for Child Development, 82,* 20–43.

Fisher, H. E. (1989). Evolution of human serial pairbonding. *American Journal of Physical Anthropology, 78,* 331–354.

Fisher, H. E. (2003, July 16). *The brain chemistry of romantic attraction and its positive effect on sexual motivation.* Paper presented at the 29th annual meeting of the International Academy of Sex Research, Bloomington, IN.

Fisher, H. E. (2004). *Why we love: The nature and chemistry of romantic love.* New York: Holt.

Fukuda, N. (1991). Women in Japan. In L. L. Adler (Ed.), *Women in cross-cultural perspective* (pp. 205–219). Westport, CT: Praeger.

Gayford, J. J. (1979). Battered wives. *British Journal of Hospital Medicine, 22,* 496, 503.

Gil, V. E. (1992). Clinical notes: The cut sleeve revisited: A brief ethnographic interview with a male homosexual in mainland China. *Journal of Sex Research, 29,* 569–577.

Glass, S. P., & Wright, T. L. (1985). Sex differences in type of extramarital involvement and marital dissatisfaction. *Sex Roles, 12,* 1101–1120.

Goode, W. J. (1959). The theoretical importance of love. *American Sociological Review, 24,* 38–47.

Goode, W. J. (1963). *World revolution and family patterns.* New York: Free Press.

Goodwin, G. (1942). *The social organization of the Western Apache.* Chicago: University of Chicago Press.

Goodwin, R. (1999). *Personal relationships across cultures.* London: Routledge.

Gouldsbury, C., & Sheane, H. (1911). *The Great Plateau of Northern Rhodesia.* London: Arnold.

Greenhouse, S. (1994, February 3). State Dept. finds widespread abuse of world's women. *The New York Times,* pp. 1A–6A.

Haavio-Mannila, E., & Kontula, O. (2003). Single and double sexual standards in Finland, Estonia, and St. Petersburg. *Journal of Sex Research, 40,* 36–49.

Harris, C. R. (2003). A review of sex differences in sexual jealousy, including self-report data, psychophysiological responses, interpersonal violence, and morbid jealousy. *Personality and Social Psychology Review, 7,* 102–128.

Hatfield, E., & Rapson, R. L. (1987). Passionate love/sexual desire: Can the same paradigm explain both? *Archives of Sexual Behavior, 16,* 259–277.

Hatfield, E., & Rapson, R. L. (1993). *Love, sex, and intimacy: Their psychology, biology, and history.* New York: HarperCollins.

Hatfield, E., & Rapson, R. L. (1996). *Love and sex: Cross-cultural perspectives.* Boston, MA: Allyn & Bacon.

Hatfield, E., & Sprecher, S. (1986). Measuring passionate love in intimate relations. *Journal of Adolescence, 9,* 383–410.

Hatfield, E., & Sprecher, S. (1996). Men's and women's mate preferences in the United States, Russia, and Japan. *Journal of Cross-Cultural Psychology, 26,* 728–750.

Hendrick, C., & Hendrick, S. S. (1989). Research on love: Does it measure up? *Journal of Personality and Social Psychology, 56,* 784–794.

Hilger, M. I. (1952). *Arapaho child life and its cultural background.* Washington, DC: U.S. Government Printing Office.

Hrdy, S. B. (1999). *The woman that never evolved.* Cambridge, MA: Harvard University Press.

Hsu, F. L. K. (1953). *Americans and Chinese: Passage to difference* (3rd ed.). Honolulu: University Press of Hawaii.

Hsu, F. L. K. (1985). The self in cross-cultural perspective. In A. J. Marsella, G. DeVos, & F. L. K. Hsu (Eds.), *Culture and self: Asian and Western perspectives* (pp. 24–55). London: Tavistock.

Hunt, M. (1959). *The natural history of love.* New York: Grove Press.

Hupka, R. B. (1981). Cultural determinants of jealousy. *Alternative Lifestyles, 4,* 310–356.

Hupka, R. B. (1991). The motive for the arousal of romantic jealousy: Its cultural origin. In P. Salovey (Ed.), *The psychology of jealousy and envy* (pp. 252–270). New York: Guilford Press.

Hupka, R. B., & Ryan, J. M. (1990). The cultural contribution to jealousy: Cross-cultural aggression in sexual jealousy situations. *Behavior Science Research, 24,* 51–71.

Hyde, J. S. (Ed.). (2005). *Biological substrates of human sexuality.* Washington, DC: American Psychological Association.

Jankowiak, W. (Ed.). (1995). *Romantic passion: A universal experience?* New York: Columbia University Press.

Jankowiak, W. R., & Fischer, E. F. (1992). A cross-cultural perspective on romantic love. *Ethology, 31,* 149–155.

Joseph, R., & Joseph, T. B. (1987). *The rose and the thorn.* Tucson: University of Arizona Press.

Kelley, H. H., Berscheid, E., Christensen, A., Harvey, J. H., Huston, T. L., Levinger, G., et al. (Eds.). (1983). *Close relationships.* New York: Freeman.

Kephart, W. M. (1967). Some correlates of romantic love. *Journal of Marriage and the Family, 29,* 470–479.

Kim, J., & Hatfield, E. (2004). Love types and subjective well being. *Social Behavior and Personality: An International Journal, 32,* 173–182.

Kitayama, S. (2002). Culture and basic psychological processes—toward a system view of culture: Comment on Oyserman et al. (2002). *Psychological Bulletin, 128,* 89–96.

Komisaruk, B. R., & Whipple, B. (1998). Love as sensory stimulation: Physiological consequences of its deprivation and expression. *Psychoneuroendocrinology, 8,* 927–944.

Landis, D., & O'Shea, W. A. O., III. (2000). Cross-cultural aspects of passionate love: An individual difference analysis. *Journal of Cross-Cultural Psychology, 31,* 754–779.

Lee, G. R., & Stone, L. H. (1980). Mate-selection systems and criteria: Variation according to family structure. *Journal of Marriage and the Family, 42,* 319–326.

Levine, R., Sato, S., Hashimoto, T., & Verma, J. (1995). Love and marriage in eleven cultures. *Journal of Cross-Cultural Psychology, 26,* 554–571.

Linton, R. (1936). *The study of man.* New York: Appleton-Century.

Luciano, E. M. C. (2003). *Caribbean love and sex: Ethnographic study of rejection and betrayal in heterosexual relationships in Puerto Rico.* Paper presented at the 29th annual meeting of the International Academy of Sex Research Meeting, Bloomington, IN.

Mace, D., & Mace, V. (1980). *Marriage: East and West.* New York: Dolphin Books.

Markus, H. R., & Kitayama, S. (1991). Culture and self: Implications for cognition, emotion, and motivation. *Psychological Review, 98,* 224–253.

Marazziti, D., Akiskal, H. S., Rossi, A., & Cassano, G. B. (1999). Alteration of the platelet serotonin transporter in romantic love. *Psychological Medicine, 29*(3), 741–745.

Marazziti, D., & Canale, D. (2004). Hormonal changes when falling in love. *Psychoneuroendocrinology, 29*(7), 931–936.

Mead, M. (1931). Jealousy: Primitive and civilized. In S. D. Schmalhausen & V. F. Calverton (Eds.), *Woman's coming of age* (pp. 35–48). New York: Liveright.

Mirsky, J. (1937). The Eskimo of Greenland. In M. Mead (Ed.), *Cooperation and competition among primitive peoples* (pp. 51–86). New York: McGraw-Hill.

Mishkin, B. (1937). The Maori of New Zealand. In M. Mead (Ed.), *Cooperation and competition among primitive peoples* (pp. 428–457). New York: McGraw-Hill.

Money, J. (1977). Peking: The sexual revolution. In J. Money & H. Musaph (Eds.), *Handbook of sexology* (pp. 543–550). Amsterdam: Excerpta Medica.

Murstein, B. I. (1974). *Love, sex, and marriage through the ages.* New York: Springer.

Nadler, A., & Dotan, I. (1992). Commitment and rival attractiveness: Their effects on male and female reactions to jealousy arousing situations. *Sex Roles, 26,* 293–310.

Nisbett, R. (2003). *The geography of thought: How Asians and Westerners think differently . . . and why.* New York: Free Press.

Oysermann, D., Kemmelmeier, M., & Coon, H. M. (2002). Cultural psychology, a new look: Reply to Bond (2002), Fiske (2002), Kitayama (2002), and Miller. *Psychological Bulletin, 128,* 110–117.

Pimentel, E. E. (2000). Just how do I love thee?: Marital relations in urban China. *Journal of Marriage and the Family, 62,* 32–47.

Prakasa, V. V., & Rao, V. N. (1979). Arranged marriages: An assessment of the attitudes of the college students in India. In G. Kurian (Ed.), *Cross-cultural perspectives of mate-selection and marriage* (pp. 11–31). Westport, CT: Greenwood Press.

Regan, P. C., & Berscheid, E. (1999). *Lust: what we know about human sexual desire.* London: Sage.

Rivers, W. H. R. (1906). *The Todas.* London: Macmillan.

Rosenblatt, P. C. (1967). Marital residence and the function of romantic love. *Ethnology, 6,* 471–480.

Rosenblatt, P. C., & Anderson, R. M. (1981). Human sexuality in cross-cultural perspective. In M. Cook (Ed.), *The bases of human sexual attraction* (pp. 215–250). London: Academic Press.

Ruan, F. F. (1991). *Sex in China: Studies in sexology in Chinese culture.* New York: Plenum Press.

Salovey, P., & Rodin, J. (1985). The heart of jealousy. *Psychology Today, 19,* 22–29.

Shaver, P. R., & Hazan, C. (1988). A biased overview of the study of love. *Journal of Social and Personal Relationships, 5,* 474–501.

Shaver, P. R., Morgan, H. J., & Wu, S. (1996). Is love a "basic" emotion? *Personal Relationships, 3,* 81–96.

Shaver, P. R., Murdaya, U., & Fraley, R. C. (2001). Structure of the Indonesian emotion lexicon. *Asian Journal of Social Psychology, 4,* 201–224.

Shaver, P. R., Wu, S., & Schwartz, J. C. (1991). Cross-cultural similarities and differences in emotion and its representation: A prototype approach. In M. S. Clark (Ed.), *Review of personality and social psychology* (Vol. 13, pp. 175–212). Newbury Park, CA: Sage.

Shostak, M. (1981). *Nisa: The life and words of a !Kung woman.* Cambridge, MA: Harvard University Press.

Simmons, C. H., Vom Kolke, A., & Shimizu, H. (1986). Attitudes toward romantic love among American, German, and Japanese students. *Journal of Social Psychology, 126,* 327–337.

Simpson, J. A., Campbell, B., & Berscheid, E. (1986). The association between romantic love and marriage: Kephart (1967) twice revisited. *Personality and Social Psychology Bulletin, 12,* 363–372.

Smith, J. C., & Hogan, B. (1983). *Criminal law* (5th ed.). London: Butterworths.

Sommer, V. (1993, November 13). *Primate origins: The hardware of human sexuality.* Paper presented at the meeting of the Society for the Scientific Study of Sex, San Diego, CA.

Soueif, A. (1999). *The map of love.* London: Bloomsbury.

Sprecher, S., Aron, A., Hatfield, E., Cortese, A., Potapova, E., & Levitskaya, A. (1994). Love: American style, Russian style, and Japanese style. *Personal Relationships, 1,* 349–369.

Sprecher, S., & Chandak, R. (1992). Attitudes about arranged marriages and dating among men and women from India. *Free Inquiry in Creative Sociology, 20*, 1–11.

Stephens, W. N. (1963). *The family in cross-cultural perspective.* New York: Holt, Rinehart & Winston.

Sternberg, R. J. (1988). Triangulating love. In R. J. Sternberg & M. L. Barnes (Eds.), *The psychology of love* (pp. 119–138). New Haven, CT: Yale University Press.

Tannahill, R. (1980). *Sex in history.* New York: Stein & Day.

Tooby, J., & Cosmides, L. (1992). The evolutionary and psychological foundations of the social sciences. In J. H. Barkow, L. Cosmides, & J. Tooby (Eds.), *The adapted mind: Evolutionary psychology and the generation of culture* (pp. 19–136). New York: Oxford University Press.

Trawick, M. (1990). *Notes on love in a Tamil family.* Berkeley: University of California Press.

Triandis, H. C., McCusker, C., & Hui, C. H. (1990). Multimethod probes of individualism and collectiv-

ism. *Journal of Personality and Social Psychology, 59*, 1006–1020.

Wallen, K. (1989). Mate selection: Economics and affection. *Behavioral and Brain Sciences, 12*, 37–38.

Weaver, S. E., & Ganong, L. W. (2004). The factor structure of the Romantic Belief Scale for African Americans and European Americans. *Journal of Social and Personal Relationships, 21*, 171–185.

White, G. L., & Mullen, P. E. (1989). *Jealousy: Theory, research, and clinical strategies.* New York: Guilford Press.

Wilson, M., & Daly, M. (1992). The man who mistook his wife for a chattel. In J. H. Barkow, L. Cosmides, & J. Tooby (Eds.), *The adapted mind: Evolutionary psychology and the generation of culture* (pp. 289–326). New York: Oxford University Press.

Wolkstein, D. (1991). *The first love stories.* New York: Harper Perennial.

Xu, X., & Whyte, M. K. (1990). Love matches and arranged marriages: A Chinese replication. *Journal of Marriage and the Family, 52*, 709–722.

CHAPTER 32

Emotion, Biology, and Culture

ROBERT W. LEVENSON
JOSE SOTO
NNAMDI POLE

In this chapter we first review theories of emotion that are most relevant to a consideration of the roles of biology and culture. We then review the existing cross-cultural and cross-ethnic research relevant to these theories, with particular emphasis on studies that have actually measured biological responses that occur during emotional reactions. We conclude by presenting a revised version of our earlier biocultural model of emotion (Levenson, 2003) that allows for both biological and cultural influences, and that is informed by existing empirical data.

EMOTION THEORY

Emotions are short-lived psychological–physiological phenomena that represent efficient modes of adaptation to changing environmental demands (Levenson, 1994). In humans, the emotion system is influenced by both biology (e.g., the availability of a facial musculature that can produce an array of appearance changes) and culture (e.g., the rules, traditions, and beliefs concerning how and when to use these muscles to reveal or conceal how we feel).

Emotion theorists have long struggled with how to account for both kinds of influence. In general, theories growing out of the evolutionary tradition embrace biological influences, viewing specific features of the emotion system as chosen by natural selection for their value in survival and reproduction. In contrast, theories growing out of the anthropological tradition embrace cultural influences, viewing emotion as created in ways that meet cultural traditions, beliefs, and values. Although most modern theories eschew extreme evolutionary and cultural construction positions, they differ greatly in terms of how they locate emotion between these poles.

Evolutionary Theories

Darwin pioneered the evolutionary view of emotions in his book *The Expression of the Emotions in Man and Animals* (1872), portraying emotional expression as a hardwired, automatic response that is integrally tied to the nervous system. A large part of his research program was devoted to documenting the existence of emotional facial expressions and gestures that were common across cultures and species—that is, to demonstrating the universality of emotional expression. Interestingly, despite recognizing the important communicative functions of emotional expression, he never focused on how individuals label their emotions. This likely reflected his commitment to a cross-species approach. Although not totally discounting the role of culture in emotion, Darwin did not afford it great importance.

Physiological Theories

Near the turn of the century, two influential theories arose that emphasized the critical role that physiological responses played in emotion. James (1884) suggested that emotions derive from the body's patterned response to challenging situations (e.g., "I feel afraid because I am trembling"). This peripheralist view envisioned autonomic and somatic nervous system activity as antecedents rather than as consequences of emotion. Cannon (1927) took a different view, believing that emotions originate in the central nervous system, with the resulting emotional experience growing out of unconscious neurological activity. Although differing in their views as to the source of emotion and the role of conscious awareness, both approaches viewed physiological changes as primary determinants of emotion. Facial expressions were not explicitly considered by James or Cannon, and neither theory was very conducive to cultural influence.

Schachter and Singer (1962) proposed another physiologically based theory of emotion that was far more amenable to cultural influence. In their view, the physiological arousal associated with emotion is essentially undifferentiated. The individual perceives this arousal and labels it as a particular emotion based on a cognitive appraisal of the current situation. From this perspective, physiology is integral to emotion, but the appraisal process is key to determining the specific emotion that occurred. Although Schachter and Singer did not explore cultural influences in any depth, their appraisal process certainly allows for culturally determined variation in how the meaning of a given situation is understood.

Social Construction Theories

In *Sex and Temperament in Three Primitive Societies* (1935), anthropologist Mead wrote: "We are forced to conclude that human nature

is almost unbelievably malleable, responding accurately and contrastingly to contrasting cultural conditions" (p. 289). This view represents one of the earliest social constructivist theories of emotion, envisioning emotions as arising from the dynamic interactions between individuals and cultures (Lutz & Abu-Lughod, 1990; Oatley, 1993; Saarni, 1993). To explicate this perspective, Oatley (1993) likens emotions to language:

> Although there is no doubt a common basis for language in all human beings, each culture has its own vocabulary, its syntactic forms, its meanings, and its range of pragmatic effects. Comparably, it is argued, that each culture has patterns of emotions that are somewhat distinctive, that derive from social practices, and that convey meanings and effects to members of that culture. (p. 341)

In sharp contrast to the theories of Darwin, James, and Cannon, social constructivists locate the core of emotion outside of the human body and squarely within cultural processes. Although some theorists in this tradition acknowledge a few innate emotional responses, they still maintain that most aspects of emotion are socially constructed. Because cultural influences have their effect on emotion over time, social constructionists often adopt a developmental view of emotion, emphasizing that emotions are socialized from childhood on (e.g., Saarni, 1993).

Lexical Theories

Lexical theorists highlight the role of language in emotion, believing that emotion is "created in, rather than shaped by, speech in the sense that it is postulated as an entity in language where its meaning to social actors is also elaborated" (Lutz & Abu-Lughod, 1990, p. 12). From this perspective, the essence of emotion lies in the ways that people label their subjective experience. For example, claims of universality for a given emotion would require it to have lexical equivalents in all natural languages:

> If lists [of emotion terms] . . . are supposed to enumerate universal human emotions, how is it that these emotions are so neatly identified by means of English words? For example, Polish does not have a word corresponding exactly to the English word disgust. What if the psychologists working

on the "fundamental human emotions" happened to be native speakers of Polish rather than English? Would it still have occurred to them to include "disgust" on their list? (Wierzbicka, 1986, p. 584)

Lexical theorists raise important methodological caveats for emotion research. For example, to get around the problem of translation equivalents between languages, Wierzbicka (1986) has advocated using "language-independent semantic metalanguage" (e.g., replacing the term *fear* with "the experience that occurs when one thinks that something bad might happen to one"). Ascribing such a key role for language in emotion provides for profound cultural influence in the ways that emotions are labeled and experienced. Lexical theories have not envisioned a major role for biological factors such as facial expression.

Appraisal Theories

Appraisal theories are based on the notion that emotions result from our conscious or unconscious cognitive evaluations of events and situations. Placing the emphasis on appraisal allows for cross-cultural and within-cultural variability in the evaluative process, without precluding some universality in biological features. In these models, subjective emotional experience is largely dependent on earlier evaluative processes: Physiological and facial reactions follow as a natural response to the felt emotion. Appraisal theories readily encompass cultural influences on emotion in terms of differences in the ways particular situations are appraised. As Scherer (2000) notes:

> Component theorists share the social constructivists' insistence on the powerful role of sociocultural determinants of emotional experiences by assuming, for example, that cultural values can strongly affect appraisal, that the regulation of the emotion depends on norms and social context, and that the subjective experience reflects the sociocultural context. (p. 152)

At the same time, these theorists are often quite comfortable with indications that a particular biological aspect of emotion (e.g., physical sensations) shows consistency across cultures (Scherer & Wallbott, 1994).

Biocultural Theories

A number of emotion theorists have attempted to integrate the roles of biology and culture, seeing both as significantly influencing emotion. In a summary of biocultural approaches to emotion, Hinton (1999) outlined four kinds of integrative theories: (1) biocultural synergy, (2) embodiment, (3) systems theory, and (4) local biology. Biocultural synergy theorists argue that biology and culture are mutually dependent and continually transform each other throughout the organism's lifetime (Changeux, 1985). Embodiment represents the commingling of physiological and mental processes, and asserts that emotion cannot be understood in isolation from the social context in which it occurs. Systems theory envisions emotions as comprising multiple components, including biology and culture, that work in parallel and are all necessary for understanding emotion. Local biology highlights the interplay between biology and culture over the lifetime of the organism and allows for the creation of new variations in the emotional system that arise from this codevelopment. At the core of these anthropologically based theories is an equal partnership between culture and biology. However, they are often articulated at a very broad level and do not specify precisely how culture and biology interact to produce the various aspects of emotion, such as facial expression, subjective experience, and peripheral physiological response. An exception to this is Ekman's "neurocultural" theory (Ekman & Friesen, 1969), which describes how emotional facial expression can have both universal features (e.g., facial configurations associated with particular emotions) and culture-specific features (e.g., "display rules" concerning when these facial configurations are shown or hidden). At the end of this chapter, we present an elaboration of our own biocultural model of emotion (Levenson, 2003), which encompasses multiple aspects of emotion and allows for different "mixtures" of biological and cultural influences.

Summary

Emotion theories run the gamut from those that view emotion as purely biological to those that envision pure cultural construction. Many theories, especially the more contemporary ones, fall between these extremes, proposing different mixtures of biological and cultural influences, different ways that these two forces interact, and different implications for the nature of emotion.

EMPIRICAL STUDIES

In this section, we examine the empirical evidence relevant to the question of whether emotions manifest themselves differently across cultures, concentrating on two biological systems prominent in emotion: facial expression and peripheral physiology. The focus of this review is on studies of emotion *production* (in which emotions are stimulated in some way and responses in these two biological systems are measured). We mention only in passing the literature on cultural influences on emotion *recognition* (in which subjects typically are asked to identify the emotion portrayed in photographs; see Elfenbein & Ambady, 2002, for a review) and on emotion-related *psychopathologies* (e.g., Pole, Best, Metzler, & Marmar, 2005; Tsai, Pole, Levenson, & Muñoz, 2003). This distinction among emotion production, emotion recognition, and emotion pathology reflects our view that these are quite different processes and are likely influenced by culture in different ways. Of the three processes, emotion production is arguably the most elemental stage upon which the intricate dance between biology and culture is performed.

Facial Expression

Given the apparent differences in facial features between ethnocultural groups, one might wonder whether their facial expressions of emotions also differ. Darwin (1872) was one of the first to examine whether facial expressions of emotions were culturally invariant. Surveying former British residents living in approximately 40 regions of the world, he found that the expressions of what are often referred to as "basic" emotions (e.g., anger, disgust, fear, happiness, sadness, surprise) were observed in all. Although his methods were crude by modern standards, this work set the stage for future studies using improved methodologies. These subsequent studies also found evidence that the basic emotions are associated with similar facial expressions in different

ethnocultural groups. For example, Ekman (reviewed in 1982) presented members of a preliterate culture in New Guinea with situations thought to elicit anger, disgust, fear, happiness, sadness, and surprise, and asked them to display the appropriate facial expression. Videotapes of these expressions were later shown to American college students, who correctly identified the emotions displayed by the New Guineans. This result suggests that facial expressions associated with these emotions are sufficiently similar in these two cultures to allow for "translation" and "backtranslation." Although there has been a great deal of controversy over how definitive the evidence is for the universality of the *recognition* of emotional facial expression (Ekman, 1994; Russell, 1994), there is certainly no consistent evidence suggesting that some cultures rewrite the basic mapping between facial expression and emotion (e.g., cultures in which happiness is associated with lowered rather than raised lip corners).

Cultural differences have been found in the *amount* and *type* of emotion shown in response to a given elicitor. Comparing two cultures, Tsai and Chentsova-Dutton (2003) found that European Americans of Scandinavian descent showed less emotional facial behavior (especially during happiness and love memories) than those of Irish descent. These findings were interpreted as reflecting the cultural traditions of emotional control in Scandinavian culture and of emotional expression in Irish culture. However, not all studies have found cultural differences. Tsai, Levenson, and Carstensen (2000) found no differences in emotional facial expressions of young and elderly Chinese American and European American participants in response to film clips designed to elicit amusement or sadness.

Comparing acculturation levels in Chinese Americans and Mexican Americans, Soto, Levenson, and Ebling (2005) found that emotional facial behavior in response to an aversive, acoustical startle stimulus mirrored ethnographic norms to the extent that participants identified strongly with their culture of origin. Specifically, they found less negative emotional expression in Chinese Americans most identified with Chinese culture (which emphasizes emotion moderation) and more negative emotional expression in Mexican Americans most identified with Mexican culture (which emphasizes emotion expression). Similarly, Tsai, Chentsova-Dutton, Freire-Bebeau, and Przymus (2002) found that Hmong Americans who were most strongly identified with Hmong culture (which emphasizes emotion moderation) showed fewer "non-Duchenne" smiles while reliving happy and proud experiences than those who were less identified with Hmong culture.

Cultural differences have also been found in the extent to which emotional facial expressions can be produced voluntarily. Levenson, Ekman, Heider, and Friesen (1992) studied voluntary facial expressions in the Minangkabau of West Sumatra (a matrilineal, Muslim culture that views emotion as interpersonally situated). Levenson et al. used a directed facial action task in which participants were given muscle-by-muscle instructions to construct prototypical emotional facial expressions without mentioning the name of the target emotion. Results revealed that Minangkabau produced lower quality expressions of fear, happiness, and sadness compared to European American controls.

Emotional facial expressions are also sensitive to cultural "display rules," which can be triggered by cues, including the presence of other members of the culture. In a classic study, Ekman and Friesen (1969; Friesen, 1972) compared emotional facial expressions of American and Japanese students watching a stressful movie. The two groups did not differ in their facial expressions when watching the films. However, when later interviewed about their emotional responses by a Japanese experimenter, Japanese participants exhibited more positive emotion than their American counterparts. The authors concluded that Japanese participants masked their negative emotions in compliance with their culture's prohibitions against displaying negative emotions in social settings. More recently, Vrana and Rollock (1998) compared African American and European American subjects as they encountered confederates of both races. They found that both groups showed more positive facial expressions during the first few seconds of an encounter with a confederate of their own ethnic background, but subsequently showed greater positive facial expressions with confederates of the other ethnic background. This could reflect an initial spontaneous positive emotional response to encountering a person of one's own ethnic group, followed by a socially prescribed positive emotional display that might indicate

cooperativeness with an ethnic outgroup member.

Cultural ingroup–outgroup influences on facial expression do not require that the other person be physically present. Roberts and Levenson (2006) found that European American, Chinese American, Mexican American, and African American participants did not differ overall in the amount of emotional facial behavior they displayed when watching emotion-eliciting film clips. However, when ethnic match between the participants and the characters in the films was considered, Chinese American and African American participants displayed more facial expressions of amusement while watching amusing films featuring their own ethnic group than those featuring the other ethnic groups. Vanman, Paul, Ito, and Miller (1997) found that European American college students showed more facial muscle activity consistent with positive emotion when they imagined working with other European Americans than with African Americans. Finally, Vrana and Rollock (2002) found that African American and European American subjects showed more emotional facial responses when imagining interaction with an African American compared to a European American.

Summary

For the "basic" emotions, we are aware of no convincing demonstration of consistent cultural differences in the particular assembly of facial muscles contracted when a given emotion is elicited. This biologically based part of the emotion system appears to be universal. Of course, subtle differences between cultures in the appearance changes that accompany these contractions are quite possible, reflecting differences in facial morphology. Cultural differences are found, however, in the amount and type of emotional expressions that occur in response to emotion elicitors. These differences often reflect cultural norms concerning emotional expression, especially in those individuals most strongly identified with that culture. In addition, the presence of a member of a culture (in person, imagined, or depicted) can result in modulation of emotional expression in culturally consistent ways. Thus, the existing research clearly indicates that the production of emotional facial behavior is influenced by both biology and culture.

Peripheral Physiology

Peripheral nervous system activity, most notably in the autonomic nervous system, plays an important role in many emotion theories, contributing to the subjective experience of emotion, alerting the organism to significant encounters, and preparing the body for action (Levenson, 2003). As with emotional facial expression, there are several fundamental issues about the influence of culture on what is basically a biological system. First, there is the question of cultural differences in the mapping of particular features of the autonomic response onto particular emotions (e.g., are there cultures in which people's blood pressures fall and their faces blanch when they become angry?). Second, there is the question of whether cultures differ in terms of the intensity of the autonomic response overall and/or of the separate organ systems (e.g., do cultures differ in the ratio of cardiac to electrodermal activation in anger?). Despite the fundamental importance of these questions, relatively few studies of cultural influences on emotion have directly measured physiological responses during emotion production. Instead, studies have assessed subjective reports of physiological responses (e.g., beliefs about what is happening in the body), cultural differences in resting or baseline physiological levels (i.e., not measured during emotion production), and physiological reactions to stressful situations (in which a specific emotional response is not identified). These kinds of studies are reviewed below. Also important, but not directly relevant to our focus in this section, are studies of the extent to which individuals in cultures somatize emotions (e.g., Heelas, 1986; Shweder, 1993) and emotional distress (e.g., Kleinman, 1977; Pole et al., 2005).

Subjective Reports of Physiological Response

Subjective reports of physiological responses are not proxies for actual physiological measurement. Research on visceral perceptions has shown that our estimates of physiological activity are often not very accurate (Katkin, Blascovich, & Goldband, 1981; Pennebaker, 1982). Nonetheless, visceral perceptions clearly exist, influence the way we talk about our emotions (Lakoff, 1987), and assume an important role in many emotion theories (Damasio, 1998; James, 1884; Levenson, 2003; Schachter & Singer, 1962).

Wallbott and Scherer (1988) surveyed respondents in 27 countries about the physiological experiences (e.g., relaxed muscles, feeling warm) they associated with anger, fear, guilt, joy, sadness and shame. They found that the amount of variance in subjective physiological responses due to the specific emotion was larger than that due to country, concluding that different cultures have similar subjective appraisals of emotion-related physiology. Other studies, however, have identified differences between cultural groups. Scherer, Wallbott, and Summerfield (1986) asked respondents from Northern and Southern Europe to indicate what bodily responses they experienced during specific emotional states (anger, fear, happiness, and sadness). Each emotion was accompanied by distinguishable bodily signs; however, sadness elicited different responses from Northern and Southern Europeans. Scherer, Wallbott, Matsumoto, and Kudoh (1988) repeated the study in a sample of U.S. and Japanese students. They found that U.S. students reported physiological states similar to those reported by European respondents in the earlier study; however, Japanese respondents reported far fewer physiological reactions. Probably the most dramatic findings of cultural variation measured by subjective physiological responses were reported by Hupka, Zbigniew, Jurgen, and Reidl (1996). Students in Mexico, Russia, Poland, Germany, and the United States rated the extent to which they felt anger, fear, jealousy, and envy in specific parts of their bodies (e.g., bones, heart). Findings suggested several cross-cultural similarities (e.g., respondents from all nations reported feeling envy and jealousy in the breath, chest, and heart) and a number of differences (e.g., only respondents from the United States reported feeling envy and jealousy in their eyes, face, stomach, and tears). Given that physiology was not directly measured in this paradigm, the authors interpreted their findings as most likely reflecting cultural stereotypes and emotion metaphors.

Resting or Baseline Physiological Levels

A number of studies have examined cultural differences in physiological states measured in the *absence* of any specific, emotion-eliciting stimuli. Depending on the research tradition, measures obtained in this manner can be described as "tonic" (vs. "phasic"), "trait" (vs.

"state"), or "resting" (vs. "reactive"). Most of these studies have compared African Americans and European Americans, in an attempt to understand the high incidence of essential hypertension (i.e., chronic high blood pressure of unknown etiology) in African Americans (Akinkube, 1985). Findings suggest that African Americans begin life with faster resting heart rates than their European American counterparts (Lee, Rosner, Gould, Lowe, & Kass, 1976; Schachter, Kerr, Wimberly, & Lachin, 1974; Schachter, Lachin, Kerr, Wimberly, & Ratey, 1976) but achieve similar heart rates to European Americans by adolescence (Schachter, Kuller, & Perfetti, 1984; Shekelle, Liu, Raynor, & Miller, 1978; Voors, Webber, & Berenson, 1982) and that this equivalency continues into older age (Persky, Dyer, Stamler, Shekelle, & Schoenberger, 1979). In addition, compared to European Americans, African Americans have been found to have lower resting skin conductance levels (L. C. Johnson & Corah, 1963; L. C. Johnson & Landon, 1965; Juniper & Dykman, 1967; Korol, Bergfield, & McLaughlin, 1975; Lieblich, Kugelmass, & Ben-Shakhar, 1973; Morell et al., 1988) and higher resting blood pressure levels (Levinson et al., 1985; Morell et al., 1988; Roberts & Rowlands, 1981). The reasons for these differences are not fully understood. For example, differences in skin conductance have been attributed to darker skin pigmentation and differences in the number of active sweat glands (Boucsein, 1992). However, these assertions have not always been supported empirically (L. C. Johnson & Landon, 1965; Korol et al., 1975).

Ethnocultural differences in resting physiological levels are not readily interpreted in terms of emotions but may reflect more enduring factors such as mood, styles of emotion regulation, and sensitivity to contextual cues. Brownley, Light, and Anderson (1996) found that high hostility levels were associated with higher blood pressure in European Americans, but lower blood pressure in African Americans. E. H. Johnson (1989) found that African American adolescents suppressed anger more frequently and had higher blood pressure than their European American counterparts. Lazarus, Tomita, Opton, and Kodoma (1966) found that Japanese participants showed higher skin conductance levels than U.S. participants, despite reporting similar levels of distress. Closer analysis of the

skin conductance data revealed that the higher skin conductance levels in the Japanese participants occurred throughout the experiment, and not just in response to the film stimuli, arguably reflecting their greater concern about the experimental situation.

Stressful Situations

In these studies, cultural groups are exposed to challenging situations. The situations are generically stressful; thus, it is difficult to know exactly which emotion(s) are being produced. Because emotion is not the primary focus of these studies, researchers typically do not query subjects about their emotional experience or measure emotional expressive behavior. As in the previous section on resting levels, the majority of these studies have compared African Americans and European Americans. Anderson, Lane, Muranaka, Williams, and Houseworth (1988) found African Americans to have greater increases in blood pressure and forearm vascular resistance, but no differences in heart rate reactivity in response to a cold stressor (ice pack applied to forehead) compared to European Americans. Alpert et al. (1981) found African Americans to have higher blood pressure reactivity than European Americans to an exercise stressor, but found no ethnic differences in heart rate reactivity. Hohn et al. (1983) found that among participants with a family history of hypertension, African American children had larger blood pressure responses than European American children to an exercise stressor. Murphy, Alpert, Moes, and Somes (1986) found that African American children had greater blood pressure reactivity than European American children to a video game. Finally, Jackson, Treiber, Turner, Davis, and Strong (1999) found that African Americans showed greater reactivity in systolic and diastolic blood pressure to a range of physical and psychological stressors, but European Americans showed greater reactivity in heart rate. Consistent with these findings, this literature is often summarized as indicating that African Americans have greater cardiovascular reactivity to stress than do European Americans. However, it is important to note the sizable number of contrary results (e.g., Anderson et al., 1988; Anderson, Lane, Taguchi, & Williams, 1989; Delehanty, Dimsdale, & Mills, 1991; Falkner & Kushner, 1989; Morell et al., 1988; Saab et al., 1997).

Emotion Production

Studies in which the influence of culture is assessed by physiological responses measured directly during emotion production are critical for understanding the interplay between culture and biology. The simplest emotional stimulus for which cultural differences have been studied in this way is the acoustic startle. Although the initial response to the startle (i.e., in approximately the first 500 milliseconds) is arguably more a reflexive defensive reaction than an emotion, it is often followed by a rich emotional response (Ekman, Friesen, & Simons, 1985). Korol et al. (1975) found that African Americans had smaller skin conductance responses to an acoustical startle than did European Americans, a finding they interpreted as related to the lower resting skin conductance levels commonly found among individuals with darker skin. Soto et al. (2005) found no physiological differences in responses to an acoustical startle between Mexican Americans and Chinese Americans. When King and Levenson (2004) expanded this study to include African Americans and European Americans, they also found no ethnic group differences in physiological response.

Studies of prejudice (see Guglielmi, 1999, for a review) often examine the emotional reaction of a person from one race to encountering someone from another race. Rankin and Campbell (1955) found that European American males had larger skin conductance responses when interacting with African American than did their European American confederates. Vrana and Rollock (1998) found that African American and European American males had larger increases in heart rate when encountering African American confederates compared to European American confederates.

Social interaction between partners in committed, intimate relationships is an extremely rich source of emotion (Gottman & Levenson, 1986). Tsai and Levenson (1997) examined physiological responses of Chinese American and European American couples in committed dating relationships as they engaged in a 15-minute discussion of an area of relationship conflict. Levels of physiological arousal provoked by the conflict did not differ between the two ethnic groups.

Only a handful of studies of cultural influences in emotion have directly measured physiology in response to well-defined stimuli de-signed to elicit specific emotions. All of the studies on emotional facial expressions from our laboratory and from the Tsai laboratory, reviewed in an earlier section, also included an extensive set of autonomic measures (typically including measures of cardiovascular, electrodermal, respiratory, and somatic activity), and most found no significant cultural differences in measures of peripheral physiological response. Levenson et al. (1992) found that physiological responses to emotional facial configurations using the directed facial action task were the same in Minangkabau participants living in West Sumatra and in European American controls. Tsai et al. (2000) found no differences in physiological response to sad and amusing films in Chinese American and European American participants. Roberts and Levenson (2006) found no overall differences in the physiological responses of African American, Chinese American, European American, and Mexican American participants in response to amusing, disgusting, and sad films. Tsai et al. (2003) found no ethnic differences in physiological response to imagined emotional scenarios in Scandinavian Americans and Irish Americans.

There are two exceptions to this general trend of no cultural differences. Tsai et al. (2002) found that Hmong Americans had smaller skin conductance responses than their European American counterparts while reliving a "love" memory. Vrana and Rollock (2002) found that African Americans had larger blood pressure responses than European Americans when imagining emotional scenarios.

Summary

The literature on cultural influences on peripheral physiological response suggests that culture may have an influence on subjective reports of physiological response, resting physiological levels, and physiological responses to generalized stress. However, in the realm of directly measured physiological response to well-defined emotional stimuli, the impact of culture appears to be relatively minimal. Nonetheless, within this scant literature, with contributions by only a few laboratories, caveats abound. Still, it does seem to be the case that for the two biological systems being considered in this review, cultural influence on peripheral physiological response is less profound than that on facial expression. This notion that cultural "penetrance" or influence varies for different aspects of emotion plays a central role in the theoretical formulation presented in the next section.

TOWARD AN EMPIRICALLY INFORMED BIOCULTURAL THEORY

One failing of most theories of emotion that have considered cultural influences is that they have treated emotion as a monolith. Thus, culture is viewed as having an effect on emotion in its entirety rather than as having more variable levels of influence depending on features of the emotion, context, and person. Viewed in this more differentiated way, cultural influences may vary for aspects of emotion (e.g., subjective experience, language, expressive behavior, peripheral physiology), type of emotion (e.g., negative emotion, positive emotion, self-conscious emotion), context (e.g., presence of culturally salient cues), and the individual (e.g., extent of identification with cultural traditions). As the body of cross-cultural and cross-ethnic empirical research on emotion has increased, it has become increasingly clear to us that the impact of culture on emotion is anything but uniform.

Components of Emotion: Differential Susceptibility to Cultural Influence

Although this chapter focuses on the impact of culture on two biological systems, facial expression and peripheral physiology, a number of studies from our laboratory and others have examined self-reported subjective emotional experience as well. Upon examination of this work in its entirety, a clear pattern emerges: (1) Self-reported subjective emotional experience is *highly* susceptible to cultural influence—often mirroring ethnographic descriptions of cultural values and mores; (2) emotional expressive behavior is *somewhat* susceptible to cultural influence; and (3) autonomic nervous system response is *minimally* susceptible to cultural influence.

The cultural malleability of self-reported emotional experience is dramatically demonstrated in our work with the directed facial action task conducted in West Sumatra with the Minangkabau (Levenson et al., 1992). When Minangkabau and European American con-

trols produced emotional facial configurations, they activated the same patterns of autonomic nervous system activity. However, the Minangkabau were *much* less likely than European Americans to report feeling the associated emotion. Even after taking into account cultural differences in the ability to produce the facial configurations, this difference in self-reported subjective experience remained. Moreover, our careful translation–backtranslation work and testing of how emotion terms were used with other emotion-eliciting tasks (not reported in the published work) indicated that translation inequivalencies were not responsible for this finding. Thus, we found members of two different cultures could produce the same emotional configurations on their faces and have the same attendant autonomic nervous system activity but report very different subjective emotional states. Our speculation as to the basis of this difference was that emotion is viewed as more of an internal state in European American culture, and as more of an interpersonal condition in Minangkabau culture. Thus, a situation in which facial and physiological aspects were activated (along with the attendant somatic and visceral sensations) would be sufficient for labeling the state as "emotion" for European Americans, but not for Minangkabau, for whom it lacked the appropriate interpersonal grounding.

The previously described research by Soto et al. (2005) also illustrates this pattern using a more "conventional" emotional elicitor. In this study, Chinese Americans reported experiencing significantly less emotion than did Mexican Americans in response to an aversive acoustical startle stimulus. This is consistent with ethnographic descriptions of Chinese culture as a culture of emotional moderation and of Mexican culture as a culture of emotional expression. However, in the realm of emotional behavior, evidence for greater emotional expression in Mexican Americans than in Chinese Americans was only found when participants who most strongly identified with their culture of origin were compared. Physiological differences among the groups were minimal. Why would this differential susceptibility to cultural influence exist? We believe it primarily reflects the extent to which these different aspects of the emotional response are amenable to voluntary control and, to some extent, the social visibility of those components.

Self-Reported Emotional Experience

We do not view the ways we label our emotional states as being predetermined by biological "hardwiring," but rather as quite malleable, reflecting factors such as situational cues, visceral sensations, cultural values and mores, and "feeling rules" (Hochschild, 1979). In most situations we are able to exert a great deal of voluntary control over what we *say* we are feeling. These emotion labels are highly socially visible events; thus, there is a strong incentive to modulate this aspect of our emotional response in culturally sanctioned ways. Arguably, when emotions are extremely intense, or when we are dealing with immediate utterances rather than retrospective reports, this modulation becomes more difficult.

Emotional Facial Expressions

We believe that the set of facial muscles that contracts for particular "basic" emotions such as anger, disgust, fear, happiness, sadness, and surprise is determined by hardwired, involuntary neural circuitry. However, the innervation of the facial muscles is such that voluntary pathways can, under some conditions, alter and override these expressions (Rinn, 1984). For example, in a series of emotional suppression studies, we found that participants can dramatically decrease and increase the amount of facial behavior produced by emotion-eliciting films and acoustic startle stimuli (Gross & Levenson, 1993; Hagemann, Levenson, & Gross, 2006; Kunzmann, Kupperbusch, & Levenson, 2005). Thus, in theory, people should be able to comply with cultural "display rules." However, the empirical evidence suggests that modulation of facial displays in culturally proscribed ways is much *less* likely to be observed than modulation of self-reported emotional experience. It is important to note that despite the huge theoretical impact the display rule notion has had on the field of emotion research, empirical tests have been quite limited. The original research on display rules (Friesen, 1972) did not find cultural difference when participants viewed films, only when they discussed them afterwards. In more contemporary studies with bicultural participants, cultural differences have often been limited to those participants with the strongest identification with their culture of origin (Soto et al., 2005; Tsai et al.,

2002). Facial expressions are clearly socially visible; nonetheless, the importance of controlling them may be lessened by several factors. For example, although people have proved to be quite good at identifying the emotional meaning of static photographs of high-intensity expressions, they may be less accurate at identifying the emotional meaning of low-intensity and brief facial expressions (Ambadar, Schooler, & Cohn, 2005). In addition, cultural conventions may place limits on attending to and labeling the facial expressions of others (e.g., Goffman, 1971). These inaccuracies, coupled with culturally proscribed neglect, may make it relatively "safer" to allow true feelings to show on the face.

Autonomic Nervous System Response

The autonomic nervous system is designed to function automatically and in general is not subject to direct voluntary control (Levenson, 1979). Although a great deal of autonomic activity is socially invisible (e.g., regulation of core temperature), the autonomic nervous system is also responsible for producing a number of highly visible, emotionally relevant appearance changes (e.g., blushing, blanching; for a comprehensive listing, see Levenson, 2003). Thus, there clearly are good reasons to try to modulate autonomic activity to conform to social norms. Nature, however, has wisely *not* provided us with the tools to override easily the essential biological functions the autonomic nervous system serves. Consistent with this, in our own work, we have found few physiological differences between cultural groups relative to those found in emotional facial expression and self-reported emotional experience. Several caveats, however, must accompany this observation. First, interpretations of failure to find differences between cultural groups must be tempered by considerations of sample size/power and the impossibility of proving null hypotheses. Second, when cultural groups appraise the eliciting situation in ways that result in different emotional states, we would expect physiological differences consistent with those states to occur (e.g., when an epithet caused Southerners to feel insulted but had little effect on Northerners, Southerners showed a larger endocrine response; Cohen, Nisbett, Bowdle, & Schwarz, 1996). These caveats notwithstanding, the lack of consistent findings of cultural differences in autonomic activity is impressive.

A Revised Biocultural Model of Emotion

The growing body of empirical data on cultural influences on emotion reviewed in this chapter suggests several revisions to our original biocultural model of emotion (Levenson, 2003). In the revised model, presented in Figure 32.1, a core system (inside the large rectangle) continuously scans incoming information in search of patterns that match one of a limited set of configurations that match prototypical challenges and opportunities (e.g., loss of support, presence of attachment object). When a match occurs, a hardwired organized set of response tendencies (i.e., an emotion) is activated. This set of response tendencies has been selected by evolution for having the highest probability of dealing successfully with that kind of situation most of the time. For simplicity, in this version, we have omitted some of the additional response systems that are recruited (e.g., perception, attention, purposeful behavior, vocalization, gross motor activity, gating of higher mental processes—see Levenson, 1999, for a more complete set). The different patterns of activation of these systems, especially the visceral and somatic sensations and proprioceptive feedback, contribute to the subjective

experience of different emotions. All of this occurs automatically, without conscious intervention. As such, it does not allow for a great deal of learned cultural influence.

In humans, the core system is encapsulated by a control system (outside the large rectangle) that influences both the input to and output from the core system. On the input side, an appraisal system can alter the extent to which an event matches a prototype, thus influencing whether an emotion is elicited by a particular event, and if so, which emotion. For example, a sudden loss of support experienced during a roller-coaster ride may be appraised in a way that makes it less life threatening; thus, it is less likely to produce fear and more likely to produce amusement or excitement. On the output side, another part of the control system alters the likelihood that a response tendency activated in the core will lead to its usual, observable response (e.g., whether a tendency to show a facial expression of disgust when viewing a decaying body results in an observable disgust expression or a neutral face; whether a particular configuration of visceral sensations is labeled as disgust or not). It should be noted that the control system can both increase and decrease the likelihood of a given event resulting

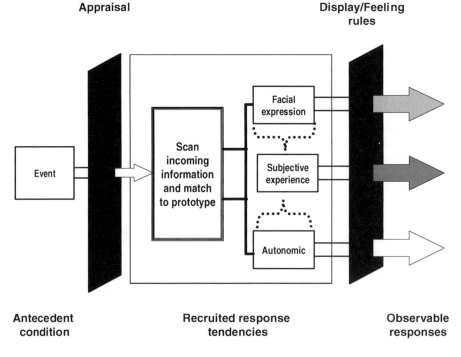

FIGURE 32.1. Revised biocultural model of emotion.

in an emotion and its typical, associated responses. Cultural influences on emotion occur in both aspects of the control system, in the ways that the world is appraised (e.g., what is dangerous, what is safe) and in the extent to which emotional response tendencies are expressed (e.g., conventions and values concerning emotional expression and experience, such as display rules and feeling rules).

In this revised model (Figure 32.1) the differential susceptibility of emotion response systems to cultural influence is depicted in the shading of the observable responses—with darker arrows indicating greater cultural influence. Thus, autonomic response tendencies pass through the control system relatively unin-

fluenced, facial expression tendencies are somewhat influenced, and self-reports of subjective emotional experience are highly susceptible to cultural conventions.

Modulating Cultural Influence

We believe that the extent of influence culture has on the various components of emotion is not fixed, but rather is modulated dynamically by a number of features of the emotion, context, and person. We present our ideas about modulators in Table 32.1 below along with empirical support where available. Should these hypotheses about the modulating influences of culture prove to be correct, they will indicate

TABLE 32.1. Moderators of Cultural Influence on Emotion

Modulator	Greater cultural influence on emotion associated with	Rationale
Acculturation/stage of ethnic identity	Stronger immersion in and identification with cultural beliefs and mores about emotion	Familiarity with cultural norms and reinforcement history of rewards for conforming to these norms increases likelihood of future conformity (Soto et al., 2005; Tsai et al., 2002).
Intensity	Less intense emotion	Strong emotion "floods" system, making voluntary control more difficult.
Timing	More gradual onset of emotion	Rapid onset cuts off opportunity to reappraise situations and to "brace" against the natural expression of the emotion.
Match to prototypical elicitor	Antecedent condition more distal from a prototypical elicitor	Species-relevant prototypical elicitors (e.g., loss of support as prototypical fear elicitor in humans) have strong evolved hardwired circuitry that is extremely difficult to modulate. Antecedents that diverge from prototypes produce weaker response tendencies that are easier to override and alter.
Class of emotion	Emotions that are more self-referential than survival-oriented	Self-referential emotions (e.g., pride, shame, guilt) are more culturally constructed (Kitayama, Markus, & Matsumoto, 1995), more directly embody cultural norms, and have less strongly evolved hardwired circuitry than survival-oriented negative emotions (e.g., fear, anger). Positive emotions likely fall somewhere in between. Emotions, such as disgust, that have not only hardwired origins but also "moral" extensions (Rozin, Lowery, Imada, & Haidt, 1999) could provide particularly interesting tests.
Social context	Presence (real or imagined) of other members of ethnic group or cultural cues	Ethnic ingroup members and other culturally relevant symbols (language, food, etc.) can cue cultural norms, making them more salient and more likely to influence emotion (Kitayama, Markus, Matsumoto, & Norasakkunkit, 1997; N. A. Roberts & Levenson, in press; Vanman, Paul, Ito, & Miller, 1997; Vrana & Rollock, 2002).

important issues for researchers to consider and control for when attempting to evaluate, compare, and aggregate findings concerning cultural influences on emotion.

FUTURE DIRECTIONS

Studying the influences that culture has on actual emotion production provides a rich and fertile direction for future research. Such research arguably provides the third essential leg of a modern empirical science of culture and emotion consisting of emotional ethnography (critical for hypothesis generation and interpretation of results); studies of emotion perception, understanding, and values (critical for understanding the ways that culture influences our thinking about emotion); and studies of emotion production (critical for discovering the influences of culture on different emotion systems as emotions unfold over time). Studies of culture and emotion production lend themselves readily to experimental designs in which cultural variables are carefully manipulated (e.g., presence of culture-salient cues) and their influence on emotional responding precisely measured. Because cultural influences on emotion production likely accumulate over time, longitudinal designs could be particularly useful in documenting how people become culturally competent in the emotional realm. Greater use of experimental and longitudinal designs in research on culture and emotion production could be quite helpful in moving this highly important area of inquiry more prominently into the scientific mainstream.

In the previous section, we suggested a number of possible modulators of the influence of culture on emotional responding, and provided some hypotheses about the nature of these modulating influences. These hypotheses are outgrowths of our notions about the nature of emotion and culture, and about their interactions. Of course, other theoretical starting points could lead to quite different predictions. What is important is that the portfolio of research on the influence of culture on emotion, which has traditionally had a strong investment in using descriptive and qualitative methods, and in measuring emotional judgments, should also have a strong investment in using experimental and quasi-experimental methods

to test falsifiable hypotheses and to explore causal, mediating, and moderating influences on actual emotion production.

CONCLUSION

In this chapter we have reviewed the literature that has considered cultural influences on two of the primary biological systems in emotion—facial expression and peripheral physiological response. Many of these studies include self-report measures of emotional experience, and these data have also been considered. Although there have been a large number of studies of cultural influences on the ability to *recognize* the emotions being expressed by others, we have given primary consideration to studies of emotion *production* in which these biological systems have been directly measured during actual emotions. Based on this body of research, we conclude that cultural influences in emotion vary depending on which aspect of emotion is being considered, with the strongest influence on self-reported emotional experience, somewhat weaker influence on emotional facial expression, and relatively minimal influence on autonomic nervous system response. These findings led us to present a revision of our earlier biocultural model of emotion (Levenson, 2003) that now explicitly reflects varying cultural influence on different aspects of emotion. We have also articulated some testable, but admittedly speculative, hypotheses about characteristics of emotion, context, and person that modulate the extent of cultural influence. These modulatory influences extend our general conclusion that the influence of culture on emotion is neither monotonic nor constant, but rather is nuanced and variable.

We recognize that some of these conclusions are based on a relatively small number of studies that met our criteria for directly measuring biological response during actual emotional episodes. We hope that additional studies of this nature will enable us to test and refine these notions. It is important that studies of cultural influences on the biology of emotion be held to the same high standards of methodology necessary for any study of cultural influence. For example, sample selection criteria are particularly important when working with "domestic" samples to ensure that they are truly representative of the cultural traditions of interest. Bicultural college students are often quite capable of "code-switching" (i.e., shifting between their culture of origin and their adopted "mainstream" culture); thus, it is important to be sensitive to the extent that the laboratory environment is providing cues as to what behavior is "appropriate" (e.g., the ethnic match between experimenters and participants). Studies assessing multiple aspects of emotion present special analytical challenges in attempts to apportion cultural influences among the measured systems (e.g., is the found cultural influence on facial expression more or less than would be expected given the found cultural influence on peripheral physiology?). Moreover, researchers need to consider factors that could modulate the impact of culture on emotion (e.g., intensity of stimuli, type of emotion, acculturation level of participants) when attempting to aggregate findings across different studies.

Emotion provides an ideal stage for studying the interplay of culture and biology, nature and nurture, and contexts and individuals. We are still at a relatively early stage in the study of cultural influences on the biology of emotion. As this research area continues to mature, we expect the theoretical and practical yield for understanding culture, emotion, and their interaction to be considerable.

REFERENCES

Akinkube, O. O. (1985). World epidemiology of hypertension in Blacks. In E. S. W. D. Hall & N. B. Shulman (Ed.), *Hypertension in Blacks: Epidemiology, pathyphysiology, and treatment* (pp. 3–16). Chicago: Yearbook.

Alpert, B. S., Dover, E. V., Booker, D. L., Martin, A. M., & Strong, W. B. (1981). Blood pressure response to dynamic exercise in healthy children—Black versus White. *Journal of Pediatrics, 99,* 556–560.

Ambadar, Z., Schooler, J. W., & Cohn, J. F. (2005). Deciphering the enigmatic face: The importance of facial dynamics in interpreting subtle facial expressions. *Psychological Science, 16*(5), 403–410.

Anderson, N. B., Lane, J. D., Muranaka, M., Williams, R. B., Jr., & Houseworth, S. J. (1988). Racial differences in blood pressure and forearm vascular responses to the cold face stimulus. *Psychosomatic Medicine, 50,* 57–63.

Anderson, N. B., Lane, J. D., Taguchi, F., & Williams, R. B., Jr. (1989). Patterns of cardiovascular responses to stress as a function of race and parental hypertension in men. *Health Psychology, 8,* 525–540.

Boucsein, W. (1992). *Electrodermal activity.* New York: Plenum Press.

Brownley, K. A., Light, K. C., & Anderson, N. B. (1996). Social support and hostility interact to influence clinic, work, and home blood pressure in Black and White men and women. *Psychophysiology, 33,* 434–445.

Cannon, W. B. (1927). The James–Lange theory of emotions: A critical examination and an alternative theory. *American Journal of Psychology, 39,* 106–124.

Changeux, J.-P. (1985). *Neuronal man: The biology of mind.* New York: Oxford University Press.

Cohen, D., Nisbett, R. E., Bowdle, B. F., & Schwarz, N. (1996). Insult, aggression, and the southern culture of honor: An "experimental ethnography." *Journal of Personality and Social Psychology, 70*(5), 945–959.

Damasio, A. (1998). The somatic marker hypothesis and the possible functions of the prefrontal cortex. In A. C. Roberts, T. W. Robbins, & L. Weiskrantz (Eds.), *The prefrontal cortex: Executive and cognitive functions* (pp. 36–50). New York: Oxford University Press.

Darwin, C. (1872). *The expression of the emotions in man and animals.* London: Murray.

Delehanty, S. G., Dimsdale, J. E., & Mills, P. (1991). Psychosocial correlates of reactivity in Black and White men. *Journal of Psychosomatic Research, 35,* 451–460.

Ekman, P. (1994). Strong evidence for universals in facial expressions: A reply to Russell's mistaken critique. *Psychological Bulletin, 115*(2), 268–287.

Ekman, P., & Friesen, W. V. (1969). The repertoire of nonverbal behavior: Categories, origins, usage, and coding. *Semiotica, 1,* 49–98.

Ekman, P., Friesen, W. V., & Ellsworth, P. (1982). What are the similarities and differences in facial behavior across cultures? In P. Ekman (Ed.), *Emotion in the human face* (pp. 128–146). Cambridge, UK: Cambridge University Press.

Ekman, P., Friesen, W. V., & Simons, R. C. (1985). Is the startle reaction an emotion? *Journal of Personality and Social Psychology, 49,* 1416–1426.

Elfenbein, H. A., & Ambady, N. (2002). On the universality and cultural specificity of emotion recognition: A meta-analysis. *Psychological Bulletin, 128,* 203–235.

Falkner, B., & Kushner, H. (1989). Race differences in stress induced reactivity in young adults. *Health Psychology, 8,* 613–627.

Friesen, W. V. (1972). *Cultural differences in facial expressions in a social situation: An experimental test of the concept of display rules.* Unpublished doctoral dissertation, University of California, San Francisco.

Goffman, E. (1971). *Relations in public; microstudies of the public order.* New York: Harper & Row.

Gottman, J. M., & Levenson, R. W. (1986). Assessing the role of emotion in marriage. *Behavioral Assessment, 8*(1), 31–48.

Gross, J. J., & Levenson, R. W. (1993). Emotional suppression: Physiology, self-report, and expressive behavior. *Journal of Personality and Social Psychology*, 64(6), 970–986.

Guglielmi, R. S. (1999). Psychophysiological assessment of prejudice: Past research, current status, and future directions. *Personality and Social Psychology Review*, 3, 123–157.

Hagemann, T., Levenson, R. W., & Gross, J. J. (2006). Expressive suppression during an acoustic startle. *Psychophysiology*, 43(1), 104–112.

Heelas, P. (1986). Emotion talk across cultures. In R. M. Harre (Ed.), *The social construction of emotions* (pp. 234–266). Oxford, UK: Blackwell.

Hinton, A. L. (1999). *Biocultural approaches to the emotions*. New York: Cambridge University Press.

Hochschild, A. R. (1979). Emotion work, feeling rules, and social structure. *American Journal of Sociology*, 84, 551–575.

Hohn, A., Riopel, D., Kiel, J., Loadhold, C., Margolius, H., Halushka, P., et al. (1983). Childhood familial and racial differences in physiologic and biochemical factors related to hypertension. *Hypertension*, 5, 56–70.

Hupka, R. B., Zbigniew, Z., Jurgen, O., & Reidl, L. (1996). Anger, envy, fear, and jealousy as felt in the body: A five-nation study. *Cross-Cultural Research*, 30, 243–264.

Jackson, R. W., Treiber, F. A., Turner, J. R., Davis, H., & Strong, W. B. (1999). Effects of race, sex, and socioeconomic status upon cardiovascular stress responsivity and recovery in youth. *International Journal of Psychophysiology*, 31, 111–119.

James, W. (1884). What is an emotion? *Mind*, 9, 188–205.

Johnson, E. H. (1989). The role of the experience and expression of anger and anxiety in elevated blood pressure among Black and White adolescents. *Journal of the National Medical Association*, 81, 573–584.

Johnson, L. C., & Corah, N. L. (1963). Racial differences in skin resistance. *Science*, 139, 766–767.

Johnson, L. C., & Landon, M. M. (1965). Eccrine sweat gland activity and racial differences in resting skin conductance. *Psychophysiology*, 1, 322–329.

Juniper, K., Jr., & Dykman, R. A. (1967). Skin resistance, sweat-gland counts, salivary flow, and gastric secretion: Age, race, and sex differences, and intercorrelations. *Psychophysiology*, 4, 216–222.

Katkin, E. S., Blascovich, J., & Goldband, S. (1981). Empirical assessment of visceral self-perception: Individual and sex differences in the acquisition of heart beat discrimination. *Journal of Personality and Social Psychology*, 40, 1095–1101.

King, A. R., & Levenson, R. W. (2004). *Individual differences in autonomic responses to stress*. Berkeley: University of California Press.

Kitayama, S., Markus, H. R., & Matsumoto, H. (1995). Culture, self, and emotion: A cultural perspective on "self-conscious" emotions. In J. P. Tangney & K. W. Fischer (Eds.), *Self-conscious emotions: The psychology of shame, guilt, embarrassment, and pride*. (pp. 439–464). New York: Guilford Press.

Kitayama, S., Markus, H. R., Matsumoto, H., & Norasakkunkit, V. (1997). Individual and collective processes in the construction of the self: self-enhancement in the United States and self-criticism in Japan. *Journal of Personality and Social Psychology*, 72(6), 1245–1267.

Kleinman, A. (1977). Depression, somatization, and the new cross-cultural psychiatry. *Social Science and Medicine*, 11, 3–10.

Korol, B., Bergfield, G. R., & McLaughlin, L. J. (1975). Skin color and autonomic nervous system measures. *Physiology and Behavior*, 14, 575–578.

Kunzmann, U., Kupperbusch, C. S., & Levenson, R. W. (2005). Behavioral inhibition and amplification during emotional arousal: A comparison of two age groups. *Psychology and Aging*, 20, 144–158.

Lakoff, G. (1987). *Women, fire, and dangerous things*. Chicago: University of Chicago Press.

Lazarus, R. S., Tomita, M., Opton, E., & Kodoma, M. (1966). A cross-cultural study of stress-reaction patterns in Japan. *Journal of Personality and Social Psychology*, 4, 622–633.

Lee, Y., Rosner, B., Gould, J., Lowe, E., & Kass, E. (1976). Familial aggregation of blood pressure in newborn infants and their mothers. *Pediatrics*, 58, 722–729.

Levenson, R. W. (1979). Cardiac–respiratory–somatic relationships and feedback effects in a multiple session heart rate control experiment. *Psychophysiology*, 16(4), 367–373.

Levenson, R. W. (1999). The intrapersonal functions of emotion. *Cognition and Emotion*, 13, 481–504.

Levenson, R. W. (2003). Blood, sweat, and fears: The autonomic architecture of emotion. In P. Ekman, J. J. Campos, R. J. Davidson, & F. B. M. de Waal (Eds.), *Emotions inside out: 130 years after Darwin's* The Expression of the Emotions in Man and Animals (pp. 348–356). New York: New York Academy of Sciences.

Levenson, R. W., Ekman, P., Heider, K., & Friesen, W. V. (1992). Emotion and autonomic nervous system activity in the Minangkabau of West Sumatra. *Journal of Personality and Social Psychology*, 62(6), 972–988.

Levinson, S., Liu, K., Stamler, J., Stamler, R., Whipple, I., Ausbrook, D., & Berkson, D. (1985). Ethnic differences in blood pressure and heart rate of Chicago school children. *American Journal of Epidemiology*, 122, 366–377.

Lieblich, I., Kugelmass, S., & Ben-Shakhar, G. (1973). Psychophysiological baselines as a function of race and origin. *Psychophysiology*, 10, 426–430.

Lutz, C. A., & Abu-Lughod, L. (Eds.). (1990). *Language and the politics of emotion*. Cambridge, UK: Cambridge University Press.

Mead, M. (1935). *Sex and temperament in three primitive societies*. Oxford, UK: Morrow.

Morell, M. A., Myers, H. F., Shapiro, D., Goldstein, I. B., & Armstrong, M. (1988). Psychophysiological reactivity to mental arithmetic stress in Black and White normotensive men. *Health Psychology, 7*(5), 479–496.

Murphy, J., Alpert, B., Moes, D., & Somes, G. (1986). Race and cardiovascular reactivity: A neglected relationship. *Hypertension, 8*, 1075–1083.

Oatley, K. (1993). Social construction in emotions. In M. Lewis & J. M. Haviland (Eds.), *Handbook of emotions* (pp. 341–352). New York: Guilford Press.

Pennebaker, J. W. (1982). *The psychology of physical symptoms*. New York: Springer-Verlag.

Persky, V., Dyer, A., Stamler, J., Shekelle, R., & Schoenberger, J. (1979). Racial patterns of heart rate in an employed adult population. *American Journal of Epidemiology, 110*, 274–280.

Pole, N., Best, S. R., Metzler, T., & Marmar, C. R. (2005). Why are Hispanics at greater risk for PTSD? *Cultural Diversity and Ethnic Minority Psychology, 11*, 144–161.

Rankin, R. E., & Campbell, D. T. (1955). Galvanic skin response to negro and white experimenters. *Journal of Abnormal and Social Psychology, 51*, 30–33.

Rinn, W. E. (1984). The neuropsychology of facial expression: A review of the neurological and psychological mechanisms for producing facial expressions. *Psychological Bulletin, 95*(1), 52–77.

Roberts, J., & Rowlands, M. (1981). *Vital and health statistics: Hypertension in adults 25–74 years of age: United States, 1971–1975* (Series 11, No. 221, DHEW Publication No. PHS 81-1671). Washington, DC: U.S. Government Printing Office.

Roberts, N. A., & Levenson, R. W. (2006). Subjective, behavioral, and physiological reactivity to ethnically matched and ethnically mismatched film clips. *Emotion, 6*(4), 635–646.

Rozin, P., Lowery, L., Imada, S., & Haidt, J. (1999). The CAD triad hypothesis: A mapping between three moral emotions (contempt, anger, disgust) and three moral codes (community, autonomy, divinity). *Journal of Personality and Social Psychology, 76*(4), 574–586.

Russell, J. A. (1994). Is there universal recognition of emotion from facial expressions?: A review of the cross-cultural studies. *Psychological Bulletin, 115*(1), 102–141.

Saab, P. G., Llabre, M. M., Schneiderman, N., Hurwitz, B. E., McDonald, P. G., Evans, J., et al. (1997). Influence of ethnicity and gender on cardiovascular responses to active coping and inhibitory-passive coping challenges. *Psychosomatic Medicine, 59*, 434–446.

Saarni, C. (1993). Socialization of emotion. In M. Lewis & J. M. Haviland (Eds.), *Handbook of emotions* (pp. 435–446). New York: Guilford Press.

Schachter, J., Kerr, J., Wimberly, E., & Lachin, J. (1974).

Heart rate levels of Black and White newborns. *Psychosomatic Medicine, 36*, 513–524.

Schachter, J., Kuller, L., & Perfetti, C. (1984). Heart rate during the first five years of life: Relation to ethnic group (Black or White) and to parental hypertension. *American Journal of Epidemiology, 119*, 554–563.

Schachter, J., Lachin, J., Kerr, J., Wimberly, E., & Ratey, J. (1976). Heart rate and blood pressure in Black newborns and in White newborns. *Pediatrics, 58*, 283–287.

Schachter, S., & Singer, J. (1962). Cognitive, social, and physiological determinants of emotional state. *Psychological Review, 69*(5), 379–399.

Scherer, K. R. (2000). Psychological models of emotion. In J. C. Borod (Ed.), *The neuropsychology of emotion* (pp. 137–162). New York: Oxford University Press.

Scherer, K. R., & Wallbott, H. G. (1994). Evidence for universality and cultural variation of differential emotion response patterning. *Journal of Personality and Social Psychology, 66*(2), 310–328.

Scherer, K. R., Wallbott, H. G., Matsumoto, D., & Kudoh, T. (1988). Emotional experience in cultural context: A comparison between Europe, Japan, and the United States. In K. R. Scherer (Ed.), *Facets of emotions* (pp. 5–30). Hillsdale, NJ: Erlbaum.

Scherer, K. R., Wallbott, H. G., & Summerfield, A. B. (1986). *Experiencing emotion: A cross-cultural study*. Cambridge, UK: Cambridge University Press.

Shekelle, R., Liu, S., Raynor, W., & Miller, R. (1978). Racial difference in mean pulse rate of children aged six to eleven years. *Pediatrics, 61*, 119–121.

Shweder, R. A. (1993). The cultural psychology of emotions. In M. Lewis & J. M. Haviland (Eds.), *Handbook of emotions* (pp. 417–431). New York: Guilford Press.

Soto, J. A., Levenson, R. W., & Ebling, R. (2005). Cultures of moderation and expression: Emotional experience, behavior, and physiology in Chinese Americans and Mexican Americans. *Emotion, 5*(2), 154–165.

Tsai, J. L., & Chentsova-Dutton, Y. (2003). Variation among European Americans in emotional facial expression. *Journal of Cross Cultural Psychology, 34*, 650–657.

Tsai, J. L., Chentsova-Dutton, Y., Freire-Bebeau, L., & Przymus, D. E. (2002). Emotional expression and physiology in European Americans and Hmong Americans. *Emotion, 2*, 380–397.

Tsai, J. L., & Levenson, R. W. (1997). Cultural influences on emotional responding: Chinese American and European American dating couples during interpersonal conflict. *Journal of Cross-Cultural Psychology, 28*, 600–625.

Tsai, J. L., Levenson, R. W., & Carstensen, L. L. (2000). Autonomic, subjective, and expressive responses to emotional films in older and younger Chinese Americans and European Americans. *Psychology and Aging, 15*, 684–693.

Tsai, J. L., Pole, N., Levenson, R. W., & Muñoz, R. F. (2003). The effects of depression on the emotional responses of Spanish-speaking Latinas. *Cultural Diversity and Ethnic Minority Psychology*, 9, 49–63.

Vanman, E., Paul, B. Y., Ito, T. A., & Miller, N. (1997). The modern face of prejudice and structural features that moderate the effect of cooperation on affect. *Journal of Personality and Social Psychology*, 73, 941–959.

Voors, A., Webber, L., & Berenson, G. (1982). Resting heart rate and pressure-rate product of children in a total biracial community: The Bogulusa Heart Study. *American Journal of Epidemiology*, 116, 276–286.

Vrana, S. R., & Rollock, D. (1998). Physiological response to a minimal social encounter: Effects of gender, ethnicity, and social context. *Psychophysiology*, 35, 462–469.

Vrana, S. R., & Rollock, D. (2002). The role of ethnicity, gender, emotional content, and contextual differences in physiological, expressive, and self-reported emotional responses to imagery. *Cognition and Emotion*, 16, 165–192.

Wallbott, H. G., & Scherer, K. R. (1988). How universal and specific is emotional experience?: Evidence from 27 countries on five continents. In K. R. Scherer (Ed.), *Facets of emotion: Recent research.* (pp. 31–56). Hillsdale, NJ: Erlbaum.

Wierzbicka, A. (1986). Human emotions: Universal or culture-specific. *American Anthropologist*, 88, 584–594.

CHAPTER 33

Culture and Psychopathology
Foundations, Issues, and Directions

ANTHONY J. MARSELLA
ANN MARIE YAMADA

Shall we write about the things
not to be spoken of?
Shall we divulge the things
not to be divulged?
Shall we pronounce the things
not to be pronounced?
—JULIAN THE APOSTATE (332–363 C.E.)
Hymn to the Mother of the Gods

After decades of relative neglect and marginalization within psychiatry, the study of the relationship between culture and psychopathology has emerged as topic of considerable interest and influence. In 1994, under pressure from ethnic minority and international psychiatric professionals, the American Psychiatric Association included new sections in the fourth edition of *Diagnostic and Statistical Manual of* *Mental Disorders* (DSM-IV) under the titles "Glossary of Culture-Bound Syndromes" and "Outline for the Cultural Formulation of Case." Though these sections appeared at the very ends of the book (pp. 843–849), they nevertheless signaled a new era in psychiatry, in which cultural factors would now be given increased attention in our understanding of the etiology, expression, assessment, diagnosis, and treatment of psychopathology. Of particular note is the warning statement inserted at the beginning of DSM-IV and DSM-IV-TR (American Psychiatric Association, 1994, p. xxiv; 2000, p. xxxiv). This statement, perhaps more than any other in psychiatry, encourages clinicians and researchers to be sensitive to cultural variations or risk serious mistakes: "A clinician who is unfamiliar with the nuances of an individual's cultural frame of reference may incorrectly judge as psychopathology those normal variations in behavior, belief, or experience that are particular to the individual's culture."

The fact that this increased responsivity to cultural variables occurred in a time when biological and other reductionistic views of psychopathology dominated professional training, clinical applications, and research adds to the significance of what occurred and emphasizes the important influence of "political" forces in our work. The mental health professions would now be asked to consider "cultural" variables in their case construction, their training curricula, and their research efforts. Even with this, a gap remains between the fields of psychiatry and psychology. This chapter provides an overview of the study of culture and psychopathology, with special emphasis on its historical development, basic assumptions, theoretical and empirical findings, and related issues.

FORCES FOR CHANGE

The forces that led to these changes are numerous and deserve to be mentioned, because they reveal how our scientific and professional knowledge and practice are often determined not by "science" but by the particular people, theoretical orientations, and ideologies that hold the power and that come to dominate a field (e.g., biological reductionism). Clearly, although there was considerable evidence of cultural and ethnic bias and abuses in psychiatric practice, cultural considerations were ignored, and pressures for change ultimately required a "political" response in which ethnic minority and international voices called for significant changes in DSM-IV (e.g., Chakraborty, 1991; Mezzich, Kleinman, Fabrega, & Parron, 1996; Rogler, 1996).

The changes were facilitated by a number of events and forces that converged between 1980 and the present:

1. Increasing numbers of ethnic minority and international psychiatrists and social scientists gave increased power to their voices. Sometimes motivated by anger, resentment, and the problem of irrelevance, these voices raised questions about the universal applicability of Western concepts of illness and health.

2. Research was seen as inadequate, because it was often limited to Western samples; when research on ethnic/minority and non-Western patients did occur, it was conducted from a Western viewpoint and knowledge base.

3. Increases occurred in political and social awareness of the pathological consequences of racism, sexism, imperialism, colonialism, and other "isms" that produce powerlessness, marginalization, and underprivileging among sizable population sectors.

4. There emerged a new awareness of the multiple and interactive determinants of psychopathology (e.g., biological, psychological, cultural, sociological, spiritual, environmental).

5. Proliferation of scientific and professional communication networks and outlets promoted interest in the topic across the world through professional societies (e.g., International Association of Cross-Cultural Psychology, World Federation for Mental Health, World Psychiatric Association), journals (e.g., *Transcultural Psychiatry, Culture, Medicine and Psychiatry, Hispanic Journal of Behavioral Sciences, Cultural Diversity and Ethnic Minority Psychology*).

6. Development of cooperative international studies of psychiatric disorders by the World Health Organization (e.g., International Pilot Study of Schizophrenia; Determinants of Outcomes of Severe Mental Disorders) not only revealed cultural variations in disorder but also trained a growing number of non-Western psychiatric professionals capable and willing to critique contemporary psychiatry. Within psychology, the pioneering work of Juris Draguns (1973, 1980, 1990; Draguns & Tanaka-Matusmo, 2003) provided systematic coverage of major issues, conceptual models, and therapeutic considerations.

HISTORICAL CONSIDERATIONS

Concern for the sociocultural determinants of psychopathology can be traced to the 18th and 19th centuries, when philosophers (e.g., Jean Jacques Rousseau, Karl Marx), and physicians (e.g., Freud, Kraepelin) raised questions about the contributions of culture to the etiology, expression, and treatment of mental disorders. Emil Kraeplein (1904), the father of our contemporary diagnostic system, suggested that cultural variables need to be considered in understanding mental disorder, and he suggested that a new specialty area be created— *Vergleichende Psychiatrie*, or comparative psychiatry. Kraepelin wrote:

> The characteristics of a people should find expression in the frequency as well as the shaping of the manifestations of mental illness in general; so that comparative psychiatry shall make it possible to gain valuable insights into the psyche of nations and shall in turn also be able to contribute to the understanding of pathological psychic processes. (1904, p. 434)

In the years that followed, a score of terms emerged as culture and psychopathology were studied in different disciplines: transcultural psychiatry, cross-cultural psychiatry, comparative psychiatry, ethnopsychiatry, cultural psychiatry, psychiatric anthropology, and even the "new" transcultural psychiatry. A detailed review of these terms and of the history of the field from its beginnings to the 1980s can be found in Marsella (1993).

RESISTANCE TO WESTERN VIEWS

Initially, many of the critiques were commentaries designed to raise consciousness about the ethnocentric biases inherent in Western psychiatry. For example, Chakraborty (1991), an Asian Indian psychiatrist, wrote:

> Even where studies were sensitive, and the aim was to show relative differences caused by culture, the ideas and tools were still derived from a circumscribed area of European thought. This difficulty still continues and, despite modifications, mainstream psychiatry remains rooted in Kraepelin's classic 19th century classification, the essence of which is the description of the two major "mental diseases" seen in mental hospitals in

his time—schizophrenia and manic depression. Research is constrained by this view of psychiatry. A central pattern of (Western) disorders is identified and taken as the standard by which other (local) patterns are seen as minor variations. Such a construct implies some inadequacy on the part of those patients who fail to reach "standard." Though few people would agree with such statements, there is evidence of biased, value-based, and often racist undercurrents in psychiatry. . . . Psychiatrists in the developing world . . . have accepted a diagnostic framework developed by Western medicine, but which does not seem to take into account the diversity of behavioral patterns they encounter. (p. 1204)

Kirmayer (1998), Editor-in-Chief of the journal *Transcultural Psychiatry*, captured the dilemma facing those supporting the "new" transcultural psychiatry and those holding traditional psychiatric medical perspectives, when he wrote:

> While cultural psychiatry aims to understand problems in context, diagnosis is essentializing: referring to decontextualized entities whose characteristics can be studied independently of the particulars of a person's life and social circumstances. The entities of the DSM implicitly situate human problems within the brain or the psychology of the individual, while many human problems brought to psychiatrists are located in patterns of interaction in families, communities, or wider social spheres. Ultimately, whatever the extent to which we can universalize the categories of the DSM by choosing suitable level of abstraction, diagnosis remains a social practice that must be studied, critiqued, and clarified by cultural analysis. (1998, p. 342)

THE CLINICAL AND RESEARCH LITERATURE

However, critical commentaries soon yielded to a widespread, implicit understanding that cultural factors are critical in shaping the onset, expression, course, and outcome of psychopathology. It was simply a case of a gathering mass of evidence combined with a new consciousness of the power of culture in shaping both normal and abnormal behavior. No single event nor publication turned the tide in favor of increased attention to cultural variables. However, certain publications are considered by many to have had a profound influence on the field. For example, within psychology, the publication of the *Handbook of Cross-Cultural Psychology: Vol. VI. Psychopathology* (Triandis & Draguns, 1981) did much to articulate the relationship between culture and various forms of psychopathology, such as depression, schizophrenia, and disorders of everyday life. In anthropology, a series of publications from the University of Hawaii/National Institute of Mental Health (NIMH) Culture and Mental Health Program (e.g., Caudill & Lin, 1969; Lebra, 1972) served to raise clinical and scientific consciousness about cultural variations in psychopathology. In psychiatry the pioneering work by Alexander Leighton and his colleagues (1959; Leighton et al., 1963) laid the sociocultural foundations of psychopathology. By the 1970s and 1980s, publications by Kleinman (1980) and Marsella and White (1982; Marsella & Higginbotham, 1984) offered theoretical foundations for understanding the role of sociocultural factors in psychopathology. In 1992, the American Psychological Association (1992) published guidelines for providers of psychological services to ethnic, linguistic, and culturally diverse populations in which the need for familiarity with the patient's background was advocated.

Of particular importance in strengthening interest in culture and psychopathology was the volume *Culture and Depression* (Kleinman & Good, 1985), which applied the ideas of the new "transcultural psychiatry" to the topic of depression. This volume emphasized the importance of "context," asserting that depressive experience and disorder could be understood apart from the cultural context in which it was embedded. Indeed, it was noted that depressive experience and disorder might not have the same meaning or implications across cultural boundaries, or the same expressions or etiologies. The widespread impact of this volume was provided by a collection of substantive chapters written by experienced clinicians and academics.

Within the last decade, a number of books have offered overviews of the culture and psychopathology field (e.g., Castillo, 1996; Cuellar & Paniagua, 2000; Mezzich & Fabrega, 2001), and topics such diagnosis/classification (e.g., Mezzich et al., 1996; Paniagua, 2001) and specific disorders such as posttraumatic stress disorder (PTSD; Marsella, Friedman, Gerrity, & Scurfield, 1996). It is notable that a topical specialization in ethnocultural variations in responsivity to medications has

also emerged, under the rubric of "ethno-psychopharmacology," in the work of Keh Ming Lin (e.g., Lin, Smith, & Ortiz, 2001). A number of books have also appeared that address cultural variations in psychopathology among specific ethnic and racial populations including minorities (e.g., Bernal, Trimble, Burlew, & Leong, 2003; Littlewood & Lipsedge, 1997), Native Americans (O'Nell, 1998), Chinese (e.g., Lin, Tseng, & Yeh, 1999; Phoon & Macindoe, 2003), and Hispanics/Latinos (e.g., Becerra, Karno, & Escobar, 1982; Carrillo & Lopez, 2001; Telles & Karno, 1994).

Yet another important event in shaping the study of culture and psychopathology came via the U.S. Department of Health and Human Services (DHHS; 2001) in its published report *Mental Health: Culture, Race, and Ethnicity*. In this report, the DHHS reached specific conclusions about the role of culture and forcefully stated, "Culture counts!" The report detailed disparities in the provision of psychiatric services to racial/ethnic minorities in the United States and called for renewed efforts to address these problems:

> The main message of this supplement is that "culture counts." The cultures that patients come from shape their mental health and affect the types of mental health services they use. Likewise, the cultures of clinician and the service system affect diagnosis, treatment, and the organization and financing of services. Cultural and social influences are not the only influences on mental health and service delivery, but they have been historically underestimated—*and they do count.* Cultural differences must be accounted for to ensure that minorities, like all Americans, receive mental health care tailored to their needs. (p. 14)

In brief, after years of limited attention, the study of culture and psychopathology has now assumed a prominent position within the professional and scientific efforts of psychiatry and the social sciences. The result is that our understanding of psychopathology will never be the same!

THE CONCEPT OF CULTURE AND ITS IMPORTANCE FOR PSYCHOPATHOLOGY

Defining Culture

If we are to understand the relationship of culture to psychopathology, it is critical that we first understand the concept of culture. Definitions of culture are numerous and varied. More than a half-century ago, Kroeber and Kluckhohn (1952) had already summarized more than 125 definitions. For our purposes, we use the following definition:

> Culture is shared, learned behavior and meanings that are socially transferred in various life-activity settings. Cultures can be (1) *transitory* (i.e., situational, for even a few minutes) or (2) *enduring* (e.g., ethnocultural lifestyles), and in all instances are (3) *dynamic* (i.e., constantly subject to change and modification). Cultures are represented (4) *internally* (i.e., values, beliefs, attitudes, images, symbols, orientations, epistemologies, consciousness levels, perceptions, expectations, personhood) and (5) *externally* (i.e., artifacts, roles, institutions, social structures). Cultures (6) *shape and construct our realities* (i.e., they contribute to our worldviews, perceptions, orientations) and, with this, frame many critical concepts (e.g., normality–abnormality, morality, aesthetics).

The virtue of this definition is that it captures the dynamic complexity of cultural experience and the fact that culture, while represented externally in artifacts, roles, and institutions, also is represented internally in the human psyche, in many forms that ultimately shape both normal and abnormal behavior (e.g., values, beliefs, epistemologies). The influence of cultural factors on psychopathology is now well accepted. That this should be the case is not surprising. The rates, etiology, diagnosis, and expression or manifestation of psychopathology are all culturally constructed and contextualized. Variations in stresses, coping resources, definitions of health and illness, and a score of cultural variables, such as language, dietary preferences, morality codes, and definitions of personhood, all converge to shape psychopathology.

Our views of reality are culturally constructed (Marsella, 1999)! Our worldviews—our cultural templates for negotiating reality—emerge from our inborn human effort after meaning, an effort that reflexively provokes us to describe, understand, predict, and control the world about us through the ordering of stimuli into complex belief and meaning systems that can guide behavior. The brain not only responds to stimuli, it also organizes, connects, and symbolizes them, and, in this process, generates patterns of explicit and implicit meanings and purposes that promote survival,

growth, and development. This process occurs through socialization and often leads us to accept the idea that our "constructed" realities are in fact realities. The "relativity" of the process and product is ignored in favor of the "certainty" provided by the assumption that our way of life is correct, righteous, and indisputable (e.g., ethnocentricity).

Sometimes, an entire cultural milieu may be pathogenic. For example, Edgerton (1992) coined the term "sick societies" to describe cultures in which ways of life have become destructive their members. Consider the possibility that certain cultures may become pathogenic by virtue of their collapse and disintegration, with dire consequences for members (e.g., an inner-city slum area in which drugs, violence, disorders abound; a national culture that advocates war, violence, hate, and destruction as a means of defining its identity).

Ethnocentricity

Our "realities" are culturally constructed (Marsella, 1999), and because of this, it is easy for us to be ethnocentric in our assumptions and practices regarding psychopathology. "Ethnocentricity" refers to a tendency or inclination to perceive reality from the vantage point of our own cultural experience. Thus, we "center" or anchor our perceptions within a "biased" viewpoint, much as the term "egocentric" describes the tendency to see things only from our limited, individual perspective. The simple fact is that we are often unaware of and/or insensitive to alternative culturally constructed realities can lead to misguided intentions and behaviors. When ethnocentricity is combined with the power to control knowledge and opinion, the results are dangerous, because we are blinded to the possibilities of differences in our construction and experience of reality.

We must recognize that current knowledge about psychopathology as reflected in the widespread use of DSM-IV-TR (American Psychiatric Association, 2000) is based on assumptions about the nature of health and disease that are embedded within Western culture. The "power" assigned to Western psychiatry because of Western economic, political, and military dominance does not mean that Western psychiatry is "accurate"; rather, it is merely dominant. The position of dominance can lead to many problems, because people from different ethnocultural groups are assessed, diagnosed, and treated according to the dominant viewpoint. Furthermore, even the research conducted is often framed with the dominant culture's assumptions and preferences for research design, data analysis, and data interpretation.

Ethnic Identity

As patients enter the Western psychiatric system as either ethnic/racial minorities or as patients within their own culture, but one dominated by a Western psychiatric system (e.g., Mexican patients in Mexico treated according to North American psychiatric approaches), the issue of ethnic identity becomes an essential consideration. The patient may belong to a particular ethnic/racial minority culture or be a resident in a mainstream culture but not be "identified" with that culture (e.g., Horvath, 1997; Yamada, 1998). Merely because the patient has a foreign last name and appearance (e.g., Japanese) does not mean he or she is not highly "Westernized" via acculturation processes (e.g., Chun, Organista, & Marin, 2002). The extent to which people are identified with a particular ethnic group, and engage in the attitudes, beliefs, and behaviors of that ethnic group, refers to their "ethnic identity" (Marsella & Kameoka, 1989). There are numerous ways to assess "ethnic identity" (see Dana, 1998; Ponterotto, Gretchen, & Chauhan, 2001; Yamada, Marsella, & Atuel, 2002). Some professionals have approached this topic from the viewpoint of "acculturation," or the extent to which a person may be embedded in a cultural context (e.g., Chun et al., 2002). It is noteworthy that DSM-IV-TR calls for an assessment of this variable in making a diagnosis as the first step in a cultural interview (American Psychiatric Association, 2000, p. 897).

CULTURAL INFLUENCES ON PSYCHOPATHOLOGY

The study of culture and psychopathology raises a number of basic questions that literally define the field:

- What is the role of cultural variables in the etiology of psychopathology?
- Are all mental disorders culture bound?
- What are the cultural variations in the rates and distribution of psychopathology? What

are some of the methodological considerations in conducting epidemiological research across cultures?
- What are the cultural variations in the classification and diagnosis of psychopathology (e.g., Mezzich et al., 1996; Paniagua, 2001)?
- What are the cultural variations in the phenomenological experience, manifestation, course and outcome of psychopathology?
- What are the cultural variations in standards of normality and abnormality?
- What psychometric factors must be considered in the assessment of psychopathology across cultures (e.g., Marsella, 2000b; Marsella & Leong, 1995)?

Space does not permit a detailed discussion of all these questions, but the first three questions are of sufficient importance to warrant discussion in this chapter.

Culture and the Etiology of Mental Disorders

Biological and Cultural Interaction

The role of cultural factors in the etiology of mental disorders is complex and varies as a function of the particular disorder and its plasticity. To the extent that a mental disorder may have a strong biological penetrance (e.g., certain forms of depressive disorders), the disorder will evidence great homogeneity across cultures because of biological similarity, and the influence may be minimal. However, to the extent that a mental disorder is influenced and shaped by learning and other contextual factors, thus having much more behavioral plasticity, acquired cultural factors may play a critical role. Expressions of a disorder may be more "homogenous" as a function of biological penetrance; yet even when the biological penetrance is extensive (e.g., Alzheimer's disease), it is still possible to see cultural variation. Figure 33.1 displays this thinking. Clearly, normal behavior is subject to the greatest cultural influence. But, even when there are severe neurological intrusions, culture still impacts the meaning, experience, and expression of disorder (Fabrega, 1995).

Cultural Factors in the Etiology of Mental Disorders

Cultural factors have been demonstrated to influence and shape mental disorders through a number of factors (Leighton & Murphy, 1961; Marsella, 1982, 1987, 2000a):

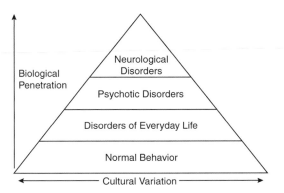

FIGURE 33.1. Cultural variations in mental disorders as a function of biological penetration and behavioral plasticity.

- Culture determines the types and parameters of physical and psychosocial stressors.
- Culture determines the types and parameters of coping mechanisms and resources used to mediate stressors.
- Culture determines basic personality patterns, including, but not limited to, self-structure, self-concept, and needs/motivational systems.
- Culture determines the language system of an individual, and it is language that assists us in the perception, classification, and organization of responses to reality.
- Culture determines the standards of normality, deviance, and health of an individual and society. It influences health ideology and attitudes, as well as treatment orientations and practices.

- Culture determines classification patterns for various disorders and diseases. In this respect, all mental disorders are culture-specific, and not simply those designated by Western professionals as exotic disorders.
- Culture determines the patterns of experience and expression of psychopathology, including factors such as onset, manifestation, course, and outcome.

Models of Cultural Etiology in Psychopathology

Among the conceptual approaches that have been advanced to explain cultural factors in the etiology of mental disorders, cultural disintegration and collapse has been advanced as a major hypothesis. This view was advocated quite early by Alexander Leighton (1959) in his classic work, *My Name is Legion*. Subsequent writings have elaborated on his contributions and suggested that general systems theory can be used to link stressors at the socioenvironmental level with the etiology of mental disorders at the individual level. Figure 33.2 displays these relationships (e.g., Marsella, Austin, & Grant, 2005).

Potential pathways between specific variables such as cultural collapse and disintegration, in which a culture's lack of coherence and integration eventually influences the mental health and well-being of members via intervening levels, are displayed in Figure 33.2. This is an important conceptual framework, because throughout the world today, as traditional cultures are faced with Westernization and other forms of rapid social change, members are left without a strong sense of ethnic identity and

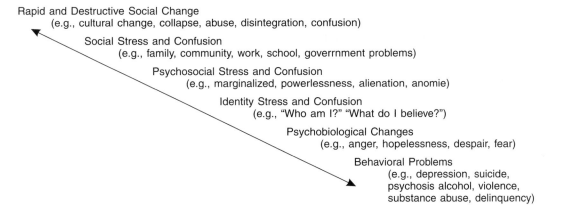

FIGURE 33.2. Sociocultural pathways to distress, deviance, and disorder.

continuity with their past, which results in conflict, confusion, and despair (e.g., Marsella et al., 2005).

Specific Sociocultural Variables Associated with Psychopathology

Numerous sociocultural variables have been posited as sources of psychopathology, including acculturation, urbanization, migration, and poverty. These variables have been primarily concerned with the etiology of psychopathology rather than its manifestations and/or courses and outcomes. All of these variables exercise their effects via stressors and stress variables. But each is unique in the specific stressors it embodies, and in the variations in the stress response that occurs. For example, acculturation and poverty stressors are both capable of eliciting stress states that can attain pathogenic levels. But each is unique in their stressor and stress-state parameters because of individual and cultural differences in coping resources. Nevertheless, they remain critical determinants of psychopathology that are rooted within cultural contexts (Marsella & Scheuer, 1993).

Acculturation

Acculturation refers to both the content and the process by which an individual from one ethnocultural group begins to assimilate and accommodate to the cultural traditions and ways of life of another—often contrasting—group. Acculturation can be a major source of stress, and as such is frequently considered a cause of maladaptation and maladjustment (Berry, 1997; Chun et al., 2002; Schmitz, 2003; Ward, 1997). The topic itself has been the subject of considerable debate and argument, especially with regard to its nature and measurement (Rudmin, 2003). Of special interest has been the yet unresolved issue of whether acculturation stress is associated with the onset of psychopathology, or whether it has little or no impact on the latter. For our purposes, we point out that the evidence is equivocal: Both sides have offered data to support their point of view.

Three things are needed at this point: (1) valid and reliable instruments for its assessment, (2) valid and reliable instruments for the assessment of psychopathology in the target groups, and (3) a clear description and understanding of the acculturative stresses involved, and a conceptual linkage to a broad spectrum of psychopathology and to adaptive patterns. In other words, for some people, the interaction between acculturation stresses and traditional ways of life are clearly disruptive and can lead to psychopathology. However, others manage acculturation in such a way that they may have multiple cultural identities, completely assimilate into the new lifestyle, or even reject both.

Thus, the question becomes which individuals are most subject to psychopathology—those who maintain a traditional identity, those who embrace multiple identities, those who assimilate, or those for whom none of these apply? Furthermore, because of measurement problems, we must consider the possibility of the discrepancy among behaviors, attitudes, and a psychological sense of who one is or chooses to be. Conclusions are still being debated.

Urbanization and Psychopathology

Urbanization and urban life have long been proposed to be sources of psychopathology because of the multiple stressors imposed on urban residents (e.g., Marsella, 1998; Caracci & Mezzich, 2001) including stressors from overstimulation involved in crowding, noise–air–visual pollution, crime and violence, homelessness, poverty, and transportation. Clearly, rural life has its own share of stressors and rural dwellers should not be thought of as being immune to psychopathology. Because most of the world will soon be living in urban settings, the risks associated with urban life must be considered. Urban life is demanding, and the difficulties may exceed the abilities of individuals and groups to cope with the pressures.

Marsella (1998), in his review of the urbanization studies in the mental health literature, claimed that urban life stressors are numerous and varied (i.e., environmental, economic, sociological, psychosocial, and psychological) and as such are connected to a broad spectrum of psychopathological responses that often do not fit the standard psychiatric nomenclature (including misery, demoralization, apathy, indifference, alienation, trauma, distress and distrust, suspicion, dissatisfaction) but are nevertheless states of serious discomfort and maladjustment. Many social deviancies (i.e., substance abuse, alcoholism, divorce, crime, gambling) also emerge within the urban life context. That these may also occur in non-urban settings does not exclude them from the pressures of urban life. Yet, even as we point this out, it is clear that urban life has many positive outcomes, including opportunities for new lifestyles, education, access to health care, and so forth. As was the case for acculturation, this topic is ripe for additional study.

Migration/Immigration

Migration/immigration has long been considered a major influence upon the onset of psychopathology (e.g., Marsella & Ring, 2003; Schmitz, 2003). Researchers have speculated about the possibility that migrants may actually be selected for particular forms of disorder or social deviancy, and this is reflected in the actual choice to migrate. Yet others have argued that the very best and strongest stock often migrates, and that the stress of the migration process and of acculturation is the source of psychopathology. The answer remains in debate. Certainly, if the pressures of migration and acculturation exceed the resources available for coping, then maladaptation and maladjustment may occur.

Culture shock, a syndrome of symptoms that includes paranoia, anxiety, somatic complaints, and a valorization of the home culture, is often found in sojourners and migrants during the early months of contact. Denial of opportunity and denigration of the migrant's self-esteem and sense of worth are also sources of discontent and distress. In our contemporary world, in which migration is now emerging as a major force for cultural contact, problems of acceptance are numerous. Ethnic and racial ghettos often develop as migrants are compelled to work for low wages and to live on the margins of acceptability and respect. This topic is in need of more research, because migration from East to West and from South to North brings millions of people from non-Western cultures to the Western world. Migrants seek hope and opportunity, but often find rejection and despair that lead to a breeding ground for anger, paranoia, and depression.

Poverty

Since the classic work on social class and mental illness by Hollingshead and Redlich (1958), it has long been accepted that lower social class individuals are at increased risk of mental illness. A recent meta-analysis of the literature (Lorant et al., 2003) supports the original conclusions. Low levels of education rather than low income per se has often been considered a key factor in these class differences. However, in a recent report on poverty and common mental disorders in developing countries, Patel and Kleinman (2003) concluded that factors such as the experience of insecurity and hopelessness, rapid social change, and risks of violence and poor physical health may better explain the vulnerability of the poor to common mental disorders. *Poverty and Psychology*, a recent volume edited by Carr and Sloan (2004), provides a detailed examination and analysis of the poverty experience, replete with its assaults on psychological and social well-being. In it, Moreira (2004) offers a specific review of the impact of poverty on mental health, including a discussion of the consequences of hegemonic globalization, marginalization, deprivation of power, trauma, low self-esteem, and nihilism. It seems clear that poverty imposes stresses of enormous proportion and frequency that exact a harsh toll on physical, mental, and spiritual health and well-being.

Culture-Specific (Culture-Bound) Disorders

The decision to list a series of "culture-bound" disorders in DSM-IV (American Psychiatric Association, 1994) called attention to a critical issue facing psychiatry and the study of psychopathology: Numerous previous publications had raised serious questions about these disorders and their implications for psychiatry (e.g., Simons & Hughes, 1985). DSM-IV (American Psychiatric Association, 1994) states the following about culture-bound disorders:

> Culture-bound syndromes are generally limited to specific societies or culture areas and are localized, folk, diagnostic categories that frame coherent meanings for certain repetitive, patterned, and troubling sets of experiences and observations. There is seldom a one-to-one equivalence of any culture-bound syndrome with a DSM diagnostic entity. (844)

But are mental disorders universal or are they a function of the cultural context in which they occur? For some, this controversy has been attenuated by the answer that both are possible. Nevertheless, the recognition that cultural factors may shape the rates and expressions of mental disorders represented a critical conceptual issue. Identifying a group of disorders with "non-Western" and "exotic" (some of these culture-bound disorders used to be called the "exotic" disorders, a testimony to our ethnocentric biases) names raised the issue of whether any disorder can escape cultural influence. And if this is the case, then is it not logical to assume that all disorders, including schizophrenia, depression, anxiety disorders, and so forth, are "culture bound." The question must be asked: Is DSM-IV-TR, with its hundreds of disorders, a culturally biased work and as such, might it actually have destructive consequences when misapplied to cultures in which it is not applicable? Table 33.1 lists some "culture-bound" disorders.

Marsella (2000b, p. 407), listed a series of questions regarding culture-bound disorders:

1. Should culture-bound disorders be considered neurotic, psychotic, or personality disorders?
2. Should these disorders be considered variants of disorders considered to be "universal" by Western scientists and professionals (e.g., *susto* [soul loss] as merely a variant of depression)?
3. Are these disorders variations of common "hysteria," "anxiety," "depression," or "psychotic" processes that arise in response to severe tension, stress, and/or fear, and present with specific culture content and expression?
4. Are there taxonomically different kinds of culture-bound syndromes (i.e., anxiety syndromes, depression syndromes, violence/anger syndromes, startle syndromes, dissociation syndromes)?

TABLE 33.1. Examples of Culture-Bound Disorders

Name	Definition and Cultural and Geographical Location
Amok	Sudden outburst of explosive and assaultive violence preceded by period of social withdrawal and apathy (Southeast Asia, Philippines).
Ataque de nervios	Uncontrollable shouting and/or crying. Verbal and physical aggression. Heat in chest rising to head. Feeling of losing control. Occasional amnesia for experience (Caribbean Latinos and South American Latinos).
Hwa-Byung	Acute panic, fear of death, fatigue, anorexia, dyspnea, palpitations, lump in upper stomach (Korea).
Latah	Startle reaction followed by echolalia and echopraxia, and sometimes coprolalia and altered consciousness (Malaysia and Indonesia).
Koro (shook yong)	Intense fear following perception that one's genitalia (men/women) or breasts (women) are withdrawing into one's body. Shame may also be present if perception is associated in time with immoral sexual activity (Chinese populations in Hong Kong and Southeast Asia).
Phii pob	Believes one is possessed by a spirit. Numbness of limbs, shouting, weeping, confused speech, shyness (Thailand).
Pissu	Burning sensations in stomach, coldness in body, hallucinations, dissociation (Ceylon).
Suchi-bai	Excessive concerns for cleanliness (changes street clothes, washes money, hops while walking to avoid dirt, washes furniture, remains immersed in holy river (Bengal, India—especially Hindu widows).
Susto (espanto)	Strong sense of fear that one has lost his or her soul. Accompanied by anorexia, weight loss, skin pallor, fatigue, lethargy, extensive thirst, untidiness, tachycardia, and withdrawal (Latinos in South and Central America, Mexico, and Latino migrants to North America).
Taijin kyofusho	Intense fear of interpersonal relations. Belief that parts of body give off offensive odors or displease others (Japan).
Tawatl ye sni	Total discouragement. Preoccupation with death, ghosts, spirits. Excessive drinking, suicide thoughts and attempts (Sioux Indians).
Uquamairineq	Hypnotic states, disturbed sleep, sleep paralysis, dissociative episodes and occasional hallucinations (Native Alaskans: Inuit, Yuit).

Note. From Marsella (2000b, p. 408). Copyright 2000 by the American Psychological Association. Reprinted by permission.

5. Do some culture-bound disorders have biological origins (e.g., *pibloktoq*—screaming and running naked in the Artic snow—has been considered to result from calcium and potassium deficiencies because of dietary restrictions; *amok* has been considered to result from febrile disorders and neurological damage)?

6. Are all disorders "culture-bound" disorders given that no disorder can escape cultural encoding, shaping, and presentation (e.g., schizophrenia, depression, anxiety disorders)?

The last question continues to arouse controversy. If the answer is "yes," then the implications for Western psychiatry are truly profound, for it indicates an inherent bias in its assumptions and practices from diagnosis to treatment. In so many ways, the culture-bound disorders issue confronts Western psychiatry with its most significant challenge.

Diagnosis and Classification

The American Psychiatric Association's (2000) DSM-IV-TR provides clear-cut guidelines for diagnosing and classifying mental disorders when cultural boundaries are a concern. DSM-IV (American Psychiatric Association, 1994, pp. 843–844) guidelines suggest five major areas be addressed:

1. *Cultural identity of the individual* (e.g., ethnocultural identity, language abilities and preferences).
2. *Cultural explanations of the individual's illness* (e.g., idioms of distress, meaning and perceived severity, any local illness categories used, perceived causes or explanatory models, current preferences for care).
3. *Cultural factors related to psychosocial environment and levels of functioning* (e.g., interpretations of social stressors, available social supports, levels of functioning and disability).
4. *Cultural elements of the relationship between the individual and the clinician* (e.g., note differences in culture and status of patient and clinician, and possible problems these differences may present, including problems regarding perceived normality, symptom expression, communication).
5. *Overall cultural assessment for diagnosis and care* (e.g., how the cultural formulation impacts diagnosis and care).

These guidelines articulate and anticipate many of the problems that one must face when seeking to diagnose and classify an individual within a cross-cultural context. The risks of error are obvious. Without understanding a person's cultural identity and experience, errors in diagnosis may lead to destructive treatments. It is necessary to have a firm understanding of the standards of normality and abnormality for that person and his or her culture and, especially, particular models of health and illness (see Alarcon, Bell, et al., 2002; Canino, Canino, & Arroyo, 1997; Mezzich et al., 1996; Mezzich & Fabrega, 2001; Paniagua, 2001; Rogler, 1997).

It is also important to note that virtually every ethnocultural group has its own diagnostic and classification system for psychopathology and social deviancies. These systems often address disorders that appear to be "similar" to Western disorders, such as PTSD (e.g., Fox, 2003). Yet we are once again faced with the challenge of "decontextualizing" a disorder when we assume that it is similar. In Hispanic culture, is *ataques de nervious* simply an anxiety disorder, or is *susto* simply a depressive disorder? In Japanese culture, is *shinkeishitsusho* simply a variant of neurasthenia, a popular 19th-century Western diagnostic category (Ohnuki-Tierney, 1984)? For example, consider the case of Samoans, who speak of four major categories of mental illness (see Clement, 1982):

1. *Ma'i o le mafaufau* (physical brain abnormalities)
2. *Ma'i aitu* (spirit possession)
3. *Ma'i valea* (strange, severe, and stupid, improper behavior)
4. Excess emotion:
   • *Ma'i ita*—anger, rage
   • *Ma'i manatu*—sadness, grief
   • *Ma'i popole*—worry

Do the apparent similarities or approximations indicate that the disorder has the same etiology, onset, expression, course, and outcome as disorders in the Western world? The answer in our opinion is "no!" The overt appearance of a disorder does not mean that the causes, experience, or pattern are the same. How can we separate a disorder from the very psyche in which it is construed and the very social context in which people respond to it?

The separation of mind and body introduces a dramatic difference in the conceptualization of psychopathology, especially with regard to its etiology and expressions. For example, in her excellent discussion of Japanese concepts and categories of mental illness, Ohnuki-Tierney (1984) wrote:

> When the Japanese postulate that *ki* (mind, spirit) is responsible for illness, they really do not mean psychogenesis. When they say *yamai wa ki kara* (illness from one's mind), they refer to physical illnesses resulting from worries and other psychological propensities that have a negative effect on the body. When they use the lable *ki no yamai*, they refer to a mild negative psychological state, such as a mild case of hypochondria. In both expressions, *ki* (mind, spirit) refers to a psychological state in the simple sense of the word. It does not refer to either "psychological problems" or "psychodynamics" as these terms are used in the United States. (p. 75)

Epidemiology of Mental Disorders

One of the most obvious questions about mental illness is whether there are cultural and international variations in the rates and distribution of mental illness. But because of the complexities involved in obtaining data to inform this question, any answers must be very tentative and subject to careful scrutiny. Even case identification, which seems like such a straightforward activity, can be filled with problems depending upon the source of the data, the measurement criteria, and the biases of the researcher. As we have pointed out, numerous issues are involved in the assessment and diagnosis of mental illness across cultures. These issues make valid data collection a difficult task. Marsella (1979) and Marsella, Sartorious, Jablensky, and Fenton (1985) listed criteria that must be met before data can be compared. They stated that the comparative epidemiological studies must do the following:

1. Use relevant ethnographic and anthropological data in designing an epidemiological study, especially in determining what constitutes a symptom or category or a case.
2. Develop glossaries of terms and definitions for symptoms and categories.
3. Derive symptom patterns and clusters using multivariate techniques rather than relying on simple a priori clinical categories.

4. Use similar/comparable case identification and validation methods.
5. Use culturally appropriate measurement methods that include a broad range of indigenous symptoms and signs that can be reliably assessed.
6. Establish frequency, severity, and duration baselines for indigenous and medical symptoms for normal and pathological populations.

These steps do not guarantee accuracy, but they do call attention to the complexities involved in conducting comparative epidemiological studies of mental illness. Failure to consider them can lead to destructive consequences for cultures under study, because they may either overestimate or underestimate actual rates leading to faulty policy decisions and misleading stereotypes.

The World Health Organization (2004) initiated a survey of the prevalence, severity, and treatment of DSM-IV mental disorders in six less developed countries and eight developed countries using door-to-door surveys of 60,463 community adults in the Americas, Europe, the Middle East, Africa, and Asia. Psychiatric assessments were conducted using the WHO world Mental Health Composite International Diagnostic Interview (WMH-CIDI), a fully structured, lay-administered psychiatric diagnostic interview. Results revealed that the prevalence of having a disorder during the previous year varied widely, from low rates of 4.3% in Shanghai, China, and 4.6% in Nigeria, to the highest rate of a 26.4% in the United States. Higher rates of anxiety were found in the United States, France, and Lebanon, and lower rates of anxiety were found Shanghai, Beijing, and Nigeria. The study also reported that 35.5–50.3% of serious cases in developed countries and 76.3–85.4% in less developed countries received no treatment in the 12 months prior to the interviews.

The profound variations in rates of disorder across developed and less developed countries raise interesting questions about the reasons for the results. Although it is possible that these rates accurately reflect differences because of a number of reasons related to stress levels, coping resources, and even genetic variations, the risk of bias in content and process of the actual interviews cannot and should not be ignored. For example, the content of the interview is clearly Western (e.g., anxiety, mood) and does not include indigenous examples of disorders. It is possible that different results might emerge if disorders were keyed to specific locations and the study examined rates of Western disorders and indigenous disorders in the less developed countries. Comparison data must meet stringent criteria for case recognition and inclusion, or one group may be seen as pathological and another as salutogenic, when the opposite may be true. The criteria listed previously for valid epidemiological studies must be considered.

Weiss (2001) proposes a culturally sensitive model of illness representations for epidemiological studies and Weiss, Cohen, and Eisenberg (2001) offer an integrative framework for cross-cultural epidemiological studies that captures both the complexity and critical consequences of epidemiological studies. In a similar vein, Alarcon et al. (2002) wrote:

> A crucial feature of the cultural epidemiologic context in relation to diagnosis is who decides on the values and priorities that transform findings into authoritative evidence. The cultural representation of mental illness requires a categorical identification but also a narrative account and a full assessment of the social context in which illness occurs. (p. 234)

CULTURE AND VARIOUS FORMS OF SERIOUS PSYCHOPATHOLOGY

Schizophrenia across Cultures

Among all the forms of mental disorder, schizophrenia has been considered to be the least influenced by cultural factors. Yet this assumption is highly questionable given the fact that there are considerable variations in the rates of schizophrenic disorders and considerable differences in its experience, course, and outcome (e.g., Jablensky et al., 1992; Marsella, Suarez, et al., 2002; Jenkins, 1998; Barrio et al., 2003; Jenkins & Barrett, 2004). The assumption is that because schizophrenia is considered to have a neurological (chemical and/or structural) basis, cultural variations should be minimal. But research indicates that that the very conceptualization of schizophrenia in the West may be a major source of impediment to understanding and curing it. Indeed, despite the fact that schizophrenia research in the West has advanced different sites of pathology, different etiologies, different expressions, and different treatment responsivities, we continue to use the

term, thus inviting confusion for both the public and professionals.

Research has shown that the expression of psychotic symptoms can be embedded in the patient's sociocultural context reflecting strongly held values and beliefs (Suhail & Cochrane, 2002). For instance, in the United States a triethnic study of psychotic symptoms assessed with a structured interview, African Americans were more likely to report higher hallucinatory behavior and suspicion scores than were European Americans, whereas European Americans exhibited more severity than African Americans in the excitement symptom score, and Latinos reported higher rates of somatic concern than both European Americans and African Americans (Barrio et al., 2003). In another triethnic study, which included a community outpatient sample, that European Americans had a more symptomatic profile than did African Americans and Latinos when assessed with standardized assessment tools (Bae, Brekke, & Bola, 2004; Brekke & Barrio, 1997). One potential explanation is that content experienced as culturally syntonic may be less likely to be reported as a distressing psychiatric complaint by certain ethnic/minority patients (Guarnaccia, Parra, Deschamps, Milstein, & Argiles, 1992).

Distinguishing between culturally appropriate and pathological content of symptoms to ensure that best practices are followed is facilitated by careful consideration of the manifestation and expression of distress (American Psychiatric Association, 1994; Gaines, 1995). Table 33.2 lists some of the sociocultural determinants of "schizophrenia" that have been advanced in the research literature, and Table 33.3 summarizes some of the many reasons why the course and outcome of schizophrenia varies across cultures (for reviews of the empirical literature, see also Jablensky et al., 1992; Marsella, Suarez, et al., 2002).

Kelly (2005) has called attention to the growing interest in the role of social, cultural, economic, and political factors in influencing clinical and outcome aspects of schizophrenic disorders:

> Despite clear evidence of a substantial biological basis to schizophrenia, there is also evidence that social, economic and political factors have considerable relevance to the clinical features, treatment and outcome of the illness. Individuals from lower socio-economic groups have an earlier age at first presentation and longer durations of untreated illness, both of which are associated with poor out-

TABLE 33.2. Some Sociocultural Determinants of Schizophrenia

1. Cultural concepts of personhood and the related implications of this for individuated versus unindividuated definitions of selfhood and reality.
2. Cultural concepts regarding the nature and causes of abnormality, discomfort, disorder, deviance, and disease, and those regarding the nature and cause of normality, health, and well-being.
3. Cultural concepts and practices regarding health, and medical care and prevention; attitudes toward illness and disease.
4. Cultural concepts and practices regarding breeding patterns and lineages.
5. Cultural concepts regarding prenatal care, birth practices, and postnatal care, especially in areas such as nutrition and disease exposure.
6. Cultural concepts and practices regarding socialization, especially family, community, and religious institutions, structures, and processes.
7. Cultural concepts and practices regarding medical and health care, especially with regard to the number and types of healers, doctors, sick-role statuses, etc.
8. Cultural stressors such as rates of sociotechnical change, sociocultural disintegration, family disintegration, migration, economic development, industrialization, and urbanization.
9. Culturally related patterns of deviance and dysfunction including trauma (PTSD), substance abuse, violence and crime, social isolation, alienation/anomie, and the creation of pathological and deviant subcultures.
10. Cultural stressors related to the clarity, conflicts, deprivations, denigrations, and discrepancies associated with particular needs, roles, values, statuses, and identities.
11. Cultural stressors related to sociopolitical factors such as racism, sexism, and ageism and the accompanying marginalization, segmentalization, and underprivileging.
12. Cultural resources and coping patterns, including institutional supports, social networks, social supports, and religious beliefs and practices.
13. Cultural exposure to various risk conditions, such as communicable diseases (e.g., viruses), toxins, dietary practices, population density, poverty, and homelessness.

TABLE 33.3. Potential Reasons for More Negative Course and Outcome of Schizophrenia (Psychotic Disorders) in Developed Countries

1. Schizophrenia is considered to be a biological disease that is relatively immutable to life circumstances.
2. Causes of schizophrenia are considered to be within the individual. Personal control and responsibility are assumed.
3. High social rejection and stigma attached to schizophrenia.
4. Individual burdens are demanding, because family resources are not often present.
5. Patient is often hospitalized and isolated from family and community. Custodial care, in disguised forms, is present.
6. Financial incentive to continue the sick role (i.e., disability payments, insurance payments) are numerous and easily available.
7. Stressors are numerous and supports are minimal.
8. Competency levels required for normal functioning are very high and very demanding upon social and intellectual skills and abilities (e.g., bank accounts, tax forms, housing, automobile maintenance, literacy skills).
9. Religious systems and spiritual concerns are often inadequate.
10. Comorbidities are numerous and complex (e.g., substance abuse, alcohol, trauma).
11. Treatments are primarily medical and invasive, with compounding iatrogenic effects (e.g., tardive dyskinesia).
12. Insensitivities to class and cultural differences between patient and professional abound with resulting communication problems.

Note. The inverse of these conditions is considered to be present in developing countries, accounting for their positive outcomes.

come. Individuals with schizophrenia are over-represented in the homeless population. Migration is associated with increased rates of mental illness, including schizophrenia, and this relationship appears to be mediated by psycho-social factors, including difficulties establishing social capital in smaller migrant groups. Individuals with schizophrenia are substantially over-represented amongst prison populations, and imprisonment increases the disability and stigma associated with mental illness, and impedes long-term recovery. The adverse effects of these social, economic and societal factors, along with the social stigma of mental illness, constitute a form of "structural violence" which impairs access to psychiatric and social services and amplifies the effects of schizophrenia in the lives of sufferers. As a result of these over-arching social and economic factors, many individuals with schizophrenia are systematically excluded from full participation in civic and social life, and are constrained to live lives that are shaped by stigma, isolation, homelessness and denial of rights. There are urgent needs for the development of enhanced aetiological models of schizophrenia, which elucidate the interactions between genetic risk and social environment, and can better inform bio-psycho-social approaches to treatment. (p. 721)

It is clear that in spite of extensive research, biological models of schizophrenic disorders continue to be inadequate in accounting for the many and varied patterns of symptomatology, course, outcome, and responsivity to treatment. The complexity of this spectrum of disorders appears to require a biopsychosocial approach in which cultural factors are considered to be a critical determinant of these clinical parameters.

Culture and Depressive Experience and Disorder

Another popular area of inquiry has been the relationship between culture and depressive experience and disorder. This topic has been the subject of extensive theoretical and clinical publications (e.g., Kleinman & Good, 1985; Marsella, Kaplan, & Suarez, 2002; Andrade et al., 2003). Marsella, Kaplan, et al. (2002) note that depression has long been a major topic of concern in Western medical history:

> Depressive experience and disorder have long been a source of concern in Western cultural traditions. Hippocrates (330–399 B.C.E.) included melancholia within his tripartite classification of disorders (i.e., mania, melancholia, phrenitis). He considered its cause to be a function of excessive

black bile. Stanley Jackson (1986), in his scholarly book on the topic, *Melancholy and Depression: From Hippocratic Times to the Present*, points out that the term "melancholy" was first used in ancient Greece to describe a disorder characterized by fear, nervous conduct, and sorrow. By the fourth century A.D., the Christian Church had begun to shape the concept of melancholy with its use of the term *acedia* to designate a cluster of feelings and behaviors associated with "dejection" (Jackson, 1986). The condition was often associated with religious fervor among monks and others that practiced isolation and self-denial. It came to mean sluggishness, lassitude, torpor, and non-caring, as well as those emotions associated with *tristitia* (i.e., sadness) and *desperatio* (i.e., despair). . . . "Melancholy" was used extensively in Europe until the 17th century when the term "depression" began to acquire currency. The promotion of "melancholy" as a major mood disorder, dysfunction, and problematic characterological orientation was assisted by the publication of Robert Burton's tome, *The Anatomy of Melancholia*, published in 1652. This book gained immediate and widespread popularity and remained a vital source of clinical insight and acumen on mood problems for subsequent centuries because of its encyclopedic coverage of the topic. (p. 50)

Emerging social conditions now suggest that depressive disorders are becoming the world's foremost psychiatric problem because of global challenges such as war, natural disasters, racism, poverty, cultural collapse, aging populations, urbanization, and rapid social and technological changes. The burdens from these challenges often exceed individual and social resources necessary for mediation (Marsella, Kaplan, et al., 2002). Some writers, such as Murray and Lopez (1996), contend that within a few decades, depression may be the greatest cause of disability worldwide. Under these circumstances, it is clear that we must make every effort to grasp the nature and consequences of this disorder(s). And it also clear that we must consider cultural contributions to depressive experience and disorder.

Marsella (1985, 1987) notes that the Western experience with depressive disorders may be a function of Western preoccupation with guilt, individualism, self-structure, self-control, personal responsibility, and an "abstract" language structure that creates distance between the person and his or her experience through language and self. In contrast, the Eastern experience of depression tends to reflect the integrated conception of mind and body as one and is portrayed through somatic symptoms rather than feelings of sadness (Marsella, Kinzie, & Gordon, 1973; Kleinman, 2004; Kleinman & Good, 1985).

In a fascinating study in Australia, Gattuso, Fullagar, and Young (2005) examined the construction of depression promoted in popular women's magazines (e.g., celebrity stories, advice columns, resource links) and contrasted this with governmental health materials promoting a "depression" literacy. They found that the latter privileges biomedical and psychological expertise and help-seeking behavior, whereas the former emphasizes self-management and biological expertise. The authors also contend the government materials do not emphasize gender differences and fail to discuss social inequities. What is so important about this study is its recognition of the critical role that communication media may play in favoring certain constructions over others and in shaping views that may or may not be held among populations—an example of cultural influences.

The very way we come to know the world about us (i.e., epistemology) becomes a mediator of depressive experience and disorder. Here, the possibility that cultural variations in the very nature of definition and construction the self (also personhood) mediates depressive experience and disorder become apparent. This viewpoint emphasizes the role of the subjective experience for psychopathology, because at this level the experiential meanings of both health and disorder become apparent (e.g., Jenkins, 1998; Jenkins & Barrett, 2004). In addition to Jenkins and Barrett (2004), many other writers acknowledge cultural variations in self, subjectivity, and emotion, and the implications this may have for behavior (e.g., Csordas, 1994; Kanagawa, Cross, & Markus, 2001; Kitayama, Markus, Matsumoto, & Norasakkunkit, 1997; Marsella, 1985; Nathan, Marsella, & Horvath, 1999).

Yet another variable that must be considered is social class and all that this implies for different racial and ethnic minorities. A recent meta-analytic review of social class by Lorant et al. (2004) concluded that depression is inversely related to social class (i.e., the lower the class, the higher the rate of depression). This is not unexpected because it highlights how certain social conditions such as poverty, racism, powerlessness, and marginalization can contribute to the onset of despair, hopelessness, and helplessness (Marsella, 1997). Marsella stated:

> Mental health is not only about biology and psychology, but also about education, economics, social structure, religion, and politics. There can be no mental health where there is *powerlessness*, because powerlessness breeds despair; there can be no mental health where there is *poverty*, because poverty breeds hopelessness; there can be no mental health where there is *inequality*, because inequality breeds anger and resentment; there can be no mental health where there is *racism*, because racism breeds low self-esteem and self denigration; and lastly, there can be no mental health where there is *cultural disintegration* and destruction, because cultural disintegration and destruction breed confusion and conflict. (Marsella, 1997, quoted in Marsella & Yamada, 2000, p. 10)

These words embody the complex challenges we face as mental health scientists and professionals. In a world in which medications have become commonplace, we must not forget the structural problems that contribute to depressive experience and disorder.

The stigma of depression can also be a cultural barrier to diagnosis and treatment in many cultures (e.g., Docherty, 1997). Despite an awareness of the urgent need for culturally sensitive interventions to address depressive disorders, relatively little research has been conducted. An NIMH-sponsored workgroup established to develop recommendations to improve access to preventive and treatment options for depression (Hollon et al., 2002) recommended increasing the involvement of minority researchers and developing user-friendly and nontraditional delivery methods to increase access of racial/ethnic minority groups to evidence-based interventions. A similar workgroup considered strategies that use social marketing research to increase access to services to ethnic and minority populations with affective disorders (Bruce, Smith, Miranda, Hoagwood, & Wells, 2002). Wells, Miranda, Bruce, Alegria, and Wallerstein (2004) also reported on an approach directed toward increasing access to mental health service interventions in diverse communities. There remains a need for special attention to disparities in access to treatments among vulnerable populations, such the youth (Richardson, DiGiuseppe, Garrison, & Christakis, 2003), older adults (Crystal, Sambamoorthi, Walkup, & Akincigil, 2003), and refugees and displaced victims of war and natural disaster (Carballo et al., 2004).

Culture, Alcoholism, and Substance Abuse

In a review of the literature on cultural aspects of alcoholism and substance abuse, Marsella (2004) noted that although the use and abuse of alcohol and various substances are quite old (e.g., mead or fermented honey may date back to 4000 B.C.E.; opium and hallucinogen use may date back to 1000 B.C.E.), misuse of both alcohol and substances has become a serious source of societal problems (e.g., Heath, 1995; Helzer & Canino, 1992; Staussner, 2001). The multiple cultural factors in alcohol and substance use include rituals (e.g., peyote cults), health and medications, religious experiences, social lubricants, occupational and group membership functions (e.g., military, police, factory workers), sensation seeking, commerce, and pleasurable states.

Cultural factors in the use and abuse of alcohol and various substances often assume location contexts that serve to reinforce and value them. For example, consider the fact that college fraternities now constitute one of the highest risk subcultures for the promotion of alcoholism and substance abuse. Other high-risk subcultures include the military, the entertainment industry, and the ubiquitous cocktail hour. These cultural activity settings often promote excesses in alcohol and substance use. American popular culture may also be considered a source for alcoholism and substance abuse, through its use of mass advertising, lobbying, and information groups supported by industries; corporations that produce alcohol and tobacco; positive portrayal of substance and alcohol use through celebrity and enter-

tainment media; the promotion of subcultures that endorse social deviancies (e.g., violent rap music cultures, bars/pubs); and the promotion of positive images of substance abuse and alcohol use (e.g., the Marlboro Man, Joe Camel, beer drinkers as macho men and sensual women, sexual images).

In addition, high-stress situations, such as being homeless, have been associated with increased rates of substance use (VanGeest & Johnson, 1997). Although immigrants as a group experience numerous daily stressors, they have been shown to misuse substances to a much lesser degree than do native-born citizens (Johnson, VanGeest, & Cho, 2002). As immigrants acculturate and adapt to the "American" lifestyle, their use and misuse of substances rises (Johnson et al., 2002; O'Hare & Van Tran, 1998). This rise in substance abuse was noted whether degree of acculturation was measured in terms of learning to speak English or length of residence (Gfroerer & Tan, 2003). Despite evidence of the negative ramifications of American popular cultural investigating the characteristics of immigrants rather than studying the components of the American way of life that may be contributing to substance abuse has remained the focus of the literature.

The complex ecology of American popular culture that supports and maintains alcoholism and substance abuse is displayed in Figure 33.3, which points out that popular cultures, much like ethnocultural groups, can also influence psychopathology in the form of various personal and social deviancies. A WHO (2004) study comparing prevalence rates of substance abuse during the previous year across 14 coun-

Ethos	Subculture	Location	Rewards
Self-Indulgence	Celebrity	Home	Addiction
Hedonism	Advertising	School/College	Pleasure
Immediacy	Parents	Parties/Proms	Escape, Drop Out
Conformity	Rock Culture	Clubs	Dulling
Macho	Teen Culture	Parks	Liberation
Sexualism	Military	Bashes	Social Acceptance
Grow-Up Quick	Drop Out	Private Rooms	Altered Conscious
Risk Behaviors	Fraternities	Concerts	Punish Parents
Competition	Sororities	Bars	Status

FIGURE 33.3. The complex ecology of alcoholism and substance abuse: Interactions/reciprocity of cultural ethos, subcultures, locations, and rewards.

tries found the Ukraine to have highest rates (6.4%) and Italy, Spain, and France to have the lowest rates (0.1–0.7%). However, we need to consider instrument and procedural bias need before we accept these results.

Based on the research and clinical literature on cultural considerations in alcoholism and substance abuse (e.g., Marsella, 2004), a number of conclusions can be reached:

- The causes and functions of alcohol and substance use and abuse vary according to culture, society, and historical period (e.g., ritual, nutrition, pleasure, economic scale).
- As alcohol and substance use and abuse become a problem (i.e., medical health, safety, economic loss) in a given setting, laws and other social restrictions and guidelines emerge to control and limit problems (e.g., prohibition, labeling a person a "drunk").
- Substantial cultural, local, and national variations characterize the patterns of use and endorsement of alcohol and substances.
- The particular kinds of alcoholic beverage and substances that emerge in a given setting and time are a function of available substances (e.g., mushrooms, rice, wheat), technology (e.g., distillation), and particular aversions and/or preferences.
- The definition and meaning of "abuse" can vary according to "legal," "medical," "moral," and/or "normative" perspectives and across cultures and settings.
- Understanding alcoholism and substance abuse may require new conceptual models that consider the complex ecology of the substance, location, people present, functions, and antecedents–consequences of use and abuse.
- As cultures and societies grow, complex laws of supply and demand emerge that may have international implications (e.g., external suppliers of cocaine) as new sources and substances become available.
- Certain types of substances may come into being for one purpose but end up serving others for which they were not intended (e.g., opium, morphine, heroin).
- Cultures often have political, economic, and social forces that encourage the use of alcohol and substances in spite of their known dangers (e.g., alcohol industry, tobacco industry). These forces, driven by profit, can shape public views of alcoholic beverages and substance abuse.

- Changes in alcohol and substance use and abuse, patterns and consequences occur so rapidly that research is often dated.

CONCLUSIONS AND SUMMARY

After many years of being ignored and marginalized, both mental health professionals and researchers have come to accept the important role of cultural factors in the etiology, expression, manifestation, distribution, course, and outcome of all forms of psychopathology and social deviancy. This acceptance is now codified in DSM-IV-TR (American Psychiatric Association, 2000) in the form of both warnings to clinicians to consider cultural variables and a diagnostic heuristic (pp. 897–903) and list of culture-bound disorders. To a large extent, this acknowledgment has led to a widespread concern about among practitioners and scientists alike about teaching and practicing cultural competence.

The facts were clear! Cultural factors had for too long been ignored at the expense of the patient's welfare and an accurate, valid portrayal and understanding of psychopathology. As the research progressed, it became clear that psychopathology, like normal behavior, evidenced considerable variations. The etiology of disorders was seem to be linked to a broad spectrum of sociocultural conditions, including cultural disintegration and collapse, poverty, crowding, rapid social change, acculturation, and a host of other forces that increased stress levels in the face of inadequate personal and collective resources. It also became clear that mental health could not be achieved apart from the sociopolitical context of life, in which forces such as racism, sexism, and political oppression fostered marginalization, powerlessness, and lack of privilege. Individuals and groups compelled to live on the margins of society would inevitably be faced with stress levels that would lead to distress, dysfunction, deviancy, and disorder.

Rates and expressions of psychopathology were also demonstrated to vary across ethnocultural boundaries; comparative studies used matched diagnoses, matched samples, international surveys, and factor-analytic research strategies. What emerged for depressive disorders was a variation in the expression that included limited guilt, existential despair, and low self-esteem, all of which were hallmarks of the disorder in the Western world. Even in the schizophrenic disorders, long considered to be universal disorders tied to genetic and biological substrates, ethnocultural and national variations emerged in rates, patterns, course, and outcome. For ethnic minorities in the United States, and for the entire international community, the consideration of cultural factors introduced a new hope that eradication of diagnostic inaccuracies and erroneous treatments would lead to improvements in the accessibility, availability, and acceptability of care and service provision.

Today the study of culture and psychopathology has emerged as a popular area of inquiry, with its own journals and books, conferences, and professional and scientific leaders. To a large extent, many of the latter are ethnic minority or international figures, and this is good, for it ensures that issues ignored for so long now inspire a new level of awareness and a new response. The fact of the matter is that the study of culture and psychopathology has revealed how our clinical knowledge and practices are often shaped not by science but by social and political forces that advance particular views based on their ethnocentric or gender biases. We are not free of this risk, but now that we are much more aware of it, we are capable of responding with corrective and preventive measures.

REFERENCES

Alarcon, R., Alegria, M., Bell, C., Boyce, C., Kirmayer, L., Lin, K. M., et al. (2002). Beyond the funhouse mirrors: Research agenda on culture and psychiatric diagnosis. In D. Kupfer, M. First, & D. Regier (Eds.), *A research agenda for DSM-V* (pp. 219–282). Washington, DC: American Psychiatric Press

American Psychiatric Association. (1994). *Diagnostic and statistical manual of mental disorders* (4th ed.). Washington, DC: Author.

American Psychiatric Association. (2000). *Diagnostic and statistical manual of mental disorders* (4th ed., text rev.). Washington, DC: Author.

American Psychological Association. (1992). Guidelines for providers of psychological services to ethnic, linguistic, and culturally diverse populations. *American Psychologist, 48,* 45–48.

Andrade, L., Caraveo-Anduaga, J., Berglund, P., Bijl, R. V., DeGraff, R., Vollebergh, W., et al. (2003). The epidemiology of major depressive episodes: Results from the International Consortium of Psychiatric Epidemiology Surveys. *International Journal of Methods in Psychiatric Research, 12,* 3–21.

Bae, S., Brekke, J., & Bola, J. (2004). Ethnicity and treatment outcome variation in schizophrenia: A longitudinal study of community-based psychosocial rehabilitation interventions. *Journal of Nervous and Mental Disease, 192,* 623–628.

Barrio, C., Yamada, A.-M., Atuel, H., Hough, R., Yee, S., Russo, P., et al. (2003). A tri-ethnic examination of symptom expression on the positive and negative syndrome scale in schizophrenia spectrum disorders. *Schizophrenia Research, 6,* 259–269.

Becerra, R., Karno, M., & Escobar, L. (Eds.). (1982). *Mental health and Hispanic-Americans: Clinical perspectives.* New York: Grune & Stratton.

Bernal, G., Trimble, J., Burlew, K., & Leong, F. (Eds.). (2003). *Handbook of racial and ethnic minority psychology.* Thousand Oaks, CA: Sage.

Berry, J. (1997). Immigration, acculturation, and adaptation. *Applied Psychology: An International Review, 46,* 5–34.

Brekke, J. S., & Barrio, C. (1997). Cross-ethnic symptom differences in schizophrenia: The influence of culture and minority status. *Schizophrenia Bulletin, 23,* 305–316.

Bruce, M., Smith, W., Miranda, J., Hoagwood, K., & Wells, K. (2002). NIMH Affective Disorders Workgroup: Community-based interventions. *Mental Health Services Research, 4,* 205–214.

Canino, G., Canino, I., & Arroyo, W. (1997). Cultural considerations in the classification of mental disorders in children and adolescents. In T. Widiger, A. Frances, H. Pincus, R. Ross, M. First, & W. Davis (Eds.), *DSM-IV sourcebook* (Vol. 3, pp. 873–883). Washington, DC: American Psychiatric Association Press.

Caracci, G., & Mezzich, J. (2001). Culture and urban mental health. In J. Mezzich & H. Fabrega (Eds.), *Cultural psychiatry: International perspectives* (pp. 581–594). Philadelphia: Saunders.

Carballo, M., Smajkic, A., Zeric, D., Dzidowska, M., Gebre-Medhin, J., & Van Halem, J. (2004). Mental health and coping in a war situation: The case of Bosnia and Herzegovina. *Journal of Biosocial Science, 36,* 463–77.

Carillo, E., & Lopez, A. (2001). *The Latino psychiatric patient: Assessment and treatment.* Washington, DC: American Psychiatric Association Press.

Carr, S., & Sloan, T. (Eds.). (2004). *Poverty and psychology: From global perspective to local practice.* New York: Kluwer Academic/Plenum Press.

Castillo, R. J. (1996). *Culture and mental illness: A client-centered approach culture and mental illness.* Los Angeles: Wadsworth.

Caudill, W., & Lin, T. (Eds.). (1969). *Mental health research in Asia and the Pacific,* Honolulu: University Press of Hawaii.

Chakraborty, A. (1991). Culture, colonialism, and psychiatry. *Lancet, 337,* 1204–1207.

Chun, K., Organista, P., & Marin, G. (2002). *Acculturation: Advances in theory, measurement, and applied research.* Washington, DC: American Psychological Association Press.

Clement, D. (1982). Samoan folk knowledge of mental disorder. In A.J. Marsella & G. White (Eds.), *Cultural conceptions of mental health and therapy* (pp. 193–213). Boston: Reidel.

Crystal, S., Sambamoorthi, U., Walkup, J., & Akincigil, A. (2003). Diagnosis and treatment of depression in the elderly medicare population: Predictors, disparities, and trends. *Journal of the American Geriatrics Society, 51*, 1718–1728.

Csordas, T. (1994). *Embodiment and experience: The existential ground of culture and self.* New York: Cambridge University Press.

Cuellar, I., & Paniagua, F. (2000). *Handbook of multicultural mental health.* New York: Academic Press.

Dana, R. (1998). *Understanding cultural identity in intervention and assessment.* Thousand Oaks, CA: Sage.

Docherty, J. (1997). Barriers to the diagnosis of depression in primary care. *Journal of Clinical Psychiatry Supplement, 158*, 5–10.

Draguns, J. (1973). Comparisons of psychopathology across cultures: Issues, findings, directions. *Journal of Cross-Cultural Psychology, , 4*, 9–47.

Draguns, J. (1980). Psychological disorders of clinical severity. In H. Triandis & J. Draguns (Eds.), *Handbook of cross-cultural psychology: Vol. 6. Psychopathology* (pp. 99–174). Boston: Allyn & Bacon.

Draguns, J. (1990). Normal and abnormal behavior in cross-cultural perspective. In J. Berman (Ed.), Nebraska Symposium on Motivation: *Cross-cultural perspectives* (pp. 235–278). Lincoln: University of Nebraska Press.

Draguns, J., & Tanaka-Matsumi, J. (2003). Assessment of psychopathology across and within cultures: Issues and findings. *Behaviour Research and Therapy, 41*, 755–776.

Edgerton, R. (1992). *Sick societies: Challenging the myth of primitive harmony.* New York: Free Press.

Fox, S. (2003). The Mandinka nosological system in the context of post-traumatic syndromes. *Transcultural Psychiatry, 4*, 488–506.

Gaines, A. (1995). Culture-specific delusions: Sense and nonsense in cultural context. *Psychiatric Clinics of North America, 18*, 281–301.

Gattuso, S., Fullagar, S., & Young, I. (2005). Speaking of women's "nameless misery": The everyday construction depression in Australia's women's magazines. *Social Science and Medicine, 61*, 1640–1648.

Gfroerer, J., & Tan, L. (2003). Substance use among foreign-born youths in the United States: Does the length of residence matter? *American Journal of Public Health, 93*, 1892–1895.

Guarnaccia, P., Parra, P., Deschamps, A., Milstein, G., & Argiles, N. (1992). *Si Dios quiere*: Hispanic families' experiences of caring for a seriously mentally ill family member. *Culture, Medicine and Psychiatry, 16*, 187–215.

Heath, D. (Ed.). (1995). *International handbook on alcohol and culture.* Westport, CT: Greenwood.

Helzer, J., & Canino, G. (Eds.). (1992). *Alcoholism in North America, Europe, and Asia.* New York: Oxford University Press.

Hollingshead, A., & Redlich, F. (1958). *Social class and mental illness: A community study.* New York: Wiley.

Hollon, S., Munoz, R., Barlow, D., Beardslee, W., Bell, C., Bernal, G., et al. (2002). Psychosocial intervention development for the prevention and treatment of depression: Promoting innovation and increasing access. *Biological Psychiatry, 52*, 610–630.

Horvath, A.-M. (1997). Ethnocultural identification and the complexities of ethnicity. In K. Cushner & R. W. Brislin (Eds.), *Improving intercultural interactions, V2: Models for cross-cultural training programs* (pp. 165–183). Thousand Oaks, CA: Sage.

Jablensky, A., Sartorius, N., Ernberg, N., Anker, M., Korten, A., Cooper, J. E., et al. (1992). Schizophrenia: Manifestations incidence, and course in different cultures: A WHO ten country study. *Psychological Medicine, 20*, 1–97. (Monograph supplement)

Jenkins, J. (1998). Diagnostic criteria for schizophrenia and related psychotic disorders: Integration and suppression of cultural evidence in DSM-IV. *Transcultural Psychiatry, 35*, 357–376.

Jenkins, J., & Barrett, R. (2004). Introduction. In *Schizophrenia, culture, and subjectivity: The edge of experience* (pp. 1–23). New York: Cambridge University Press.

Johnson, T., VanGeest, J., & Cho, Y. (2002). Migration and substance use: Evidence from the U.S. National Health Interview Survey. *Substance Use and Misuse, 37*, 941–972.

Kanagawa, C., Cross, S., & Markus, H. (2001). "Who am I?": The cultural psychology of the conceptual self. *Personality and Social Psychology Bulletin, 27*, 90–103.

Kelly, B. (2005). Structural violence and schizophrenia. *Social Science and Medicine, 61*, 721–730.

Kirmayer, L. (1998). Editorial: The fate of culture in DSM-IV. *Transcultural Psychiatry, 35*, 339–343.

Kitayama, S., Markus, H., Matsumoto, H., & Norasakkunkit, V. (1997). Individual and collective processes in the construction of the self: Self-enhancement in the United States and self-criticism in Japan. *Journal of Personality and Social Psychology, 72*, 1245–1267.

Kleinman, A. (1980). *Patients and healers in the context of culture: An exploration of the borderland between anthropology, medicine, and psychiatry.* Berkeley: University of California Press.

Kleinman, A. (2004). Culture and depression. *New England Journal of Medicine, 351*, 951–953.

Kleinman, A., & Good, B. (Eds.). (1985). *Culture and depression.* Berkeley: University of California Press.

Kraepelin, E. (1904). *Vergleichende psychaitrie* [Comparative psychiatry]. *Zentralblatt für Nervenheilkunde und Psychiatrie, 15*, 433–437.

Kroeber, A., & Kluckhohn, C. (1952). *Culture: A critical review of concepts and definitions.* Cambridge, MA: Peabody Museum.

Lebra, W. (Ed.). (1972). *Transcultural research in mental health.* Honolulu: University Press of Hawaii.

Leighton, A. (1959). *My name is legion: Foundations for a theory of man in relation to culture.* New York: Basic Books.

Leighton, A., Lambo, A., Hughes, C., Leighton, D., Murphy, J., & Macklin, D. (1963). *Psychiatric disorder among the Yoruba.* Ithaca, NY: Cornell University Press.

Leighton, A., & Murphy, J. (1961). Cultures as causative of mental disorder. *Milbank Memorial Fund Quarterly, 38,* 341–383.

Lin, K. M., Smith, M., & Ortiz, V. (2001). Culture and psychopharmacology. In J. Mezzich & H. Fabrega (Eds.), *Cultural psychiatry: International perspectives* (pp. 523–538). Philadelphia: Saunders.

Lin, T., Tseng, W., & Yeh, E. (1995). *Chinese societies and mental health.* New York: Oxford University Press.

Littlewood, R., & Lipsedge, M. (1997). *Aliens and alienists: Ethnic minorities and psychiatry.* London: Routledge.

Lorant, V., Deliege, D., Eaton, W., Robert, A., Philippot, P., & Ansseau, M. (2004). Socioeconomic inequalities in depression: A meta-analysis. *American Journal of Epidemiology, 157,* 98–112.

Marsella, A. J. (1979). Cross-cultural studies of mental disorders. In A. J. Marsella, R. Tharp, & T. Ciborowski (Eds.), *Perspectives on cross-cultural psychology* (pp. 233–264). New York: Academic Press.

Marsella, A. J. (1982). Culture and mental health: An overview. In A. J. Marsella & G. White (Eds.), *Cultural conceptions of mental health and therapy* (pp. 359–388). Boston: Reidel/Kluwer.

Marsella, A. J. (1985). Culture, self, and mental disorder. In A. J. Marsella, G. DeVos, & F. Hsu (Eds.), *Culture and self: Asian and Western perspectives* (pp. 281–308). London: Tavistock Press.

Marsella, A. J. (1987). The measurement of depressive experience and disorder across cultures. In A. J. Marsella, R. Hirtschfeld, & M. Katz (Eds.), *The measurement of depression* (pp. 376–397). New York: Guilford Press.

Marsella, A. J. (1993). Sociocultural foundations of psychopathology: A pre-1970 historical overview. *Transcultural Psychiatric Research and Review, 30,* 97–142.

Marsella, A. J. (1997, February 15). *The plight of the Native Hawaiians.* Paper presented at the Native Hawaiian Identity and Acculturation, Union of Polynesian Nations Conference, Honolulu, HI.

Marsella, A. J. (1998). Urbanization, mental health, and social deviancy: A review of issues and research. *American Psychologist, 53,* 624–634.

Marsella, A. J. (1999). In search of meaning: Some thoughts on belief, doubt, and well being. *International Journal of Transpersonal Studies, 18,* 41–52.

Marsella, A. J. (2000a). Culture and psychopathology. In A. Kazdin (Ed.), *The encyclopedia of psychology.*

Washington, DC: American Psychological Association Press.

Marsella, A. J. (2000b). Culture-bound disorders. In A. Kazdin (Ed.), *The encyclopedia of psychology* (pp. 407–410). Washington, DC: American Psychological Association Press.

Marsella, A. J. (2004, October). *Culture, alcoholism, and substance abuse.* Workshop presentation at the Hawaii Psychological Association Annual Meeting, Honolulu.

Marsella, A. J., Austin, A., & Grant, B. (Eds.). (2005). *Cultures in transition: Social change and well-being in the Pacific Islands.* New York: Springer.

Marsella, A. J., Friedman, M., Gerrity, E., & Scurfield, R. (1996). *Ethnocultural aspects of PTSD.* Washington, DC: American Psychological Association Press.

Marsella, A. J., & Higginbotham, H. (1984). Traditional Asian medicine: Applications to psychiatric services in developing nations. In P. Pedersen, N. Sartorius, & A. J. Marsella (Eds.), *Mental health services: The cross-cultural context* (pp. 175–197). Beverly Hills, CA: Sage.

Marsella, A. J., & Kameoka, V. (1989). Ethnocultural issues in the assessment of psychopathology. In S. Wetzler (Ed.), *Measuring mental illness: Psychometric assessment for clinicians* (pp. 231–256). Washington, DC: American Psychiatric Press.

Marsella, A. J., Kaplan, A., & Suarez, E. (2002). Cultural considerations for understanding, assessing, and treating depressive experience and disorders. In M. Reinecke & J. Cohler (Eds.), *Comparative treatments of depression* (pp. 47–78). New York: Springer.

Marsella, A. J., Kinzie, D., & Gordon, P. (1973). Ethnocultural variations in the expression of depression. *Journal of Cross-Cultural Psychology, 4,* 435–458.

Marsella, A. J., & Leong, F. (1995). Cross-cultural assessment of personality and career decisions. *Journal of Career Assessment, 3,* 202–218.

Marsella, A. J., & Ring, E (2003). Human migration and immigration: An overview. In L. Adler & U. Gielen (Eds.), *Migration: Immigration and emigration in international perspective* (pp. 3–22). Westport, CT: Praeger.

Marsella, A. J., Sartorius, N., Jablensky, A., & Fenton, R. (1985). Culture and depressive disorders. In A. Kleinman & B. Good (Eds.), *Culture and depression* (pp. 299–324). Berkeley: University of California Press.

Marsella, A. J., & Scheuer, A. (1993). Coping: Definitions, conceptualizations, and issues. *Integrative Psychiatry, 9,* 124–134.

Marsella, A. J., Suarez, E., Leland, T., Morse, H., Digman, B., & Scheuer, A. (2002). *Culture and schizophrenia: An overview of the research and clinical literature.* In H. Bot, M. Braakman, L. Preijde, & W. Wassink (Eds.), *Culturen op de vlucht* [Cultures in transition and change]. Amsterdam: Afdeling Phoenix.

Marsella, A. J., & White, G. (Eds.). (1982). *Cultural conceptions of mental health and therapy.* Boston: Reidel.

Marsella, A. J., & Yamada, A. (2000). Culture and mental health: An overview. In I. Cuellar & F. Paniagua (Eds.), *Handbook of multicultural mental health: Assessment and treatment of diverse populations* (pp. 3–26). New York: Academic Press.

Mezzich, J., & Fabrega, H. (2001). *Cultural psychiatry: International perspectives.* Philadelphia: Saunders.

Mezzich, J., Kleinman, A., Fabrega, H., & Parron, D. (Eds.). (1996). *Culture and psychiatric diagnosis: A DSM-IV perspective.* Washington, DC: American Psychiatric Press.

Moreira, V. (2004). Poverty and psychopathology. In S. Carr & T. Sloan (Eds.), *Poverty and psychology: From global perspective to local practice* (pp. 69–86). New York: Kluwer Academic/Plenum Press.

Murray, C., & Lopez, A. (Eds.). (1996). *Quantifying global health risks: The burden of disease attributable to selected risk factors in 1990 and projected to 2020.* Cambridge, MA: Harvard University Press.

Nathan, J., Marsella, A. J., & Horvath, A. (1999). An ethnosemantic analysis of the concepts of self and group among Caucasians, Japanese-Americans, and Japanese Nationals. *International Journal of Intercultural Relation, 23,* 711–725.

O'Hare, T., & Van Tran, T. (1998). Substance abuse among Southeast Asians in the U.S.: Implications for practice and research. *Social Work and Health Care, 26,* 69–80.

Ohnuki-Tierney, E. (1984). *Illness and culture in contemporary Japan: An anthropological view.* New York: Cambridge University Press.

O'Nell, T. (1998). *Disciplined hearts: Hearts, identity and depression in an American Indian community.* Los Angeles: University of California Press.

Paniagua, F. (2001). *Diagnosis in a multicultural context.* Thousand Oaks, CA: Sage.

Patel, V., & Kleinman, A. (2003). Poverty and common mental disorders in developing countries. *Bulletin of the World Health Organization, 81,* 609–613.

Phoon, W., & Macindoe, I. (Eds.). (2003). *Untangling the threads: Perspectives on mental health in Chinese communities.* Parramatta, Australia: Transcultural Mental Health Centre.

Ponterotto, J., Gretchen, D., & Chauhan, R. (2001). Cultural identity and multicultural assessment: Quantitative and qualitative tools for the clinician In L. Suzuki & J. Ponterotto, et al. (Eds.), *Handbook of multicultural assessment: Clinical, psychological, and educational applications* (2nd ed., pp. 67–99). San Francisco: Jossey-Bass.

Richardson, L., DiGiuseppe, D., Garrison, M., & Christakis, D. (2003). Depression in Medicaid-covered youth: Differences by race and ethnicity. *Archives of Pediatric and Adolescent Medicine, 157,* 984–989.

Rogler, L. (1997). Framing research on culture in psychiatric diagnosis: The case of the DSM-IV. *Psychiatry, 59,* 145–155.

Rudmin, F. (2003). Critical history of the acculturation, psychology of assimilation, separation, integration, and marginalization. *Review of General Psychology, 7,* 3–37.

Schmitz, P. (2003). Psychosocial factors of immigration and emigration: An introduction. In L. Adler & U. Gielen (Eds.), *Migration: Immigration and emigration in international perspective* (pp. 23–50). Westport, CT: Praeger.

Simons, R., & Hughes, C. (Eds.). (1985). *The culture-bound syndromes.* Boston: Reidel/Kluwer.

Straussner, S. (Ed.). (2001). *Ethnocultural factors in substance abuse.* New York: Guilford Press.

Suhail, K., & Cochrane, R. (2002). Effect of culture and environment on the phenomenology of delusions and hallucinations. *International Journal of Social Psychiatry, 48,* 126–138.

Telles, M., & Karno, M. (Eds.). (1994). *Latino mental health: Current research and policy perspectives.* Los Angeles: Neuropsychiatric Institute, University of California at Los Angeles.

Triandis, H., & Draguns, J. (Eds.). (1981). *Handbook of cross-cultural psychology: Vol. 6. Psychopathology.* Boston: Allyn & Bacon.

U.S. Department of Health and Human Services. (2001). *Mental health: Culture, race, and ethnicity* (DHHS, Public Health Service, Office of the Surgeon General). Rockville, MD: U.S. Government Printing Office.

VanGeest, J., & Johnson, T. (1997). Substance use patterns among homeless migrants and nonmigrants in Chicago. *Substance Use and Misuse, 32,* 877–907.

Ward, C. (1997). Culture learning, acculturative stress, and psychopathology: Three perspectives on acculturation. *Applied Psychology: An International Review, 46,* 58–62.

Weiss, M. (2001). Cultural epidemiology: An introduction and overview. *Anthropology and Medicine, 8,* 5–29.

Wells, K., Miranda, J., Bruce, M., Alegria, M., & Wallerstein, N. (2004). Bridging community intervention and mental health services research. *American Journal of Psychiatry, 161,* 955–963.

World Health Organization World Mental Health Consortium. (2004). Prevalence, severity, and unmet need for treatment of mental disorders in the WHO World Mental Health Surveys. *Journal of the American Medical Association, 291,* 2581–2590.

Yamada, A-M. (1998). Multidimensional identification. In T. Singelis (Ed.), *Teaching about culture, ethnicity, and diversity* (pp. 141–149). Thousand Oaks, CA: Sage.

Yamada, A-M., Marsella, A. J., & Atuel, H. (2002). Development of a Cultural Identification Battery for Asian and Pacific Islander Americans in Hawai'i. *Asian Psychologist, 3,* 11–20.

PART VII

COMMENTARIES FROM TWO PERSPECTIVES

CHAPTER 34

An Anthropological Perspective
The Revival of Cultural Psychology—
Some Premonitions and Reflections

RICHARD A. SHWEDER

The publication of this handbook is of historical importance for the field of cultural psychology, and it is a fitting and useful form of acknowledgment of an intellectual revival or take-off of interdisciplinary research interests that began about 25 years ago. It is also a welcome opportunity to take stock and imagine future possibilities for creative investigations of diversity in human mentalities (the different things people know, think, want, feel, and value) across distinguishable culture-dependent groups. Although the volume is surely going to become a canonical text for anyone who has been engaged in or wishes to become part of the lively ongoing conversation that began to emerge in the early 1980s at the interface of social psychology and anthropology, it will certainly also interest developmental psychologists, cognitive psychologists, philosophers, and even linguists. Robert LeVine's chapter (Chapter 2, this volume) tells a story of academic ancestry that must read like ancient history to contemporary social psychologists doing work in cultural psychology (and an even deeper history going back many centuries, one

that all of us should know, can be found in Gustav Jahoda's [1993] *Crossroads between Culture and Mind*). So it is a very old conversation, but a new one as well, and one that has grown in depth and intensity over the past couple of decades.

Increasingly, this renewed conversation has been gaining widespread recognition. One is actually heartened to read the five-paragraph entry under "Cultural Psychology" that appears in Wikipedia, not only because that consensus-seeking online encyclopedia acknowledges the discipline but also because they more or less get it right. Here is all or part of the lead sentence from each of the five paragraphs: "Cultural psychology is a field of psychology which contains the idea that culture and mind are inseparable"; "Cultural psychology has its roots in the 1960s and 1970s but became more prominent in the 1980s and 1990s"; "Cultural psychology is distinct from cross-cultural psychology in that cross-cultural psychologists generally use culture as a means of testing the universality of psychological processes rather than determining how local cultural practices shape psychological processes"; "Cultural psychology research informs several fields within psychology, including social psychology, developmental psychology, and cognitive psychology"; "One of the most significant themes in recent years has been cultural differences between East Asian and North Americans in attention (Masuda & Nisbett, 2001), perception (Kitayama, Duffy, Kawamura, & Larsen, 2003), cognition (Nisbett, Peng, Choi, & Norenzayan, 2001) and social-psychological phenomena such as the self (Markus & Kitayama, 1991)." They also write: "So whereas a cross-cultural psychologist might ask whether Piaget's stages of development are universal across a variety of cultures, a cultural psychologist would be interested in how the social practices of a particular set of cultures shape the development of cognitive processes in different ways." Perhaps the authors of the entry do go a bit overboard in associating cultural psychology with the view that "there are no universal laws for how the mind works," but for the most part they get the point.

Indeed, my own earliest anticipation of a cultural psychology revival—at the time it was little more than a premonition—does go back to the 1960s. In 1964 the anthropologists A. Kimball Romney and Roy D'Andrade published an influential special issue of the *American Anthropologist* titled "Transcultural Studies in Cognition." That collection of essays, originally prepared for an interdisciplinary Social Science Research Council conference on culture and intellective processes held in Mexico in the spring of 1963, was an intimation that something new and interdisciplinary—on the frontiers of anthropology, psychology and linguistics—might soon be in the air. Best of all, the publication included a "Summary of Participants' Discussion," which contained some rather eye-opening (and even entertaining) transcripts of verbal exchanges (and sallies) between several social psychologists and several cultural anthropologists. Comments and quips included:

> In using the semantic differential, people are forced to evaluate objects, and apparently there is consistency in the way in which they respond. I don't understand what the meaning of this consistency is in terms of the culture in which it occurred. And until I understand it, I don't see any point in comparing across cultures. You say that these factors are related to "visceral reactions"—then perhaps what this consistency means is that

cultural differences have been wiped out and only a common animal reaction remains. —anthropologist William Sturtevant, critiquing psychologist Charles Osgood (p. 238)

No, just the reverse. We are trying to find a framework of similarities within which we can observe more meaningfully and more rigorously real differences. Then we can be sure that these are real differences and not just artifacts of the language being used. —psychologist Charles Osgood (p. 238)

If you did investigate which adjectives went together in a language and culture which you know, do you doubt seriously that you would find three dimensions similar to evaluation, potency, and activity? —psychologist Fred Strodtbeck, addressing anthropologist Sturtevant (p. 238)

I don't know. And the reason it bothers me is that it seems so artificial to force people to tell you whether "Wednesday" is "good" or "bad." And I don't understand what significance any consistency you may get in forced tasks such as this has for understanding a culture. —anthropologist William Sturtevant (p. 238)

Why is it more arbitrary to employ the probes used in the semantic differential than it is to employ the "kind of" or "part of" questions [Charles] Frake uses? What is there unique about one kind of questioning which makes it arbitrary? —psychologist Charles Osgood (p. 238)

I think we are doing the same things for different reasons. We are both asking people questions and getting answers. But one difference is that if people laugh at one of my questions, I throw away the question. If people laugh at what you ask, you force an answer and say, "Come on, boys, now this is serious." What I would like to know is, "How much force is legitimate, and is the amount of force a variable to be taken into consideration?" —anthropologist Charles Frake (p. 238)

This is the narrow line we have tried hard to walk. That is, in order to get comparability, we have had to use enough control over the general context in which the data is elicited to obtain some reasonable security of equivalence. The problem, then, is to make sure that the kind of control that is exercised for that purpose can in no way influence the substantive relationships within the material. . . . —psychologist Charles Osgood (p. 238)

In their summary of the conversations among the conference participants, the editors Roy D'Andrade and Kim Romney (two very multidisciplinary graduates of the Harvard University Department of Social Relations) tried to comprehend the disciplinary tensions between the anthropologists and the psychologists by drawing a distinction between the study of "codes" (associated with anthropological research) and the study of "intellectual processes" (associated with psychological research). They imagined a hypothetical research project in which anthropologists and psychologists go off together hand in hand to study ordinary game-playing behavior in games such as chess, checkers, or baseball, but end up parting ways by asking very different questions (e.g., "What are the rules of this game?" vs. "Which intellectual abilities differentiate winning players from losing players?") and end up developing two very different theories of psychological functioning and methods of research. D'Andrade and Romney elaborated on this imagined contrast. Anthropologists, they suggested, tend to study socially learned codes, rules, and meanings for the interpretation of a behavior (remember Clifford Geertz's [1973] famous example of the "blink [or was it a 'wink'?] of an eye"); and for the anthropologist "behavior" is treated as a symbol or message that requires interpretation of its meaning, often in relation to codes, rules or norms of some sort. Psychologists, on the other hand, tend to study intellectual processes such as categorization, inference, or memory and view socially learned codes, rules, and meanings as mere content (or even as "noise") that should be ignored or filtered out in any study of the basic elements of mental functioning.

Yet D'Andrade and Romney also made the following crucial observation, which I take to be a central tenet of cultural psychology, namely, that what you think about and with (the meaning or content of ones thinking) can be decisive for how you think and that culture and psyche make each other up. This is their key remark:

> The relationship between the codes an individual learns and the intellective processes of the individual is apparently very complex. Such processes as categorization and inference, for example, appear to be built into codes, providing the individual with a ready-made set of categories and inferences for use. However, to allow the individual to use these cognitive maps which are built into codes also demands the exercise of other complex intellective processes. (p. 231)

They also pointed out that in any interdisciplinary research project on game-playing behavior around the world an anthropologist "would probably come to distrust generalizations made about human behavior across all classes of games, since for him most behavior is 'determined' by the code in use, which varies by the game" (p. 232). I'll return to this point later in a brief discussion of cross-cultural research in experimental economics, where behavior in the "ultimatum game" varies widely and in some counterintuitive ways (given our own culturally shaped intuitions) across cultural groups, which seems to be related to the way the game (which is itself a cultural product whose rules and meanings have been defined by the researchers) gets assimilated to local codes, rules, and meanings when transported abroad and presented to subjects in another culture. Here I simply want to note one of the lessons I took away from my 1960s reading of "Transcultural Studies in Cognition," namely, that research designed to discover the empirically uniform features of human mentalities is likely to bracket the existence of (and hence underestimate the behavioral significance of) the local, socially learned "codes" that define social life in human groups and dismiss them as mere content, thereby ignoring one of the great sources of mental differences between the members of different code-dependent groups (cultures).

That gathering of anthropologists, psychologists and linguists in the Yucatán in Mexico in 1963 was one of many such meetings that took place in the 1960s and 1970s, premised on the article of faith that interdisciplinary conversation can be a good thing. Historical precursors and personal premonitions aside, however, I suppose I really associate the current and rather dramatic revival of cultural psychology as a vibrant and visible academic discipline with a few key academic events in the 1980s and 1990s and several nonacademic contemporary trends on the domestic and international scene.

One of those academic events was of huge import for the rebirth of an interest in higher-order units of analysis (such as culture, ethnicity, and race) among mainstream social psychologists, namely, the ongoing seminar on cultural psychology organized and run for several years in the early 1990s by Hazel Markus and Richard Nisbett at the University of Michigan. (It was a time when the reductive tendencies within psychology were apparent and social psychology was at risk of becoming a branch of cognitive psychology, which, it has now become apparent, was itself at risk of becoming a branch of neuroscience.) During that period, interdisciplinary visitors came from all over the world to Ann Arbor, old but profound formulations in anthropology and psychology were reexamined and revived (e.g., the work of John Whiting and Irvin Child on the "custom complex" and of Harry Triandis on "individualism" and "collectivism"), and the University of Michigan and later Stanford University put themselves on the map as leading centers of research on cultural psychology, ultimately resulting in the creation of the Center for Culture and Cognition at the University of Michigan (whose vibrant voices and critical intelligences have included psychologists Phoebe Ellsworth and Shinobu Kitayama and anthropologists Lawrence Hirschfeld and Scott Atran). One should not be surprised that so many of the most active and creative social psychologists who now call themselves cultural psychologists or sociocultural psychologists (including the two editors of this volume) have ancestral connections to either the University of Michigan or Stanford University, although there are now several other leading psychology department-based centers of excellence in cultural psychology (University of California, Berkeley; University of British Columbia; University of California, Los Angeles; University of Illinois; and others). And of course there are several other centers for training and research in cultural psychology that are based in either anthropology departments (UCLA; Emory University; Duke University; University of California, San Diego) or interdisciplinary departments such as the Department for Comparative Human Development at the University of Chicago (where for nearly 70 years anthropologists and psychologists have been colleagues in the same program).

The second academic event I would mention is the Culture Theory Conference held in the spring of 1981 and subsequently published in the book *Culture Theory: Essays on Mind, Self, and Emotion* (Shweder & LeVine, 1984). Perhaps this is an all too personal and autobiographical recollection of the history of the growing interest in cultural psychology. Robert LeVine's chapter in this volume brings us up to date and puts contemporary practitioners of cultural psychology in touch with some of their relatively recent anthropological ancestors, but it stops just short of 1984, when (at least from my biased point of view) at least some of the current action began. It began with the publication of LeVine's own coedited volume *Culture Theory* (which, with characteristic modesty, he never mentions). The "Culture Theory" project was an attempt to draw out the implications of a symbols- and meaning-centered or interpretive conception of culture for the study of mental functioning across groups, with special attention to certain key formulations, for example, the work of Geertz on local forms of mental functioning and culturally parochial ideas about the self. Had LeVine added just one more page to his narrative he might well have turned his attention to the conception and birth of the Social Science Research Council's Culture Theory project, in which he played a major role and for which I was his coconspirator. It was at that conference that several anthropologists began to articulate once again (and with new ethnographic and linguistic evidence) some of the definitive and provocative ancient propositions of cultural psychology—for example, that when it comes to the study of human consciousness (including human self-consciousness) there are multiple diverse psychologies out there rather than a single psychology; and that many of those distinctive mental qualities of individuals are acquired, activated, maintained, or lost by virtue of participation in the way of life (including the linguistic life) of particular ancestral groups.

At the 1963 Romney and D'Andrade culture and cognition conference, the psychologists in attendance included Roger Brown, Jerome Kagan, William Kessen, Charles Osgood, and Fred Strodtbeck, and the anthropologists included Brent Berlin, Roy D'Andrade, Charles Frake, Dell Hymes, A. Kimball Romney, and William Sturtevant. It was the era of the cognitive revolution and "ethnoscience" was a hot topic in cultural anthropology. At the 1981 Culture Theory conference the psychologists in attendance included Jerome Bruner, Cal Izard, Martin Hoffman, Howard Gardner, Catherine Snow, and Elliot Turiel, and the anthropologists included Robbins Burling, Roy D'Andrade, Michael Fischer, Clifford Geertz, Paul Kay, Robert LeVine, Robert Levy, John Lucy, Michele Rosaldo, Bambi Scheiffelin, David Schneider, Richard Shweder, Michael Silverstein, and Melford Spiro. Jürgen Habermas attended and served as the general discussant. It was an era when the cognitive revolution was no longer hegemonic and studies of self and emotion were back at center stage; one of the major aims of the conference was to critically examine the "symbolic" or "interpretative" approach to culture (as the socially inherited goals, values, and pictures of the world that are distinctive of members of different groups and made manifest in their behavioral norms), as well as the implications of that approach for research on psychological development (including research on self, emotion, moral reasoning, and language acquisition). As I recall, it was LeVine who had the prescience to recognize the potential value of Geertz's conception of culture for the study of psychological development. At the conference we brought together anthropologists (who at the time were actively debating and trying to make sense of a Geertzian conception of culture) and psychologists (who at the time were struggling with, and resisting, the reductive and restrictive implications of the "cognitive revolution" for the study of the mental life). Many psychologists at that time were interested in going beyond the structural analysis of human perceptual and reasoning processes to the study of human wants, feelings, and values; the anthropologists believed they had something to contribute by virtue of their ethnographic research on the more revelatory and meaning-laden aspects of daily experience and the socially inherited goals, values, and pictures of reality that lead individuals to commit to a particular way of life. While there was disagreement among the conference participants about whether the "cognitive revolution" had been a blessing or a curse for the study of language, culture, and mental functioning, there was a notable level of expressed concern about the negative influence of the cognitive revolution on anthropology and psychology: concern about the apparent prestige associated with cognitive research; concern about the lack of attention to social practices and higher order units of analysis among cognitive researchers; concern about the tendency to put everything inside the head. The following fascinating exchange took place between Roy D'Andrade and Clifford Geertz (see Shweder & LeVine, 1984). This particular give-and-take raises far more issues than I can address here (for example, the direct or indirect influence of the philosophies of the early versus late Ludwig Wittgenstein on the formulations offered below; the metaphysical status of a "conceptual structure" that is not "in the head"; the way an

"interpretive approach" to culture might successfully join the study of behavior with the study of ideas), but this exchange does give a sense of how, by the early 1980s, the cognitive revolution was already "breaking up":

Roy D'Andrade: When I was a graduate student, one imagined people *in* a culture; ten years later culture was all in their heads. The thing went from something out there and very large to something that got placed inside. Culture became a branch of cognitive psychology. We went from "let's try to look at behavior and describe it" to "let's try to look at ideas." Now, how you were to look at ideas was a bit of a problem and some people said, "Well, look at language." That notion, that you look at idea systems, was extremely general in the social sciences. On, I think, the same afternoon in 1957 you have papers by Chomsky and Miller and in anthropology, Ward Goodenough. All signal an end to the era of "Let's look at behavior and see what they do." Before 1957 the definition of culture was primarily a behavioral one – culture was patterns of behavior, actions, and customs. The same behavioral emphasis was there in linguistics and psychology. The idea that cognition is where it is at struck all three fields at the same time—it has a slightly different trajectory in each discipline—whether you do experiments or whether you look for intuitions or whether you talk to informants. I think it was a nice replacement. But the thing is now breaking—that force set in motion in the late fifties .. . and we each have different ideas about how it is breaking up.

Clifford Geertz: At the same time the revolution was going on where people were putting things inside people's heads a counterrevolution was going the other way—criticizing the whole myth of inner reality, the whole myth of private language. The one thing that anthropologists hadn't said about culture is that it is a conceptual structure. What does it mean to say that? Take, for example, the theory of infant damnation. To know what it is you have to, first of all, conceptualize it historically and with other beliefs of this type. Then you can discuss the incidence of it, and how people got it, and how they got rid of it, and what determined all these things. But what the cultural element is, is the structure of meanings, ideas or significances that that particular religious ideology contained. The reason I am against putting things in people's heads is that it reduces the tension between cultural analysis and psychological analysis. By psychologizing things you don't have the kind of problematic where you can ask what is the impact of a conceptual structure or system of ideas such as the theory of infant damnation during the Reformation. What psychological effect did it have on different people in different contexts? That tends to get lost because the theory is identified as a psychological phenomenon in the first place. It's a conceptual structure—and that is what the whole depsychologizing of the concept of sense, of meaning, was all about and still is about. (pp. 7–8)

I believe it was about that time, in the early 1980s, as I prepared for the Culture Theory conference, that I began to recognize the connection between the interpretive or symbolic approach to culture and some of the tenets of the historical Romantic rebellion against the Enlightenment; and I even tried to comprehend some of the tensions that emerged at the conference in those terms (see Shweder, 1984). Even now, as I think about the intellectual foundations of cultural psychology as a discipline, I resonate to the observation by the political and moral philosopher Isaiah Berlin, in which he contrasted enlightenment figures such as Voltaire and Condorcet with Johann Herder, one of the great Romantic rebels (and a founder of cultural psychology). Berlin (1976, quoted in Gray, 1996) wrote:

> For Voltaire, Diderot, Helvetius, Holbach, Condorcet, there is only one universal civilization, of which now one nation, now another, represents the richest flowering. For Herder there is a plurality of incommensurable cultures. To belong to a given community, to be connected with its members by indissoluble and impalpable ties of a common language, historical memory, habit, tradition and feeling, is a basic human need no less natural than that for food or drink or security or procreation. One nation can understand and sympathize with the institutions of another only because it knows how much its own mean to itself. Cosmopolitanism is the shedding of all that makes one most human, most oneself. (p. 122)

Perhaps that last sentence will seem shocking to some readers, especially those who live or idealize a cosmopolitan way of life. Nevertheless, the Romantic rebellion was in large part an act of intellectual resistance to the Enlightenment. It was a rejection of the Enlightenment ideal for a "modern self," with its highly individualistic image of a fully realized human person as one who has become liberated or emancipated from all traditions, from all revelations or faith-based attachments to groups, from all commitments to received values or pictures of the world other than those that can be univer-

sally justified or grounded in logic or science. It is that "enlightened" cosmopolitan vision of the liberated individual (who is at home nowhere in particular or feels at home only when detached from all groups and loyal to none of them) that Johann Herder opposed and viewed as the shedding all that makes us most human. One trusts it is a message that many social psychologists will readily understand.

When reflecting on the contemporary psychological sciences, it is tempting to draw an analogous contrast. On the one hand, psychology aims to describe a universal psychology, and, in pursuit of that universal psychology, ends up investigating the cosmopolitan college student subject as its richest flowering and adduces an account of that psychology that is largely devoid of all mention of historical memory, local language, distinctive communal attachments, group traditions, or the parochial mental states that make us what we are. On the other hand, cultural psychology, as Herder might have envisioned it, is the investigation of those distinctive and several (or multiple) psychologies that make it possible for each of us to be and feel at home in some particular group.

Now I do not mean to suggest that any one, two, or three academic events should be fully credited with the revival of interest in cultural psychology. The organized efforts, including this monumental handbook project, to move the field forward have been many. One welcomes all of these efforts and looks forward to the day when the recent history of cultural psychology as a reemerging discipline is systematically documented. Any such history, one imagines, will surely also point to events and processes outside the academy that have created a favorable environment for the growth of a field that is so deeply concerned with questions of cultural difference. I have in mind, of course, changes in the U.S. immigration laws in the 1960s that prepared the way for increased levels of Asian, African, and South and Middle American migration; the international pendulum swing in the direction of economic globalization, which eroded national barriers to the flow of goods, information, capital, and labor (including students and scholars) all over the world; the emergence of identity politics, social justice consciousness, and affirmative action policies and their beneficial consequences for funding research or researcher training with regard to ethnic and racial minority groups; and the various and numerous conflicts and competitions between nations and groups over the past decades (from the Japanese success in the world economy to the current war in Iraq and the tensions between Islam and Christianity in Europe) which have made it increasingly apparent that cultural differences not only are here to stay but also need to be understood for the sake of domestic and international tranquility, and for everyone's general well-being.

By now it should be apparent that I use the expression "cultural psychology" (as does Wikipedia) in a sense that is much narrower than the usage implied by the very broad reach of the preceding 33 chapters in this volume. Breadth of coverage is a good thing for a handbook, and it is a fact of life and sign of healthy intellectual activity that scholars who do comparative research on mental states and processes across code-dependent (i.e., cultural) groups do so with many different types of aims and agendas, most of which are important and legitimate. Nevertheless, not all of them are doing cultural psychology in the sense I have been describing. What is that sense?

Here I draw upon several earlier formulations in which I have tried to imagine a field of study called cultural psychology (Shweder 1990, 1991, 1993, 1999, 2003a, 2003b, and the other entries in the reference section under my name; Shweder & Sullivan, 1990). That field has a distinctive subject matter (psychological diversity, rather than psychological uniformity); it aims to reassess the uniformitarian principle of psychic unity and develop a credible theory of psychological pluralism. One does hope that it goes without saying by now that any theory of psychological pluralism would lack credibility if it staunchly denied the existence of any and all universals. That is why a credible theory of psychological pluralism, one that honors our true, deep, and significant differences, cannot and does not entail the denial of all universals. Cultural psychology presupposes many universals, including a theory of mind according to which to be a "person" is to have the capacity to initiate action; to construct a picture of the world; and to display the features of creative intelligence in the generic sense, which include the abilities to imagine the future, know things, want things, feel things, and value things (see Shweder et al., 2006). Nevertheless, as I use the expression, cultural psychology refers to the study of ethnic and cultural sources of *diversity* in emotional and

somatic functioning, self-organization, moral evaluation, social cognition, and human development.

The field also has a particular conception of the proper units of analysis for comparative research on psychological facts. It calls for the study of human "mentalities" (in the plural) as conceptualized by Johann Herder (that 18th-century Romantic German philosopher), whose central premise was that "to be a member of a group is to think and act in a certain way, in the light of particular goals, values, and pictures of the world; and to think and act so is to belong to a group" (Berlin, 1976). According to this approach to cultural psychology, the idea of "goals" includes wants, preferences, and motives of various kinds. The idea of "values" includes emotional reactions as well as "goods" and "ends" that are thought to be "preference-worthy" or morally desirable. The idea of "pictures of the world" includes local definitions and categorizations, beliefs about means–ends connections and causal connections and metaphysical and existential premises of various kinds. To describe a "mentality" (e.g., the "mentality" of Oriya Hindu Brahmans or Mandarin Chinese or liberal American middle-class anticlerical cosmopolites) is to get specific about the particular conceptual contents (the "ideas") that have actually been cognized and activated by such persons or peoples, where to "cognize" refers to any process that enables human beings to represent "ideas" (conceptual content) and to attain knowledge by deriving or computing their implications. In other words, cultural psychology is the study of the specific conceptual content that renders meaning-full behavior (or "actions") intelligible.

I have not counted how many of the chapters in this volume are prototypes or even instances of cultural psychology in that sense of the field. However, what does strike me as noteworthy is the breadth of the collection and how the expression "cultural psychology" has come to encompass so many very different types of intellectual traditions. Reading through reference sections when I first received the chapters for this volume, I had the impression that the authors were inspired by very different canonical texts and did not really share common intellectual ancestors, although for the most part, all the chapter authors have some kind of interest in research that in some sense or other is "cross-cultural." In order to be a bit more objective about the sharing or nonsharing of canonical texts and intellectual ancestors every cited author and every cited written work in each of the chapters was entered into a database (the data analyzed were nearly complete at the time of the analysis, although a few citations that were either added or dropped during the final editorial process may have been overlooked). This made it possible to derive pairwise similarity measures for all of the chapters based on the degree of overlap either in the specific authors or in the specific works cited in their chapters and to conduct cluster and multi-dimensional scaling analyses on the co-citation or similarity structures of the chapters themselves (similarity or proximity measures were used that did not treat the joint noncitation of an author or text as a measure of sharing or similarity). It also made it possible to determine which authors and texts were the most cited and to what degree.[1]

One basic fact about the citations in this volume is this: The vast majority of both cited authors (approximately 77%) and cited written works (approximately 88%) are cited in some single chapter only, and not mentioned in any other chapter in the book (see Figures 34.1 and 34.2). In other words, most citations are unique; hence, the "J" shape of the curve of the distributions in the graphs is dramatic, and it reveals that, for both researchers and texts, if you are cited at all you probably are cited in only one of the chapters. Of the 3,560 written works cited herein, there is only one—Hazel Markus and Shinobu Kitayama's (1991) *Psychological Review* article "Culture and the Self"—that is cited in even half of the chapters, and it is an outlier. Of 4,057 authors, only seven are widely cited, in the sense of being cited in at least half of the chapters. Gustav Jahoda's useful primer on the history of theory and research on culture and mind (which I pointed to earlier) does inform the historically oriented chapter by Harry Triandis but is not mentioned in any of the other chapters.

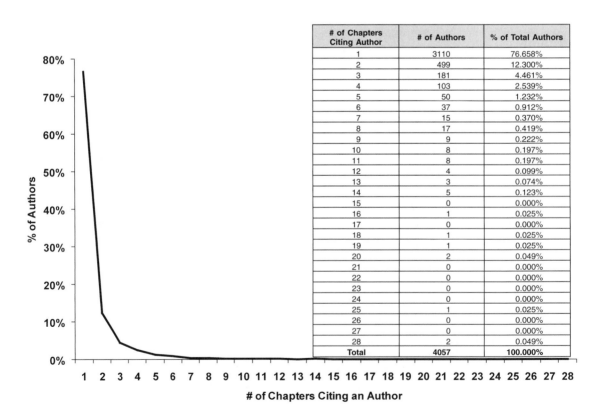

# of Chapters Citing Author	# of Authors	% of Total Authors
1	3110	76.658%
2	499	12.300%
3	181	4.461%
4	103	2.539%
5	50	1.232%
6	37	0.912%
7	15	0.370%
8	17	0.419%
9	9	0.222%
10	8	0.197%
11	8	0.197%
12	4	0.099%
13	3	0.074%
14	5	0.123%
15	0	0.000%
16	1	0.025%
17	0	0.000%
18	1	0.025%
19	1	0.025%
20	2	0.049%
21	0	0.000%
22	0	0.000%
23	0	0.000%
24	0	0.000%
25	1	0.025%
26	0	0.000%
27	0	0.000%
28	2	0.049%
Total	**4057**	**100.000%**

FIGURE 34.1. Citing trend of authors.

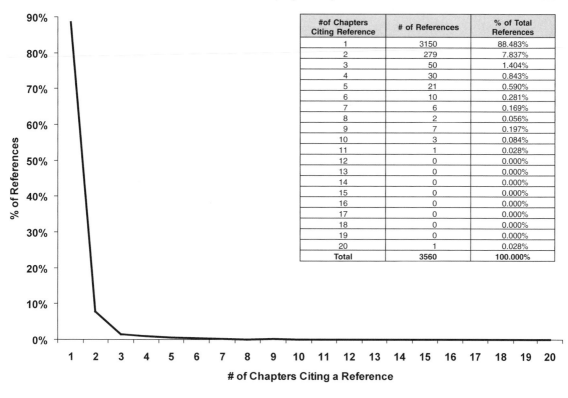

#of Chapters Citing Reference	# of References	% of Total References
1	3150	88.483%
2	279	7.837%
3	50	1.404%
4	30	0.843%
5	21	0.590%
6	10	0.281%
7	6	0.169%
8	2	0.056%
9	7	0.197%
10	3	0.084%
11	1	0.028%
12	0	0.000%
13	0	0.000%
14	0	0.000%
15	0	0.000%
16	0	0.000%
17	0	0.000%
18	0	0.000%
19	0	0.000%
20	1	0.028%
Total	3560	100.000%

FIGURE 34.2. Citing trend of particular works.

I realize, of course, that it is hazardous to interpret the significance of this basic fact. Perhaps the relative lack of common intellectual reference points (including historical reference points) is a feature of every subfield in the social sciences. But it does give the impression that "cultural psychology," at least in this particular usage of the expression in a *handbook of cultural psychology*, is a cover phrase for a wide range of intellectual programs and research agendas. Figure 34.3 lists the 62 most-cited authors across the chapters, where the inclusion criterion is citation in at least 8 of the preceding 33 chapters. Figure 34.4 lists the 51 most-cited written works, where the inclusion criterion is citation in at least 5 of the preceding 33 chapters. When inspecting these figures, two things seem apparent. First, the field of cultural psychology, at least among academic social psychologists, has been riding a wave associated with East/West comparisons and especially a small set of almost personality-trait-like theoretical contrasts between individualistic versus collectivist societies, independent versus interdependent selves, and analytic versus holistic thinking. Secondly, the most widely cited articles are those published in a very small set of mainstream psychological journals, for example, the *Journal of Personality and Social Psychology, Psychological Review, Psychological Bulletin,* and the *American Psychologist.* Relevant articles on cultural psychology published in the journals of other disciplines (anthropology, philosophy, linguistics) are not widely cited, although three books about culture written by anthropologists (Geertz, Sperber, and Kroeber & Kluckhohn) and one written by a sociologist (by Weber) are acknowledged in at least 5 or more of the 33 preceding chapters.

Reading through this volume, the overall or general impression one gets is of the following: (1) one big idea organizing a coherent research agenda for a subset of social psychology authors interested in psychological diversity but framed very much as a debate about the scope or generality of fundamental intellectual processes and researched in a way that parallels the logic of personality-trait psychology at the level of groups and fits the format of main-

Author Cited	# of Chapters Citing Author	CH 1 Markus, Hamedani	CH 2 LeVine	CH 3 Triandis	CH 4 Konner	CH 5 Cole, Hatano	CH 6 Kitayama, Duffy, Uchida	CH 7 Mendoza-Denton, Mischel	CH 8 Cohen	CH 9 Chiao, Ambady	CH 10 Oyserman, Lee	CH 11 Fiske, Fiske	CH 12 Brewer, Yuki	CH 13 Hong, Wan, No, Chiu	CH 14 Sanchez-Burks, Lee	CH 15 Schooler	CH 16 Rozin	CH 17 Atran	CH 18 Newson, Richerson, Boyd	CH 19 Miller	CH 20 Morelli, Rothbaum	CH 21 Li	CH 22 Sternberg	CH 23 Norenzayan, Choi, Peng	CH 24 Miller, Fung, Koven	CH 25 Medin, Unsworth, Hirschfeld	CH 26 Wang, Ross	CH 27 Chiu, Leung, Kwan	CH 28 Tov, Diener	CH 29 Heine	CH 30 Mesquita, Leu	CH 31 Hatfield, Rapson, Martel	CH 32 Levenson, Soto, Pole	CH 33 Marsella, Yamada
Kitayama, S.	28	X	X	X	X		X	X	X	X	X	X	X	X						X	X	X	X	X	X	X	X	X	X	X	X	X	X	X
Markus, H. R.	28	X	X	X	X	X	X	X	X	X	X	X	X	X						X	X	X	X	X	X	X	X	X	X	X	X	X	X	X
Nisbett, R. E.	25	X		X	X	X	X	X	X	X	X	X		X	X					X	X	X	X	X		X	X	X		X	X	X	X	X
Lehman, D. R.	20	X		X	X		X	X	X	X	X	X	X	X						X				X		X	X	X		X	X	X		X
Shweder, R. A.	20	X	X	X		X	X	X	X	X	X						X			X	X			X	X	X	X	X	X	X			X	
Cohen, D.	19	X		X		X	X	X	X	X	X			X			X			X				X		X	X			X		X	X	X
Triandis, H. C.	18	X		X	X		X	X	X		X		X	X	X					X				X		X	X		X	X		X	X	
Heine, S. J.	16	X				X	X	X	X		X	X	X							X				X		X	X		X	X	X	X		
Chiu, C.	14	X		X	X		X	X	X		X			X	X					X				X			X		X	X	X	X		
Choi, I.	14	X		X		X	X	X	X	X		X								X				X			X		X	X	X	X		
Hong, Y.	14	X		X			X	X	X		X			X	X	X				X				X			X		X	X	X	X		
Norenzayan, A.	14	X		X		X	X		X	X									X			X	X				X		X	X	X			
Peng, K.	14	X		X		X	X	X	X	X				X						X		X	X				X			X		X		
Bond, M. H.	13	X				X			X	X	X	X								X	X			X			X			X				
LeVine, R. A.	13	X	X	X	X	X			X			X		X						X	X			X			X		X		X			X
Morris, M. W.	13	X		X			X	X	X	X	X		X			X	X			X				X			X	X		X				
Berry, J. W.	12	X		X			X	X	X		X		X	X						X			X	X			X			X				X
Miller, J. G.	12	X		X			X	X	X	X		X	X			X				X	X			X			X				X			
Oyserman, D.	12	X					X		X	X	X	X	X							X				X		X				X		X		
Sperber, D.	12	X	X	X	X		X					X			X			X	X				X			X			X					
Bruner, J. S.	11	X		X	X		X													X			X		X		X		X		X	X		
Coon, H. M.	11	X					X		X			X	X	X		X								X		X				X		X	X	
D'Andrade, R. G.	11	X	X	X	X	X		X												X			X			X			X		X			
Fiske, A. P.	11	X		X			X			X			X	X			X			X				X		X			X		X			
Geertz, C.	11	X	X	X	X		X	X				X								X			X	X			X		X		X			
Kemmelmeier, M.	11	X					X		X			X	X	X		X								X		X				X		X	X	
Norasakkunkit, V.	11	X		X			X	X	X					X														X	X	X		X	X	X
Rogoff, B.	11	X		X	X	X	X											X		X		X	X	X	X	X								
Baumeister, R. F.	10	X		X			X				X	X								X			X						X		X	X		
Benet-Martinez, V.	10	X		X			X	X	X			X	X							X				X					X		X			
Cole, M.	10	X		X			X	X	X											X		X	X	X	X									
Kroeber, A.L.	10	X	X	X	X	X	X										X		X					X										X
Matsumoto, H.	10	X		X			X	X	X			X												X			X			X	X		X	X
Smith, P. B.	10	X		X			X		X			X	X											X			X			X	X			
Tomascello, M.	10	X			X	X												X	X			X	X			X			X		X			
Vygotsky, L. S.	10	X		X	X	X														X	X	X	X			X								
Cavalli-Sforza, L.	9	X			X			X	X					X		X		X						X				X						
Cosmides, L.	9	X		X	X				X						X	X				X			X						X		X	X		
Diener, E.	9			X			X		X				X							X	X			X	X		X	X		X	X			
Fung, H. H.	9	X																		X	X			X		X	X	X	X	X	X			
Kashima, Y.	9	X		X			X	X			X		X	X						X				X			X			X				
Kim, H. S.	9	X		X			X		X				X							X				X			X			X	X	X		
Miller, P. J.	9	X			X															X	X			X			X			X	X	X	X	
Schaller, M.	9	X		X	X		X			X			X							X				X			X			X				
Tooby, J.	9			X	X				X									X	X				X			X			X		X	X		
Atran, S.	8	X			X			X		X								X						X	X	X			X					
Boyd, R.	8	X		X			X		X									X	X				X			X			X					
Gardner, W. L.	8	X					X		X		X		X	X						X				X			X			X				
Greenfield, P. M.	8	X		X	X	X	X		X			X									X		X			X	X	X		X	X			
Hatano, G.	8	X			X																X	X	X		X	X	X	X						
Hofstede, G.	8	X		X			X				X	X	X		X					X				X			X			X				
Iyengar, S. S.	8	X		X			X	X					X		X									X						X	X			
Leung, K.	8	X					X		X			X		X	X									X						X	X			
Masuda, T.	8	X					X		X	X														X			X			X	X			
Mead, M.	8			X	X									X		X					X				X			X				X	X	X
Medin, D. L.	8	X				X												X						X	X	X	X	X						
Miyamoto, Y.	8	X					X		X	X	X		X										X			X				X			X	
Oishi, S.	8						X		X			X	X											X			X		X	X	X	X		
Poortinga, Y.H.	8	X		X			X	X	X					X						X				X			X							
Ross, M.	8						X	X	X		X		X	X										X						X	X			
Singelis, T. M.	8			X			X		X			X	X		X	X														X	X			
Trafimow, D.	8	X					X		X			X	X		X	X														X	X			
# of Frequently Cited Authors per Chapter		54	8	42	21	19	48	23	39	17	35	16	25	22	19	4	3	12	8	16	21	14	18	36	13	28	31	17	22	34	24	12	8	7

FIGURE 34.3. Most frequently cited authors.

stream psychological science methodologies; and (2) a diverse set of research agendas—some more interested in evolutionary psychology than cultural psychology; some more interested in universal psychology than cultural psychology; some more interested in biological realities than ideational or linguistic realities; some more interested in a sociohistorical Vygotskian approach to contextual psychology than a Geertzian approach to meaning systems—but all willing to say something interesting about how their particular research specialty thinks about either culture or behavior across groups.

Whether this is good enough for the future of the field is an open question. I suspect, however, that the future health of the discipline is going to depend, at least in part, on our capacity to shift a few gears and move in a few new directions. For example, I have long thought that there is wisdom in Kuo-shu Yang's (2000) vision of ways to "indigenize" psychological research. Here I allude to three of Yang's proposed virtues for the aspiring indigenous psychologist of China:

FIGURE 34.4. Most frequently cited works.

WORK CITED	# of Chapters Citing Reference
Markus, H. R., & Kitayama, S. (1991)	20
Kitayama, S., Markus, H. R., Matsumoto, H., & Norasakkunkit, V. (1997)	11
Geertz, C. (1973)	10
Heine, S. J., Lehman, D. R., Markus, H. R., & Kitayama, S. (1999)	10
Sperber, D. (1996)	10
Cole, M. (1996)	9
Hong, Y., Morris, M. W., Chiu, C., & Benet-Martinez, V. (2000)	9
Nisbett, R. E. (2003)	9
Nisbett, R. E., Peng, K., Choi, I., & Norenzayan, A. (2001)	9
Oyserman, D., Coon, H. M., & Kemmelmeier, M. (2002)	9
Triandis, H. C. (1995)	9
Vygotsky, L. S. (1978)	9
Bruner, J. (1990)	8
Fiske, A. P., Kitayama, S., Markus, H. R., & Nisbett, R. E. (1998)	8
Cohen, D. (2001)	7
Hofstede, G. (1980)	7
Kitayama, S., Duffy, S., Kawamura, T., & Larsen, J. T. (2003)	7
Miller, J. G. (1984)	7
Tomasello, M. (1999)	7
Trafimow, D., Triandis, H. C., & Goto, S. G. (1991)	7
Cohen, D., Nisbett, R. E., Bowdle, B. F., & Schwarz, N. (1996)	6
Heine, S. J., Lehman, D. R., Peng, K., & Greenholtz, J. (2002)	6
Kroeber, A. L. & Kluckhohn, C. (1952)	6
Lehman, D. R., Chiu, C., & Schaller, M. (2004)	6
Masuda, T., & Nisbett, R. E. (2001)	6
Peng, K., Nisbett, R. E., & Wong, N. Y. C. (1997)	6
Rogoff, B. (1990)	6
Shweder, R. A. (1990a)	6
Shweder, R. A., Much, N. C., Mahapatra, M., & Park, L. (1997)	6
Triandis, H. C. (1989)	6
Atran, S., Medin, D. L., & Ross, N. O. (2005)	5
Barkow, G., Cosmides, L., & Tooby, J. (Eds.) (1992)	5
Berry, J. W., Poortinga, Y. H., Segall, M. H., & Dasen, P. R. (1992/2002)	5
Choi, I., Nisbett, R. E., & Norenzayan, A. (1999)	5
Cohen, D., & Nisbett, R. E. (1997)	5
Gardner, W., Gabriel, S., & Lee, A. (1999)	5
Heine, S. J., & Lehman, D. R. (1997)	5
Kim, H. S., & Markus, H. R. (1999)	5
Kitayama, S. (2002)	5
Kitayama, S., & Markus, H. R. (1999)	5
Kitayama, S., Markus, H. R., & Kurokawa, M. (2000)	5
Kühnen, U., & Oyserman, D. (2002)	5
Markus, H. R., Mullally, P. R., & Kitayama, S. (1997)	5
Medin, D. L, & Atran, S. (2004)	5
Miller, P. J., Wiley, A. R., Fung, H., & Liang, C.-H. (1997)	5
Miyamoto, Y., Nisbett, R. E. & Masuda, T. (2006)	5
Morris, M. W., & Peng, K. (1994)	5
Ross, M., Xun, W. Q. E., & Wilson, A. E. (2002)	5
Sanchez-Burks, J. (2002)	5
Shweder, R. A., Goodnow, J., Hatano, G., LeVine, R. A., Markus, H., & Miller, P. J. (2006)	5
Weber, M. (1904/1930)	5

# of Frequently Cited Works per Chapter

1. Give priority to the study of culturally unique psychological and behavioral phenomena or characteristics of the Chinese people.
2. Investigate both the specific content and the involved process of the phenomenon.
3. Make it a rule to begin any research with a thorough immersion into the natural, concrete details of the phenomenon to be studied.

Speaking as an anthropologist, this emphasis on starting one's research in cultural psychology with an immersion experience makes great sense and places some emphasis on field research, the observation of real-world practices and behavior (including language use), and the investigation of the native's point of view (content, meaning, and context). It also might have the effect of getting researchers in cultural psychology to rethink the dubious and hence vulnerable assumption that cultural variability can be indexed by census categories such as nationality, race, or ethnicity. Indeed it might help to free the discipline from its heavy reliance on cosmopolitan college student subjects who happen to come from different national, racial, or ethnic groups.

The advantage of taking this step can be seen in the field of experimental economics, which has for many years relied on college student subjects but has recently transported its "comparable stimuli" (its experimental games) to rural and "third-world" field settings and to the type of small-scale societies that are familiar to anthropologists. Lo and behold, they have discovered substantially greater variability in bargaining behavior in experimental game situations than previously discovered with student populations. The variability across groups that has been discovered lends itself to explanation by reference to local socially learned codes, norms, and meanings associated with social interaction in everyday life in this or that particular cultural group (Henrich et al., 2005). This research is carried forward very much in the interdisciplinary spirit of cultural psychology, with a good deal of reliance on ethnographic knowledge to build a model of a cultural mentality that helps in the interpretation of behavior in an experimental game situation (the meaning of which it is not possible for the experimenters to fully control precisely because there are cultural differences in the significance of the stimulus situation).

Consider, for example, the "ultimatum game" as defined in the experimental econom-

ics literature and described by Henrich et al. (2005):

> In this game, subjects are paired, and the first player, often called the "proposer," is provisionally allotted a divisible "pie" (usually money). The proposer then offers a portion of the total pie to a second person, called the "responder." The responder, knowing both the offer and the amount of the pie, can then either accept or reject the proposer's offer. If the responder accepts, he receives the offer and the proposer gets the remainder (the pie minus the offer). If the responder rejects the offer, then neither receives anything. In either case the game ends; the two players receive their winnings and depart. Players are typically paid in cash and are anonymous to other players. . . . (p. 798)

In the comparative field-based research reported by Henrich et al. substantial amounts of money (in local currencies) were involved, and the "players" were kept anonymous to each other.

From the point of view of cultural psychology almost everything interesting about this type of experimental approach turns on understanding how the "stimulus situation," or experimental game, is understood and given meaning from the "native point of view" of members of different groups. The challenge for a cultural psychologist is to engage in the type of "thick description" of the mentality of local "game players" so as to understand precisely how and why the stimulus situation is, in fact, not the same or equivalent as it is transported from one code-dependent world to another. That is what "thick description" amounts to: specifying the local goals, values, and pictures of the world that render apparently identical stimuli (e.g., the experimenter-defined rules of the "ultimatum game") nonequivalent. Consider this possible picture of the world: Imagine a society of strangers in which all persons are motivated mainly by material rewards and hold to the premise that more is always better than less, and hence interpret the stimulus situation (the "ultimatum game") in such a way that they conclude that any proposed offer, however small, should be accepted, given the constraints of the game (because if you refuse the offer no one gets anything), leading to the shared expectation that proposers should and will offer very little and responders should and will accept it. Apparently, not even "first-world" cosmopolitan college student subjects picture the world that way or construe the stimulus situation in those terms; the typical offer among college student subjects over many studies is around 45–50% of the original pie and college student responders typically reject low offers, even though they end up with nothing. These results have been shown to be reliable and robust across variations in the details of the experimental procedure.

More important, as one moves into rural field settings away from the "first world," all sorts of astonishing and variable patterns of behavior emerge. This variation in "bargaining behavior" is independent of such individual characteristics of the subjects as their age, education, or wealth, and seems to be related specifically to group membership and to the particular picture of persons and social relationships shared by members of one's group. As Henrich et al. (2005) note, "In some groups, rejection rates are extremely rare, even in the presence of low offers, while in others rejection rates are substantial, including frequent rejections of offers above 50%" (pp. 801–802). Consider, for example, the experimental game behavior of the Au and Gnau peoples of Papua New Guinea, where many "proposers" offered more than 50% of the available currency and many of these offers were turned down by the "responder," leaving both "players" with nothing.

What thick description of goals, values, and pictures of the world can help us comprehend what the stimulus situation actually meant to these subjects? Henrich et al. offer the following explanation:

> The rejection of seemingly generous offers, of more than half, may have a parallel in the culture of status-seeking through gift-giving found in Au and Gnau villages, and throughout Melanesia. In these societies, accepting gifts, even unsolicited ones, implies a strong obligation to reciprocate at some future time. Unrepaid debts accumulate, and place the received in a subordinate status. Further, the giver may demand repayment at times, or in forms (political alliances), not to the receiver's liking—but the receiver is still strongly obliged to respond. As a consequence, excessively large gifts, especially unsolicited ones, will be refused. (p. 811)

The main (and perhaps obvious) point to be made here is that there are many different pictures of the world or cultural mentalities that might be brought to the table when "playing an experimental game" (of course, that very way of describing the interaction or event is itself a discretionary and not mandatory way of understanding the stimulus situation), and "thick description" is a way of rendering behavior intelligible in terms of local and socially shared meanings.

I think something like that form of explanation—thick description of local meanings—is pretty much what D'Andrade and Romney (1964) had in mind when they wrote:

> The relationship between the codes an individual learns and the intellective processes of the individual is apparently very complex. Such processes as categorization and inference, for example, appear to be built into codes, providing the individual with a ready-made set of categories and inferences for use. (p. 231)

Indeed, that may be one of the primary reasons for cultural group based variations in bargaining behavior in the "ultimatum game."

Although I have raised some questions about heterogeneity of coverage, the publication of this volume is a monumental achievement and marks a new stage in the revival of the field. Back in 1964 it was not obvious that in the coming decades so many mainstream social psychologists would embrace the notion of cross-cultural research and run with it in so many fascinating directions, or that so many would become suspicious of strong claims about psychic unity and seriously entertain the possibility that mentalities are not uniform around the world. Nor, might I add in conclusion, was it obvious back then that work in experimental economics would simultaneously force us to recognize the importance of ethnographic fieldwork with diverse groups, deepen our appreciation of the psychological significance of social learned cultural codes, and lend support to the central notion of cultural psychology that culture and psyche make each other up.

NOTE

1. I am most grateful to Michele Wittels and Jacob Hickman for assisting me in these analyses. Any detailed presentations and discussion of the taxonomic structure of the Handbook chapters based on their cocitation patterns will have to wait for another occasion. Here in this commentary I just want to make a few brief observations about the breadth of this volume and raise a question or two about the future of the field.

ACKNOWLEDGMENT

I wish to thank Jacob Hickman and Michele Wittels for their research assistance in the preparation of this commentary and the Carnegie Foundation of New York and the Russell Sage Foundation for their support of my research in cultural psychology.

REFERENCES

Atran, S., Medin, D. L., & Ross, N. O. (2005). The cultural mind: Environmental decision making and cultural modeling within and across populations. *Psychological Review, 112,* 774–776.

Barkow, G., Cosmides, L., & Tooby, J. (Eds.). (1992). *The adapted mind: Evolutionary psychology and the generation of culture.* New York: Oxford University Press.

Berlin, I. (1976). *Vico and Herder: Two studies in the history of ideas.* London: Hogarth Press.

Berry, J. W., Poortinga, Y. H., Segall, M. H., & Dasen, P. R. (2002). *Cross-cultural psychology: Research and applications* (2nd ed.). New York: Cambridge University Press.

Bruner, J. S. (1990). *Acts of meaning.* Cambridge, MA: Harvard University Press.

Choi, I., Nisbett, R. E., & Norenzayan, A. (1999). Causal attribution across cultures: Variation and universality. *Psychological Bulletin, 125,* 47–63.

Cohen, D. (2001). Cultural variation: Considerations and implications. *Psychological Bulletin, 127,* 451–471.

Cohen, D., & Nisbett, R. E. (1997). Field experiments examining the culture of honor: The role of institutions in perpetuating norms about violence. *Personality and Social Psychology Bulletin, 23,* 1188–1199.

Cohen, D., Nisbett, R. E., Bowdle, B. F., & Schwarz, N. (1996). Insult, aggression, and the southern culture of honor: An "experimental ethnography." *Journal of Personality and Social Psychology, 70,* 945–960.

Cole, M. (1996). *Cultural psychology: A once and future discipline.* Cambridge, MA: Belknap Press of Harvard University Press.

Fiske, A. P., Kitayama, S., Markus, H. R., & Nisbett, R. E. (1998). The cultural matrix of social psychology. In D. T. Gilbert, S. T. Fiske, & G. Lindzey (Eds.), *Handbook of social psychology* (4th ed., pp. 915–981). Boston: McGraw-Hill.

Gardner, W. L., Gabriel, S., & Lee, A. Y. (1999). "I" value freedom, but "we" value relationships: Self-construal priming mirrors cultural differences in judgment. *Psychological Science, 10,* 321–326.

Geertz, C. (1973). *The interpretation of cultures.* New York: Basic Books.

Gray, J. (1996). *Isaiah Berlin.* Princeton, NJ: Princeton University Press.

Heine, S. J., & Lehman, D. R. (1997). Culture, dissonance, and self-affirmation. *Personality and Social Psychology Bulletin, 23,* 389–400.

Heine, S. J., Lehman, D. R., Markus, H. R., & Kitayama, S. (1999). Is there a universal need for positive self-regard? *Psychological Review, 106,* 766–794.

Heine, S. J., Lehman, D. R., Peng, K., & Greenholtz, J. (2002). What's wrong with cross-cultural comparisons of subjective Likert scales? The reference-group effect. *Journal of personality and Social Psychology, 82,* 903–918.

Henrich, J., Boyd, R., Bowles, S., Camerer, C., Fehr, E., Gintis, H., et al. (2005). "Economic Man" in cross-cultural perspective: Behavioral experiments in 15 small-scale societies. *Behavioral and Brain Sciences, 28*(6), 795–815.

Hofstede, G. (1980). *Culture's consequences: International differences in work-related values.* Beverly Hills, CA: Sage.

Hong, Y., Morris, M. W., Chiu, C., & Benet-Martínez, V. (2000). Multicultural minds: A dynamic constructivist approach to culture and cognition. *American Psychologist, 55,* 709–720.

Jahoda, G. (1993). *Crossroads between culture and mind: Continuities and change in theories of human nature.* London: Harvester Wheatsheaf, and Cambridge, MA: Harvard University Press.

Kim, H. S., & Markus, H. R. (1999). Deviance or uniqueness, harmony or conformity?: A cultural analysis. *Journal of Personality and Social Psychology, 77,* 785–800.

Kitayama, S. (2002). Cultural and basic psychological processes-toward a system view of culture: Comment on Oyserman et al. *Psychological Bulletin, 128,* 189–196.

Kitayama, S., & Markus, H. R. (1999). Yin and yang of the Japanese self: The cultural psychology of personality coherence. In D. Cervone & Y. Shoda (Eds.), *The coherence of personality: Social cognitive bases of personality consistency, variability, and organization* (pp. 242–302). New York: Guilford Press.

Kitayama, S., Duffy, S., Kawamura, T., & Larsen, J. (2003). Perceiving an object and its context in different cultures: A cultural look at new look. *Psychological Science, 14,* 201–206.

Kitayama, S., Markus, H. R., & Kurokawa, M. (2000). Culture, emotion and well-being: Good feelings in Japan and the U.S. *Cognition and Emotion, 14*(1), 93–124.

Kitayama, S., Markus, H. R., Matsumoto, H., & Norasakkunkit, V. (1997). Individual and collective processes in the construction of the self: Self-enhancement in the United States and self-criticism in Japan. *Journal of Personality and Social Psychology, 72,* 1245–1267.

Kroeber, A. L., & Kluckhohn, C. (1966). *Culture: A critical review of concepts and definitions.* New York: Vintage. (Original work published 1952)

Kühnen, U., & Oyserman, D. (2002). Thinking about the self influences thinking in general: Cognitive consequences of salient self-concept. *Journal of Experimental Social Psychology, 38,* 492–499.

Lehman, D. R., Chiu, C., & Schaller, M. (2004). Psychology and culture. *Annual Review of Psychology*, *55*, 689–714.

Markus, H. R., Mullally, P. R., & Kitayama, S. (1997). Selfways: Diversity in modes of cultural participation. In U. Neisser & D. Jopling (Eds.), *The conceptual self in context: Culture, experience, self-understanding* (pp. 13–62). Cambridge, UK: Cambridge University Press.

Markus, H., & Kitayama, S. (1991). Culture and the self: Implications for cognition, emotion, and motivation. *Psychological Review*, *98*, 224–253.

Masuda, T., & Nisbett, R. E. (2001). Attending holistically versus analytically: Comparing the context sensitivity of Japanese and Americans. *Journal of Personality and Social Psychology*, *81*, 922–934.

Medin, D. L., & Atran, S. (2004). The native mind: Biological categorization and reasoning in development and across cultures. *Psychological Review*, *111*, 960–983.

Miller, J. G. (1984). Culture and the development of everyday social explanation. *Journal of Personality and Social Psychology*, *46*, 961–978.

Miller, P., Wiley, A. R., Fung, H., & Liang, C-h. (1997). Personal storytelling as a medium of socialization in Chinese and American families. *Child Development*, *68*, 557–568.

Miyamoto, Y., Nisbett, R. E., & Masuda, T. (2006). Culture and the physical environment: Holistic versus analytic perceptual affordances. *Psychological Science*, *17*, 113–119.

Morris, M., & Peng, K. (1994). Culture and cause: American and Chinese attributions for social and physical events. *Journal of Personality and Social Psychology*, *67*, 949–971.

Nisbett, R. E. (2003). *The geography of thought: Why we think the way we do*. New York: Free Press.

Nisbett, R. E., Peng, K., Choi, I., & Norenzayan, A. (2001). Culture and systems of thought: Holistic vs. analytic cognition. *Psychological Review*, *108*, 291–310.

Oyserman, D., Coon, H. M., & Kemmelmeier, M. (2002). Rethinking individualism and collectivism: Evaluation of theoretical and assumptions and meta-analyses. *Psychological Bulletin*, *128*, 3–72.

Peng, K., Nisbett, R. E., & Wong, N. (1997). Validity problems of cross-cultural value comparison and possible solutions. *Psychological Methods*, *2*, 329–341.

Rogoff, B. (1990). *Apprenticeship in thinking: Cognitive development in social context*. New York: Oxford University Press.

Romney, A. K., & D'Andrade, R. (Eds.). (1964). Transcultural studies in cognition [Special issue]. *American Anthropologist*, *66*(3).

Ross, M., Xun, W. Q. E., & Wilson, A. E. (2002). Language and the bicultural self. *Personality and Social Psychology Bulletin*, *28*, 1040–1050.

Sanchez-Burks, J. (2002). Protestant relational ideology and (in) attention to relational cues in work settings.

Journal of Personality and Social Psychology, *83*, 919.

Shweder, R. A. (1984). Anthropology's romantic rebellion against the enlightenment, or, there is more to thinking than reason and evidence. In R. A. Shweder & R. A. LeVine (Eds.), *Culture theory: Essays on mind, self, and emotion* (pp. 27–66). New York: Cambridge University Press.

Shweder, R. A. (1990a). Cultural psychology: What is it? In J. W. Stigler, R. A. Shweder, & G. Herdt (Eds.), *Cultural psychology: Essays on comparative human development*. Cambridge, UK: Cambridge University Press.

Shweder, R. A. (1990b). In defense of moral realism. *Child Development*, *61*, 2060–2067.

Shweder, R. A. (1991). *Thinking through cultures: Expeditions in cultural psychology*. Cambridge, MA: Harvard University Press.

Shweder, R. A. (1992). Ghost busters in anthropology. In C. Strauss & R. G. D'Andrade (Eds.), *Human motives and cultural models* (pp. 45–58). New York: Cambridge University Press.

Shweder, R. A. (1996). True ethnography: The lore, the law and the lure. In R. Jessor, A. Colby, & R. A. Shweder (Eds.), *Ethnography and human development: Context and meaning in social inquiry*. Chicago: University of Chicago Press.

Shweder, R. A. (1999). Why cultural psychology? *Ethos: Journal of the Society for Psychological Anthropology*, *27*, 62–73.

Shweder, R. A. (2003a). Toward a deep cultural psychology of shame. *Social Research*, *70*, 1401–1422.

Shweder, R. A. (2003b). *Why do men barbecue? Recipes for cultural psychology*. Cambridge, MA: Harvard University Press.

Shweder, R. A. (2004). Deconstructing the emotions for the sake of comparative research. In A. S. R. Manstead, N. Frijda, & A. Fischer (Eds.), *Feelings and emotions: The Amsterdam Symposium* (pp. 81–97). Cambridge, UK: Cambridge University Press.

Shweder, R. A., & Bourne, L. (1984). Does the concept of the person vary cross-culturally? In R. A. Shweder & R. A. LeVine (Eds.), *Culture theory: Essays on mind, self, and emotion* (pp. 158–199). New York: Cambridge University Press.

Shweder, R. A., Balle-Jensen, L., & Goldstein, W. (1995). Who sleeps by whom revisited: A method for extracting the moral goods implicit in praxis. In J. J. Goodnow, P. J. Miller, & F. Kessell (Eds.), *Cultural practices as contexts for development: New directions for child development*. San Francisco: Jossey-Bass.

Shweder, R. A., Goodnow, J., Hatano, G., LeVine, R., Markus, H., & Miller, P. (2006). The cultural psychology of development: One mind, many mentalities. In R. Lerner (Ed.), *Handbook of child psychology: Vol. 1. Theoretical models of human development* (6th ed., pp. 716–792). New York: Wiley.

Shweder, R. A., & Haidt, J. (2000). The cultural psychology of the emotions: Ancient and new. In M. Lewis & J. M. Haviland (Eds.), *Handbook of emotions* (pp. 397–414). New York: Guilford Press.

Shweder, R. A., & LeVine, R. A. (Eds.). (1984). *Culture theory: Essays on mind, self, and emotion.* New York: Cambridge University Press.

Shweder, R. A., Mahapatra, M., & Miller, J. G. (1990). Culture and moral development. In J. Stigler, R. A. Shweder, & G. Herdt (Eds.), *Cultural psychology: Essays on comparative human development* (pp. 138–204). New York: Cambridge University Press.

Shweder, R. A., & Much, N. C. (1987). Determinants of meaning: Discourse and moral socialization. In W. Kurtines & J. Gewirtz (Eds.), *Moral development through social interaction* (pp. 245–280). New York: Wiley.

Shweder, R. A., Much, N. C., Mahapatra, M., & Park, L. (1997). The big three of morality (autonomy, community, divinity) and the big three explanations of suffering. In A. Brandt & P. Rozin (Eds.), *Morality and health* (pp. 119–169). New York: Routledge & Kegan Paul.

Shweder, R. A., & Sullivan, M. (1990). The semiotic subject of cultural psychology. In L. Pervin (Ed.), *Handbook of personality: Theory and research* (pp. 399–416). New York: Guilford Press.

Shweder, R. A., & Sullivan, M. (1993). Cultural psychology: Who needs it? *Annual Review of Psychology, 44,* 497–523.

Sperber, D. (1996). *Explaining culture: A naturalistic approach.* London: Blackwell.

Tomasello, M. (1999). *The cultural origins of human cognition.* Cambridge, MA: Harvard University Press.

Trafimow, D., Triandis, H. C., & Goto, S. G. (1991). Some tests of the distinction between the private self and the collective self. *Journal of Personality and Social Psychology, 60,* 649–655.

Triandis, H. C. (1989). The self and social behavior in differing cultural-contexts. *Psychological Review, 96,* 506–520.

Triandis, H. C. (1990). Cross-cultural studies of individualism and collectivism. In J. Berman (Ed.), *Nebraska Symposium on Motivation, 1989* (pp. 41–133). Lincoln: University of Nebraska Press.

Triandis, H. C. (1995). Individualism and collectivism. Boulder, CO: Westview Press.

Vygotsky, L. S. (1978). *Mind in society: The development of higher psychological processes* (M. Cole, V. John-Steiner, S. Scribner & E. Souberman, Eds.). Cambridge, MA: Harvard University Press.

Weber, M. (1930). *Protestant ethic and the spirit of capitalism.* Winchester, MA: Allen & Unwin. (Original work published 1904)

Whiting, J. W. M., & Child, I. (1953). *Child training and personality.* New Haven, CT: Yale University Press.

Yang, K.-S. (2000). Monocultural and cross-cultural indigenous approaches: The royal road to the development of a balanced global human psychology. *Asian Journal of Social Psychology, 3,* 241–263.

CHAPTER 35

A Psychological Perspective
Cultural Psychology—Past, Present, and Future

RICHARD E. NISBETT

People who are unaware of the history of cultural psychology are surprised to learn that the founder of experimental psychology, Wilhelm Wundt, was also a cultural psychologist. He believed that one could not understand behavior by just looking at what people were doing in laboratories. One also had to know history and culture. Kurt Lewin, the founder of the field of experimental social psychology, was also a student of collectives of all sorts. He actually wrote one important ethnography comparing Germany and the United States. And there was always a fundamental concern with history and culture and collective issues on the part of the Soviet psychologists, notably Vygotsky and Luria. Through at least the 1950s, plenty of psychologists—especially social psychologists—were concerned with societal and collective and cultural issues.

But a very dramatic shift away from concern with culture occurred roughly in the mid-60s. I have two theories about why this happened. I think it was partly because culture in the 1940s and 1950s was studied in the context of what was called the "culture and personality movement." Unfortunately,

this movement operated with the two predominant theories in the behavioral sciences, and these were not well suited for studying culture. One of these, Freudian theory, is perfectly good for some things, including, for example, the theory of "preperception" in attention. But Freudian theory just is not very good for studying culture. Cultures do not differ from one another because of when they do their toilet training or how they resolve their Oedipus complexes. The other orientation that guided research was learning theory. When applied to human behavior, the theory was rarely used in an explanatory or predictive, as opposed to a purely circular, fashion. Why do people do what they do? Well, because they are being reinforced for it. And how do we know that they are being reinforced for it? Well, because they are doing it. As Robert Abelson pointed out, social psychology, which is the fountainhead of contemporary cultural psychology, is the only field of psychology that was never behaviorized. It was always clear to social psychologists that cognitive structures in people's heads were doing the work, although it was not until the late 1960s that people began to get some idea of what those cognitive structures might look like.

Another important factor in the shift away from collective phenomena is that, roughly in the early 1960s, it began to be clear that social psychologists were doing science. When dissonance research was starting to be done, it was very exciting to people to realize that one could do things that were replicable, surprising, and incontrovertible. The social psychologists of the 1960s were able to demonstrate interesting and surprising phenomena in the laboratory, and they had good theories as to why the phenomena occurred. Dissonance theory was followed by attribution theory, which was similar in many ways in that the experiments were difficult to refute and the theories were well grounded. But studies of collective phenomena, including culture, just did not have that ring of science. The methods were sufficiently weak that if a piece of research turned up something that seemed implausible, one was not inclined to trust the research over a prior opinion. Given a choice between science and journalism, the field stampeded toward science.

Still another reason for the movement away from collective phenomena may have to do with the center of gravity of psychology shifting so completely from Europe to North America. And we North Americans are so individualistic in our orientation that that stance carried over into the discipline, including our understanding of how to look at things and what things are interesting to look at. Social psychology began to become the study of the individual—or, to be more precise, of the individual's thoughts about the world. There is real discomfort on the part of Europeans with what is called "methodological individualism." I have an acquaintance, a German political scientist, who tells me that when he goes back to Germany for a conference, it is like going into a room where there is sufficient oxygen. He feels very weighed down by the necessity to communicate with his American colleagues, who tend to insist that all phenomena are rightly understood at the individual level rather than, at least sometimes, having to go to some higher, broader level of analysis. This is something I'm very sympathetic with now, but I would not really have understood the complaint not so long ago.

So, for about 30 years, I'd say Harry Triandis, Michael Bond, John Berry, Michael Cole, and only a few others were among the small cadre of people doing cultural psychology in a way that spoke to the scientist. Like many people, I was paying some attention to what they were saying. But they did not really influence what most social psychologists thought they should be doing. My own attitude toward their work, and the work of the Soviet cultural psychologists, was that there was probably some truth to what they were saying, but the claims of cultural differences were probably exaggerated and at any rate were peripheral to my concerns.

What really got the attention of the field—certainly of those of us working in attribution research and convinced of the universality of the fundamental attribution error—was Joan Miller's (1984) dissertation. I think our convictions about universality were far from being unexamined assumptions. We could have given excellent reasons for why the fundamental attribution error had to be universal and equally strong in all cultures. The primary reason for this for me, at least, was that I believed that the error was at base a perceptual phenomenon. And I still think that is essentially correct. It is just that it would have been hard to guess how much perception is influenced by culture. Miller's research made it abundantly clear that the fundamental attribution error was much more prevalent for some peoples than for others. The work was so well done and so convincing that I experienced a certain exhilaration when I first read the paper, though basically I was not pleased to see the results. I suppose I was like the wife of the Bishop of Worcester after Darwin's theory of evolution was explained to her: "My dear, let us hope that it is not true, but if it is, let us pray that it will not become generally known."

Miller's work did not immediately spawn other research in cultural psychology, but after 7 or 8 years psychologists all over North America suddenly began thinking about cultural differences, and within short order began producing the sort of work that fills this volume. Personally, I was quite surprised to see so many people working in the field so quickly. As Daniel Dennett has said, you think you are original, and then you realize you've just been floating on the Zeitgeist. And the Zeitgeist has just continued to shift in the direction of cultural psychology. More and more people want to know whether the phenomena they are been investigating look the same in cultures different from their own.

Why did the shift take place, and why does it remain largely a North American phenomenon? One reason I think is that it suddenly dawned on psychologists that not everybody is North American. This had been obvious to Europeans. There was once an article by a Frenchman on American social psychology, with an amusing title, something like "The Social Psychology of the Nice Guy" (whom he regarded with the disdain the French reserve for Americans). Perhaps the flattening of the world had something to do with the emergence of cultural psychology. The world started shrinking and there was increasing immigration to the United States and to Canada. There was competition from Japan, which obviously did all kinds of things drastically differently from the way we did. Suddenly American academics realized they could not ignore the other 96% of the world.

But I think a major ingredient in the move toward cultural research has to do with our realization that the strong inference techniques that we have honed, experimental techniques in particular, can be applied to cultural phenomena. We stopped being interested in collective questions in part because we found that we could make so much more progress with questions at the individual level. But then, starting about 15 years ago or so, people began realizing that the methodology developed over the preceding 20–30 years was adequate to speak in a thoroughly scientific way to collective questions. And once we started doing it, and realizing that the inferences were really as tight as elsewhere in psychology, it was a big thrill.

As this volume shows, what we have now is an absolute flood of research. And I do not think it is like any prior movement in social psychology. It is substantially bigger and qualitatively different from dissonance or attribution, or person memory or judgment and decision making. It is not a topic that in 6 or 7 years will no longer interest people. It is a new way of doing business. I do not think we can (or, at any rate, should) make assertions about human behavior anymore without having in the back of our minds, "How would this play through in other cultures?"

Another striking thing is that psychology is going to be reshaped by ideas from outside the Western tradition. East Asians are particularly well placed to play a creative role because of the very different nature of their societies and the capacity to draw on intellectual traditions

that are thousands of years old. In one case, by the way, a social science field has already been totally transformed by East Asians—primatology. Thirty years ago, Western primatologists could not see anything larger than a dyadic relationship among primates. But Japanese primatologists insisted that the relationships are extremely complex. There are coalitions that involve many individuals and that shift over time. The reaction to this on the part of Western primatologists was derision at first. *Nature* magazine published a condescending, early critique of Japanese primatology that maintained the culture of the Japanese had colored their view of the relationships among primates. Indeed. Now the entire field shares the Japanese assumptions about the nature and complexity of primate relationships.

As to the future, I do not pretend to know what will happen, but there are several things I would like to see happen. Some of them have to do with my own confusions.

First, should we think about culture as traits? For some kinds of behaviors, that analogy seems very powerful and largely correct, at least to a first approximation. Individualism versus collectivism, or independence versus interdependence, clearly can be thought of very much like a trait dimension. In fact, Harry Triandis (1995) has argued, successfully in my view, that there are traits at the level of individuals within a culture that mimic those poles, namely, idiocentrism and allocentrism. The same thing is true of dominance behavior, aggressive behavior, and extraversion. It makes sense to think of cultures as being relatively extraverted or relatively introverted. The Finns like to say that the difference between a Finnish introvert and a Finnish extravert is that the introvert looks at his shoes when he talks to you and the extravert looks at your shoes. And I think it is fair to say that Americans as a group compared to, say, the English or the Japanese, are rather extraverted.

On the other hand, sometimes it makes more sense to look at culture as a chronic situation, or set of situations. Lee Ross has a nice anecdote that provides a helpful way to think about the way material aspects of situations both reflect and sustain cultures. He spent 1 or 2 weeks at an academic institution in Spain. Hanging around with the faculty and graduate students he had a wonderful time, going out to tapas bars, having wine and conversations late at night, and walking along the streets to the parks. It was all marvelous and Lee found he fit right in. He thought to himself, "I'd like to bring as much of this as possible to Stanford. I'm going to shift Palo Alto culture, or at least my part of it in the social psychology program, toward Spanish academic culture." But it turns out there are some problems with that. For starters, there are not any tapas bars in Palo Alto. And a person can't go from one place to any other place in Palo Alto without getting into a car. And that sort of breaks the rhythm: "You take the Volkswagen and I'll take the SUV, and we'll get everybody downtown." You're not in the Mediterranean any more if you're having to do that. Beyond that is the fact that one tapas bar would not do the trick. The institution is tapas bar *hopping*, not just plopping down in *a* tapas bar. Work and sleep schedules are sufficiently different in Palo Alto than those in the Mediterranean that even a cluster of tapas bars would not really sustain the culture. Climate would also conspire. It can get cold at night in Palo Alto, and then there is the rainy season to contend with, and so on. Lee did not get very far with his desire to create a Spanish academic culture at Stanford.

So actual physical setups determine what kinds of cultural attributes are possible. Hazel Markus and I, in our first cultural psychology seminar, had students write a brief ethnography. One of the most insightful, and sad, was by Susan Cross, who grew up in Houston. She recounted the profound change in the nature of social life that was produced by the introduction of the air conditioner. Previously a great deal of social life was oriented around the porch, where people would sit in the evening to cool off and invite people strolling along the sidewalk to come up for a visit. But the advent of the air conditioner changed all that. No longer was it necessary to sit on the porch to cool off, and no longer was there a motive to stroll the sidewalks during an evening. Social life withered into the connectionless accumulations of people in malls and Astrodomes and bowlers bowling alone.

A second set of questions concerns the triggering of cultural phenomena, notably, how long it takes to adopt the social and cognitive habits of a host culture and the degree to which priming of certain orientations can mimic the effects of culture. The "framed line" findings of Kitayama, Duffy, Kawamura, and Larson (2003) are extremely thought provoking, in that they suggest that living in a new environ-ment even for a relatively brief amount of time can produce a shift in perception that is influenced by culture, namely, attention to a focal object versus attention to the field. Americans living in Japan are moved substantially toward the Japanese pattern of greater ability to reproduce the length of a line relative to its surrounding square compared to ability to reproduce the absolute length of the line. Japanese living in America are nearly identical to Americans in their tendency to be equally adept at both productions. Of course it is possible that those Japanese living in the United States were just self-selected because they were very American from the start. And maybe the Americans who went to Japan were pretty Japanese from the start. But it seems equally likely that something is happening chronically to people in the two cultures that makes them have certain kinds of perceptual orientations. One possibility is that the society is different with respect to some important social practices. The practices direct attention differently, either specifically to objects and one's goals in relation to them in the case of the West, or toward the social environment and, consequently, the environment more generally in the case of the East (Markus & Kitayama, 1991). The Kitayama et al. (2003) findings suggest that if we reverse the chronic orientation for a modest period of time, we may reverse the perceptual habits as well.

But it may be possible to produce "cultural" shifts with far less exposure to culture-relevant stimuli. There is evidence that even brief exposures to stimuli that trigger interdependent versus independent orientations (e.g., having people think about the ways in which they are similar to others vs. the ways in which they are different from others) have effects on social cognition and even on attentional processes (Gardner, Gabriel, & Lee, 1999; Haberstroh, Kühnen, Oyserman, & Schwarz, 2000; Hong, Morris, Chiu, & Benet-Martinez, 2000; Kühnen, Hannover, & Schubert, 2001; Kühnen & Oyserman, 2002; Trafimow, Triandis, & Goto, 1991). Because everyone has moments when attention is directed toward individual objects (including themselves), and moments when their attention is directed toward contexts (including other people), there can be acute analogues to chronic cultural states. Everyone can be relatively interdependent or independent. Consequently everyone can be deflected toward objects and goals or toward looking more broadly at the environment.

The priming studies raise another important question for the future: What is modifiable in the short term and what is not? Can we turn anybody into a member of another culture just by priming procedures? It is astonishing (to me, at least) that just circling first-person plural pronouns (*we, us, ourselves*) in a paragraph makes people less capable of solving embedded figures problems than they are after circling first-person plural pronouns (*I, me, mine*). Hannah Chua, Julie Boland, and I (Chua, Boland, & Nisbett, 2005) have found that in the first second of looking at a picture Americans focus on the object for an average of 600 milliseconds compared to 40 milliseconds for Chinese—a finding that helps to explain why Americans are more likely to attribute events to objects, and Asians to attribute to contexts. Would the pronoun prime affect whether a person's eye movements focus more on backgrounds rather than objects? Would the pronoun prime make people more likely to reason in dialectical ways (Peng & Nisbett, 1999)? Less likely to apply logic to everyday problems (Norenzayan, Smith, Kim, & Nisbett, 2002)? More likely to organize objects and events on the basis of relationships rather than categories (Chiu, 1972; Ji, Zhang, & Nisbett, 2004)? Less able to realize that they should be surprised by some unusual fact they have just been told (Choi, 1998; Choi & Nisbett, 2000)? Obtaining the latter effects would suggest that perceptual differences are more closely tied to cognitive ones than is currently assumed to be the case, and that the two are linked more tightly to culture than is assumed. Most importantly, such results would suggest that independence and interdependence serve as major coordinates organizing a wide variety of mental functions. And if priming procedures could produce such broad and general components of different cultures, what other sorts of cultural differences can be primed by similar manipulations?

There is evidence that environments in which people live habitually, as well as the environments to which they are exposed acutely, can affect the nature of perception. There are myriad sights on the East Asian street, whereas American environments are relatively simple. Yuri Miyamoto, Taka Masuda, and I (Miyamoto, Nisbett, & Masuda, 2006) have found that Japanese urban environments are just much more complex than American ones. Whereas objects stand out against relatively empty backgrounds in American environ-

ments, everything is context in Japanese environments. There are three important consequences:

1. Americans tend to see objects when they look at a scene; Japanese tend to see backgrounds and relationships among objects.
2. Both Americans and Japanese, when looking at American scenes, tend to see objects; and both groups, when looking at Japanese scenes, tend to see backgrounds and relationships.
3. Even brief exposure to Japanese scenes makes both Japanese and Americans more likely subsequently to focus on contexts rather than objects as compared to brief exposure to American scenes.

Here, again, is an instance of producing culture-like differences on an acute timescale that resemble those produced by chronic conditions.

Some cultural differences are not like chronic situations and not like temporary states, and not like personality traits, but something like what Harry Triandis refers to as cultural syndromes and others refer to as culture complexes. In some Arab cultures, for example, every man knows that it is an incredible infraction to look directly at his wife's face. They just know that—it is not as if this is an individual difference we could sensibly examine in their culture, let alone in ours. People in New Jersey just do not differ in the degree to which they see the world in that respect; no Jerseyites feel that way.

I can tell two anecdotes about furniture that each tapping into culture complexes that are impenetrable to me. Michael Morris tells about his sister, who worked for many years in Japan. Early on she went to some friends' apartment and saw a desk that they had. She said, "Gee, that's a lovely desk." The next day, to her mortification, the desk was delivered to her home, and every month its former owners would come back and polish it for her. Contrast that with the wealthy English gentleman who invited an American to his home. The American made the apparently ghastly mistake of complimenting the man's dining room chairs. "My gosh, those are gorgeous Chippendale chairs." And the English gentleman threw him out of his house. "Damn fellow thinks he can praise my chairs." It would probably take me hours to learn to give a coherent verbal account of what is going on in these furniture episodes, and years to understand them in some deep intuitive way.

Then there are culture complexes I have worked on myself, including the culture of honor I researched with Dov Cohen (Cohen, Nisbett, Bowdle, & Schwarz, 1996; Nisbett & Cohen, 1996). There is a syndrome of believing that you have to protect yourself, your home, and your family without the aid of the law, that violence, or the threat of it, is a necessary response to an insult, and that you have to be terribly polite to people yet frank and direct when necessary to avoid conflict. This is not best thought of as a personality variable. It is a syndrome, and in a culture like that you are going to participate in that syndrome to one degree or another. But there is not a comparable syndrome in other cultures, so there cannot be individual differences in it. The pieces are not united in the same way in other cultures. Cohen actually has evidence of this in recent work showing that various attitudes and behaviors hang together in the South in ways that they do not in the North (see, e.g., Leung & Cohen, 2006; Cohen, Vandello, Puente, & Rantilla, 1999). Most importantly, the sorts of things that predict honor-related violence are quite different in the North than in the South. Endorsement of honor-related aggression in the North is associated with social disruption and anomie—higher divorce rates, more moving around, and so on. But endorsement of honor-related aggression in the South is associated with social cohesion and organization—lower divorce rates, more stable residence patterns, and so on (Cohen, 1998). Violence in the North, in other words, is in part the result of social pathology. Violence in the South is learned at Mother's knee.

Or take a cultural syndrome that is even more clearly a conglomeration rather than a trait, namely, the Calvinist Protestant ethic complex. There are people who think they have got to work hard all the time and be thrifty, that they should never buy a car better than a Chevrolet because that would be too showy, that they should not enjoy eating or any of the other pleasures of the flesh too much, or incur obligations to people, that they should not get too emotionally close to people, and that everybody has a calling or should have—not just a job, but a calling. Well, it would be preposterous to talk about this dog's breakfast of attributes as a personality trait. Instead, it is some kind of syndrome or culture complex. People in a given Calvinist subculture may differ to one degree or another in the extent to which they participate in the syndrome: It may "take" to different degrees in different people, but it would be absurd to think that the attributes would hang together for people not part of such a culture. Actually, there is reason to doubt that the attributes of such complexes correlate all that well even in cultures that have them. Cohen (2006, Chapter 8, this volume) did not find a coherent, underlying factor of Jewish religious observance. To one person, being Jewish means doing X; to another, being Jewish means doing Y; and for yet another person it means doing Z. Cohen (2006) looked at eight religious behaviors—keeping kosher, fasting on Yom Kippur, having a seder, lighting Shabbat candles, and so on. After excluding the Orthodox individuals whose very strong ideology requires following all the practices, and the purely secular, who follow none, they found that the correlation between following any two practices ranged from .1 to .2.

So when is it best to think about some cultural fact in one way and when in another? I believe we will be making a lot of progress on this question in the near future.

I believe that some culture complexes will turn out to be "unprimable." I doubt that there is a simple prime that can make a Northern, suburban Jewish boy behave like a Southern, rural Baptist kid by insulting him. You could get the Northerner mad, even mad enough to take a swing at somebody else, but I doubt whether you could get him to think that he was *obligated* to inflict physical harm to maintain his reputation for toughness. Still less would you be able to get him to think that the *only appropriate* way to respond to an insult is through physical violence. I also doubt that you could prime a Spanish Catholic to think that she must really discover her calling by getting her to think about luxury goods.

How long do you have to live in a culture before you think habitually like a native? Before your socioemotional reactions are like those of a native? As an example of my own bias, I suspect some aspects of cognition, and perhaps habitual aspects of attention, can change at a fairly late point to a fairly marked degree, perhaps in late adolescence or even early adulthood. (And David Liu, Jan Leu, and I have some preliminary data indicating that this is actually the case for Asian immigrants to America.) But like many developmental psychologists, I suspect socioemotional attributes cannot change much past late childhood. I left Texas at 17, and I used to think of myself as a standard-issue liberal pacifist, but after I started studying the culture of honor I realized that I was very much imbued with that culture. You can take the boy off the ranch, but you can't take the ranch out of the boy. Similarly, I used to think I was a completely fallen-away Methodist, but reading Weber was a revelation to me. I am a Calvinist almost to the core: I could not live with myself if I did not think I had a true calling and, at least until I grew fat and sleek-headed under the influence of my adored, sybaritic spouse, was compulsively thrifty and luxury-avoidant.

Still other questions for the future have to do with what is universal after all. We have an interesting case history of universality lost and near-universality regained for cognitive dissonance. It looked for quite a while as if we would be unable to find dissonance effects in Asia in either the forced compliance or the free choice paradigm (Heine & Lehman, 1997). It is now clear that we can get dissonance effects with Asians; it is just that very different conditions are required to elicit them than is the case for Westerners. Westerners worry about whether they are competent decision makers, thus showing dissonance effects even when they are by themselves. Asians are more worried about what other people will think about their choices and show dissonance reduction effects only when they are primed to think about other people while they are making their decisions (Kitayama, Snibbe, Markus, & Suzuki, 2004). The same is true for the fundamental attribution error; that is to say, it is alive and well in the East, just more easily avoided there than in the West because of greater Eastern sensitivity to situational factors (Choi & Nisbett, 1998; Norenzayan & Nisbett, 2000). We do not have to give up either of these staples of social psychology—though we are going to have to think about them in very different ways than in the past.

In fact, I think we will have to think about all psychological phenomena—down to the level of allegedly cognitively impenetrable perception—in very different ways. We can no longer assume that everybody thinks, feels, and sees in the same way—even when they are placed in what appears to the observer to be identical situations.

ACKNOWLEDGMENT

A version of this chapter appeared in Nisbett (2005). Copyright 2005 by Lawrence Erlbaum Associates. Adapted by permission.

REFERENCES

Chiu, L.-H. (1972). A cross-cultural comparison of cognitive styles in Chinese and American children. *International Journal of Psychology, 7*, 235–242.

Choi, I. (1998). *The cultural psychology of surprise: Holistic theories, contradiction, and epistemic curiosity.* Unpublished doctoral dissertation, University of Michigan, Ann Arbor.

Choi, I., & Nisbett, R. E. (1998). Situational salience and cultural differences in the correspondence bias and in the actor–observer bias. *Personality and Social Psychology Bulletin, 24*, 949–960.

Choi, I., & Nisbett, R. E. (2000). The cultural psychology of surprise: Holistic theories and recognition of contradiction. *Journal of Personality and Social Psychology, 9*, 890–905.

Chua, H. F., Boland, J. E., & Nisbett, R. E. (2005). Cultural variation in eye movements during scene perception. *Proceedings of the National Academy of Science of the USA, 102*, 12629–12633.

Cohen, D. (1998). Culture, social organization, and patterns of violence. *Journal of Personality and Social Psychology, 75*, 408–419.

Cohen, D. (2006). *Tradition's thread.* Unpublished manuscript, University of Illinois, Urbana–Champaign.

Cohen, D., Nisbett, R. E., Bowdle, B., & Schwarz, N. (1996). Insult, aggression, and the Southern culture of honor: An "experimental ethnography." *Journal of Personality and Social Psychology, 70*, 945–960.

Cohen, D., Vandello, J., Puente, S., & Rantilla, A. (1999). "When you call me that, smile!" *Social Psychology Quarterly, 62*, 257–275.

Gardner, W. L., Gabriel, S., & Lee, A. Y. (1999). "I" value freedom, but "we" value relationships: Self-construal priming mirrors cultural differences in judgment. *Psychological Science, 10*, 321–326.

Haberstroh, S., Kühnen, U., Oyserman, D., & Schwarz, N. (2000). Is the interdependent self a better communicator than the independent self?: Self-construal and the observation of conversational norms. Heidelberg: University of Heidelberg.

Heine, S. J., & Lehman, D. R. (1997). Culture, dissonance, and self-affirmation. Personality and Social Psychology Bulletin, *81*, 599–615.

Hong, Y.-Y., Morris, M. W., Chiu, C.-Y., & Benet-Martinez, V. (2000). Multicultural minds: A dynamic constructivist approach to culture and cognition. *American Psychologist, 55*, 709–720.

Ji, L.-J., Zhang, Z., & Nisbett, R. E. (2004). Is it culture or is it language?: Examination of language effects in cross-cultural research on categorization. *Journal of Personality and Social Psychology, 87*, 57–65.

Kitayama, S., Duffy, S., Kawamura, T., & Larson, J. T. (2003). Perceiving an object and its context in different cultures: A cultural look at New Look. *Psychological Science, 14*, 201–206.

Kühnen, U., Hannover, B., & Schubert, B. (2001). The semantic–procedural interface model of the self: The role of self-knowledge for context-dependent versus context-independent modes of thinking. *Journal of Personality and Social Psychology, 80*, 397–409.

Kühnen, U., & Oyserman, D. (2002). Thinking about the self influences thinking in general: Cognitive consequences of salient self-concept. *Journal of Experimental Social Psychology, 38*, 492–499.

Leung, A. & Cohen, D. (2006). *Honor, face, and dignity: Ideal types and experiments.* Unpublished manuscript, University of Illinois, Urbana–champaign.

Markus, H. R., & Kitayama, S. (1991). Culture and the self: Implications for cognition, emotion, and motivation. *Psychological Review, 98*, 224–253.

Masuda, T., & Nisbett, R. E. (2001). Attending holistically vs. analytically: Comparing the context sensitivity of Japanese and Americans. *Journal of Personality and Social Psychology, 81*, 922–934.

Miller, J. G. (1984). Culture and the development of everyday social explanation. *Journal of Personality and Social Psychology, 46*, 961–978.

Miyamoto, Y., Nisbett, R. E., & Masuda, T. (2006). Culture and physical environment: Holistic versus analytic perceptual affordances. *Psychological Science, 17*, 113–119.

Nisbett, R. E. (2005). The ghosts of cultural psychology. In R. Sorrentino, D. Cohen, J. Olson, & M. P. Zanna (Eds.), *Culture and social behavior: The tenth Ontario Symposium.* Hillsdale, NJ: Erlbaum.

Nisbett, R. E., & Cohen, D. (1996). *Culture of honor: The psychology of violence in the South.* Boulder, CO: Westview Press.

Norenzayan, A., & Nisbett, R. E. (2000). Culture and causal cognition. *Current Directions in Psychological Science, 9*, 132–135.

Norenzayan, A., Smith, E. E., Kim, B. J., & Nisbett, R. E. (2002). Cultural preferences for formal versus intuitive reasoning. *Cognitive Science, 26*, 653–684.

Peng, K., & Nisbett, R. E. (1999). Culture, dialectics, and reasoning about contradiction. *American Psychologist, 54*, 741–754.

Trafimow, D., Triandis, H. C., & Goto, S. G. (1991). Some tests of the distinction between the private self and the collective self. *Journal of Personality and Social Psychology, 60*, 649–655.

Triandis, H. C. (1995). *Individualism and collectivism.* Boulder, CO: Westview Press.

PART VIII

EPILOGUE

CHAPTER 36

Cultural Psychology
This Stanza and the Next

DOV COHEN
SHINOBU KITAYAMA

"Universalism without the uniformity" may be a good way to describe cultural psychology (see Shweder, Chapter 34, this volume). And perhaps it is a decent way to describe this handbook as well. The chapters in this volume have a great deal in common, but they also illustrate the many ways one can be a cultural psychologist.

As a final word, we briefly try to sum up some themes that emerged in this book and what they may point us toward in the future. One can readily identify four themes that give some unity to the emerging field. Cultural psychologists tend to regard culture as a dynamic system of practices and meanings (a definitional tenet of the field); they regard content and process of the mind as inseparable (a theoretical tenet); and they tend to rely heavily on "thick experimentation" (a methodological tenet). In addition, cultural psychologists tend to regard Westernization as only one rather limited social force that is influencing the non-Western world today. Each of these points can be traced back to a variety of different intellectual traditions such as experimental psychology, social psychology, and anthropology

among others. Yet in combination they establish cultural psychology as a relatively unified field that is well positioned to grow.

1. A definitional tenet of cultural psychology says that culture is composed of a rich network of practices, meanings, and attendant psychological habits and experiences. In this respect, cultural psychology is somewhat different from older, more traditional approaches to culture in psychology, which tended to focus on abstract values or national character.

Cultural psychologists believe, to use Einstein's famous phrase, that culture does not work through "spooky action at a distance." It works through the quotidian—the way we tell stories, eat, speak, cook, socialize, make love, act, sleep, remember, perceive, comport our bodies and so on (see, e.g., Brewer & Yuki, Chapter 12; Chiu, Leung, & Kwan, Chapter 27; Fiske & Fiske, Chapter 11; Hatfield, Rapson, & Martel, Chapter 31; Mesquita & Leu, Chapter 30; J. Miller, Chapter 19; P. Miller, Fung, & Koven, Chapter 24; Rozin, Chapter 16; Sanchez-Burks & Lee, Chapter 14; Schooler, Chapter 15; Wang & Ross, Chapter 26, all this volume; see also Kim, 2002; Konner, 2002; Shweder, 1993; Tsai, Louie, Chen, & Uchida, 2007). It gets instantiated in the everyday practices of our world. The point might seem obvious at first. However, this way of thinking would make it clear that culture is not separable from the mind. Instead, it is a dynamic system of which a mind is part. Moreover, the idea of culture as a dynamic system is central to the *methodology* of cultural psychologists who tend to focus on processes that *re-create* culture in the everyday—rather than, say, on the measurement of abstract values, personality traits, or macro-level indicators (see Markus & Hamedani, Chapter 1 this volume).

This re-creation is an active process that people engage in. Culture is not the dead weight of history, carried forward through inertia (Moore, 1966). It is remade daily in the quotidian.

2. A theoretical tenet of the field holds that processes of the mind are inseparable from the content that makes up the mind. The "old" division in psychology was between *how* human beings thought and *what* they thought about. The first was the really interesting stuff that was the purview of "real" psychologists. The latter was . . . not. Even if one initially accepted this dubious and territorial belief, cultural psychology has redrawn the map and has shown how the *what* and the *how* are fundamentally inseparable. The work on independence versus interdependence and holistic versus analytic cognition makes this clear (Oyserman & Lee, Chapter 10; Kitayama, Duffy, & Uchida, Chapter 6; Norenzayan, Choi, & Peng, Chapter 23; Nisbett, Chapter 35, all this volume; also Cohen, Hoshino-Browne, & Leung, 2007; Leung & Cohen, in press), but the point about content and process being inseparable is also implicit in other places as well (see, e.g., Marsella & Yamada, Chapter 33, this volume, on psychopathology, and Chiu et al., Chapter 27, on language). *What* we think affects *how* we think, and *how* we think affects *what* we think.

3. A methodological corner stone of the field lies in what one may call "thick experimentation." As Shweder (Chapter 34, this volume) notes, the discovery of meaning is central to the mission of cultural psychology. Fieldwork that produced "thick description" was the path to the discovery of meaning. However, with some notable exceptions (see, e.g., J.

Miller, Chapter 19; P. Miller et al., Chapter 24; Morelli & Rothbaum, Chapter 20, all this volume), the field has been a little thin on "thick description." Most cultural psychologists (at least, most in this book) are still *psychologists*, and most have retained their general disciplinary bias toward more quantitative analysis.

Meaning is still central, however, and one of the advances has been the development of a type of "thick experimentation" that uses the tools of traditional psychology to discern meaning and even provide nuance and texture. Research programs on the meaning of choice and on the role of self-enhancement and self-criticism in the United States and Japan are two such examples (Kitayama et al., Chapter 6; Heine, Chapter 29; Markus & Hamedani, Chapter 1, all this volume; Hoshino-Browne, et al., 2005; Snibbe & Markus, 2005; Kitayama & Markus, 1999; Heine, Lehman, Markus, & Kitayama, 1999; see also Mendoza-Denton & Mischel, Chapter 7, this volume, for an individual differences approach that highlights the psychological meanings of events).

"Science," it has been said, "is the search for better and better control conditions." In this light, researchers have focused on the situations *when* an effect occurs to understand *why* an effect occurs. Rozin's elaborate program of research on disgust, eating, and contamination is another example of how controlled experiments can tease apart the meaning of stimuli and reveal the laws of sympathetic magic that transform a basic disgust reaction into a culturally elaborated emotion of moral significance (see Rozin, Chapter 16, this volume; Rozin, Haidt, & McCauley, 2000).

Of course, to set appropriate control conditions requires substantial ethnographic knowledge informed by an insider's point of view (Geertz, 1973). This is the case because cultural meaning systems must be understood from the logic of the inside, and not from the vantage point of some presumed "universal cultural logic." Thus, for example, it requires thinking like an insider to understand why a belief in fatalism or predestination can result in (a) economic languor in one culture and (b) the strict, austere Calvinist work ethic in another (Sanchez-Burks & Lee, Chapter 14; Heine, Chapter 29; J. Miller, Chapter 19, all this volume; see also Bond et al., 2004). Thus we believe that work in cultural psychology should be informed by both thorough, first-hand knowledge about the culture at hand (e.g., ethnography) and careful experimentation designed to elucidate the underlying meaning systems.

4. Cultural psychologists are skeptical of the notion of uniform Westernization. Contemporary American rhetoric regards Western values as the ideal that all rational people would and will aspire to (once they become sufficiently educated, wealthy, or cured of their delusions). It professes an almost magical belief that drinking American soda pop, wearing "American" jeans (actually made in a "third-world" country), and having a TV satellite dish are enough to transform people into Americans (Huntington, 1996). And it regards every blip of convergence or similarity in public opinion as proof positive that a new era (an era of modern Western values) has arrived.

Cultural psychologists regard all these claims with suspicion. The belief in an inevitable Westernization (a) ignores the way cultures often adapt each others' customs for their own ends, (b) seems contradicted by the empirical record of the long duree (Braudel, 1980), and (c) assumes dubiously that Western values are universal values.

With respect to the first point, globalization may indeed internationalize some customs. However, these customs are often adapted to local practices (Hong, Wan, No, & Chiu, Chapter 13, this volume), and non-Western peoples are no less adept than Westerners at collectively reinventing the meaning of what they import from elsewhere. Because culture is composed of a system of meanings and practices that are interlocking and often redundant with one another (see Schooler, Chapter 15, this volume), new practices, tools, and ideas from elsewhere are more likely to be assimilated than accommodated.

Second, empirically, technological change and its accompanying affluence and affordance of possibilities seems to have led to more cultural divergence rather than less across the long duree. Braudel (1980) asks us to engage in a thought experiment: "Turn the problem around . . . and note the unity of earlier times . . . . Should the historian turn toward those past ages. . . , he will perceive as many astonishing resemblances and analogous rhythms working independently thousands of miles apart. [Ming China] was assuredly closer to the France of the Valois than the China of Mao Tse-tung is to the France of the Fifth Republic" (p. 213).

Finally—and this is mostly a matter of faith—cultural diversity seems to be an inevitable part of the human condition, because cultures must necessarily make trade-offs between different values (Shweder, 2000). And whereas cultures may all universally regard values such as autonomy, purity, community, mercy, justice, and social order as good things, cultures will differ in (a) how they conceive of these values as being implemented and (b) how much they are willing to trade-off one value for another when these values inevitably conflict (hence Shweder's [2000, p. 164] "universalism without the uniformity"). We may all agree that "vice is virtue to excess" or "everything in moderation," but what is "excess" and what is "moderation"?

These four tenets of cultural psychology seem to make up the "family resemblance" of work here: (1) Culture works through the quotidian, rather than through "spooky action at a distance"; (2) culture is both content and process and the two are fundamentally linked; (3) "thick experimentation" and observation can be used for the important task of uncovering meaning and understanding cultural logics from the inside; and (4) non-Western people are not simply Westerners "in disguise"—their values must be taken seriously and have an enduring appeal that may resist Westernization. There may be more core tenets. There may be fewer (all are, after all, *empirical* claims and are thus subject to revision). Nevertheless, this handful seems a reasonable starting point.

The chapters of this volume make it obvious that these four tenets can comprise no more than a "family resemblance" (rather than a strict definition) because there is a fair amount of variation in how researchers go about studying cultural psychology. However, where there is deviation from these four tenets also shows us where the field has room to grow. Below, we list three areas that may merit further exploration.

1. Individuals are active participants in their culture (see point 1, above), and that means they are free to contest, reject, or react against the culture they are in. Cultural psychology has tended to focus on the re-creation of cultural patterns, so it has tended to focus on stability rather than change and prototypical behavior rather than variation (cf. Newson, Richerson, & Boyd, Chapter 18, this volume). There has

been some research examining individual differences (see, e.g., work summarized in Cohen, Chapter 8; Tov & Diener, Chapter 28; Medin, Unsworth, & Hirschfeld, Chapter 25; Mendoza-Denton & Mischel, Chapter 7; Nisbett, Chapter 35, all this volume; Leung & Cohen, 2007; Fu et al., in press; Kitayama, Markus, Matsumoto, & Norasakkunkit, 1997). However, for the most part, cultural psychologists have focused on prototypes rather than patterns of within-culture variability.

As Konner (Chapter 4, this volume; see also LeVine, 2001, Chapter 2, this volume; Triandis, Chapter 3, this volume) notes, a single prototype focus was one of the factors that doomed studies of "national character" and one faction of the old "culture and personality" movement: "Individual variation . . . is great in every known culture. . . . At best there is perhaps a 'modal personality,' shared by a substantial minority of a culture's members . . . and in any case a culture must derive its distinctiveness from the particular mutual articulation of its various personality types, and the opportunities it provides for their expression, rather than from fundamental tendencies shared by a majority—a sort of symphony orchestra model of culture and personality, in which each culture provides a series of scores" (Konner, Chapter 4, this volume, p. 79). A study of *patterns* of variation rather than *prototypes* provides one important way for the field to grow theoretically and avoid degenerating into caricature.

2. The study of culture and evolution can be integrated. As has been observed, what begins as heresy ends as common sense. No longer is E. O. Wilson vilified for the suggestion that evolution may have shaped human psychology. Cultural psychologists not only need to make their peace with evolution but also must integrate this knowledge into our understanding of culture. As a whole, the field has yet to do so, but it is starting to confront the issue seriously (see Konner, 2002, Chapter 4, this volume; Atran, Chapter 17; Chiao & Amabady, Chapter 9; Cole & Hatano, Chapter 5; Levenson, Soto, & Pole, Chapter 32; Li, Chapter 21; Newson et al., Chapter 18, all this volume; Norenzayan & Heine, 2005). Similarly, biological research represents another way we can enrich our field, provided we do serious work and not simply "ooh and ahh" whenever we find out that some psychological process is reflected in—surprise!—the brain (Chiao & Ambady,

Chapter 9, this volume; see also discussions by Harmon-Jones & Winkielman, 2007, and the special issue of the *Journal of Personality and Social Psychology* edited by Harmon-Jones & Devine, October 2003).

3. There is still plenty of unexplored territory in terms of populations and phenomena to be studied (see Rozin, Chapter 16, and Shweder, Chapter 34, both this volume). Psychology is more than just the study of upper-middle-class white Americans, and cultural psychology is more than just the study of upper-middle-class white Americans and Asians. By far, these are the two dominant groups that cultural psychologists have examined (cf. Sternberg, Chapter 22, and Hatfield et al., Chapter 31, both this volume). However, we must take our own critique of mainstream psychology seriously and expand the samples we study. Our job is *not* to take on the Sisyphean task of cataloging the world's cultures. But obviously, if we take seriously our own argument that human psychology shapes and is shaped by culture, then there is still plenty about human psychology that has yet to be discovered and *cannot* be discovered without expanding the range of populations we study.

Expanding our samples and the phenomena we study is necessary for our theories and for understanding some of the real issues that present themselves in the world today. These include issues such as the vexing problem of race in America; the friction between secularism and religion in the West and the frictions between different religions in the West and Middle East; the increased immigration that will occur as ageing "first-world" countries try to recruit productive young workers from abroad; environmental problems that will require cooperation from both developed and developing countries; the persistent poverty of underdeveloped nations; and so on. As the salience of these issues grows, avenues of research in cultural psychology will expand.

In summary, we hope that the work in this handbook marks a beginning—or, more properly, a renewal of psychology's interest in culture (Markus & Hamedani, Chapter 1; Nisbett, Chapter 35; Shweder, Chapter 34; Triandis, Chapter 3, all this volume). We hope this current generation of research can add something to the long line of work that has come before it. Mark Twain is often (and perhaps apocryphally) credited with saying, "His-

tory does not repeat itself, but it does rhyme."
Our hope is that this handbook can add another stanza to this long history of the study of
culture and psychology.

REFERENCES

Bond, M., Leung, K., Au, A., Tong, K., De Carrasquel, S., Murakami, F., et al. (2004). Cultural dimensions of social axioms and their correlates across 41 cultures. *Journal of Cross-Cultural Psychology, 35,* 548–570.

Braudel, F. (1980). *On history.* Chicago: University of Chicago Press.

Cohen, D., Hoshino-Browne, E., & Leung, A. K.-y. (2007). Culture and the structure of personal experience: Insider and outsider phenomenologies of the self and social world. In M. Zanna (Ed.), *Advances in experimental social psychology* (pp. 1–67). San Diego: Academic Press.

Fu, J., Morris, M., Lee, S., Chao, M., Chiu, C. Y., & Hong, Y.-y. (in press). Epistemic motives and cultural conformity. *Journal of Personality and Social Psychology.*

Geertz, C. (1973). *The interpretation of cultures.* New York: Basic Books.

Harmon-Jones, E. & Winkielman, P. (2007). A brief overview of social neuroscience. In E. Harmon-Jones & P. Winkielman (Eds.), *Social neuroscience: Integrating biological and psychological explanations of social behavior* (pp. 3–11). New York: Guilford Press.

Heine, S., Lehman, D., Markus, H., & Kitayama, S. (1999). Is there a universal need for positive self-regard? *Psychological Review, 106,* 766–794.

Hoshino-Browne, E., Zanna, A. S., Spencer, S. J., Zanna, M. P., Kitayama, S., & Lackenbauer, S. (2005). On the cultural guises of cognitive dissonance. *Journal of Personality and Social Psychology, 89,* 294–310.

Huntington, S. P. (1996). *The clash of civilizations and the remaking of world order.* New York: Simon & Schuster.

Kim, H. (2002). We talk, therefore we think? *Journal of Personality and Social Psychology, 83,* 828–842.

Kitayama, S., & Markus, H. (1999). Yin and yang of the Japanese self. In D. Cervone & Y. Shoda (Eds.), *The coherence of personality: Social-cognitive bases of consistency, variability, and organization* (pp. 242–302). New York: Guilford Press.

Kitayama, S., Markus, H., Matsumoto, H., & Norasakkunkit, V. (1997). Individual and collective processes in the construction of the self. *Journal of Personality and Social Psychology, 72,* 1245–1267.

Konner, M. (2002). *The tangled wing.* New York: Holt.

Leung, A. K-y. & Cohen, D. (2007). *Within- and between-culture variation.* Unpublished manuscript, University of Illinois.

Leung, A. K-y., & Cohen, D. (in press). The soft embodiment of culture. *Psychological Science.*

LeVine, R. (2001). Culture and personality studies, 1918–1960: Myths and history. *Journal of Personality, 69,* 803–818.

Moore, B. (1966). *Social origins of dictatorship and democracy.* New York: Beacon.

Norenzayan, A., & Heine, S. J. (2005). Psychological universals: What are they and how can we know? *Psychological Bulletin, 131,* 763–784.

Rozin, P., Haidt, J., & McCauley, C. (2000). Disgust. In M. Lewis & J. Haviland (Eds.), *The Handbook of Emotions* (2nd ed., pp. 637–653). New York: Guilford Press.

Shweder, R. (1993). "Why do men barbeque" and other postmodern ironies of growing up in the decade of ethnicity. *Daedalus, 122,* 279–308.

Shweder, R. (2000). Moral maps, "first world" conceits, and the new evangelists. In L. Harrison & S. Huntington (Eds.), *Culture matters* (pp. 158–176). New York: Basic Books.

Snibbe, A. C., & Markus, H. R. (2005). You can't always get what you want: Educational attainment, agency, and choice. *Journal of Personality and Social Psychology, 88,* 703–720.

Tsai, J., Louie, J., Chen, E., & Uchida, Y. (2007). Learning what feelings to desire. *Personality and Social Psychology Bulletin, 33,* 17–30.

Author Index

852

Subject Index

Abacus expertise
    cultural practices amplification,
        127–130
    neuronal changes, 128
Absolutist view of culture and
    psychology, 66
Abstract verb phrases
    vs. concrete verb phrases, 684
    in outgroup behavior descriptions,
        684
Academic achievement
    and life satisfaction, 702
    socioeconomic status effects, 377
Accessibility effects, and priming, 263
Accountability, in moral reasoning,
    486–487
Acculturation
    definition, 65
    developmental perspective, 329–
        330
    psychological adjustment, 331–332
    and psychopathology, 804
Aché culture, childhood model, 86–
    87
Achievement motivation, and
    religion, 168, 715–718
Acoustic startle
    autonomic effects, 787, 788
    cultural effects susceptibility, 788
Acquiescence bias, 141, 166, 219,
    706
Action readiness, 742–746
    cultural context link, 745–746
    cultural themes, 743
    in emotional experience, 736, 742–
        746
    and general somatic activity, 743
    and happiness, 743–744
    Northern vs. Southern U.S. men,
        745
    in shame reactions, 744

Action regulation, 139–153
    and health and well-being, 152–
        153
    independent vs. interdependent
        cultures, 142–153
    motivational consequences, 151–
        152
    principle of, 142–143
    and social relations, 139–145
    style of, emotional consequences,
        151
Activity theory. See Cultural–
    historical activity theory
Adaptation
    and cultural diversity, 458–459
    environmental context, 64
    myth of, 208
    religion theory, 422–426
Adjustment style
    and depression, 749
    East Asians vs. North Americans,
        145–147, 748
    ideal affect link, 748
    vs. influence style, 145–147, 748
Adult Attachment Interview, 518
Adultery. See Sexual infidelity
Advertisements, East–West
    differences, 164, 222, 326,
        684, 728
Advertising, research samples, 215
Affordances. See Cultural affordances
African Americans
    baseline autonomic physiology, 786
    emotion production studies, 787
    facial expression, 784
    fantasy narratives, 600, 610
    individualism vs. collectivism effect
        sizes, 258–260
    schizophrenic symptoms, 809
    storytelling, young children, 600
    stress reactions, physiology, 786

Africans
    collectivism vs. individualism, 258–
        259
    context-related intellectual abilities,
        557–559
    intelligence conception, 551–553
Agemate relationships, 288
Agency, 723–727. See also
    Supernatural agents
    appraisal effects of, 742
    in choice making, 725–727
    and control, 723–727
    East Asian vs. Western culture, 29,
        723–727
    independent vs. interdependent
        mode of being, 138, 143–145
    lay theories, 149–150
    sociocultural influences on, 29,
        143–145
Aggregate behaviors, in cultural
    products, 222
Aggression
    behavioral concomitants, 746
    sex differences, universality, 91
Aging, and memory decline, 662
Agricultural societies
    and cultural diversity pattern, 470–
        471
    and culture's rate of conformity,
        206–207
Agta culture, childhood model, 86–
    87
Aka culture, childhood model, 86–87
Alcoholism, 804, 813–814
    popular culture role, 813
    prevalence, 813–814
ALFRED, 243, 251n1
Allocentrism
    as cultural trait, 822, 839
    personality pattern, 69
    and self-descriptions, 313

About the Editors

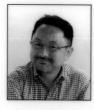

Shinobu Kitayama, PhD, is Professor of Psychology and Director of the Culture and Cognition Program at the University of Michigan. He received his doctorate from the University of Michigan, where he has been teaching since 2003. Prior to joining the faculty there, Dr. Kitayama taught at the Universities of Oregon and Chicago and at Kyoto University. He serves as an Associate Editor of the *Personality and Social Psychology Bulletin.* Throughout his career Dr. Kitayama has studied cultural variations of self, emotion, and cognition, and has presented his work in the books *Culture and Emotion: The Study of Mutual Influences* (with Hazel Markus) and *The Heart's Eye: Emotional Influences in Perception and Attention,* as well as in such leading journals as *Psychological Review, Psychological Science,* and the *Journal of Personality and Social Psychology.*

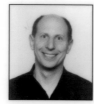

Dov Cohen, PhD, received his doctorate from the University of Michigan and taught at the University of Waterloo, Ontario, Canada, and the University of Illinois, where he is currently a faculty member. His research interests relate to cultural continuity and change, within-culture variability, and the way people position themselves with respect to dominant cultural ideals. Dr. Cohen has conducted research on the cultural syndromes of honor, dignity, and face, as well as on cross-cultural similarities and differences in the experience of self. He coauthored the book *Culture of Honor* (with Richard Nisbett) and coedited *Culture and Social Behavior* (with Richard Sorrentino, James Olson, and Mark Zanna).